Cardiac therapy

Cardiac therapy

Edited by
MICHAEL R. ROSEN, M.D. and BRIAN F. HOFFMAN, M.D.
Columbia University, New York

1983 **MARTINUS NIJHOFF PUBLISHERS**
a member of the KLUWER ACADEMIC PUBLISHERS GROUP
BOSTON / THE HAGUE / DORDRECHT / LANCASTER

Distributors

for the United States and Canada: Kluwer Boston, Inc., 190 Old Derby Street, Hingham, MA 02043, USA
for all other countries: Kluwer Academic Publishers Group, Distribution Center, P.O. Box 322, 3300 AH Dordrecht, The Netherlands

Library of Congress Cataloging in Publication Data

Library of Congress Cataloging in Publication Data
Main entry under title:

Cardiac therapy.

    1. Heart--Diseases--Treatment. I. Rosen,
Michael R. II. Hoffman, Brian F. [DNLM: 1. Heart
diseases--Therapy. WG 200 C267]
RC683.8.C37 1983   616.1'206   82-18814

ISBN 0-89838-564-4

First printing 1983
Second printing 1984

Preface

Cardiac therapy has become ever more complex during the past quarter century. For example, 25 years ago, the therapy of cardiac failure was largely limited to digitalis, a very few diuretics, salt restriction, and general supportive measures. Antiarrhythmic therapy involved – in the main – quinidine, procainamide, and digitalis, and questions such as which arrhythmia to treat and how to measure drug efficacy had been addressed in elementary fashion only. Cardiac surgery was limited largely to congenital and valvular heart disease; the areas of cardiac pacemaker therapy, defibrillation and other forms of electrical diagnosis and therapy were rudimentary.

The expansion of support of cardiovascular research by the National Institutes of Health as well as by institutional sources following World War II has led to major successes in clinical health care delivery and improved technology made available to clinical investigators. In reviewing progress over the past 25 years, we have been particularly impressed by one observation: this is the important interaction that has developed between studies of pathophysiology and the delivery of appropriate cardiac therapy. Whether one is considering vasodilator therapy, the use of electrophysiologic techniques for diagnosis and treatment, the actions of beta-blocking and slow-channel-blocking drugs – or many other examples – it is clear that an understanding of the physiology of the cardiovascular system, its interaction with important modifiers such as the autonomic nervous system, and its responses to pathologic processes all play an important role in helping the investigator to design protocols for testing therapeutic modalities, to decide which types of therapy to select, and to understand the effects – or lack of efficacy – of particular therapeutic interventions.

In planning the content of this volume, we did so with the above-mentioned observation in mind: We therefore decided to include, first, information on normal physiology and pathophysiology of various forms of cardiac disease, and, then, to include chapters in which the approach to therapy would relate to mechanisms of action of the therapeutic interventions as well as to an understanding of normal and of pathologic physiology.

It is our hope that, as a result of this approach, in this volume the reader will be able to learn not only what the 'state of the art' is with respect to the modalities of cardiac therapy discussed, but also will learn what the basis is for the approach to therapy selected, and how the therapeutic modality is related to the pathophysiology of the disease process. We hope that the volume will go beyond explaining 'what to do' in particular instances, but will provide answers to the equally important question of 'why.' It is only by answering the question 'why' that those individuals interested in the delivery of cardiac therapy can move beyond empiricism (which although important in its own right is often inadequate) to a rational basis for delivery of therapy.

We would like to express our gratitude to many individuals for their contributions to this volume: first to the authors of the individual sections. All are involved in cardiac investigation as clinical and/or basic scientists and all have contributed significantly to the fields about which they have written. The meticulous care they have taken and the promptness of most is gratefully acknowledged. We also express our gratitude to Dr. Julian Frieden and Mr. Jeffrey K. Smith who encouraged us to take on this project, to Mrs. Cynthia

Brandt for her aid in preparing the volume, and to Mrs. Sivia Brodsky for her editorial assistance. Finally, we thank our families, with whom our time was limited even more by the hours spent in preparing the volume, and whose unselfish support was – as always – essential.

Michael R. Rosen, M.D.
Departments of Pharmacology and Pediatrics
Columbia University, New York

Brian F. Hoffman, M.D.
Department of Pharmacology
Columbia University, New York

Table of contents

PART FOUR: THERAPY OF CARDIAC FAILURE AND ISCHEMIA

Contributors

Penelope A. Boyden, Ph.D., Department of Pharmacology, Columbia University, College of Physicians and Surgeons, 630 W. 168th St., New York, NY 10032

Paul J. Cannon, M.D., Professor of Medicine, Columbia University, College of Physicians and Surgeons, 630 W. 168th St., New York, NY 10032

Charles Fisch, M.D., Professor of Medicine, Indiana University School of Medicine, University Hospital Room 485, 1100 W. Michigan St., Indianapolis, IN 46202

James R. Foster, M.D., Associate Professor, Department of Medicine, University of North Carolina at Chapel Hill, 349 Clinical Sciences Building, Chapel Hill, NC 27514

Leonard S. Gettes, M.D., Director, Division of Cardiology, Department of Medicine, University of North Carolina at Chapel Hill, 349 Clinical Sciences Building 229-H, Chapel Hill, NC 27514

Alden H. Harken, M.D., Department of Surgery, 4 Silverstein, Box 649, Hospital University of Pennsylvania, Philadelphia, PA 19104

Brian F. Hoffman, M.D., David Hosack Professor of Pharmacology and Chairman of the Department, Columbia University, College of Physicians and Surgeons, 630 W. 168th St. New York, NY 10032

Mark Josephson, M.D., Department of Medicine, Section of Cardiology, Hospital of University of Pennsylvania, 3400 Spruce St., Philadelphia, PA 19104

Nicholas T. Kouchoukas, M.D., Department of Medicine, University of Alabama Medical Center, University Station, Birmingham, AL 35274

Matthew N. Levy, M.D., Chief, Investigative Medicine, The Mt. Sinai Hospital of Cleveland, University Circle, Cleveland, OH 44106

Alan S. Nies, M.D., Head, Division of Clinical Pharmacology, C-237, University of Colorado Medical School, 4200 E. 9th Ave, Denver, CO 80220

Dr. Gwynn Neufeld, University of Colorado Medical School, 4200 E. 9th Ave, Denver, Co 80220

John A. Oates, M.D., Professor of Pharmacology and Medicine, Head, Clinical Pharmacology, Vanderbilt University, Nashville, TN 37232

William W. Parmley, M.D., Professor of Medicine, Chief, Cardiovascular Division, University of California at San Francisco, San Francisco, CA 94143

Charles E. Rackley, M.D., Department of Medicine, University of Alabama Medical Center, University Station, Birmingham, AL 35294

David Robertson, M.D., Assistant Professor, Departments of Pharmacology and Medicine, Vanderbilt University, Nashville, TN 37232

Michael R. Rosen, M.D., Professor, Departments of Pharmacology and Pediatrics, Columbia University, College of Physicians and Surgeons, 630 W. 168th St., New York, NY 10032

John Ross, Jr., M.D., Department of Medicine M-013, University of California at San Diego, La Jolla, CA 92093

Richard O. Russell, Jr., M.D., Professor of Medicine, University of Alabama Medical Center, University Station, Birmingham, AL 35294

Ross J. Simpson, Jr., M.D., Assistant Professor, Department of Medicine, University of North Carolina at Chapel Hill, 349 Clinical Sciences Building, Chapel Hill, NC 27514

Burton E. Sobel, M.D., Professor of Medicine, Director, Cardiovascular Division, Washington University School of Medicine, Barnes and Wohl Hospitals, 660 S. Euclid Ave., St. Louis, MO 63110

David W. Snyder, M.D., Cardiovascular Division, Washington University School of Medicine, 660 S. Euclid Ave., St. Louis, MO 63110

Albert L. Waldo, M.D., University of Alabama Medical Center, University Station, Birmingham, AL 35294

August M. Watanabe, M.D., Indiana University School of Medicine, 1100 W. Michigan St., Indianapolis, IN 46202

Eric S. Williams, M.D., Associate Professor, Department of Medicine, Indiana University School of Medicine, 1100 W. Michigan St., Indianapolis, IN 46202

Andrew L. Wit, Ph.D., Professor, Department of Pharmacology, Columbia University, College of Physicians and Surgeons, 630 W. 168th St., New York, NY 10032

Alastair Wood, M.D., Assistant Professor, Departments of Pharmacology and Medicine, Vanderbilt University, Nashville, TN 37232

Raymond L. Woosley, M.D., Ph.D., Associate Professor, Departments of Clinical Pharmacology and Medicine, Vanderbilt University, A-5213, Nashville, TN 37232

CHAPTER 1

Electrophysiologic determinants of normal cardiac rhythms and arrhythmias

MICHAEL R. ROSEN and BRIAN F. HOFFMAN

The purpose of this chapter is to review the mechanisms responsible for normal impulse initiation and propagation, as well as the mechanisms for cardiac arrhythmias. We hope not only to provide an understanding of the pathophysiology of cardiac arrhythmias but – in addition – to provide a basis for the discussion of antiarrhythmic drug actions and antiarrhythmic therapy that will follow. The approach to be taken will rely heavily on cellular electrophysiology. By referring to data obtained from the single cardiac cell that is the final common denominator of cardiac electrical activity, as well as the interactions among groups of cells, we can describe the cellular electrophysiologic mechanisms responsible for normal electrical activity as well as arrhythmogenesis.

Electrical activity in the normal heart

The transmembrane potential

The cardiac cell membrane can be conceived of as having a series of 'channels' traversing it that control the influx and efflux of ions. Either inward or outward currents can flow across the cell membrane through these channels. Inward currents can be the result of either the influx of positively charged ions or the efflux of negatively charged ions, whereas outward currents are induced by the efflux of positively charged or the influx of negatively charged ions. Inward currents depolarize the membrane and outward currents hyperpolarize it. The distribution of ions across the membrane at any time and the relative permeabilities to those ions

are the major determinants of the membrane potential.

The transmembrane resting potential of fibers in the Purkinje system is approximately –90 mV. This potential is the result of a concentration gradient for potassium across the cell membrane such that the ratio of intracellular to extracellular potassium concentration ($[K^+]$) is about 30:1. The transmembrane K^+ ion gradient is established by the enzyme Na-K ATPase which pumps sodium out of and potassium into the cell. The transport of Na^+ and K^+ is electrogenic in nature, in that more Na^+ is pumped out than K^+ pumped in (approximately a 3:2 Na–K ratio); active transport thereby provides an outward current that contributes to the resting potential and influences the time-course of the action potential and phase 4 depolarization [1]. Potassium ions move passively across the membrane (providing an outward current) down the concentration gradient until the transmembrane potential is approximately equal to the potassium equilibrium potential, E_K.

$$E_K = \frac{RT}{F} \ln \frac{[K^+]_o}{[K^+]_i}, \text{ where} \qquad (1)$$

R = the gas constant
T = temperature (absolute)
F = the Faraday.

Because the resting membrane is much more permeable to K^+ than to other ions, the contribution of other ions to the resting potential is much smaller than that of K^+.

As extracellular $[K^+]$ is increased, the resting potential changes in a manner approximated by the

Rosen, M. R. and Hoffman, B. F. (eds.), Cardiac Therapy. ISBN 0-89838-564-4.
© 1983, Martinus Nijhoff Publishers, Boston, The Hague, Dordrecht, Lancaster. Printed in the Netherlands.

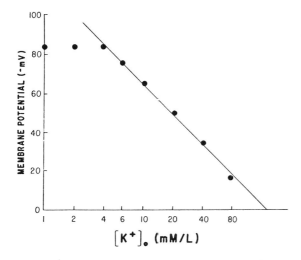

Figure 1. Relationship of resting membrane potential to extracellular potassium concentration of a human ventricular fiber. The circles indicate experimental data points; the line, the expected relationship between [K$^+$] and membrane potential assuming the Nernst relationship (see text) (reprinted from Dangman et al., Circulation (in press), by permission of the Am Heart Assoc, Inc).

Nernst equation (Equation 1). As a result, over a wide range of extracellular K$^+$ concentrations membrane potential decreases linearly as a function of the natural logarithm of [K$^+$]$_o$ [2,3] (see Figure 1).

The transition from rest to activity results from the effects of membrane potential on the permeability of the membrane to ions. The current carried by an ion depends on the conductance for that specific ion, i.e., the ease with which it can cross the membrane, and can be represented as follows:

$$i_i = \bar{g}_i s (E - E_i), \qquad (2)$$

where $\bar{g}$ is the maximum value of the conductance, s is a variable that changes with transmembrane potential and time, and the term $(E - E_i)$ represents the driving force and is the difference between the actual transmembrane potential and the equilibrium potential for the ion [4].

As a depolarizing stimulus changes the transmembrane potential, the conductance for Na$^+$ and inward Na$^+$ current increase (Figure 2A). A subthreshold stimulus will not increase sodium current enough to exceed K$^+$ current; thus, at the end of the stimulus, net ionic current will be outward and the membrane will repolarize. A threshold stimulus, in contrast, is one that increases $\bar{g}_{Na}$ until net ionic current is inward. Under this condition the depolarization becomes self-sustaining or regenerative and the upstroke (phase 0) of the action potential is inscribed (Figure 2B). The inward sodium current shifts transmembrane potential toward the sodium equilibrium potential, E_{Na}. The transmembrane potential at the peak of the action potential upstroke

(A)

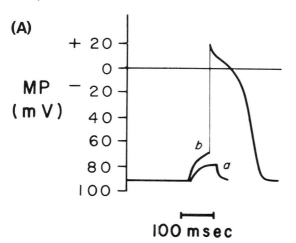

(B)

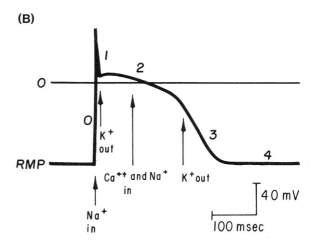

Figure 2: (A) Threshold potential of a Purkinje fiber: 'a' represents a depolarizing stimulus that does not attain threshold; 'b' a stimulus that reaches threshold potential and induces the fast inward current and an action potential (reprinted from Rosen MR: Electrophysiology of the cardiac specialized conduction system. In: Narula O (ed) His Bundle Electrocardiography and Clinical Electrophysiology. F. A. Davis Co, Philadelphia, 1975, p 23, by permission of the publisher). (B) Transmembrane action potential of a Purkinje fiber; RMP = resting membrane potential. The major ionic currents responsible for the action potential during phases 0 (rapid upstroke), 1 (initial repolarization), 2 (plateau), and 3 (repolarization) are indicated. For further description of these and of phase 4, see text.

does not attain E_{Na}, however, because the conductance of the sodium channels is governed by two variables, m and h. The sodium current thus is:

$$i_{Na} = \overline{g}_{Na}\, m^3\, h\, (E - E_{Na}). \tag{3}$$

The value of m increases very rapidly with depolarization whereas h increases somewhat more slowly. An increase in m *opens* sodium channels and an increase in h *closes* them [5]. The former process is called *activation* and the latter *inactivation*. The channels thus change between three states [6]:

resting → open → inactivated.

Inactivated channels, on repolarization, return to the resting state. Because the channels that open to permit an inward current and cause the action potential upstroke respond quickly to a change in transmembrane potential they are called *fast inward channels*, to contrast with the kinetics of other channels subserving an inward current and described below.

Depolarization during the action potential upstroke influences the conductance of several other types of channels. There is a decrease in the conductance of the K^+ channels that dominate resting permeability, g_{k_1}, and thus outward or repolarizing current through them is limited. In contrast a different K^+ channel, in combination with inactivation of the fast sodium channel, causes the prompt partial repolarization shown by phase 1 of the transmembrane action potential [7]. This phase is succeeded by a prolonged phase of depolarization known as phase 2, or the plateau. The plateau results because depolarization slowly opens another channel, g_{si}, that permits an inward current of calcium and sodium [8]. The inward current in this *slow inward channel* is much smaller than the fast inward current and just sufficient to balance outward K^+ currents. With time the slow inward channel closes partially and another K^+ channel, $g_{x,l}$, opens [9]. The net current becomes outward and the membrane potential shifts to the resting value.

The above-mentioned characteristics are typical of Purkinje fibers. Fibers at other sites in the heart have electrophysiologic properties that differ to a varying extent from those of Purkinje fibers. For example, whereas atrial specialized fibers have transmembrane potentials quite similar to those of Purkinje fibers, fibers in the atrial and ventricular myocardium tend to have less negative resting potentials (–80 to –85 mV), lower action potential amplitudes and slower rates of phase 0 depolarization. In all these cell types the basis for the resting potential and action potential upstroke is the same as in Purkinje fibers, with resting potential depending on the K^+ permeability of the membrane and phase 0 resulting from opening of fast channels and an inward Na^+ current. Slow inward channels also are present in all these fibers and current in them causes the plateau of the transmembrane action potential as well as providing the calcium for excitation–contraction coupling. Phase 3 repolarization in all fiber types is the result of an outward K^+ current. It is to be emphasized that the kinetics of this current differ markedly amongst various cardiac tissues, resulting in very different voltage–time courses of repolarization. As an example, the duration of the Purkinje fiber action potential exceeds that of ventricular myocardium; similarly the repolarization process is faster in atrial myocardial than in specialized fibers.

Cells in the sinus and AV nodes and the atrial surfaces of the AV valves have quite low resting membrane potentials (in the range of –60 to –70 mV) and very slowly rising action potentials (Figure 3). For nodal fibers there is no well-defined phase 1, and phases 2 and 3 of repolarization are not clearly demarcated as in the Purkinje system. The specialized cells of the sinus and AV node (N region) are unique in that under normal conditions the inward current causing the action potential upstroke flows in slow inward channels [10, 11]. The rate of change of membrane potential during phase 0 thus is quite low compared to that in other types of cardiac cells. Action potential generation in these cells hence is

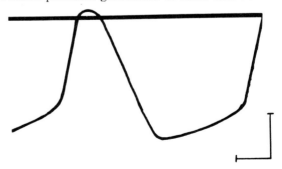

Figure 3. Transmembrane potential of rabbit sinus node fiber. Note low resting potential as compared to that of Purkinje fiber in Figure 2 (vertical calibration, 20 mV; horizontal, 100 msec).

insensitive to tetrodotoxin, which blocks fast inward channels, but quite sensitive to verapamil and other agents that block slow channels.

One further point deserves emphasis in contrasting action potentials resulting from currents in fast and slow channels. Inactivation of fast channels is removed quite rapidly when transmembrane potential attains the normal resting potential. In contrast, inactivation of slow channels is removed less rapidly. For this reason refractoriness of Purkinje fibers and atrial and ventricular muscle fibers ends soon after repolarization, whereas in sinus and AV nodes refractoriness and incomplete recovery of responsiveness usually persist for some time after the end of phase 3 [12].

In addition to their role in the genesis of sinus and AV nodal action potentials and the plateau phase of other action potentials, the slow inward channels can provide the current for a unique type of response in all cardiac fibers, the *slow response* [12]. If the resting transmembrane potential is reduced enough to cause complete or almost complete inactivation of fast channels (–50 to –55 mV), sodium current can not contribute to action potential generation. At such values of transmembrane potential, however, the slow channels still are available for activation. If extracellular calcium concentration is elevated or if catecholamines are present to increase the current in slow channels, all cardiac cells can generate action potentials for which the depolarizing current is carried by these channels. These slow responses propagate very slowly and have a very low margin of safety. They are thought to be important in the generation of certain arrhythmias as will be described later.

Impulse initiation

All cardiac cells are excitable; that is, they respond to a stimulus that is sufficient to bring them to threshold by generating an action potential. Certain cardiac fibers are *automatic* as well; on cessation of extrinsic stimulation they can depolarize spontaneously and initiate an action potential. In the normally functioning heart automaticity of the sinus node controls rate and rhythm. Should normal sinus function cease, then specialized fibers in the atrium, the AV junction and the ventricular specialized conducting system can depolarize spontaneously and function as automatic pacemakers.

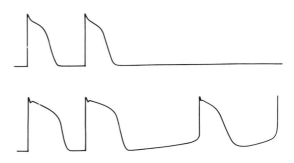

Figure 4 (schematic). Upper panel: a myocardial fiber is stimulated for the first two cycles. The stimulus then is discontinued and the fiber remains quiescent. Lower panel: a Purkinje fiber is stimulated for the first two cycles; the stimulus then is discontinued and the fiber depolarizes during phase 4, establishing an automatic rhythm.

Such pacemakers tend to develop slower rates than does the sinus node, although – as shall be noted below – there are exceptions to this. Moreover, in specific experimental situations – as well as in cardiac disease – working myocardial fibers also can generate automatic rhythms. These, too, will be discussed below.

Figure 4 provides an example of a normal automatic pacemaker, and compares its behavior to that of a muscle fiber that is excitable, but not automatic. In Figure 4, upper panel, a normal myocardial fiber is being stimulated by an electrical pulse for the first two cycles. Each stimulus provides sufficient current to depolarize the membrane to threshold potential. After the second cycle the extrinsic stimulus is discontinued and the cell remains quiescent. Working myocardial fibers in the atria and ventricles do not generate automatic rhythms at normal levels of membrane potential.

Figure 4, lower panel, shows the transmembrane potential of a Purkinje fiber that is being driven by an extrinsic stimulus. On discontinuation of the stimulus after the second action potential the fiber depolarizes gradually until at the threshold potential an automatic impulse is generated. The slow depolarization that lowers transmembrane potential is called slow diastolic or phase 4 depolarization. The change in transmembrane potential that is responsible for normal automaticity of the sinus node pacemaker resembles that diagrammed for the Purkinje fiber.

One characteristic of normal automaticity should

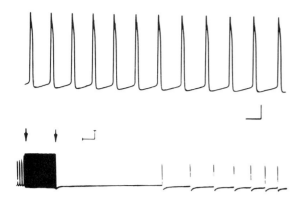

Figure 5. Overdrive suppression of normal automatic pacemaker. Upper panel: phase 4 depolarization and automaticity (vertical calibration = 20 mV; horizontal = 1 sec). Lower panel: at slower sweep speed, fiber is overdriven (between two arrows). On discontinuation of drive there is a long period of quiescence before automaticity recommences (vertical calibration = 30 mV; horizontal = 6 sec) (reprinted from Rosen M, Reder R: Does triggered activity have a role in the genesis of cardiac arrhythmias. Ann Int Med 94:795, 1981, by permission of the Am College of Physicians).

be emphasized at this time. This is the response to stimulation at a rate more rapid than the intrinsic rate of the potential pacemaker (Figure 5). The effect of overdrive on an automatic or potentially automatic cell is to suppress its automaticity [13, 14]. This phenomenon is called overdrive suppression and is the mechanism that permits the most rapid automatic cell to serve as the cardiac pacemaker. Overdrive suppression occurs in the following way: during a rapid rhythm Na^+ enters the cell during each action potential and causes $[Na^+]_i$ to increase. This, in turn, stimulates Na^+ for K^+ exchange. Because the exchange process is electrogenic there is an augmented outward current that hyperpolarizes the membrane and suppresses phase 4 depolarization. Since, in the sinus node, the depolarizing current during the action potential upstroke is carried mainly by Ca^{2+} rather than Na^+ [10], overdrive suppression of sinus node pacemakers is less marked than for ectopic pacemakers demonstrating normal automaticity.

When, in a subsequent section, we discuss abnormal mechanisms for impulse initiation we will note that one of the major differentiators of normal and abnormal impulse initiation is the response to overdrive pacing. Whereas normal pacemakers can be relied on to respond consistently to overdrive by being suppressed, the abnormal mechanisms for impulse initiation are less readily or not at all suppressed by short periods of overdrive. In some instances they may show increases in pacemaker rate as a result of overdrive [15].

The ionic mechanisms responsible for automaticity are complex [16]. In automatic sinus node cells phase 4 depolarization results from an inward current that is activated on repolarization. As the outward currents causing repolarization during phase 3 decrease, the inward current causes slow depolarization during phase 4 and lowers transmembrane potential to threshold.

In the case of Purkinje fibers it was thought for some time that the cause of phase 4 depolarization was the time- and voltage-dependent decrease of an outward potassium current, i_{k_2}, that had been activated during the preceding action potential [17]. More recent data indicate that this concept was incorrect and that the pacemaker current is an increasing inward current carried mainly by Na^+ [18]. The important concept is the following: during phase 3 the net ionic current is outward and transmembrane potential becomes more negative. At the resting potential the repolarizing current, i_{x_1}, decreases and membrane potential is sustained at the resting potential by potassium current in the g_{k_1} channels. In automatic cells an additional inward current is activated by depolarization and during phase 4 slowly shifts membrane potential towards the threshold value.

Impulse propagation

The propagation of the cardiac impulse depends on both the passive properties (that is, the ability to function as electrical cables) and the active properties of cardiac tissues. In considering passive properties, it generally is assumed that cardiac tissue behaves as a uniform cable, although in terms of the anatomy of cardiac fibers, this is an oversimplification. The conduction velocity of the cardiac impulse is determined by the flow of electrical current from sites that have been stimulated (and are generating action potentials) to sites that are still in the resting state. The flow of electrical current, in turn, is determined by factors such as the resistance and capacitance of the membrane, the cytoplasmic and extracellular resistances, the dimensions of the cable, and ionic current flow across the membrane.

5

The total membrane current can be defined as follows [19]:

$$i_m = i_c + i_i;$$ (4)

that is, the membrane current (i_m) is the sum of the capacitative current (i_c) as well as the ionic currents (i_i). The capacitative current is induced by the movement of positive charge inward across the cell membrane. This tends to depolarize the membrane. During phase 0 the ionic current is the rapid inward Na^+ current, which depolarizes the membrane by carrying positive charge into the cell.

Both the capacitative and ionic currents vary with the area of the membrane. As area increases so does conduction velocity. Because of the relationship between area and fiber radius, the conduction velocity (θ) can be considered in terms of radius (r) as follows: $\theta \propto \sqrt{r}$; in other words, the velocity of conduction will tend to increase with the square root of the radius.

Another important determinant of conduction velocity is the threshold potential of a cardiac fiber. Threshold potential is that level of potential that must be attained for the inward ionic current responsible for phase 0 depolarization to be initiated. The time required to depolarize the membrane to its threshold potential will – in part – determine the velocity of conduction. For example, depolarizing Purkinje or ventricular myocardial fibers by a few mV (by elevating $[K^+]_0$ from 4 to 5.5 mM) has been shown to result in an increase in conduction velocity [20]. The major determinant of this increase in velocity appears to be the closer relationship between resting and threshold potentials than existed prior to depolarization.

Once a cell has been brought to threshold potential, the characteristics of the action potential upstroke still further modify conduction. For example, in cells with rapid phase 0 upstroke velocities, there usually is more rapid conduction than in cells that have slowly rising action potentials (Figure 6).

In sum, then, it is the interaction of a number of membrane properties that determines conduction velocity. The passive properties of the membrane, the level of threshold potential, and the maximum upstroke velocity of the action potential all play a role here.

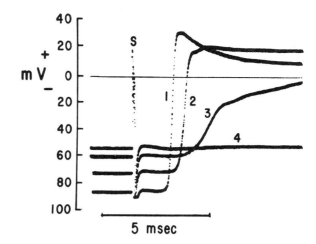

Figure 6. Relationship of phase 0 upstroke to membrane potential and conduction time: S = stimulus artifact, 1–4 indicate traces recorded at successively less negative membrane potentials. Conduction time can be estimated by measuring the interval from 'S' to the action potential upstrokes 1, 2, and 3 (reprinted from Rosen M, Hordof A: Mechanisms of arrhythmias. In: Roberts N, Gelband H (eds) Cardiac Arrhythmias in the Neonate, Infant and Child. Appleton-Century-Crofts, New York, 1977, p 118, by permission of the publisher).

Refractoriness

If a premature stimulus is applied at varying intervals after the action potential upstroke the response will be a function of the stimulus strength and the time after the upstroke [1]. Until the end of the plateau even a very strong stimulus will not elicit a premature response, because the fast channels are inactivated. During phase 3, as repolarization progressively removes inactivation, strong stimuli may elicit local responses that fail to propagate. When the membrane has repolarized enough the premature response will propagate and this moment signifies the end of the *effective refractory period* (Figure 7). The effective refractory period is particularly important because it is the duration of this period that can limit the propagation of premature impulses to a local site in the cardiac conducting system. Ectopic impulses arriving at a site before termination of the effective refractory period will be unable to propagate beyond that site.

The premature responses elicited during phase 3 are abnormal in terms of the rate of depolarization during phase 0 and the amplitude and duration of the premature action potential. They may propa-

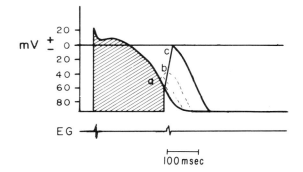

Figure 7. Effective refractory period. Upper trace is a Purkinje fiber action potential; the lower a recording from a surface electrogram (EG) distal to the site at which the action potential is recorded. Following excitation, the fiber is refractory and will not propagate premature impulses (crosshatched area). Premature impulse c is the first that propagates distally, and its upstroke indicates the termination of the effective refractory period (modified after Rosen M: Cellular electrophysiologic basis for cardiac arrhythmias. Angiology 28:294, 1977).

gate less rapidly than normal responses and are more prone to block. The recovery of the ability to respond by generating an action potential has been used as a measure of the responsiveness of the tissue. Usually this is quantified in terms of the maximum rate of depolarization during phase 0 of the premature action potential [21].

Although increased outward current (i_{x_1}) contributes to the reduced excitability and reduced responsiveness during phase 3, the main cause of the alterations in excitability and responsiveness is inactivation of fast inward channels. In fibers with normal resting potentials in the range of –85 to –95 mV inactivation is removed fairly rapidly and thus normal excitability and responsiveness are restored soon after the end of repolarization. If resting potential is reduced, however, inactivation is removed less rapidly and less completely and under these conditions the control excitability and responsiveness may not be restored until some time after the end of repolarization.

As mentioned above, in cells of the sinus and AV nodes, in which slow channels are responsible for action potential generation, refractoriness and reduced responsiveness typically outlast the action potential because removal of slow channel inactivation is slow. When other types of fibers are partially depolarized and generating slow responses their refractoriness resembles that of nodal cells.

Autonomic effects on normal cardiac fibers*

Parasympathetic effects

Parasympathetic innervation is far more dense in supraventricular than in ventricular tissue, and the effects of parasympathetic stimulation and of acetylcholine differ markedly in different areas of the heart. In the sinus node and atrium, acetylcholine increases potassium conductance, resulting in hyperpolarization [22], and blocks the slow inward current (i_{s_1}) [23]. In those fibers in which phase 4 depolarization is taking place, the slope of phase 4 is decreased by acetylcholine and automatic rate slows. All these effects of acetylcholine are blocked by atropine. In the AV node the major effect of acetylcholine is to decrease both the amplitude and upstroke velocity of the action potential, primarily in the upper and midnodal regions, to slow conduction and to prolong refractoriness [1]. At sufficiently high acetylcholine concentrations there is complete AV conduction block. Recently, it has been shown that acetylcholine not only increases the K conductance of cardiac fibers, but that it depresses the slow inward (Ca^{++}) current [23]. This effect would tend to reduce the amplitude and upstroke velocity of the AV nodal action potential and would contribute to the slowing of the conduction that occurs.

In the canine ventricular specialized conducting system acetylcholine even in quite high concentrations (10^{-5}–10^{-4} M) has only minor effects on repolarization, accelerating its voltage–time course [24]. However, moderate concentrations of acetylcholine ($\geq 10^{-7}$ M) induce a concentration-dependent decrease in the slope of phase 4 depolarization and in automaticity [25, 26]. This action is blocked by atropine.

Although acetylcholine slows normal pacemaker rate in the ventricle as well as in the sinus node and atrium, this information should not be interpreted to indicate that the effects of vagal stimulation will alter pacemaker function equivalently throughout the heart. The vagal innervation of the heart is such that the sinus node, atrium and AV junction receive a rich cholinergic nerve supply [27]. In the ventricle cholinergic innervation is relatively dense in the region of the proximal bundle branches (especially

* Detailed discussions of this subject are presented in Chapter 4; only a brief review will be incorporated here.

on the left) but its density decreases peripherally [28].

Experiments concerning the effects of vagal stimulation on ventricular automaticity in dogs were conducted by Vassalle et al. [29, 30]. They found that whereas vagal stimulation induced AV nodal block, the actual suppression of ventricular automaticity was determined by atrial impulse initiation occurring prior to block. In other words, the suppression of automaticity that occurred on vagal stimulation occurred as the result of atrial overdrive of the ventricle and *not* as the result of a direct vagal effect on the automatic pacemaker.

In clinical studies of sustained ventricular tachycardia, Waxman et al. were able to terminate this arrhythmia by elevating blood pressure with phenylephrine [31, 32]. The antiarrhythmic action of phenylephrine was blocked by atropine, suggesting that the vagus might well play an important role in terminating such arrhythmias. However, their subsequent studies of nonsustained tachycardias have emphasized the importance of atrial rate changes in modifying arrhythmogenesis (M. Waxman, personal communication). In pointing out the important effect of cardiac rate as opposed to the vagus in modifying ventricular arrhythmias these observations of Waxman et al. complement those of Vassalle et al. in experimental animals [29, 30].

Sympathetic effects
Both alpha and beta adrenergic effects of catecholamines on cardiac fibers have been demonstrated. In normal sinus node and Purkinje fibers, beta adrenergic stimulation increases the slope of phase 4 depolarization and increases spontaneous pacemaker rate. In depolarized Purkinje and myocardial fibers, beta adrenergic stimulation may induce hyperpolarization, which is thought to result from stimulation of electrogenic pumping [33]. The hyperpolarization and the increase in slope of phase 4 and automaticity all can be blocked by beta adrenergic blocking agents. In myocardial and Purkinje fibers, beta adrenergic stimulation also increases inward calcium current and plateau height and increases the slope of phase 3 repolarization.

The alpha adrenergic effects of catecholamines on the heart have been described more recently. Whereas beta adrenergic stimulation accelerates the voltage–time course of repolarization of myocardial fibers, alpha adrenergic amines have been reported to show the opposite effect [34]. Moreover, they have little or no effect on maximum diastolic potential but decrease the slope of phase 4 depolarization and the rate of impulse initiation of pacemaker fibers in both the normal Purkinje system and atrium [35–37]. Hence, whereas beta adrenergic stimulation increases the rate at which normal Purkinje fiber and atrial pacemakers initiate impulses, alpha adrenergic stimulation decreases the rate of impulse initiation. Whether an alpha adrenergic effect occurs on the sinus node has not as yet been demonstrated.

Some recent studies have considered the role of alpha adrenergic stimulation in myocardial ischemia and infarction. These have demonstrated an increased α_1 adrenergic receptor number in feline myocardium subjected to coronary occlusion and reperfusion [38]. Occurring, as well, in this model are ventricular premature depolarizations and fibrillation that can be prevented or reduced by the α_1 blocker, prazosin, but not by the β blocker, propranolol [39]. Other studies of the effects of adrenergic amines on automaticity of depolarized ventricular myocardium in the guinea pig have shown that α agonists do not depress automaticity at low membrane potentials [40]. In sum, it appears that α adrenergic inhibition of impulse initiation is – at least in part – membrane potential dependent and that the currents that induce pacemaker activity at low levels of membrane potential respond differently to α agonists than those at high levels of membrane potential.

Mechanisms of arrhythmias

In the presence of cardiac disease – whether spontaneous or experimentally induced – a variety of changes have been described in the cardiac transmembrane potential. In studies of the human ventricle [41, 42] it has been shown that infarction and ventricular dilatation are accompanied by depolarization of the cell membrane, depression of the action potential upstroke and a slowing of conduction. In human atrium, cellular electrophysiologic studies have demonstrated an association between marked chamber dilatation, the occurrence of slow response action potentials in cells having a low resting membrane potential, and the occurrence of paroxysmal atrial tachyarrhythmias [43]. It also has been shown that even in the presence of marked chamber dilatation and chronic arrhythmias such as atrial fibrillation, the slow response does not invariably occur [44, 45]. In other words, both the slow response and depressed conduction in fibers having the fast response are compatible with arrhythmogenesis.

A number of *in vitro* models have been used to mimic pathological conditions and to permit the study of resultant action potentials. Some of these depend on the depolarizaton of cardiac fibers. As a fiber is depolarized, the amplitude of its action potential decreases, the action potential upstroke velocity diminishes and, often, conduction velocity is slowed. At sufficiently low levels of membrane potential (i.e., < -50 mV), the inward Na^+ current responsible for phase 0 of the normal action potential no longer is activated (Figure 8). Instead there is a slowly propagating action potential that has been referred to as the 'slow response.' The slow response has been identified in experiments on fibers depolarized with solutions containing a high $[K^+]$ and epinephrine [46], and in fibers superfused with a Na^+-free, Ca^{++}-rich solution [47]. The latter experiment showed that in the complete absence of Na^+, an action potential still could occur, the upstroke of which resulted entirely from a Ca^{++} current. In subsequent studies of different cardiac tissues (atrium, Purkinje fiber, ventricle) under a variety of conditions (e.g., infarction, chamber dila-

tation, depolarization induced by drugs or by K^+), slow response action potentials were shown to occur [41–43]. It is likely that in most of these instances (the only definite exception being the Na^+-free solution), the action potentials are not solely the result of slow inward current. Rather it appears that Na^+ entering through the same 'slow' channel as calcium contributes to their occurrence as well [48]. Moreover, a number of tissues – even in the normal state – have action potentials similar to the slow response and evince slow conduction, including the sinus and AV nodes, and fibers in the AV valves. By providing a mechanism for very slow conduction, the slow response fulfills an important criterion for conduction delay in reentrant rhythms. This will be discussed below.

We must stress that, although slow responses (defined as those that have no tetrodotoxin-sensitive fast inward current and are the result of a verapamil-sensitive slow inward current) are demonstrable in tissues from human and animal hearts, it is likely that in many instances of arrhythmogenesis the action potential is a 'mixed' fast-channel- and slow-channel-dependent response. Studies of myocardial infarction in dogs have demonstrated that current in a fast channel contributed to the action potential even when there was marked depression of the upstroke and very slow propagation [49]. This highlights the heterogeneity of transmembrane potential changes that occur in the presence of cardiac disease. In the following pages we will categorize these abnormalities under the general headings of abnormal impulse initiation and abnormal impulse propagation.

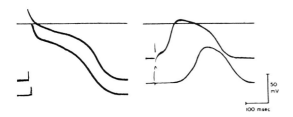

Figure 8. Fast and slow response action potentials. Two transmembrane action potentials recorded from a single unbranched Purkinje fiber bundle. On left, 'fast response' fibers have a high resting potential, rapid upstroke (not seen at this sweep speed) and propagate rapidly. On right, same two cells while superfusing the preparation with a solution containing a high K^+ concentration (16 mM) and epinephrine. The fibers have depolarized, upstroke velocity is low and conduction is slow. Note: 0 reference line refers to upper trace in each panel only (reprinted from Wit et al.: Electrophysiology and pharmacology of cardiac arrhythmias: Am Heart J 88:516, 1974, by permission of CV Mosby Co).

Abnormal impulse initiation

Automaticity
Abnormal impulse initiation may occur as the result of the abnormal expression of normal automatic mechanisms or, alternatively, as a result of the occurrence of abnormal automaticity either competing with or replacing the normal pacemaker. To define abnormal automaticity, we shall use normal automaticity as a point of reference. In the Purkinje system, normal automaticity occurs in fibers having a high maximum diastolic potential (i.e., > -90 mV) in which the automatic rhythm responds to overdrive by being suppressed. In the sinus node, al-

though membrane potential is low, the normal pacemaker also is suppressed by overdrive. Hence, the major descriptor we can provide for a normal automatic pacemaker is one which occurs in a fiber whose membrane potential is in the normal range and whose pacemaker currents are normal for that type of tissue (i.e., Purkinje fiber, sinus node, etc.) and which is overdrive suppressible.

We can best conceive of a normal pacemaker inducing ectopic activity when the sinus node pacemaker is unable to overdrive suppress it. Situations in which sinus nodal exit block or complete AV conduction block occur are settings in which a pacemaker fiber functioning normally at another site in the heart may induce an arrhythmia. In these instances, the emergence of such pacemaker function at a site outside the sinus node provides impulse initiation for the heart. As an alternative, under circumstances such as stress and adrenal or autonomic catecholamine release, subsidiary pacemakers having normal mechanisms for impulse initiation might attain a rate faster than that of the sinus node, giving rise to a tachycardia.

In addition to this normal automatic mechanism, there is an abnormal type of automaticity, the characteristics of which are very different [50, 51]. Abnormal automaticity occurs in specialized conducting or myocardial fibers that have been depolarized to low membrane potentials ($\sim$ –60 mV). At these membrane potentials, the ionic currents responsible for normal pacemaker function in the Purkinje system appear to be inactivated. Although the currents that induce abnormal automaticity at low membrane potentials are not yet characterized, much work has been done in this area. In muscle or Purkinje fibers depolarized using Ba^{++} or Cs^{++}, there is a decrease in membrane K^+ conductance which reduces maximum diastolic potential [52, 53]. At this reduced level of membrane potential an increase in membrane Na^+ conductance and/or a time- and voltage-dependent decrease in the repolarizing current, i_{x_1}, may be responsible for phase 4 depolarization [53, 54]. Others have suggested that an inward Ca^{++} current may play a role here as well [55].

An important characteristic of abnormal automaticity is that it is not as readily subject to overdrive suppression by short periods of pacing as is normal automaticity. Using the Purkinje fiber as an example, pacemakers that are readily overdrive

suppressed at high membrane potentials become less affected by overdrive as membrane potential is decreased [56]. At very low levels of membrane potential ($<$ –60 mV) overdrive can even result in speeding up and attainment of the overdrive rate by the abnormal pacemaker (Figure 9) [15, 56]. Such

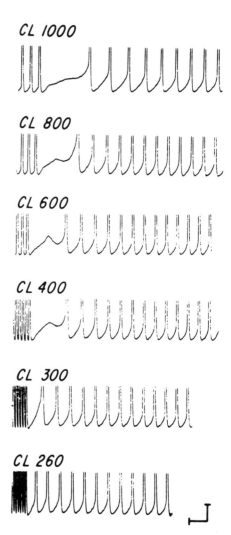

Figure 9. Abnormal automaticity induced by ouabain. On the left in each panel the preparation is driven at successively shorter cycle lengths. The stimulus then is discontinued. As drive cycle length decreases the escape interval from the last driven to the first spontaneous beat decreases. In addition, the cycle length of the automatic rhythm shortens to some extent as well: vertical calibration = 15 mV; horizontal = 2 sec (from Rosen MR, Danilo P: Effects of TTX, lidocaine, verapamil and AHR-2666 on ouabain-induced delayed afterdepolarizations in canine Purkinje fibers. Circ Res 46:121, 1980, reprinted by permission of the Am Heart Assoc, Inc).

10

abnormal automatic activity, which is not readily suppressed by overdrive, also should not easily be suppressed by the sinus node and should be able to induce automatic rhythms even in the presence of normal sinus node function.

The effect of overdrive pacing on abnormal automaticity is complex. As already stated, short periods of overdrive (i.e., $< \sim 15$ sec) will not suppress the pacemaker and may even increase its rate [56]. However, long periods of overdrive ($> \sim 120$ sec) often suppress it. Extrapolating this information to the intact heart, the suppression of a pacemaker by overdrive would not categorically mean that it is a 'normal' pacemaker. If it responds to brief periods of overdrive, then the likelihood is good that the mechanism is normal automaticity; however, if long periods of overdrive are required, the rhythm may well be an abnormal form of automaticity.

It is important to reemphasize that abnormal automaticity does not occur only in specialized cardiac fibers. Depolarization of myocardium to –60 mV or less also can result in abnormal automaticity [57, 58]. Hence, whereas normal automatic mechanisms are peculiar only to certain of the specialized fibers of the heart, abnormal automaticity can be seen in muscle fibers as well, under appropriate circumstances.

Afterdepolarizations

Afterdepolarizations are oscillations in membrane potential that occur during or following repolarization. The relationship between afterdepolarizations and action potentials is a complex one, wherein the afterdepolarization can modify the action potential and at the same time the action potential can modify the afterdepolarization. To facilitate our consideration of the relationship of afterdepolarizations to action potentials, we will consider two types of afterdepolarizations consecutively, starting with those which occur during repolarization.

Following initiation of an action potential, phases 2 and/or 3 of repolarization may be interrupted by oscillations which are either followed by further repolarization or by initiation of action potentials (Figure 10). In the latter instance the resultant rhythmic activity may persist for varying periods of time at a low level of membrane potential. This type of oscillation has been referred to by Cranefield as an early afterdepolarization [12]. Its characteristics are that it requires an action potential to induce it (i.e., it cannot arise *de novo*) and it occurs before full repolarization.

Delayed afterdepolarizations (Figures 10 and 11A) are oscillations that occur after the cell has repolarized to its maximum diastolic potential. They can be induced by digitalis toxicity [59–62] by catecholamines or by myocardial infarction [42]. They occur in normal coronary sinus [63] and AV valvular tissue [64], as well as in diseased tissues from human atrium [65, 66] and ventricle [42]. When induced by digitalis toxicity, delayed afterdepolarizations can occur in sequences of 2, 3, or more; in other instances, such as epinephrine-induced delayed afterdepolarizations in coronary sinus fibers, there tend to be single oscillations only. The characteristic of delayed afterdepolarizations that is most notable in terms of arrhythmogenesis is their marked dependence on the rate of impulse

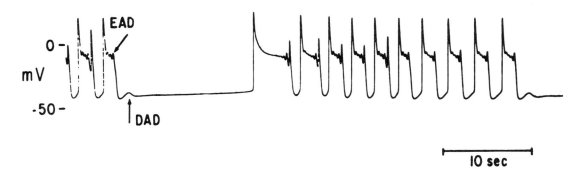

Figure 10. Early (EAD) and delayed (DAD) afterdepolarizations in canine Purkinje fibers superfused with cesium, 20 mM. See text for description (reprinted from Hoffman B, Rosen M: Cellular mechanisms for cardiac arrhythmias, Circ Res 49:6, 1981, by permission of the Am Heart Assoc, Inc).

initiation in the preparation in which they are occurring [61]. As the spontaneous rate of a preparation increases, the amplitude of delayed afterdepolarizations concomitantly increases and their coupling interval to the action potential which induces them shortens. At appropriately short cycle lengths delayed afterdepolarizations can attain threshold potential and induce rhythms whose rate is equal to or faster than the rate that induced them. It is important to stress that the relationship between the basic cycle length and both the amplitude of delayed afterdepolarizations and the cycle lengths of the rhythms they induce is a complex one. The model we will use to demonstrate this is the digitalis-induced delayed afterdepolarization, as shown in Figure 11. As drive cycle length decreases, the amplitude of the first delayed afterdepolarization increases, reaches a peak at a CL of about 600 msec [60], and then decreases. For the second delayed afterdepolarization, amplitude increases nearly exponentially. This suggests the following: for the first delayed afterdepolarization in a sequence, peak amplitude will be attained at a drive cycle length of about 500–700 msec. At this drive cycle length it will be most likely to initiate arrhythmias, whose coupling intervals will equal or be slightly shorter than the drive cycle length. An individual having such an arrhythmia intermittently would be most likely to experience it when his heart rate – for whatever reason – is about 100–120/min. At faster heart rates, the same arrhythmia would not occur, but another one might supervene, induced by the second delayed afterdepolarization.

Whereas early afterdepolarizations are thought to result from the slow inward (Ca^{++}) current the mechanism for delayed afterdepolarizations is uncertain. Tsien and associates [67–69] have suggested the following hypothesis for the genesis of digitalis-induced delayed afterdepolarizations. As a result of Na-K ATPase poisoning by digitalis, the fiber accumulates Na^+ intracellularly (i.e., the Na–K exchange mechanism is depressed by digitalis). The accumulation of Na^+ results in an alteration of the Na^+–Ca^{++} exchange, causing an increase in $[Ca^{++}]_i$. As $[Ca^{++}]_i$ increases, this induces an oscillatory release of Ca^{++} by the sarcoplasmic reticulum. This in turn increases membrane monovalent cation conductance, resulting in a transient inward current that is carried by Na^+. It is the latter current that is presumably responsible for

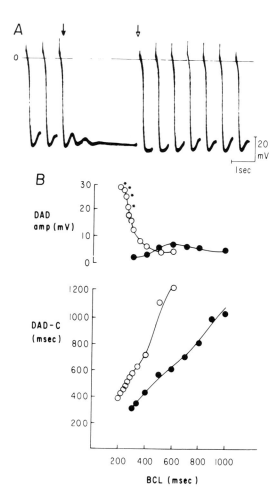

Figure 11. (A) Delayed afterdepolarizations induced by digitalis. On discontinuation of drive (filled arrow) two delayed afterdepolarizations occur in sequence followed by quiescence until the drive is reinitiated (unfilled arrow). (B) The relationship between the amplitude (amp) and coupling interval (DAD-C) of the first (filled circles) and second (unfilled circles) delayed afterdepolarizations in a sequence to drive cycle length. Asterisks indicate the afterdepolarizations that attain threshold and induce a tachyarrhythmia (panel A from Rosen et al.: Mechanisms of digitalis toxicity, Circulation 47:684, 1973, by permission of the Am Heart Assoc, Inc; panel B from Rosen M, Danilo P: Digitalis-induced delayed afterdepolarizations. In: Zipes D, Bailey J, Elharrar V (eds) The Slow Inward Current, Martinus Nijhoff, The Hague, 1980, p 421, by permission of the publisher).

delayed afterdepolarizations.

In considering afterdepolarizations, abnormal automaticity, and normal automaticity, we appear to be dealing with a continuum. On the one hand in normal automaticity we have a mechanism that is readily overdrive suppressed; at the other extreme with delayed afterdepolarizations the mechanism responds to rapid drive by showing an increase in the rate of the resultant arrhythmia (although when driven at very short cycle lengths [i.e., $<\sim 250$ msec] delayed afterdepolarization-induced rhythms can be overdrive suppressed). In terms of its response to overdrive, abnormal automaticity appears to lie somewhere between these two extremes.

Considering the means to differentiate among these mechanisms, both normal and abnormal automaticity can be suppressed by overdrive pacing (the latter only if long periods of pacing are used). Both would tend to be either reset or unaffected by premature stimulation. In contrast, arrhythmias induced by delayed afterdepolarizations will tend to increase in their rate following periods of overdrive stimulation, although at very short cycle lengths (e.g., ~ 250 msec or less for digitalis-induced delayed afterdepolarizations), overdrive may terminate these rhythms as well. The response of delayed afterdepolarization-induced rhythms to single premature stimuli is quite variable: premature stimulation may accelerate the rate of an afterdepolarization-induced rhythm, may reset it, or may terminate it.

It is likely that in the intact heart all of these mechanisms can play a role in different pathologic conditions. In addition it has been demonstrated that the occurrence of one mechanism does not rule out another mechanism occurring simultaneously in the same cell [66]. Hence, abnormal impulse initiation is complex and requires further investigation before we can identify which mechanisms are responsible for particular arrhythmias. In studies of the *in situ* heart, nonetheless, some headway has been made in identifying arrhythmias resulting from delayed afterdepolarizations. For example, it appears that digitalis-induced repetitive ventricular responses in the dog [70] are readily explained by this mechanism. This will be reviewed in a subsequent section of this chapter.

Abnormal conduction

Perhaps the simplest forms of abnormal conduction are slowing and complete block. These occur most frequently if a portion of the conducting system is rendered inexcitable. Such an event may occur transiently or may be persistent. An example

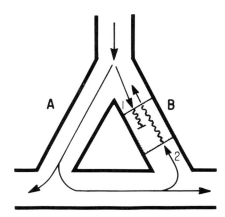

Figure 12. A Purkinje fiber bundle is depicted with its two terminal branches (A and B) and attached ventricular muscle. An impulse propagating antegrade through the bundle (arrows) is blocked by depolarized tissue in limb 'B' (stippled area) but conducts through limb 'A' to the myocardium and enters the depolarized area retrogradely at 2. It propagates through this site and reenters the proximal conducting system at 1 (reprinted from Hoffman BF, Rosen M: Cellular mechanisms for cardiac arrhythmias. Circ Res 49:9, 1981, by permission of the Am Heart Assoc, Inc).

of the former is the occurrence of varying degrees of AV block secondary to vagal stimulation or digitalis effect on the AV node. An example of the latter is interruption of one or both bundle branches as a result of infarction.

Conduction abnormalities are responsible for a variety of arrhythmias beyond the simple manifestations of conduction block. The first arrhythmia we will consider is that of reentry which was well described for the heart by Schmitt and Erlanger in 1928 [71]. As shown in Figure 12 local depolarization and antegrade conduction block have occurred in one branch of the distal Purkinje system. Although antegrade propagation has failed, conduction proceeds through the normal limb of the Purkinje system and the normal myocardium and then retrogradely to the site of conduction block. Several events then are possible: retrograde conduction can be blocked just as antegrade conduction was, in which case there is an area of bidirectional conduction block, but no arrhythmia. Alternatively, retrograde propagation can occur slowly and – if this impulse arrives at the interface with normal tissue after termination of the effective refractory period of the latter – activation of the proximal system may occur. The result would be either a single reentrant beat or the onset of a reentrant tachyarrhythmia.

In this model for reentry there are several requisites: (a) block of an impulse at a site in the conducting system; (b) a site of slow retrograde conduction; (c) sufficiently delayed activation such that refractoriness proximal to the block terminates; and (d) reexcitation of tissue proximal to the block [72, 73]. For some time, a major reservation concerning this description of reentry was related to the need for slow conduction. However, the description of the slow response action potential provided a mechanism for conduction sufficiently slow to permit reentry [12]. This is not to suggest that the slow response is the only means whereby reentry may occur. For example, studies of infarcted canine myocardium have demonstrated the occurrence of depressed action potentials that still are dependent on the fast response mechanism [49]. These propagate very slowly and are seen in settings in which reentry occurs. Moreover, the occurrence of reentry has been demonstrated in isolated tissues that contain an inexcitable segment. Here, the spread of electrotonic potentials may provide a sufficient stimulus for excitation of adjacent normal tissues, and thereby may induce reentry [74, 75].

It also has been shown that reentrant rhythms can occur in nonbranched segments of the conducting system as a result of 'reflection' [12]. In this instance, the electrical activity that occurs in the depressed segment is not the result of its excitation, but rather, is the passive effect of an active response in tissues beyond the area of depressed excitability. That is, the electrical activity induced in the depressed segment is not an action potential, but an electrotonic response. When conditions are appropriate these electrotonic potentials can reexcite the fibers that carried the impulse to the depressed segment.

Allessie, Bonke, and their associates have studied reentry in the isolated rabbit left atrium and their experiments have given rise to a 'leading circle' hypothesis for reentry [76, 77]. Preparations were paced regularly and premature stimuli were applied after every 20th paced beat. Under appropriate circumstances, a critically timed premature impulse would reproducibly initiate rapid, repetitive activity. In the circumstances of the arrhythmia they found the following: (a) a circular pathway for the tachycardia could be mapped; (b) for this to occur

the premature impulse had to be conducted in one direction but blocked in the other; and (c) for this to occur the site of block of the premature impulse had to be activated sufficiently late that the fibers proximal to the site of block no longer were refractory and could again be excited. A necessary accompaniment of this phenomenon was nonuniformity of the recovery of excitability which – in turn – was associated with dispersion of repolarization and refractoriness. The leading circle hypothesis also suggests that the rate of the tachycardia will be determined by the reentrant circuit with the smallest dimensions and that the dimensions of the circuit are determined by the refractory periods of the tissues, by conduction velocity, and by the effectiveness of the activation wave in stimulating tissues into which it is propagating.

One of the crucial factors in the leading circle concept is the dispersion of refractoriness amongst tissues. Such dispersion of refractoriness also is important in the genesis of other reentrant arrhythmias. It has long been suggested that, as a result of dispersion of refractoriness, tissues quite near one another anatomically might have very different levels of membrane potential [78]. For example, in the situation of myocardial infarction, cells in infarcted and adjacent normal tissues may repolarize at different rates. At the time the infarcted cell has repolarized, the normal one may be at a more positive membrane potential. Such a situation would permit current to flow between the two cells, and, if this were of sufficient magnitude, the fully repolarized cell might be brought to its level of threshold potential, giving rise to a premature action potential. In recent experiments, Janse et al. [79] have measured current flow between normal and infarcted regions in the pig heart and have demonstrated the occurrence of such current flow. Hence, it is feasible to suggest that such a mechanism might contribute to the occurrence of reentry in the intact heart.

Another mechanism that may cause reentrant rhythms is summation [80]. As shown in Figure 13 an impulse initiated at point A propagates a variable distance into a depressed segment and fails to propagate further. The same outcome is seen if an impulse is initiated at point C, only. However, if the initiation of impulses at points A and C is timed appropriately they can summate within the depressed segment producing a larger response than

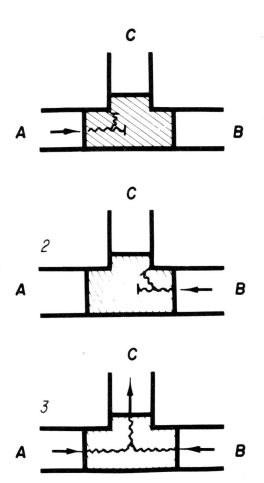

Figure 13. Summation in the Purkinje system. A branching segment of Purkinje fibers is shown with a central depressed area. See text for discussion (reprinted from Hoffman B, Rosen M: Cellular mechanisms for cardiac arrhythmias. Circ Res 49: 11, 1981, by permission of the Am Heart Assoc, Inc).

occurs following impulse initiation at one site only. This can propagate through branch B and initiate a reentrant arrhythmia.

Combined abnormal impulse initiation and propagation

An example of this type of arrhythmia is parasystole. Let us assume that at a particular site depolarized fibers encircle an area of normal specialized conducting tissue. These normal specialized conducting fibers ordinarily would be excited by the sinus node pacemaker and be overdrive suppressed.

However, because the depolarized fibers around them provide a site of conduction block (or 'entry block'), the normal fibers are 'protected' from overdrive by the sinus pacemaker. As a result, the protected fibers generate phase 4 depolarization and initiate an automatic rhythm. If conditions are appropriate in the depolarized fibers surrounding this ectopic pacemaker, its impulses can propagate into the normal myocardium and induce premature depolarizations. The frequency with which dysrhythmic beats occur will be determined by the extent of the exit block in the fibers surrounding the parasystolic pacemaker, by the rate of impulse initiation in both the parasystolic pacemaker and the normal cardiac pacemaker and by the duration of the refractory period. The impulses that propagate beyond the site of entry block then can compete with the normal cardiac pacemaker. Such a parasystolic pacemaker may have as its mechanism either normal or abnormal automaticity.

A model of parasystole has been studied by Jalife and Moe [81, 82]. They studied Purkinje fibers, the central segments of which were superfused with sucrose to prevent propagation of the action potential. One end of the fiber bundle was stimulated electrically, the other was permitted to develop an automatic rhythm. They stimulated one end of the preparation at various cycle lengths and determined the effects of electrotonic potentials spreading through the sucrose-superfused tissue on pacemaker function at the other end of the preparation. Using this model they showed that electrotonus in tissues adjacent to the parasystolic focus may have considerable influence on the focus. The interaction between the normal pacemaker site, the surrounding segment and the parasystolic focus can be appreciated by referring to Figure 14. This shows that an action potential occurring during the first half of phase 4 will reset the pacemaker such that a longer time is required for the next impulse to be initiated. Alternatively, depolarizing current delivered late in phase 4 will tend to depolarize the preparation more rapidly and cause it to fire early. Applying this model to the heart, the normal sinus pacemaker function can induce electrotonic potentials in depolarized tissues surrounding the parasystolic focus. Depending on the sinus rate, the presence of electrotonic potentials induced by the sinus mechanism can modify the rate of impulse initiation by the parasystolic pacemaker.

15

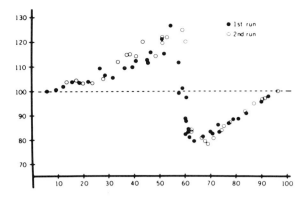

Figure 14. Electrotonic effect on spontaneous cycle length of a pacemaker fiber (induced by premature beat applied every 10–15 cycles). Vertical axis: test cycle length as percent of control (control = 100). Horizontal axis: test stimulus interval expressed as percent of change of spontaneous cycle length. There are early delay, and late acceleration of the spontaneous pacemaker (reprinted from Jalife J, Moe G: Effects of electrotonic potentials on pacemaker activity of canine Purkinje fibers in relation to parasystole. Circ Res 39:804, 1976, by permission of the Am Heart Assoc, Inc).

Arrhythmias in the in situ heart

It is important not only to describe the mechanisms studied in isolated tissues that may be arrhythmogenic but to attempt whenever possible to relate them to cardiac arrhythmias that occur in the intact heart. One model for such an arrhythmia is the repetitive ventricular response that was described by Lown and associates in dogs that were digitalis toxic [83]. They noted that prior to digitalis toxicity a single premature stimulus (applied after the termination of the vulnerable period on ECG) would result in a single premature QRS complex. They also found that with increasing doses of acetylstrophanthidin there was a diminished stimulus requirement for induction of a premature beat and – rather than single prematures occurring in response to the premature stimuli – trains of premature QRS complexes arose, leading to ventricular tachycardia. This model for digitalis toxic tachyarrhythmias in the intact dog can be explained by observations made of delayed afterdepolarizations in isolated cardiac tissues [70]. As the digitalis concentration is increased or exposure to a given concentration increases in isolated tissues then delayed afterdepolarizations occur. As the amplitude of these delayed afterdepolarizations increases, the amount of cur-

rent that must be injected into a cardiac fiber to bring them to threshold potential diminishes. Finally, with further toxicity, sustained tachyarrhythmias can occur.

A mechanism for arrhythmias that is even more readily demonstrable in the intact heart is that which contributes to preexcitation in the Wolff-Parkinson-White syndrome. The presence of an area of slow conduction, usually in this case the AV node, as well as an anatomic bypass tract offers a classic example of reentry as described above in isolated cardiac preparations [84, 85]. Other examples of reentry occurring in the intact ventricle have been provided in studies of human subjects [86–88]. Finally, studies of atrial flutter in the human heart by Waldo and associates have been suggestive of reentry as well [89].

There is at least one instance in which cellular electrophysiologic studies have led us to question the mechanism to which a specific clinical arrhythmia has long been attributed. For some time, it was believed that bigeminal rhythms were a classic example of reentry. However, Jalife and Moe have shown that, as a result of electrotonic effects on parasystolic pacemakers, this automatic rhythm can give the electrocardiographic appearance of bigeminy [82]. Hence, it probably is not appropriate to state *de facto* that bigeminal rhythms are reentrant.

Apart from these examples it is difficult to relate cellular mechanisms to clinical arrhythmias. We should mention that attempts have been made to relate accelerated ventricular [90, 91] and junctional [92] rhythms to delayed afterdepolarizations as a mechanism. Although the hypotheses and the evidence presented for these have been provocative, no final proof of the association of either arrhythmia with afterdepolarizations exists.

Conclusions

We have presented a brief overview of the mechanisms responsible for both normal and abnormal impulse initiation in the heart. It is apparent from our discussion that much of the information we have still is preliminary. Nonetheless, it now is possible to relate specific mechanisms for arrhythmias to at least some arrhythmias that occur in the intact heart. As we learn more about the association be-

16

tween mechanism and arrhythmia, it is anticipated that we will improve our abilities to diagnose and to treat clinical cardiac arrhythmias.

Acknowledgments

Certain of the experiments referred to were supported in part by USPHS-NHLBI grants HL-12738, HL-08508 and HL-28223.

References

1. Hoffman BF, Cranefield PF: Electrophysiology of the Heart. McGraw-Hill, New York, 1960.
2. Burgen ASV, Terroux, KG: The membrane resting and action potentials of cat auricle. J Physiol 119:139–152, 1953.
3. Hoffman BF: Electrophysiology of single cardiac cells. Bull NY Acad Med 35:689–706, 1959.
4. Hodgkin AL, Huxley AF: A quantitative description of membrane current and its application to conduction and excitation in nerve. J Physiol 117:500–544, 1952.
5. Jack JJB, Noble D, Tsien RW: Electric Current Flow in Excitable Cells. Clarendon Press, Oxford, 1975.
6. Hondeghem L, Katzung B: Time and voltage dependent interactions of antiarrhythmic drugs with cardiac sodium channels. Biochem Biophys Acta 472:373–398, 1977.
7. Kenyon JL, Gibbons WR: Influence of chloride, potassium and tetraethylammonium on the early outward current of sheep cardiac Purkinje fibers. J Gen Physiol 73:117–138, 1979.
8. Reuter H: Divalent cations as charge carriers in excitable membranes. In: Butler JAV, Noble D (eds) Progress in Biophysics and Molecular Biology. Pergamon Press, New York, 1973, pp 3–43.
9. McAllister RE, Noble D, Tsien RW: Reconstruction of the electrical activity of cardiac Purkinje fibers. J Physiol 251:1–59, 1975.
10. Irisawa H, Yanagihara K: The slow inward current of the rabbit sino-atrial nodal cells. In: Zipes DP, Bailey JC, Elharrar V (eds) The Slow Inward Current and Cardiac Arrhythmias. Martinus Nijhoff, The Hague, 1980, pp 265–284.
11. Noma A, Irasawa H, Kokobun S, Kotake H, Nishimura M, Watanabe Y: Slow current systems in the A-V node of the rabbit heart. Nature 285:228–229, 1980.
12. Cranefield PF: The Conduction of the Cardiac Impulse: The Slow Response and Cardiac Arrhythmias. Futura Press, Mt. Kisco, 1975.
13. Vassalle M: Electrogenic suppression of automaticity in sheep and dog Purkinje fibers. Circ Res 27:361–377, 1970.
14. Vassalle M: The relationship among cardiac pacemakers: overdrive suppression. Circ Res 41:269–277, 1977.
15. Rosen MR, Danilo P: Effects of tetrodotoxin, lidocaine, verapamil and AHR-2666 on ouabain-induced delayed afterdepolarization in canine Purkinje fibers. Circ Res 46:117–124, 1980.
16. Noma A, Irasawa H: A time- and voltage-dependent potassium current in the rabbit sinoatrial node cell. Pflugers Arch 366:251–258, 1976.
17. Noble D, Tsien RW: The kinetics and rectifier properties of the slow potassium current in cardiac Purkinje fibers. J Physiol 195:185–214, 1968.
18. DiFrancesco D: A new interpretation of the pace-maker current in calf Purkinje fibers. J Physiol 314:359–376, 1981.
19. Noble D: The Initiation of the Heart Beat. Clarendon Press, Oxford, 1975.
20. Dominguez G, Fozzard HA: Influence of extracellular K^+ concentration on cable properties and excitability of sheep cardiac Purkinje fibers. Circ Res 26:565, 1970.
21. Weidmann S: The effect of the cardiac membrane potential on the rapid availability of the sodium carrying system. J Physiol 127:213–214, 1955.
22. Trautwein W, Kuffler SW, Edward C: Changes in membrane characteristics of heart muscle during inhibition. J Gen Physiol 40:135–145, 1956.
23. Giles W, Noble SJ: Changes in membrane currents in bullfrog atrium produced by acetylcholine; J Physiol (Lond) 261:103–123, 1976.
24. Gadsby DC, Wit AL, Cranefield PF: The effects of acetylcholine on the electrical activity of canine cardiac Purkinje fibers. Circ Res 43:29–35, 1978.
25. Bailey JC, Greenspan K, Elizari MV, Anderson GJ, Fisch C: Effects of acetylcholine on automaticity and conduction in the proximal portion of the His-Purkinje system in the dog. Circ Res 30:210–216, 1972.
26. Danilo P, Rosen MR, Hordof AJ: Effects of acetylcholine on the ventricular specialized conducting system of neonatal and adult dogs. Circ Res 43:777–784, 1978.
27. Randall WC, Armour JA: Gross and microscopic anatomy of the cardiac innervation. In: Randall WC (ed) Neural Regulation of the Heart. Oxford Univ Press, New York, 1977, pp 13–41.
28. Kent KM, Epstein SE, Cooper T, Jacobowitz DC: Cholinergic innervation of the canine and human ventricular conducting system, anatomic and electrophysiologic correlations. Circulation 50:948–955, 1975.
29. Vassalle M, Vagnini FJ, Gourin A, Stuckey JH: Suppression and initiation of idioventricular automaticity during vagal stimulation. Am J Physiol 212:1–7, 1967.
30. Vassalle M, Caress DL, Slovin AJ, Stuckey JH: On the cause of ventricular asystole during vagal stimulation. Circ Res 20:228–241, 1967.
31. Waxman MB, Downar E, Berman ND, Felderhof CH: Phenylephrine (neo-synephrine) terminated ventricular tachycardia. Circulation 50:656–664, 1974.
32. Waxman MB, Wald RW: Termination of ventricular tachycardia by an increase in cardiac vagal drive. Circulation 56:385–391, 1977.
33. Vassalle M, Barnabei O: Norepinephrine and potassium fluxes in cardiac fibers. Pflugers Arch 322:287–303, 1971.
34. Giotti A, Ledda F, Mannaioni PF: Effects of noradrenaline and isoprenaline, in combination with α- and β-receptor blocking substances, on the action potential of cardiac Purkinje fibers. J Physiol 229:99–113, 1973.

35. Posner P, Farrar E, Lambert C: Inhibitory effects of catecholamines in canine cardiac Purkinje fibers. Am J Physiol 231:1415–1420, 1976.

36. Rosen MR, Hordof AJ, Ilvento JP, Danilo P Jr.: Effects of adrenergic amines on electrophysiological properties and automaticity of neonatal and adult canine Purkinje fibers: evidence for alpha and beta adrenergic actions. Circ Res 40:390–400, 1977.

37. Mary-Rabine L, Hordof A, Bowman F, Malm J, Rosen MR: Alpha and beta adrenergic effects on human atrial specialized conducting fibers. Circulation 57:84–90, 1978.

38. Corr PB, Shayman JA, Kramer JB, Kipnis RJ: Increased α-adrenergic receptors in ischemic cat myocardium. J Clin Invest 67:1232–1236, 1981.

39. Sheriden DJ, Penkoske PA, Sobel BE, Corr PB: Alpha adrenergic contributions to dysrhythmia during myocardial ischemia and reperfusion in cats. J Clin Invest 65:161–171, 1980.

40. Hume JR, Katzung BG: The effects of α and β adrenergic agonists upon depolarization induced ventricular automaticity. Proc West Pharmacol Soc 21:77–81, 1978.

41. Spear J, Horowitz L, Hodess A, MacVaugh H, Moore E: Cellular electrophysiology of human myocardial infarction. I. Abnormalities of cellular activation. Circulation 59:247–256, 1979.

42. Dangman KH, Danilo P Jr, Hordof AJ, Mary-Rabine L, Reder R, Rosen MR: Electrophysiologic characteristics of human ventricular and Purkinje fibers. Circulation 65:362–368, 1982.

43. Hordof A, Edie R, Malm J, Hoffman B, Rosen M: Electrophysiologic properties and response to pharmacologic agents of fibers from diseased human atria. Circulation 54:774–779, 1976.

44. Boyden PA, Tilley LP, Pham TD, Liu SK, Fenoglio JJ, Wit AL: Effects of left atrial enlargement on atrial transmembrane potentials and structure in dogs with mitral valve fibrosis. Am J Cardiol 49:1896–1908, 1982.

45. Rosen M, Bowman FO, Mary-Rabine L: Atrial fibrillation: The relationship between cellular electrophysiologic and clinical data. In: Kulbertus HE, Olsson SB, Schlepper M (eds) Atrial Fibrillation. Hassle, Molndal, 1982, pp 62–69.

46. Cranefield PF, Klein HO, Hoffman BF: Conduction of the cardiac impulse. I. Delay, block and one-way block in the depressed Purkinje fibers. Circ Res 28:199–219, 1971.

47. Aronson RS, Cranefield PF: The electrical activity of canine cardiac Purkinje fibers in sodium-free, calcium-rich solutions. J Gen Physiol 61:786–808, 1973.

48. Shigenobu K, Schneider JA, Sperelakis N: Verapamil blockade of slow Na^+ and Ca^{++} responses in myocardial cells. J Pharmacol Exp Ther 190:280–288, 1974.

49. El-Sherif N, Scherlag BJ, Lazzara R, Hope R: Reentrant ventricular arrhythmias in the late myocardial infarction period. Circulation 56:395–402, 1977.

50. Friedman PL, Stewart JR, Wit A: Spontaneous and induced cardiac arrhythmias in subendocardial Purkinje fibers surviving extensive myocardial infarction in dogs. Circ Res 33:612–626, 1973.

51. Lazarra R, El-Sherif N, Scherlag BJ: Electrophysiological properties of canine Purkinje cells in one-day-old myocardial infarction. Circ Res 33:722–734, 1979.

52. Reid A, Hecht HH: Barium-induced automaticity in right ventricular muscle in the dog. Circ Res 21:849–856, 1967.

53. Isenberg J: Cardiac Purkinje fibers: (Ca^{2+}) controls the potassium permeability via the conductance components gK_1 and gK_2. Pflugers Arch 371:77–85, 1977.

54. Dangman K, Hoffman B: Effects of nifedipine on electrical activity of cardiac cells. Am J Cardiol 46:1059–1067, 1980.

55. Toda N: Barium-induced automaticity in relation to calcium ions and norepinephrine in the rabbit left atrium. Circ Res 27:45–57, 1970.

56. Hoffman B, Dangman K: Are arrhythmias caused by automatic impulse generation? In: Paes de Carvalho P, Lieberman M, Hoffman B (eds) Normal and Abnormal Conduction in the Heart. Futura Press, New York, 1982, pp 429–448.

57. Katzung BO, Morgenstern JA: Effects of extracellular potassium on ventricular automaticity and evidence for a pacemaker current in mammalian ventricular myocardium. Circ Res 40:105–111, 1977.

58. Surawicz B, Imanishi S: Automatic activity in depolarized guinea pig ventricular myocardium: characteristics and mechanisms. Circ Res 39:751–759, 1976.

59. Davis LD: Effects of changes in cycle length on diastolic depolarization produced by ouabain in canine Purkinje fibers. Circ Res 32:206–214, 1973.

60. Ferrier GR: Digitalis arrhythmias: role of oscillatory afterpotentials. Prog Cardiovasc Dis 19:459–474, 1977.

61. Ferrier GR, Saunders J, Mendez C: Cellular mechanism for the generation of ventricular arrhythmias by acetylstrophanthidin. Circ Res 32:610–617, 1973.

62. Rosen MR, Merker C, Gelband H, Hoffman BF: Effects of ouabain on phase 4 of Purkinje fiber transmembrane potential. Circulation 47:681–689, 1973.

63. Wit AL, Cranefield PF: Triggered and automatic activity in the canine coronary sinus. Circ Res 41:435–445, 1977.

64. Wit AL, Cranefield PF: Triggered activity in cardiac muscle fibers of the simian mitral valve. Circ Res 38:85–98, 1976.

65. Hordof A, Spotnitz H, Mary-Rabine L, Edie R, Rosen M: The cellular electrophysiologic effects of digitalis on human atrial fibers. Circulation 57:223–229, 1978.

66. Mary-Rabine L, Hordof AJ, Danilo P, Malm JR, Rosen MR: Mechanisms for impulse initiation in isolated human atrial fibers. Circ Res 47:267–277, 1980.

67. Kass RS, Tsien RW, Weingart R: Ionic basis of transient inward currents induced by strophanthidin in cardiac Purkinje fibers. J Physiol (Lond) 281:209–226, 1978.

68. Tsien RW, Carpenter DO: Ionic mechanisms of pacemaker activity in cardiac Purkinje fibers. Fed Proc 37:2127–2131, 1978.

69. Lederer WJ, Tsien RW: Transient inward current underlying arrhythmogenic effects of cardiotonic steroids in Purkinje fibers. J Physiol 263:73–100, 1976.

70. Rosen MR, Reder RF: Does triggered activity have a role in the genesis of cardiac arrhythmias? Ann Intern Med 94:794–801, 1981.

71. Schmitt FO, Erlanger J: Directional differences in the conduction of the impulse through heart muscle and their possible relation to extrasystolic and fibrillary contractions. Am J Physiol 87:326–347, 1967.

72. Moe GK: Evidence for reentry as a mechanism for cardiac arrhythmias. Rev Physiol Biochem Pharmacol 72:56–66, 1975.

73. Wit AL, Cranefield PF: Reentrant excitation as a cause of cardiac arrhythmias. Am J Physiol 235:H1–H17, 1978.

74. Wennemark JR, Ruesta VJ, Brody DA: Microelectrode study of delayed conduction in the canine right bundle branch. Circ Res 23:753–769, 1968.

75. Antzelevitch C, Jalife J, Moe GK: Characteristics of reflection as a mechanism of reentrant arrhythmias and its relationship to parasystole. Circulation 61:182–191, 1980.

76. Allessie MA, Bonke FIM, Schopman F: Circus movement in rabbit atrial muscle as a mechanism of tachycardia. Circ Res 33:54–62, 1973.

77. Allessie MA, Bonke FIM, Schopman FJG: Circus movement in rabbit atrial muscle as a mechanism of tachycardia. III. The 'leading circle' concept: a new model of circus movement in cardiac tissue without the involvement of an anatomical obstacle. Circ Res 41:9–18, 1977.

78. Moe GK, Mendez C: Physiological basis of premature beats and sustained tachycardia. N Engl J Med 288:250–254, 1973.

79. Janse MJ, van Capelle F, Morsink H, Kleber AG, Wilms-Schopman F, Cardinal R, Naumann d'Alnoncourt C, Durrer D: Flow of 'injury' current and patterns of excitation during early ventricular arrhythmias in acute regional myocardial ischemia in isolated porcine and canine hearts. Circ Res 47:151–165, 1980.

80. Cranefield PF, Hoffman BF: Conduction of the cardiac impulse. II. Summation and inhibition. Circ Res 28:220–233, 1971.

81. Jalife J, Moe GK: Effects of electrotonic potentials on pacemaker activity of canine Purkinje fibers in relation to parasystole. Circ Res 39:801–809, 1976.

82. Jalife J, Moe GK: A biologic model of parasystole. Am J Cardiol 43:761–772, 1979.

83. Lown B, Cannon RL III, Rossi MA: Electrical stimulation and digitalis drugs: repetitive response in digitalis. Proc Soc Exp Biol Med 126:698–701, 1967.

84. Durrer D, Roos JP: Epicardial excitation of the ventricles in a patient with Wolff-Parkinson-White Syndrome (type B). Circulation 35:15–21, 1967.

85. Burchell HB, Frye RL, Anderson MW, McGoon DC: Atrioventricular and ventriculoatrial excitation in Wolff-Parkinson-White Syndrome (Type B): transitory ablation at surgery. Circulation 36:663–672, 1967.

86. Wellens HJJ, Schuilenberg RM, Durrer D: Electrical stimulation of the heart in patients with ventricular tachycardia. Circulation 46:216–226, 1974.

87. Denes P, Wu D, Dhingra RC, Wyndham C, Mautner RK, Rosen KM: Electrophysiologic studies in patients with chronic recurrent ventricular tachycardia. Circulation 54:229–236, 1976.

88. Fontaine G, Guiraudon G, Frank R, Vedel J, Grosgogeat Y, Cabrel C, Facquet J: Stimulation studies and epicardial mapping in ventricular tachycardia: study of mechanisms and selection for surgery. In: Kulbertus H (ed) Reentrant Arrhythmias: Mechanisms and Treatment. MTP Press, Lancaster, 1977, pp 334–350.

89. Wells JL Jr, MacLean WAH, James TN, Waldo AL: Characterization of atrial flutter: studies in patients after open heart surgery using fixed electrodes. Circulation 60:665–673, 1979.

90. Josephson M, Horowitz L, Farshidi A: Continuous local electrical activity: a mechanism of recurrent ventricular tachycardia. Circulation 57:659–665, 1978.

91. Zipes DP, Foster PR, Trays PJ, Pedersen DH: Atrial induction of ventricular tachycardia: re-entry versus triggered automaticity. Am J Cardiol 44:1–8, 1979.

92. Rosen MR, Fisch C, Hoffman BF, Danilo P, Lovelace PE, Knoebel SB: Can accelerated atrioventricular junctional escape rhythms be explained by delayed afterdepolarizations? Am J Cardiol 45:1272–1284, 1980.

CHAPTER 2

Cardiac failure

WILLIAM W. PARMLEY

Introduction

Congestive heart failure is a common syndrome which accompanies all forms of cardiac disease. It is generally accompanied by two major symptom complexes (shortness of breath and fatigue), which relate to the primary physiologic derangements. As the contractile abilities of the myocardium decrease, the heart has difficulty ejecting the blood that returns to it. This results in an increase in the venous pressures filling the two sides of the heart. On the left side of the heart this leads to the signs and symptoms of pulmonary congestion with *shortness of breath* as the major symptom. On the right side of the heart this leads to the signs and symptoms of systemic venous congestion. The second major symptom complex in patients with heart failure is *fatigue* secondary to low cardiac output. This is particularly manifest during exertion. Although the heart may be able to supply enough blood to peripheral tissues to meet resting demands, it may be totally inadequate to supply the needs of the body associated with vigorous exercise.

The purpose of this chapter is to review first the physiology of normal cardiovascular function, and then to describe those derangements which lead to the syndrome of congestive heart failure. There will be little discussion of the effects of cardiac ischemia (the most common cause of heart failure), since this subject will be discussed in detail in Chapter 3. In discussing the pathophysiology of congestive heart failure, we will concentrate particularly on those principles which form the basis for various therapeutic interventions. Since other chapters discuss, in detail, pharmacologic agents which can be used

for the management of heart failure, they will be considered only briefly in this chapter in relation to their effects on the pathophysiology and manifestations of heart failure. We shall begin by first considering the functional anatomy of the heart.

Normal cardiac structure and function

Cellular and subcellular structure

Individual myocardial cells or fibers are approximately 50–100 μ in length and about 10–20 μ in diameter. Cells are bounded by intercalated discs in a branching arrangement as conceptually illustrated in Figure 1A. In contrast to skeletal muscle which has multiple, peripherally placed nuclei, cardiac muscle has a single centrally placed nucleus. Each cell or fiber is made up of fibrils as illustrated in Figure 1B. These fibrils can be thought of as a long train in which the sarcomeres (the fundamental unit of contraction) represent individual cars. A sarcomere, which is bounded by Z lines, is schematically illustrated in Figure 1C. In the middle it contains thick myosin filaments (about 1.5 μ long), which are interdigitated with thin actin filaments (approximately 1 μ long). The overall length of the sarcomere at its optimum is approximately 2.2 μ. Actin filaments are attached to the Z lines and extend to or beyond the center of the sarcomere during contraction.

Also shown in Figure 1B is the sarcolemma or outer membrane of each fiber. The sarcolemma has transverse inward extensions called the transverse T system. This tubular system extends to individual

Rosen, M. R. and Hoffman, B. F. (eds.), Cardiac Therapy. ISBN 0-89838-564-4.
© 1983, Martinus Nijhoff Publishers, Boston, The Hague, Dordrecht, Lancaster. Printed in the Netherlands.

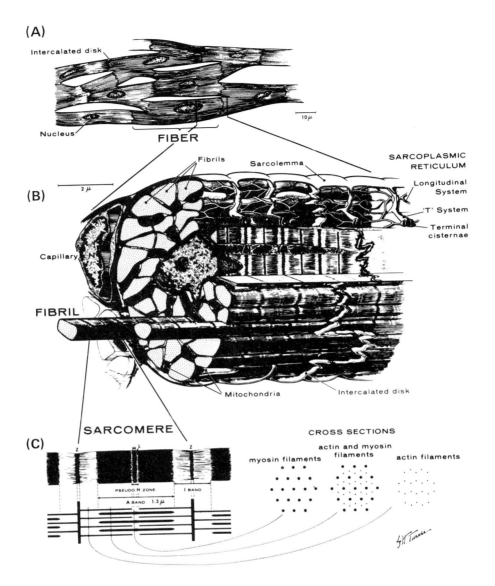

(A)

Intercalated disk

Nucleus

FIBER

10μ

(B)

2μ

Fibrils

Sarcolemma

SARCOPLASMIC
RETICULUM

Longitudinal
System

'T' System

Terminal
cisternae

Capillary

FIBRIL

Mitochondria

Intercalated disk

SARCOMERE

(C)

CROSS SECTIONS

actin and myosin
filaments

myosin filaments

actin filaments

Z   M   Z

PSEUDO H ZONE   I BAND

A BAND 1.5μ

Figure 1. Microscopic structure of heart muscle: (A) The branching interconnected myocardial fibers are illustrated; (B) reconstruction of a myocardial cell or fiber showing the relationship of the fibrils to the other subcellular structure; (C) representation of an individual sarcomere, the fundamental unit of contraction. The schematic arrangement of the thin and thick filaments is illustrated below (reproduced with permission [34]).

sarcomeres at the Z line. As the wave of depolarization, initiated by the action potential, sweeps across the muscle, this signal is carried inward along the transverse tubular system. Calcium crosses the sarcolemma during the action potential and triggers the additional release of calcium stored in the sarcoplasmic reticulum, especially the lateral or terminal cisternae [1]. Calcium, in turn, attaches to the protein troponin, which is located on the actin filament at periodic intervals of 429 Å (Figure 2). This interaction uncovers an active site at which the myosin cross bridges can attach to actin to initiate the process of contraction. Contraction is ended when calcium is taken up by the sarcoplasmic reticular system which is the longitudinal network of tubules seen in Figure 1B. This system is interwoven

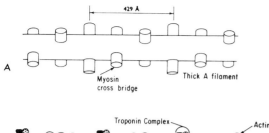

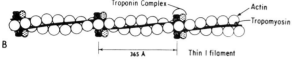

Figure 2. Relation of the structure of the thick myosin filaments to the thin actin filaments: (A) The extension of the heavy meromyosin cross bridges from the central myosin filament are shown; (B) the relation of the troponin complex (where calcium attaches) to the tropomyosin backbone and double-stranded actin helix (reproduced by permission [35]).

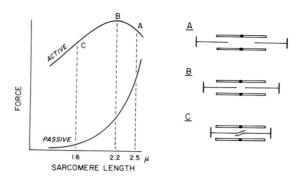

Figure 3. Relation of myocardial sarcomere length to the passive and active length–tension curves of isolated heart muscle: As muscle is passively stretched, there is an increase in resting force. When the muscle is stimulated at each sarcomere length, the level of developed force is indicated by the active curve. The optimum sarcomere length for force development is 2.2μ. A representation of sarcomeres at points A, B, and C is illustrated on the right. Optimum overlap exists at L_{max}, point B. Overstretching of the sarcomere, point A, reduces the number of cross bridges that can be formed. At sarcomere lengths shorter than 2.2μ, point C, actin filaments cross through the center of the sarcomere and interfere with each other's attachment to the cross bridges. Sarcomeres normally work between points B and C.

with, but distinct from, the transverse system. ATP is required for the uptake of calcium by the sarcoplasmic reticulum.

The relationship between sarcomere length and the ability of heart muscle to develop force is illustrated in Figure 3. This figure is representative of studies of isolated heart muscle *in vitro* [2]. The passive and active length tension curves of such a muscle are illustrated on the left side of Figure 3. If one passively stretches the strip of muscle, the rise in resting force becomes progressively steep as one passes beyond sarcomere lengths of 2.2μ (passive curve). This increasing stiffness of cardiac muscle is an important protective mechanism to prevent overdilation of the heart with acute heart failure. The upper (active) curve represents the force which can be developed at each sarcomere length. It reaches a peak at approximately 2.2μ with a short descending limb thereafter. This increase in force over the ascending limb of the curve is named the Frank-Starling mechanism after the two men who described it. At points A, B, and C schematic representations of sarcomere length are shown on the right-hand side of Figure 3. At the optimum length of 2.2μ (B) the actin filaments extend close to the center of the myosin filament, thus providing an opportunity for optimal overlap of thin and thick filaments and, therefore, attachment of a maximum number of cross bridges. This is the probable mechanism responsible for maximum force development at that length. In overstretched sarcomeres (2.5μ) as shown in panel A, the actin filaments are pulled out from the myosin filaments resulting in decreased force because of the reduced ability of cross bridges to form. It should be emphasized, however, that it is extremely difficult to stretch sarcomeres much beyond their optimal length. When chronic dilation occurs, sarcomeres are added in series, with replication perhaps occurring at intercalated discs [3]. Even in enormously dilated hearts, however, individual sarcomere lengths remain close to the optimal length of 2.2μ [4]. The normal operating range of the sarcomere is to the left of B. The decrease in force produced at point C is presumably due to the fact that filaments have crossed through the center of the sarcomere and interfere with each other in forming cross bridge attachments. Over the normal range of the Frank-Starling mechanism sarcomeres are operating at diastolic lengths between 1.8 and 2.2μ.

23

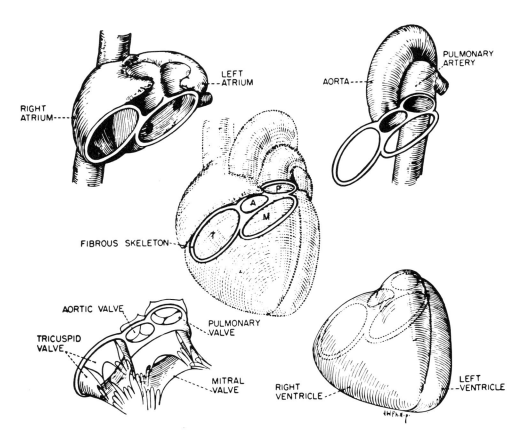

Figure 4. Anatomical arrangement of the heart: The relation of the chambers, valves, and great vessels to the central fibrous skeletal rings are illustrated (reproduced with permission [5]).

Whole heart

The normal heart weighs approximately 250–300 g in the adult. The general arrangement of the four chambers and great vessels is illustrated in Figure 4. The fibrous skeleton consists of the four valve rings which are joined together and separate the atria above from the ventricles below [5]. The atria are thin-walled, shallow cups which function as follows: When the atrio-ventricular (A-V) valves are closed during ventricular systole, the atria collect blood from the two venous systems. When the A-V valves open, there is rapid filling of the ventricles in early diastole. The valves remain partially open during mid-diastole so that the atria serve as a conduit between the veins and the ventricles. During late diastole, active atrial contraction ejects an additional portion of blood into each ventricle just prior to ventricular contraction. A properly timed atrial contribution to ventricular filling is very helpful in maintaining an appropriate cardiac output.

The right ventricle is a relatively thin-walled volume pump which operates against the relatively low resistance of the pulmonary artery. The left ventricle is a more thick-walled pressure pump as it operates against the higher aortic pressure. The thick interventricular septum is more closely associated with the pumping action of the left ventricle for which it forms the medial wall. Ejection of blood is accomplished primarily by constriction of the chamber with only slight shortening from apex to base. In the left ventricle there is a constantly changing direction of muscle fibers. The predominant muscle bundles are the circumferential fibers in the middle layers of the ventricle which are oriented perpendicularly to the long axis of the ventricle. These fibers constrict the chamber and account for most of the blood volume ejected.

24

Pericardium

The pericardium is a fibroserous sac that surrounds the heart in the middle mediastinum. Under normal circumstances the pericardial sac contains only a few cubic centimeters of fluid. The pericardium is a relatively stiff structure which helps the heart resist sudden dilatation associated with acute heart failure. Recent studies have pointed out how this stiff pericardium also can affect the passive pressure–volume relationship of the left ventricle in the failing heart [6]. This will be discussed later. Large collections of fluid inside the pericardium, with tamponade, can obviously produce severe hemodynamic consequences. Similar deleterious effects are produced by constrictive pericarditis, wherein the thickened, fibrous pericardium greatly limits cardiac filling.

Biochemical control of contraction

Calcium is the ion responsible for the activation of cardiac muscle during the process of excitation–contraction coupling. The calcium concentration around the myofilaments is 10^{-7} M or less during diastole and rises to about 5×10^{-6} M during the full activation of actomyosin. Whereas skeletal muscle has major stores of internal calcium in its sarcoplasmic reticulum, and is less dependent on extracellular calcium, cardiac muscle is dependent on a continuous source of external calcium to maintain contractile tension. For example, if heart muscle is perfused with solutions containing no calcium, contractile tension falls with a half-time of approximately 1 min or less [7]. In skeletal muscle, the half-time for this decline in tension is 20 min or more. During depolarization by the action potential, calcium both crosses the membrane and is released from internal storage sites to raise calcium to an appropriate level for contraction. Calcium attaches to troponin C on the actin filament which normally inhibits the active site of cross bridge formation. Calcium attachment to troponin reverses this repression and uncovers the active site, which then becomes available for attachment of the myosin cross bridge (Figure 2). Cross bridge attachment, movement, and detachment, in a rowing fashion, pull the actin filaments in towards the center of the sarcomere and thus are responsible for the development of force and shortening. Active up-take of calcium by the sarcoplasmic reticulum, an energy requiring (ATP) process, reduces calcium below the critical level of activation and results in relaxation and the diastolic phase. The heavy meromyosin cross bridge, when attached to actin, has enzymatic activity (ATPase) which results in the splitting of high energy phosphate ATP so that the released energy can be used for the contractile process. An interesting relation between the mechanics of contraction and actomyosin ATPase activity has been noted. There is a relatively direct correlation between maximum velocity of muscle shortening, (V_{max}), and actomyosin ATPase activity [8]. This relationship also holds with the development of congestive heart failure, in that both the maximum velocity of shortening and the actomyosin ATPase activity are reduced [9].

There are two primary mechanisms whereby cardiac muscle can alter its force development. The first is by changing initial length, i.e., the Frank-Starling mechanism as illustrated in Figure 3. The second is by increasing contractile state. All interventions which increase contractile state appear to do so by increasing the availability of calcium ion [7]. For example, changes in external calcium concentration will increase the amount of calcium available to heart muscle and thus increase contractility. Increases in heart rate will also increase the calcium flux across the sarcolemma and produce a slight increase in cardiac contractility. Paired electrical stimulation also makes more calcium available to the myofilaments by coupling two depolarizations close together in time. Catecholamines or increased sympathetic tone also result in an increase in calcium as the final pathway for their inotropic effect. Digitalis also increases intracellular calcium by inhibiting a sodium potassium ATPase which is involved in sodium-potassium exchange across the sarcolemma. By inhibiting sodium-potassium exchange there is an enhancement of sodium-calcium exchange, thus making more calcium available to the myofilaments.

Although increased calcium availability to the myofilaments is related to all acute interventions which increase contractile state, it is not clear whether decreased calcium availability is the mechanism for all interventions which acutely decrease contractility. Thus, the precise mechanisms for acute depression with antiarrhythmic drugs, hypoxia, or acidosis are less certain.

Although distinction is usually made between increases in muscle performance produced by increased preload or contractility, these two mechanisms may not be as separate as formerly thought. Recent evidence suggests that length-dependent activation of muscle may be as important as degree of filament overlap in producing the Frank-Starling mechanism [10]. This length-dependent activation is presumably mediated by the availability of differing amounts of calcium to the myofilaments.

The only energy source which heart muscle can use for contraction is ATP. Depletion of ATP will markedly impair myocardial performance. Creatine phosphate (CP) is another high energy phosphate found in the myocardium, but must be interchanged with ATP before its high energy phosphate bonding (in ATP) can be released for contraction:

$$CP + ADP = ATP + C$$

Depletion of high energy phosphates is not the primary cause for reduced intrinsic contractility in heart failure [11].

Coronary circulation

The large coronary arteries lie on the epicardial surface. As they distribute across the surface of the heart, small intramural branches splay out through and within the myocardium to provide blood to all portions of the heart. The coronary veins, for the most part, lie next to their arterial counterparts. Approximately 70% of the coronary blood flow supplies the left ventricular myocardium and is collected via the coronary veins for return via the coronary sinus. The great cardiac vein generally collects blood from the anterior portion of the heart, primarily reflecting left anterior descending blood flow. Venous return from the right ventricular myocardium flows into anterior cardiac veins which drain more directly into the right-sided chambers through thebesian veins.

Normal coronary flow is about 75 ml per 100 g heart muscle. In general the heart receives about 5% of the cardiac output, whereas the kidneys receive approximately 20–25% of the total cardiac output. Despite this difference, the heart consumes nearly twice as much oxygen as the kidneys.

In general, coronary blood flow occurs primarily in diastole, since the wall tension developed by the heart during systole tends to limit coronary flow during that period of the cardiac cycle, particularly to the left ventricle. There are powerful autoregulatory factors which control the arteriolar tone in coronary blood vessels [12]. The most important of these regulatory factors are local metabolic products, particularly adenosine. Levels of pO_2 and pCO_2 may also be important. In addition, stimulation of the alpha and beta receptors in the coronary vessels is responsible for some superimposed vasoconstriction and vasodilation. When coronary perfusion pressure falls to about 60–70 mmHg autoregulation of coronary flow ceases, since the vessels are nearly maximally dilated. Flow at that level becomes pressure dependent. Further reductions of pressure will result in a reduction of flow which produces ischemia. Because of a large demand for continuous O_2 delivery, the myocardium tends to maximally extract the O_2 from the blood flowing through the coronary arteries. Thus, increasing arteriovenous oxygen extraction is not an important mechanism whereby the heart can receive increased oxygen. Rather, changes in oxygen delivery to the myocardium are dependent on changes in coronary blood flow. If one occludes a coronary artery in an experimental animal, there is a reduction in force development in the affected myocardium, and force development will cease within 1 min. This emphasizes the importance of a continuous delivery of oxygen to the myocardium, since heart muscle cannot develop an oxygen debt as does skeletal muscle.

The regulation of coronary blood flow is closely related to the oxygen demands of the myocardium. There are four primary determinants of myocardial oxygen demand. These include heart rate, pressure development, heart size, and contractile state. Heart rate is an obvious determinant of oxygen consumption, in that oxygen will be required in proportion to the number of times per minute the heart contracts. Pressure development is also a major determinant of myocardial oxygen consumption. It is of great interest that heart muscle shortening does not require much oxygen, but rather that most of the oxygen required is related to the development of pressure. In terms of oxygen consumption, therefore, pressure work is very costly to the heart, whereas flow work is not. The third major determinant of oxygen consumption is heart size. This relates to the fact that wall tension in the heart is related to the intraventricular pressure and geometry by the La-Place relation. In simple terms: wall tension = pressure × radius. Thus, for a given intraventricular pressure, the oxygen requirements of the heart will be increased if the heart dilates. This points out the importance of reducing heart size in patients with congestive heart failure by the appropriate administration of diuretics, vasodilators, or inotropic agents. The LaPlace relation also helps us to understand the reason for a different wall thickness in different parts of the heart. In general, wall stress (force per cross-sectional area) tends to remain relatively constant throughout the heart. A simplified formula for the LaPlace relation is:

$$\text{Wall stress (force/cross-sectional area)} = \frac{PR}{2h},$$

where P = intraventricular pressure, R = radius of curvature, and h is wall thickness. Thus, at the apex of the heart, where the radius of curvature is quite short, the wall can be much thinner and still maintain a constant wall stress. In the lateral ventricular wall, the radius of curvature is much larger, thus requiring a much thicker wall in order to maintain a constant wall stress.

The absolute oxygen requirements of the heart also are dependent on the mass of heart muscle and are increased with hypertrophy. When hypertrophy becomes extreme there is difficulty supplying enough coronary flow, especially to the endocardium. This may be related to problems in delivering blood from the epicardial vessels, through perforating vessels, to the subendocardium. There may be inadequate vessel formation in proportion to the hypertrophy that occurs. It also appears that wall stress is highest in the subendocardium and that the blood supply to that area is at jeopardy because of this high demand. It is not unexpected, therefore, that subendocardial ischemia is extremely common, as manifest by ST segment depression in the electrocardiogram.

Pump function of the left ventricle

A number of indices of cardiac performance have been derived. Some of these describe the hydraulic performance of the heart in terms of pressure and flow, whereas others describe the contractile properties of cardiac muscle in terms of force development, shortening, and velocity of shortening. In general, those indices which describe the pump performance of the heart have been more useful clinically, and accordingly are the only ones which will be described in this chapter. A recent review of both pump and muscle function indices is recommended for the interested reader [13].

There are four primary determinants of cardiovascular performance: preload, afterload, heart rate, and contractile state [14]. These will be described individually. In studies of isolated heart muscle, preload represents the force stretching the muscle to an initial length prior to contraction. If one directly extrapolated this concept to the intact heart, preload would represent end-diastolic wall stress. To calculate this from the LaPlace relation, one would need to know left ventricular end-diastolic pressure, wall thickness, and radius of curvature. Because these usually are not available for such a complex calculation, several indices of preload have come into common use. The first is left ventricular end-diastolic pressure alone, which can be measured with a catheter in the left ventricle. In a similar sense, left ventricular end-diastolic volume may be used as an index of the diastolic length of the muscle fibers. End-diastolic pressure and volume, however, represent only a given point on the passive pressure–volume relation of the left ventricle. Acute shifts in the passive pressure–volume relation alter this relationship so that end-diastolic pressure no longer can be used to predict end-diastolic volume [6]. Under these circumstances end-diastolic volume is a better index of diastolic stretch.

In patients in special care units, balloon tip catheters have been used to measure pulmonary capillary wedge pressure, as an indirect measure of left atrial pressure. This pressure, by definition, represents the filling pressure of the left ventricle and has been clinically useful. Not only does left ventricular filling pressure help describe left ventricular function, but it also represents the pressure responsible for fluid transudation in the pulmonary capillaries. Thus, reduction in an elevated pulmonary capillary wedge pressure is important in managing the signs and symptoms of left heart failure. Although emphasis is placed on left ventricular function in this chapter, similar concepts apply to the right ventricle, in which preload is represented by right ventricular end-diastolic pressure or right atrial pressure.

Afterload was a term initially used in studies of isolated heart muscle to reflect the additional load above the preload that a muscle had to develop in order to shorten [14]. Analogous measurements in the intact heart would be the wall stress developed during systolic contraction. In accord with the La-Place relation, afterload would be constantly changing, since left ventricular pressure, wall thickness, and radius of curvature are continually changing during systole. In addition to the difficulties of such calculations, these measurements are not routinely available. Thus, other indices are used in clinical situations. One index of the afterload of the left ventricle would be aortic pressure, which represents the pressure which the ventricle must develop in order to eject blood. Another index of afterload is aortic impedance, i.e., the instantaneous relationship of pressure divided by flow. Unfortunately, calculations of impedance require the calculation of a series of harmonics which do not lend themselves to practical routine application [15]. Often it is helpful to measure systemic vascular resistance; i.e., mean aortic pressure divided by flow. Whatever the measurement utilized, all of these indices are potentially valuable in describing the 'afterload' of the heart and in evaluating the effects of various therapeutic interventions, particularly the class of vasodilator drugs which reduce afterload.

Contractile state refers to the intrinsic contractile abilities of the heart which can be altered with various inotropic interventions. As we have noted, contractile state is ultimately changed by making more calcium available. An increase in contractile state generally results in an increased rate of pressure development and an increased rate of ejection.

Now that we have briefly described the four determinants of cardiac function, we will next integrate these into an overall scheme of contraction. A useful format for describing cardiac contraction is to describe the pressure–volume relation as illustrated in Figure 5. The broken line at the bottom represents the passive pressure–volume relation. Beginning at the lower left-hand corner of the pressure–volume loop, the cardiac cycle begins with opening of the mitral valve and filling of the ventricle along the passive pressure–volume relation (segment 1). Filling is initially passive, until late diastole, when left atrial contraction adds an additional increment in volume. The lower right-hand point of the loop, therefore, represents end-diastol-

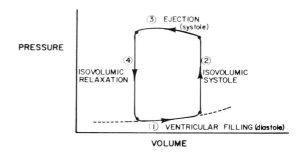

Figure 5. Pressure volume loop of the left ventricle: The broken line at the bottom represents the passive pressure–volume relationship of the left ventricle. The four cycles include the following: (1) passive and active ventricular filling during diastole, (2) isovolumic pressure development, (3) ejection of blood into the aorta during systole, and (4) isovolumic relaxation.

ic pressure and end-diastolic volume (the preload). Segment 2 represents isovolumic systole, during which the ventricle is developing pressure but has not yet opened the aortic valve. The upper right-hand corner of the loop represents the point of opening of the aortic valve (aortic diastolic pressure) and initiates the ejection phase [3]. The upper left-hand corner of the loop represents dicrotic notch aortic pressure (closing of the aortic valve) and end-systolic volume. Phase 4, or isovolumic relaxation, next occurs with a decrease in pressure, but no change in volume until the mitral valve opens again to begin the next cycle.

In physics, pressure–volume loops of this type have been used to describe the work of engines. By definition, the area inside such a counterclockwise loop represents the work done by that engine. By analogy, the area inside the counterclockwise pressure–volume loop represents the stroke work done by the left ventricle. The magnitude of left ventricular stroke work has important prognostic and functional implications as will be detailed later.

Alterations in the pressure–volume loop with changes in preload and afterload [16] are understood by considering Figure 6. First of all, we perform a series of experimental contractions, where we prevent any ejection of blood from the left ventricle by clamping the aorta just above the aortic valve. The pressure which the ventricle could develop at each volume is represented by a series of points which form a straight line, designated as the isovolumic pressure line (Figure 6). This represents the maximum ability of the ventricle to develop

28

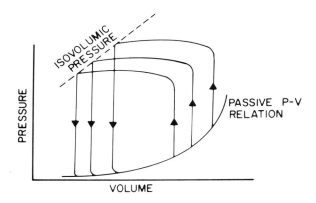

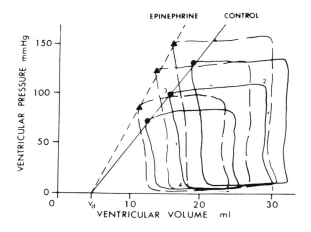

Figure 6. Alterations in the pressure–volume loop with changes in preload and afterload: The isovolumic pressure line was determined by having the ventricle contract at different end-diastolic volumes, but preventing ejection by clamping the aorta. Thus, the isovolumic pressure line represents the maximum pressure developed at each preload. Subsequent to calculation of the isovolumic pressure line, the aortic clamp is released. Illustrated are three different pressure–volume loops, beginning at different preloads and facing different afterloads. Note that the upper left-hand corner of each loop ends on the isovolumic pressure line.

Figure 7. Pressure–volume loops following a change in contractile state: The control pressure–volume loop is illustrated, together with three control pressure–volume loops at different preloads and afterloads. Contractile state was increased by infusing epinephrine 2 μg/kg/min. The isovolumic pressure line was shifted up and to the left, although the volume intercept (V_d) remained unchanged. Three pressure–volume loops at the higher contractile state are illustrated (broken lines) (reproduced by permission of the Am Heart Assoc, Inc [16]).

pressure at a given level of contractile state, when not ejecting blood. Also illustrated in Figure 6 are three pressure–volume loops, each of which begins at a different preload and each of which is working against a different aortic pressure. Note, however, that despite differing preloads and afterloads, the upper left-hand corner of each pressure–volume loop falls on the isovolumic pressure line. Recall that the upper left-hand corner of the loop represents dicrotic notch aortic pressure and end-systolic volume. Thus, despite changes in preload and afterload, the end point of contraction falls on the isovolumic pressure line. This line, therefore, represents a unique way of describing the state of the heart at a given contractile state independent of changes in preload and afterload.

If we now alter contractile state, the alterations in the isovolumic pressure line and pressure–volume loops are illustrated in Figure 7. Note that an increase in contractile state produced by epinephrine shifts the isovolumic pressure line up and to the left, although the intercept on the volume axis (V_d) remains about the same. At any given preload and afterload the heart can eject more blood (the width of the loop is stroke volume). Thus, the isovolumic pressure line is a way of characterizing the contrac-

tile state of an individual heart at any point in time. Furthermore, any given isovolumic pressure line describes the end point of contraction independent of preload or afterload.

Because of the difficulty in continuously measuring left ventricular pressure and volume, this type of approach is only recently being utilized to describe left ventricular function. Preliminary studies, however, suggest that it will be a valuable approach in characterizing the response of patients to various interventions [17].

A more commonly used technique for describing left ventricular function is the ventricular function curve, illustrated in Figure 8. Some measure of left ventricular performance, such as stroke work (area inside the pressure–volume loop), or stroke volume (width of the pressure–volume loop) is plotted as a function of the preload. In cardiac care units, the preload is commonly estimated by measuring the pulmonary capillary wedge pressure (using balloon tip catheters) as an indirect measure of the filling pressure (left atrial pressure) of the left ventricle [18]. There is an ascending limb of the ventricular function curve which reaches a plateau at approximately 15 mmHg. This information is extremely

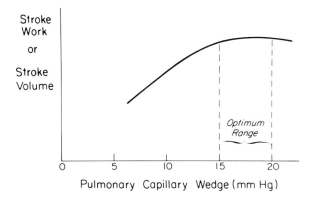

Figure 8. Left ventricular function curve: Some measure of left ventricular performance (stroke work or stroke volume) is plotted as a measure of left ventricular filling pressure (pulmonary capillary wedge pressure). The ventricular function curve has an ascending limb until pulmonary capillary wedge pressure reaches about 15 mmHg. Thereafter, the curve is relatively flat or slightly descending (reproduced with permission [32]).

valuable in adjusting the volume status of patients with heart disease, to optimize left ventricular performance, particularly in patients who are hypotensive, or who have low cardiac outputs.

Alterations in preload move the heart up or down its ventricular function curve. Shifts in the ventricular function curve reflect important alterations in performance. Shifts up and to the left, in general, represent an improvement in ventricular performance; whereas shifts down and to the right represent worsening of ventricular performance, such as occurs with congestive heart failure. Three different interventions can shift the ventricular function curve. Shifts up and to the left can be produced by (a) increasing contractile state, (b) decreasing afterload as with vasodilator drugs, and (c) increasing the compliance of the left ventricle by acutely changing the passive pressure–volume relation. Shifts down and to the right occur with a decrease in contractile state, an increase in afterload, and decreased compliance of the left ventricle.

The effects of compliance on the left ventricular function curve operate as follows: left ventricular end-diastolic volume, not end-diastolic pressure, is the primary determinant of stroke volume. If one acutely shifts the passive pressure–volume relation to the right, i.e., end-diastolic volume becomes larger at a given pulmonary capillary wedge pressure, stroke volume will go up at the same pulmonary capillary wedge pressure. Thus, if one is plotting a ventricular function curve, where pulmonary capillary wedge pressure represents the preload axis, there will be a shift to the left of the ventricular function curve, which is unrelated to changes in contractile state. Several interventions can acutely shift the left ventricular pressure–volume relation including vasodilator drugs, which dramatically alter peripheral hemodynamics, and myocardial ischemia. These have been described elsewhere [6] and will not be discussed in detail. Briefly, the mechanism of these shifts appears to be related to the interaction of the right and left ventricles inside a stiff pericardial sac. In general, vasodilator drugs, which decrease afterload, tend to shift the ventricular function curve up and to the left, both by a decrease of afterload and an increase in the compliance of the left ventricle. Vasoconstrictor drugs may shift the ventricular function curve down and to the right by increasing afterload, which reduces stroke volume, and also by shifting the passive pressure–volume curve to the left with a decrease in end-diastolic volume at a given end-diastolic pressure.

Another useful index of cardiovascular function is the ejection fraction which, by definition, is the stroke volume divided by the end-diastolic volume. A normal ejection fraction is approximately 66% whereas ejection fractions below 50% are abnormal. In patients with severe heart failure, the ejection fraction may go as low as 10%, although moderate heart failure is accompanied by an ejection fraction in the range of 30%. Figure 9 illustrates the fact that ejection fraction is a single number which can be used to describe a ventricular function curve. If one plots stroke volume on the vertical axis and end-diastolic volume on the horizontal axis, then the slope of the line connecting zero with the point at which any patient is on the ventricular function curve is, by definition, the ejection fraction. In Figure 9, note that as the ventricular function curves are shifted down and to the right, there is also a shift down and to the right in ejection fraction (the slope of the line from the origin to the point in question).

Regulation of cardiac output

In general, the cardiac output is determined by the requirements of the body. In a sense, therefore, the heart is relatively unimportant as a determinant of

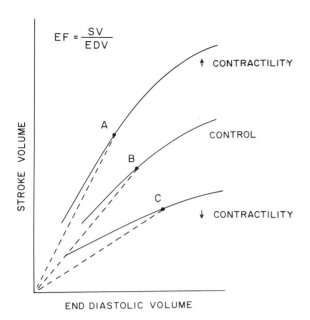

$$EF = \frac{SV}{EDV}$$

STROKE VOLUME

↑ CONTRACTILITY

A

B

CONTROL

C

↓ CONTRACTILITY

END DIASTOLIC VOLUME

Figure 9. Ejection fraction as a measure of ventricular function: By definition, ejection fraction equals stroke volume divided by end-diastolic volume. If one uses these two variables to construct a ventricular function curve, then the slope of the line connecting the origin to a specific point on a ventricular function curve is, by definition, the ejection fraction. Note that a shift in ventricular function down and to the right (A to B to C), is associated with a reduction in the slope of the line (ejection fraction).

resting cardiac output. It merely pumps out all of the blood that is returned to it. Thus, cardiac output is generally determined by the venous return to the heart. During exercise, for example, peripheral vasodilation increases flow to skeletal muscle which, in turn, increases the venous return and the cardiac output. Furthermore, the pumping action of skeletal muscles also helps to maintain venous return so as to maintain an appropriate cardiac output.

Catecholamine influences during exercise also constrict the venous bed and this additionally can enhance the return of blood to the heart by augmenting venous return. In general, therefore, the activities of the peripheral vascular system are far more important in determining the cardiac output than the heart itself which is a more passive part of the system. Only at maximal exercise, or when the heart begins to fail, does it become a limiting factor in this scheme. At that point, alterations in preload, afterload, contractile state, and heart rate become extremely important in determining the level of

cardiovascular function. Furthermore, alterations in these four variables form the basis for therapeutic interventions designed to improve cardiac function.

Regulation of arterial pressure

Individuals can carry out a wide range of activities with a reasonably constant arterial pressure; this is indicative of a regulatory system of some diversity. Consider the following formula:

Blood pressure = Cardiac output ×
Systemic vascular resistance.

It is clear from this equation that blood pressure can be increased by an increase in cardiac output, although, in general, this is less important than increasing resistance. The principal factor responsible for altering arterial pressure is a change in peripheral vascular resistance, generally through neurogenic arteriolar constriction or dilation. Normally, arteriolar dilation or constriction occurs in response to either autoregulation or neurogenic regulation. Autoregulation is produced by two opposing mechanisms. Stretching of the vascular smooth muscle increases its spontaneous activity and thus initiates progressive vasoconstriction. On the other hand, accumulation of tissue metabolites exerts a local vasodilator influence, so that the opposing effects of pressure-induced vasoconstriction and metabolite-induced vasodilation tend to maintain flow at a level appropriate to the needs of the tissue.

A schematic representation of the circulatory system is illustrated in Figure 10. The percent of cardiac output going to various organ systems is shown in the upper portion of the figure. Several regulatory systems are available to maintain blood pressure at approximately the same level. Some of the best studied are the carotid and aortic baroreceptors and chemoreceptors which are in the middle of Figure 10. One of these pressure-sensitive receptors, the carotid body, is located at the junction of the common carotid artery with its internal and external branches. Pressure sensitive nerve endings in the wall of the receptor alter their discharge rate according to the pressure that is applied. At high pressures, the discharge rate is increased. These impulses pass through the cardiovasculator regula-

31

FACTORS AFFECTING
EXTRACELLULAR
FLUID AND BLOOD
VOLUME

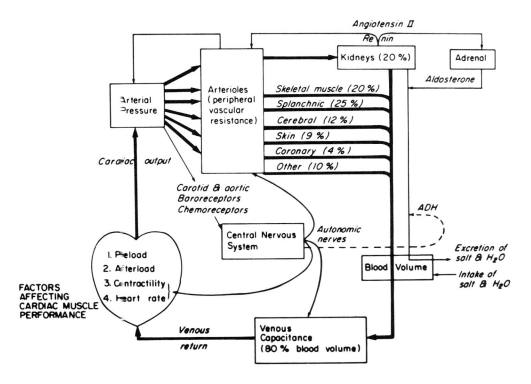

Figure 10. Schematic representation of the circulation system: The four factors affecting cardiac performance are shown inside the heart at the lower left. The distribution of cardiac output to major organ systems is shown in the upper right, with central nervous system reflexes in the center of the diagram. On the right-hand side of the diagram are those factors affecting extracellular fluid and blood volume. (See text for further details) (reproduced by permission [36]).

tory centers in the medulla which then alter the relative magnitude of parasympathetic and sympathetic tone. Sympathetic tone via the autonomic nervous system regulates peripheral vascular resistance by producing arteriolar constriction or vasodilation. The sympathetic nervous system also may affect cardiac contractility and heart rate, and alter venous capacitance.

Despite an increase in sympathetic tone in heart failure, baroreceptor function tends to be blunted [19]. Thus, alterations in arterial pressure do not lead to the same reflex changes in heart rate or sympathetic tone, as in a normal person. This phenomenon is especially evident during the administration of vasodilator drugs to patients with chronic heart failure. There is far less reflex tachycardia in

these patients as compared to patients with normal ventricular function who receive the drugs for the management of hypertension.

Chemoreceptors, lying near the carotid bifurcation and in the aortic arch, respond to changes in pH, pCO_2 and pO_2. Reduced oxygen, increased CO_2, or lowered pH stimulate the chemoreceptors and lead to an elevation of systemic arterial pressure.

There is considerable fluctuation in blood pressure during the day as influenced by factors such as posture, emotion, exercise, stress, and sleep. For example, exercise generally causes an increase in both systolic and diastolic pressure which persists for some time after the termination of exercise. Sleep, on the other hand, usually results in a reduc-

32

tion of blood pressure, although intense dreaming may produce an elevation of both heart rate and blood pressure.

The arterial system represents the conduit for delivery of blood to all parts of the body. Blood pressure remains constant in this system up to the level of the terminal arteries and arterioles, where there is an 80% drop in pressure. The subsequent cross-sectional area of the capillaries is enormous, to provide for exchange of oxygen and other substances. The relatively large velocity of blood in the aorta (40–50 cm/sec) is reduced to about 0.07 cm/sec in the capillaries.

The venous system serves as the capacitance reservoir of the circulatory system. At any one time, approximately 75–80% of the blood volume is in the peripheral veins. Thus, vasoconstriction or dilation of these veins can produce marked shifts in blood from the central to the peripheral circulation. Catecholamine-induced venoconstriction during exercise is an important way of increasing venous return and cardiac output. Similarly, drug-induced venodilation during congestive heart failure, as, for example, with nitroglycerin, is an important way of redistributing blood away from the chest into the peripheral system, and thus reducing the signs and symptoms of pulmonary congestion.

Regulation of blood volume

The right-hand side of Figure 10 shows some of the factors responsible for regulating extracellular fluid and blood volume. Excretion of salt and water by the kidney, in general, tends to balance intake of salt and water to maintain a relatively constant fluid volume. ADH secretion from the central nervous system, caused by a decrease in plasma volume, also helps to decrease the amount of water excretion. Decreased arterial flow to the kidneys causes release of renin from the juxtaglomerular apparatus and this promotes the formation of angiotensin II from angiotensin I, an alpha 2 globulin synthesized in the liver. Angiotensin II has potent vasoconstricting effects on the arterioles, although its primary effect may be in the adrenal gland where it promotes the release of aldosterone, which increases the reabsorption of salt and water. With normal renal and cardiovascular function, these compensatory mechanisms provide for a relatively constant arterial pressure, and salt and water bal-

ance, despite considerable changes in heart rate and cardiac output.

Cardiac reserve

An important principle related to the cardiovascular system is the concept of cardiac reserve. Although it is important to make measurements of cardiovascular function at rest, much more information about the reserve capabilities of the heart can be obtained by subjecting the cardiovascular system to some form of stress. This is certainly helpful in characterizing the degree and type of impairment in patients with coronary artery disease or heart failure.

Two different types of stress have been used to evaluate the cardiovascular system. That most commonly used is exercise such as walking on a treadmill. This is a form of isotonic stress, i.e., there is considerable motion against a small constant load. The other form of stress which has been utilized is the so-called isometric exercise, which implies little change in the length of exercising skeletal muscles as they exert considerable force against a relatively stationary object. An example of this form of stress is weight lifting. Both forms of stress have been used to evaluate cardiovascular reserve. Figure 11 illustrates a study of two patients employing isometric exercise (hand grip) [20]. Isometric exercise is accompanied by a reflex increase in arterial pressure due to an increase in sympathetic tone and arteriolar constriction. Presumably this increase in arterial pressure is designed to maintain perfusion of blood to exercising muscles. This increase in arterial pressure provides a large increase in afterload, which makes it more difficult for the heart to eject blood. The differing responses of the two patients to isometric exercise are schematically illustrated in Figure 11. In the middle of the figure are two points representing the similar ventricular function of patients A and B. In response to isometric exercise produced by hand grip, there is a rise in arterial pressure, which tends to reduce stroke volume. This is countered by an increase in contractile state, which tends to increase cardiovascular performance. Patient A shows a normal integrated response to this increase in arterial pressure, by increasing his stroke work with little change in left ventricular end-diastolic pressure. On the other hand, patient B exhibits a substantial reduction in

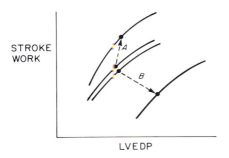

STROKE WORK

LVEDP

Figure 11. Effects of increased arterial pressure on ventricular function: Hand-grip isometric exercise was used to stress the left ventricles of two patients with relatively similar function. The response of patient A is an increase in stroke work with little change in left ventricular end-diastolic pressure – a relatively normal response. Patient B showed a substantial reduction in stroke work, together with an elevation of end-diastolic pressure, indicative of poor ventricular reserve.

stroke work, together with a rise in left ventricular end-diastolic pressure. This shift in the ventricular function curve down and to the right is indicative of poor ventricular reserve and far worse cardiovascular decompensation than in patient A. Thus, even though resting ventricular function was similar in these two patients, their ventricular reserve was markedly different. This figure illustrates the additional information about ventricular function which can be obtained by imposing a stress and making repeated quantitative measurements of ventricular function.

Cardiac failure

Introduction

The general term congestive heart failure is used to describe the constellation of symptoms and physical signs associated with four syndromes. These include (a) failure of the left ventricle as a pump, (b) failure of the right ventricle, (c) pulmonary venous hypertension, and (d) systemic venous hypertension. These syndromes often exist in combination but should be distinguished in defining the etiology of the symptoms and signs of heart failure. Heart failure is associated with an elevated preload. On the left side of the heart this results in elevated left ventricular end-diastolic, left atrial, and pulmonary venous pressures which produce pulmonary con-

gestion and dyspnea. Right heart failure is associated with elevated right ventricular end-diastolic pressure and right atrial and systemic venous pressures which produce passive congestion of organs like the liver and peripheral edema. Although the most common cause of right heart failure is left heart failure, right heart failure can occur in the absence of left heart failure as, for example, in patients with chronic obstructive lung disease and pulmonary hypertension. The prototype example of pulmonary venous hypertension is mitral stenosis. By increasing left atrial pressure, there is a concomitant increase in pulmonary artery pressure, which increases the afterload of the right ventricle, and in time can lead to right heart failure. The prototype example of systemic venous hypertension is that produced by pericardial constriction or tamponade.

A useful definition of heart failure is that state which results from the inability of the heart to pump sufficient blood to the body tissues to meet ordinary metabolic demands. When this occurs under resting conditions, ventricular performance is usually markedly depressed. Lesser degrees of heart failure result only in an inability to meet peripheral demands during times of stress such as exercise. The common symptoms associated with left heart failure include dyspnea on exertion, orthopnea, and paroxysmal nocturnal dyspnea. Occasionally, elevated pulmonary venous pressures can result in an asthma-like syndrome with severe bronchial constriction. At other times, troublesome cough may be the only evidence for elevated pulmonary venous pressures. Symptoms associated with right heart failure include peripheral edema, or abdominal distension associated with enlargement of the liver and spleen, and the accumulation of ascitic fluid. Right subcostal pain may result from distension of the hepatic capsule. Decreased cardiac output may lead to weight gain and reversal of the diurnal urinary excretion pattern, thus producing nocturia. Weakness and fatigue are primary symptoms of reduced cardiac output. In patients with reduced arterial pressure, dizziness, light headedness, or fainting may ensue.

Signs of left heart failure include the presence of basilar rales, or wheezing. A third heart sound is common with either left or right failure. With the development of right heart failure, jugular venous distension, hepatojugular reflux, hepatomegaly, pleural effusion, ascites, and peripheral edema may be quite prominent. Pulsus alternans is a relatively specific indication of left ventricular dysfunction.

Years ago the terms forward heart failure and backward heart failure were used to describe the pathophysiology of heart failure and its primary manifestations. This distinction is no longer important, since the two tend to occur together, and the mechanisms invoked in both of these forms of heart failure may be similar. The concept of backward heart failure reflects the fact that as the left ventricle fails there is an elevation of pulmonary venous and arterial pressure, which, in turn, leads to right heart failure, and associated systemic venous congestion. Certainly, this sequence is a common and important one in the pathophysiology of heart failure. In the concept of forward heart failure, inadequate delivery of blood to the periphery is the primary responsible mechanism. Thus, reduction of flow to the kidneys leads to sodium and water retention, which, in turn, produces the congestion found in heart failure. It is clear that the primary value of these two terms at present is descriptive, since they are but two facets of a complex interaction which produces all the signs and symptoms that we associate with heart failure.

Etiology

Several different mechanisms are responsible for left heart failure. A common cause includes loss of muscle as with acute myocardial infarction. This decrease in muscle mass with scar formation obviously decreases the pumping ability of the heart. Furthermore, ischemic muscle is also noncontractile, so that episodes of angina pectoris may produce transient left heart failure with its accompanying signs and symptoms.

Decreased function of heart muscle commonly occurs in several situations. Pressure overload of the left ventricle such as with severe aortic stenosis or end-stage hypertensive heart disease is a common cause of this phenomenon. Initially, the heart hypertrophies in an attempt to meet the increased pressure demands of an elevated aortic pressure. Gradually, however, irreversible changes occur in the myocardium which lead to a decrease in the intrinsic capacity of the heart muscle to develop pressure and shorten. These irreversible changes are accompanied by a decrease in ejection velocity

and actomyosin ATPase activity. Over a wide range of species, maximum velocity of muscle shortening is correlated with actomyosin ATPase activity [8]. It is not surprising, therefore, that a reduction in velocity of shortening of failing heart muscle is accompanied by a reduction in actomyosin ATPase activity [9]. With hypertrophy there is an increase in collagen content in the myocardium. There is also a decrease in catecholamine stores. This occurs both because of increased sympathetic secretion from storage sites in terminal nerve endings and also because of decreased synthesis of cardiac catecholamines [21]. Similar changes occur with long-standing volume overload, which can be produced by severe mitral regurgitation or aortic regurgitation. Decreases in intrinsic muscle performance tend to be irreversible and lead to worsening heart failure. These changes emphasize the need for early intervention in an attempt to relieve volume or pressure overload prior to irreversible myocardial changes.

Pericardial or endocardial disease can also produce the signs and symptoms of heart failure, primarily by limiting inflow into the heart. The elevation of venous pressure and its consequent passive congestion of organs, and peripheral edema, may be prominent signs and symptoms of this disorder.

Although most types of heart failure are associated with a low cardiac output, there are a few situations in which high cardiac output can aggravate or precipitate heart failure in certain patients. Important etiologic factors which have been associated with high output failure include fever, arteriovenous fistula, thyrotoxicosis, anemia, beri-beri, Paget's disease of the bone, and pregnancy. High output cardiac failure is a form of volume overload, and in some sense is similar to mitral regurgitation or aortic insufficiency. In general, such volume overload states tend to be tolerated for a considerable time by a heart with relatively normal intrinsic contractility. With time, however, the prolonged need for high output can lead to the commonly recognized signs and symptoms of heart failure. The most important therapy in such patients is to reduce the need for high cardiac output. This might result from reduction of fever, correction of anemia, correction of thyrotoxicosis, obliteration of an arterio-venous fistula, and delivery of the baby in the case of pregnancy. Only when the primary cause for high output failure is appropriately corrected does the usual therapy for congestive heart failure need to be employed, since it may be relatively ineffective until the underlying cause is corrected.

Circulatory adjustments in congestive heart failure

The cardiovascular system makes several adjustments which help to maintain function during the development of heart failure. One compensatory mechanism utilized by the ventricle is to dilate in order to increase cardiac output according to the Frank-Starling mechanism. As indicated, however, this reserve function is exhausted when pulmonary capillary wedge pressure reaches the range of 15 to 20 mmHG (Figure 8). Any further increase in filling pressures will not result in an increase in performance, but in some cases will result in a slight decrease in ventricular performance. Another compensatory mechanism is an increase in sympathetic tone and circulating catecholamines. In patients with severe heart failure, catecholamines are increased considerably [22]. The increases in heart rate and cardiac contractile state produced by catecholamines are important mechanisms for maintaining cardiac compensation. This fact underlies the potential danger of giving beta adrenergic blocking drugs to these patients. By blocking the effects of catecholamines on beta 1 receptors in the heart, one limits the increase in contractility and heart rate produced by catecholamines, and thus may worsen congestive heart failure.

An increase in heart rate is a particularly important compensatory mechanism. Cardiac output is the product of heart rate and stroke volume. As the ventricular function curve shifts down and to the right and the patient moves on to the plateau of a depressed ventricular function curve, stroke volume becomes relatively fixed. Therefore, any increase in cardiac output must be produced by an increase in heart rate. A marked tachycardia is often a sign of the severity of heart failure, in that it implies an extremely low, fixed stroke volume with an inability to increase cardiac output by any mechanisms other than heart rate.

Increasing muscle mass is an important mechanism for maintaining the ability of the heart to increase its pressure development in response to an increased load. In pressure-overloaded ventricles, hypertrophy tends to be considerable with no change or an actual reduction in the end-diastolic volume. In patients with volume-overloaded ventricles, hypertrophy is less and the end-diastolic volume is markedly increased. These changes, however, occur in such a way as to maintain a relatively constant systolic wall stress, in accord with the LaPlace relation. Thus, in the pressure-overloaded heart the greater wall thickness and smaller radius of curvature all counterbalance the increased pressure developed, so that wall stress remains relatively constant. In the volume-overloaded heart, developed pressure is relatively normal, so that the increase in wall thickness only needs to counteract the increase in radius of curvature. As long as wall stress remains relatively normal, the hearts of such patients tend to be compensated. When wall stress becomes greater than normal because of inadequate hypertrophy or excessive dilatation, however, the heart begins to fail and irreversible changes occur in the contractile abilities of the myocardium [23]. Even following surgical correction of the valvular problems responsible for pressure or volume overload, and despite clinical improvement in patients because of the reduced loading factors, the intrinsic contractile properties of the heart muscle may never return to normal. This emphasizes the importance of intervening in such patients before irreversible changes in contractile state occur due to excessive wall stress.

Another compensatory mechanism utilized in congestive heart failure is the ability of peripheral tissues to increase the extraction of oxygen from hemoglobin. This shift in the oxygen–hemoglobin dissociation curve allows the blood to give up more oxygen at a given pO_2, and thus enhances oxygen delivery. The shift in the hemoglobin dissociation curve occurs in part because of a decreased pH (Bohr effect). Overall, however, this is a modest compensatory effect and cannot counteract a major reduction in cardiac output.

One consequence of severe chronic heart failure is decreased renal perfusion. Decreased renal blood flow results in decreased urine output with a consequent retention of salt and water. Furthermore, a reduction in renal perfusion (reduced pressure and flow) is sensed by the juxtaglomerular apparatus which releases renin. Increased sympathetic tone and low blood sodium also trigger the release of renin from the juxtaglomerular apparatus. Renin subsequently promotes the formation of angiotensin I to angiotensin II. Angiotensin II is a powerful vasoconstrictor and also increases aldosterone secretion from the adrenal glands. Aldosterone promotes the retention of salt and water in the renal tubule by increasing sodium-potassium exchange. This increases the blood volume and the total body salt and water content. Aldosterone levels are usually increased in severe heart failure, secondary both to reduced renal perfusion and to decreased metabolism of aldosterone in the liver. These increased aldosterone levels form the basis for the use of aldosterone antagonists as diuretic agents. Vascular regions, such as the skin and splanchnic bed, also become vasoconstricted so that blood may be preferentially shunted to more vital organs. On the other hand, regional circulations such as the cerebral or coronary circulations have powerful autoregulatory capabilities so that blood flow can be maintained, despite a moderate reduction in arterial pressure and cardiac output. With exercise there is an increase in flow to skeletal muscles. With heart failure, however, the absolute increase in flow to skeletal muscles is far less than that found in a normal person during exercise.

The vicious cycle of chronic heart failure

During the process of heart failure there is an inevitable reduction in cardiac output. The body, however, attempts to maintain arterial pressure within reasonable levels in order to perfuse vital organs. Therefore, as cardiac output falls, there is a reflex increase in peripheral vascular resistance, mediated mostly by the increase in sympathetic tone. Other factors, however, also contribute to this increase in systemic vascular resistance. The direct effects of angiotensin II produce vasoconstriction. In addition, salt and water retention lead to increased sodium content of the arterioles and decrease their ability to dilate. In patients with heart failure, it has been noted that the posthyperemic response following transient limb occlusion is markedly blunted, suggesting an inability of these vessels to dilate to the same extent as normal [24]. This increase in peripheral vascular resistance is responsible for a vicious cycle in heart failure. This is illustrated schematically in Figure 12. As shown, a decrease in cardiac output leads to a reflex increase in systemic vascular resistance by the mechanisms indicated. In turn, this increased systemic vascular resistance acts as an increased afterload to the left ventricle

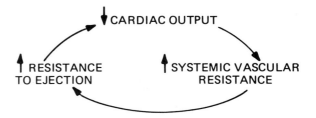

Figure 12. The vicious cycle of chronic heart failure is illustrated: With a decrease in cardiac output there is a reflex and neurohumeral increase in systemic vascular resistance in an attempt to maintain arterial blood pressure. This increased resistance further reduces ejection of blood from the heart, thus reducing cardiac output further. Patients spiral down this vicious cycle until they reach a new low steady state level, where cardiac output is lower and systemic vascular resistance is higher for optimal patient function (reproduced by permission [32]).

and thus further reduces stroke volume and cardiac output. Patients tend to spiral down this cycle until they reach a new low steady state level, at which cardiac output is lower and systemic vascular resistance higher than is optimal for the patient.

There is striking pharmacologic evidence for the existence of such a vicious cycle in chronic heart failure. For example, the administration of hydralazine, a relatively pure arteriolar dilator, to patients with severe Class III and Class IV (New York Heart Association) heart failure, results in a 50% increase in cardiac output [25]. In general, there are no changes in heart rate, arterial pressure, or left or right atrial pressure. Since this occurs in patients who are already being optimally treated with digitalis and diuretics, these data provide the basis for the use of arteriolar dilators in patients with severe chronic heart failure.

There is also considerable venoconstriction in patients with heart failure, presumably related to increased sympathetic tone and circulating catecholamines. This fact provides the basis for the use of venodilators such as nitroglycerin [26]. By dilating these constricted veins one can increase their volume, thus redistributing blood in the circulatory system. With more blood in the peripheral veins and less blood in the chest, there is a marked reduction in right and left atrial pressures, which results in a reduction of the signs and symptoms of right and left heart failure. In general, however, venodilators do not alter cardiac output. Thus, combination arteriolar dilators and venodilators are extremely helpful in increasing cardiac output and reducing right and left heart filling pressures.

Therapeutic considerations

These general considerations of the pathophysiology of heart failure point out that alterations in preload, afterload, contractile state and heart rate provide the basis for most of the therapeutic interventions employed. In patients with moderate heart failure, appropriate modification of preload and contractile state may be beneficial. This concept is illustrated in Figure 13. Point A represents cardiac function on a normal ventricular function curve. As the heart goes into failure, the ventricular function curve is shifted down and to the right and the preload is increased from B to C as the heart dilates. At point C, with an elevated preload, the patient received diuretics to reduce preload to point D. This would help relieve the signs and symptoms of pul-

monary congestion, although it would have little effect on cardiac output. To counteract the marked decrease in intrinsic contractility, digitalis was given to shift the curve up and to the left to point E on a more compensated curve. Even though stroke volume was still lower, and filling pressure higher than normal, the patient could function at a better level because of the reduced preload and increased contractile state. If digitalis and diuretics are insufficient to maintain compensation, there is generally a substantial decrease in cardiac output, accompanied by a marked elevation of systemic vascular resistance. As previously described, this sets up a vicious cycle which further reduces cardiac output and sets the stage for the use of vasodilators.

The use of vasodilator drugs in chronic congestive heart failure is an excellent illustration of the appropriate manipulation of preload and afterload. Reduction in preload is produced primarily by peripheral venodilation. When a venodilator, such as one of the nitrates, is given to patients with severe heart failure, the peripheral venodilation increases the capacitance of this system for blood. Accordingly, more blood is located in the peripheral veins at any one time and less blood is located in the central chest. This reduces right and left atrial pressures and relieves the signs and symptoms of pulmonary congestion. An increase in cardiac output is produced primarily by arteriolar dilators, which reduce systemic vascular resistance and increase forward flow. Figure 14 is an example of a patient with severe chronic congestive heart failure who was treated with combined arteriolar and venodilation. Control hemodynamic studies showed a pulmonary capillary wedge pressure of 30 mmHg and a stroke work index of 28 g–m/m². Following administration of oral hydralazine, the ventricular function curve was shifted upwards with primarily an increase in stroke work, and only a slight fall in pulmonary capillary wedge pressure. The addition of nitrates to hydralazine therapy shifted the curve leftwards, with a reduction in pulmonary capillary wedge pressure, but no further increase in stroke work index. Thus, the combined administration of arteriolar and venodilators shifts the ventricular function curve up and to the left and this is beneficial to patients with chronic heart failure. A number of different vasodilator drugs are available to produce these changes. These drugs will not be described in detail here, since they are discussed in Chapter 13.

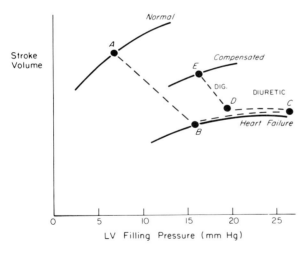

Figure 13. Effects of digitalis and diuretics in heart failure: Conceptually illustrated are the changes that occur during the development and therapy of congestive heart failure. Initially, the patient is at point A on a normal ventricular function curve. With the onset of heart failure the curve shifts down and to the right. The patient moves to point B and with further cardiac dilation to point C. The administration of a diuretic, which reduces intravascular volume, reduces left ventricular filling pressure and moves the patient from point C to point D. The addition of digitalis improves contractility and shifts the ventricular function curve up and to the left so that the patient moves from point D to E, to a relatively compensated position.

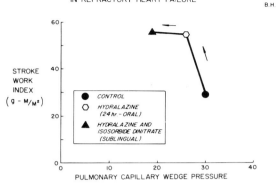

Figure 14. Effects of veno- and arteriolar dilators in chronic congestive heart failure: The control measurements of hemodynamic function are from a patient with severe chronic congestive heart failure unresponsive to digitalis and diuretics. The administration of hydralazine increases stroke work with only a slight reduction in pulmonary capillary wedge pressure. The further addition of nitrates shifts function leftward with a reduction in pulmonary capillary wedge pressure, although there is no change in stroke work index. Combined administration of hydralazine and nitrates to reduce preload and afterload shifts function in a beneficial direction up and to the left (reproduced by permission [25]).

When one gives vasodilators that reduce both preload and afterload, the resultant effect on stroke volume will depend on the final level of left ventricular filling pressure reached. This important principle is illustrated in Figure 15. Shown in the middle is a control ventricular function curve which plots stroke volume as a function of left ventricular filling pressure. If a patient begins at a left ventricular filling pressure of 20 mmHg, the shift in ventricular function (line A) in response to sodium nitroprusside is illustrated. Sodium nitroprusside is a balanced veno- and arteriolar dilator, and thus produces both a reduction in preload and a reduction in afterload. The reduction in afterload (decreased impedance) shifts function upwards, whereas the reduction in preload shifts function leftwards. The resultant effect (line A) is a shift in function up and to the left, which would be a beneficial hemodynamic response in this patient. If, prior to the administration of nitroprusside, however, the patient were given potent diuretics to a point at which ventricular filling pressure was 10 mmHg, then de-

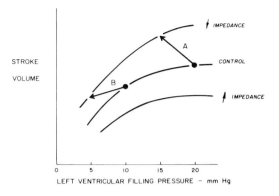

Figure 15. Effects of preload and afterload on ventricular function: The middle ventricular function curve represents the control curve of a patient in severe heart failure relatively unresponsive to digitalis and diuretics. The response to the administration of sodium nitroprusside, a combined veno- and arteriolar dilator, shifts function up and to the left along line A to a higher ventricular function curve, representing an improvement in performance. If potent diuretics had been used to reduce filling pressure from 20 mmHg to 10 mmHg, the administration of nitroprusside would have produced a slight reduction in stroke volume (line B). Although function moves to the new curve, it is down the ascending limb. This reduction in ventricular function may be associated with hypotension and tachycardia (reproduced by permission [32]).

leterious effects might result from the administration of nitroprusside (line B). In response to the drug there is a shift to the new curve, but the accompanying reduction in preload produces an actual reduction in stroke volume because the curve is now on the ascending limb of the Frank-Starling mechanism. This reduction in preload and stroke volume might be accompanied by hypotension and reflex tachycardia, all unfavorable effects of the drug. Besides withdrawing the vasodilator, one could volume load the patient to bring the filling pressure up to the optimal level of about 15 mmHg. In this case the patient would have the same beneficial response indicated in line A. This illustration emphasizes the importance of considering simultaneous changes in preload and afterload when using drugs which produce both arteriolar dilation and venodilation. It further emphasizes the importance of maintaining the preload near 15 mmHg in patients with heart failure, if one wishes to achieve optimal ventricular performance, while at the same time reducing pulmonary congestion.

One of the difficult clinical decisions related to the manifestations of worsening heart failure is to determine whether or not the progression is due to a precipitating cause or due to progression of the underlying disease. In general, precipitating causes are an extremely common reason for worsening heart failure and should be carefully sought prior to assuming that a change in the heart failure state represents progression of the disease. There are multiple reasons for worsening heart failure in the category of precipitating causes. One of the most common is poor patient compliance with the medical regimen. This may mean excessive sodium intake or failure to take appropriate diuretics, digitalis, or vasodilator drugs.

An increase in the need for cardiac output can also exacerbate heart failure. This could occur in patients who develop infection, anemia, fever or who undergo excessive, prolonged exertion, or exposure to a hot, humid climate. Any of the causes mentioned above for high output states may also worsen congestive heart failure. Patients with heart failure are particularly susceptible to a decrease in pulmonary function as a cause of worsening heart failure. For example, unrecognized pulmonary emboli are a commonly overlooked reason for worsening heart failure. Any bronchial or pulmonary infection can also markedly worsen the symptoms of congestive heart failure. In considering associated cardiac causes for worsening heart failure, endocarditis superimposed on diseased valves must be carefully sought. Arrhythmias superimposed on a poorly compensated heart may dramatically worsen the signs and symptoms of heart failure. A prime example of this is the patient with severe hypertrophy who develops atrial fibrillation. With the loss of the atrial contribution to ventricular filling, there may be a dramatic worsening of symptoms associated with reduced cardiac output and elevated left ventricular filling pressures. Other arrythmias may also worsen the heart failure state.

It also is possible for patients to develop additional forms of heart disease. The development of coronary artery disease, with ischemia or myocardial infarction superimposed on other forms of heart failure, may greatly worsen the heart failure. If myocardial infarction is silent, this may make it extremely difficult to detect this superimposed problem unless it is carefully sought.

Management of acute heart failure

It is outside the scope of this chapter to review the various clinical settings in which heart failure is recognized and treated. It is appropriate, however, to consider one example to illustrate the application of the principles which have been discussed.

A dramatic example of a patient with left ventricular failure is one with the syndrome of acute pulmonary edema. The characteristic clinical picture of this syndrome is virtually unmistakable. The patient is acutely anxious, agitated, and is using the accessory muscles of respiration. He is coughing pink, foamy, sputum and wet rales are heard all over the front and back of the lungs. There is usually a tachycardia with peripheral vasoconstriction and sweating due to increased sympathetic tone. The blood pressure may be elevated initially, although it may be reduced to low levels with prolonged pulmonary edema, or in patients in cardiogenic shock.

The most important goal in such patients is to lower the preload as rapidly as possible. Some ways of affecting the preload are illustrated below as techniques for improving function in patients with left heart failure. Putting the patient in the erect sitting posture will make him more comfortable because of the tendency of blood to pool in the extremities and also because of an increase in vital capacity in the erect posture. Rotating tourniquets on the limbs are effective in pooling blood and, therefore, redistributing it away from the chest. Similarly, administration of nitrates, such as sublingual nitroglycerin, is extremely effective in producing venodilation and distributing blood away from the chest. Intravenous morphine sulphate has been an extremely effective drug in pulmonary edema. It has transient arteriolar and venodilating effects which may help to reduce both the preload and afterload of the heart. Much of the beneficial effect of morphine may be due to relief of anxiety. In turn, this reduces sympathetic tone and peripheral vascular resistance, thus decreasing afterload. Potent diuretics, like furosemide, also are beneficial. When given intravenously furosemide rapidly dilates veins and thus pools blood peripherally, resulting in a rapid drop in left atrial pressure [27]. The subsequent diuresis further reduces left atrial pressure. If the blood pressure is elevated due to a marked increase in circulating catecholamines, reduction of blood pressure (relief of afterload) with vasodilators will help the heart empty more effectively and thus reduce the left atrial pressure and pulmonary congestion. In patients with a normal hematocrit, rapid removal of a unit of blood by phlebotomy also may be effective in rapidly reducing intravascular volume and the level of left atrial pressure.

The role of acute digitalization in patients with acute pulmonary edema is less certain. Because of the marked increase in sympathetic tone which these patients have, they tend to have an increase in contractile state due to the circulating catecholamines. It is unclear whether a further beneficial increase in contractility can be produced by digitalis. In patients with pulmonary edema and cardiogenic shock following acute myocardial infarction, for example, digitalis has been uniformly disappointing in producing any kind of beneficial hemodynamic effect [28]. In patients with atrial fibrillation, digitalis is extremely effective in reducing the ventricular rate by increasing A-V block. This is true particularly in patients with mitral stenosis as the cause of their acute pulmonary edema.

Some inotropic agents may be helpful in patients with acute pulmonary edema. Two drugs commonly employed are dopamine and dobutamine. Although somewhat similar in their actions, there are important differences between them which should be considered in selecting one or the other. Both drugs increase heart rate and cardiac contractility. At progressively higher doses, dopamine produces vasoconstriction and increases blood pressure, whereas dobutamine has little effect on arterial pressure. With similar increases in cardiac output, dobutamine lowers filling pressure more than dopamine [29]. This occurs because dopamine increases arterial pressure (afterload), thus making it more difficult for the ventricle to empty, and thereby keeping the filling pressure higher. In general, therefore, dopamine is preferred if one wants to increase cardiac output *and* increase arterial pressure in a very hypotensive patient. If arterial pressure is adequate and the primary goal is to increase cardiac output and lower left ventricular filling pressure, then dobutamine would be the preferred drug. The use of inotropic agents in patients with

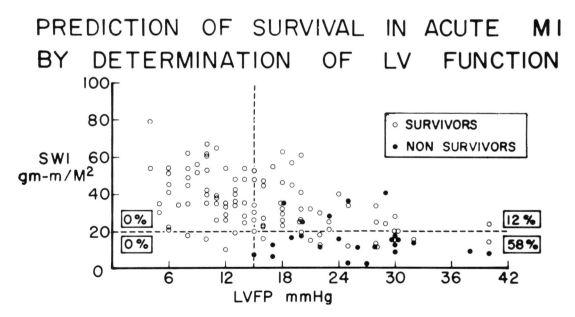

Figure 16. Hemodynamic determinants of survival following acute myocardial infarction: Hemodynamic measurements in patients with acute myocardial infarction, obtained shortly after admission, illustrate the prognostic significance of the data. The broken lines are drawn arbitrarily to divide the patients into four quadrants with the appropriate in-hospital mortality figures in each quadrant. In patients with function shifted down and to the right (stroke work index less than 20 g–m/ m² and left ventricular filling pressure greater than 15 mmHg), there is an excessively high mortality. There are no deaths in the patient group with a filling pressure less than 15 mmHg (reproduced with permission [30]).

coronary artery disease may produce undesirable side effects by increasing myocardial oxygen demand. If flow is limited by coronary stenosis this leads to further ischemia, and may produce serious arrhythmias.

Another important principle in the management of both acute and chronic failure is the fact that vasodilator and inotropic drugs have additive effects on cardiac output. This occurs because they work by different mechanisms. Inotropic drugs increase the force of contraction, whereas vasodilators reduce the load against which the heart is working. Combined therapy, therefore, should always be considered in severe heart failure.

Prognostic value of hemodynamic measurements

In patients with both acute and chronic heart failure, their survival is closely linked to the level of ventricular dysfunction. An example of the acute predictive value of such measurements in patients with acute myocardial infarction is illustrated in Figure 16. The hemodynamic status of each patient is plotted, shortly after admission to the coronary care unit with an acute myocardial infarction [30]. Left ventricular stroke work index (area of the pressure–volume loop) is plotted as a function of the left ventricular filling pressure (pulmonary capillary wedge pressure). The unfilled circles represent patients who survived to leave the hospital. The filled circles represent patients who died in the hospital. Note that mortality is progressively increased as ventricular function is shifted down and to the right, with a decrease in stroke work index and an increase in left ventricular filling pressure. The broken lines are arbitrarily drawn to divide the patients into four groups, with the appropriate mortality percentages indicated in each of the four quadrants. Note that those patients with a stroke work index less than 20 g–m/m^2 and a left ventricular filling pressure greater than 15 mmHg had a high mortality. Patients with a stroke work index less than 20 g–m/m^2 but a filling pressure less than 15 mmHg tended to be relatively hypovolemic, and thus could be treated appropriately with volume administration which raised their stroke work index as they moved up the ventricular function curve. In surviving patients with a low stroke work index, the subsequent mortality after discharge from the hospital was also extremely high [31].

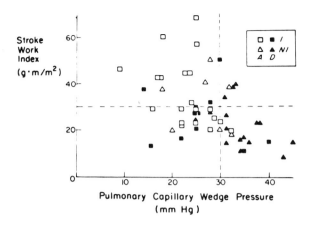

RELATIONSHIP OF PRE-TREATMENT SWI AND PCW TO OUTCOME

Figure 17. Hemodynamic determinants of survival in chronic congestive heart failure: In 56 patients with severe heart failure unresponsive to digitalis and diuretics, control hemodynamics are shown prior to the initiation of vasodilator therapy. The status of the patients at an average follow-up of 13 months is indicated by the appropriate symbols. Unfilled symbols represent living patients; filled symbols are those who died. The squares are clinically improved patients, and the triangles are those not clinically improved. The broken lines are drawn to separate the patients into four quadrants. In general, patients in the lower right-hand quadrant did not improve clinically and did not survive. Patients in the upper left-hand quadrant were clinically improved and alive at the time of follow-up. Patients in between the two quadrants represented a mixture of these two extremes (reproduced by permission [33]).

Similar hemodynamic measurements have important prognostic implications in patients with chronic refractory congestive heart failure. We have had considerable experience with a variety of vasodilator drugs [32]. Despite acute hemodynamic improvement in many of these patients, the 50% survival time is only about 15 months. In 56 such patients that we have followed [33], their baseline hemodynamic measurements (on digitalis and diuretics, but prior to vasodilator therapy) are illustrated in Figure 17. Most of these patients had underlying coronary artery disease as the basis for their heart failure. Note that the lower right-hand quadrant (stroke work index less than 30 g–m/m^2 and pulmonary capillary wedge pressure greater than 30 mmHg) contains mostly filled triangles, i.e., patients who did not improve clinically and who did not survive. Note that the upper left-hand quadrant contains mostly unfilled symbols (primarily squares), i.e., patients who improved clinically and who were alive at the time of follow-up. Between these two quadrants is an intermediate group of patients. Note, in particular, that a wedge pressure greater than 30 mmHg, despite optimal digitalis and diuretic therapy, was an extremely poor prognostic sign. In general, therefore, it is clear that these patients improved and survived in proportion to the initial level of their ventricular function. Those with extremely poor ventricular function had a high mortality, whereas those with good ventricular function had a much better survival rate.

Although the level of baseline ventricular function is an important determinant of prognosis, it is unclear whether improvement of ventricular function improves the prognosis appropriate to the new level of function. This question is analogous to the prognostic implications of a given serum cholesterol level. Although it is clear that the risk of developing coronary artery disease is proportional to the serum cholesterol, it is less clear whether reduction of the serum level improves the risk proportionally. One fact that is clear, however, is that appropriate therapy of such patients can often relieve the symptoms and signs of heart failure. Thus, reduction of pulmonary capillary wedge pressure with diuretics and vasodilators can markedly reduce the signs and symptoms of pulmonary congestion. Similarly, augmentation of cardiac output by digitalis or vasodilator drugs can increase the exercise tolerance of some patients and thus improve their functional ability. Even if there is no increase in longevity these functional improvements alone represent important goals for the practicing physician. The important question of whether or not various therapies prolong life can be answered only by clinical studies with substantial numbers of patients randomized to different treatment groups.

References

1. Fabiato A, Fabiato F: Calcium and cardiac excitation-contraction coupling. Ann Rev Physiol 41:473–484, 1979.
2. Sonnenblick EH: Force–velocity relations in mammalian heart muscle. Am J Physiol 202:931–939, 1962.
3. Adomian G, Laks M, Morady F, Swan HJC: Significance of the multiple intercalated disc in the hypertrophied canine heart. J Mol Cell Cardiol 6:105–109, 1974.
4. Sonnenblick EH, Ross J Jr, Covell JW, Spotnitz HM, Spiro D: Ultrastructure of the heart in systole and diastole. Circ Res 21:423–431, 1967.
5. Rushmer RF: Cardiovascular Dynamics, 4th Ed. Saunders, Philadelphia, 1976.
6. Glantz SA, Parmley WW: Factors which affect the diastolic pressure–volume curve. Circ Res 42:171–180, 1978.
7. Winegrad S: Electromechanical coupling in heart muscle. In: Berne RM (ed) Handbook of Physiology. Section 2: The Cardiovascular System, vol 1. Am Physiol Soc, Bethesda, 1979, pp 393–428.
8. Barany M: ATPase activity of myosin correlated with speed, muscle shortening. J Gen Physiol 50:197–202, 1967.
9. Chandler BM, Sonnenblick EH, Spann JR Jr, Pool PE: Association of depressed myofibrillar adenosine triphosphatase and reduced contractility in experimental heart failure. Circ Res 21:717–725, 1967.
10. Jewell BR: Brief reviews: a re-examination of the influence of muscle length on myocardial performance. Circ Res 40:221–230, 1977.
11. Pool PE, Spann JF Jr, Buccino RA, Sonnenblick EJ, Braunwald E: Myocardial high energy phosphate stores in cardiac hypertrophy and heart failure. Circ Res 21:365–373, 1967.
12. Berne RM, Rubio R: Coronary circulation. In: Berne RM (ed) Handbook of Physiology. Section 2: The Cardiovascular System, vol 1. Am Physiol Soc, Bethesda, 1979, pp 873–952.
13. Braunwald E, Ross J Jr: Control of cardiac performance. In: Berne RM (ed) Handbook of Physiology. Section 2: The Cardiovascular System, vol 1. Am Physiol Soc, Bethesda, 1979, pp 533–580.
14. Braunwald E, Ross J Jr, Sonnenblick EH: Mechanics of isolated heart muscle. In: Mechanisms of Contraction of the Normal and Failing Heart. Little, Brown and Co, Boston, 1968, pp 31–48.
15. Milnor WR: Arterial impedance as ventricular afterload. Circ Res 36:565–570, 1975.
16. Suga H, Sagawa K, Shoukas AA: Load independence of the instantaneous pressure–volume ratio of the canine left ventricle and effects of epinephrine and heart rate on the ratio. Circ Res 32:314–322, 1973.
17. Grossman W, Braunwald E, Mann T, McLaurin L, Green L: Contractile state of the left ventricle in man as evaluated from end-systolic pressure–volume relation. Circulation 56:845–850, 1977.
18. Swan HJC, Ganz W, Forrester J, Marcus H, Diamond G, Chonette D: Catheterization of the heart in man with the use of a flow-directed balloon-tipped catheter. N Engl J Med 283:447–451, 1970.
19. Abboud FM, Schmid PG: Circulatory adjustments to heart failure. In: Fishman AP (ed) Heart Failure. Hemisphere Publ Co, Washington-London, 1978, pp 249–260.
20. Kivowitz C, Parmley WW, Donoso R, Marcus H, Ganz W, Swan HJC: Effects of isometric exercise on cardiac performance: the grip test. Circulation 44:994–1002, 1971.
21. Braunwald E: Pathophysiology of heart failure. In: Braunwald E (ed) Heart Disease. Saunders, Philadelphia, 1980, pp 453–471.
22. Thomas JA, Marks BH: Plasma norepinephrine in conges-

tive heart failure. Am J Cardiol 41:233–243, 1978.

23. Grossman W, Jones D, McLaurin LP: Wall stress and patterns of hypertrophy in the human left ventricle. J Clin Invest 56:56–64, 1975.

24. Zelis R, Flaim SF, Nellis S, Longhurst J, Moskowitz R: Autonomic adjustments to congestive heart failure and their consequences. In: Fishman AP (ed) Heart Failure, Hemisphere Publ Co, Washington-London, 1978, pp 237–247.

25. Chatterjee K, Parmley WW, Massie B, Greenberg B, Werner J, Klausner S, Norman A: Oral hydralazine therapy for chronic refractory heart failure. Circulation 54:879–883, 1976.

26. Franciosa JA, Mikulic E, Cohn JN: Hemodynamic effect of orally administered isosorbide dinitrate in patients with congestive heart failure. Circulation 50:1020–1024, 1974.

27. Dikshit K, Vyden JK, Forrester JS, Chatterjee K, Prakash R, Swan HJC: Renal and extrarenal hemodynamic effects of furosemide in congestive failure after acute myocardial infarction. N Engl J Med 288:1087–1096, 1973.

28. Forrester J, Bezdek W, Chatterjee K, Levin P, Parmley WW, Swan HJC: Hemodynamic effects of digitalis in acute myocardial infarction. Ann Intern Med 76:863–864, 1972.

29. Loeb HS, Bredakis J, Gunnar RM: Superiority of dobutamine over dopamine for augmentation of cardiac output in patients with chronic low output cardiac failure. Circulation 55:375–381, 1977.

30. Forrester JS, Diamond G, Chatterjee K, Swan HJC: Hemodynamic therapy of acute myocardial infarction, Parts I and II. N Engl J Med 295:1356–1362; 295:1404–1413, 1976.

31. Chatterjee K, Swan HJC, Kaushik VS, Jobin G, Magnusson P, Forrester JS: Effects of vasodilator therapy for severe pump failure in acute myocardial infarction on short term and late prognosis. Circulation 53:797–802, 1976.

32. Chatterjee K, Parmley WW: The role of vasodilator therapy in heart failure. Prog Cardiovasc Dis 19:301–325, 1977.

33. Massie B, Ports T, Chatterjee K, Ostlund J, O'Young J, Haughbom F, Parmley WW: Long-term vasodilator therapy for heart failure: clinical response and its relationship to hemodynamic measurements. Circulation 63: 269–278, 1981.

34. Braunwald E, Ross J Jr, Sonnenblick EH: Structure of the myocardium. In: Mechanisms of Contraction of the Normal and Failing Heart. Little, Brown and Co, Boston, 1968, pp 1–19.

35. Perry SV: Control of muscular contraction. Symp Soc Exp Biol 27:531–550, 1973.

36. Parmley WW: Circulatory function and control. In: Beeson PB, McDermott W, Wyngaarden JB (eds) Cecil Textbook of Medicine. Saunders, Philadelphia, 1979, pp 1903–1072.

CHAPTER 3

Myocardial ischemia

JOHN ROSS, Jr.

This chapter will be concerned primarily with experimental studies on the relation between insufficiency of local coronary blood flow and regional cardiac contractile function, and its implications for human disease. The consequences of reduced coronary blood flow are complex, however, and before analyzing its effects on the dynamics of regional and overall cardiac contraction, it will be useful to consider briefly general mechanisms which reduce coronary blood flow, as well as the overall effects of ischemia on cardiac metabolism structure, and function.

General effects of ischemia on the heart

Causes of cardiac ischemia

The most common clinical setting for ischemia is atherosclerotic narrowing of one or more coronary arteries, a process which can gradually lead to a degree of coronary stenosis that limits coronary blood flow during stress. Typically, when a 70–75% reduction of cross-sectional diameter of the vessel is present, reactive hyperemia is eliminated [1], and the increase in blood flow that ordinarily accompanies muscular exercise cannot occur. Symptoms and signs of local ischemia may then appear during such stress, including angina pectoris, repolarization abnormalities on the electrocardiogram, or evidence of a left ventricular contraction disorder by radionuclide angiography or on echocardiography. Of course, if narrowing of the coronary artery is abrupt and complete, as when hemorrhage into an atherosclerotic plaque or thrombosis of an ulcerat-

ed plaque occur [2], acute mycocardial infarction usually ensues. Whether or not ischemia or infarction occur as a result of rapid or gradual coronary obstruction is importantly influenced by variable development of the coronary collateral circulation [3]. The collateral circulation has been studied in a variety of animal species. In the dog, there is usually a substantial epicardial collateral network even without the stimulus of ischemia; in the pig, collaterals are much less prominent [3], and the baboon tends to have very few subendocardial collateral vessels [4]. The coronary collateral circulation in the normal human heart tends to resemble that in the baboon [3], but it is well recognized that in patients with coronary heart disease a variable degree of collateral formation occurs. Such collateral channels may significantly modify or prevent the development of ischemia [5] and they can even prevent the development of myocardial infarction in the presence of total occlusion of a coronary artery. However, the lack of reliable methods for measuring collateral blood flow in human subjects has limited our understanding of the functional significance of the collateral circulation in clinical coronary heart disease.

In general, when sufficient coronary stenosis is present to cause lowered perfusion pressure in the artery distal to the stenosis, insufficient blood flow to that region ensues. Thus, it has been shown experimentally that coronary autoregulation maintains coronary blood flow constant in a separately perfused coronary artery over a wide range of perfusion pressures (provided the work of the heart is maintained constant), with maximal coronary vasodilation (loss of autoregulation) occurring at a

Rosen, M. R. and Hoffman, B. F. (eds.), Cardiac Therapy. ISBN 0-89838-564-4.
© 1983, Martinus Nijhoff Publishers, Boston, The Hague, Dordrecht, Lancaster. Printed in the Netherlands.

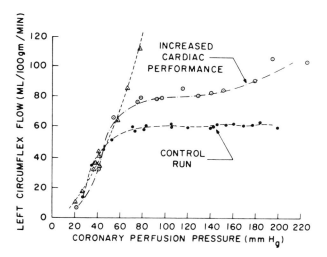

Figure 1. Pressure-flow curves in the separately perfused coronary artery of the dog at a control level (filled circles) and at an increased level of cardiac performance (unfilled circles) showing autoregulation. The instantaneous relation between pressure and flow in the dilated bed from a perfusion pressure of 40 mmHg is indicated by the dashed line through the triangles (reproduced from [1] by permission of the Am Heart Assoc, Inc).

mean perfusion pressure of about 60 mmHg or below [6]. At that point, coronary blood flow becomes pressure-dependent and the pressure–flow relation exhibits the characteristics of a maximally dilated vascular bed [7] (Figure 1). In the presence of a fixed coronary artery stenosis, increased myocardial oxygen consumption ($M\dot{V}O_2$) during exercise consequent to tachycardia, elevated systolic arterial pressure, and enhanced contractility contribute to ischemia by producing increased demand for blood flow through the stenotic vessel. Since the vascular bed beyond the stenosis may be nearly maximally dilated at rest, the lack of vasodilator reserve and increased metabolic demands, coupled with decreased time for diastolic coronary perfusion due to the tachycardia [8], further promote the development of ischemia.

Considerable evidence now indicates that another important mechanism for ischemia and angina pectoris in the clinical setting is relatively common; that is, reduced myocardial oxygen supply in the absence of increased demands. Perhaps most instances of angina pectoris occurring at rest, including the variant anginal syndrome of Prinzmetal (in which transmural ischemia is suggested by elevated S-T segments during pain [9]), result from functional spasm of one or more coronary arteries [10]. Such coronary artery spasms may occur at the site of a significant fixed atherosclerotic lesion, or in an entirely normal coronary artery [10, 11], and rarely is it of sufficient severity and duration to produce myocardial infarction [12]. The mechanisms responsible for initiating coronary artery spasm have not yet been defined, although proposed causes include altered alpha-adrenergic tone to the coronary arteries [13], endogenous prostaglandin release and/or release of thromboxane A_2 from platelets [14]. Formation of platelet thrombi on atherosclerotic plaques, with or without accompanying coronary artery spasm, also has been described experimentally [15].

The basic setting for cardiac ischemia, therefore, is either increased oxygen demand, reduced oxygen supply, or both. This has led to a variety of therapeutic approaches for the relief of cardiac ischemia and angina pectoris, including drugs to decrease myocardial oxygen consumption (beta-blockers; nitrates), agents to relieve coronary artery spasm (nitrates; calcium antagonists), and measures to increase myocardial blood flow (coronary vasodilators such as the nitrates; coronary artery bypass grafting).

Metabolic consequences of cardiac ischemia

Mammalian cardiac muscle, unlike skeletal muscle, cannot develop a sizable oxygen debt during contractile activity, to be repaid later during a period of rest. The heart is a continuously active organ which, under normal conditions, relies almost exclusively on sustained aerobic metabolism. The oxygen consumption of the myocardium is relatively high, most of the energy requirements being related to the pumping activity of the left ventricle; this chamber comprises less than 0.5% of the body weight in man, but it accounts for about 7% of the total basal oxygen consumption of the body. Cardiac muscle uses primarily fatty acids and glucose to generate ATP but lactate, pyruvate, ketone bodies, and even amino acids also can be utilized [16]. Fatty acids are oxidized in preference to carbohydrates and account for 60–70% of oxidative metabolism, but glucose is also important, intermediates formed during glycolysis being used by the citric acid cycle [16].

When the heart is subjected to ischemia, oxidative production of high energy phosphates falls as

46

use of fatty acids is inhibited, ATP production by glycolysis becomes important and lactate is produced [17, 18]. During hypoxia and/or mild ischemia, increased glucose transport is observed, and anaerobic glycolysis is stimulated. There are several key control points in the main glycolytic pathway, each of which is regulated by feedback control mechanisms [17]. For example, phosphofructokinase is the enzyme involved in the first irreversible step in the glycolytic pathway, and during normal myocardial metabolism (when ATP and citrate concentrations are high) it is inhibited. When oxidative phosphorylation is limited, this enzyme is activated by decreased ATP concentrations as well as by increased levels of $5'$-AMP, inorganic phosphate, ADP, and other factors. However, H^+ accumulation as ischemia progresses leads to inhibition of this enzyme [19], thereby slowing glycolysis. The accumulation of glucose-6-phosphate inhibits hexokinase, further decreasing glucose phosphorylation [2]. Under anaerobic conditions another key enzyme, glyceraldehyde-3-phosphate dehydrogenase, is inhibited by NADH accumulation [20], but, if pyruvate can be converted to lactate, NADH produced at this step can be oxidized and glycolytic production of ATP will continue [17]. Again, however, with the low flow conditions of ischemia, metabolic products rapidly accumulate, and further impairment of the glycolytic pathway ensues.

When the heart is completely deprived of oxygen during ischemia, glycogen stores are depleted rapidly and the rate of ATP production by glycolysis is not sufficient to maintain normal creatine phosphate and ATP concentrations; if the ischemic insult is prolonged, even cell-maintenance levels of ATP cannot be generated by glycolysis [19]. At the point of irreversible myocardial damage, generally after 40–60 min of complete ischemia, ATP is reduced below $2\,\mu$ moles/g [21], the adenine nucleotide pool is depleted, and there is evidence of structural mitochondrial damage [19, 22].

Myocardial contraction is depressed very early after the onset of ischemia. The precise metabolic events causing this rapid reduction of contractility are unknown, but it occurs well before critical reduction of high energy phosphate levels. The accumulation of H^+ ion has been implicated [23, 24], and there is evidence that decreased contractility is related to both extracellular and intracellular acidosis [25].

Functional consequences of cardiac ischemia

The earliest physiologic consequence readily detected in an area subjected to acute coronary stenosis or occlusion is reduction of regional contractile function [26]. As the contractile defect persists and becomes more severe, repolarization abnormalities appear on the local electrogram (S-T segment elevation or depression, and T-wave changes) [27], followed by similar changes on the body surface electrocardiogram [28]. If the zone of ischemia is sufficiently large, changes in overall hemodynamic function of the left ventricle rapidly ensue, including elevation of the left ventricular end-diastolic pressure, reduction of peak left ventricular dP/dt, and sometimes a fall in peak systolic pressure [29]. Such hemodynamic changes have been found to precede electrocardiographic changes and chest pain during coronary artery spasm [10]. When angina pectoris occurs during cardiac catheterization, it is often accompanied by an increase of the left ventricular filling pressure [30, 31], and a fall in the left ventricular ejection fraction during spontaneous angina pectoris has been documented by radionuclide angiography [32]. Acute myocardial infarction is accompanied by a wide spectrum of effects on left ventricular function [33]; if the infarct is small, hemodynamic impairment may be brief and mild, whereas in patients with extensive prior myocardial infarction or a very large new area of myocardial damage (generally over 40% of the left ventricle [34]), the cardiogenic shock or 'power failure' syndrome is seen [33].

Following experimental coronary artery occlusion in various animal species, ventricular dysrhythmias including ventricular tachycardia and ventricular fibrillation are common. These have been related to several mechanisms involving changes in membrane potentials in the ischemic zone (see Chapter 1), and such dysrhythmias are very common in humans following acute coronary occlusion, as discussed in Chapter 15. Conduction disturbances including complete heart block also are relatively common. Even during acute severe ischemia without infarction (such as in variant angina pectoris), a variety of ventricular or atrial dysrhythmias and conduction disturbances have been described [35]. Severe dysrhythmias often are responsible for very early death after coronary occlusion.

With prolonged persistent ischemia leading to infarction, changes also occur in the coronary vessels and microvasculature. Increased capillary permeability may lead to tissue edema and further impairment of regional perfusion [36]. Also, by about 90 min after the onset of coronary occlusion in experimental animals, reperfusion of the coronary bed may result in the 'no reflow' phenomenon, a lack of blood flow to the involved region due to increased local vascular resistance resulting from vascular damage and edema [37].

Effects of myocardial ischemia on regional cardiac function

A variety of methods has been used in the experimental setting to assess local cardiac contraction [29, 38–43]. Since the time of Tennant and Wiggers [26], it has been known that in fully ischemic regions regional systolic shortening is replaced by holosystolic elongation of the muscle. We have examined such responses in several regions of the heart simultaneously by ultrasound using implanted piezoelectric crystals [29]. With this approach, a pair of small (2 mm) crystals is placed about 10–20 mm apart in the inner wall of the left ventricle in a zone to be rendered ischemic by stenosis or occlusion of a coronary artery; other pairs of crystals are implanted in the border zone, and in a distant normal region [29, 43]. Alternatively, pairs of crystals are placed across the wall to measure the dynamics of regional wall thickening [44], a technique which may more closely reflect overall wall motion abnormalities as measured by angiography in human subjects.

Regional myocardial contraction during coronary occlusion or stenosis

The rapid sequence of events which follows abrupt occlusion of a coronary artery in a chronically instrumented, conscious dog is illustrated in Figure 2.

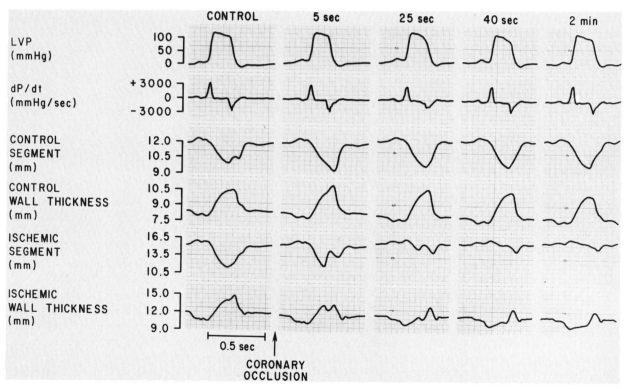

Figure 2. Effects of acute coronary occlusion in the conscious dog on left ventricular pressure (LVP), its first derivative (d*P*/d*t*), and segment lengths and wall thicknesses in both control and ischemic areas. The time of occlusion is indicated by an arrow. Note the mirror image relations between wall thickness and subendocardial segment length in the ischemic zone (reproduced from [44] by permission of the Am Heart Assoc, Inc).

Within a few cardiac cycles, reduced shortening of the subendocardial segment occurs and shortly thereafter late systolic elongation develops in that region; subsequently, there is further loss of active shortening and then gradual development of holosystolic elongation over the course of 30 seconds to one or two minutes, indicating passive stretch of the subendocardial region [29]. When regional wall thickness is measured in the central ischemic zone under similar circumstances, normal systolic wall thickening of about 30% [44] is rapidly replaced by reduced systolic thickening and late systolic wall thickening, later by akinesia, and then holosystolic wall thinning (Figure 2) [27, 33]. In the conscious animal, reflex tachycardia mediated by both the sympathetic and parasympathetic systems [45] is observed within 15–30 sec of coronary occlusion (Figure 3), a response not seen in the open-chest animal [29].

Simultaneously, in the normal regions there is a very early increase in systolic segment shortening (decreased end-systolic length) without an increase of resting fiber length, which is associated with development of the systolic bulge in the ischemic region (dyskinesia). This sequence is followed by an increase in resting fiber length in the normal segments, often with some compensatory use of the Frank-Starling mechanism [29] (Figure 3). As expected, diastolic wall thinning and increased systolic wall thickening also occur in the normal regions [29]. Border zones, in which the crystals in the subendocardial segments tend to straddle both ischemic and normal tissue, show reduced function (hypokinesia) (Figure 3) [29].

Partial obstruction of a coronary artery in the dog by means of an implanted hydraulic cuff occluder results in varying degrees of hypofunction in the involved regions ranging from mild hypokinesia to severe dyskinesia, depending on the degree of stenosis and the extent of coronary collateral supply [46]. In the conscious dog, reflex tachycardia also accompanies partial stenosis [46].

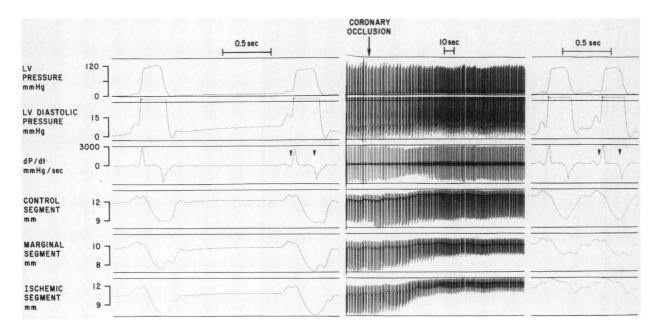

Figure 3. Direct recording from a resting, unanesthetized dog in which left ventricular pressure and three segment dimensions are recorded simultaneously. Control tracings before coronary occlusion are shown on the left, and changes induced by a rapid cuff inflation (indicated by the arrow at coronary occlusion) are shown at slow paper speed in the central panel. On the right are tracings obtained at the same paper speed as the left panel about 2 min after the occlusion, during the reflex tachycardia. Measurements of end-diastolic dimensions are taken at the nadir of pressure following atrial contraction (at the time dP/dt crosses zero). End-systolic dimensions are taken 20 msec prior to the nadir of negative dP/dt. These points are indicated by arrows (reproduced from [43] by permission of the Am Heart Assoc, Inc).

Following permanent coronary occlusion in the dog, subendocardial scar formation over the course of several weeks results in a progressive decrease in distance between the crystals in the central ischemic zone, and there is little return of systolic function [47]. In the normal region there is compensatory diastolic elongation with hyperfunction of involved segments [47]. Overall wall function, as assessed by systolic wall thickening in the ischemic zone after permanent coronary occlusion in the dog, tends to show more return of function over several weeks than function measured only in the subendocardial region; moreover, there is lack of wall thinning despite loss of tissue with scarring in the subendo-cardium [48]. These responses may be due to compensatory hypertrophy of outer myocardial layers, due to the rich epicardial collateral blood supply which develops in the dog [48].

In the baboon, a species with a sparse collateral circulation [4], rapid development of marked holo-systolic expansion occurs in the ischemic zone, accompanied by marked systolic wall thinning, and often serious ventricular dysrhythmias [4]. Following permanent coronary artery occlusion in the baboon, in contrast with the dog, there is often late, persistent holosystolic bulging in the infarcted zone (Figure 4), which is associated with transmural scar and wall thinning at postmortem examination and presumably reflects the lack of collateral blood supply to the ischemic region [4]. This setting may relate to aneurysm formation after acute myocardial infarction in some patients.

A few observations have been made on regional contractile function in patients during acute myocardial infarction. In early studies, radarkymography was employed to show the development of outward wall motion) dyskinesia in some regions of the left ventricle within one or two hours after the onset of symptoms of acute myocardial infarction [49]. More recently, echocardiography has documented regional dyskinesia and wall thinning early after coronary occlusion [50]. In chronic coronary heart disease, cine left ventriculography has been widely employed to document regional wall motion

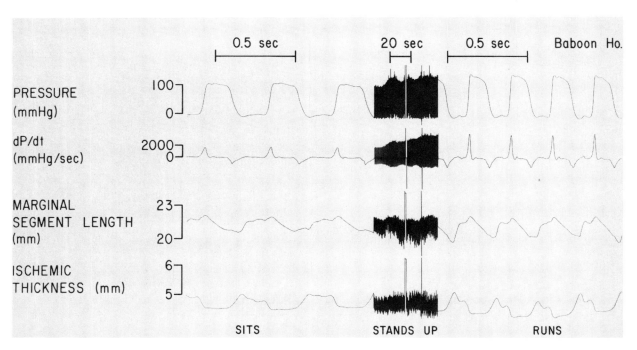

Figure 4. Study obtained by telemetry in a conscious baboon 1 week after acute anterior descending coronary occlusion. Left ventricular pressure and its first derivative (dP/dt) are shown in two upper tracings. Regional function obtained with ultrasonic crystals is shown in a marginal segment, and wall thickness is measured in the ischemic region. While the animal is sitting at rest, the high-speed tracings on the left show reduced shortening in the marginal region with holosystolic wall thinning in the ischemic segment. When the animal stands up and then runs about the cage, there is a substantial increase in left ventricular systolic pressure and dP/dt, while systolic thinning of the wall increases slightly during the activity (reproduced by permission from [4]).

abnormalities due to prior myocardial infarction [51], and this approach has also documented the development of regional wall motion abnormalities consequent to pacing-induced ischemia [52]. With the cineangiographic approach, normal inward motion or abnormal contraction patterns in various regions of the ventricle can be evaluated precisely (Figure 5), along with assessment of global ventricular function by calculation of the left ventricular ejection fraction. Radionuclide angiography can also be used to detect overall impairment of ventricular function by calculation of the ejection fraction [53], and techniques are improving for the study of regional wall motion abnormalities by this approach [54].

Relations between electrocardiographic and mechanical events

After experimental coronary occlusion, regional contractile dysfunction is known to precede the development of electrocardiographic abnormalities [27]. Regional myocardial function (wall thicken-

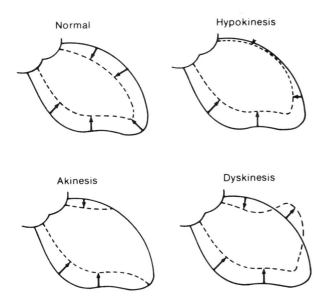

Normal   Hypokinesis

Akinesis   Dyskinesis

Figure 5. Diagrams of cineangiographic outlines of the left ventricle demonstrating various wall motion abnormalities in coronary heart disease (reproduced by permission from Ross and Peterson: Cardiac Catheterization and Angiography. In: Isselbacher KJ, Adams RD, Braunwald E, Petersdorf RG, Wilson JD (eds) Harrison's Principles of Internal Medicine, 9th Ed. McGraw-Hill Book Co, New York, 1980, pp 1018–1025).

ing by ultrasonic crystals), local electrograms, and a surface VCG array (XYZ leads) have been measured during acute coronary stenosis and occlusion in conscious, chronically instrumented dogs [28]. In this study, as expected, loss of systolic wall thickening occurred before any electrical changes; with complete coronary occlusions, surface ECG changes tended to precede those measured from the local subendocardial electrogram. However, during mild coronary stenosis (sufficient to produce a decrease of approximately 25% in systolic wall thickening) it was possible in a number of animals to maintain stable regional contractile dysfunction for at least 10 min without any detectable changes in the surface electrocardiogram [28]; changes in the local electrogram did occur, however (Figure 6). These findings indicate that regional contractile dysfunction provides a more sensitive indicator of regional ischemia than the surface ECG. Since mild contractile dysfunction is associated with reduced coronary blood flow, as discussed below, these findings provide a basis for the sensitive detection of latent coronary stenosis by measurements of regional or global ventricular contractile function in humans.

Relations between regional myocardial blood flow and regional function

Studies in experimental animals have shown a general relation between reductions of coronary inflow, measured by a flowmeter, and changes in local cardiac function [55, 56]. In addition, use of the radioactive microsphere technique, in conjunction with implanted ultrasonic dimension gauges, has allowed correlation of changes in transmural myocardial blood flow distribution with regional contractile function. In experiments in open-chest animals, changes in regional contractile function were measured during various degrees of coronary artery stenosis and a linear correlaton between subendocardial regional blood flow and function was found (Figure 7) [56]. In conscious dogs, Vatner has described an exponential relation between subendocardial blood flow and function [57], initial reductions in blood flow causing less marked changes in function than found in the open-chest animal. Correlations between regional wall thickening dynamics and transmural blood flow in the anesthetized dog indicate that reduction of subendocardial flow produces regional hypokinesia of the entire

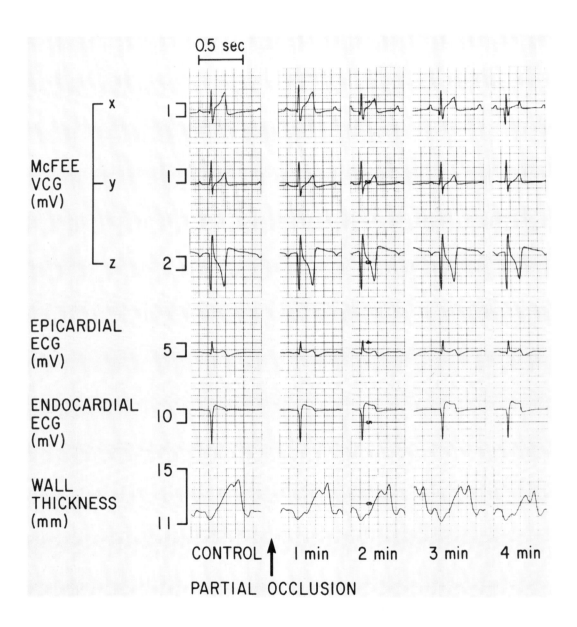

Figure 6. Tracings from a dog in which partial coronary stenosis was induced to produce about 30% reduction of systolic wall thickening and maintained at a relatively stable state for 4 min. ST-segment changes in the local electrograms precede minimal changes on surface X, Y, Z ECG leads, and both are preceded by regional myocardial dysfunction; VCG = vectorcardiogram (reproduced from [28] by permission of the Am Heart Assoc, Inc).

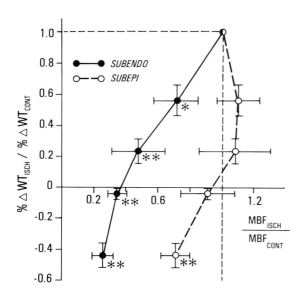

Figure 7. Relative changes in subendocardial (layer 1) and subepicardial (layer 4) myocardial blood flow versus relative changes in systolic wall thickening in anesthetized dogs. Significant changes in blood flow are indicated with asterisks (* = p < 0.05, ** = p < 0.01). Subendocardial blood flow was closely related to reductions in wall thickening, but subepicardial blood flow was decreased significantly only with severe stenosis (reproduced from [56] by permission of the Am Heart Assoc, Inc).

wall [56]; even with akinesia of the wall, blood flow to the epicardial regions of the wall is well preserved, and with transmural reductions of blood flow (most marked in the subendocardium), holosystolic wall thinning occurs [56]. These observations indicate a close coupling in the resting state between reductions of blood flow and impairment of contractile function.

Diastolic compliance after coronary occlusion or stenosis

After permanent experimental coronary occlusion, a decrease in regional compliance (increased stiffness) occurs over several days, presumably secondary to edema and inflammation [58]. Subsequently the involved segments show further marked increases in stiffness, as progressive scarring occurs [47, 58]. However, the immediate effect of acute ischemia on diastolic compliance has been less clear, and left ventricular chamber stiffness has been reported to increase, decrease, or exhibit no change in dogs subjected to acute coronary occlu-

sion [59–61]. In most clinical studies, rapid pacing has been employed to induce ischemia in patients with coronary heart disease, and the responses following sudden cessation of pacing have been analyzed. There is a marked depression of systolic cardiac function during and after pacing, and the left ventricular end-diastolic pressure often rises markedly [32, 52]. Studies on the pressure–volume relation of the ventricle analyzed during single cardiac cycles in the period after pacing have shown a shift of this relation upward and to the left [62, 63], suggesting decreased chamber compliance. Minor changes in right ventricular diastolic pressure during this period have suggested that the effects of the pericardium [64] on ventricular interaction may not be primarily responsible for the observed shifts in the left ventricular pressure–volume curve [65]. Myocardial stress–strain relations have not been analyzed in the clinical setting, however.

Experimental studies on left ventricular diastolic pressure–volume relations have confirmed the shift upward and to the left during postpacing ischemia. The shift upward, suggesting increased chamber stiffness, occurs in the absence of the pericardium [66, 67], and it was therefore suggested that it is myocardial in origin [66]. On the other hand, such a shift does not appear to occur during partial coronary stenosis sufficient to produce regional hypokinesia [67]. Moreover, although it is observed during complete coronary occlusion in the absence of the pericardium, when right ventricular filling is reduced by partial inferior vena caval occlusion, the shift is not observed [67]; the latter observation suggests that ventricular interaction may play a role in this response [64, 67]. An increase in the time constant for ventricular relaxation during myocardial ischemia, derived from the rate of change of left ventricular pressure during isovolumetric relaxation, has been described [68], and it has been suggested that such delayed relaxation may be responsible for impaired early diastolic filling which, in turn, affects the passive pressure–volume relation [66, 69].

The relations between left ventricular diastolic pressure and segment lengths in normal and ischemic regions have been examined in open-chest and conscious dogs following acute coronary occlusion [29, 47]. Under these conditions, an increase in ventricular end-diastolic pressure occurs, but in normal zones there is no change in the relationship

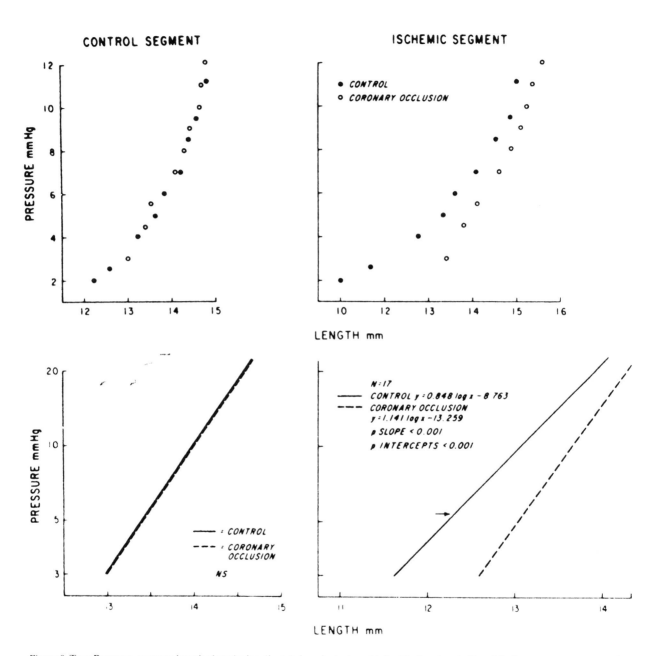

Figure 8. Top: Pressure–segment length plots during diastole in a single dog obtained before (control) and during coronary artery occlusion in the control segment (left) and the ischemic segment (right). Bottom: Average semilogarithmic pressure–length plots before (control, solid lines) and during coronary artery occlusion (dashed lines) (reproduced from [29] by permission of the Am Heart Assoc, Inc).

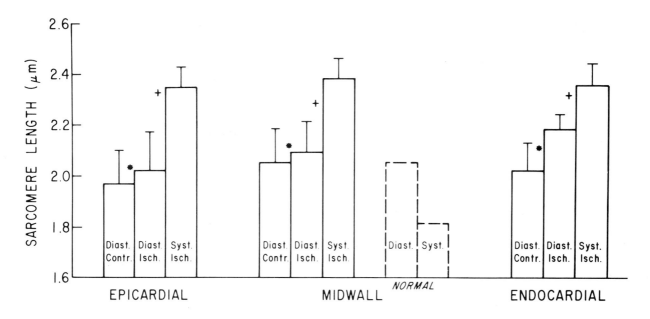

Figure 9. Sarcomere lengths in four hearts fixed after 15 min of coronary artery occlusion: Contr. = control segments; Isch. = ischemic segments; Diast. = fixation at end-diastole; Syst. Isch. = fixation at maximum systolic length of ischemic segments. Normal (---) shows midwall sarcomere lengths from previous studies with fixation of the normal diastolic heart at 6 mmHg and at end-systole. Bars indicate standard deviations. * Significant difference (p < 0.001) between control and ischemic segment sarcomeres fixed at end-diastole; + significant difference (p < 0.001) between ischemic segment sarcomeres fixed at end-diastole and those fixed at maximum systolic length. Note that sarcomere lengths in the ischemic segment are elongated across the wall (reproduced by permission from [70]).

between regional segment length and ventricular diastolic pressure throughout single diastolic cycles. In ischemic zones, however, there is a shift to the right and steepening of this relationship over the course of several minutes, which accompanies the development of regional holosystolic lengthening (Figure 8) [29, 47]. This finding suggested that segment compliance was reduced [29]. We have attributed this displacement of the regional diastolic pressure–segment length relation to repeated systolic overstretch of the sarcomeres in the ischemic region associated with the regional dysknesia, and in other studies systolic overstretch during ischemia has been shown to produce progressive elongation of the sarcomeres in the ischemic zone (Figure 9) [70].

Diastolic stress–strain relations of the myocardium during ischemia have also been examined in conscious dogs with the pericardium open. The left ventricular major and minor axes were measured with ultrasonic dimension gauges, together with wall thickness both in ischemic and normal zones, during complete and partial coronary artery steno-

ses; the zero intercepts for left ventricular diastolic pressure were determined by transient inferior vena caval occlusions, providing a common zero reference pressure during these interventions [67]. During partial coronary stenoses, which produced systolic hypoknesia or akinesia without holosystolic expansion, no significant changes in chamber or myocardial stiffness occurred [67]. However, after 3 min of complete coronary occlusion, left ventricular chamber stiffness (assessed by the diastolic pressure–volume relation) was augmented, and myocardial wall stiffness (assessed by the stress–strain relation) increased [67] (Figure 10). During complete coronary occlusions, there was a consistently larger ventricular volume at the zero pressure intercept (termed creep) during complete coronary occlusions, which did not occur during partial coronary stenoses. Therefore, these studies suggested that creep occurring in severely ischemic regions was important in causing increased myocardial stiffness during severe ischemia, since in the absence of this phenomenon myocardial properties were not significantly changed [67]. Further studies will be

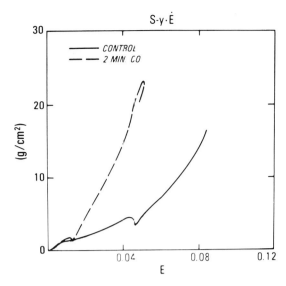

Figure 10. Stress–strain relationship of the left ventricle in a dog during control and at 2 min of complete coronary occlusion. The stress–strain relationship is steeper during occlusion. $S - y \cdot \dot{E}$: Left ventricular circumferential wall stress minus the product of myocardial viscosity and strain rate; E = Midwall strain.

needed to characterize fully the relative contributions of various factors to increased wall stiffness (delayed relaxation, creep) and to shifts of the pressure–volume relation in humans (increased wall stiffness, elevated intrapericardial pressure, ventricular interaction) [64].

Effects of selected pharmacologic agents and other stimuli during acute coronary occlusion

The effects of a number of interventions on regional function during acute experimental coronary artery occlusion have been studied both in open-chest animals and in conscious, chronically instrumented dogs.

Beta-adrenergic blockade
The effects of propanolol during acute coronary occlusion have been evaluated by comparing regional myocardial function during a control coronary occlusion with that during a repeat occlusion following intravenous propanolol administration.

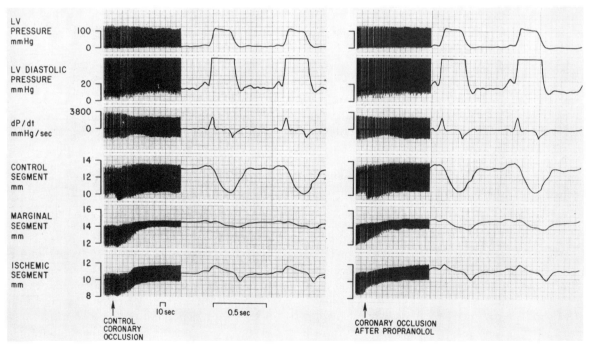

Figure 11. Left ventricular (LV) pressure and its first derivative (dP/dt) with tracings from segments in three regions of the left ventricular myocardium of a conscious dog during a control coronary occlusion (left panel) and in the same dog after the administration of propranolol intravenously (right panel). Note the somewhat slower heart rate in the right panel and the increased shortening, which is particularly evident in the marginal segment (reproduced by permission from Ross J Jr et al. In: Schwartz PJ, Brown AM, Malliani A, Zanchetti A (eds) Neural Mechanisms in Cardiac Arrhythmias. Raven Press, New York, 1978, pp 401–418).

56

Typical results in such an experiment in the anesthetized dog are shown in Figure 11. After propranolol, the heart rate before coronary occlusion is lower and regional function in all zones, as well as peak LV dP/dt, are depressed compared to the control study. Despite decreased function in the normal regions secondary to beta–adrenergic blockade, the extent of systolic shortening in the border zones is improved during coronary occlusion, compared to that during the control occlusion [29, 71]. This finding suggests that decreased oxygen demands in that zone (slower heart rate and reduced contractility) due to propanolol resulted in a more favorable oxygen supply–demand ratio; increased myocardial oxygen supply may also have contributed (increased time for diastolic subendocardial perfusion) [6, 72]. Results in the conscious, chronically instrumented animal are similar [43]. These findings may explain the improvement of hemodynamic function sometimes observed in humans when propanolol is administered following acute myocardial infarction [73].

Positive inotropic stimulation

When isoproterenol is administered following experimental coronary occlusion there is initial improvement of contraction in normal and border zones due to the positive inotropic and chronotropic properties of this drug; however, as the drug infusion is continued, deterioration of function occurs in the border zones [29]. This response is presumably due to an oxygen supply–demand imbalance in those regions resulting from the increased heart rate and contractility, decreased time for diastolic perfusion, and a fall in coronary artery perfusion pressure secondary to the peripheral vasodilating effects of isoproterenol.

In studies in conscious dogs, it has been found that acute administration of a digitalis preparation after coronary occlusion causes sustained improvement of overall cardiac function and regional function in marginal zones, together with improvement of blood flow to those regions [74]. When catecholamines were administered to produce a rise in blood pressure without a substantial change in

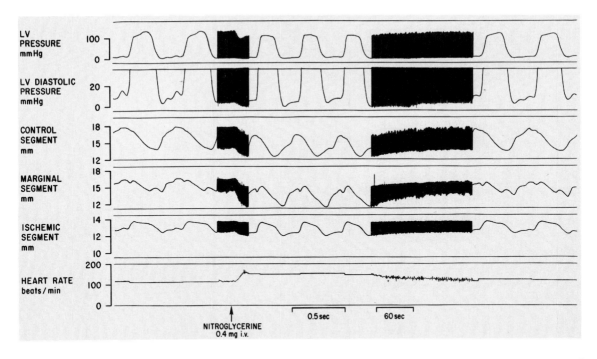

Figure 12. Left ventricular (LV) pressure and dimensions in three segments of the left ventricular myocardium in a conscious dog before and during administration of nitroglycerin in the presence of acute coronary artery occlusion. Note the drop in systolic and end-diastolic left ventricular pressures and the considerable reduction of end-diastolic segment length in the control segment. There is marked improvement of shortening, particularly in the marginal segment, with only a small effect on the fully ischemic segment (reproduced from [43] by permission from the Am Heart Assoc, Inc).

57

heart rate, overall cardiac function and contractility in marginally perfused zones also improved and subendocardial blood flow increased [75]; however, after several minutes of isoproterenol infusion, which lowered mean blood pressure and increased heart rate, regional contraction in marginally perfused areas decreased, as observed in the open-chest animal [29], together with reduction of blood flow to those zones [87], supporting the view that an oxygen supply–demand imbalance was induced. Similar unfavorable effects of isoproterenol have been documented by hemodynamic and metabolic studies in patients with acute myocardial infarction [76].

Nitroglycerin

The effects of intravenously administered nitroglycerin following experimental coronary artery occlusion in the dog are shown in Figure 12. A prompt fall in systemic arterial pressure followed by some reflex tachycardia are generally noted, with considerable improvement in shortening of border regions [29, 43]. The holosystolic elongation in ischemic zones generally is not abolished, although its contour may be modified suggesting lessening of systolic elongation during late systole (Figure 12) which could result from reduced heart size and lessened systolic loading conditions.

Postextrasystolic potentiation

The effects of postextrasystolic potentiation have been studied following acute coronary artery occlusion in dogs using implanted ultrasonic crystals [77]. Increased shortening is observed in normal zones during the postextrasystolic beat (increase about 45%) and was unchanged before and after coronary occlusion (Figure 13); fully ischemic zones (holosystolic expansion) showed rapid loss of active shortening produced by postextrasystolic potentiation over the course of two or three minutes, which persisted over the subsequent two hours (Figure 13), although modification of the degree of systolic expansion was observed. In marginal zones, the degree of postextrasystolic potentiation was attenuated (Figure 13), but significant potentiation persisted throughout the 2-hr observation period [77]. Others, using epicardial mercury-in-rubber gauges for measuring regional function have reported some persistence of potentiation in fully ischemic zones, without significant attenuation of

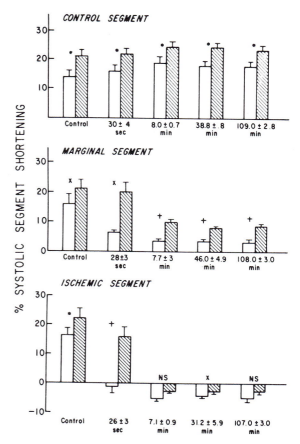

Figure 13. Averaged data showing evolution of postextrasystolic potentiation in the dog before (control) and serially at several time points after coronary occlusion in control, marginal, and ischemic segments: Systolic segment shortening is expressed as percent shortening or lengthening (mean ± SEM): unfilled bars = control beats, hatched bars = potentiated beats; * = p < 0.001, + = p < 0.01, x = p < 0.05 (reproduced by permission from [77]).

postextrasystolic potentiation in border zones despite marked reduction of function [78]. In long-term studies in which postextrasystolic potentiation was measured using regional wall thickening dynamics, persistence of potentiation in border zones was found for several weeks after coronary occlusion [79].

In the dog, the border zone subtended by crystals consists of both normal myocardium and ischemic fibers [29, 43, 47], and a narrow serpigenous boundary has been described by some investigators [80]. The improved function in border zones described above during positive inotropic stimulation and during nitroglycerin administration may be related to several mechanisms. For example, during nitroglycerin administration, the decrease in arterial pressure and heart size caused by the peripheral vasodilatation [81] may cause reduced systolic loading (lowered afterload) allowing both normal or partially ischemic fibers in the border zone to shorten more completely; in addition, it is possible that improved collateral blood flow to the border zone may be produced by nitroglycerin. In the case of postextrasystolic potentiation, it is possible that the stimulus is acting predominantly on normal fibers in the border zone to enhance their contractility, with relatively little effect on ischemic fibers; thus, the degree of potentiation could depend on the relative volume of normally perfused and ischemic fibers in the zone measured. The degree of systolic expansion in fully ischemic regions could be affected by reduced ventricular volume due to the enhanced stroke volume of the postextrasystolic beat, rather than to a direct effect on the contractility of ischemic fibers. Further studies are needed, however, to elucidate fully the mechanisms involved.

Stimulation or unloading of abnormally contracting regions in hearts of patients with chronic coronary artery disease by postextrasystolic potentiation or nitroglycerin have been proposed as methods for identifying zones of partial ischemia that might revert to normal function after coronary artery bypass grafting, as discussed in a subsequent section.

Stress-induced myocardial ischemia

Models for partial coronary stenosis

Many of the manifestations of acute ischemia in humans, including angina pectoris, occur in the setting of partial coronary artery narrowing. In the conscious animal, acute coronary stenosis can be produced by means of hydraulic occluders implanted around one or more coronary arteries while left ventricular pressure and regional myocardial dimensions are monitored. This approach has been useful for studying effects of several interventions, including exercise. With this approach it is difficult to maintain or to reproduce the degree of coronary stenosis, however, and therefore it has limited applicability for comparing the effects of interventions, such as the functional responses to exercise before and after administration of a pharmacologic agent. Another approach has involved the development of a chronic model for partial, chronic coronary artery stenosis by implanting an ameroid constrictor which gradually occludes the coronary artery [81–83]. In the dog, implantation of such a device around the circumflex coronary artery causes gradual narrowing of the vessel over three to four weeks; during that time, the progressive development of collateral vessels is indicated by the differing responses to brief coronary occlusions produced by means of a hydraulic cuff placed on the same vessel as the ameroid constrictor [83]. Early (one week) after ameroid implantation there is marked regional dyskinesia during a brief coronary occlusion (Figure 14), but as the constrictor narrows the response becomes less marked; eventually, there is no effect of brief coronary occlusions on regional contractile function, indicating that gradual narrowing of the coronary artery has stimulated the development of sufficient collateral blood flow to completely supply metabolic needs in the resting state (Figure 14) [83]. During this phase of coronary artery stenosis (about three weeks), however, collateral development is still incomplete. Therefore, it is possible to induce regional myocardial ischemia by a stress such as exercise, and to analyze the effects of experimental therapy in this setting, as discussed further below. In the dog, little or no myocardial infarction results during such gradual coronary artery narrowing, although in the pig, a species in which the collateral circulation is initially less well developed [3], myocardial infarction frequently occurs after implantation of an ameroid device.

Acute partial coronary stenosis

As discussed earlier, progressive acute stenosis of a coronary artery by means of a hydraulic cuff results in progressive regional dysfunction that is closely related to the accompanying reduction of regional coronary blood flow. Acute coronary stenosis in the conscious dog produces a reflex tachycardia, and administration of propanolol intravenously under such conditions results in slowing of the heart rate and prompt improvement of regional wall thickening in the ischemic zone, together with improvement of total coronary blood flow to that

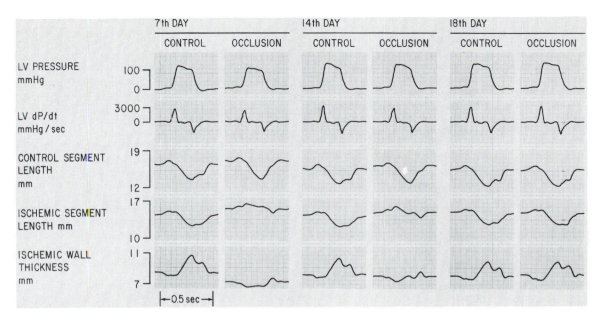

	7th DAY		14th DAY		18th DAY	
	CONTROL	OCCLUSION	CONTROL	OCCLUSION	CONTROL	OCCLUSION

LV PRESSURE mmHg — 100 / 0

LV dP/dt mmHg/sec — 3000 / 0

CONTROL SEGMENT LENGTH mm — 19 / 12

ISCHEMIC SEGMENT LENGTH mm — 17 / 10

ISCHEMIC WALL THICKNESS mm — 11 / 7

|←0.5 sec→|

Figure 14. Responses to abrupt coronary occlusions during progressive coronary stenosis induced by an ameroid coronary constrictor in the conscious dog. Left ventricular pressure, dP/dt, regional segment lengths in control and ischemic areas are shown, together with wall thickness in the ischemic zone, on the 7th, 14th, and 18th day after ameroid implantation. Basal conditions are shown to the left (control) and conditions 1 min after coronary occlusion on the right at each time. In this representative dog, an ischemic functional response was marked at the 7th day with increased end-diastolic length and holosystolic lengthening during ejection; the response was less marked on the 14th day and disappeared on the 18th day indicating collateral development (reproduced by permission from [83]).

region measured with an ultrasonic flowmeter [46]. Such effects may relate predominantly to the slowing of heart rate produced by propanolol, although an additional effect of the drug may be postulated, since improved function persists even when the heart rate is returned by atrial pacing to the level existing prior to propanolol [46].

Isoproterenol-stress
Under conditions of global ischemia in the conscious dog (stenosis of the left main coronary artery), infusion of isoproterenol produces rapid further deterioration of myocardial function [84]. Isoproterenol also has been studied in the conscious dog in the presence of acute partial coronary stenosis which is not sufficient to produce regional myocardial dysfunction at rest. Regional contractile dysfunction (depression of systolic wall thickening) develops rapidly after the onset of isoproterenol infusion (Figure 15), and local and surface electrocardiographic repolarization abnormalities occur somewhat later [84]. Such studies indicate that isoproterenol stress might be useful as a method of

detecting latent coronary artery stenosis, as suggested by electrocardiographic findings in older clinical studies [85, 86].

Regional myocardial blood flow also has been measured together with regional function during isoproterenol stress in the conscious, chronically instrumented animal under conditions of partial coronary stenosis, and a state of 'relative' myocardial ischemia has been characterized [87]. With moderate left circumflex coronary artery stenosis, isoproterenol infusion (0.2 μg/kg/min) produced a considerable decrease in regional wall thickening in the circumflex-supplied zone, whereas contractile function increased in normal regions; regional myocardial flow rose strikingly in normal zones, while in the ischemic zone total transmural flow failed to rise, being maintained at normal resting levels, due to a slight increase in epicardial flow and an insignificant reduction in subendocardial flow [87]. This finding clearly indicated relative myocardial ischemia, in which regional flow was maintained while ischemia was evidenced by a reduction of regional myocardial contraction. With more se-

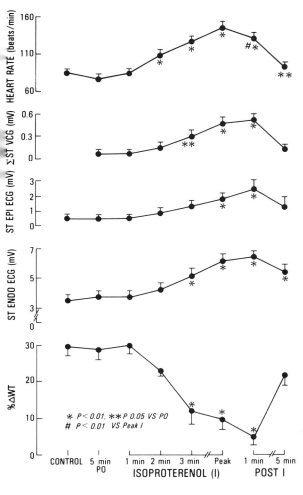

Figure 15. The mean ± SE in eight dogs of the percentage wall thickening (%ΔWT), endocardial ST segment (ST ENDO ECG), epicardial ST segment (ST EPI ECG), the sum of X, Y, Z VCG ST segments (ΣST VCG), and heart rate at control, 5 min after producing partial coronary occlusion (PO), during isoproterenol infusion and after stopping the infusion (Post 1). At 3 min the dose in all dogs was 0.02 μg/kg/min (reproduced by permission from [84]).

vere coronary artery stenosis, isoproterenol infusion produced a marked regional contractile defect, and a reduction of subendocardial blood flow to below resting levels [87]. This stress-induced reduction of absolute flow was undoubtedly a consequence of the tachycardia and lowering of coronary perfusion pressure, as well as increased oxygen demands produced by isoproterenol. Somewhat similar responses have been found in border zones after complete coronary occlusions [88].

Exercise

Overall impairment of left ventricular function during exercise has been shown to occur during exercise in dogs subjected to partial coronary stenosis, with reversion of the abnormal function following cessation of the exercise [89]. More recently, hemodynamic and regional functional responses to severe exercise before and after acute partial coronary stenosis have been examined in chronically instrumented dogs studied by telemetry during unrestrained exercise behind a mobile van [90]. Under control conditions without coronary stenosis, exercise resulted in substantial increases in left ventricular systolic pressure, dP/dt, subendocardial segment shortening extent and velocity in all regions of the left ventricle (Figure 16). Following production of acute coronary stenosis that was not sufficient to cause significant depression of regional myocardial function prior to exercise, strenuous exercise (average heart rate 285/min) produced rapid and severe regional myocardial dysfunction, sometimes associated with holosystolic segment lengthening (Figure 16) [90]. Following cessation of exercise, this effect subsided over the course of several minutes. Accompanying the regional dysfunction was impairment of overall hemodynamic function of the left ventricle, evidenced by reduced increases in left ventricular systolic pressure and dP/dt, and by an abnormal rise in the left ventricular end-diastolic pressure during exercise [90].

Gallagher et al. have documented a linear relation between reductions in regional systolic wall thickening and reductions in transmural coronary blood flow in that zone during isoproterenol infusion [87]. This finding documents the close coupling between flow and function under stress conditions, and further verifies the sensitivity of regional contractile function to ischemia.

Such exercise-induced regional myocardial dysfunction has a clinical counterpart in patients with angina pectoris, in whom radionuclide techniques have shown that the ejection fraction often falls during exercise from a normal resting value [53]; regional wall motion abnormalities may also be identified by this technique [54]. In addition, two-dimensional echocardiography allows detection of overall and regional contraction abnormalities of the left ventricle during exercise in patients with chronic coronary heart disease [91, 92].

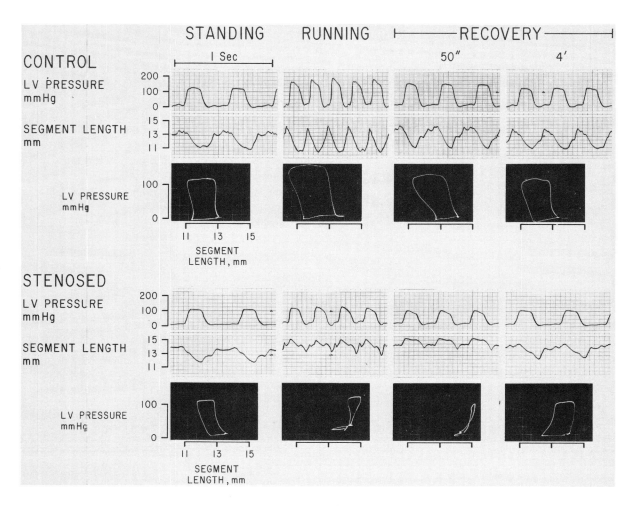

Figure 16. Left ventricular (LV) pressure, segment length, and photographs of length–pressure loops in a conscious dog during standing, running, and recovery in a control run and in a run during partial coronary constriction. During the control run, LVSP pressure rises, segment shortening increases, and the length–pressure loop opens widely but without a gross change in configuration. After coronary artery constriction, the percent shortening and area of the loop at rest are slightly reduced. During running (30 sec of exercise), regional segment dysfunction becomes extreme, LV pressure is lower than in the control run, and there is a marked reduction in the area of the length–pressure loop, which becomes more marked immediately after exercise (reproduced from [90] by permission of the Am Heart Assoc, Inc).

Cardiac pacing

When acute partial coronary stenosis is produced in the conscious dog to cause little or no regional contractile dysfunction at rest, rapid pacing of the heart produces regional myocardial dysfunction which is then followed by postpacing depression of regional contraction in the involved zone [93]. The average responses to such stimulation in a group of conscious dogs is shown in Figure 17. In normal regions, dysfunction does not develop during pacing, and following cessation of pacing there is initial enhancement of contraction (poststimulation potentiation), followed by a minimal fall of regional shortening and rapid return to normal (Figure 17). In contrast, in the zone supplied by the partially stenotic vessel, normal contraction is replaced by ischemic dysfunction during pacing. Following cessation of pacing, despite an initial slight increase in contraction due to poststimulation potentiation, a rapid fall of systolic shortening ensues which is sustained for two to three minutes (Figure 17). This postpacing depression of regional function may re-

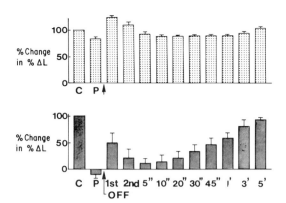

Figure 17. Percentage changes in regional myocardial shortening expressed as percent segment shortening (%ΔL) at various times after electrical pacing (resting state = 100%), expressed as mean ± SEM. Upper panel shows average responses of segments to be rendered ischemic prior to coronary stenosis, and lower panel shows responses with coronary stenosis: C = control period prior to pacing, P = responses at maximum pacing rate, arrow (off) = cessation of pacing. The first and second beats and subsequent responses are plotted; N = 6 (reproduced from [93] by permission of the Am Heart Assoc, Inc).

late to several mechanisms, including loss of post-stimulation potentiation, increased loading on the ischemic region due to abrupt slowing of the heart rate with a rise in systolic arterial pressure and, most importantly, to the persistence of ischemia due to the prior pacing stress [93].

This response has a clinical counterpart in patients with chronic coronary artery disease. In some patients following cessation of pacing there is a marked rise in the left ventricular end-diastolic pressure which may be accompanied by a shift upward of the diastolic pressure–volume relation of the ventricle, as discussed above. Using 'intervention left ventriculography,' regional wall motion abnormalities also have been described in the human left ventricle during rapid cardiac pacing in patients with coronary heart disease [52].

Chronic coronary artery stenosis

In the early weeks after implantation of an ameroid constrictor, antegrade flow through the vessel may be markedly diminished or absent, although collateral development prevents the occurrence of ischemia at rest, as discussed above. This situation may mimic the setting of single vessel high-grade coro-

nary artery stenosis in man when the development of collateral vessels is sparse. In both settings, the imposition of a stress can induce ischemia.

Exercise and pacing stress

When exercise is carried out in the dog about three weeks after implantation of an ameroid constrictor (either free-running or on a treadmill), there is rapid development of varying degrees of ischemic dysfunction, as assessed by decreased subendocardial systolic shortening or diminished systolic wall thickening in the zones supplied by the stenotic circumflex artery [81, 82, 83a]. The ischemic effect is transient and rapidly reverts to normal within two or three minutes following cessation of the exercise. Similarly, if rapid cardiac pacing is carried out at the same point in time after implantation of the ameroid constrictor, there is development of ischemic dysfunction during and after pacing [83a].

In the dog, further development of collateral channels occurs, and by about eight weeks after implantation of an ameroid constrictor the post-pacing response has returned to normal (maximum pacing rate of 210), whereas exercise at approximately the same heart rate continues to produce regional ischemic dysfunction during the exercise stress [83a]. This finding indicates that exercise provides a more reliable means than pacing of detecting latent coronary insufficiency, and suggests that the added burden of increased systemic arterial pressure and enhanced contractility produced by exercise imposes an additional oxygen supply–demand imbalance on the involved region [83a].

If exercise is carried out several months after implantation of an ameroid constrictor, complete collateral development has been reported in the dog; that is, regional myocardial blood flow at rest and during exercise in the involved zone is entirely normal and comparable to the increase measured in normal regions [94].

Propranolol and exercise

In the presence of chronic coronary artery stenosis in conscious dogs, when exercise produces severe regional myocardial dysfunction, if propranolol is administered intravenously (0.50 mg/kg) and an identical exercise bout repeated 2 hr later, the dysfunction is prevented [82]. The usual exercise-induced increase of regional function in normal zones was lessened by propranolol, but no decrease of function occurred in the previously is-chemic zone [82]. At the lower heart rate produced by propranolol, there were less marked increases in arterial pressure and dP/dt during exercise and a reduced rise in left ventricular end-diastolic pressure, suggesting amelioration of an oxygen supply–demand imbalance [82].

Such a protective effect of propranolol has been shown to occur in humans as well. Thus, in patients with angina pectoris who were studied by radionuclide angiography at rest and exercise both on and off chronic propanolol therapy, propranolol diminished or prevented the decrease in ejection fraction which occurred in the absence of the drug [95].

Isosorbide dinitrate and exercise
Under conditions of chronic coronary stenosis similar to those described above with propranolol, exercise was repeated before and after the administration of 60 mg of isosorbide dinitrate orally, 15 min before exercise [81]. The hemodynamic and regional functional responses to exercise during the control periods were similar to those described above prior to propranolol administration, namely, increases in heart rate, systolic blood pressure, and dP/dt, accompanied by marked regional dysfunction. Following isosorbide dinitrate, in contrast to propranolol the heart rate and dP/dt responses were not reduced during exercise, and responses in the control regions were similar to those during the control exercise period. However, as with propranolol, no significant deterioration of subendocardial segment shortening or regional wall thickening occurred in the involved zone during exercise (Figure 18) [81]. These findings suggest that isosorbide dinitrate prevented or ameliorated exercise-induced regional myocardial ischemia by mechanisms quite different from those associated with propranolol. The left ventricular end-diastolic pressures and end-diastolic dimensions were significantly lower compared to the control values before and during exercise after isosorbide dinitrate (Figure 18); therefore, it may be postulated that improved subendocardial perfusion, and perhaps improved collateral blood flow, combined with decreased myocardial oxygen requirements secondary to the diminished afterload (decreased heart size and systolic pressure) were responsible for the improved regional function [81]. Precise determination of the mechanisms of such drug actions, however, await

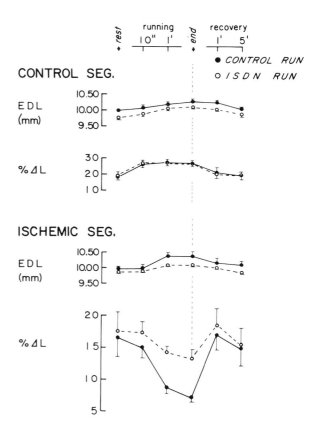

Figure 18. Summary of control and ischemic segment length responses to exercise before and after isosorbide dinitrate (ISDN) in conscious dogs with chronic coronary stenosis: EDL = end-diastolic length; %ΔL = percent shortening of segments (mean ± SEM). Note that there is prevention of severe ischemic dysfunction during exercise by the drug (reproduced by permission from [81]).

measurements of regional myocardial blood flow. It has been reported in patients with exercise-induced angina pectoris that isosorbide dinitrate improves the ejection fraction and regional wall motion during exercise [96].

Verapamil and exercise
Administration of the calcium antagonist verapamil also has been shown to lessen regional myocardial dysfunction during exercise in dogs with chronic coronary artery stenosis [97]. This effect was accompanied by a mild reduction of the maximum heart rate during exercise, but there was no impairment of exercise-induced increases in blood pressure or maximum dP/dt, and overall heart size

was not significantly affected [97]. The mechanism of this beneficial effect remains to be established.

Reversibility of the effects of sustained coronary occlusion

Effects of reperfusion after sustained coronary artery occlusion

Coronary artery reperfusion after a period of occlusion has provided an experimental model for determining whether or not myocardial tissue can be salvaged in evolving myocardial infarction [98]. A number of years ago, Blumgart et al. [99] studied the effects of reperfusion on myocardial structure, and these and later experiments attempted to determine whether or not reperfusion could prevent myocardial infarction [100, 101]. It was found that infarction occurred if the coronary occlusion was maintained beyond 45 min, but the question of whether or not the size of the damaged area could be reduced by coronary artery reflow was not addressed. Initial studies on this subject in our laboratory involved dogs that were subjected to 3 hr of coronary artery occlusion followed by reperfusion, and these animals were compared to dogs having permanent coronary occlusions. It was shown that, despite similar average S-T segment elevations and S-T segment areas in the two groups at 15 min after coronary occlusion, the reperfused hearts exhibited considerably smaller infarct sizes at one week as determined by gross and histologic examinations (Figure 19) [102]. The myocardial creatine kinase values in control animals also were much lower, substantial preservation of enzyme activity being demonstrated in the ischemic areas in the reperfused group both at 24 hr and one week [102, 103]. These experiments in the dog demonstrated, therefore, that it was possible to salvage tissue with an occlusion far longer than the 45-min period commonly thought to represent the maximum time limit. Others have confirmed these findings in the dog [104, 105], and it has been shown that reperfusion also can salvage myocardium in the baboon [106]. Intramyocardial hemorrhage occurs in some dogs when reperfusion is carried out after prolonged periods of coronary occlusion of 5 hr or more [107]. It is likely that studies showing tissue salvage in the dog differ from the findings in experiments limited

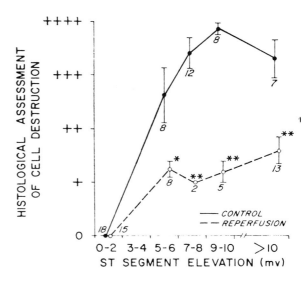

Figure 19. Comparison between ST segment elevation 15 min after occlusion and the histological assessment of cell destruction at the same sites one week later in control dog hearts subjected to permanent occlusion (solid upper line) and in reperfused hearts (broken lower line). The numbers next to each symbol represent the number of specimens at each level of ST segment elevation. The difference between control and reperfusion at any given ST segment elevation (mean ± SEM) is statistically significant (* P < 0.05, ** P < 0.01) (reproduced by permission from [102]).

to the posterior papillary muscle of the dog, where there is little collateral circulation [108]; thus, when larger ischemic zones of the free wall are investigated, zones are included in which ischemia is incomplete due to collateral blood flow.

Whether or not myocardial infarction could actually be prevented during coronary occlusion was also examined in dogs [109]. A group of animals was treated with a combination of arterial counterpulsation, propranolol, and hypothermia during a 3-hr period of coronary occlusion, followed by reperfusion. One week later, myocardial damage was difficult to demonstrate. Most of the dogs showed no gross infarction, and there were minimal histologic changes. A group of control animals with permanent coronary occlusion for one week showed extensive myocardial damage [109].

Changes in regional myocardial function during coronary artery occlusion and reperfusion were then investigated using ultrasonic crystals implanted in the zone to be rendered ischemic, in a border zone, and a control region. Conscious dogs were

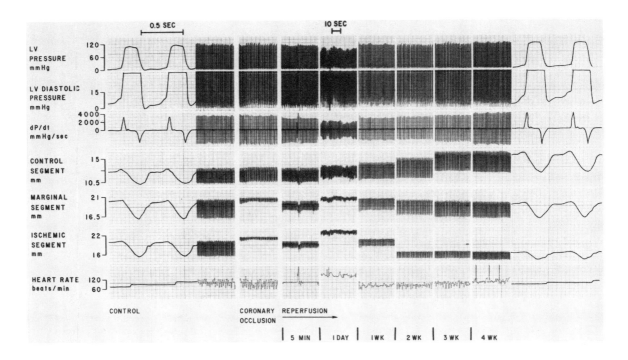

Figure 20. Serial responses in three segments of the myocardium of the left ventricle (LV) in a conscious dog subjected to 2 hr of occlusion of the left circumflex coronary artery and subsequent reperfusion. Rapid speed tracings are shown for the control period and four weeks after reperfusion, with slow tracings showing intermediate periods: dP/dt = rate of rise of left ventricular pressure (reproduced by permission from [110]).

subjected either to permanent coronary occlusion [47, 110] or to circumflex coronary artery occlusion for 2 hr followed by reperfusion [110]. As discussed earlier, the typical response to permanent coronary occlusion was complete loss of shortening in the central ischemic zone, with systolic expansion early after the occlusion, followed by tissue loss and slight restoration of function over a one-month follow-up period; in border zones, marked hypokinesia was noted immediately after the occlusion with some recovery of function over the one-month period (Figure 20) [110]. In the dogs subjected to reperfusion after a 2-hr period of occlusion, initial deterioration in the central ischemic segments which lasted two or three days was followed by a modest recovery of function. However, in the border segments, following transient deterioration of function for several days, marked recovery of function occurred, and by one month systolic shortening did not differ significantly from control (Figure 20) [110]. Thus, late recovery of myocardial function in border areas occurred over several weeks after coronary artery reperfusion [110].

In the clinical area there has been interest in early surgical revascularization after acute coronary occlusion [111], and recently successful recanalization of acutely thrombosed coronary arteries early after the onset of acute myocardial infarction has been accomplished by the intracoronary infusion of antistreptolysin [112, 113]. However, effects on myocardial function and infarct size have not yet been evaluated in humans.

Reversibility of chronic regional dysfunction
When persistent left ventricular dysfunction is present in the resting state, the degree to which it is due to previous myocardial infarction or to potentially reversible ischemic dysfunction has remained uncertain. Thus, in the patient who is found to have persistent regional or global myocardial dysfunction, operation is sometimes considered not only for the relief of angina pectoris but also for possible beneficial effects of myocardial revascularization on left ventricular function. In some patients with stable or unstable angina pectoris who have not had prior myocardial infarction, marked improvement

in regional wall motion and the ejection fraction have been reported within two weeks of operation, even when extensive regional wall motion abnormalities existed preoperatively [114]. On the other hand, most studies at about six months following coronary artery bypass grafting indicate that many zones of regional dysfunction fail to show improvement after operation, whereas others exhibit enhanced shortening, and a few show decreased function. Although average ventricular function (as assessed by the ejection fraction) usually has not changed significantly following myocardial revascularization [115–120], more recent studies suggest that overall improvement of ventricular function can occur [121]. There appears to be a correlation between the adequacy of revascularization and recovery of resting function [115, 117], as well as with improvement of the ejection fraction during exercise [120].

Experimental and clinical evidence suggest that it may be possible to identify preoperatively those zones which will show improvement following coronary artery bypass operations [29, 77, 122–125]. Myocardial biopsies taken at the time of operation in patients with coronary heart disease indicate that regions which preoperatively showed improved wall motion following nitroglycerin or postextrasystolic potentiation exhibit only a small amount of scar, and such regions may show improved function on ventriculographic studies some months later [126]. However, whether the original response was due to potentiation of a uniform population of myocardial cells which are partially ischemic, or an admixture of scarred cells and normal cells in which only the normal cells are potentiated, is not clear. Moreover, it remains to be clarified whether or not such improved function after operation reflects correction of 'chronic ischemia,' or whether revascularization allows compensatory hypertrophy of adjacent regions of myocardium, or both.

References

1. Gallagher KP, Folts JD, Shebuski RJ, Rankin JHG, Rowe GG: Subepicardial vasodilator reserve in the presence of critical coronary stenosis in dogs. Am J Cardiol 46:67–73, 1980.
2. Baroldi G, Radice F, Schmid G, Leone A: Morphology of acute myocardial infarction in relation to coronary thrombosis. Am Heart J 87:65–75, 1974.
3. Schaper W: Collateral Circulation of the Heart. North Holland Publ, Amsterdam, 1971.
4. Crozatier B, Ross J Jr, Franklin D, Bloor CM, White FC, Tomoike H, McKown DP: Myocardial infarction in the baboon: regional function and the collateral circulation. Am J Physiol 235:H413–H421, 1978.
5. Fuster V, Frye RL, Kennedy MA, Connolly DC, Mankin HT: The role of collateral circulation in the various coronary syndromes. Circulation 59:1137–1144, 1979.
6. Mosher P, Ross J Jr, McFate PA, Shaw RF: Control of coronary blood flow by an autoregulatory mechanism. Circ Res 14:250–259, 1964.
7. Sonnenblick EH, Ross J Jr, Braunwald E: Oxygen consumption of the heart: newer concepts of its multifactoral determination. Am J Cardiol 22:328–336, 1968.
8. Hoffman JIE, Buckberg GD: Transmural variations in myocardial perfusion. In: Yu PN, Goodwin JF (eds) Progress in Cardiology, vol 5. Lea and Febiger, Philadelphia, 1976, pp 37–89.
9. Dhurandar RW, Watt DL, Silver MD, Trimble AS, Adelman AG: Prinzmetal's variant form of angina with arteriographic evidence of coronary arterial spasm. Am J Cardiol 30:902–905, 1972.
10. Maseri A, Pesola A, Marzilli M, Severi S, Parodi O. L'Abate A, Ballestra AM, Maltinti G, DeMes DM, Biagini A: Coronary vasospasm in angina pectoris. Lancet 1:713–721, 1977.
11. Johnson AD, Stroud HA, Vieweg WVR, Ross J Jr: Variant angina pectoris: clinical presentations, coronary angiographic patterns, and the results of medical and surgical management in 42 consecutive patients. Chest 73:786–794, 1978.
12. Oliva PB, Breckinridge JC, Goolsby JP: Demonstration of coronary arterial spasm in acute myocardial infarction. Cathet Cardiovasc Diagn 3:195–197, 1977.
13. Levene DL, Freeman MR: Alpha-adrenoreceptor-mediated coronary artery spasm. J Am Med Assoc 236:1018–1022, 1976.
14. Ellis EF, Oelz O, Roberts LJ II, Payne NA, Sweetman BJ, Nies AS, Oates JA: Coronary arterial smooth muscle contraction by a substance released from platelets: evidence that it is thromboxane A_2. Science 193:1135–1137, 1976.
15. El-Maraghi N, Genton E: The relevance of platelet and fibrin thromboembolism of the coronary microcirculation, with special reference to sudden cardiac death. Circulation 62:936–944, 1980.
16. Neely JR, Rovetto MJ, Oram JF: Myocardial utilization of carbohydrate and lipids. Prog Cardiovasc Dis 15:289–329, 1972.
17. Neely JR, Morgan HE: Relationship between carbohydrate and lipid metabolism and the energy balance of heart muscle. Ann Rev Physiol 36:413–459, 1974.
18. Ross J Jr, Sobel BE: Regulation of cardiac contraction. Ann Rev Physiol 34:47–90, 1972.
19. Kubler W, Spieckermann PG: Regulation of glycolysis in the ischemic and the anoxic myocardium. J Mol Cell Cardiol 1:351–377, 1970.
20. Rovetto MJ, Lamberton WF, Neely JR: Mechanisms of glycolytic inhibition in ischemic rat hearts. Circ Res 37:742–751, 1975.

21. Williamson JR, Steenbergen C, Rich T, Deleeuw G, Barlow C, Chance B: The nature of ischemic injury in cardiac tissue. In: Lefer AM, Kelliher GJ, Rovetto MJ (eds) Pathophysiology and Therapeutics of Myocardial Ischemia. Spectrum Publ, Inc, New York, 1977, p 193.

22. Jennings RB: Discussion – relationship of acute ischemia to functional defects and irreversibility. Circulation 53: I-26-I-29, 1976.

23. Williamson JR, Safer B, Rich T, Schafter SW, Kobayashi K: Effects of acidosis on myocardial contractility and metabolism. Acta Med Scand Suppl 587:95–111, 1975.

24. Katz AM, Hecht HH: The early 'pump' failure of the ischemic heart. Am J Med 47:497–502, 1969.

25. Steenbergen C, Deleeuw G, Rich T, Williamson JR: Effects of acidosis and ischemia on contractility and intracellular pH of rat heart. Circ Res 41:849–858, 1977.

26. Tennant R, Wiggers CJ: Effect of coronary occlusion on myocardial contraction. Am J Physiol 112:351–361, 1935.

27. Ross J Jr, Franklin D: Analysis of regional myocardial function, dimensions, and wall thickness in the characterization of myocardial ischemia and infarction. Circulation (Suppl I) 53:88–92, 1976.

28. Battler A, Froelicher V, Gallagher KP, Kemper S, Ross J Jr: Dissociation between regional myocardial dysfunction and ECG changes during ischemia in the conscious dog. Circulation 62:735–744, 1980.

29. Theroux P, Franklin D, Ross J Jr, Kemper WS: Regional myocardial function during acute coronary artery occlusion and its modification by pharmacologic agents in the dog. Circ Res 35:896–908, 1974.

30. Müller O, Rørvik K: Haemodynamic consequences of coronary heart disease with observations during anginal pain and on the effect of nitroglycerine. Br Heart J 20:302–310, 1958.

31. Parker JO, Ledwich JR, West RO, Case MD: Reversible cardiac failure during angina pectoris. Hemodynamic effects of atrial pacing in coronary artery disease. Circulation 39:745–757, 1969.

32. Slutsky R, Curtis G, Froelicher V, Batler A, Ross J Jr, Gordon D, Ashburn W, Karliner J: The effect of sublingual nitroglycerin on left ventricular function at rest and during spontaneous angina pectoris assessment by a new radionuclide approach. Am J Cardiol 44:1365–1370, 1979.

33. Karliner JS, Ross J Jr: Left ventricular performance after acute myocardial infarction. Prog Cardiovasc Dis 13: 374–391, 1971; Prog Patol Cardiovasc 14:197–219, 1971.

34. Page DL, Caulfield JB, Kastor JA, DeSanctis RW, Saunders CA: Myocardial changes associated with cardiogenic shock. N Engl J Med 285:133–137, 1971.

35. Kerin NZ, Rubenfire M, Naini M, Wajszczuk WJ, Patamat A, Cascade PN: Arrhythmias in variant angina pectoris. Relationship of arrhythmias to ST-segment elevation and R-wave changes. Circulation 60:1343–1350, 1979.

36. Kloner RA, Rude RE, Carlson N, Maroko PR, DeBoer LWV, Braunwald E: Ultrastructural evidence of microvascular damage and myocardial cell injury after coronary artery occlusion: which comes first? Circulation 62:945–952, 1980.

37. Kloner RA, Ganote CE, Jennings RB: The 'no-reflow' phenomenon after temporary coronary occlusion in the dog. J Clin Invest 54:1496–1508, 1974.

38. Hood WB, Covelli VH, Abelmann WH, Norman JC: Persistence of contractile behaviour in acutely ischaemic myocardium. Cardiovasc Res 3:249–260, 1969.

39. Heikkila J, Tabakin BS, Hugenholtz PG: Quantification of function in normal and infarcted regions of the left ventricle. Cardiovasc Res 6:516–531, 1972.

40. Kerber RE, Abboud FM: Echocardiographic detection of regional myocardial infarction: an experimental study. Circulation 47:997–1005, 1973.

41. Tyberg JV, Forrester JS, Wyatt HL, Goldner SJ, Parmley WW, Swan HJC: Analysis of segmental ischemic dysfunction utilizing the pressure–length loop. Circulation 44: 748–754, 1974.

42. Schelbert HR, Covell JW, Burns JW, Maroko PR, Ross J Jr: Observations on factors affecting local forces in the left ventricular wall during acute myocardial ischemia. Circ Res 29:306–316, 1971.

43. Theroux P, Ross J Jr, Franklin D, Kemper WS, Sasayama S: Regional myocardial function in the conscious dog during acute coronary occlusion and responses to morphine, propranolol, nitroglycerin, and lidocaine. Circulation 53: 302–314, 1976.

44. Sasayama S, Franklin D, Ross J Jr, Kemper WS, McKown D: Dynamic changes in left ventricular wall thickness and their use in analyzing cardiac function in the conscious dog. Am J Cardiol 38:870–879, 1976.

45. Peterson DF, Kaspar RL, Bishop VS: Reflex tachycardia due to temperary coronary occlusion in the conscious dog. Circ Res 32:652–659, 1973.

46. Tomoike H, Ross J Jr, Franklin D, Crozatier B, McKown D, Kemper WS: Improvement by propranolol of regional myocardial dysfunction and abnormal coronary flow pattern in conscious dogs with coronary narrowing. Am J Cardiol 41:689–696, 1978.

47. Theroux P, Ross J Jr, Franklin D, Covell JW, Bloor CM, Sasayama S: Regional myocardial function and dimensions early and late after myocardial infarction in the unanesthetized dog. Circ Res 40:158–165, 1977.

48. Sasayama S, Gallagher KP, Kemper WS, Franklin D, Ross J Jr: Regional left ventricular wall thickness early and late after coronary occlusion in the conscious dog. Am J Physiol 240:H293–H299, 1981.

49. Kazamias TM, Gander MP, Ross J Jr, Braunwald E: Detection of left-ventricular-wall motion disorders in coronary artery disease by radarkymography. N Engl J Med 285:63–71, 1971.

50. Corya BC, Rasmussen S, Knoebel SB, Feigenbaum H: Echocardiography in acute myocardial infarction. Am J Cardiol 36:1–10, 1975.

51. Klein MD, Herman MV, Gorlin R: Hemodynamic study of left ventricular aneurysm. Circulation 35:614–630, 1967.

52. Pasternac A, Gorlin R, Sonnenblick EH, Haft JI, Kemp HG: Abnormalities of ventricular motion induced by atrial pacing in coronary artery disease. Circulaton 45:1195–1205, 1972.

53. Ashburn WL, Schelbert HR, Verba JW: Left ventricular ejection fraction – a review of several radionuclide angiographic approaches using the scintillation camera. Prog Cardiovasc Dis 20:267–284, 1978.

54. Bodenheimer MM, Banka VS, Helfant RH: Nuclear cardiology. I. Radionuclide angiographic assessment of left ventricular contraction: uses, limitations and future directions. Am J Cardiol 45:661–673, 1980.

55. Waters DD, da Luz P, Wyatt HL, Swann HJC, Forrester JS: Early changes in regional and global left ventricular function induced by graded reductions in regional coronary perfusion. Am J Cardiol 39:537–543, 1977.

56. Gallagher KP, Kumada T, Koziol JA, McKown MD, Kemper WS, Ross J Jr: Significance of regional wall thickening abnormalities relative to transmural myocardial perfusion in anesthetized dogs. Circulation 62:1266–1274, 1980.

57. Vatner SF: Correlation between acute reductions in myocardial blood flow and function in conscious dogs. Circ Res 47:201–207, 1980.

58. Hood WB Jr, Bianco JA, Kumar R, Whiting RB: Experimental myocardial infarction. IV. Reduction of left ventricular compliance in the healing phase. J Clin Invest 49:1316–1323. 1970.

59. Tyberg JV, Forrester JS, Wyatt HL, Goldner SJ, Parmley WW, Swan HJC: An analysis of segmental ischemic dysfunction utilizing the pressure–length loop. Circulation 49:748–754, 1974.

60. Palacios I, Johnson RA, Newell JB, Powell WJ Jr: Left ventricular end-diastolic pressure–volume relationship with experimental acute global ischemia. Circulation 53:428–436, 1976.

61. Wong BYS, Toyama M, Reis RL, Goodyer AVN: Sequential changes in left ventricular compliance during acute coronary occlusion in the isovolumic working canine heart. Circ Res 43:274–286, 1978.

62. Barry WH, Brooker JZ, Alderman EL, Harrison DC: Changes in diastolic stiffness and tone of the left ventricle during angina pectoris. Circulation 49:255–263, 1974.

63. McLaurin LP, Rolett EL, Grossman W: Impaired left ventricular relaxation during pacing-induced ischemia. Am J Cardiol 32:751–757, 1973.

64. Ross J Jr: Editorial. Acute displacement of the diastolic pressure–volume curve of the left ventricle: role of the pericardium and the right ventricle. Circulation 59:32–37, 1979.

65. Mann T, Goldberg S, Mudge GH, Grossman W: Factors contributing to altered left ventricular diastolic properties during angina pectoris. Circulation 59:14–20, 1979.

66. Serizawa T, Carabello BA, Grossman W: Effect of pacing-induced ischemia on left ventricular diastolic pressure–volume relations in dogs with coronary stenoses. Circ Res 46:430–439, 1980.

67. Hess OM, Osakada G, Lavelle JF, Kemper WS, Ross J Jr: Diastolic myocardial wall stiffness during partial and complete coronary occlusion. Cir Res (in press).

68. Kumada T, Karliner JS, Pouleur H, Gallagher K, Shirato K, Ross J Jr: Effects of coronary occlusion on early ventricular diastolic events in conscious dogs. Am J Physiol 6:H542–H549, 1979.

69. Weisfeldt ML, Frederiksen JW, Yin FCP, Weiss JL: Evidence of incomplete left ventricular relaxation in the dog. J Clin Invest 62:1296–1302, 1978.

70. Crozatier B, Ashraf M, Franklin D, Ross J Jr: Sarcomere length in experimental myocardial infarction: evidence for sarcomere overstretch in dyskinetic ventricular regions. J Mol Cell Cardiol 9:785–797, 1977.

71. Ross J Jr, Higginson L, Franklin D, Tomoike H: Beta-adrenergic blockade in experimental myocardial ischemia and infarction: effects on regional myocardial function and dysrhythmias. In: Schwartz PJ, Brown AM, Malliani A, Zanchetti A (eds) Neural Mechanisms in Cardiac Arrhythmias. Raven Press, New York, 1978.

72. Bache RJ, Cobb FR: Effect of maximal coronary vasodilation on transmural myocardial perfusion during tachycardia in the awake dog. Circ Res 41:648–653, 1977.

73. Mueller HS, Ayres SM, Regila A, Evans RG: Propranolol in the treatment of acute myocardial infarction. Effect on myocardial oxygenation and hemodynamics. Circulation 49:1078–1087, 1974.

74. Vatner SF: Correlaton between acute reductions in myocardial blood flow and function in conscious dogs. Circ Res 47:201–207, 1980.

75. Vatner SF, Baig H: Importance of heart rate in determining the effects of sympathomimetic amines on regional myocardial function and blood flow in conscious dogs with acute myocardial ischemia. Circ Res 45:793–803, 1980.

76. Mueller H, Ayers SM, Gregory JJ, Giannelli S, Grace WJ: Hemodynamics, coronary blood flow, and myocardial metabolism in coronary shock: response to l-Norepinephrine and isoproterenol. J Clin Invest 49:1885–1902, 1970.

77. Crozatier B, Franklin D, Theroux P, Tomoike H, Sasayama S, Ross J Jr: Loss of regional ventricular postextrasystolic potentiation after coronary occlusion in dogs. Am J Physiol 233:H392–H398, 1977.

78. Boden WE, Chang-seng L, Hood WB: Postextrasystolic potentiation of regional mechanical performance during prolonged myocardial ischemia in the dog. Circulation 61:1063–1075, 1980.

79. Dyke SH, Urschel CW, Sonnenblick EH, Gorlin R, Cohn PF: Detection of latent function in acutely ischemic myocardium in the dog: comparison of pharmacologic inotropic stimulation and postextrasystolic potentiation. Circ Res 36:490–497, 1975.

80. Hirzel HO, Sonnenblick EH, Kirk ES: Absence of a lateral border zone of intermediate creatine phosphokinase depletion surrounding a central infarct 24 hours after acute coronary occlusion in the dog. Circ Res 41:673–683, 1977.

81. Kumada T, Gallagher KP, Miller M, McKown M, White F, McKown D, Kemper WS, Ross J Jr: Improvement by isosorbide dinitrate of exercise-induced regional myocardial dysfunction in the dog. Am J Physiol 239:H399–H405, 1980.

82. Kumada T, Gallagher K, Shirato K, McKown D, Miller M, Kemper WS, White F, Ross J Jr: Reduction of exercise-induced regional myocardial dysfunction by propranolol: studies in a canine model of chronic coronary artery stenosis. Circ Res 46:190–200, 1980.

83. Tomoike H, Franklin D, Kemper WS, McKown D, Ross J Jr: Functional evaluation of coronary collateral develop-

ment in conscious dogs. Am J Physiol (in press).

83a. Kumada T, Gallagher KP, Battler A, White F, Kemper WS, Ross J Jr: Comparison of post-pacing and exercise-induced myocardial dysfunction during collateral development in conscious dogs. Circulation 65:1178–1185, 1982.

84. Battler A, Gallagher KP, Froelicher VF, Kmada T, Kemper WS, Ross J Jr: Detection of latent coronary stenosis in conscious dogs: regional functional and electrocardiographic responses to isoprenaline. Cardiovasc Res 14: 476–481, 1980.

85. Wexler H, Kuaity J, Simonson E: Electrocardiographic effects of isoprenaline in normal subjects and patients with coronary atherosclerosis. Br Heart J 33:759–764, 1971.

86. Combs DT, Martin CM: Evaluation of isoproterenol as a method of stress testing. Am Heart J 87:711–715, 1974.

87. Gallagher KP, Kumada T, Battler A, Kemper WS, Ross J Jr: Isoproterenol-induced myocardial dysfunction in dogs with coronary stenosis. Am J Physiol 242:H260–H267, 1982.

88. Vatner SF, Millard RW, Patrick TA, Heyndrickx GR: Effects of isoproterenol on regional myocardial function, electrogram, and blood flow in conscious dogs with myocardial ischemia. J Clin Invest 57:1261–1271, 1976.

89. Horwitz LE, Peterson DF, Bishop VS: Effect of regional myocardial ischemia on cardiac pump performance during exercise. Am J Physiol 234:H157–H162, 1978.

90. Tomoike H, Franklin D, McKown D, Kemper WS, Guberek M, Ross J Jr: Regional myocardial dysfunction and hemodynamic abnormalities during strenuous exercise in dogs with limited coronary flow. Circ Res 42:487–496, 1978.

91. Sugishita Y, Koseki S: Dynamic exercise echocardiography. Circulation 60:743–752, 1979.

92. Wann LS, Faris JV, Childress RH, Dillon JC, Weyman AE, Feigenbaum H: Exercise cross-sectional echocardiography in ischemic heart disease. Circulation 60:1300–1308, 1979.

93. Tomoike H, Franklin D, Ross J Jr: Detection of myocardial ischemia by regional dysfunction during and after rapid pacing in conscious dogs. Circulation 58:48–56, 1978.

94. Lambert PR, Hess DS, Bache RJ: Effect of exercise on perfusion of collateral-dependent myocardium in dogs with chronic coronary artery occlusion. J Clin Invest 59:1–7, 1977.

95. Battler A, Ross J Jr, Slutsky R, Pfisterer M, Ashburn W, Froelicher V: Improvement of exercise-induced left ventricular dysfunction with oral propranolol in patients with coronary heart disease. Am J Cardiol 44:318–324, 1979.

96. Steele PP, Rainwater J, Jensen D, Vogel RA, Battock D: Isosorbide dinitrate-induced improvement in left ventricular ejection fraction during exercise in coronary arterial disease. Chest 74:526–530, 1978.

97. Osakada G, Kumada T, Gallagher KP, Kemper WS, Ross J Jr: Reduction of exercise-induced regional myocardial dysfunction by verapamil in conscious dogs. Am Heart J 101:707–712, 1981.

98. Ross J Jr: Early revascularization after coronary occlusion. An editorial. Circulation 50:1061–1062, 1974.

99. Blumgart HL, Gilligan OR, Schlesinger MJ: Experimental studies on the effect of temporary occlusion of coronary arteries. Am Heart J 22:374–389, 1941.

100. Yabuki S, Gumersildo B, Imbriglia JE, Bentivoglio L, Bailey CP: Time studies of acute reversible coronary occlusion in dogs. J Thorac Cardiovasc Surg 38:40–45, 1959.

101. Bolooki H, Rooks JJ, Visra CE, Smith B, Mobin-Uddin K, Lombardo CR, Jude JR: Comparison of the effect of temporary or permanent myocardial ischemia on cardiac function and pathology. J Thorac Cardiovasc Surg 56:590–598, 1968.

102. Ginks WR, Sybers HD, Maroko PR, Covell JW, Sobel BE, Ross J Jr: Coronary artery reperfusion II: reduction of myocardial infarct size one week after the coronary occlusion. J Clin Invest 51:2717–2723, 1972.

103. Maroko PR, Libby P, Ginks WR, Bloor CM, Shell WE, Sobel BE, Ross J Jr: Coronary artery reperfusion I: Early effects on local myocardial function and the extent of myocardial necrosis. J Clin Invest 51:2710–2716, 1972.

104. Costantini C, Corday E, Lang TW, Meerbaum S, Brasch J, Kaplan L, Rubins S, Gold H, Osher J: Revascularization after 3 hours of coronary arterial occlusion: effects on regional cardiac metabolic function and infarct size. Am J Cardiol 36:368–384, 1975.

105. Bolooki H: Myocardial revascularization after acute infarction. Am J Cardiol 36:395–406, 1975.

106. Smith GT, Soeter JR, Haston HH, McNamara JJ: Coronary reperfusion in primates: serial electrocardiographic and histologic assessment. J Clin Invest 54:1420–1427, 1974.

107. Bresnahan GF, Roberts R, Shell WE, Ross J Jr, Sobel BE: Deleterious effects due to hemorrhage after myocardial reperfusion. Am J Cardiol 33:82–86, 1974.

108. Jennings RB, Ganote CE, Reimer KA: Ischemic tissue injury. Am J Pathol 81:179–198, 1975.

109. Ginks W, Ross J Jr, Sybers HD: Prevention of gross myocardial infarction in the canine heart. Arch Pathol 97:380–384, 1974.

110. Theroux P, Ross J Jr, Franklin D, Kemper WS, Sasayama S: Coronary arterial reperfusion. III. Early and late effects on regional myocardial function and dimensions in conscious dogs. Am J Cardiol 38:599–606, 1976.

111. Phillips SJ, Kongtahworn C, Zeff RH, Benson M, Iannone L, Brown T, Gordon DF: Emergency coronary artery revascularization: a possible therapy for acute myocardial infarction. Circulation 60:241–250, 1979.

112. Mathey DG, Kuck KH, Tilsner V, Krebber HJ, Bleifeld W: Nonsurgical coronary artery recanalization in acute transmural myocardial infarction. Circulation 63:489–497, 1981.

113. Ganz W, Buchbinder N, Marcus H, Mondkar A, Maddahi J, Charuzi Y, O'Connor L, Schell W, Fishbein MC, Kass R, Miyamoto A, Swan HJC: Intracoronary thrombolysis in evolving myocardial infarction. Am Heart J 101:4, 1981.

114. Chatterjee K, Swan HJC, Parmley WW, Sustaita H, Marcus HS, Matloff J: Influence of direct myocardial revascularization on left ventricular asynergy and function in patients with coronary heart disease. Circulation 47:276–286, 1973.

115. Arbogast R, Solignac A, Bourassa MG: Influence of aortocoronary saphenous vein bypass surgery on left ventricu-

lar volumes and ejection fraction. Comparison before and one year after surgery in 51 patients. Am J Med 54:290–296, 1973.

116. Achuff SC, Griffith LSC, Conti CR, Humphries JO, Brawley RK, Gott VL, Ross RS: The 'angina-producing' myocardial segment: an approach to the interpretation of results of coronary bypass surgery. Am J Cardiol 36:723–733, 1975.

117. Levine JA, Bechtel DJ, Cohn PF, Herman MV, Gorlin R, Cohn LH, Colins JJ Jr: Ventricular function before and after direct revascularization surgery, a proposal for an index of vascularization to correlate angiographic and ventriculographic findings. Circulation 51:1071–1078, 1975.

118. Righetti A, Crawford MH, O'Rourke RA, Schelbert H, Daily PO, Ross J Jr: Interventricular septal motion and left ventricular function after coronary bypass surgery. Am J Cardiol 39:372–377, 1977.

119. Zir LM, Dinsmore R, Vexeridis M, Singh JB, Harthorne JW, Daggett WM: Effects of coronary bypass grafting on resting left ventricular contraction in patients studied 1 to 2 years after operation. Am J Cardiol 44:601–606, 1979.

120. Kent KM, Borer JS, Green MV, Bachrach SL, McIntosh CL, Conkle DM, Epstein SE: Effects of coronary-artery bypass on global and regional left ventricular function during exercise. N Engl J med 298:1434–1441, 1978.

121. Hellman C, Schmidt DH, Kamath L, Anholm J, Balu F, Johnson WD: Bypass graft surgery in severe left ventricular dysfunction. Circulation 62: 1103, 1980.

122. Helfant RH, Pine R, Meister SG, Feldman MS, Trout RG, Banka VS: Nitroglycerin to unmask reversible asynergy: correlation with post coronary bypass ventriculography. Circulation 50:108–113, 1974.

123. McAnulty JH, Hattenbauer MT, Rosch J, Kloster FE, Rahimtoola SH: Improvement in left ventricular wall motion abnormalities after nitroglycerin. Circulation 51:140–145, 1975.

124. Banka VS, Bodenheimer MM, Shah R, Helfant RH: Intervention ventriculography, comparative value of nitroglycerin, postextrasystolic potentiation and nitroglycerin plus postextrasystolic potentiation. Circulation 53: 632–637, 1976.

125. Komer RR, Edalji A, Hood WB: Effects of nitroglycerin on echocardiographic measurements of left ventricular wall thickness and regional myocardial performance during acute coronary ischemia. Circulation 59:926–937, 1979.

126. Bodenheimer MM, Banka VS, Hermann GA, Trout RG, Pasdar H, Helfant RH: Reversible asynergy. Circulation 53:792–796, 1976.

CHAPTER 4

Neural control of cardiac rhythm and contraction

MATTHEW N. LEVY

In this chapter, I will present the anatomy of the cardiac innervation, the effects of the cardiac nerves on various aspects of cardiac function, and a description of some of the important cardiovascular reflexes.

Cardiac innervation

Sympathetic pathways

The cell bodies of the preganglionic neurons of the cardiac sympathetic nerves are located in the intermediolateral columns of the upper seven or eight thoracic segments of the spinal cord. The preganglionic axons enter the paravertebral chains of ganglia via the white rami communicantes (Figure 1). The course of the sympathetic fibers to the heart varies considerably among mammalian species. In the dog, which has been studied most extensively [1, 2], the preganglionic cardiac fibers ascend in the paravertebral chains and funnel through the stellate ganglia [3]. They traverse either the dorsal or ventral limbs of the ansae subclaviae and finally synapse with postganglionic neurons in the caudal cervical ganglia [4, 5]. In many other species, such as the cat, the synapses occur mainly in the stellate ganglia [6], and the efferent fibers in the ansae subclaviae are largely postganglionic.

Parasympathetic pathways

The precise location of the preganglionic vagal neurons in the medulla varies among mammalian species. In the cat, the neurons are located almost exclusively in the nucleus ambiguus [7]. In the rab-

bit, however, they occur mainly in the dorsal motor nucleus [8], whereas in the dog, they are situated in both of these nuclei [9, 10]. The preganglionic vagal fibers exit from the skull and travel caudally through the neck in the carotid sheaths. In the dog

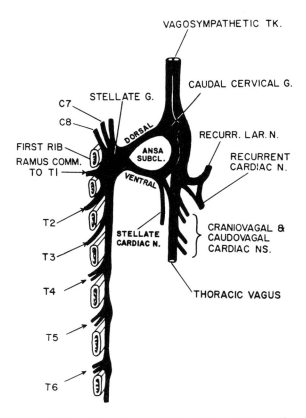

Figure 1. Upper thoracic sympathetic chain and the cardiac autonomic nerves on the right side in the dog (modified from [1]).

Rosen, M. R. and Hoffman, B. F. (eds.), Cardiac Therapy. ISBN 0-89838-564-4.

and certain other mammals, the vagal and sympathetic fibers on each side of the neck join to form two common nerve bundles, the right and left vagosympathetic trunks (Figure 1). As the vagal fibers enter the superior region of the chest, they pass close to the caudal cervical ganglia. Vagal and sympathetic fibers combine to form a plexus of mixed nerve trunks that innervate the various cardiac structures (Figure 1).

Control by higher centers

In addition to the vagal nuclei described in the preceding section, there are other centers in the medulla that regulate the sympathetic nervous activity to the cardiovascular system. Neurons distributed within the reticular formation in the brainstem are not organized into anatomically discrete nuclei. Stimulation of certain broad regions within such a 'vasomotor center' augments sympathetic activity, whereas stimulation of other regions reduces sympathetic tone [11].

It was originally believed that the sympatho-adrenal system was organized largely for mass action [12]. It is now apparent, however, that the autonomic control of the cardiovascular system involves complex, highly differentiated response patterns [13]. Inputs from centers in the pons, midbrain, cerebellum, diencephalon, and cerebral cortex interact in the central nervous system at numerous sites. Stimulation of certain sites in the diencephalon, such as the H2 fields of Forel, initiate a series of changes in circulatory function, such as tachycardia, increased cardiac output, and elevated arterial pressure [14]. These alterations closely resemble those observed during muscular exercise. Furthermore, destruction of these hypothalamic regions markedly attenuates these circulatory responses to exercise. Stimulation in another region of the hypothalamus evokes a different pattern of responses, which has been termed the 'defense reaction' [13]. Augmentations of heart rate, cardiac output, and blood pressure are also observed in this reaction, but they are accompanied by a characteristic redistribution of blood flow. The cutaneous, renal, and intestinal resistance vessels constrict, but the arterioles in the skeletal muscles dilate. These changes mimic the pattern that develops spontaneously in the 'fight or flight' response to a threatening event [13].

74

Sino-atrial node

Electrophysiological characteristics

The transmembrane potential changes recorded from pacemaker cells in the S-A node (Figure 2) differ in several important respects from those recorded from ventricular and atrial myocardial fibers [15]. In automatic cells in the S-A node and elsewhere in the heart, there is a slow diastolic depolarization during phase 4 (middle panel). When the threshold potential is attained, the upstroke (phase 0) of the next action potential begins. In nonautomatic fibers (top and bottom panels), the potential remains constant during phase 4. In the

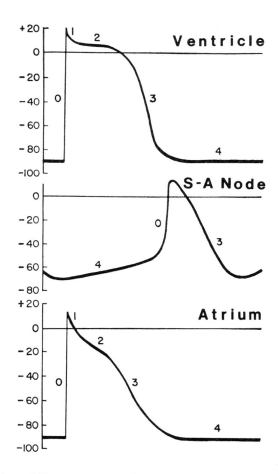

Figure 2. Transmembrane action potentials recorded from a ventricular myocardial cell, an S-A nodal pacemaker cell, and an atrial myocardial cell. The sweep speed in the middle panel is one-half that in the other two panels (modified from [15], with permission of McGraw-Hill).

typical S-A node cell (middle panel) the potentials recorded during phase 4 are considerably less negative and the upstroke velocities (i.e., the time rate of change of potential, dV/dt) during phase 0 are much lower than are those in atrial and ventricular fibers (top and bottom panels). In normal atrial and ventricular fibers the action potential upstroke is produced by the rapid influx of Na through 'fast channels' in the membrane. In the S-A node, on the other hand, the upstroke reflects the influx of Ca^{2+} and Na^+ through slow membrane channels. Furthermore, in the S-A node, the initial, brief phase of rapid repolarization (phase 1) is absent, and the plateau (phase 2) is much less prominent than in action potentials recorded from atrial and ventricular fibers.

Adrenergic effects

Adrenergic agonists increase the slope of phase 4 depolarization (Figure 3) in S-A nodal cells [15–18]. However, there is also some tendency for the maximum diastolic potential (i.e., the potential just after completion of repolarization) to become more negative, for the slope of the upstroke to increase, and for the amplitude of the action potential to become greater under the influence of adrenergic agents (Figure 3).

The ionic basis for the slow diastolic depolarization in the pacemaker cells during phase 4 is not known. In automatic Purkinje fibers, the principal change in the cell membrane that accounts for the slow diastolic depolarization is a progressive reduction in K conductance [16, 18]. Recent evidence indicates that a similar change in K conductance does not occur in the automatic cells in the S-A node [19, 20]. The progressive change in membrane

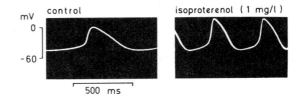

Figure 3. The effect of isoproterenol (1 mg/l) on the action potentials recorded from an S-A nodal cell in an isolated atrial preparation from a rabbit (from [17]).

potential in the S-A nodal cells during phase 4 probably reflects a net influx of certain cations, notably Na and Ca [16–18, 20]. The rate of impulse initiation of the S-A node is sensitive to changes in the external Ca^{2+} concentration, but relatively insensitive to changes in the external Na concentration. Slow-channel blocking agents, such as verapamil, diminish the firing rate of S-A nodal pacemaker cells [17, 21], principally by diminishing the slope of phase 4 (Figure 4). Concomitantly, such blocking agents markedly decrease the slope of the upstroke and the action potential amplitude, and may suppress automaticity entirely (Figure 4). Catecholamines probably act to augment the influx of Ca during phase 4 [16]. Therefore, they tend to increase the slope of diastolic depolarization (Figure 3) and hence the firing rate of the automatic cell.

Sympathetic activity

Increased sympathetic activity produces a positive chronotropic effect by the mechanisms described in the preceding section. When a tonic stimulus is applied to the cardiac sympathetic nerves at a constant frequency of stimulation, the heart rate in-

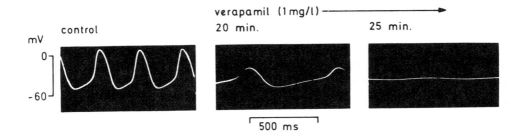

Figure 4. The effect of verapamil (1 mg/l) on the action potentials recorded from an S-A nodal cell in an isolated atrial preparation from a rabbit (modified from [17]).

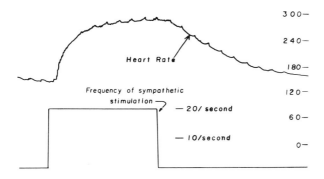

Figure 5. Heart rate response of an anesthetized dog to steady stimulation of the cardiac sympathetic nerves at a frequency of 20 Hz for 30 sec (from [20]).

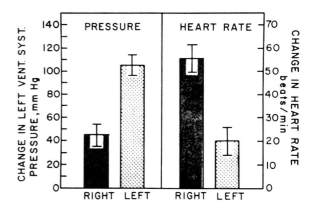

Figure 6. The effects of right and left stellate ganglion stimulation on left ventricular systolic pressure and heart rate in canine isovolumetric left ventricle preparations. Left ventricular systolic pressure is an index of myocardial contractility in that preparation. The bars represent the mean values (± SEM) from eight preparations (from [3], with permission from the Am Heart Assoc, Inc).

creases rapidly at first (Figure 5), but more than 30 sec are required to attain the new steady-state value [22]. When the stimulus is discontinued, the heart rate returns slowly to its resting level. The norepinephrine released at the sympathetic nerve terminals is dissipated by two main mechanisms; namely, reuptake by the nerve terminals and diffusion into the nearby capillaries [23, 24]. These processes are relatively slow, especially in comparison with the speed (cf., Figure 8) at which the parasympathetic neurotransmitter is hydrolyzed by acetylcholinesterase.

The distribution of the sympathetic nerve fibers to the heart is asymmetrical [1–3, 25–27]. The right-sided sympathetic nerves have a much greater chronotropic effect than do those on the left side, whereas the nerves of the left side predominate in the control of ventricular contractility (Figure 6) and of A-V conduction.

Cholinergic effects

Cholinergic agents produce their negative chronotropic effects (Figure 7) through membrane hyperpolarization and diminution of the rate of diastolic depolarization [15, 16, 18, 28–32]. Such hyperpolarization is achieved by a substantial increase in potassium conductance [33]. The ionic mechanism responsible for the diminished slope of diastolic depolarization is not clearly established. Diastolic depolarization in S-A nodal cells is achieved in part by the influx of Ca through the slow membrane channels [16–18]. It is likely that cholinergic agents

reduce the Ca conductance through such channels [30].

Vagal activity

When the vagus nerves are tonically stimulated, the heart rate decreases abruptly (Figure 8). The new steady-state rate is achieved much more quickly (cf., Figure 5) with vagal stimulation than with cardiac sympathetic stimulation [22]. When stimulation is discontinued, the heart rate quickly returns to its control level. The swiftness of this return to the control state is accomplished by the rapid hydrolysis of the acetylcholine released at the vagal endings in the S-A node. There is a high concentration of acetylcholinesterase in the nodal structures in the heart [34, 35], which accounts for the rapid termination of the vagal effect.

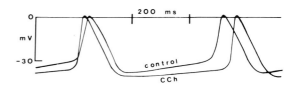

Figure 7. Transmembrane potentials recorded from a pacemaker cell in the rabbit S-A node in the presence and absence of carbamylcholine (CCH), 10^{-8} M (modified from [28]).

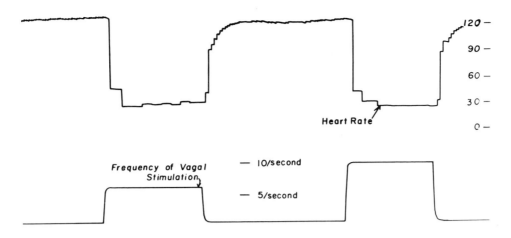

Figure 8. The changes in heart rate in an anesthetized dog produced by stimulating the right vagus nerve for about 20 sec at frequencies of 7 and 10 Hz (from [20]).

When a very brief stimulus is given to the vagus nerves, the time course of the negative chronotropic response consists of two inhibitory phases (Figure 9, ABC and EFG), separated by a transient phase (CDE) of relative or actual cardiac acceleration [31, 32, 36–38]. Recent electrophysiological studies [31, 32] have elucidated some of the mechanisms that underly the different phases of this response. The initial deceleratory phase (ABC, Figure 9) is associated with a transient period of hyperpolarization, as shown in Figure 10 (after the arrow). Most of the released acetylcholine is probably dissipated by the end of this period of hyperpolarization [31, 32]. The secondary phase of cardiac deceleration (EFG) is

associated with no detectable hyperpolarization, but with a diminished slope of diastolic depolarization (Figure 10). Studies with a potassium-sensitive electrode [31] have shown that the prolongations of the cardiac cycle length are closely paralleled by an elevation of the tissue K concentrations in the S-A node. It remains to be established whether this change in interstitial K concentration directly or indirectly influences the sinus rate [31], or whether

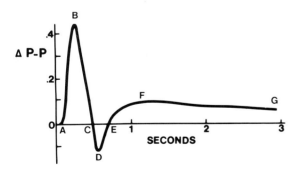

Figure 9. The time course of the chronotropic response to a brief burst of vagal stimuli in an anesthetized dog. The response is expressed as the fractional change in cardiac cycle length (P–P interval) (modified from [38]).

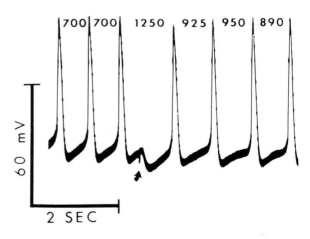

Figure 10. The changes in transmembrane potential in an S-A nodal pacemaker cell evoked by a brief burst of vagal stimuli (at the arrow) in an isolated right atrial preparation from a cat. The cardiac cycle lengths (in msec) are denoted by the numbers at the top (modified from [32], with permission from the Am Heart Assoc, Inc).

77

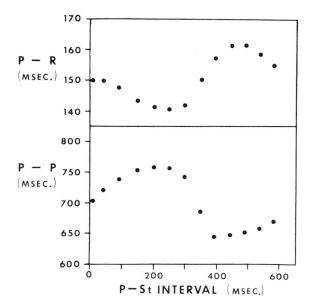

Figure 11. The changes in A-V conduction time (P–R interval) and in cardiac cycle length (P–P interval) produced by one vagal stimulus per cardiac cycle in an anesthetized dog. The time (P–St interval) from the beginning of atrial depolarization (P wave) till the vagal stimulus (St) was varied systematically (from [40], with permission from the Am Heart Assoc, Inc).

concentrations of acetylcholine too low to evoke hyperpolarization are still adequate to depress Ca conductance [30] and thereby to alter the sinus rate.

The time within the cardiac cycle at which a vagal impulse arrives at the S-A node is an important determinant of the efficacy of that impulse. When one vagal stimulus is given each cardiac cycle, but the time within the cycle is varied systematically, the negative chronotropic effect can be related to the phase of the cardiac cycle [27, 39–41]. In the experiment shown in Figure 11, the P–St interval represents the time from the beginning of a given atrial depolarization (P wave) till the time that a stimulus (St) was given to the cervical vagus nerves in an anesthetized dog [40]. In that experiment, the P–P interval was 390 msec when the vagus nerves were not being stimulated. When one vagal stimulus was given each cardiac cycle, and each stimulus was delivered at the beginning of atrial depolarization (P–St = 0), the P–P interval was about 700 msec (Figure 11, bottom panel). As the stimuli were given progressively later in the cycle, the P–P interval gradually increased, until the maximum nega-

tive chronotropic response was reached at a P–St interval of about 225 msec. Thereafter, the chronotropic effect became attenuated, and the minimum response was attained at a P–St interval of about 400 msec. The P–P interval then became greater again as the stimuli were applied still later in the cardiac cycle. The top panel shows that the A-V conduction time (P–R interval) also varied with the time of vagal stimulation; this will be discussed below, in the section on vagal activity.

Atrioventricular junction

Electrophysiological characteristics

The atrioventricular (A-V) node may be subdivided into three functional regions: the A-N, or upper portion; the N, or middle portion; and the N-H, or lower portion. Action potentials recorded from all three regions have the low amplitudes and slow conduction velocities characteristic of slow responses [15, 21, 42–45]. In the N region (Figure 12C),

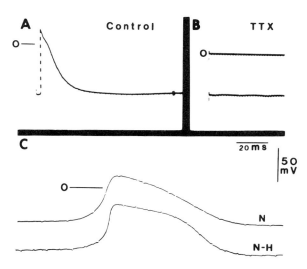

Figure 12. Transmembrane action potentials recorded from atrial and A-V nodal cells in a rabbit heart: (A) control atrial action potential; (B) effect of tetrodotoxin (TTX), 5×10^{-6} g/ml. Upper trace denotes zero potential and lower trace, resting membrane potential; (C) action potentials from an N cell (upper trace) and an N-H cell (lower trace); TTX, 5×10^{-6} g/ml, had virtually no effect on these action potentials. Zero mV line in panel C applies only to N fiber. Calibrations: vertical, 50 mV for all panels; horizontal, 100 msec for A, 200 msec for B, and 20 msec for C (from [43], with permission from the Am Heart Assoc, Inc).

the resting membrane potential is less negative and the amplitude, the rate of rise of the upstroke, and the conduction velocity are less than in the A-N or N-H regions. In the A-N region, the characteristics approach those of atrial myocardial action potentials, whereas in the N-H region (Figure 12C), they approach those of His bundle fibers. In common with other cardiac fibers that display slow response action potentials, the nodal cells are insensitive to the effects of tetrodotoxin (TTX). Conversely, fast response action potentials, such as those in atrial myocardial cells, are abolished by TTX (Figure 12, A and B).

Slow-channel blocking agents, such as verapamil, have a pronounced inhibitory effect on A-V conduction however [21, 42–45]. Verapamil greatly prolongs the effective (ERP) and functional (FRP) refractory periods (Figure 13) of the A-V node [44]. The ERP is the shortest interval between two atrial depolarizations (A1–A2) that can be conducted

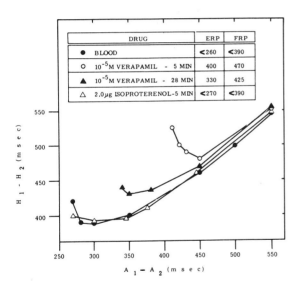

Figure 13. The changes in effective (ERP) and functional (FRP) refractory periods of the A-V node in an anesthetized dog produced by a brief infusion of verapamil (10^{-5} M) into the posterior septal artery. The unfilled circles and filled triangles show the changes 5 and 28 min, respectively, after the verapamil infusion. When a bolus of isoproterenol (2 ml, 1.0 μg/ml) was injected (unfilled triangles) 5 min after the verapamil, the ERP and FRP transiently became equal to the control values (filled circles). The A1–A2 intervals (abscissae) are the cycle lengths of prematurely induced atrial extrasystoles; the H1–H2 intervals are the corresponding intervals between His-bundle deflections (from [44], with permission from the Am Heart Assoc, Inc).

through the A-V node. The abscissal value at the left end of any curve in Figure 13 denotes the ERP for the corresponding experimental condition. The FRP is the minimum interval (H1–H2) between two His bundle depolarizations that can be achieved at a given basic atrial driving interval. For a given curve in the figure, the FRP is the smallest ordinate value for that curve.

Certain cells in the A-V node have the characteristics of automatic fibers. They are located mainly in the lower (N-H) regions of the node, and have electrophysiological and pharmacological characteristics that resemble those of S-A nodal pacemaker cells [46, 47].

Adrenergic effects

Catecholamines increase the amplitude and the upstroke velocity of cells in the A-N and N regions of the A-V node without altering the resting potentials [48]. They also enhance the impulse propagation velocity throughout the node [48], and diminish the refractory periods [49]. Furthermore, when the refractory periods are prolonged by slow-channel blocking agents (Figure 13), catecholamines restore normal refractoriness [44]. Cells in the N-H region of the node are relatively unaffected by catecholamines, except for those cells that display slow diastolic depolarization. Catecholamines increase the slope of phase 4 depolarization in such automatic cells, and thereby increase their rates of spontaneous firing [48].

Sympathetic activity

Increases in sympathetic activity reduce the A-V conduction time (Figure 14), as assessed by the P–R interval of the electrocardiogram [50]. The A–H interval is curtailed by sympathetic stimulation, whereas the H–V interval is not significantly affected [51–53]; hence, the principal effect on A-V transmission occurs in the A-V node. The left-sided sympathetic nerves have a somewhat greater dromotropic effect on the A-V junction than do those on the right side [51, 53]. The effects on A-V conduction of a very brief sympathetic stimulus will persist for about 20 sec, whereas the effects of a similar, brief vagal stimulus will be dissipated in less than 2 sec [53].

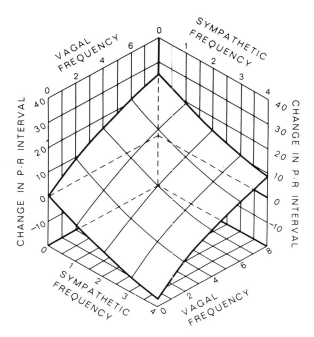

Figure 14. The changes in A-V conduction time (P–R interval) produced by simultaneous stimulation of the cardiac sympathetic and vagal nerves at different frequencies. The response surface was derived from data obtained from six dogs (from [50]).

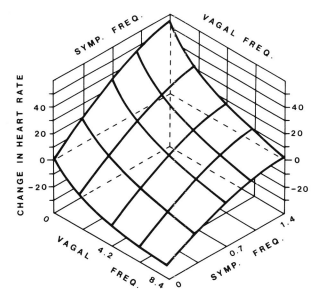

Figure 15. The mean changes in heart rate (beats/min) evoked by simultaneous stimulation of the cardiac sympathetic and vagal nerves in a group of seven dogs with an A-V junctional rhythm. The sinus node had been suppressed by injecting pentobarbital into the sinus node artery (from [55]).

The automatic cells in the A-V node also are influenced by changes in sympathetic activity [53–56]. The positive chronotropic effect of sympathetic stimulation varies with the stimulation frequency (Figure 15) in dogs in which an A-V junctional rhythm has been induced [55]. The magnitude of the chronotropic effect also depends on the prevailing level of vagal activity. When the changes in heart rate evoked by sympathetic stimulation are calculated as a fractional change from the basal rate, the chronotropic effect on the A-V junction is greater than that on the S-A node [55].

Cholinergic effects

The principal influence of acetylcholine (ACh) and other cholinergic agents on A-V nodal conducting fibers is to diminish the upstroke velocity and the amplitude of the action potential, and hence to reduce the impulse propagation velocity through the node [15, 27, 42, 45, 57]. The refractory periods are also prolonged. Higher concentrations of ACh lead to second- or third-degree blocks. Cells in the A-N and N regions are principally affected by cholinergic compounds; cells in the N-H region are relatively unaffected.

Vagal activity

Vagal stimulation has a negative dromotropic effect on the A-V junction [27, 48, 53, 57, 58]. There is a progressive increase in the A-V conduction time (Figure 14) as the frequency of vagal stimulation is increased [50]. The change in the A-V conduction time evoked by a given vagal stimulus (Figure 14) appears to be independent of the background level of sympathetic activity [50]. The timing of a vagal stimulus within the cardiac cycle (Figure 11, top panel) does have an appreciable influence on the dromotropic response [40].

The frequency with which cardiac impulses arrive at the A-V node is an important determinant of the A-V conduction time. In general, the faster the sinus rate, the longer the conduction time. The influence of a given level of vagal activity on the A-V conduction system varies, therefore, with the prevailing heart rate.

Changes in vagal activity influence both the S-A and the A-V nodes. The acetylcholine released at the vagal endings in the A-V node acts *directly* on the conducting fibers to retard conduction. Vagal

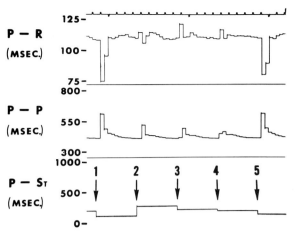

Figure 16. Changes in P–R and P–P intervals produced by five vagal stimuli, 5 sec apart, in an anesthetized dog. The P–St interval is the time from the beginning of atrial depolarization (P wave) to the time of vagal stimulation (St) (from [37]).

activity also acts on the S-A nodal pacemaker cells to diminish the heart rate. The resultant cardiac deceleration acts *indirectly* to facilitate A-V conduction. In response to an increase in vagal activity, therefore, the actual change in A-V conduction time is the resultant of these direct and indirect influences. In the experiment illustrated in Figure 16, five identical electrical pulses were delivered to the vagus nerves exactly 5 sec apart [37]. The stimuli all occurred at different times (P–St intervals) in the cardiac cycle. When the stimuli (arrows 3 and 4) elicited only a slight prolongation of the cardiac cycle (P–P interval), the A-V conduction time (P–R interval) was prolonged. However when greater increases in the P–P intervals were evoked by the vagal stimuli (arrows 1 and 5), the P–R intervals were shortened substantially. The interactions between heart rate changes and the direct vagal influence on the A-V conducting fibers have been studied extensively [27, 57, 59], and they are highly nonlinear.

The automatic cells in the A-V node are under parasympathetic control [53, 55, 56]. The negative chronotropic effect of vagal stimulation (Figure 15) varies with the frequency of stimulation and with the prevailing level of sympathetic activity [55]. Furthermore, the timing of vagal activity relative to the phase of the cardiac cycle has just as great an influence on the automatic cells in the A-V node as it does on those in the S-A node [60].

Ventricular specialized conduction system

After the cardiac impulse has been propagated through the A-V node, it enters the bundle of His, which constitutes the beginning of the 'ventricular conduction system.' The impulse proceeds down the right and left bundle branches, and then through the extensive Purkinje fiber network, which ramifies throughout the endocardial surfaces of both ventricles.

Electrophysiological characteristics

Transmembrane action potentials recorded from cells throughout the ventricular specialized conduction system all have similar characteristics, except that the durations vary with the location [15, 42, 61, 62]. The effective refractory periods (ERP) parallel the action potential durations [15, 42, 61]. Hence those Purkinje fibers with the longest action potentials are sometimes referred to as 'gate' cells [42, 61, 62]. In the slow to normal range of heart rates, a premature atrial depolarization is often blocked at such gates, because they have the longest ERP in the path between atria and ventricles. As the sinus rate increases, the A-V nodal ERP progressively increases and the Purkinje fiber ERP diminishes. Hence, at rapid heart rates, the site of block is more likely to be in the A-V node itself.

Action potentials recorded from the specialized conduction fibers are in many ways similar to those from ventricular myocardial fibers (Figure 2). However, the action potential durations of the specialized conduction fibers are longer [15] and the phase 0 upstroke velocity and conduction velocity are higher in the Purkinje fibers. The upstrokes of these action potentials depend on the rapid influx of Na through the fast membrane channels. Hence, conduction in such fibers is impaired by fast-channel blocking agents, such as tetrodotoxin.

Except under unusual experimental conditions, myocardial fibers do not display the property of automaticity [63]. However, fibers in the specialized conduction system do possess this attribute [15, 18, 42, 63, 64]. Ordinarily, the sinus rate is high enough to suppress automaticity in these specialized conducting fibers [18, 63]. In the absence of such 'overdrive suppression,' however, gradual phase 4 depolarization will appear. When the threshold potential is reached, the fast Na channels are activated, and the upstroke of the action potential is initiated.

Adrenergic effects

The principal effect of catecholamines on spontaneously depolarizing Purkinje fibers is to increase the slope of the pacemaker potential, and hence to increase the frequency of firing of these automatic cells [18, 63–65]. The mechanism by which catecholamines exert this positive chronotropic effect appears to involve specific channels through which K leaves the cells during diastolic depolarization [63].

Catecholamines shift the voltage dependence of the deactivation of the K channels [63], such that virtually all of them are closed when the membrane potential reaches −80 mV. Catecholamines do not affect the inward leakage of Na during phase 4. Hence, adrenergic agents exaggerate the disparity between the relatively constant influx of Na and the progressively decreasing efflux of K, and thereby accelerate the depolarization process during phase 4.

When Purkinje fibers are driven electrically at a rate sufficient to suppress their automaticity, beta-receptor agonists tend to decrease the action potential duration [65, 66]. In the experiment illustrated in Figure 17, the duration of the Purkinje fiber action potential was considerably less after (panel B) than before (panel A) the addition of isoproterenol [66].

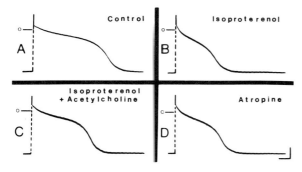

Figure 17. The antagonistic effects of acetylcholine and isoproterenol on the duration of the action potentials in a canine Purkinje fiber: (A) control tracing; (B) addition of isoproterenol (10^{-7} M); (C) addition of acetylcholine (10^{-6} M) to the bath already containing isoproterenol; (D) addition of atropine (10^{-6} M). The addition of acetylcholine (10^{-6} M) in the absence of isoproterenol had no detectable effect on the action potential (from [66], with permission of the Am Heart Assoc, Inc).

Sympathetic activity

Very little information is available concerning the sympathetic regulation of the His-Purkinje system, but it is likely that the effects of sympathetic neural activity are similar to those evoked by exogenous catecholamines. When complete A-V block is induced in experimental animals, sympathetic stimulation does accelerate the idioventricular rate [67, 68].

Cholinergic effects

Cholinergic agents have a variable effect on the action potentials of Purkinje fibers, depending on the species being studied and on other experimental conditions. In electrically driven preparations obtained from sheep, ACh caused a slight hyperpolarization during phase 4, and the action potential was slightly prolonged [69]. In certain studies of canine Purkinje fibers, ACh also hyperpolarized the cell membrane, but it shortened the action potential [70]. In other studies on canine Purkinje fibers, however, ACh had no detectable effect when it was added alone to the tissue bath [66]. It did, however, antagonize the action of isoproterenol (Figure 17C). This antagonistic action of ACh was blocked by atropine (Figure 17D).

When Purkinje fibers are permitted to depolarize spontaneously, ACh increases the maximum diastolic potential and diminishes the slope of diastolic depolarization [70–72]. Hence, ACh reduces the spontaneous firing rate of these automatic cells.

Vagal activity

In anesthetized dogs, vagal stimulation does not affect significantly the His-Purkinje conduction time, as assessed by the H–V interval of the His-bundle electrogram [73]. In dogs with experimentally induced complete A-V block, vagal stimulation does slow the idioventricular rate however [67, 74].

Atrial and ventricular myocardium

Adrenergic effects

The effects of beta-receptor agonists on the electrical and mechanical properties of myocardial fibers

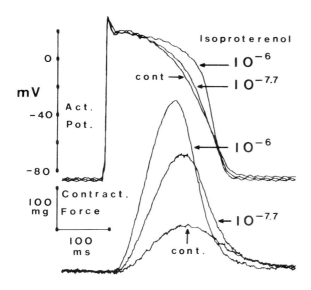

Figure 18. Computer-reproduced traces of the action potentials and contractions recorded from canine papillary muscles under control conditions and in the presence of $10^{-7.7}$ and 10^{-6} M isoproterenol (2.5×10^{-9} M) A Ca-sensitive bioluminescent pro-

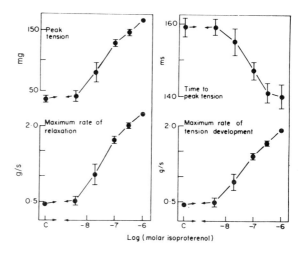

Figure 19. Dose–response curves for the effects of isoproterenol on four indices of the isometric contractions of canine papillary muscles (with permission from [75]).

[75] are summarized in Figures 18 and 19. The effects are qualitatively similar for atrial and ventricular fibers. Adrenergic agents have a pronounced positive inotropic effect on cardiac muscle. In a dose-dependent fashion, they increase the peak developed tension, the maximum rate of tension development, and the maximum rate of relaxation, and they decrease the time required to reach the peak tension.

Cathecholamines have only slight effects on the action potentials of normally polarized myocardial fibers. The transmembrane potential tends to be more positive during the plateau, the plateau tends to remain at positive potentials for a longer time and the maximum rate of repolarization is increased (Figure 18).

The duration of the plateau is determined mainly by the balance between an inward and an outward ionic current. The principal ionic influx is the so-called 'slow inward current' carried by Ca and Na, whereas a concomitant, gradual increase in K conductance during the plateau leads to an efflux of K. The plateau persists as long as these two currents are approximately equal. Toward the end of the plateau, the efflux of K begins to exceed the influx of Ca and Na, and the membrane begins to repolar-

ize. The K conductance increases as the membrane becomes more negative, which further accelerates the efflux of K. Hence, the repolarization process (phase 3) is a 'regenerative' one; that is, an increased K conductance tends to make the transmembrane potential more negative, and in turn the more negative potential augments the K conductance.

The principal direct effect of beta-receptor agonists on the myocardial cell membrane is to increase the slow inward current of Ca and Na [75–79]. Such adrenergic compounds probably act on the cell membrane to increase the number of open channels through which the slow inward current flows [79]. Consequently, the intracellular stores of Ca are increased, and more Ca is available to activate the contractile proteins. The increased Ca content has been demonstrated experimentally by injecting a Ca-sensitive luminescent protein, aequorin, into atrial myocardial cells of frogs [80]. The luminescent signal is much greater after isoproterenol than before (Figure 20).

The augmentation of the intracellular content of Ca is probably the principal mechanism by which the catecholamines exert their potent positive inotropic influence. This increased inward current of Ca and Na is probably also the reason why the transmembrane potential tends to be more positive during the plateau in the presence of adrenergic agents (Figure 18).

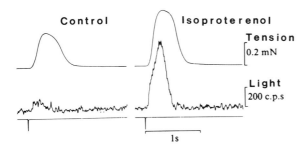

Control   Isoproterenol

Tension
[0.2 mN

Light
[200 c.p.s

1s

Figure 20. The tension (top tracing) and light signal (bottom tracing) recorded during the contraction of a frog atrial trabecula before (left panel) and after (right panel) the addition of isoproterenol (2.5×10^{-9} M). A Ca-sensitive bioluminescent protein, aequorin, was injected intracellularly. The light signal, in photon counts per sec, reflects the intracellular Ca content (modified with permission from [80]).

This augmentation of the slow inward current by catecholamines would, by itself, tend to prolong the plateau of the action potential. Yet, catecholamines are found to shorten action potentials under certain conditions and to prolong them under other conditions [77, 78]. The change in action potential duration evoked by beta-receptor agonists probably is the result of a direct and an indirect influence [78]. The direct effect of the increase in slow inward current is to extend the plateau. However, the rise in intracellular Ca content evoked by catecholamines acts indirectly to increase K conductance toward the end of the plateau and during phase 3. This indirect effect tends to enhance the efflux of K, which would terminate the plateau and accelerate repolarization (Figure 18), and thereby shorten the action potential. The resultant action potential duration under a given set of experimental conditions would depend, therefore, on the balance between these direct and indirect influences.

The effects of catecholamines on myocardial cell action potentials are much more pronounced when the cells are partially depolarized, either by high external K concentrations or by voltage clamping. In the experiment shown in Figure 21, the resting membrane potential of a ventricular myocardial cell was reduced to –40 mV (panel a) by voltage clamping [81]. The amplitude and upstroke velocity of the resultant slow response were increased by isoproterenol, and the duration was prolonged sub-

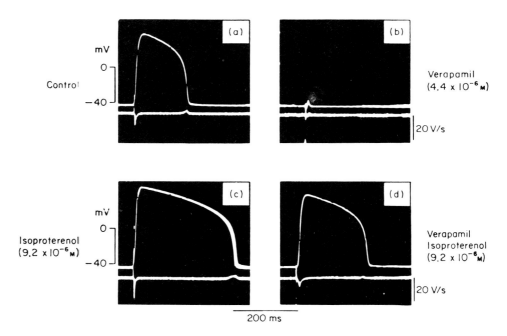

Figure 21. Slow response action potential (a) recorded from papillary muscle in which the resting potential was reduced to –40 mV by voltage clamping. Isoproterenol (c) increased the amplitude, upstroke velocity, and duration of the action potential, whereas verapamil (b) abolished it. The effect of verapamil was overcome by the addition of isoproterenol (d) (with permission from [81]; copyright by Academic Press, Inc).

stantially (panel c). The slow response was abolished by verapamil (panel b), but it was restored by isoproterenol (panel d).

Sympathetic activity

Increased sympathetic activity has a pronounced positive inotropic effect on atrial and ventricular myocardial fibers. The norepinephrine released at the postganglionic sympathetic nerve endings interacts with beta-receptors on the myocardial cell surfaces, evoking electrophysiological and mechanical effects similar to those elicited by exogenous catecholamines. Extensive reviews have recently been published on this subject [27, 82], and therefore only a brief summary will be given here.

Pressure pulse analysis [82] discloses that increased sympathetic activity augments the peak ventricular and aortic pressures, abridges the duration of ventricular systole, increases the rate of change of intraventricular pressure (dP/dt) during contraction and relaxation, and enhances the stroke volume and the maximum rate of ventricular ejection (Figure 22). The augmentation of cardiac output produced by cardiac sympathetic nerve stimulation (Figure 23) is accompanied by a reduction in mean right and left atrial pressures [83]. The diminution in atrial pressures is ascribable to a redistribution of the blood volume from the venous to the arterial segments of the circulation [84]. The augmented arterial blood volume is reflected by the substantial elevation of aortic pressure.

The sympathetic innervation of the ventricles is highly asymmetrical [1–3, 25–27, 82]. The left-sided nerves exert a much greater positive inotropic effect on the left ventricular myocardium than do the right-sided nerves (Figure 6). Stellate ganglionectomy prolongs the functional refractory period of the ventricles [85]. Right-sided ganglionectomy has its greatest influence over the anterior surface of the ventricles, whereas excision of the left ganglion affects mainly the posterior surface.

Cholinergic effects

Atria
Acetylcholine (ACh) and other cholinergic substances have pronounced effects on atrial myocardial fibers, but their influence on the ventricles is much more subtle [27, 29, 86]. ACh markedly re-

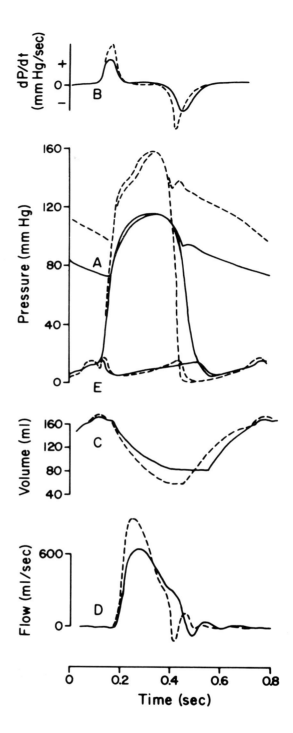

Figure 22. Left ventricular and aortic pressures (A), left ventricular dP/dt (B), left ventricular volume (C), aortic flow (D), and left atrial pressure (E) before (continuous lines) and during (dashed lines) stimulation of the cardiac sympathetic nerves (from [82]).

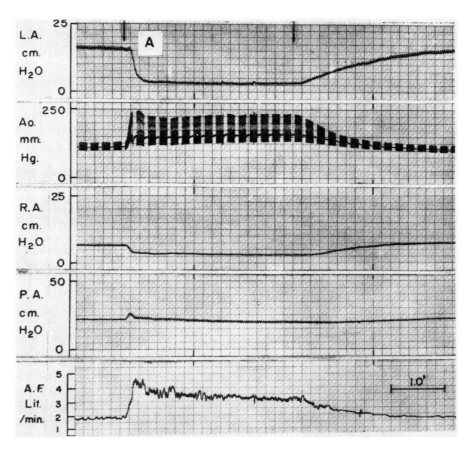

Figure 23. The changes in left atrial (L.A.), aortic (Ao.), right atrial (R.A.), and pulmonary arterial (P.A.) pressures, and in aortic flow (A.F.) produced by left stellate ganglion stimulation (5 Hz, between the arrows) (modified from [83], with permission of the Am Heart Assoc, Inc).

duces the action potential duration of atrial myocardial fibers (Figure 24) and hyperpolarizes the membrane during phase 4 [87]. Concomitantly, the force of contraction is severely depressed. This negative inotropic effect is achieved through two main

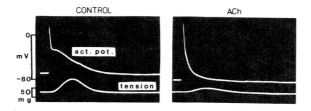

Figure 24. The action potential (upper tracing) and contractile force (lower tracing) recorded from a canine atrial fiber under control conditions (left panel) and in the presence of acetylcholine (ACh) 2×10^{-6} M (modified from [87]).

mechanisms, the relative importance of which appears to depend on the species. In mammalian hearts at relatively low ACh concentrations, the major mechanism is probably the reduction in action potential duration which is evoked by an increase in outward K current. This efflux of K terminates the plateau prematurely, and thereby curtails the slow inward current of Ca simply by abridging the time over which Ca influx can take place [87]. At higher ACh concentrations, the slow inward current is also suppressed directly, presumably through an effect on the slow membrane channels. In frog atrial fibers, this direct effect on the slow channels appears to be more important, even at relatively low ACh concentrations [88].

ACh has variable effects on intra-atrial conduction [29]. When it causes substantial hyperpolarization of previously depolarized fibers, ACh will tend to enhance atrial conduction, presumably by increasing the number of fast Na channels that are available to be activated during phase 0. However, in previously normal tissues it is likely that the hyperpolarization induced by ACh will have little effect on conduction. Moreover, ACh tends to decrease the space constant and, at high concentrations, the action potential amplitude [29]. These factors would tend to impair conduction.

Ventricles

Cholinergic agents have much less influence on ventricular than on atrial myocardial cells. In general, ACh has a slight negative inotropic effect on the ventricles [27, 86, 89, 90], although, under certain conditions, positive inotropic responses may be elicited [91]. An example of the response to a brief infusion of ACh into a coronary artery in a canine isovolumetric left ventricle preparation is shown in Figure 25B. The ACh elicited a substantial increase in coronary blood flow, and the left ventricular contractile force was reduced by about 30% during the infusion [90]. After termination of the infusion, there was a brief positive inotropic rebound. The negative inotropic effect observed during the infusion becomes much more pronounced if the ACh is given in the presence of a substantial background of adrenergic activity [89].

The electrophysiological effects of ACh on the normal ventricular myocardium are negligible [92]. However, if the myocardial fibers are partially depolarized and rendered inexcitable by high K concentrations and then restored by isoproterenol, the resultant slow response action potentials are indeed suppressed by ACh [93]. It is likely that ACh curtails the increase in slow inward current induced by beta-receptor agonists.

Vagal activity

Atria

The potent depressant effect of vagal activity on the atria has been appreciated for over 60 years [94, 95]. Increased vagal tone diminishes the atrial contribution to ventricular filling [83, 96] and interferes with the normal closure of the A-V valves [97, 98]. When the A-V conduction time is normal, atrial relaxation begins shortly before the start of ventricular contraction. The resultant, abrupt decline in atrial pressure causes the A-V valves to move toward the closed position just before ventricular contraction begins. If increased vagal activity suppresses atrial contraction sufficiently, this 'preclosure' of the A-V valves will fail to occur. Furthermore, if the A-V conduction time is unduly prolonged by the augmented vagal activity, if the valves do preclose, they then tend to swing open again before the onset of the retarded ventricular contraction.

The negative inotropic effects of vagal stimulation on the atria depend on the background level of sympathetic activity (Figure 26A). Also, the vagal effects are prepotent over the prevailing sympathetic influence [99]. In the experiment illustrated in Figure 26, the positive inotropic effect evoked by sympathetic stimulation (panel B) was virtually abolished by vagal stimulation at a frequency of 1.2

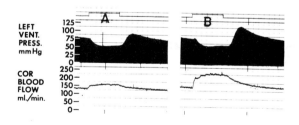

Figure 25. The changes in left ventricular pressure and coronary blood flow evoked by supramaximal vagal stimulation for 1 min (event mark A) at a frequency of 20 Hz and by an acetylcholine infusion at 18 μg/min for 1 min (event mark B) in a canine isovolumetric left ventricle preparation. Pressure was recorded from a balloon in the left ventricle; the balloon contained a fixed volume of liquid. Heart was paced at a constant rate of 165 beats/min (modified from [90]).

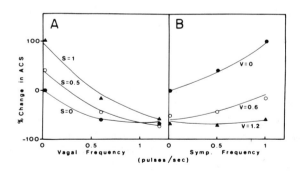

Figure 26. The changes in atrial contractile strength (ACS) produced by various combinations of frequencies of vagal and sympathetic stimulation in an anesthetized dog. The numbers along the curves denote the frequencies (in Hz) of vagal (V) and sympathetic (S) stimulation (from [99]).

Hz. In the absence of vagal activity (V = 0), on the other hand, such sympathetic stimulation evoked a 100% increase in atrial contractile strength. This predominance of vagal control reflects the tendency for the neurally released ACh to antagonize the adrenergically induced increase in slow inward current [93], as described in the preceding section.

Ventricles

In mammals the negative inotropic effects of vagal stimulation are much less pronounced on the ventricles than on the atria. Consequently, until about 15 years ago, it was generally considered that the mammalian ventricles are not parasympathetically innervated. Since that time, abundant evidence to the contrary has been adduced [27, 86, 100–104].

The depressant effect of vagal stimulation on ventricular contractility (Figure 25A) resembles the response to an intracoronary injection of ACh (Figure 25B), except that the ACh injection evokes a greater increase in coronary blood flow. The depressant effect of vagal stimulation is more pronounced the greater the background level of adrenergic activity. At times, vagal stimulation alone evokes an almost undetectable response [103], as illustrated by vagal stimuli A and C in Figure 27. However, when the cardiac sympathetic nerves are also being stimulated (between marks 1 and 2), the same vagal stimulus (B) exerts a pronounced depressant effect; it virtually neutralizes the facilitatory influence of the concomitant sympathetic activity. It is likely that the ACh released from the vagal nerve endings exerts much of its effect on ventricular contractility either by antagonizing the increased slow inward current induced by concurrent sympathetic activity [93] or by curtailing the quantity of norepinephrine that is released from neighboring

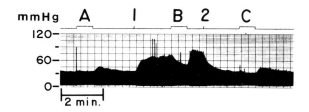

mmHg

120–

60–

0–

2 min.

Figure 27. Changes in left ventricular pressure in a canine isovolumetric left ventricle preparation evoked by supramaximal vagal stimulation (20 Hz) before (A), during (B), and after (C) left stellate ganglion stimulation (2 Hz, between marks 1 and 2) (from [103]).

sympathetic nerve terminals [27, 86, 100, 104]. This subject is discussed in greater detail in Chapter 5.

Similar neural antagonisms have been observed with respect to the excitability of the ventricles. Vagal stimulation prolongs the effective refractory period (ERP) of the ventricular myocardium, whereas sympathetic stimulation shortens it [105]. However, the vagally induced prolongation of the ERP becomes more pronounced when sympathetic tone has been augmented. Also, vagal stimulation alone is without significant effect on the vulnerability to ventricular fibrillation [106]. However, in the presence of increased sympatho-adrenal activity, the same vagal stimulation exerts a substantial protective effect [106].

Cardiac reflexes

The reflex control of the heart has been studied extensively, and several comprehensive reviews have recently appeared [13, 107–112]. Only a brief description of the three most important reflexes will be presented here; namely, the baroreceptor, Bainbridge, and chemoreceptor reflexes.

Baroreceptor reflex

Baroreceptors are arterial stretch receptors that are located in the carotid sinuses and aortic arch [107, 112]. Afferent impulses from the carotid sinus receptors travel to the brain in the carotid sinus nerves, which are branches of the glossopharyngeal, or ninth cranial, nerves. Impulses from the aortic baroreceptors ascend to the brain via the aortic nerves, which are branches of the vagus, or tenth cranial, nerves. The afferent fibers from the carotid sinus and aortic baroreceptors synapse with neurons located in the nucleus tractus solitarius, in the medulla oblongata. Sympathetic and parasympathetic (vagal) fibers constitute the efferent limbs of the baroreceptor reflex.

The arterial baroreceptors discharge impulses at an increasing frequency as the mean arterial pressure rises in the carotid sinuses and aortic arch. The discharge frequency also increases when the rate of change of arterial pressure rises. An increased frequency of impulses in the carotid sinus and aortic nerves diminishes the neural activity in efferent sympathetic fibers and augments the activity in efferent vagal fibers. The decreased sympathetic activity results in a reduction in vasomotor tone in resistance (arterioles) and capacitance (venules and veins) vessels throughout the body.

With respect to the control of cardiac function, a rise in afferent activity in the baroreceptor nerves evokes a reciprocal effect in efferent cardiac sympathetic and parasympathetic fibers. Sympathetic activity diminishes and vagal activity increases, thereby reducing heart rate, prolonging A-V conduction, and depressing atrial and ventricular contractility. This reciprocal action usually takes place only at arterial pressures within or near the normal range of pressures. If the arterial blood pressure is acutely reduced to abnormally low levels, vagal tone disappears completely; the gradation of reflex control is then achieved solely by variations in efferent sympathetic activity. Conversely, if the arterial blood pressure is acutely elevated to abnormally high levels, sympathetic tone is completely suppressed; the gradation of reflex control is then accomplished by alterations in efferent vagal activity.

The cardiac deceleration reflexly evoked by an elevation of the arterial blood pressure has been used to assess the efficacy (or gain) of the baroreceptor reflex [113]. An alpha-receptor agonist, such as phenylephrine, is injected intravenously, and the slope of the regression line relating the cardiac cycle length to the systolic blood pressure is taken as an index of 'baroreceptor sensitivity.' The slope of such a regression line is much less in animals in heart failure than in normal animals (Figure 28), reflecting the impairment of reflex cardiovascular control that prevails in heart failure [114].

Bainbridge reflex

Bainbridge noted in 1915 that when he infused blood or saline into anesthetized animals, the heart rate increased, even though the arterial blood pressure also might have risen [115]. Cardiac acceleration was correlated with an increase in central venous pressure and was abolished by bilateral vagotomy. Bainbridge postulated that the reflex was initiated by distension of the right side of the heart, and that the afferent impulses were carried in the vagi.

The Bainbridge reflex has been controversial since its original description. Other reflexes, notably the baroreceptor reflex, are also invoked by a

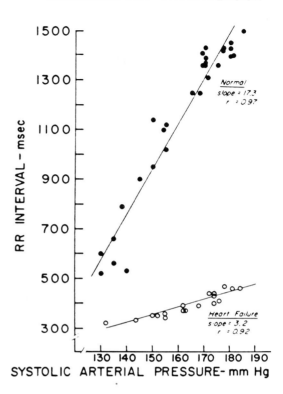

Figure 28. The relationship between cardiac cycle length (R–R interval) and the systolic blood pressure during the preceding heart beat, in normal conscious dogs and in dogs in congestive heart failure. The slope of this relationship is considered to be an index of baroreflex sensitivity (from [114]).

change in blood volume. Hence, the directional change in heart rate elicited by an alteration of blood volume will be the resultant of opposing reflex influences. Frequently, infusions of fluid cause cardiac acceleration when the prevailing basal heart rate is slow, but they induce a diminished heart rate when the basal rate is rapid.

In a recent study in unanesthetized dogs [116], volume loading with blood produced substantial increases in cardiac output and arterial blood pressure. The heart rate increased in proportion to the cardiac output (Figure 29), despite a concomitant elevation of blood pressure. Hence, the Bainbridge reflex must have predominated over the baroreceptor reflex in these animals during volume expansion. Conversely, volume depletion caused a reduction in cardiac output and arterial blood pressure.

89

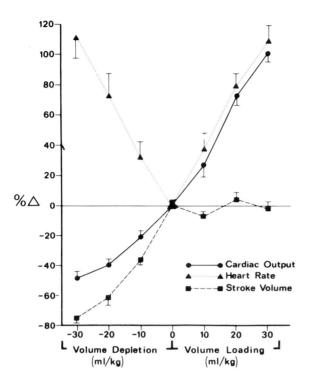

Figure 29. Effects of blood transfusion and of bleeding on cardiac output, heart rate, and stroke volume in unanesthetized dogs (from [116], with permission of the Am Heart Assoc, Inc).

Heart rate increased as the blood pressure and cardiac output diminished (Figure 29). Therefore, the baroreceptor reflex must have predominated over the Bainbridge reflex under these conditions of volume depletion.

Chemoreceptor reflex

The peripheral arterial chemoreceptors respond to reductions in arterial pO_2 and pH and to elevations in arterial pCO_2. The chemoreceptors are located in the aortic arch and in the carotid bodies, which are adjacent to the carotid sinuses. Arterial chemoreceptor stimulation induces pulmonary hyperventilation. It also tends to evoke vasoconstriction and bradycardia, but the magnitude of these cardiovascular responses depends on the extent of the concomitant change in pulmonary ventilation [111, 117]. For example, if a given chemoreceptor stimulus evokes only a mild degree of hyperventilation, the cardiac response tends to be bradycardia. Conversely, if the chemoreceptor stimulus leads to intense hyperventilation, the heart rate is likely to increase.

An extreme example of this reflex respiratory–circulatory interaction is the dramatic cardiac response that may ensue when hyperventilation fails

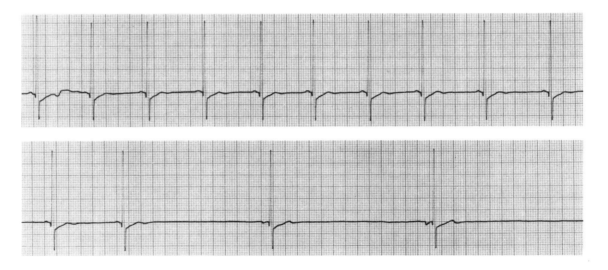

Figure 30. Electrocardiogram of a quadriplegic patient who required tracheal intubation and artificial respiration; the two strips are continuous. At the beginning of the top strip, the tracheal catheter was disconnected to permit nursing care. In less than 10 sec, the patient's heart rate decreased from 65 to about 20 beats/min (adapted from [118]).

90

to occur in response to chemoreceptor stimulation. In experimental animals, when ventilation is controlled by an artificial respirator, carotid chemoreceptor stimulation evokes an intense vagal discharge, which induces a pronounced bradycardia and an impairment of A-V conduction [111, 117]. Similar changes have been reported in quadriplegic patients who are dependent on mechanical respirators [117, 118]. Briefly disconnecting the tracheal catheter from a respirator in order to permit tracheal aspiration promptly induced a profound bradycardia in a quadriplegic patient (Figure 30). His heart rate dropped from 65 to 20 beats/min within 10 sec after cessation of artificial respiration. This bradycardia could be retarded by hyperventilating the patient prior to disconnecting the tracheal catheter, and it could be prevented by administering atropine. The abrupt reduction in heart rate undoubtedly reflects the primary reflex cardiac response to arterial chemoreceptor excitation in a patient in whom the secondary effects of hyperventilation were not able to develop.

References

1. Mizeres NJ: The origin and course of the cardioaccelerator fibers in the dog. Anat Rec 132:261–279, 1958.
2. Randall WC, Armour JA: Gross and microscopic anatomy of the cardiac innervation. In: Randall WC (ed) Neural Regulation of the Heart. Oxford Univ Press, New York, 1977, pp 13–41.
3. Levy MN, Ng ML, Zieske H: Functional distribution of the peripheral cardiac sympathetic pathways. Circ Res 19:650–661, 1966.
4. Wacksman J, Farr WC, Grupp G: Localization of the cardiac sympathetic synapses in the dog. Proc Soc Exp Biol Med 131:336–339, 1969.
5. Wechsler JS, Pace JB, Goldberg JM, Randall WC: Location of synaptic connections in canine sympathetic cardiac innervation. Am J Physiol 217:1789–1794, 1969.
6. Aiken JW, Reit E: Stimulation of the cat stellate ganglion by angiotensin. J Pharmacol Exp Ther 159:107–114, 1968.
7. McAllen RM, Spyer KM: The location of cardiac vagal preganglionic motoneurones in the medulla of the cat. J Physiol (Lond) 258:187–204, 1976.
8. Schwaber J, Schneiderman N: Aortic nerve activated cardio-inhibitory neurons and interneurons. Am J Physiol 229:783–789, 1975.
9. Gunn CG, Sevelius G, Puiggari MJ, Myers FK: Vagal cardiomotor mechanisms in the hindbrain of the dog and cat. Am J Physiol 214:258–262, 1968.
10. Weiss GK, Priola DV: Brainstem sites for activation of vagal cardioaccelerator fibers in the dog. Am J Physiol 223:300–304, 1972.
11. Alexander RS: Tonic and reflex functions of medullary sympathetic cardiovascular centers. J Neurophysiol 9:205–217, 1946.
12. Cannon WB: Bodily Changes in Pain, Hunger, Fear, and Rage, 2nd Ed. Appleton, New York, 1929.
13. Korner PI: Central nervous control of autonomic cardiovascular function. In: Berne RM (ed) Handbook of Physiology. Section 2: The Cardiovascular System, vol 1. Am Physiol Soc, Bethesda, 1979, pp 691–739.
14. Rushmer RF, Smith OA Jr: Cardiac control. Physiol Rev 39:41–68, 1959.
15. Hoffman BF, Cranefield PF: Electrophysiology of the Heart. McGraw-Hill, New York, 1960.
16. Noble D: The Initiation of the Heartbeat, 2nd Ed. Clarendon Press, Oxford, 1979.
17. Kohlhardt M, Figulla HR, Tripathi O: The slow membrane channel as the predominant mediator of the excitation process of the sinoatrial pacemaker cell. Basic Res Cardiol 71:17–26, 1976.
18. Vassalle M: Cardiac automaticity and its control. Am J Physiol 233:H625–H634, 1977.
19. Di Francesco D, Ojeda C: Properties of the current i_f in the sino-atrial node of the rabbit compared with those of the current i_{K_2} in Purkinje fibres. J Physiol (Lond) 308:353–367, 1980.
20. Maylie J, Morad M, Weiss J: A study of pacemaker potential in rabbit sino-atrial node: measurement of potassium activity under voltage-clamp conditions. J Physiol (Lond) 311:161–178, 1981.
21. Wit AL, Cranefield PF: Effect of verapamil on the sino-atrial and atrioventricular nodes of the rabbit and the mechanism by which it arrests reentrant atrioventricular nodal tachycardia. Circ Res 35:413–425, 1974.
22. Warner HR, Cox A: A mathematical model of heart rate control by sympathetic and vagus efferent information. J Appl Physiol 17:349–355, 1962.
23. Kopin IJ, Hertting G, Gordon EK: Fate of norepinephrine-H3 in the isolated perfused rat heart. J Pharmacol Exp Ther 138:38–40, 1962.
24. Wennmalm A: Quantitative evaluation of release and reuptake of adrenergic transmitter in the rabbit heart. Acta Physiol Scand 82:532–538, 1971.
25. Pannier R: Contribution à l'innervation sympathique du coeur. Les nerfs cardioaccélérateurs. Arch Intern Pharmacodyn 73:193–259, 1946.
26. Randall WC, Priola DV, Ulmer RH: A functional study of the distribution of cardiac sympathetic nerves. Am J Physiol 205:1227–1231, 1963.
27. Levy MN, Martin PJ: Neural control of the heart. In: Berne RM (ed) Handbook of Physiology. Section 2: The Cardiovascular System, vol 1. Am Physiol Soc, Bethesda, 1979, pp 581–620.
28. Kreitner D: Evidence for the existence of a rapid sodium channel in the membrane of rabbit sinoatrial cells. J Mol Cell Cardiol 7:655–662, 1975.
29. Strauss HC, Prystowsky EN, Scheinman MM: Sino-atrial and atrial electrogenesis. Prog Cardiovasc Dis 19:385–404, 1977.
30. Brown H, Noble D, Noble S: The initiation of the heartbeat

and its control by autonomic transmitters. In: Dickinson CJ, Marks J (eds) Developments in Cardiovascular Medicine. Univ Park Press, Baltimore, 1978, pp 31–51.

31. Spear JF, Kronhaus KD, Moore EN, Kline RP: The effect of brief vagal stimulation on the isolated rabbit sinus node. Circ Res 44:75–88, 1979.

32. Jalife J, Moe GK: Phasic effects of vagal stimulation on pacemaker activity of the isolated sinus node of the young cat. Circ Res 45:595–607, 1979.

33. Hutter OF: Mode of action of autonomic transmitters on the heart. Br Med Bull 13:176–180, 1957.

34. Bielecki K, Lewartowski B: The influence of hemicholinium no. 3 and vagus stimulation on acetylcholine distribution in the cat's heart. Pflugers Arch 279:149–155, 1964.

35. Brown OM: Cat heart acetylcholine: structural proof and distribution. Am J Physiol 231:781–785, 1976.

36. Brown GL, Eccles JE: The action of a single vagal volley on the rhythm of the heart beat. J Physiol (Lond) 82:211–240, 1934.

37. Levy MN, Martin PJ, Iano T, Zieske H: Effects of single vagal stimuli on heart rate and atrioventricular conduction. Am J Physiol 218:1256–1262, 1970.

38. Iano TL, Levy MN, Lee MH: An acceleratory component of the parasympathetic control of heart rate. Am J Physiol 224:997–1005, 1973.

39. Stuesse SL, Levy MN, Zieske H: Phase-related sensitivity of the sinoatrial node to vagal stimuli in the isolated rat atrium. Circ Res 43:217–224, 1978.

40. Levy MN, Martin PJ, Iano T, Zieske H: Paradoxical effect of vagus nerve stimulation on heart rate in dogs. Circ Res 25:303–314, 1969.

41. Levy MN, Iano T, Zieske H: Effects of repetitive bursts of vagal activity on heart rate. Circ Res 30:186–195, 1972.

42. Mendez C, Moe GK: Atrioventricular transmission. In: DeMello WC (ed) Electrical Phenomena in the Heart. Academic Press, New York, 1972, pp 263–291.

43. Zipes DP, Mendez C: Action of manganese ions and tetrodotoxin on atrioventricular nodal transmembrane potentials in isolated rabbit hearts. Circ Res 32:447–454, 1973.

44. Zipes DP, Fischer JC: Effects of agents which inhibit the slow channel on sinus node automaticity and atrioventricular conduction in the dog. Circ Res 34:184–192, 1974.

45. Cranefield PF: The Conduction of the Cardiac Impulse. Futura Publ Co, Mt Kisco, NY, 1975.

46. Wit, AL, Rosen MR, Hoffman BF: Electrophysiology and pharmacology of cardiac arrhythmias. II. Relationship of normal and abnormal electrical activity of cardiac fibers to the genesis of arrhythmias. Am Heart J 88:515–524, 1974.

47. Childers R: The AV node: normal and abnormal physiology. Prog Cardiovasc Dis 19:361–384, 1977.

48. Wit AL, Hoffman BF, Rosen MR: Electrophysiology and pharmacology of cardiac arrhythmias. IX. Cardiac electrophysiologic effects of beta-adrenergic receptor stimulation and blockade. Part A. Am Heart J 90:521–533, 1975.

49. Krayer O, Mandoki JJ, Mendez C: Studies on veratrum alkaloids. XVI. The action of epinephrine and of veratrine on the functional refractory period of the auriculo-ventricular transmission in the heart–lung preparation of the dog. J Pharmacol Exp Ther 103:412–419, 1951.

50. Levy MN, Zieske H: Autonomic control of cardiac pacemaker activity and atrioventricular transmission. J Appl Physiol 27:465–470, 1969.

51. Goldberg JM, Randall WC: Dromotropic effects of stellate stimulation on the AV node and internodal pathways. Proc Soc Exp Biol Med 143:623–628, 1973.

52. Priola DV: Effects of beta receptor stimulation and blockade on A-V nodal and bundle branch conduction in the canine heart. Am J Cardiol 31:35–40, 1973.

53. Spear JF, Moore EN: Influence of brief vagal and stellate nerve stimulation on pacemaker activity and conduction within the atrioventricular conduction system of the dog. Circ Res 32:27–41, 1973.

54. Geesbreght JM, Randall WC: Area localization of shifting cardiac pacemakers during sympathetic stimulation. Am J Physiol 220:1522–1527, 1971.

55. Wallick DW, Felder D, Levy MN: Autonomic control of pacemaker activity in the atrioventricular junction of the dog. Am J Physiol 235:H308–H313, 1978.

56. Tanahashi Y, Toyama J, Ito A, Sawada K, Ito T, Tsuzuki J, Hattori M, Ishikawa S, Yasui S: Effect of the autonomic blockade on the automaticity of the A-V junctional pacemaker in awake dogs. J Electrocardiol 12:77–81, 1979.

57. Martin PJ: The influence of the parasympathetic nervous system on atrioventricular conduction. Circ Res 41:593–599, 1977.

58. Hamlin RL, Smith CR: Effects of vagal stimulation on S-A and A-V nodes. Am J Physiol 215:560–568, 1968.

59. Martin PJ: Paradoxical dynamic interaction of heart period and vagal activity on atrioventricular conduction in the dog. Circ Res 40:81–89, 1977.

60. Wallick DW, Levy MN, Felder DS, Zieske H: Effects of repetitive bursts of vagal activity on atrioventricular junctional rate in dogs. Am J Physiol 237:H275–H281, 1979.

61. Lazzara R, El-Sherif N, Befeler B, Scherlag BJ: Regional refractoriness within the ventricular conduction system. An evaluation of the 'gate' hypothesis. Circ Res 39:254–262, 1976.

62. Gautier P, Coraboeuf E: The site of gating in the ventricular conducting system of rabbit, dog and monkey hearts. Experientia 36:431–433, 1980.

63. Vassalle M: Electrogenesis of the plateau and pacemaker potential. Ann Rev Physiol 41:425–440, 1979.

64. Tsien RW, Carpenter DO: Ionic mechanisms of pacemaker activity in cardiac Purkinje fibers. Fed Proc 37:2127–2131, 1978.

65. Rosen MR, Hordof AJ, Ilvento JP, Danilo P Jr: Effects of adrenergic amines on electrophysiological properties and automaticity of neonatal and adult canine Purkinje fibers. Circ Res 40:390–400, 1977.

66. Bailey JC, Watanabe AM, Besch HR Jr, Lathrop DA: Acetylcholine antagonism of the electrophysiological effects of isoproterenol on canine cardiac Purkinje fibers. Circ Res 44:378–383, 1979.

67. González-Serrato H, Alanís J: La acción de los nervios cardíacos y de la acetilcolina sobre el automatismo del corazón. Acta Physiol Lat Am 12:139–152, 1962.

68. Vassalle M, Levine MJ, Stuckey JH: On the sympathetic control of ventricular automaticity. Circ Res 23:249–258, 1968.

69. Lipsius SL, Gibbons WR: Acetylcholine lengthens action potentials of sheep cardiac Purkinje fibers. Am J Physiol 238:H237–H243, 1980.

70. Gadsby DC, Wit AL, Cranefield PF: The effects of acetylcholine on the electrical activity of canine cardiac Purkinje fibers. Circ Res 43:29–35, 1978.

71. Danilo P, Rosen MR, Hordof AJ: Effects of acetylcholine on the ventricular specialized conducting system of neonatal and adult dogs. Circ Res 43:777–784, 1978.

72. Tse WW, Han J, Yoon MS: Effect of acetylcholine on automaticity of canine Purkinje fibers. Am J Physiol 230:116–119, 1976.

73. Varghese PJ, Damato AN, Lau SH, Akhtar M, Bobb GA: The effect of heart rate, acetylcholine, and vagal stimulation on antegrade and retrograde His-Purkinje conductions in the intact heart. Am Heart J 86:203–210, 1973.

74. Eliakim M, Bellet S, Tawil E, Muller O: Effect of vagal stimulation and acetylcholine on the ventricle. Circ Res 9:1372–1379, 1961.

75. Nathan D, Beeler GW Jr: Electrophysiologic correlates of the inotropic effects of isoproterenol in canine myocardium. J Mol Cell Cardiol 7:1–15, 1975.

76. Vassort G, Rougier O, Garnier D, Sauviat MP, Coraboeuf E, Gargouil YM: Effects of adrenaline on membrane inward currents during the cardiac action potential. Pflugers Arch 309:70–81, 1969.

77. Quadbeck J, Reiter M: Cardiac action potential and inotropic effect of noradrenaline and calcium. Naunyn Schmiedebergs Arch Pharmacol 286:337–351, 1975.

78. Boyett MR: An analysis of the effect of the rate of stimulation and adrenaline on the duration of the cardiac action potential. Pflugers Arch 377:155–166, 1978.

79. Reuter H: Properties of two inward membrane currents in the heart. Ann Rev Physiol 41:413–424, 1979.

80. Allen DG, Blinks JR: Calcium transients in aequorin-injected frog cardiac muscle. Nature 273:509–513, 1978.

81. Kohlhardt M, Mnich Z: Studies on the inhibitory effect of verapamil on the slow inward current in mammalian ventricular myocardium. J Mol Cell Cardiol 10:1037–1052, 1978.

82. Randall WC: Sympathetic control of the heart. In: Randall WC (ed) Neural Regulation of the Heart. Oxford University Press, New York, 1977, pp 43–94.

83. Sarnoff SJ, Brockman SK, Gilmore JP, Linden RJ, Mitchell JH: Regulation of ventricular contraction: influence of cardiac sympathetic and vagal nerve stimulation on atrial and ventricular dynamics. Circ Res 8:1108–1122, 1960.

84. Levy MN: The cardiac and vascular factors that determine systemic blood flow. Circ Res 44:739–746, 1979.

85. Yanowitz F, Preston JB, Abildskov JA: Functional distribution of right and left stellate innervation to the ventricles: production of neurogenic electrocardiographic changes by unilateral alteration of sympathetic tone. Circ Res 18:416–428, 1966.

86. Higgins CB, Vatner SF, Braunwald E: Parasympathetic control of the heart. Pharmacol Rev 25:120–155, 1973.

87. Ten Eick R, Nawrath H, McDonald TF, Trautwein W: On the mechanism of the negative inotropic effect of acetylcholine. Pflugers Arch 361:207–213, 1976.

88. Giles W, Noble SJ: Changes in membrane currents in bullfrog atrium produced by acetylcholine. J Physiol (Lond) 261:103–123, 1976.

89. Hollenberg M, Carriere S, Barger AC: Biphasic action of acetylcholine on ventricular myocardium. Circ Res 16:527–536, 1965.

90. Levy MN, Zieske H: Comparison of the cardiac effects of vagus nerve stimulation and of acetylcholine infusions. Am J Physiol 216:890–897, 1969.

91. Buccino RA, Sonnenblick EH, Cooper T, Braunwald E: Direct positive inotropic effect of acetylcholine on myocardium. Evidence for multiple cholinergic receptors in the heart. Circ Res 11:1097–1108, 1966.

92. Hoffman BF, Suckling EE: Cardiac cellular potentials: effect of vagal stimulation and acetylcholine. Am J Physiol 173:312–320, 1953.

93. Inui J, Imamura H: Effects of acetylcholine on calcium-dependent electrical and mechanical responses in the guinea-pig papillary muscle partially depolarized by potassium. Naunyn Schmiedebergs Arch Pharmacol 299:1–7, 1977.

94. Gesell RA: Cardiodynamics in heart block as affected by auricular systole, auricular fibrillation and stimulation of the vagus nerve. Am J Physiol 40:267–313, 1916.

95. Wiggers CJ: The physiology of the mammalian auricle. II. The influence of the vagus nerves on the fractionate contraction of the right auricle. Am J Physiol 42:133–140, 1917.

96. Mitchell JH, Gilmore JP, Sarnoff SJ: The transport function of the atrium. Am J Cardiol 9:237–247, 1962.

97. Sarnoff SJ, Gilmore JP, Mitchell JH: Influence of atrial contraction and relaxation on closure of mitral valve. Circ Res 11:26–35, 1962.

98. Zaky A, Steinmetz E, Feigenbaum H: Role of atrium in closure of mitral valve in man. Am J Physiol 217:1652–1659, 1969.

99. Stuesse SL, Wallick DW, Levy MN: Autonomic control of right atrial contractile strength in the dog. Am J Physiol 236:H860–H865, 1979.

100. Duchêne-Marullaz P: Effets de l'innervation cholinergique sur le coeur de mammifère. Le tonus cardiomodérateur. J Physiol (Paris) 66:373–397, 1973.

101. Levy MN: Sympathetic–parasympathetic interactions in the heart. Circ Res 29:437–445, 1971.

102. Levy MN: Parasympathetic control of the heart. In: Randall WC (ed) Neural Regulation of the Heart. Oxford Univ Press, New York, 1976, pp 97–129.

103. Levy MN: Neural control of the heart: sympathetic–vagal interactions. In: Baan J, Noordergraaf A, Raines J (eds) Cardiovascular System Dynamics. MIT Press, Cambridge, 1978, pp 365–370.

104. Vanhoutte PM, Levy MN: Prejunctional cholinergic modulation of adrenergic neurotransmission in the cardiovascular system. Am J Physiol 238:H275–H281, 1980.

105. Martins JB, Zipes DP: Effects of sympathetic and vagal nerves on recovery properties of the endocardium and epicardium of the canine left ventricle. Circ Res 46:100–110, 1980.

106. Verrier RJ, Lown B: Sympathetic–parasympathetic interactions and ventricular electrical stability. In: Schwartz PJ, Brown AM, Malliani A, Zanchetti A (eds) Neural

Mechanisms in Cardiac Arrhythmias. Raven Press, New York, 1978, pp 75–85.

107. Kirchheim HR: Systemic arterial baroreceptor reflexes. Physiol Rev 56:100–176, 1976.

108. Thorén PN, Donald DE, Shepherd JT: Role of heart and lung receptors with nonmedullated vagal afferents in circulatory control. Circ Res 38 (Suppl II):2–9, 1976.

109. Armour JA, Wurster RD, Randall WC: Cardiac reflexes. In: Randall WC (ed) Neural Regulation of the Heart. Oxford Univ Press, New York, 1977, pp 157–186.

110. Brown AM: Cardiac reflexes. In: Handbook of Physiology. Section 2: The Cardiovascular System, vol 1. Am Physiol Soc, Bethesda, 1979, pp 677–690.

111. Coleridge JCG, Coleridge HM: Chemoreflex of the heart. In: Handbook of Physiology. Section 2: The Cardiovascular System, vol 1. Am Physiol Soc, Bethesda, 1979, pp 653–676.

112. Downing SE: Baroreceptor regulation of the heart. In: Handbook of Physiology. Section 2: The Cardiovascular System, vol 1. Am Physiol Soc, Bethesda, 1979, pp 621–652.

113. Bristow JD, Honour AJ, Pickering GW, Sleight P, Smyth HS: Diminished baroreflex sensitivity in high blood pressure. Circulation 39:48–54, 1969.

114. Higgins CB, Vatner SF, Eckberg DL, Braunwald E: Alterations in the baroreceptor reflex in experimental heart failure in the conscious dog. J Clin Invest 51:715–724, 1972.

115. Bainbridge FA: The influence of venous filling upon the rate of the heart. J Physiol (Lond) 50:65–84, 1915.

116. Vatner SF, Boettcher DH: Regulation of cardiac output by stroke volume and heart rate in conscious dogs. Circ Res 42:557–561, 1978.

117. Daly M de B, Angell-James JE, Elsner R: Role of carotid-body chemoreceptors and their reflex interactions in bradycardia and cardiac arrest. Lancet 1:764–767, 1979.

118. Berk JL, Levy MN: Profound reflex bradycardia produced by transient hypoxia or hypercapnia in man. Eur Surg Res 9:75–84, 1977.

CHAPTER 5

Cholinergic agonists and antagonists

AUGUST M. WATANABE

This chapter reviews the effects of the parasympathetic nervous system on the physiological properties of the cardiovascular system and the mechanisms by which these effects are produced. In the context of this background, the cardiovascular effects of agents that augment and antagonize parasympathetic nervous system activity will be discussed.

Physiological and biochemical background

Parasympathetic innervation of the heart

The location of the cell bodies of preganglionic vagus nerves in the central nervous system (CNS) and the anatomical pathways of vagus nerves leading from the CNS to the heart have been reviewed in Chapter 4. In the present discussion, the vagus innervation of the heart will be reviewed briefly with emphases on informaton relevant to understanding the pharmacology of drugs that modify parasympathetic nervous system function and on certain newer areas of information which may still be associated with some controversy (e.g., vagus innervation of ventricular tissues).

Vagus innervation of the sinoatrial node, atria, and atrioventricular node is firmly established and generally accepted, based on abundant and longstanding physiological data regarding the effects of vagus nerve stimulation on the function of these tissues and on histological, histochemical, and enzymatic evidence demonstrating directly the presence of the nerves or enzymes known to be localized to parasympathetic nerves (see Chapter 4). On the

other hand, it had been believed for many years that the vagus nerves did not innervate the ventricles, probably because modification of ventricular function in response to vagus nerve stimulation was more difficult to demonstrate than modification of the function of supraventricular structures. However, evidence accumulated during the past two decades clearly establishes that there is vagus innervation of ventricular tissues (myocardium, specialized conducting tissues and coronary arteries) and that this innervation probably has physiological and pathophysiological significance [1]. The direct evidence will be reviewed briefly here and the indirect (functional) evidence will be discussed in the section on cardiovascular effects of parasympathetic nerve activity.

The direct evidence for vagus innervation of ventricular tissues includes histological data, identification and quantification of enzymes known to be localized to parasympathetic nerves, and measurement of acetylcholine levels. Electron microscopic studies of normal canine ventricles revealed neural elements (C fibers) which persisted after total extrinsic cardiac denervation [2]. These fibers were by definition intrinsic and presumably represented parasympathetic fibers whose ganglia were located within the ventricles [3]. That some of these intrinsic neural fibers were parasympathetic was subsequently confirmed by histochemical studies which demonstrated in dog, cat, and human hearts that some of the fibers contained acetylcholinesterase [4–6]. The enzyme acetylcholinesterase is known to be concentrated in cholinergic fibers. The parasympathetic innervation of ventricular myocardium is sparse, particularly compared to the innerva-

Rosen, M. R. and Hoffman, B. F. (eds.), Cardiac Therapy. ISBN 0-89838-564-4.
© 1983, Martinus Nijhoff Publishers, Boston, The Hague, Dordrecht, Lancaster. Printed in the Netherlands.

tion of supraventricular structures. However, the specialized ventricular conducting system is richly innervated by parasympathetic fibers [6]. In one of the few studies in which direct histochemical measurements were correlated with functional assessments, the presence of parasympathetic innervation (demonstrated by acetylcholinesterase staining) of ventricular tissues was associated with vagus nerve stimulation-induced increases in ventricular fibrillation threshold (VFT) in dogs [6]. Injection of vinblastine (a neurotoxin) into parasympathetic nerve pathways at the base of the aorta markedly reduced acetylcholinesterase staining in the ventricles and concomitantly abolished vagus nerve stimulation-induced changes in VFT [6]. These results were interpreted as showing vagus nerve regulation of electrophysiological properties of the ventricles, presumably by effects on the properties of the specialized conducting system.

Another enzyme which has been studied to assess parasympathetic innervation of the heart is choline acetyltransferase (CAT) which catalyses the synthesis of acetylcholine from choline and acetyl coenzyme A. CAT activity has been measured in atria, ventricles, and the specialized nodal and conducting tissues of guinea pigs and rats [7–10]. Generally, the conclusions based on measurement of CAT activity are compatible with those based on measurement of acetylcholinesterase activity. That is, parasympathetic innervation of supraventricular structures and specialized ventricular conducting tissues were rich whereas the innervation of the ventricular free walls was relatively less abundant [7–10]. Extrinsic denervation of the heart decreased CAT activity consistent with the extrinsic parasympathetic innervation of the heart [10]. Acetylcholine has also been measured directly in cat hearts [11]. Consistent with the histochemical stu-

dies, atria contained greater amounts of acetylcholine than ventricles, and specialized Purkinje fibers appeared to contain very high amounts of the choline ester [11]. Vagotomy reduced acetylcholine content in the various cardiac tissues [11].

To summarize, assessment of parasympathetic innervation by several different means leads to generally consistent conclusions (Table 1). The data are acceptably consistent in view of the fundamental differences in the methods of assessing parasympathetic innervation and the probable differences in methods of dissecting the heart. These data indicate that the nodal tissues and specialized ventricular conducting tissues are most richly innervated by vagus nerves, the atria are the next most richly innervated, and the ventricles are the least richly innervated (Table 1). However, although the ventricles are less richly innervated than the other tissues, they are innervated and, as will be discussed in more detail in the section on cardiovascular effects of parasympathetic nerve activity, the innervation is probably physiologically significant.

Biosynthesis, storage and metabolism of acetylcholine

According to the theory of neurohumoral transmission, parasympathetic nerves transmit impulses across synapses and neuroeffector junctions by releasing the neurohumoral transmitter acetylcholine which interacts with postsynaptic nicotinic receptors in ganglia and with postjunctional nicotinic and muscarinic receptors located on the plasma membrane of innervated cells. The biosynthesis, storage, and release of acetylcholine have been reviewed extensively in the past several years and will not be covered in detail here [12–15].

Acetylcholine is synthesized in the region of the

Table 1. Chemical, histochemical, and enzymatic assessment of parasympathetic innervation of various regions of the heart.

	SAN	AVN	RA	LA	RV	LV	Purk	References
CAT	187	153	137	64	67	56	133–179	[7–10]
ACh			16.8	11.3	5.0	2.0	~65	[11]
AChE	4+	3+			1+	1+	3+	[2, 4–6]

CAT: choline acetyltransferase activity expressed as nmol g^{-1}hr^{-1}; ACh: acetylcholine expressed as nmol g^{-1}; AChE: acetylcholinesterase expressed by an arbitrary grading system of 0–4+ with 0 being complete absence of activity and 4+ being dense innervation. SAN: sinoatrial node, AVN: atrioventricular node, RA: right atrium, LA: left atrium, RV: right ventricle, LV: left ventricle, Purk: Purkinje fibers and specialized ventricular conduction system. Numbers in brackets refer to references from which data were taken.

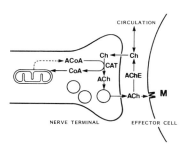

Figure 1. Diagrammatic representation of a parasympathetic nerve terminal and the components involved in the synthesis and metabolism of acetylcholine: ACoA = acetyl coenzyme A; CoA = coenzyme A; Ch = choline; CAT = choline acetyl transferase; ACh = acetylcholine; AChE = acetylcholinesterase; M = muscarinic receptor.

parasympathetic nerve terminals from choline and acetyl coenzyme A, a reaction catalyzed by CAT [7–10, 13–15] (Figure 1). Acetylcholine molecules thus synthesized are stored within synaptic vesicles in the nerve terminals. The evidence for storage of acetylcholine within vesicles is based on physiological (the observation that acetylcholine is released from nerve endings in quanta) and morphological (electron microscopic visualization of synaptic vesicles in nerve terminals) data [16, 17]. The concentration of acetylcholine within nerve terminals appears to remain relatively constant, regardless of the rate at which the neurotransmitter is released with nerve activity [14]. Thus, the rate of synthesis of acetylcholine can normally keep pace with the rate of release. The factors that regulate the rate of acetylcholine synthesis are still being elucidated, but probably include rate of choline uptake across nerve terminal membranes and the free cytoplasmic acetylcholine concentration [14, 16].

Upon activation of the parasympathetic nerves, action potentials travel along the nerves to the terminals leading to depolarization of terminal membranes. This membrane depolarization allows influx of calcium (Ca^{2+}) ions into the nerve terminals and subsequently there is fusion of the vesicular and axonal membranes and extrusion of the contents of the vesicles (acetylcholine) into the extracellular space [12, 16, 18]. Acetylcholine thus released interacts with muscarinic receptors located on the plasma membrane of innervated myocardial cells [19] (Figure 1).

The actions of released acetylcholine are termin-

ated by the enzyme acetylcholinesterase which rapidly hydrolyses acetylcholine to choline and acetic acid (Figure 1). Histochemical studies have shown the enzyme to be concentrated in cholinergic fibers (postganglionic parasympathetic, preganglionic autonomic and somatic motor) [2,4–6, 20] and at the postjunctional membrane [2], presumably in the vicinity of muscarinic receptors [19]. Thus, acetylcholinesterase appears to be located in critical regions where the enzyme and its substrate acetylcholine can readily interact for optimal physiological regulation of the effects of the neurotransmitter. The choline formed from the hydrolysis of acetylcholine can be washed away in the circulation or be recycled by being taken up by the terminal membrane for possible reuse in the biosynthesis of acetylcholine [14] (Figure 1).

Cardiovascular effects of parasympathetic nerve activity

The parasympathetic nervous system exerts its action on the heart by both direct effects and indirect effects mediated via parasympathetic modulation of the actions of the sympathetic nervous system. These two types of mediation of the effects of the parasympathetic nervous system will be discussed separately in this section.

Direct parasympathetic nervous system effects on cardiac function
The direct effects of parasympathetic nerve activity on the functional (electrophysiological and inotropic) properties of supraventricular structures are easily demonstrated, and therefore the effects are well known and established, and the physiological mechanisms for these effects well described [21]. These effects have been reviewed in Chapter 4 and in other comprehensive reviews [1, 22–24]. In general, the parasympathetic effects are inhibitory and functionally opposite to sympathetic effects (Table 2): (A) there is a negative chronotropic effect because of hyperpolarization and reduction in rate of diastolic depolarization of sinoatrial nodal cells; (B) there is a decrease in the rate of conduction of impulses across the atrioventricular node; and (C) there is marked shortening of action potential duration, hyperpolarization of the membrane and decrease in refractory period, associated with pronounced negative inotropic effects in atrial myo-

Table 2. Direct cardiac effects of vagal innervation.

Tissue	Physiological effects
Sino-atrial node	Decreased spontaneous pacing rate (Negative chronotropic effect)
Atrioventricular node	Decreased conduction velocity (negative dromotropic effect)
Atrial myocardium	Marked negative inotropic effect; Shortened action potential duration
Ventricular myocardium	Small negative inotropic effect; Altered repolarization pattern; Decreased tendency to fibrillate
Purkinje fibers	Decreased spontaneous automaticity
Coronary arteries	Vasodilation

thetic nervous system does regulate ventricular function [1, 24].

The effects of the parasympathetic nervous system on ventricular function can be demonstrated by direct electrical stimulation of vagus nerves or by modifying reflexly parasympathetic nervous tone. In whole animals, vagus nerve stimulation has been shown to produce clear-cut negative inotropic effects on ventricles [25–32] (Table 2, Figure 2). In some experiments, the negative inotropic effect has been observed to be quite potent [26] (Figure 2), whereas in others it has been observed to be 'small but significant' [30]. In the majority of the studies, it has been found that vagus nerve stimulation produces less pronounced negative inotropic effects on ventricular than on atrial muscle. Parasympathetic tone can also be activated reflexly in whole animals, for example by carotid chemoreceptor stimulation [33] or by activation of carotid sinuses by experimentally induced hypertension [34]. These maneuvers to activate reflexly vagus nerve activity produced clear-cut albeit small negative inotropic effects [33, 34] (Figure 3). The negative inotropic

cardium. In contrast to supraventricular structures, the effects of parasympathetic nervous system activity on the physiological properties of ventricular function have been relatively more difficult to demonstrate [21], and only within the past two decades has it become widely accepted that the parasympa-

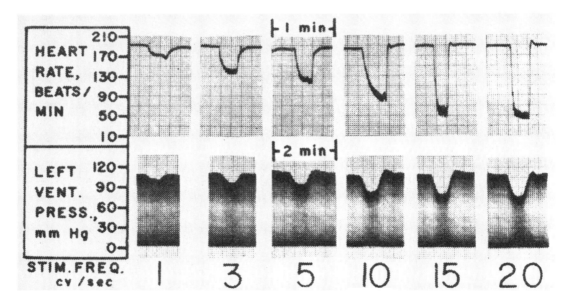

Figure 2. Effects of electrical stimulation of decentralized right vagus nerve on spontaneous heart rate (upper) and systolic left ventricular pressure (lower) in an isovolumetric canine left ventricular preparation. For ventricular pressure measurements, atria and ventricles were paced simultaneously at a rate of 210 beats/min. Coronary perfusion pressure: 130 mmHg. Vagus nerve stimulation: 10 V, 5 msec at frequencies indicated at bottom of figure. Duration of stimulation: 15 sec in unpaced heart, 30 sec in paced heart. Sequence of stimuli: in unpaced heart, 10, 1, 5, 15, 3, 20 cycles/sec; in paced heart, 1, 10, 3, 15, 5, 20 cycles/sec (reprinted with permission from [26]).

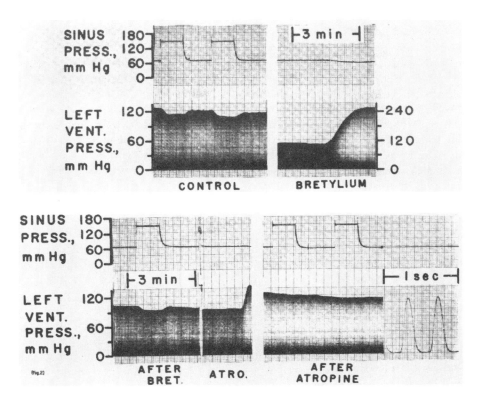

Figure 3. Left ventricular pressure responses in a paced, isovolumetric canine left ventricular preparation. Carotid sinuses were isolated to allow control of intrasinus pressure. Note that sudden elevations in sinus pressure reduce left ventricular pressure, by reflex activation of vagus nerve tone. Atropine sulfate (4.0 mg) per se increases left ventricular pressure, presumably by removing tonic vagus nerve restraint, and blocks the sinus hypertension-induced negative inotropic effect (reprinted with permission from [34]).

effects of vagus nerve activity, increased either by direct electrical stimulation of nerves or reflexly, were abolished by atropine (Figure 3). In some animal experiments, results suggest that spontaneous or tonic vagus nerve activity (in the absence of nerve stimulation) exerts a restraining or negative inotropic influence on ventricular function. Blocking vagus nerve effects per se, by administration of atropine or cooling the vagus nerve, produced positive inotropic effects [34] (Figure 3). Denervation experiments with canine hearts support the foregoing results and also provide functional evidence for the location of vagus nerve cell bodies as well as nerve terminals within the heart and, specifically, within the ventricles [35, 36]. Following total cardiac denervation, administration of nicotine produced negative inotropic effects on both atria and ventricles which were blocked by atropine [35, 36]. It was concluded that nicotine acted on ganglia located within the ventricular myocardium. The

nicotinic effect on ganglia induced release of acetylcholine from the terminals of the intrinsic parasympathetic nerves [35, 36].

The negative inotropic effects of the parasympathetic nervous system can also be demonstrated by administration of the neurotransmitter acetylcholine. Such studies done in whole animals yield results compatible with those from vagus nerve stimulation experiments. Acetylcholine produced negative inotropic effects on ventricles [25, 35, 36] which were enhanced by coadministration of neostigmine [25] and blocked by atropine [25, 35]. When acetylcholine was administered directly to isolated whole ventricles or ventricular strips in vitro, the negative inotropic effects were either absent or very small [37–39]. These results suggest that, in the whole animal studies mentioned earlier, a component of the negative inotropic effects of vagus nerve stimulation or acetylcholine may have been related to parasympathetic modulation of tonic sympathetic activity. Basal spontaneous sympathetic activity was less likely to have been present in isolated tissue studies. This will be discussed in more detail in the next section.

As mentioned earlier, whereas parasympathetic innervation of ventricular myocardium is less than that of supraventricular structures, innervation of specialized ventricular conducting tissues is rich (Table 1) [6–11]. Moreover, cellular electrophysiological studies have shown that acetylcholine suppresses spontaneous automaticity of isolated canine cardiac Purkinje fibers [40, 41] (Table 2). These histochemical and cellular electrophysiologic data indicate that vagus nerve terminals reach specialized conducting tissues in the ventricles and that acetylcholine released from these terminals might exert important effects on the electrophysiological properties of these tissues.

This conclusion is supported by studies in whole animals and in humans. Vagus nerve stimulation slowed spontaneous ventricular rate in dogs with experimentally induced complete atrioventricular block [25, 42] (Table 2, Figure 4). In the example in the bottom panel of Figure 4, vagus nerve stimulation during complete heart block slowed the rate of the ventricular ectopic pacemaker in dogs. The effect of vagus nerve stimulation on ventricular automaticity was mimicked by acetylcholine [25]. The depressant effect of acetylcholine was enhanced by the coadministration of neostigmine and blocked by atropine [25]. Vagus nerve stimulation altered ventricular repolarization in dogs, as assessed by changes in the configuration of the T-wave on the electrocardiogram [43] (Table 2). This effect was also mimicked by acetylcholine [44]. These effects of enhanced parasympathetic activity on ventricular repolarization could not be accounted for by changes in heart rate, but rather suggested a direct effect of the parasympathetic nervous system on repolarization of ventricles. Vagus nerve stimulation increased VFT in normally perfused (nonischemic) hearts of dogs [6]. Ablation of vagus nerves to the ventricles with a neurotoxin abolished this vagal-induced increase in VFT and eliminated ventricular staining for acetylcholinesterase in the same hearts [6]. Acetylcholine administered to spontaneously contracting rabbit and rat ventricles significantly slowed the spontaneous rate of these tissues [45]. This effect was augmented by physostigmine and blocked by atropine [45]. Thus, a variety of studies in whole animals and in isolated tissues suggest that parasympathetic activity influences the electrophysiological properties of ventricles.

Enhanced parasympathetic activity also may play an important role in influencing the electrophysiological properties of ischemic myocardium (Table 2). This could occur by parasympathetic diminution of ischemia (by slowing heart rate, decreasing contractility and/or increasing coronary blood flow), by parasympathetic antagonism of

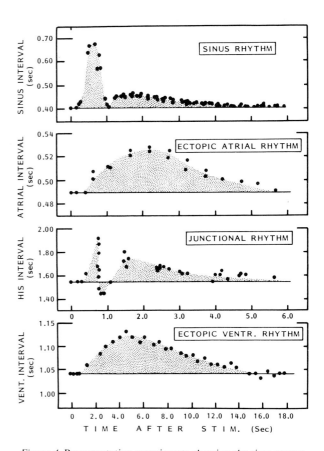

Figure 4. Representative experiments showing the time course of the changes in basic cycle length of canine hearts under control of the sino-atrial node (sinus rhythm) and various ectopic pacemakers. Each panel represents an individual experiment. A 100-msec burst of stimuli was delivered to the vagus (right vagus in top three and left in bottom panel) at time zero. Propranolol (1.0 mg/kg) was present for the sinus and junctional rhythm experiments. Complete atrioventricular block was produced to allow assessment of vagus nerve effects on the ectopic ventricular rhythm (bottom panel). Notice that in a dog with complete heart block (bottom panel), left vagus nerve stimulation slows the ectopic ventricular pacemaker rate (adapted with permission from [42]).

100

sympathetic arrhythmogenic effects (to be discussed in more detail in the following section), or by direct electrophysiological effects of vagus nerves. Evidence for the latter comes from studies of acute ischemia in dogs and cats [46–48]. Ischemia increased the disparity of refractory periods in contiguous areas of ventricles [46], and decreased the ventricular fibrillation threshold [46] and the time to onset of spontaneous ventricular fibrillation [46, 48]. Vagus nerve stimulation attenuated the ischemia-induced reduction in VFT [46] and delayed the onset of spontaneous ventricular fibrillation and death [47, 48]. That these protective effects of vagus nerve stimulation were mediated by released acetylcholine was supported by other studies which showed that edrophonium reversed ischemia-induced reductions in VFT [49].

Although limited in number, a few studies suggest parasympathetic influences on the electrophysiological properties of ventricles in humans. Activation of the baroreceptor reflex by carotid sinus pressure has been described either to suppress or promote ventricular arrhythmias [50–52]. In one clinical study, a series of cases was described in which carotid sinus massage eliminated ventricular ectopic depolarizations [51]. On the other hand, a case was reported in which carotid sinus massage was thought to induce ventricular fibrillation [50]. If the parasympathetic nervous system does regulate the electrophysiological properties of ventricles, either antiarrhythmic or arrhythmogenic effects of activating vagus nerve tone can be rationalized. Depending on the environment in which the alterations in vagus nerve tone are produced (presence or absence of ischemia, coexistent sympathetic tone, electrolyte concentrations), and the uniformity throughout the ventricles of the vagus nerve effect, increased vagus nerve activity theoretically could either reduce or enhance the vulnerability to fibrillation [43, 44, 53]. The previously mentioned clinical studies did not include enough evidence to prove that the effects of carotid sinus pressure were in fact mediated by efferent vagus nerve activity [50, 51]. It is possible that carotid sinus massage caused a withdrawal of sympathetic activity and thus decreased ventricular ectopy [51]. Alternatively, the effects of carotid sinus pressure on ventricular ectopy may have been secondary to changes in hemodynamics (e.g. decreased heart rate, decreased atrial contractility) [51]. In one clinical study, it seems

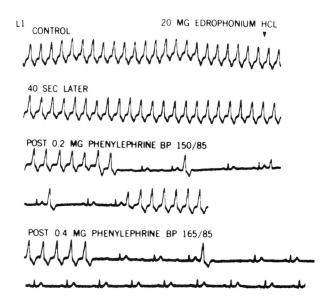

Figure 5. Lead I of electrocardiogram of a patient with ventricular tachycardia. Control rate was 180 beats/min which slowed to 150 beats/min after edrophonium. The middle and bottom pairs of tracings were recorded after edrophonium administration. 0.2 mg phenylephrine temporarily converts rhythm to normal sinus rhythm (middle tracings) and 0.4 mg permanently terminates ventricular tachycardia (bottom tracings) (reprinted with permission from [52]).

well established that increased parasympathetic nerve activity reversed ventricular tachycardia [52]. In a group of patients with recurrent, spontaneous ventricular tachycardia, reflexly increased vagus nerve activity by drug-induced hypertension or carotid sinus massage reversed ventricular tachycardia [52] (Figure 5). The efficacy of these maneuvers was enhanced by edrophonium, and the antiarrhythmic effects of increased vagus nerve activity were abolished by atropine [52] (Figure 5). Recently performed clinical electrophysiological studies also provide evidence for parasympathetic influences on the electrophysiological properties of ventricles. Ventricular functional and effective refractory periods were measured with programmed stimulation combined with direct intraventricular catheter recordings of ventricular electrograms [54]. Administration of atropine to the human subjects significantly shortened ventricular refractory periods, suggesting that in the basal, untreated state vagus nerve tone was exerting an effect on refractoriness [54].

Parasympathetic nerve activity also regulates the vascular tone of coronary arteries. Electrical stimulation of vagus nerves increased coronary blood flow in dogs [55]. Reflexly increased vagus nerve activity by injection of veratrum alkaloids into the coronary artery (Bezold-Jarisch reflex) produced coronary vasodilation [56]. These vagus nerve effects on coronary vascular tone were abolished by vagotomy or administration of atropine [55, 56]. Other determinants of coronary flow (aortic pressure, myocardial systolic compression, myocardial metabolic changes) were controlled or accounted for, so it was clearly established that the reduced coronary resistance was due to increased parasympathetic activity [55, 56].

Indirect parasympathetic nervous system effects on cardiac function: sympathetic–parasympathetic interaction

It is now well established that the parasympathetic nervous system regulates cardiovascular function not only by direct effects but also by means of parasympathetic modulation of sympathetic effects on the cardiovascular system. The anatomical and molecular bases for sympathetic–parasympathetic interactions in regulating cardiac function are well established. In the heart, sympathetic and vagus nerve terminals have been found to lie in close apposition to one another and even to be enclosed by the same Schwann cell [4, 57]. There is biochemical evidence that muscarinic receptors are located on prejunctional sympathetic nerve terminals [58] and that both muscarinic and beta-adrenergic receptors are located on the sarcolemma of myocardial cells [19, 59]. Thus, the anatomy of the nerves and the location of the neurotransmitter receptors are compatible with physical interaction between these two systems. The interaction between the sympathetic and parasympathetic nervous systems occurs at two levels, interneuronally and intracellularly [1, 24, 39, 60–64] (Figure 6).

The interneuronal interaction between the sympathetic and parasympathetic nervous systems first was shown by observing the effect of acetylcholine infusions on norepinephrine output from isolated perfused rabbit hearts [65]. Electrical stimulation of postganglionic sympathetic nerves increased norepinephrine output. Acetylcholine caused a concentration-dependent inhibition of this output and these cholinergic effects were blocked by atro-

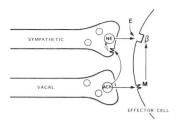

Figure 6. Diagrammatic representation of sympathetic and vagus nerve terminals and interaction between them. Acetylcholine (ACh) released from vagus nerve endings activates muscarinic receptors (M) on prejunctional sympathetic nerve endings. This results in inhibition of norepinephrine (NE) release. In addition, acetylcholine activates muscarinic receptors on postjunctional effector cells and this activation can modulate the cellular response to beta receptor activation by catecholamines: E = the circulating catecholamin, epinephrine.

pine [65]. Subsequent studies showed that endogenous acetylcholine released from vagal nerve terminals also could inhibit norepinephrine release from sympathetic nerve terminals [66–68] (Figure 7). The vagal inhibition of norepinephrine release was blocked by atropine [67, 68] and mimicked by methacholine [68]. Furthermore, in these studies the physiological importance of the vagal inhibition of norepinephrine release was demonstrated. Catecholamine output into the coronary sinus correlated with measured hemodynamic parameters [67, 68], when sympathetic nerves were stimulated alone or simultaneously with vagus nerve stimulation (Figures 7 and 8). When vagus nerves were stimulated catecholamine output was attenuated and the hemodynamic response to sympathetic nerve stimulation was blunted (Figure 8). One of these latter studies also provided further evidence for vagus nerve innervation of ventricular structures and for the physiological relevance of this innervation [67]. The contractile parameters measured were ventricular and most of the norepinephrine output was of ventricular origin [67].

Parasympathetic nervous activity also modulates sympathetic effects on vascular tone in those vessels which are innervated by both systems. Vagus nerve stimulation or administration of acetylcholine inhibited sympathetic nerve stimulation-induced vasoconstriction [69, 70] and associated release of norepinephrine from sympathetic nerves [71].

Thus, one important mechanism by which the parasympathetic nervous system modulates the ef-

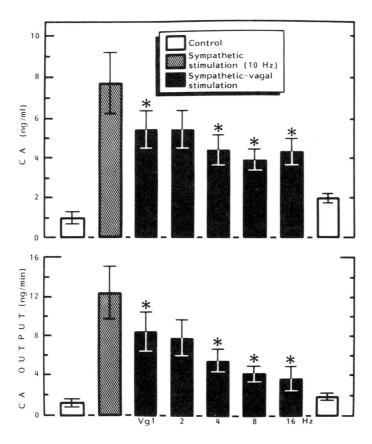

Figure 7. Effect of vagus nerve stimulation in dogs on coronary sinus catecholamine (CA) concentration (upper panel) and catecholamine output (lower panel, value corrected for changes in coronary flow) during control condition, and during sympathetic stimulation alone or simultaneously with vagus nerve stimulation. Note that sympathetic stimulation markedly increases catecholamine output and that this increase is blunted by simultaneous vagus nerve stimulation. The numbers below the bars indicate frequency of vagus nerve stimulation. Values are means ± SEM from seven dogs. Asterisks indicate significant difference from value obtained with sympathetic stimulation alone (p < 0.05) (adapted with permission from [68]).

fects of the sympathetic nervous system is by regulating the release of norepinephrine from sympathetic nerve terminals (Figure 6). The mechanism by which this occurs at the level of the sympathetic terminal membrane remains unknown. Possibilities include a muscarinic cholinergic interference with the Ca^{2+}-dependent excitation–secretion coupling or muscarinic-induced hyperpolarization of the terminal membrane [62].

The interneuronal interaction between the sympathetic and parasympathetic nervous systems cannot account entirely for the parasympathetic modulation of the cardiovascular effects of sympathetic stimulation [1, 24, 60, 64]. Studies in intact animals clearly demonstrate that vagus nerve activity attenuates the cardiac effects of circulating catecholamines. In conscious, chronically instrumented dogs, blockade of muscarinic receptors with atropine markedly augmented the positive inotropic effects of the catecholamines norepinephrine, isoproterenol, and dopamine [72] (Figure 9). The atropine-induced enhancement of catecholamine effects was abolished by vagotomy [72]. These results were interpreted as showing a vagal antagonism of the inotropic effects of circulating catecholamines. In the intact animal, tonic vagus nerve activity restrained the response of the myocardium to beta receptor stimulation by circulating catecholamines. Blockade of postjunctional muscarinic receptors removed this vagal restraint. Vagotomy also re-

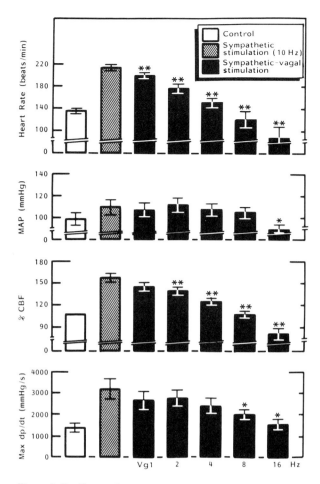

Figure 8. Cardiovascular responses to sympathetic stimulation alone or simultaneously with vagus nerve stimulation (frequency of vagus stimulation indicated by the numbers below the bars). Note the vagal attenuation of the cardiac effects of sympathetic stimulation and the good correlation of this attenuation with the reduction in catecholamine output shown in Figure 7. Values are mean ± SEM from seven dogs. Statistical significance of differences from sympathetic stimulation alone indicated by asterisks (*p < 0.05, **p < 0.01) (adapted with permission from [68]).

moved the vagal restraint so that in vagotomized animals muscarinic blockade became ineffective. These results in conscious animals also provide functional evidence for vagal innervation of the ventricles and suggest physiological relevance for this innervation. These results are consistent with earlier studies in anesthetized dogs which showed that intracoronary administration of acetylcholine attenuated the inotropic effects of catecholamines infused into coronary arteries [73].

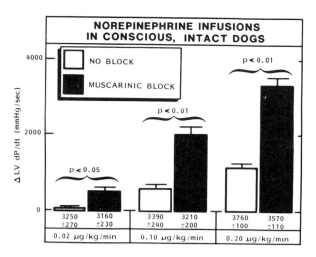

Figure 9. Effect of muscarinic blockade with atropine (0.1 mg/kg) on steady-state positive inotropic effects of three doses of norepinephrine in intact conscious dogs. Measurements were taken after 10 min of intravenous infusion. Control values are shown at the base of the bars (adapted with permission from [72]).

The intracellular (postjunctional) interaction between the sympathetic and parasympathetic nervous systems has been documented by a wide variety of studies with isolated organs and tissues. In cardiac preparations from various mammalian species (guinea pig, rabbit, cat, dog, and rat), it has been clearly shown that choline esters antagonize the positive inotropic effects of beta receptor agonists [37–39, 74–78] (Figure 10). This antiadrenergic effect of choline esters was blocked by atropine, thus verifying that the effect was mediated via muscarinic receptors presumably located on the sarcolemma of myocardial cells [38, 74, 75]. In most of these studies with isolated tissues, the negative inotropic effects of muscarinic agonists given alone were prominent and easily detectable in atria [38, 78], but were small in ventricles [38, 39, 74, 76, 77]. Muscarinic antagonism of the positive inotropic effects of catecholamines was seen in both atria and ventricles. Thus, it appears that in atrial tissues muscarinic agonists produce negative inotropic effects both by a direct action and by antagonizing the effects of the beta receptor agonists. By contrast, in ventricles the predominant muscarinic effect appears to be inhibition of the inotropic effects of beta agonists. In the previously mentioned studies of whole animals, which appeared to demon-

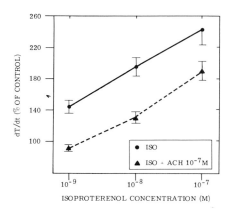

Figure 10. Effect of acetylcholine (ACh) (10^{-7} M) on the positive inotropic effect of isoproterenol (Iso) in isolated, perfused guinea pig ventricles. Measurements were taken after hearts had reached a stable level of contractions after 2 min of continuous drug infusion. Note that the inotropic response to isoproterenol is markedly attenuated by acetylcholine. Values are means ± SEM for 7–15 hearts (reprinted with permission from [39]).

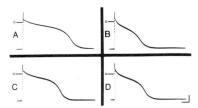

Figure 11. Effect of acetylcholine on the shortening of action potential duration produced by isoproterenol in a canine cardiac Purkinje fiber. (A) A control cardiac Purkinje fiber action potential. (B) Action potential duration shortening produced by isoproterenol (10^{-7} M). (C) The addition of acetylcholine (10^{-6} M) partially reversed the shortening of action potential duration effected by isoproterenol. (D) Atropine (10^{-6} M) attenuated the effects of acetylcholine, resulting in an action potential duration resembling that produced by the superfusion of isoproterenol alone. Zero potential indicated in each panel. Calibrations: horizontal bar = 50 msec; vertical bar = 25 mV (reprinted with permission from [85]).

strate a direct negative inotropic effect of vagus nerve stimulation on ventricles, it is possible that there was simultaneous stimulation of beta-adrenergic receptors by circulating catecholamines and/or norepinephrine released from tonically active sympathetic nerves. Thus, part of what appeared to be a direct negative inotropic effect may in fact have represented parasympathetic modulation of sympathetic effects. Stimulation of beta receptors by endogenous catecholamines would be less likely to occur in isolated preparations. In ventricular tissue, endogenous acetylcholine released from the tissue by field stimulation also antagonized the positive inotropic effects of catecholamines [79, 80]. Such results have also been obtained in human papillary muscles [80]. These results provided indirect evidence for vagus innervation of human ventricles [80].

In isolated cardiac preparations, muscarinic agonists also antagonize the electrophysiological effects of catecholamines. Choline esters attenuated the positive chronotropic effects of catecholamines on isolated atrial preparations [81–83], presumably by antagonizing the catecholamine-induced increase in spontaneous phase 4 depolarization [84]. Muscarinic agonists antagonize the electrophysiological effects of catecholamines on isolated Purkinje fibers or ventricular muscle. Acetylcholine

inhibited isoproterenol-induced shortening of action potential duration in normally polarized, paced cardiac Purkinje fibers [85] (Figure 11). Acetylcholine also abolished isoproterenol-dependent slow responses in cardiac Purkinje fibers or guinea pig papillary muscles [85, 86]. Muscarinic agonists also exerted antiarrhythmic effects in cats or dogs treated with a combination of hydrocarbon anesthetics and epinephrine [87, 88].

Activation of muscarinic receptors also modulates the cardiac metabolic effects of beta-adrenergic receptor stimulation. Acetylcholine completely antagonized the glycogenolytic effect of epinephrine in isolated perfused guinea pig hearts [89]. Subsequent studies showed that this was due to a muscarinic antagonism of beta-adrenergic activation of glycogen phosphorylase [37, 77, 90, 91] (Figure 12). Acetylcholine also antagonized norepinephrine-induced stimulation of lipase in dog myocardium [92].

Thus, in isolated cardiac preparations there is abundant evidence for intracellular interaction between activation of beta-adrenergic and muscarinic receptors (Figure 6). In isolated ventricular tissues, it appears that modulation of sympathetic effects is a major mechanism by which the parasympathetic nervous system exerts its effect. Choline esters alone produced little or no change in the inotropic [37–39], electrophysiologic [85] or metabolic [37, 89, 91] properties of isolated ventricular tissues.

105

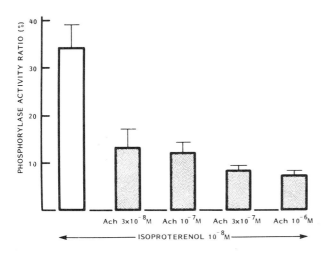

Figure 12. Muscarinic cholinergic antagonism of isoproterenol activation of glycogen phosphorylase in isolated perfused hearts taken from hyperthyroid rats. Basal phosphorylase activity ratio was 8%. Values were mean ± SEM of 6–8 hearts.

Only when these physiological or metabolic responses were altered by beta-adrenergic agonists did muscarinic cholinergic effects become readily apparent. In this situation, muscarinic agonists potently antagonized the beta-adrenergic alteration of these properties [37– 39, 85, 89, 91]. The mechanisms for the intracellular interaction between the components of the sympathetic and parasympathetic systems will be discussed in the section on intracellular effectors coupled to muscarinic receptors.

In intact animals and in humans, it is likely that parasympathetic nervous system activity regulates the cardiovascular effects of the sympathetic nervous system at both the interneuronal and intracellular levels. Acetylcholine released from vagus nerve terminals regulates the release of norepinephrine from sympathetic terminals (Figure 6). Acetylcholine also interacts with postjunctional muscarinic receptors on the cells of innervated organs to modulate the effects of catecholamines (both norepinephrine released from nerve terminals and circulating epinephrine) acting on beta-adrenergic receptors (Figure 6). The intracellular level of interaction is the only type that can occur with circulating catecholamines such as epinephrine (Figure 6).

The revelation of mechanisms (interneuronal and intracellular) for parasympathetic modulation of sympathetic effects on the heart helps to explain a large body of physiological data regarding autonomic nervous system control of cardiac function. For example, it has been known for many years that heart rate in an intact animal in response to simultaneous sympathetic–parasympathetic stimulation is not simply the algebraic sum of that rate which would result from separate sympathetic and parasympathetic stimulation [93]. Rather, it was observed that parasympathetic activity predominated over sympathetic activity in regulating heart rate [93]. These early observations were confirmed and subjected to mathematical analysis by other investigators [94, 95]. With strong vagus stimulation, sympathetic effects on heart rate were abolished [95].

This sympathetic–parasympathetic interaction also has been observed in the autonomic regulation of atrioventricular nodal pacemaker activity [96], and atrial [97] and ventricular [98, 99] contractility. As in the case of sinoatrial automaticity, sympathetic effects on atrioventricular automaticity and atrial contractility virtually could be abolished by strong vagus nerve stimulation [96, 97]. The interneuronal and intracellular interactions described above probably account for this dominating effect of vagus nerve activity over sympathetic activity. Even though the sympathetic nervous system may be stimulated to high levels of activity, strong vagus stimulation can override sympathetic effects by inhibiting norepinephrine release (interneuronal) and by antagonizing the intracellular effects of catecholamines that reach beta-adrenergic receptors on effector cells (Figure 6).

In parasympathetic regulation of certain ventricular properties, the effects appear to occur predominantly by means of sympathetic–parasympathetic interaction. As stated earlier, in isolated ventricular tissues muscarinic agonists have minimal effects on contractility [37–39], metabolic properties [37, 89, 91] or certain electrophysiological properties [85]. Even in intact animals the negative inotropic effects of vagus nerve stimulation or acetylcholine generally are small [26–30]. However, if sympathetic nervous system activity is increased (by stimulating sympathetic nerves in intact animals or administering catecholamines to isolated tissues) the effect of increasing parasympathetic nervous activity (by stimulating vagus nerves or administration of choline esters) becomes prominent [1, 24, 37–39, 60, 73, 85, 98, 99].

Sympathetic–parasympathetic interaction is probably also involved in autonomic influences on the electrical stability of ventricles. Vagus nerve stimulation in dogs shifted the strength–interval curve (a measure of ventricular excitability) later into electrical diastole [100]. This vagal effect was abolished by pretreatment of the animals with propranolol. It was concluded that the vagal effect on ventricular excitability was mediated via vagus nerve opposition of tonic sympathetic tone [100]. Vagus nerve stimulation prolonged ventricular effective refractory periods (ERP) in dogs, whereas sympathetic stimulation shortened ERP [101]. ERP prolongation by vagus nerve stimulation was attenuated markedly after sympathectomy and abolished by propranolol [101], thus suggesting that the vagus nerve effects on ERP were largely mediated via vagus modulation of sympathetic effects. In contrast to a previously mentioned study [6], one study in dogs suggested that vagus effects on VFT were not direct but rather mediated via vagal modulation of sympathetic effects on VFT [102]. In the absence of sympathetic stimulation, vagus nerve stimulation had no effect on VFT [102]. During stellate ganglion stimulation, however, vagus nerve stimulation increased VFT [102]. It was concluded that increased sympathetic activity was a required precondition for vagus nerve effects on VFT. The reason for the differences in these two studies of vagus nerve effects on VFT are not clear [6, 102]. However, it is possible that in the earlier study [6], tonic sympathetic activity and circulating epinephrine were modifying the vulnerability of the ventricles to fibrillation. Part of the vagus nerve effect observed could have resulted from vagal modulation of tonic sympathetic effects.

Biochemistry of muscarinic cholinergic receptors

A large body of information regarding the physiology and pharmacology of muscarinic receptors has come from classical pharmacologic studies, based on physiological experiments combined with analysis of structure-activity relationships [103]. These studies have yielded physiological evidence for tissue distribution of muscarinic receptors (see preceding section), evidence regarding the topology of muscarinic receptors, and the determinants of

agonist and antagonist activity in drugs that interact with the receptor [103]. The recent development of radioligand binding assays, which allows the direct study of muscarinic receptors, has resulted in major new discoveries regarding the biochemistry and molecular pharmacology of muscarinic receptors [104–109]. New information resulting from radioligand binding studies of muscarinic receptors has been reviewed recently [105–109]. This section will review some of the major findings which are particularly relevant to the cardiovascular pharmacology of drugs that modify parasympathetic nervous system function.

Radioligand binding studies of muscarinic receptors were first performed by Paton and Rang who studied the interaction of [^{3}H]-atropine with muscarinic receptors on guinea pig gastrointestinal smooth muscle [110]. Subsequently, a number of investigators have used a variety of antagonist ligands to study muscarinic receptors in various tissues ·[106–108]. [^{3}H]-quinuclidinyl benzilate ([^{3}H]-QNB) is the ligand that has been most widely used to study cardiac muscarinic receptors [111–118]. [^{3}H]-benzilyl-choline mustard, an alkylating agent, has been used to label muscarinic receptors irreversibly. The irreversibility of binding of this alkylating agent allows performance of certain studies which would be difficult or impossible with reversibly binding ligands [120]. For example, with radiolabeled alkylating ligands it is possible to label the receptor and subsequently solubilize the membranes while maintaining labeling of the receptor [120]. Fewer agonist ligands have been utilized to study muscarinic receptors than antagonist ligands [106, 107, 119, 121]. Agonist ligands have the disadvantages, compared to available antagonist ligands, of having lower affinity for the receptor and more nonspecific binding.

Three major criteria are generally applied to radioligand binding studies to establish that binding of the ligand represents specific interaction with the receptor. These criteria are saturability, specificity, and localization of binding. Receptors exist in a finite number so specific binding should saturate with increasing concentrations of the radioligand (Figure 13A). If radioligands are binding to true muscarinic receptors, this binding should be inhibited by appropriate concentrations of drugs known from physiological studies to interact with the receptor and should not be modified by drugs which

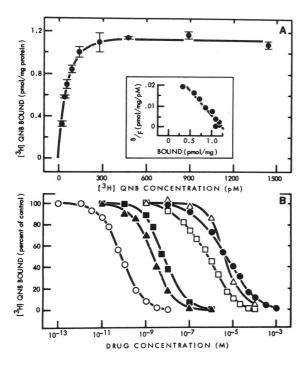

Figure 13. Saturation of [³H]QNB binding (A) and agonist and antagonist competition curves for [³H]QNB binding (B) to muscarinic receptors in membrane vesicles derived from canine ventricular myocardium. Inset in panel A is a Scatchard plot of the saturation data. In panel B, data from separate experiments performed in purified membrane preparations are presented, with binding expressed as a percent of control binding in the absence of competing drug. For all curves, [³H]QNB concentration was approximately 80 pM. Drugs are QNB (○), dexetimide (▲), atropine (■), oxotremorine (□), methacholine (●), and levetimide (△) (reprinted with permission from [117]).

do not interact with the receptor; i.e., the binding should fulfill the criterion of pharmacologic specificity (Figure 13B). Finally, saturable binding of muscarinic radioligands should occur only in tissues known from pharmacologic studies to possess muscarinic receptors. Each of these criteria has been fulfilled in radioligand binding studies of muscarinic receptors in cardiac tissues [106, 107, 112–118].

From classical pharmacological analysis in intact tissues or whole animals, muscarinic receptors in the heart are thought to be located postjunctionally on the innervated tissues and also on prejunctional sympathetic nerve terminals (see preceding section) (Figure 6). Although the presence of muscarinic receptors on prejunctional sympathetic nerve ter-

minals has been strongly suggested by physiological experiments [65–68] (Figures 7 and 8), the few studies that have attempted to demonstrate this directly by radioligand binding assays have not been in agreement [58, 122, 123]. Three different groups have attempted to demonstrate with binding assays the presence of prejunctional muscarinic receptors by comparing the density of specific binding sites in hearts from normal animals with the density in hearts from animals subjected to chemical sympathectomy with 6-OH-dopamine. One study showed a 30% reduction in specific binding of [³H]-QNB in particulate fractions derived from hearts of 6-OH-dopamine-treated animals [58]. The conclusion was that in hearts from untreated animals [³H]-QNB was binding both to postjunctional muscarinic receptors on myocardial cell membranes and to receptors on prejunctional sympathetic nerve terminals. The 30% reduction in [³H]-QNB binding after sympathectomy was thought to reflect loss of those sites originally on sympathetic nerve terminals [58]. However, two other studies that used the same method of sympathectomy did not show any change in the number of [³H]-QNB binding sites in the heart [122, 123]. The reasons for this discrepancy are not apparent. However, the presence of muscarinic receptors on prejunctional sympathetic nerve terminals seems clear from intact tissue and whole animal studies [65–68]. The inability as yet to verify this conclusively with binding studies may reflect limits of the sensitivity of the assay and/or problems with the method of sympathectomy. Perhaps the percentage contribution of neural binding sites to total cardiac binding sites is so small that the assay cannot detect the loss of sites resulting from destruction of sympathetic nerves. Alternatively, 6-OH-dopamine may produce nonspecific effects to alter the total number of binding sites and thus obscure any change that may have been produced by denervation.

Muscarinic receptors have been demonstrated in various regions of the heart by radioligand binding studies. The localization of these receptors by binding assays agrees well with physiological evidence for their distribution [124]. Binding studies of muscarinic receptors in various organs indicate that the receptors are membrane associated and probably predominantly or exclusively located in the plasma membrane [19, 59, 113, 124–127] (Figure 14). Sarcolemma and sarcoplasmic reticulum were isolated

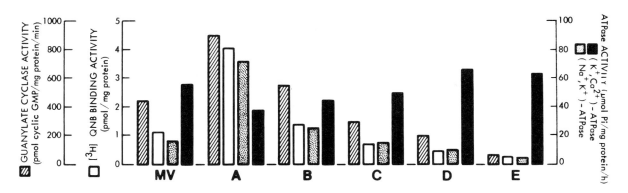

Figure 14. Copurification of particulate guanylate cyclase activity and [^{3}H]QNB binding activity with sarcolemmal (S1) Na$^+$, K$^+$-ATPase activity. Ca^{2+}-ATPase activity, the marker for sarcoplasmic reticulum (SR) membranes, is also shown. MV-membrane visicles which contain both sarcolemmal and sarcoplasmic reticulum membranes. This relatively crude MV fraction was then preloaded with Ca^{2+}-oxalate to increase selectively the density of SR vesicles, and the MV was subfractionated by density gradient centrifugation as described previously [59]. Fraction A is most enriched in Na$^+$,K$^+$-ATPase activity, with remaining fractions having progressively less enrichment [59]. By contrast, Ca^{2+}-ATPase activity progressively increases to maximal levels in fractions D and E [59]. Guanylate cyclase and [^{3}H]QNB binding activities copurify with Na$^+$,K$^+$-ATPase activity. All enzyme activities were in the presence of activating agents: sodium dodecyl sulfate for Na$^+$,K$^+$-ATPase, lubrol PX for guanylate cyclase and A23187 for Ca^{2+}-ATPase (adapted with permission from [19]).

and purified from dog hearts. [^{3}H]-QNB binding activity copurified with Na$^+$, K$^+$-ATPase activity and away from Ca^{2+}-ATPase activity (Figure 14). Furthermore, [^{3}H]-dihydroalprenolol binding activity also copurified with Na$^+$, K$^+$-ATPase activity [105]. Therefore, both beta-adrenergic and muscarinic receptors are localized to the sarcolemma in dog myocardium. Such a location would be optimal for accessibility of neurotransmitters and for intracellular interaction between the two branches of the autonomic nervous system. In cardiac muscle, muscarinic receptors are randomly distributed on the myocyte surface and are not concentrated in sites directly opposite prejunctional parasympathetic nerve terminals [125]. Because of this diffuse and random distribution of receptors on the cell surface, cardiac muscle fibers are uniformly sensitive to acetylcholine over their entire surface, as demonstrated by iontophoretic application of the choline ester to discrete regions of fibers [125].

The affinity of muscarinic receptors for antagonists appears to be similar in a wide variety of tissues from various mammalian species [106]. The affinity constants determined by antagonist binding assays agree well with those derived from classical pharmacological analyses of antagonism of whole tissue responses to muscarinic stimulation.

Antagonists bind to a single, homogeneous class of muscarinic receptors [106].

In contrast to analyses of antagonist–receptor interactions, the assessment of agonist interaction with muscarinic receptors by binding studies is much more complex [105–107]. The pharmacologic efficacy of an agonist in evoking a response in intact functioning tissues may not necessarily correspond to the affinity of the receptor for that agonist. Among the reasons for this is the likely presence of multiple intervening steps, each of which might be regulatable, between agonist interaction with the receptor and the measured physiological response. In addition, binding studies have revealed that muscarinic receptors exist in multiple states in terms of their interaction with agonists [106, 107, 119–121]. The same binding sites (i.e., muscarinic receptors) with which antagonists interact in a uniform manner, interact with agonists heterogeneously. This was first recognized by analysis of the curves relating the occupancy of muscarinic receptors to the concentration of muscarinic agonists added to the receptors. The binding curves relating antagonist occupation of receptors to antagonist concentration are of the form predicted by the application of the law of mass action to the interaction of a ligand with a uniform set of binding sites [106]

(Figure 13B). In contrast, the patterns of agonist binding curves deviate substantially from this simple mass action relationship [106, 107, 119] (Figure 13B). These curves are shallower than antagonist binding curves (Figure 13B). Several alternative explanations for this anomalous binding pattern for agonists have been considered [119]. The most plausible explanation appears to be that muscarinic receptors exist in multiple conformations in terms of their interaction with agonists [105–107, 119]. Three different classes of muscarinic binding sites, each with different affinities for agonists, have been described in rat brain membranes [119]. At least two binding sites (high and low affinity) for agonists have been described in several other organs including the heart [128–132]. These different affinity binding sites are noninterconvertible in the binding assay, and therefore the slopes describing occupancy as a function of agonist concentration represent the sum of the interaction of ligand with multiple binding sites.

The beginnings of an explanation for this phenomenon have come from studies of the regulation of muscarinic receptors by guanine nucleotides. It has been discovered recently that cardiac muscarinic receptors, like beta- and alpha-adrenergic and dopaminergic and opiate receptors, can be regulated by guanine nucleotides [128–132]. Study of muscarinic receptors in cardiac membrane preparations, from which endogenous guanine nucleotides have been removed, yields the shallow binding curves described above (Figure 13B). However, if exogenous guanine nucleotides are added, the curves shift to a steeper form, a pattern compatible with the interaction of ligand with a single, homogeneous class of binding sites [133]. At the same time the affinity of the receptor for agonists is reduced substantially [128–132]. These data have been interpreted as showing a guanine nucleotide-induced conversion of receptors in a high affinity state for agonists into a low affinity state [133], analogous to the situation with guanine nucleotide regulation of beta-adrenergic receptors [105, 134]. Thus, with added guanine nucleotides binding curves are steeper (representing a single class of binding sites) and shifted to the right because most or all of the receptors are in a low affinity state. The physiological significance of these phenomena regarding muscarinic receptors—multiple agonist states, regulation by guanine nucleotides – remains to

be elucidated. It has been suggested that the different agonist affinity states of the receptor are coupled to different membrane responses [106] – e.g., altered cation fluxes, altered phospholipid turnover, inhibition of adenylate cyclase – or that the different states represent varying degrees of receptor–effector coupling, the low affinity state being 'coupled' to an effector such as a guanine nucleotide binding protein [133].

The in vitro properties of muscarinic receptors as assessed by binding studies also can be shown to be modified by cations. Divalent cations (Mg^{2+} or Ca^{2+}) increased the affinity of muscarinic receptors for agonists and magnified the guanine nucleotide-induced decrease in receptor affinity for agonists [132]. The effects of both guanine nucleotides and divalent cations were abolished by treatment of membranes with N-ethylmaleimide, suggesting the involvement of sulfhydryl groups in the effects of these agents [132]. Monovalent cations decreased the affinity of muscarinic receptors for agonists [129, 133, 135]. This effect of monovalent cations is small and appears to be related primarily to ionic strength rather than reflecting any specific regulatory interaction of monovalent cations with the receptor [135].

The density of cardiac muscarinic receptors varies in response to the ambient concentrations of muscarinic agonists. This was first demonstrated in cultured chick embryo heart cells exposed to carbamylcholine for various durations [118]. Cultured heart cells exposed to the choline ester had a diminished negative chronotropic response to muscarinic agonists associated with a substantial reduction in receptor density [118]. More detailed analysis revealed a biphasic pattern to this agonist-induced receptor alteration, a rapid phase (occurring over 1 min) associated with a reduced affinity of receptors for agonists followed by a slower phase (occurring over several hours) reflecting a true reduction in measurable receptor binding [131]. The agonist-induced reduction in cardiac muscarinic receptor density has been confirmed in studies in vivo. Carbachol was administered to chicks in ovo. The negative chronotropic response to carbachol of hearts removed from these chicks was diminished compared to hearts from control chicks, and the density of muscarinic receptors in homogenates of these hearts was reduced markedly [136]. In another study, rats were treated chronically with methacholine in varying concentrations [137]. After various durations of treatment, hearts were removed and membranes prepared for binding assays of muscarinic receptors. In a time- and concentration-dependent manner, methacholine treatment of the intact animal induced a modest reduction in cardiac muscarinic receptor density without altering the affinity of receptors for the antagonist [3H]-QNB [137].

As has been observed with beta-adrenergic receptors [134, 138], muscarinic receptors can be heterotropically regulated. That is, hormones or neurotransmitters other than acetylcholine may modify the properties of muscarinic receptors. Thyroidectomy increased the density of cardiac muscarinic receptors as assessed by [3H]-QNB binding [139]. On the other hand, treatment with triiodothyronine resulted in a modest decrease in density of receptors [139]. These effects of thyroid state on muscarinic receptors are exactly the opposite of the effects on beta-adrenergic receptors. Hyperthyroidism increases the density [138] whereas hypothyroidism decreases [140] the density of beta-adrenergic receptors in cardiac tissues. Thus the tachycardia of hyperthyroid animals and the bradycardia of hypothyroid animals may reflect in part a reciprocal alteration in the density of receptors of both limbs of the autonomic nervous system. When interaction between the sympathetic and parasympathetic nervous systems in regulating cardiac function is considered, these reciprocal changes in autonomic receptor density become even more important. For example, in hyperthyroidism not only is beta-adrenergic receptor density increased, but muscarinic receptor density is decreased. Thus, some of the cardiovascular changes seen with hyperthyroidism may reflect not only increased sympathetic activity (because of increased beta receptor density) but also reduced parasympathetic restraint of sympathetic effects (because of diminished muscarinic receptor density).

To summarize this section, a substantial amount of new information about the biochemistry and the biochemical and molecular pharmacology of muscarinic receptors has already resulted from radioligand binding assays. These observations confirm and are complementary to conclusions based on physiological and classical pharmacological approaches. However, many fundamental questions remain to be answered. For example, the nature of the coupling of muscarinic receptors to intracellular effectors and the nature and identity of intracellular messengers that mediate the effects of muscarinic activation remain either unknown or only partially understood, as will be discussed in the next section. The application of radioligand binding assays in combination with other biochemical and molecular approaches will yield further insight into these areas of investigation.

Intracellular effectors coupled to muscarinic receptors

The intracellular mechanisms by which activation of muscarinic receptors leads to alterations in cardiovascular function have been only partially elucidated. It has been known for years, based on electrophysiological and radioisotopic studies, that activation of muscarinic receptors in cardiac tissues results in an augmentation of outward currents carried by K^+ [141]. However, it is not known if the muscarinic receptor is linked directly to K^+ channels or if intermediary steps occur between the receptor and K^+ channels. Moreover, what these intermediary steps are remain to be established. Similarly, the intracellular mediators for the other cardiac effects (e.g., negative inotropic effects, antiadrenergic effects) of muscarinic agonists are unknown. Some of the candidates for intracellular mediators of muscarinic effects are cyclic GMP, cyclic AMP, and inositol phospholipids. Although there is substantial evidence in noncardiac tissues for a role of inositol phospholipids in mediating some effects of muscarinic agonists [142], no studies have yet demonstrated this in cardiac tissues. The discussion in this section will be limited to cation channels and the cyclic nucleotides.

Cation channels
As already suggested throughout this chapter, the tissues of the mammalian heart show marked variability in response to muscarinic receptor activation [1, 21–24]. These differences are also manifest in the electrophysiological and biochemical responses of supraventricular (nodal tissues and atria) and ventricular structures. Activation of muscarinic receptors in atria caused marked shortening of action potential duration associated with negative inotropic effects [22, 53, 141, 143]. By contrast, muscarinic activation alone produced lit-

tle or no effect on action potential duration [85] or contractility [39] of isolated ventricles. The electrophysiological and inotropic effects of muscarinic activation of mammalian atria are associated with an increase in outward current carried by K^+ [141, 143, 144]. This increase in K^+ outward current results in earlier repolarization of the membrane and thus shortening of action potential duration and decreases in contractility [143]. The reduction in contractility is thought to be due to a secondary diminution in the slow inward current (I_{si}) [143]. Because action potential duration is shortened by increased outward currents, the plateau phase of the action potential during which time I_{si} occurs is abbreviated [143]. Whether this electrophysiological mechanism can account entirely for the negative inotropic effects of muscarinic activation or whether additional mechanisms (to be discussed in later parts of this section) are operative remains to be established. Also, it is not known whether muscarinic receptors are coupled directly to K^+ channels or if intermediary steps (e.g., altered phospholipid turnover, increased cyclic GMP levels) must occur between activation of the receptors and increased K^+ current.

In mammalian atria, the effects of muscarinic activation on cation channels appear to depend on the concentration of muscarinic agonist used. With low concentrations of acetylcholine (sufficient to reduce twitch tension by 30–40%), the previously described effects of muscarinic activation on K^+ currents occurred [143]. At this concentration of acetylcholine the changes in I_{si} were secondary or 'indirect'; i.e., these changes resulted from the shortening in plateau duration. With higher concentrations of acetylcholine (sufficient to reduce twitch tension by 70–90%) a direct effect on I_{si} also was observed with voltage clamp studies [143]. Thus, with high concentrations of muscarinic agonists, K^+ outward currents increased and I_{si} also decreased. These dual actions on ion flux would be expected to produce strong negative inotropic effects. As in the case of K^+ channels, the nature of the coupling between muscarinic receptors and I_{si} channels remains unknown.

Tissue differences also exist in muscarinic effects on I_{si}. In mammalian atria high concentrations of acetylcholine directly reduced I_{si} [143]. However, in mammalian ventricular tissues activation of muscarinic receptors even with high concentrations of acetylcholine did not appear to produce a direct effect on I_{si} [85, 86].

There is also species variability in muscarinic effects on cation channels. All of the foregoing observations regarding the relationship between muscarinic receptors and ion channels came from studies in mammals. Acetylcholine appeared to have a more potent effect on I_{si} in frog atrium [145] than in mammalian atria. Chick ventricular tissue behaved like either mammalian atria or ventricles, depending upon the stage of development of the chick. Ventricles taken from embryonic chicks behaved like mammalian ventricles; i.e., muscarinic agonists did not have a direct effect on I_{si} [146]. By contrast, ventricles taken from hatched chicks behaved like mammalian atria – muscarinic agonists directly reduced I_{si} [146].

Thus, one well-established effect of muscarinic activation is alteration in ion channels located in the sarcolemma of myocardial cells. It seems unlikely that these changes that occur in the sarcolemma can account entirely for the multiple intracellular effects of muscarinic receptor activation. Other possible mediators will be discussed in the remainder of this section.

Cyclic GMP
It was first shown in cardiac tissue that cyclic GMP levels could be elevated by activation of muscarinic cholinergic receptors [147]. Subsequently, many studies in a variety of different tissues have shown that activation of muscarinic receptors leads to increases in the tissue concentration of cyclic GMP [148]. However, the role, if any, of cyclic GMP in modifying the physiological properties of these tissues has not yet been firmly established [148] (Table 3). Moreover, the biochemical mechanisms by which changes in tissue cyclic GMP levels might alter function are not yet fully understood [148].

The original observation of muscarinic-induced increases in cyclic GMP levels in cardiac tissues [147] was confirmed and extended by multiple subsequent studies done in hearts from a variety of different species [39, 90, 149–154]. Thus, there is no question that under appropriate conditions (particularly in the presence of adequate Ca^{2+} in the extracellular medium) activation of muscarinic receptors can result in increases in myocardial tissue cyclic GMP levels. However, whether this muscarinic-induced elevation in cyclic GMP levels has any

Table 3. Evidence regarding a role for cyclic GMP in cardiac regulation.

Evidence in support of a role for cyclic GMP	References
Analogs of cyclic GMP mimicked the direct effects of muscarinic agonists by causing:	
Slowing of spontaneous beating rate of cultured heart cells	[160]
Decreased automaticity of sinoatrial nodal cells	[161]
Inhibition of atrial slow response action potentials	[162]
Negative inotropic effects on atria	[162, 163]
Decreased Ca^{2+}-uptake by atria	[163]
Negative inotropic effects on ventricles	[164, 166]
Analogs of cyclic GMP mimicked the indirect (antiadrenergic) effects of muscarinic agonists by antagonizing:	
Positive inotropic effects of catecholamines	[39, 91, 155, 165]
Positive chronotropic effects of catecholamines	[167]
Metabolic effects of catecholamines	[91]
The Ca^{2+} ionophore elevated cyclic GMP levels which antagonized intracellular effects of cyclic AMP	[168]
Acetylcholine increased cyclic GMP levels and activated cyclic GMP-dependent protein kinase	[158, 170]

Evidence against a role for cyclic GMP	
Muscarinic agonists produced a negative inotropic or electrophysiological effect without increasing cyclic GMP	[152, 172]
Muscarinic agonists produced antiadrenergic effects without increasing cyclic GMP	[78, 178]
Na nitroprusside increased cyclic GMP levels but did not mimic the following effects of muscarinic agonists:	
Negative inotropic	[155, 173, 174]
Electrophysiological	[152, 153]
Metabolic	[174]
Antiadrenergic	[78, 170, 174]

Numbers refer to reference citations.

physiological role remains an issue of controversy [155].

When assessing the possible role of an intracellular mediator of muscarinic effects, it must be considered that muscarinic receptors might be coupled to multiple cellular effectors which may or may not interact directly with each other. As mentioned, there is good evidence that muscarinic receptors are somehow coupled with K^+ and I_{si} channels [142–145]. As will be discussed in detail subsequently, muscarinic receptors are coupled to adenylate cyclase [64]. Muscarinic agonists also can antagonize the intracellular effects of cyclic AMP by a, as yet unexplained, mechanism [64]. In noncardiac tissues, activation of muscarinic receptors results in changes in the rate of turnover of phosphotidylinositol [156]. Therefore, before a role for cyclic GMP in mediating muscarinic effects can be ruled in or out, each of the specific known effectors of muscarinic activation must be examined. It is possible, for example, that cyclic GMP is involved only in muscarinic regulation of I_{si} and not in any of the other

effects of muscarinic activation. It is also possible that there are tissue differences in the role of cyclic GMP in muscarinic effects. For example, perhaps cyclic GMP regulates I_{si} channels in mammalian atria but not in mammalian ventricles, and perhaps this is the reason why muscarinic activation produces direct effects on I_{si} in atria but not in ventricles. These comments are all speculative. They are made only to illustrate the complexities that must be considered when attempting to establish or eliminate a role for cyclic GMP in regulating cardiac function.

The original studies which purported to demonstrate a physiological role for cyclic GMP attempted to correlate a physiological response (e.g., contractile state) with tissue cyclic GMP levels. In these studies, acetylcholine was given to cardiac preparations in various concentrations for different durations, the mechanical or electrophysiological responses of the hearts were observed and cyclic GMP levels determined in the same tissues [147, 151, 153, 157, 158]. Although there appeared to be a fairly good correlation between tissue cyclic GMP levels and the measured physiological response [151, 158], these studies could be criticized as being inconclusive because a sufficiently detailed concentration-response analysis was not performed [151, 155]. In addition, as mentioned earlier the direct negative inotropic effects of muscarinic stimulation are in general small, although the rat heart may be an exception to this rule [147, 151, 158].

The bulk of the additional evidence supporting a role for cyclic GMP in mediating some of the physiological effects of muscarinic activation comes from studies utilizing analogs of cyclic GMP to attempt to increase directly the intracellular levels of the nucleotide (Table 3). Analogs (e.g., dibutyryl cyclic GMP or 8-bromocyclic GMP) are used because they are less susceptible to degradation during superfusion or perfusion, and because they are thought to penetrate the sarcolemma more readily than cyclic GMP. It is reasoned that if intracellular cyclic GMP levels can be increased directly with these agents, and if these agents mimic the action of acetylcholine, then this is evidence that cyclic GMP mediates that action of acetylcholine. A similar rationale has been applied to studies utilizing analogs of cyclic AMP to establish the role of this nucleotide in mediating a given effect of a hormone or neurotransmitter [159]. When using analogs of either cyclic nucleotide, the results have to be interpreted with caution, because the time course of action of these agents is generally slower than that of neurotransmitters and because relatively large concentrations are needed (in view of the low endogenous concentrations of these cyclic nucleotides) to produce the expected physiological effects. Nevertheless, by using these analogs many different laboratories have generated substantial data bearing on the question of the role of cyclic GMP in cardiac regulation (Table 3).

Analogs of cyclic GMP have been shown to mimic certain of the electrophysiological effects of acetylcholine. Dibutyryl cyclic GMP slowed the spontaneous beating rate of isolated cultured rat heart cells [160]. Dibutyryl cyclic AMP increased spontaneous beating rate [160]. Importantly, control experiments were performed with various nucleotides and butyrate, and none of these agents significantly changed beating rate [160]. Cyclic GMP injected directly into sinoatrial nodal cells by iontophoresis decreased the slope of spontaneous diastolic depolarization [161]. Acetylcholine administ-

ered by this same route was without effect, presumably because the choline ester must interact with muscarinic receptors on the outside of the sarcolemma to produce its effects [161]. Like acetylcholine, 8-bromo-cyclic GMP inhibited atrial slow response action potentials [162]. The inward current of such action potentials is thought to be carried primarily by Ca^{2+} through I_{si} channels, so this model is an indirect assessment of I_{si}. Associated with this inhibition of the slow response action potential there was a negative inotropic effect [162]. 8-bromo-cyclic GMP mimicked the effects of acetylcholine on action potential configuration and contractile state of rat atria [163]. In this same study, 8-bromo-cyclic GMP decreased Ca^{2+} uptake by beating atrial preparations but had no effect on K^+ content [163]. It was concluded that cyclic GMP might mediate the effects of muscarinic activation on I_{si} but not on K^+ channels [163]. These results have been cited by other authors as showing a dissociation between cyclic GMP action and that of acetylcholine [155]. However, this interpretation does not seem valid. It seems plausible that muscarinic receptors could be coupled to different ion channels in different ways. Perhaps cyclic GMP is involved in coupling only I_{si} channels to muscarinic receptors, whereas K^+ channels are directly coupled or regulated by other factors. The observation that muscarinic agonists have a dual effect on ion flux depending on the concentration of agonist used is consistent with such a hypothesis [143]. It could be reasoned that with low concentrations of agonist only K^+ channels which are more directly coupled to muscarinic receptors are activated. With higher concentrations of agonist, cyclic GMP levels are increased and with this I_{si} channels are functionally altered. 8-bromo-cyclic GMP would then be expected to mimic only this latter effect.

Cyclic GMP has also been shown to mimic the negative inotropic effects of acetylcholine. Fibers of mouse ventricle in which the sarcolemma was chemically disrupted were used to study the inotropic effects of cyclic GMP [164]. Cyclic GMP applied to such fibers markedly reduced both the force and frequency of contractions [164].

Analogs of cyclic GMP have also been used extensively in assessing the role of cyclic GMP in the antiadrenergic effects of acetylcholine. Dibutyryl cyclic GMP mimicked the effect of acetylcholine and antagonized the positive inotropic effects of

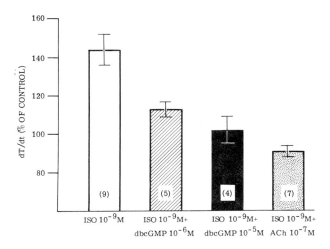

Figure 15. Effect of dibutyryl cyclic GMP (dbcGMP) on iso-proterenol (ISO)-induced increases in contractility (dT/dt). Dibutyryl cyclic GMP was perfused for 15 min prior to the administration of isoproterenol. The effect of isoproterenol on contractility was measured after 2 min of its infusion (dibutyryl cyclic GMP infusion was also continued). Values are means ± SE for the number of hearts noted at the bottom of the bars (ACh = acetylcholine) (reprinted with permission from [39]).

catecholamines in isolated cardiac tissues [39, 155, 165] (Figure 15; see also Figure 10). Like acetylcholine, dibutyryl cyclic GMP also attenuated the positive inotropic effects of isoproterenol in hearts from hyperthyroid rats [91]. In this latter study, rats were made hyperthyroid because of the apparent hyper-adrenergic state of the cardiovascular system in hyperthyroid animals. It was of interest to evaluate the efficacy of muscarinic antagonism of sympathetic effects in such hearts. Dibutyryl cyclic GMP antagonized the positive inotropic effects of dibutyryl cyclic AMP in isolated kitten papillary muscles [166]. These results were interpreted as showing an intracellular antagonism between the two cyclic nucleotides [166], similar to previous suggestions of an intracellular interaction between the two systems [39]. Cyclic GMP analogs also mimic acetylcholine in antagonizing certain of the electrophysiological effects of catecholamines or cyclic AMP. Isoproterenol antagonized the inhibition by 8-bromocyclic GMP of slow responses in guinea pig atria [162]. This can be thought of as the reciprocal of cyclic GMP antagonism of isoproterenol-induced augmentation of slow responses. Dibutyryl cyclic GMP antagonized norepinephrine and dibu-

tyryl cyclic AMP induced increases in beating rate of cultured mouse myocardial cells [167]. Cyclic GMP analogs also mimicked the cholinergic antagonism of the cardiac metabolic effects of catecholamines [91]. Hearts from hyperthyroid rats were hyper-responsive to the metabolic effects of beta agonists compared to those from euthyroid animals [91]. Acetylcholine antagonized isoproterenol-induced activation of phosphorylase in such hearts [91] (Figure 12). Dibutyryl cyclic GMP mimicked these effects of acetylcholine without lowering cyclic AMP levels [91] (Figure 16), Thus, it has been shown that analogs of cyclic GMP can mimic the effects of acetylcholine in antagonizing the electrophysiological, inotropic, and metabolic actions of beta agonists.

Cardiac cyclic GMP levels can be increased independently of stimulating muscarinic receptors by means other than administration of analogs of cyclic GMP. One agent widely used to accomplish this is Na nitroprusside. Results with this drug will be discussed subsequently. Another agent that has been used to elevate cardiac cyclic GMP levels is the divalent cation ionophore A23187 [168]. This drug produces complex effects on guinea pig ventricles. When given alone A23187 caused histamine release presumably from tissue mast cells. The net result of A23187 administration was therefore elevation in cyclic AMP levels (presumably from histamine stimulation of H_2 receptors) and increases in cyclic GMP levels (presumably from the ionophore-induced transport of Ca^{2+} to guanylate cyclase) (Figure 17). The increase in cyclic AMP levels could be blunted substantially by blockade of H_2 receptors with metiamide (Figure 17). The noteworthy finding from these studies was that a given level of cyclic AMP seemed to be relatively ineffective in causing positive inotropic effects or activating phosphorylase. Cyclic AMP levels had to exceed 1.0 pmol/mg wet weight before contractility or percent phosphorylase a were increased (Figure 17). This is in marked contrast to the efficacy of a given level of cyclic AMP when the levels are increased by catecholamines or agents such as histamine. In such cases, increasing cyclic AMP levels to 0.6 or 0.7 pmol/mg wet weight produced prominent inotropic [169] and metabolic [91] effects. One possible explanation for this apparent lack of efficacy of cyclic AMP was the fact that cyclic GMP levels in the same hearts were markedly elevated (Figure 17).

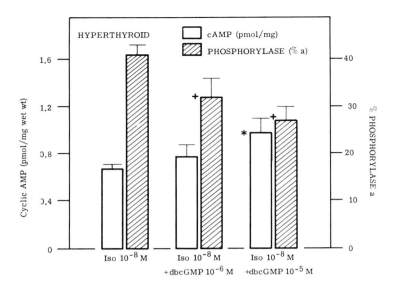

Figure 16. Effect of dibutyryl cyclic GMP (dbcGMP) on isoproterenol-induced increases in cyclic AMP levels and activation of phosphorylase in hearts from hyperthyroid rats. Note that dbcGMP attenuates isoproterenol activation of phosphorylase without lowering cyclic AMP levels. Values represent means ± SEM of 4–6 hearts. Symbols indicate significance of difference from values with isoproterenol alone, +p < 0.01, *p < 0.05 (reprinted with permission from [91]).

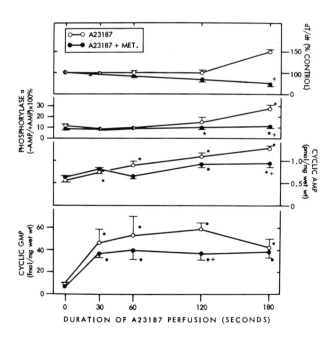

Figure 17. Effect of 1.0 μM A23187 alone and combined with metiamide (10 μM) on the contractile and biochemical properties of isolated guinea pig ventricles. Values are means ± SEM of 4–6 hearts: *p < 0.05 compared to basal; +p < 0.05 compared to absence of metiamide (adapted with permission from [169]).

Thus, it was hypothesized that cyclic GMP generated in response to the direct ionophoric effects of A23187 antagonized the intracellular effects of cyclic AMP generated in response to H_2-receptor activation [169]. Rat hearts do not possess H_2 receptors so the effects of A23187 in hearts from this species are less complicated than in hearts from guinea pigs. In hearts from rats, A23187 produced only a negative inotropic effect which appeared to correlate temporally with the increase in cyclic GMP levels (Figure 18). These results with A23187 support a physiological role for cyclic GMP in cardiac tissues: (a) cyclic GMP antagonism of the intracellular effects of cyclic AMP in guinea pig hearts and (b) a negative inotropic effect of cyclic GMP in rat hearts.

If cyclic GMP is involved in mediating some of the effects of muscarinic receptor stimulation in the heart, the biochemical mechanism by which this occurs remains unknown. One hypothesis is that, analogous to the cyclic AMP-protein kinase system, cyclic GMP interacts with a specific protein kinase which in turn phosphorylates certain substrates to alter protein function. A cyclic GMP-dependent protein kinase has been identified in various tissues including the heart [149, 158, 170]. Recently, an assay has been developed for studying

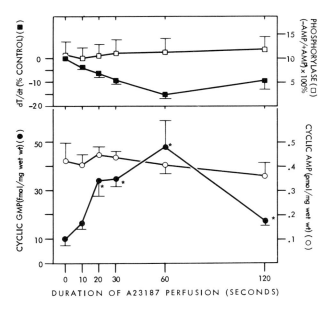

Figure 18. Time course of contractile and metabolic effects of 30 μM A23187 in isolated ventricles obtained from reserpine-pretreated rats. Values are means ± SE from 5-8 hearts: *P ± 0.05 compared to basal (adapted with permission from [169]).

the activity of cyclic GMP-dependent protein kinase in cardiac tissues [158, 170]. With this assay, it has been shown for the first time that administration of acetylcholine to an intact rat heart results in increases in cyclic GMP-dependent protein kinase activity ratios associated with elevations in cyclic GMP levels [158, 170] (Figure 19A and C). Both of these biochemical responses were associated with a negative inotropic effect in the same hearts (Figure 19D). Na nitroprusside also increased cyclic GMP levels, in fact to much greater levels than that caused by acetylcholine. However, Na nitroprusside did not increase cyclic GMP-dependent protein kinase activity ratios nor did it change the force of contraction [158, 170] (Figure 19). These results allow several conclusions: (a) they suggest a possible mechanism by which cyclic GMP, the levels of which are altered in response to muscarinic stimulation, might modify protein function and the physiological properties of the heart; (b) they support the notion, already suggested by others [171], that cyclic GMP and its intracellular effectors might be compartmentalized; and (c) they demonstrate the hazards of using agents other than muscarinic ago-

nists to elevate cyclic GMP levels and then drawing conclusions about the role of cyclic GMP if these agents do not mimic choline esters [155].

There is a body of evidence that has been interpreted to show that cyclic GMP does not have any as yet defined physiological role in cardiac regulation [155] (Table 3). One concentration-response study showed a dissociation between inotropic and cyclic GMP elevating effects of low concentrations of carbachol [172]. Low concentrations of carbachol (0.03-1.0 μM) decreased contractility whereas only high concentrations (2 or 10 μM) elevated cyclic GMP levels [172]. Also, by using a low concentration of carbachol (which had already been shown not to elevate cyclic GMP levels), a dissociation in time course of response was demonstrated. With 0.3 μM carbachol contractility fell, whereas cyclic GMP levels did not change [172]. These data were interpreted as showing that cyclic GMP does not have a role in regulating the contractile state of atria. However, another possible interpretation is that the contractile state of atria, as modified by muscarinic agonists, is determined by more than one factor, and cyclic GMP regulates only one of those factors. It was shown by voltage clamp studies that low concentrations of acetylcholine increased K^+ outward currents whereas high concentrations reduced I_{si} as well as increased outward currents in mammalian atria [143]. Even low concentrations (that only modified K^+ currents) produced negative inotropic effects, presumably because I_{si} was indirectly abbreviated owing to the shortened duration of the action potential [143]. High concentrations produced more marked negative inotropic effects presumably because I_{si} was directly inhibited as well as being abbreviated due to the shortened action potential duration. Thus, it is possible that, with low concentrations of muscarinic agonists, negative inotropic effects occur independently of cyclic GMP and with high concentrations a second mechanism (inhibition of I_{si}) becomes operative and that this second mechanism involves cyclic GMP. Such a conclusion would be compatible with studies that showed that cyclic GMP modulates I_{si} or slow responses [162, 163].

Another approach to test the cyclic GMP hypothesis has been to elevate cyclic GMP with drugs which do not interact with muscarinic receptors. Because of its potency in elevating tissue cyclic GMP levels, Na nitroprusside has been a popular

117

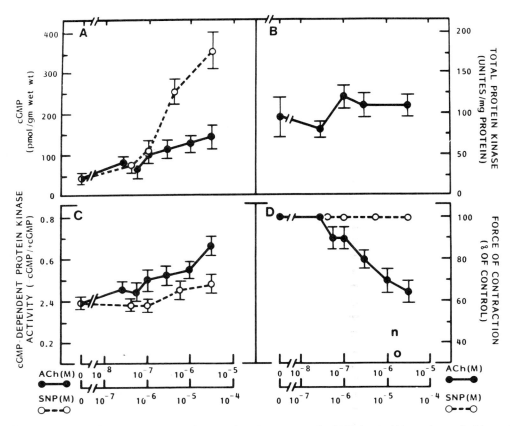

Figure 19. Effects of acetylcholine (ACh) and Na nitroprusside (SNP) on cyclic GMP levels (A), total protein kinase (B), cyclic GMP-dependent protein kinase activity (C), and force of contraction (D) of isolated perfused rat hearts. Hearts were frozen after perfusion of the various concentrations of ACh or SNP for 1 min. Each point in panels A, C, and, D represents means ± SEM of 8–10 hearts; data in panel B were taken from three hearts (adapted with permission from [170]).

agent to use for such studies (Table 3). It has been shown that Na nitroprusside did not mimic the inotropic [155, 173, 174], electrophysiological [152, 153], metabolic [174], or antiandrenergic [78, 170, 174] effects of acetylcholine, even though it markedly increased cyclic GMP levels [152, 155, 170, 173, 175]. However, the conclusion based on these results that cyclic GMP has no role in mediating these effects of acetylcholine must be questioned because of the immunohistochemical evidence in noncardiac [171] and cardiac [176] tissues that cyclic GMP can be compartmentalized within the cell and that muscarinic agonists and Na nitroprusside affect the concentrations of this nucleotide in different compartments. The recent observations that acetylcholine, but not Na nitroprusside, activates cyclic GMP-dependent protein kinase in rat hearts provide further evidence for different compart-

ments or pools of cyclic GMP, each of which can be selectively regulated and which have different intracellular effectors [158, 170] (Figure 19). Analogous evidence has been provided for compartmentation of cyclic AMP and differential regulation of cyclic AMP levels in different pools in myocardial cells [177].

Perhaps the most convincing evidence against a role for cyclic GMP, at least in mediating certain physiological effects, are the observations that over a range of concentrations of muscarinic agonist certain physiological effects can be induced without changing tissue cyclic GMP levels (Table 3). Acetylcholine decreased automaticity and shortened action potential duration of guinea pig atria and these changes appeared to occur without any relationship to tissue cyclic GMP levels [152]. Muscarinic agonists antagonized the positive inotropic effects of agents that elevate cyclic AMP levels (catecholamines, phosphodiesterase inhibitors, cholera toxin) without elevating cyclic GMP levels [78, 178]. These results could be interpreted as eliminating a role for cyclic GMP in the electrophysiological or antiadrenergic effects of muscarinic agonists. However, the following caveats are reiterated: (a) muscarinic receptors might be linked to multiple responses only one or a few of which are regulated by cyclic GMP; each of these must be examined carefully before ruling out in a blanket fashion any physiological role for cyclic GMP; (b) cyclic GMP might be compartmentalized and small undetectable (by available assays) changes in levels might have occurred in experiments that appeared to show no change in the levels of the nucleotide.

In arguing against a physiological role for cyclic GMP in the antiadrenergic effects of muscarinic agonists, the data with analogs of cyclic GMP have been discounted because other agents such as verapamil also have antiadrenergic effects [155]. This conclusion is fallacious. Simply because a given negative inotropic agent produces antiadrenergic effects by a nonspecific or generalized negative inotropic mechanism does not justify the conclusion that cyclic GMP analogs also act in such a nonspecific or generalized manner. Agents such as verapamil antagonize the positive inotropic effects of various interventions in addition to catecholamines. Before discarding on the basis of nonspecific effects the results using cyclic GMP analogs, which have come from many different laboratories during a period of several years, it must be shown that cyclic GMP analogs are indeed as nonspecific in their antiadrenergic action as agents such as verapamil [155].

To summarize, substantial evidence exists both in support of and against the concept that cyclic GMP plays a role in mediating certain cardiac effects of muscarinic receptor stimulation (Table 3). It seems clear that this remains an unresolved issue. Further experiments must be done to establish or completely eliminate a role for this cyclic nucleotide in cardiac regulation. This should be a fruitful area of future research in cardiac physiology and biochemistry.

Cyclic GMP levels are regulated by two enzymes: guanylate cyclase and cyclic GMP phosphodiesterase [148]. Guanylate cyclase occurs as both a membrane-associated and soluble enzyme in cardi-

ac tissues [19] (Figure 14). The two forms of the enzyme in cardiac muscle are differentially regulated: nonionic detergents stimulated the particulate enzyme without modifying the activity of the soluble enzyme, whereas Na nitroprusside stimulated only the soluble enzyme [19, 179]. These results showing both particulate and soluble forms of the enzyme and differential activation of the two forms of the enzyme provide further support for the notion of different intracellular pools of cyclic GMP which can be modified selectively by certain agents. Acetylcholine presumably increases cyclic GMP levels by stimulating guanylate cyclase. However, except for rare reports [180], most investigators have failed to show any effect of muscarinic agonists on guanylate cyclase activity in broken cell preparations [148]. In intact tissues Ca^{2+} is required for muscarinic-induced elevations in cyclic GMP levels [152, 181]. The divalent cation ionophore A23187 increased cyclic GMP levels in guinea pig ventricles presumably by elevating Ca^{2+} in certain critical areas of the myocardial cell [168] (Figure 17). Ca^{2+} has been shown to stimulate particulate guanylate cyclase activity [182]. Based on these types of results, it has been suggested that Ca^{2+} might in some way function as an intermediary between the muscarinic receptor and guanylate cyclase. However this conclusion remains to be established. Other studies have shown Ca^{2+} inhibition of guanylate cyclase [183, 184]. In cardiac muscle, although Ca^{2+} is required for muscarinic increases in cyclic GMP levels, the physiological response to muscarinic stimulation is either no change or a decrease in contractile state [152, 168]. Thus, muscarinic agonists do not appear to produce a generalized increase in intracellular Ca^{2+} concentration. If activation of muscarinic receptors leads to mobilization of Ca^{2+}, this must occur in discrete intracellular pools (presumably in the region of guanylate cyclase) because contractile proteins and other intracellular enzymes (e.g., phosphorylase kinase) do not appear to be affected.

Adenylate cyclase – cyclic AMP – cyclic AMP-dependent protein kinase

As described in detail in an earlier section, one important mechanism by which muscarinic agonists regulate cardiac function is by modulating the effects of the sympathetic nervous system. One level of interaction between the parasympathetic and sympathetic nervous systems is postjunctional, wherein muscarinic agonists are able to modulate the effects of beta-adrenergic agonists on myocardial cells [64] (Figure 6). In this section will be discussed the evidence regarding the involvement of the adenylate cyclase – cyclic AMP – cyclic AMP-dependent protein kinase system in this postjunctional interaction.

Substantial evidence supports the notion that cyclic AMP mediates at least some of the physiological and metabolic effects of beta-adrenergic agonists on the heart [64, 185, 186]. If muscarinic agonists produce some or all of their antiadrenergic effects by modifying the cyclic AMP system, they could theoretically do so by acting at one or more of the steps in the cascade of reactions that mediate the intracellular effects of beta agonists (Figure 20). Available evidence regarding effects of muscarinic agonists at each of these steps will be considered.

A number of investigators using different types of cardiac preparations from various species have shown that muscarinic agonists can attenuate beta agonist-induced increases in steady state tissue cyclic AMP levels [38, 78, 90, 91, 146, 154, 175, 187–190]. When physiological or metabolic responses were measured, the muscarinic attenuation of cyclic AMP generation paralleled the inhibition of the myocardial response to catecholamines. Muscarinic agonists inhibited catecholamine-induced increases in cyclic AMP levels and concomitantly attenuated the positive inotropic effects [38, 78, 146, 154, 188–190]. Muscarinic agonists also antagonized catecholamine-induced activation of phosphorylase while inhibiting cyclic AMP generation [90, 91, 188]. These results are consistent with the conclusion that the muscarinic inhibition of cyclic AMP generation is physiologically and metabolically important in cardiac cells and that attenuation of cyclic AMP generation might be a contributing mechanism for the antiadrenergic effects of muscarinic agonists.

The mechanism for muscarinic attenuation of

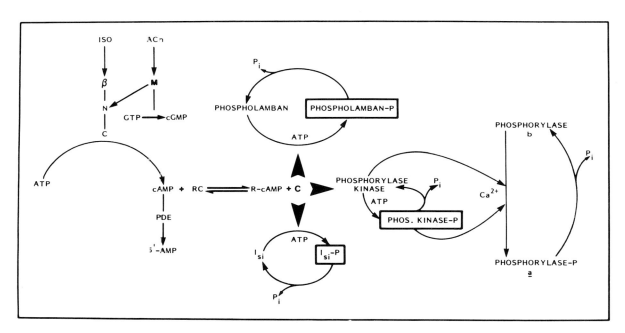

Figure 20. Flow diagram of reactions which are thought to mediate intracellular effects of autonomic receptor stimulation. Catecholamines (ISO) activate beta-adrenergic (β) receptors which leads via a regulatory protein (N) to activation of the catalytic subunit (C) of adenylate cyclase. Cyclic AMP thereby generated interacts with cyclic AMP-dependent protein kinase (RC) to release the catalytic unit (C) which, in turn, catalyzes the phosphorylation of a variety of proteins, including phospholamban, phosphorylase kinase and, possibly, slow inward current channels (I_{si}). One or more of these phosphorylation reactions may contribute to the inotropic and electrophysiologic effects of beta agonists. Acetylcholine stimulates muscarinic receptors to inhibit adenylate cyclase activity. This reaction appears to occur via the N protein. In addition, muscarinic agonists can increase cyclic GMP levels and also block the effects of beta agonists at some point beyond cyclic AMP by as yet unknown mechanisms.

120

catecholamine-induced cyclic AMP generation involves inhibition of adenylate cyclase activity. It was first shown two decades ago, prior to any detailed knowledge regarding regulation of adenylate cyclase, that muscarinic agonists inhibited adenylate cyclase activity in crude preparations of dog myocardium [191]. Carbachol added to these preparations inhibited both basal- and epinephrine-stimulated adenylate cyclase activity [191]. These results were confirmed in similar experiments which again used a crude myocardial preparation from rabbit hearts [38]. The biochemical mechanism for this muscarinic inhibition of adenylate cyclase activity began to be elucidated after substantial information regarding regulation of adenylate cyclase had been obtained from other systems [192]. Studies done largely in model systems revealed that hormone-stimulated adenylate cyclase is comprised of at least three distinct components: the hormone receptor, the catalytic subunit, and a third component which 'couples' the receptor to the catalytic subunit [192] (Figure 20). The third component has been referred to as the G/F or N protein because it possesses binding sites for and is regulated by guanine nucleotides such as GTP. In relatively purified membrane preparations devoid of endogenous GTP, exogenous guanine nucleotides must be added to the system to demonstrate hormone stimulation of adenylate cyclase activity [192]. Thus, guanine nucleotides must interact with the N protein in order for the receptor to activate the catalytic subunit. In some tissues such as myocardium, guanine nucleotides can directly activate catalytic activity of adenylate cyclase even in the absence of hormone [193]. Guanine nucleotides acting on the N protein also can modulate the affinity of receptors for agonists. This is true for a variety of receptors including beta-adrenergic [104, 105] and muscarinic [128–132] receptors (see also the section on the biochemistry of muscarinic cholinergic receptors). It has been theorized that this dual regulation by guanine nucleotides and the N protein of both the receptor and catalytic subunit is involved in mediating the receptor activation of adenylate cyclase [104, 192]. Another property associated with the N protein is a GTPase activity which is thought to regulate GTP effects by hydrolyzing the guanine nucleotide to GDP [192].

As is the case with virtually all systems studied, adenylate cyclase activity in purified membranes from myocardial cells is not stimulated by hormones unless exogenous guanine nucleotides are added. Addition of exogenous guanine nucleotides stimulated the enzyme directly as well as facilitating hormone stimulation of the enzyme [193] (Figure 21). Thus, guanine nucleotides can activate adenylate cyclase directly and are required for hormone activation of the enzyme. In purified membrane preparations, muscarinic agonists had no effect on basal adenylate cyclase activity, i.e., that activity in the absence of added guanine nucleotides [193]. If GTP was added to the enzyme preparation, muscarinic agonists inhibited adenylate cyclase activity (Figure 21, left panel). This was true whether GTP was added alone or together with a catecholamine (Figure 21, left panel). In the earlier studies cited [38, 191], it is likely that endogenous GTP was present because the membrane preparations were crude. Thus, in these earlier studies it is likely that muscarinic effects on adenylate cyclase activity were also dependent on GTP. This dependency of the muscarinic inhibitory effect on GTP was specific for this guanine nucleotide. Cardiac adenylate cyclase activity was also increased by the nonhydrolyzable guanine nucleotide Gpp(NH)p (Figure 21, right panel). However, muscarinic agonists had no effect on enzyme activity in the presence of this nucleotide [193] (Figure 21, right panel). Similarly, muscarinic agonists did not modify NaF stimulation of adenylate cyclase activity [193]. The effects of muscarinic agonists were blocked by atropine [193]. It was concluded that the interaction of both muscarinic and beta-adrenergic receptors with adenylate cyclase was regulated by the naturally occurring guanine nucleotide GTP. These studies have been subsequently confirmed [195]. Based on these findings and the data that show guanine nucleotide regulation of muscarinic receptor affinity for agonists [128–132], it is reasonable to hypothesize that an N protein, with which GTP interacts, is involved in 'coupling' inhibitory muscarinic receptors to adenylate cyclase. Whether this is the same N protein that couples stimulatory receptors to the enzyme is unknown. The detailed biochemical mechanism by which activation of muscarinic receptors leads to reduction of the efficacy of GTP is also unknown. The fact that this inhibition does not occur when the nonhydrolyzable analog Gpp(NH)p is the guanine nucleotide present suggests the hypothesis that muscarinic agonists increase the activ-

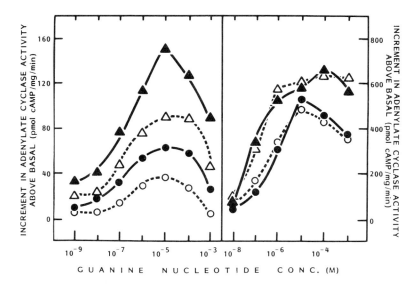

Figure 21. Guanine nucleotide stimulation of adenylate cyclase activity in canine cardiac membrane vesicles. Guanine nucleotide added was GTP in left panel and Gpp(NH)p in right panel. Circles are values with guanine nucleotides alone and triangles with guanine nucleotide plus 10^{-7} M isoproterenol. Unfilled symbols designate the presence of 10^{-5} M methacholine in addition to guanine nucleotide alone or with isoproterenol. Note that methacholine significantly inhibits GTP or GTP plus isoproterenol activation of adenylate cyclase (left panel) but does not affect adenylate cyclase activity when the guanine nucleotide added is Gpp(NH)p (right panel).

ity of an adenylate cyclase-associated GTPase. It has been shown in another system that muscarinic agonists can activate adenylate cyclase-associated GTPase activity [194]. Other mechanisms are also possible instead of or in addition to that postulated. Thus, the specific details regarding the biochemical and molecular mechanisms by which activation of muscarinic receptors inhibits adenylate cyclase remain to be elucidated. Nevertheless, it seems clear that muscarinic agonists can diminish tissue cyclic AMP levels by inhibiting catecholamine stimulation of adenylate cyclase.

Theoretically, muscarinic agonists could reduce steady-state tissue levels of cyclic AMP by activating phosphodiesterase (Figure 20). Although the studies are limited, this possibility has been examined by a few laboratories [38, 175, 196]. With the experimental approaches used, these studies failed to demonstrate any effect of muscarinic agonists on phosphodiesterase activity from myocardium [38, 175, 196].

The muscarinic attenuation of catecholamine-induced cyclic AMP generation cannot account entirely for the muscarinic antagonism of the cardiac effects of beta agonists. Under certain conditions,

perhaps determined by species and buffer conditions (e.g., Ca^{2+} concentration), muscarinic agonists can potently inhibit the physiological and metabolic effects of catecholamines without changing cyclic AMP levels. Acetylcholine markedly antagonized the positive inotropic effects of isoproterenol in isolated perfused guinea pig ventricles [39] (Figure 10). Cyclic GMP levels in the acetylcholine-treated hearts were markedly elevated (Figure 22). However, cyclic AMP levels in hearts receiving both acetylcholine and isoproterenol were not significantly different from those in hearts receiving isoproterenol alone [39] (Figure 22). These results have subsequently been confirmed by several other investigators. It has been shown that either muscarinic agonists attenuated a physiological or metabolic response to catecholamines out of proportion to the magnitude of reduction in cyclic AMP [188, 190] or that the inhibition of physiological response occurred without any change in cyclic AMP levels [78]. Additional evidence for muscarinic antagonism of catecholamine effects by mechanisms independent of cyclic AMP reduction comes from studies in which cyclic AMP levels are increased independently of stimulation of beta receptors. It

122

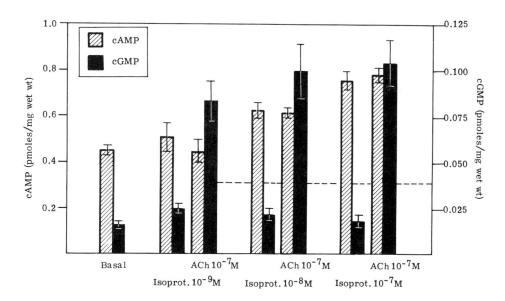

Figure 22. Cyclic nucleotide levels in hearts receiving isoproterenol (Isoprot.) alone or combined with acetylcholine (ACh) for 2 min of continuous infusion. Values are means ± SE for 7–16 hearts. The horizontal broken line is the mean value of cyclic GMP found in hearts receiving 10^{-7} M acetylcholine alone for 2 min (reprinted with permission from [39]).

was observed many years ago that acetylcholine blocked the positive inotropic effects of both epinephrine and theophylline in isolated turtle hearts [74]. Although cyclic AMP levels were not measured, it is reasonable to conclude that the positive inotropic effects of both epinephrine and theophylline were mediated at least partially by cyclic AMP [74]. Subsequently, several investigators have utilized phosphodiesterase inhibitors to produce positive inotropic effects and elevate cyclic AMP levels in cardiac preparations and then examine the effects of muscarinic agonists on these parameters. Methylisobutylxanthine (MIX) elevated cyclic AMP levels and augmented Ca^{2+}-dependent action potentials and contraction in chick ventricles [196]. Acetylcholine (10^{-6} M) abolished the MIX-induced increase in tension without reducing tissue cyclic AMP levels [196]. In isolated rat left atria, methacholine antagonized the positive inotropic effects of MIX without changing cyclic AMP levels [78]. Myocardial cyclic AMP levels also can be increased by treating the intact tissue with cholera toxin [175, 178, 189]. The presumed mechanism is that cholera toxin inhibits the adenylate cyclase-associated GTPase. Thus, the GTP concentration in the vicinity of the N protein is increased and adenylate cy-

clase thereby activated. Cholera toxin elevated cyclic AMP levels [175, 178, 189] and increased contractions [178] of intact cardiac preparations. Muscarinic agonists inhibited the positive inotropic effect of cholera toxin without reducing cyclic AMP levels [178]. These results thus provide additional evidence that muscarinic agonists can antagonize the effects of cyclic AMP within the myocardial cell.

There are several potential sites beyond cyclic AMP where muscarinic agonists could act to interfere with the intracellular effects of the nucleotide (Figure 20). One of these is cyclic AMP activation of cyclic AMP-dependent protein kinase. This has been examined in only a limited manner. However, the studies that have attempted to examine the relationship between cyclic AMP levels and activation of cyclic AMP-dependent protein kinase have failed to reveal any effect of acetylcholine on this relationship [188, 190]. That is, for a given level of cyclic AMP, cyclic AMP-dependent protein kinase was proportionately activated in the presence or absence of muscarinic agonists. Muscarinic agonists thus do not appear to interfere with cyclic AMP activation of protein kinase.

Another potential site where muscarinic agonists

Figure 23. Autoradiogram of guinea pig ventricles perfused with $^{32}P_i$ and then treated with isoproterenol (10^{-8} M) alone or isoproterenol plus acetylcholine (10^{-7} M) for 20, 40, and 60 sec. After perfusion with drugs for respective durations, ventricles were freeze-clamped and then membrane vesicles were prepared. Vesicles were subjected to gel electrophoresis and this autoradiogram was subsequently obtained. Acetylcholine was perfused simultaneously with and for the same duration as isoproterenol. Hearts in lanes 1, 3, and 5 received isoproterenol plus acetylcholine. Heart in lane 7 received atropine in addition to isoproterenol and acetylcholine, and heart in lane 8 received propranolol in addition to isoproterenol. Note that isoproterenol produces a time-dependent increase in ^{32}P incorporation into the 22,000- and 8,000- to 11,000-M_r proteins (lanes 1, 3 and 5). Propranolol antagonizes this effect of isoproterenol (lane 8). Acetylcholine clearly attenuates the isoproterenol-induced increase in ^{32}P incorporation (lanes 2, 4, and 6). Atropine reverses the effect of acetylcholine (lane 7) (reprinted with permission from [64]).

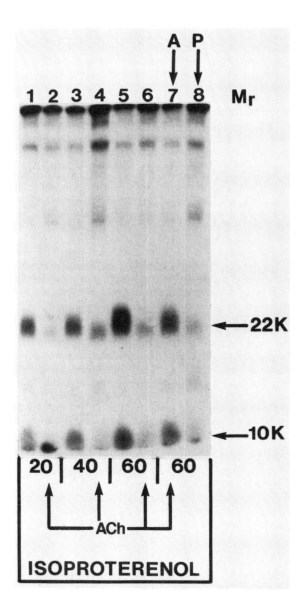

might interfere with the intracellular effects of cyclic AMP is at the level of phosphorylation of proteins which are thought to mediate the effects of hormones or drugs that elevate cyclic AMP concentrations. Several proteins, including troponin I (TN-1) [197], phosphorylase kinase [198], and phospholamban [64] have been shown to be phosphorylated in intact hearts with administration of beta-adrenergic agonists. It has been hypothesized, but not yet demonstrated, that slow inward current channels (I_{si}) are also phosphorylated when cyclic AMP levels are increased by catecholamines [186]. Isoproterenol administered to isolated perfused guinea pig hearts which had been preperfused with $^{32}P_i$ produced characteristic positive inotropic effects [64]. The hearts were then freeze-clamped, membranes prepared and then subjected to polyacrylamide gel electrophoresis. The incorporation of ^{32}P was assessed by autoradiography. Isoproterenol produced a time-dependent increase in ^{32}P incorporation into proteins with apparent molecular weights of 22,000 and 8,000 to 10,000 [64] (Figure 23). On the basis of a variety of additional information, it is felt that the 22,000-molecular-weight protein is phospholamban and the lower-molecular-weight protein is a component (perhaps a monomer) of phospholamban. The ^{32}P incorporation correlated very well temporally with the positive inotropic effects of isoproterenol. The muscarinic agonist acetylcholine potently attenuated the isoproterenol-induced increase in ^{32}P incorporation into phospholamban and also antagonized the pos-

itive inotropic effects of the catecholamine [64] (Figure 23). Thus, muscarinic agonists can potently antagonize catecholamine-induced phosphorylation of a myocardial cell protein which may be involved in mediating the positive inotropic effects of catecholamines. It is not yet known whether this attenuation of protein phosphorylation can be accounted for by muscarinic reduction in cyclic AMP levels and in protein kinase activity. In view of the studies mentioned earlier, this seems unlikely. Rather, it seems more likely that cyclic AMP may have been reduced somewhat but that some additional mechanism was also operative to produce the ultimate observed inhibition of ^{32}P incorporation. One reasonable hypothesis is that muscarinic agonists somehow activate a protein phosphatase (Figure 20). There are, however, not yet any data that address this question.

Thus, muscarinic agonists appear to act at more than one level in the cascade of reactions mediating the intracellular effects of beta receptor stimulation. They can inhibit adenylate cyclase activity by somehow reducing the efficacy of GTP. In addition, they appear to be able to interfere with the intracellular effects of cyclic AMP. The mechanism for this latter effect is as yet unknown.

Drugs that result in activation of muscarinic cholinergic receptors

This section will consider the cardiovascular effects of drugs that share the property of causing activation of muscarinic receptors at cardiovascular neuroeffector junctions. A number of these agents and some of their pharmacologic properties have been referred to already in the earlier discussions regarding parasympathetic nervous system regulation of cardiovascular function. In this section the pharmacological effects of these agents in intact systems (whole animals and humans) will be stressed. The drugs that lead to activation of muscarinic cholinergic receptors do so by one of three major mechanisms (Figure 24): (a) by direct activation of muscarinic receptors; (b) by preventing the hydrolysis of endogenous released acetylcholine; or (c) by activating parasympathetic ganglia and thereby causing release of acetylcholine from parasympathetic nerve terminals. Although all three of these classes of agents lead ultimately to activation of muscarinic receptors at cardiovascular neuroeffector junctions, their cardiovascular effects in intact animals can vary substantially because of the differences in their mechanisms of action (Figure 24). Muscarinic agonists produce effects on all organs or tissues that possess muscarinic receptors, whether or not these organs or tissues are innervated by parasympathetic nerve terminals (Figure 24). By contrast, acetylcholinesterase inhibitors depend for their action upon parasympathetic innervation from which endogenous acetylcholine is released (Figure 24). Ganglionic stimulants produce complex effects be-

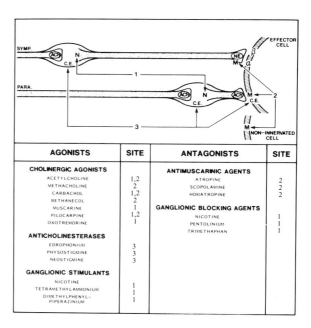

AGONISTS	SITE	ANTAGONISTS	SITE
CHOLINERGIC AGONISTS		**ANTIMUSCARINIC AGENTS**	
ACETYLCHOLINE	1,2	ATROPINE	2
METHACHOLINE	2	SCOPOLAMINE	2
CARBACHOL	1,2	HOMATROPINE	2
BETHANECOL	2		
MUSCARINE	1	**GANGLIONIC BLOCKING AGENTS**	
PILOCARPINE	1,2	NICOTINE	1
OXOTREMORINE	1	PENTOLINIUM	1
		TRIMETHAPHAN	1
ANTICHOLINESTERASES			
EDROPHONIUM	3		
PHYSOSTIGMINE	3		
NEOSTIGMINE	3		
GANGLIONIC STIMULANTS			
NICOTINE	1		
TETRAMETHYLAMMONIUM	1		
DIMETHYLPHENYL- PIPERAZINIUM	1		

Figure 24. Schematic representation of sympathetic (symp) and parasympathetic (para) nerves and potential sites of action of drugs. N = nicotinic receptor, C.E. = acetylcholinesterase, β = beta-adrenergic receptor, α = alpha-adrenergic receptor, M = muscarinic cholinergic receptor. Numbers in table correspond to sites of action of drugs in figure above table.

cause they stimulate both parasympathetic and sympathetic ganglia (Figure 24). These differences will be elaborated upon in this section.

Cholinergic agonists

Mechanism of action
The drugs in this group interact directly with muscarinic cholinergic receptors in organs or tissues which possess these receptors. These receptors are found in autonomic neuroeffector sites innervated by parasympathetic nerve terminals, other organs or tissues (e.g., arteriolar smooth muscle) which are not innervated by parasympathetic nerves, sympathetic and parasympathetic ganglion cells, the adrenal medulla, innervated skeletal muscle motor end plates, and certain CNS synapses (Figure 24). Consequently, these agonists theoretically can activate any of these systems when administered to the intact animal. These drugs can be divided into two major groups, the choline esters and the naturally occurring cholinomimetic plant alkaloids. The car-

Table 4. Properties of choline esters.

Choline ester	Structural formula	Susceptibility to cholinesterase	Muscarinic action	Nicotinic action
Acetylcholine chloride	$(CH_3)_3\overset{+}{N}CH_2CH_2O\overset{\displaystyle O}{\overset{\|}{C}}CH_3$ Cl^-	++++	+++	+++
Methacholine chloride	$(CH_3)_3\overset{+}{N}CH_2\underset{CH_3}{CH}O\overset{\displaystyle O}{\overset{\|}{C}}CH_3$ Cl^-	+	++++	+
Carbachol chloride	$(CH_3)_3\overset{+}{N}CH_2CH_2O\overset{\displaystyle O}{\overset{\|}{C}}NH_2$ Cl^-	–	++	+++
Bethanecol chloride	$(CH_3)_3\overset{+}{N}CH_2\underset{CH_3}{CH}O\overset{\displaystyle O}{\overset{\|}{C}}NH_2$ Cl^-	–	++	–

diovascular effects of these agents are qualitatively similar, the effects varying primarily in the efficacy of a given dose and duration of action. The choline esters to be considered here are acetylcholine, methacholine, carbachol, and bethanecol (Table 4). As detailed in an earlier section the physiological effects of acetylcholine are terminated by the actions of acetylcholinesterase and in some species (such as dogs) by nonspecific or pseudocholinesterases [20]. A major difference between acetylcholine and the synthetic choline esters is the relative resistance of the synthetic choline esters to hydrolysis by acetylcholinesterase (Table 4). Thus, the duration of action and the efficacy of a given dose of these synthetic agents is greater than that of acetylcholine in intact animals, even though the affinity of these compounds for muscarinic receptors does not vary markedly from that of acetylcholine [117]. Methacholine and bethanecol differ also from the other choline esters in having greater selectivity for muscarinic as compared to nicotinic receptors [199] (Table 4, Figure 24). Carbachol stimulates both muscarinic receptors on effector organs and nicotinic receptors in ganglia. Therefore, its action depends on both direct stimulation of muscarinic receptors and release of endogenous acetylcholine from parasympathetic nerve terminals (Table 4, Figure 24).

The naturally occurring cholinomimetic alkaloids that have been most extensively studied are muscarine, pilocarpine, and arecoline. Oxotremorine is a synthetic compound which is unique in its extreme potency as a muscarinic agonist. Muscarine is highly selective in its action on muscarinic receptors, whereas pilocarpine and arecoline stimulate both muscarinic and nicotinic receptors [199] (Figure 24).

Cardiovascular effects
The cardiovascular effects of muscarinic agonists in intact animals are complex as the net observed hemodynamic effects may represent the action of the drugs on both the heart and vasculature as well as autonomic ganglia of nerves that innervate the heart. Also, in view of the interaction between the sympathetic and parasympathetic nervous systems (discussed in a previous section), the effects of muscarinic agonists depend in part on the prevailing sympathetic tone. If sympathetic tone is low, little of the muscarinic effects would be manifested by modulation of sympathetic activity. On the other hand, if sympathetic activity is high, muscarinic

agonists exert effects by modifying both parasympathetic and sympathetic function. In ventricular tissue, the prevailing sympathetic tone is particularly important because of the relatively small direct parasympathetic effects on ventricular function (see the section on sympathetic–parasympathetic interaction). Muscarinic agonists modify the effects of sympathetic activity both by modulating release of norepinephrine (at the prejunctional level) and by modulating the intracellular effects of acetylcholine (Figures 6 and 24). Thus, the state of the autonomic nervous system, particularly the activity of the sympathetic limb, can determine the magnitude of muscarinic effects on ventricles [73].

The primary and most easily observable cardiovascular effects of muscarinic cholinergic agonists are reductions in blood pressure and changes in heart rate. The intravenous injection of low doses of acetylcholine to anesthetized animals produces a transient fall in blood pressure, sometimes accompanied by a reflex increase in heart rate [199]. Intravenous infusions of low doses in humans (e.g., 20–50 μg/min) produce reductions in blood pressure due to vasodilation [199]. In both animals and humans larger doses of acetylcholine produce bradycardia and decreased conduction velocity through the atrioventricular node in addition to the hypotensive effect [199]. In humans, intravenous infusions of 90–140 μg/min produces marked bradycardia, sometimes associated with heart block and hypotension [199].

In intact animals and in humans, these cardiovascular effects are due to the actions of muscarinic agonists on the sinoatrial node (negative chronotropic effect), the atrioventricular node (negative dromotropic effect), peripheral vasculature (vasodilation), and the atrial and ventricular myocardium [1, 21–24]. The reduction in blood pressure results from both the vasodilation and the negative inotropic effects of muscarinic agonists on the heart. The atria are most prominently influenced by these muscarinic negative inotropic effects [21]. Ventricular function is influenced by decreased ventricular filling resulting from the reduced contractile state of the atria and by the effects of muscarinic agonists on the ventricles per se [25, 35, 36]. These latter effects are mediated largely by muscarinic modulation of the positive inotropic effects of the sympathetic nervous system [37–39, 66–68, 74–78].

The cardiovascular effects in intact animals or in humans of the other choline esters are generally similar to those of acetylcholine, the main difference being in the efficacy and duration of action of a given dose [199]. Because of the relative resistance of methacholine, carbachol, and bethanecol to acetylcholinesterase, substantially lower doses (1/200) given intravenously are required to produce effects similar to acetylcholine and the duration of action of these synthetic choline esters is longer. The cardiovascular effects of the cholinomimetic natural alkaloids and synthetic analogs are also generally similar to those of acetylcholine, the main differences again being in efficacy of a given dose and duration of action. Intravenous injection of muscarine (0.01–0.03 μg/kg) produces hypotension, bradycardia, and sometimes atrioventricular block or asystole [199].

The cardiovascular effects of muscarinic agonists in intact animals are not necessarily identical to those of vagal nerve activation, which may occur physiologically or in the experimental setting as a result of nerve stimulation. The cardiovascular effects of muscarinic agonists are more generalized or diffuse than those of vagal nerve stimulation. The reasons for this are that muscarinic agonists can activate components of both the parasympathetic and sympathetic nervous systems (Figure 24) and also can stimulate organs or tissues that may not be innervated by parasympathetic nerves but which contain muscarinic receptors. For example, in dogs, vagal nerve stimulation and acetylcholine infusions, which were equi-effective in terms of reducing ventricular contractility, had quantitatively different effects on heart rate and coronary blood flow [200]. Vagal nerve stimulation reduced heart rate much more than did acetylcholine but had much less effect on coronary blood flow [200]. Presumably with vagal nerve stimulation muscarinic receptors on sinoatrial nodal cells were exposed to higher concentrations of acetylcholine than when acetylcholine was given by infusion, perhaps because of density of vagal innervation and differences in susceptibility of released versus infused actylcholine to cholinesterase. On the other hand, coronary arteries are not heavily innervated by vagal nerves but possess muscarinic receptors so changes in coronary vascular tone were greater with acetylcholine infusion.

The sites of action of these cholinergic agonists have been defined in experimental studies in which the agonists are given simultaneously with a receptor blocking agent. When acetylcholine and carbachol are given with agents such as atropine that selectively block muscarinic receptors (site 2 in Figure 24) their cardiovascular effects become stimulatory as a result of their activation of nicotinic receptors (site 1 in Figure 24) in sympathetic ganglia and the adrenal medulla, which then leads to release of norepinephrine and epinephrine [201] (Figure 24). Nicotinic receptors in parasympathetic ganglia are also stimulated in the presence of atropine, but no parasympathetic response is elicited because of blockade of muscarinic receptors on the effector cells. When nicotinic receptors are blocked by agents such as nicotine or hexamethonium (site 1 in Figure 24), the effects of all cholinergic agonists (even those with mixed muscarinic and nicotinic activity) are manifested only on muscarinic receptors (site 2 in Figure 24).

Noncardiovascular pharmacologic effects
The noncardiovascular effects of cholinergic agonists are manifestations of the activation of muscarinic receptors on smooth muscle and certain glands. Peristalsis and secretory activity of the stomach and intestines are increased and thus nausea and vomiting, abdominal pain and defecation may occur with administration of these drugs [199]. The effect on the urinary tract is to stimulate urination by contracting the detrusor muscle of the bladder and relaxing the trigone and external sphincter [199]. Muscarinic agonists can produce bronchoconstriction. Intraocular administration of muscarinic agonists produces pupillary constriction (miosis). All glands that are innervated by parasympathetic nerves are stimulated by muscarinic agonists, including the lacrimal, tracheobronchial, salivary, digestive, and exocrine sweat glands.

Cardiovascular therapeutic uses
There are no cardiovascular therapeutic uses of cholinergic agonists.

Acetylcholinesterase inhibitors

Mechanism of action
The anticholinesterase agents modify the effects of acetylcholine by inhibiting its hydrolysis by cholinesterases. Thus, these agents theoretically can exert effects at all synapses and neuroeffector junctions where acetylcholine is a neurotransmitter. These include effector organs innervated by parasympathetic nerves, autonomic ganglia, skeletal muscle motor end plates and the CNS (Figure 24). The diffuseness of the effects of anticholinesterases, however, is highly variable depending on the specific agent, the dose given, and the physiological regulation of specific organ systems by parasympathetic nerves. For example, compounds containing quaternary ammonium groups do not readily cross cell membranes and therefore are poorly absorbed from the gastrointestinal tract and do not readily pass the blood–brain barrier. These compounds act relatively selectively at neuromuscular junctions. By contrast, the lipid soluble agents such as tertiary amines and organophosphorous compounds are well absorbed from the gastrointestinal tract and have generalized effects at both peripheral and central cholinergic sites. Because the anticholinesterase agents work ultimately via released endogenous acetylcholine, their effects will depend upon the level of parasympathetic activity in regulating a given organ system. If tonic parasympathetic activity to a given organ is low, anticholinesterases will not change substantially the function of that organ. In contrast, if tonic parasympathetic activity is high and large amounts of endogenous acetylcholine are being released the effects of anticholinesterases may be marked. Anticholinesterases will not have any effect on organs or tissues which possess muscarinic receptors but are not innervated by parasympathetic nerves.

Although all anticholinesterases exert their pharmacological effects ultimately by increasing the concentration of acetylcholine in the vicinity of acetylcholine receptors, the molecular mechanisms, at the level of acetylcholinesterase by which these agents act, differ. Quaternary compounds such as edrophonium bind reversibly to the active site of acetylcholinesterase and thus prevent access of acetylcholine to these sites [202]. Drugs such as physostigmine and neostigmine which have carbamyl ester linkages, bind to and act as substrates for acetylcholinesterase, resulting in a carbamylated form of the enzyme which then is not available for hydrolysis of acetylcholine [202]. The carbamylated enzyme is slowly hydrolyzed to yield regenerated acetylcholinesterase. However, during this slow process acetylcholinesterase is prevented from interacting with its normal substrate acetylcholine. The irreversible organophosphorous inhibitors also bind to the enzyme and serve as substrate, thus leading to phosphorylation of the active site [202]. This phosphorylated complex is extremely stable so that the acetylcholinesterase is in effect irreversibly inhibited. After inhibition with organophosphates, return of acetylcholinesterase activity depends on synthesis of new enzyme molecules.

Cardiovascular effects
Theoretically, the cardiovascular effects of anticholinesterases could be very complex because of the multiple potential sites of action of these agents on autonomic nerves. Anticholinesterases could theoretically lead to activation of nicotinic receptors at both parasympathetic and sympathetic ganglia and of muscarinic receptors on neuroeffector junctions and prejunctional sympathetic terminals (Figure 24). In intact animals and humans the effects on the parasympathetic limb predominate. Thus, administration of cholinesterase inhibitors such as edrophonium, physostigmine, or neostigmine leads to effects which in general mimic the effects of vagal nerve activation [202]. Heart rate decreases, conduction velocity through the atrioventricular junction diminishes, atrial contractility decreases, and cardiac output falls. The fall in cardiac output is contributed to by the bradycardia, decreased atrial contractility, and also reduction in ventricular contractility. The latter effect probably occurs predominantly via muscarinic restraint of sympathetic activity.

Of the cardiovascular effects of acetylcholinesterase inhibitors, electrophysiological effects have been studied most extensively. In animals and humans, acetylcholinesterase inhibitors have been shown to modify the electrophysiological properties of both supraventricular and ventricular structures. Edrophonium increased the ventricular fibrillation threshold and prolonged the time to death in dogs with experimentally induced myocardial ischemia [49]. Edrophonium slowed heart rate, prolonged A–H intervals and increased atrioventricular nodal functional refractory periods in human subjects [203]. This anticholinesterase administered in the same manner did not change the foregoing electrophysiological properties in patients who had undergone cardiac transplantation [203]. These results in humans indicate that the effects of edrophonium are dependent on endogenous acetylcholine released from vagal nerves. The hearts of transplant recipients were denervated and therefore did not respond to anticholinesterase therapy. Large doses of edrophonium combined with carotid sinus massage or phenylephrine infusion terminated ventricular tachycardia in patients with ventricular tachycardia [52] (Figure 5).

The effects of anticholinesterase on blood pressure are less marked than those of muscarinic agonists. The reasons are that anticholinesterases modify tone of only those vessels that are innervated by parasympathetic nerves and that the net effects on vascular tone may represent activation of both the parasympathetic and sympathetic nervous systems. Whereas activation of the parasympathetic system (at ganglia and neuroeffector junctions) would tend to lower vascular resistance and blood pressure, activation of sympathetic ganglia would tend to oppose these hypotensive effects. Even when administered in low or moderate doses, likely to activate primarily the parasympathetic nervous system, anticholinesterases exert part of their effect in intact animals by modulating sympathetic nerve activity (see the section on sympathetic–parasympathetic interaction). Inhibition of acetylcholinesterase would be expected to increase acetylcholine levels in the vicinity of prejunctional muscarinic receptors on sympathetic nerve terminals as well as postjunctional receptors on effector cells (Figure 24). When large doses of anticholinesterases are given the net hemodynamic effects are the result of complex interactions. Acetylcholinesterase in ganglia (site 3 in Figure 24) would be inhibited as well as at neuroeffector junctional sites. The activation of sympathetic ganglia would tend to increase sympathetic activity and thus stimulate the heart. Simultaneously, activation of parasympathetic ganglia and augmentation of the effects of acetylcholine released from nerve terminals would be expected to produce powerful parasympathetic restraint (at both the pre-and postjunctional level) of the sympathetic effects. The net hemodynamic response of the animal would reflect these complex interactions.

The effects of anticholinesterases are blocked by appropriate receptor blockers. Antimuscarinic agents block their effects at neuroeffector junctions [49] (site 2 in Figure 24). If large doses of anticholinesterase are administered simultaneously with antimuscarinic agents, cardiovascular stimulation may ensue from unrestrained activation of the sympathetic nervous system. Ganglionic receptor blockers inhibit anticholinesterase activation of both parasympathetic and sympathetic ganglia (site 3 in Figure 24). Muscarinic effects at postjunctional receptors would still occur so that with ganglionic blockade anticholinesterases would continue to exert an inhibitory effect on cardiovascular function.

Noncardiovascular pharmacologic effects

The noncardiovascular pharmacologic effects of anticholinesterases generally can be predicted based on knowledge on sites of action of acetylcholine and the physiological effects of activating acetylcholine receptors [202]. Smooth muscle of the gastrointestinal tract, genitourinary tract, and bronchioles are stimulated. Accordingly, gastric and intestinal motility are increased and subjects may have nausea, abdominal pain, vomiting, or diarrhea. Bronchospasm may develop and subjects may have the urge to micturate. Innervated glands, including those in the gastrointestinal tract, bronchioles, and salivary glands will be stimulated to secrete. When applied locally into the eye pupillary constriction occurs.

Cardiovascular therapeutic uses

Edrophonium has been used for treatment of supraventricular tachyarrhythmias, particularly paroxysmal supraventricular tachycardia [204] (Table 5). By potentiating the effects of released endogeneous acetylcholine at the atrioventricular junction, atrioventricular conduction velocity is diminished, and the number of supraventricular impulses conducted into the ventricles may be reduced and therefore ventricular rate slowed. Edrophonium may also convert the abnormal supraventricular tachyarrhythmia into normal sinus rhythm. Edrophonium usually is given intravenously in a dose of 5–10 mg (0.15 mg/kg) administered over 30 sec. Carotid sinus massage should be performed after giving the drug. As noted earlier, acetylcholinesterase inhibition alone or combined with carotid sinus massage has been shown to terminate ventricular tachycardia in humans [52]. However, the relatively large dose used, the need to combine this with carotid sinus massage and/or a pressor agent, the lack of generally proven efficacy of this approach in all patients with ventricular tachycardia, and the usually emergent and life-threatening nature of this arrhythmia have prevented the use of anticholinesterases as a standard approach to therapy for ventricular arrhythmias. Other pharmacologic (e.g., lidocaine) approaches or cardioversion are the treatments of choice for ventricular tachycardia [205]. The value of the cited study is not in offering an alternative therapeutic approach but rather in providing evidence regarding the role of vagal innervation in regulating the electrophysiological properties of ventricles in humans.

Ganglionic stimulating agents

Ganglionic stimulants activate nicotinic receptors in both parasympathetic and sympathetic ganglia (Figure 24). The stimulation of nicotinic receptors then lends to activation of postganglionic sympathetic and parasympathetic nerves with release of the respective neurotransmitters from the nerve terminals. The ganglionic stimulating agents include nicotine, lobeline, tetramethylammonium, and 1,1-dimethyl-4-phenylpiperazinium. Nicotine stimulates, in addition to ganglia, the adrenal medulla and receptors within the CNS. The effects of

Table 5. Cardiovascular therapeutic uses of cholinergic agonists and antagonists.

Drug	Mechanism of action	Clinical use	Average dose
Edrophonium	Acetylcholinesterase inhibitor	Paroxysmal atrial tachycardia	5–10 mg I.V.
Atropine	Muscarinic receptor blocker	Sick sinus syndrome (syncope); Symptomatic bradycardia in acute myocardial infarction; Sinus bradycardia or atrio-ventricular block associated with digitalis intoxication	0.5–1.0 mg I.V.
Trimethaphan	Ganglionic blocker	Malignant hypertension; Dissecting aortic aneurysm	1–4 mg/min infusion

See text for details regarding indications and methods of administration.

nicotine on ganglia are biphasic, an initial transient stimulation followed by a longer lasting inhibition.

Because ganglionic stimulants activate nicotinic receptors in both parasympathetic and sympathetic ganglia, the cardiovascular effects of these agents are complex [206]. The cardiovascular effects of nicotine represent the net hemodynamic effects of combined parasympathetic and sympathetic nerve stimulation. When given rapidly by the intravenous route to an intact animal, such as a dog, the nicotinic stimulatory effects on the two limbs of the autonomic nervous system can be separated temporally. The earliest cardiovascular response is marked sinus bradycardia, occasionally asystole for a few seconds, and sometimes atrioventricular block, perhaps associated with ventricular escape rhythms. Associated with these electrophysiological changes is hypotension due to both reduced cardiac output and arteriolar vasodilation. These cardiovascular effects reflect activation of nicotinic receptors in parasympathetic ganglia with resultant release of acetylcholine from vagal nerve terminals. This depressant effect is followed in a few seconds by a rapidly developing stimulation of the cardiovascular system. Heart rate and blood pressure increase, and the animal soon develops tachycardia and hypertension. Frequently, abnormal cardiac rhythms including multiple ventricular premature systoles or ventricular tachycardia ensue. The stimulatory effect, which reflects activation of sympathetic ganglia and the adrenal medulla, may persist for several minutes and then gradually dissipate with the cardiovascular properties returning toward pretreatment levels. Nicotine also stimulates chemoreceptors in the aorta and carotid bodies, and this activates reflexes which contribute to the sympathomimetic cardiovascular effects of the alkaloid.

The fact that nicotinic ganglionic stimulants activate both parasympathetic and sympathetic nerves can be verified by the coadministration of selective postjunctional blocking agents. Administration of atropine or tetrodotoxin (which blocks release of acetylcholine from nerve terminals) blocks the depressant cardiovascular effects of nicotine while allowing the manifestations of the stimulatory effects [35, 36]. On the other hand, blockade of beta-adrenergic receptors eliminates the stimulatory effects but allows the depressant effects to persist [207].

The noncardiovascular effects of nicotinic agents

include CNS stimulation with resultant tremors followed by convulsions (with high doses), stimulation followed by depression of respiration, increased gastrointestinal motility sometimes associated with nausea and vomiting, and stimulation of glandular (salivary and bronchial) secretion [206].

There are no cardiovascular therapeutic uses of nicotine.

Drugs that antagonize the action of acetylcholine on muscarinic receptors

The drugs to be discussed in this section share the property of interfering with the function of postganglionic parasympathetic nerves. One group of these agents interferes with the ability of acetylcholine, released from parasympathetic nerve endings, to interact with muscarinic receptors on cardiovascular neuroeffector junctions. These agents produce this interference by interacting directly with postjunctional muscarinic receptors and thereby impeding access of acetylcholine to the receptor (Figures 13 and 24). A second group of agents impairs the function of postganglionic parasympathetic nerves by inhibiting parasympathetic ganglia (Figure 24). In the former group are included the classical antimuscarinic agents and a number of other drugs whose primary activity is directed towards other systems but which also possess significant antimuscarinic activity. These different types of drugs will be discussed separately.

Antimuscarinic agents

Mechanism of action
Antimuscarinic agents bind specifically to muscarinic receptors without activating the receptors; i.e., they do not possess agonist activity. However, by interacting with muscarinic receptors they interfere with the access of the normal neurotransmitter to the receptors (Figure 13). Accordingly, their pharmacologic effects depend on and are determined by the prevailing level of parasympathetic tone in the animal or subject administered the drugs. Their effects are determined by the distribution of parasympathetic innervation and the level of tonic parasympathetic activity. Antimuscarinic agents will not modify the properties of organs or tissues that are not innervated by parasympathetic nerves or

which are not under the influence of tonic parasympathetic activity. On the other hand, the physiological properties of organs which are under predominant parasympathetic control will be altered markedly by agents that block muscarinic receptors. The magnitude of effect of antimuscarinic agents may vary markedly between individuals or within a given individual depending on his or her state of health or level of physical activity or emotional state when the agent is administered. For example, a healthy, athletic young person at rest would be expected to have a high level of vagal control of cardiovascular function, as reflected by a relatively slow resting heart rate. Administration of an antimuscarinic agent to such an individual would be expected to increase heart rate substantially. On the other hand, the same dose of an antimuscarinic agent would not be expected to change heart rate much if the drug were administered to the individual during physical exertion or emotional excitement. Older subjects or individuals with certain cardiovascular diseases such as heart failure may have relatively little vagal tone even at rest. Antimuscarinic agents would not be expected to change heart rate much in such individuals. Thus, the quantitative effects of agents that block muscarinic receptors will be influenced importantly by the state of the animal or subject given the drug.

Muscarinic antagonists also will augment the effects of the sympathetic nervous system by interfering with muscarinic inhibition of sympathetic activity (Figures 6 and 24). Acetylcholine released from parasympathetic nerve terminals inhibits release of norepinephrine from sympathetic nerve terminals and also modulates the cellular effects of catecholamines that interact with beta-adrenergic receptors. Antimuscarinic agents block effects of acetylcholine at both the prejunctional and postjunctional level of sympathetic–parasympathetic interaction.

A large number of synthetic antimuscarinic compounds have been synthesized in attempts to obtain agents that would selectively block muscarinic receptors only in certain organ systems. These attempts have met with limited success, and none of these synthetic compounds is used clinically in cardiovascular therapeutics. Of the naturally occurring plant alkaloids, atropine and scopolamine, and the semisynthetic derivative homatropine have been studied most extensively [208]. Atropine is the prototype of this group and continues to be the most widely used antimuscarinic agent in clinical cardiology.

Cardiovascular effects
As mentioned, the cardiovascular effects of antimuscarinic agents such as atropine are dependent on the prevailing tonic activity of both the parasympathetic and sympathetic nervous systems. In addition, the effects of atropine are dose dependent. Low doses (e.g., 0.3–0.6 mg) given to human subjects may produce a transient, paradoxical slowing of heart rate [208]. This effect, which is usually small, is presumably due to actions of atropine in the CNS leading to increased efferent vagal nerve activity [208]. Within a few seconds peripheral muscarinic receptor blockade is established and heart rate increases. With larger doses (0.6–1.2 mg) heart rate immediately increases, the magnitude of change depending on the level of tonic parasympathetic activity. Conduction velocity through the atrioventricular node is increased. This effect occurs independently of changes in heart rate as can be demonstrated by measuring A–H intervals while maintaining heart rate constant by atrial pacing. In the intact animal or human, atropine administration increases cardiac output (Figure 9). This effect is due to increased heart rate as well as increased atrial and ventricular contractility, although the changes in contractility are difficult to measure in the intact animal or in a clinical setting. Atropine may decrease the electrical stability of ventricles particularly in the setting of myocardial ischemia [47, 49]. This effect of atropine presumably is due both to increased myocardial ischemia secondary to increased heart rate and to removal of antifibrillatory vagal effects per se.

Atropine blocks vagally mediated cardiovascular reflexes such as bradycardia secondary to carotid sinus massage or application of pressure on the eyeballs. Atropine also abolishes respiratory cycle-related sinus arrhythmia.

Because of the phenomenon of sympathetic–parasympathetic interaction, a significant portion of the action of atropine is mediated via enhanced sympathetic activation of the heart. Therefore, not only does atropine antagonize vagal effects on the heart, but, by so doing, it augments sympathetic effects on the heart (Figure 9). That is, by blocking prejunctional muscarinic receptors on sympathetic nerve terminals, atropine augments norepinephrine release from sympathetic nerves (Figures 6 and 24). By blocking postjunctional muscarinic receptors on effector cells (such as cells in the sinoatrial node) atropine augments the cellular response to beta-adrenergic receptor stimulation by neurally released norepinephrine or circulatory epinephrine (Figure 9). Thus, the cardiac effects of atropine are the results of both removal of parasympathetic activity and simultaneous augmentation of sympathetic activity on the heart. This is true in terms of the electrophysiological effects (increased heart rate and atrioventricular conduction) and increases in myocardial contractility [72]. The sympathetic mediation of the antimuscarinic stimulatory effects is particularly important in the ventricles because of the relatively small direct effects of vagus nerve activity on ventricular function.

Noncardiovascular effects

The different belladonna alkaloids have qualitatively different effects on the CNS [208]. In clinical doses (e.g., 0.6–1.2 mg intravenously) atropine can stimulate CNS centers causing restlessness, irritability, delirium, or hallucinations. On the other hand, scopolamine in therapeutic doses usually causes sedation, and, for this reason, it frequently is used as a preanesthetic medication or as an adjunct to anesthetics in surgery.

The peripheral noncardiovascular effects of atropine are predictable from an understanding of the normal physiological effects of the parasympathetic nervous system. The effects are generally opposite those of agents that cause activation of muscarinic receptors [208]. Smooth muscle activity generally is inhibited by atropine: gastrointestinal motility is reduced sometimes to the point of causing ileus; contractions of the ureter and bladder are reduced and patients, particularly elderly males, frequently develop urinary retention; bronchiolar smooth muscle is relaxed. Atropine also interferes with parasympathetic activation of glands. Salivary secretion is inhibited causing dry mouth and sometimes diffulty in swallowing. Secretions of the nose, mouth, pharynx, and bronchi also are inhibited. This is one of the desired effects for which antimuscarinic agents are used in preanesthetic treatment. The volume and acid content of gastric secretion is reduced by antimuscarinics. Atropine, particularly when administered intraocularly, dilates the pupil (mydriasis) and causes paralysis of accomodation (cyclopegia). The usual clinical doses of atropine given systemically do not produce these ocular effects. Scopolamine, on the other hand, even in usual clinical doses frequently causes mydriasis and cyclopegia.

Cardiovascular therapeutic uses

Atropine is the antimuscarinic agent most widely used in clinical cardiology, and in this setting it is administered parenterally (intravenously, intramuscularly, or subcutaneously) and generally used only in acute emergency situations until the patient recovers from his/her acute problem or other more long-term (e.g., temporary pacing) therapeutic interventions have been instituted. The use of atropine in specific clinical situations will be discussed (Table 5).

Sick sinus syndrome. The so-called sick sinus syndrome is a clinical syndrome that includes patients with a wide array of problems involving the pacemaking and/or specialized conducting tissues of the heart [209]. Characteristically, the sinoatrial node functions abnormally and exhibits depressed automaticity (abnormally slow rate) or inability to activate the rest of the atrium (exit block). Frequently, abnormalities of other components of the electrophysiological system are present. Thus, these patients may also exhibit abnormal atrioventricular automaticity and conduction (heart block) and bundle branch block. One of the clinical symptoms of sick sinus syndrome, due to depressed sinoatrial node automaticity and/or heart block, is syncope. If this should occur while the patient is under medical care (e.g., in hospital) atropine (intravenously 0.5–1.0 mg) may relieve symptoms until more long-term therapy (e.g., pacemaking) can be instituted.

Acute myocardial infarction. Sinus bradycardia is the most common arrhythmia seen during acute myocardial infarction [210]. This arrhythmia is particularly common with inferior infarction, possibly because the infarction in the inferior region of the heart leads to stimulation of cardiac vagal afferent receptors, which are particularly dense in this area of the heart. The activation of vagal afferent receptors is thought to result in increased efferent vagal nerve activity and thus bradycardia. The bradycardia may sometimes be associated with atrioventricular block of varying degrees: first-degree AV block; second-degree AV block (most commonly Mobitz type I or Wenkebach block); and, occasionally complete heart block [210].

If the patient is not having hemodynamic difficulties (e.g., hypotension) or other problems, such as ventricular arrhythmias with the sinus bradycardia, the bradycardia probably does not require treatment, but the patient should be carefully monitored in a coronary care unit [210]. There is experimental evidence that bradycardia during myocardial ischemia may actually be beneficial in protecting against ventricular arrhythmias. This protection appears to result from the slow heart rate itself and from vagal tone which produces the slow heart rate [46-48]. Bradycardia might be expected to be beneficial during myocardial ischemia by limiting cardiac oxygen demand and thereby limiting infarct size.

On the other hand, sinus bradycardia sometimes is associated with hypotension and/or increased ventricular arrhythmias (which clearly seem to be related to the bradycardia) [210]. The hypotension may sometimes be associated with evidence of increased myocardial ischemia, as manifested by recurrent chest pain or elevation in ST segments on the electrocardiogram. In such situations the bradyarrhythmia should be treated. Atropine should be given carefully in doses of 0.3-0.6 mg intravenously every 3-5 min with the total dose not exceeding 2 mg [211]. The objective is to increase heart rate gradually to approximately 60-75 beats/min thereby restoring blood pressure. The improved hemodynamic state and the increased heart rate should help eliminate evidence of ischemia and ventricular ectopy. Heart rate should not be increased excessively nor vagal tone abolished completely. If tachycardia results from excessive muscarinic blockade, myocardial ischemia may be increased because of excessive myocardial oxygen demand. Moreover, in view of the evidence that vagal tone per se may protect against lethal ventricular arrhythmias during myocardial ischemia [46-48], excessive muscarinic blockade may actually promote ventricular arrhythmias. If clinical problems (hypotension, ventricular arrhythmias, chest pain) from sinus bradycardia persist or recur, temporary transvenous pacemaking should be instituted for longer-term management of the patient.

Second-degree (Mobitz type I) heart block in the setting of acute myocardial infarction can also be treated acutely with atropine. If ventricular rate is adequate and hypotension, ventricular arrhythmias, or chest pain are absent, no specific therapy is required [212]. However, if any of these complications occur, the patient should be treated with atropine and consideration made for temporary transvenous pacemaking.

Intravenous atropine (0.5-1.0 mg) is often effective in reversing bradycardia sometimes seen after defibrillation of individuals who have suffered cardiac arrest.

Digitalis intoxication. Occasionally patients with digitalis intoxication will develop marked sinus bradycardia sometimes associated with atrioventricular conduction disturbances. If this is associated with other complications such as hypotension, ventricular irritability (clearly associated with the bradycardia), chest pain, or heart failure, the bradyarrhythmia should be treated. For acute treatment intravenous atropine (0.5-1.0 mg) is effective. This can be repeated every 3-4 hr if needed, but if the problem does not resolve promptly temporary transvenous pacing should be considered.

Ganglionic blocking agents

The drugs in this category interact with nicotinic receptors in autonomic ganglia and thereby prevent them from being activated by the normal transmitter acetylcholine. Ganglionic blocking agents can be divided into two groups based on their mechanism of action. The first group, typified by nicotine, produces a biphasic effect on ganglia, initially causing stimulation and subsequently blockade by persistent depolarization of the synaptic membrane [206]. The second group of drugs, of which hexamethonium is the prototype, does not produce any stimulation, rather only blockade of ganglia, presumably by competing with acetylcholine for access to nicotinic receptor sites [206]. These agents block ganglia of both the parasympathetic and sympathetic nervous systems so with appropriate doses of these agents the treated animal is in effect autonomically denervated (Figure 24). The effects on a given organ system depend on whether the system is dually innervated (by both limbs of the autonomic nervous system) and on which system predominates.

The effects of ganglionic blocking agents on the cardiovascular system are determined by which limb (parasympathetic or sympathetic) of the autonomic nervous system is exerting predominant control and by the physiological demands placed on the autonomic nervous system. Ganglionic blockers usually increase heart rate in humans, because, at rest, heart rate is predominantly under vagal control. Thus, with blockade of both parasympathetic and sympathetic ganglia, the change in vagal tone will be greater and the net change in heart rate will be an increase. Cardiac output is usually decreased by ganglionic blockers, in spite of the increase in heart rate. This is because venous tone is predominantly under sympathetic control. Abolition of sympathetic activity reduces venous tone and thus diminishes venous filling of the atria. Peripheral vascular resistance falls because of removal of sympathetic control of arterial tone. This results in a fall in blood pressure, which may not be too marked in recumbent normotensive individuals. However, when these same individuals stand – i.e., when they place physiological demands on sympathetic activity – blood pressure may fall dramatically even to the point of causing syncope.

The noncardiovascular effects of ganglionic blockers also reflect autonomic innervation and which limb of the autonomic nervous system predominantly controls function [206]. Clinical effects include constipation and sometimes paralytic ileus, urinary retention, visual disturbances, and dry mouth.

Trimethaphan (Arfonad) is the ganglionic blocker which has gained widest usage in the clinical setting (Table 5). In past years, trimethaphan was the only generally available agent for treatment of malignant hypertension. However, other agents, which are equally effective and have fewer side effects and are perhaps easier to use, have supplanted the use of trimethaphan in many patients with this clinical problem. Trimethaphan remains the treatment of choice in patients with hypertension and dissecting aortic aneurysms. The vasodilator agents, such as Na nitroprusside or diazoxide, may increase reflexly sympathetic activity and thus myocardial contractility and the rate of change of intraaortic pressure (dP/dt). This could theoretically cause progression of the dissection. By contrast, trimethaphan reduces blood pressure and at the same time decreases myocardial contractility by

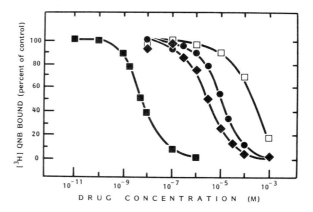

Figure 25. Curves describing competition of atropine (■), (⊥) disopyramide (♦), quinidine (●), and procainamide (□) with [3H]QNB for binding to muscarinic receptors in guinea pig right atrium. Each point is the mean of values obtained from triplicate determinations in three separate experiments with SE ≤ 5%. [3H]QNB concentration was approximately 80 pM (reprinted with permission from [117]).

blocking sympathetic stimulation of the heart. Trimethaphan is given by continuous intravenous infusion, initially at a rate of 1 mg/min and increasing to a rate of as much as 3–4 mg/min. The dose is titrated against the blood pressure, which should be monitored continuously.

Other agents which block muscarinic receptors

The antiarrhythmic agents, disopyramide and quinidine, are known to produce significant anticholinergic effects when given to intact animals and humans [213–216]. Direct binding studies utilizing [3H]-QNB have verified that these anticholinergic effects of disopyramide and quinidine are due to the interaction of these agents with muscarinic receptors [117]. As shown in Figure 25, both disopyramide and quinidine effectively competed with [3H]-QNB for binding to muscarinic receptors, the derived inhibition constants (K_i) being 8.5×10^{-7} M for disopyramide and 2.5×10^{-6} M for quinidine (for comparison the K_i for atropine was 1.2×10^{-9} M) [117]. Because of this antimuscarinic activity, the prevailing level of autonomic nervous system activity can influence qualitatively the response of cardiac tissues to these antiarrhythmic agents. One of the direct effects of disopyramide and quinidine on cardiac tissues is to depress automaticity [217]. These agents decreased the spon-

135

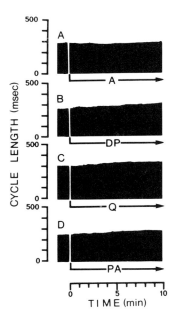

Figure 26. Effects of atropine, disopyramide, quinidine, and procainamide alone on spontaneous cycle length of guinea pig right atria. Cycle length (msec) is plotted on the vertical axis, and time (minutes) is plotted on the horizontal axis. The initial portion of each tachometer recording represents the last 2 min of the 15-min control period. The interruption of the tachometer recording after control is the time when drug infusion was initiated. (A) Atropine 1×10^{-6} M; (B) disopyramide 7×10^{-6} M; (C) quinidine 1×10^{-5} M; (D) procainamide 2×10^{-5} M (reprinted with permission from [218]).

taneous rate of isolated guinea pig right atria [218] (Figure 26). By contrast, if muscarinic receptors in atria were activated, disopyramide and quinidine increased spontaneous rate just as did atropine [218] (Figure 27). That is, in the setting of muscarinic receptor activation, the antimuscarinic effects of disopyramide and quinidine predominated over the direct depressant effects and spontaneous rate increased. The situation is more complex in ventricular tissues where muscarinic effects are largely mediated through modulation of sympathetic effects. Disopyramide and quinidine prolonged action potential duration of paced canine cardiac Purkinje fibers [218] (Figure 28), as has been shown previously [217]. When the environment of the fibers was changed to simulate in vivo autonomic tone, disopyramide and quinidine shortened action potential duration of paced Purkinje fibers [218]. Stimulation of beta receptors with isoproterenol

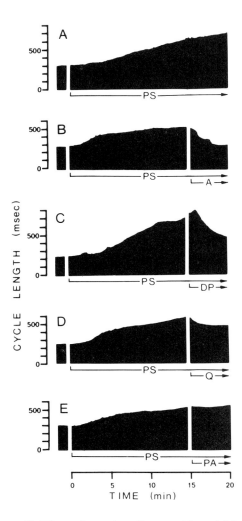

Figure 27. Effects of atropine, disopyramide, quinidine, and procainamide on spontaneous cycle length of guinea pig right atria pretreated with physostigmine. Cycle length (msec) is plotted on the vertical axis, and time (minutes) is plotted on the horizontal axis. The initial portion of each tachometer recording represents the last 1 min of the 15-min control period. The first interruption of the tachometer recording is the point at which physostigmine infusion was initiated, and the second interruption is the time point at which antiarrhythmic drug infusion was initiated. (A) Physostigmine (1×10^{-6} M) superfused alone slows spontaneous rate; (B) atropine (1×10^{-6} M) administered to an atrial preparation treated with physostigmine accelerates spontaneous rate; (C) disopyramide (7×10^{-6} M) administered to a physostigmine-pretreated preparation accelerates spontaneous rate; (D) quinidine (1×10^{-5} M) administered to a right atrial preparation which is treated with physostigmine elicits a positive chronotropic response; (E) procainamide (2×10^{-5} M) administered to a right atrial preparation treated with physostigmine produces a negative chronotropic response, similar to the response observed with procainamide alone (reprinted with permission from [218]).

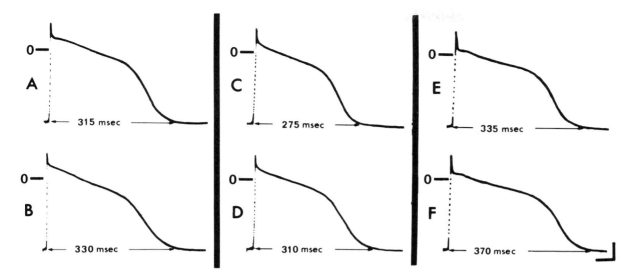

Figure 28. Effects of dysopyramide, quinidine, and procainamide administered alone on action potential duration of canine cardiac Purkinje fibers. A: Control for B; B: disopyramide (7×10^{-6} M) superfused alone for 5 min; C: control for D; D: quinidine (2×10^{-5} M) superfused alone for 5 min; E: control for F; F: procainamide (2×10^{-5} M) superfused alone for 5 min. Zero potential is indicated in each panel. Calibrations: horizontal bar = 50 msec; vertical bar = 25 mV (reprinted with permission from [218]).

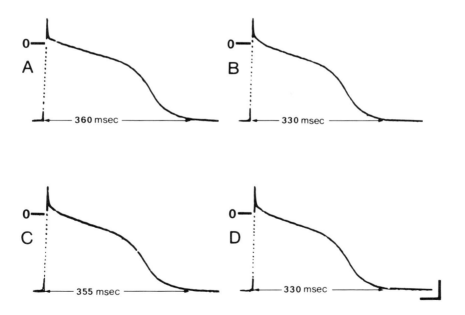

Figure 29. Effects of disopyramide on action potential duration of a Purkinje fiber treated with isoproterenol and acetylcholine. (A) control; (B) isoproterenol (1×10^{-7} M) superfused for 5 min; (C) acetylcholine (3×10^{-7}) added to the superfusate for 5 min; (D) disopyramide (7×10^{-6} M) administered for 5 min with continued superfusion of isoproterenol and acetylcholine. Zero potentials and calibrations as in Figure 28 (reprinted with permission from [218]).

137

alone shortened action potential (Figure 29B). Muscarinic agonists antagonized this beta-induced shortening of action potential duration (Figure 29C). When disopyramide was added, action potential duration again shortened, presumably because of the antimuscarinic activity of disopyramide which blocked the effects of acetylcholine (Figure 29D). Quinidine produced effects similar to those of disopyramide [218]. Thus, in both atrial and ventricular tissues, disopyramide and quinidine produce qualitatively different electrophysiological effects depending on the prevailing activity of the autonomic nervous system. In intact animals and in humans, in whom autonomic activity (i.e., both sympathetic and parasympathetic) is present and constantly changing, it seems likely that parasympathetic activity modulates the sympathetic effects on the electrophysiological properties of the heart. In this setting, the antimuscarinic activity of disopyramide and quinidine might contribute to the antiarrhythmic and/or arrhythmogenic effects of these agents.

The tricyclic antidepressants produce prominent cardiovascular effects which are similar to those of antimuscarinic agents [219]. Cardiovascular reflexes which are mediated via the parasympathetic nervous system such as the carotid occlusion reflex and the Bezold-Jarisch reflex are blunted. Tachycardia commonly is associated with therapy. Noncardiovascular side effects also are suggestive of antimuscarinic activity. Patients may have blurred vision, dry mouth, constipation, and urinary retention. That these effects are mediated by interaction of tricyclic antidepressants with muscarinic receptors has been verified directly with ligand binding assays [115]. Imipramine quite effectively inhibited [^{3}H]-QNB binding to muscarinic receptors in rabbit heart homogenates, with a K_i of 1.7×10^{-7} M [115]. This antimuscarinic activity of tricyclic antidepressants must be considered when the drugs are administered to patients with cardiovascular disease.

Acknowledgment

I gratefully acknowledge the excellent secretarial assistance of Terri Butcher and Carleen Mueller.

References

1. Levy MN, Martin PJ: Neural control of the heart. In: Berne RM (ed) Handbook of Physiology. Section 2: The Cardiovascular System, vol 1. Am Physiol Soc, Bethesda, 1979, pp 581–620.
2. Napolitano L, Willman VL, Hanlon CR, Cooper T: Intrinsic innervation of the heart. Am J Physiol 208:455–458, 1975.
3. Priola DV, Spurgeon HA, Geis WP: The intrinsic innervation of the canine heart: a functional study. Circ Res 40:50–56, 1977.
4. Jacobowitz D, Cooper T, Barner HB: Histochemical and chemical studies of the localization of adrenergic and cholinergic nerves in normal and denervated cat hearts. Circ Res 20:289–298, 1967.
5. Khaisman EB, Fedorova LG: Cholinergic and adrenergic neural structures of the ventricular epicardium. Acta Anat 82:145–158, 1972.
6. Kent KM, Epstein SE, Cooper T, Jacobowitz DM: Cholinergic innervation of the canine and human ventricular conducting system: anatomic and electrophysiologic correlations. Circulation 50:948–955, 1974.
7. Roskoski R Jr, Mayer HE, Schmid PG: Choline acetyltransferase activity in guinea-pig heart in vitro. J Neurochem 23:1197–1200, 1974.
8. Roskoski R Jr, Schmid PG, Mayer HE, Abboud FM: In vitro acetylcholine biosynthesis in normal and failing guinea pig hearts. Circ Res 36:547–552, 1975.
9. Schmid PG, Greif BJ, Lund DD, Roskoski R Jr: Regional choline acetyltransferase activity in the guinea pig heart. Circ Res 42:657–660, 1978.
10. Lund DD, Schmid PG, Kelley SE, Corry RJ, Roskoski R Jr: Choline acetyltransferase activity in rat heart after transplantation. Am J Physiol 235:H367–H371, 1978.
11. Brown OM: Cat heart acetylcholine: structural proof and distribution. Am J Physiol 231:781–785, 1976.
12. Hall ZW: Release of neurotransmitters and their interaction with receptors. Ann Rev Biochem 41:925–952, 1972.
13. Hebb C: Biosynthesis of acetylcholine in nervous tissue. Physiol Rev 52:918–957, 1972.
14. Dowdall MJ: Synthesis and storage of acetylcholine in cholinergic nerve terminals. In: Berl S (ed) Metabolic Compartmentation and Neurotransmission. Plenum Press, New York, 1975, pp 585–607.
15. Nachmanson D: Chemical and Molecular Basis of Nerve Activity. Academic Press, Inc, New York, 1959.
16. Potter LT: Synthesis, storage and release of acetylcholine from nerve terminals. In: Bourne GH (ed) The Structure and Function of Nervous Tissue. Academic Press, Inc, New York, 1972, pp 105–128.
17. DeRobertis E, Bennett HS: Some features of the submicroscopic morphology of synapses in frog and earthworm. J Physiol Biochem Cytol 1:47–58, 1955.
18. Cooke JD, Okamoto K, Quastel DMJ: The role of calcium in depolarization–secretion coupling at the motor nerve terminal. J Physiol (Lond) 223: 459–497, 1973.
19. Revtyak G, Manalan AS, Watanabe AM, Besch HR Jr, Jones LR: Subcellular distribution of guanylate cyclase

activity and muscarinic receptors in canine ventricular myocardium (in preparation).

20. Koelle GB: Microanatomy and pharmacology of cholinergic synapses. In: Tower DB (ed) The Nervous System, vol 1. Raven Press, New York, 1975, pp 363–371.
21. Sarnoff SJ, Brockman SK, Gilmore JP, Linden RJ, Mitchell JH: Regulation of ventricular contraction: influence of cardiac sympathetic and vagal nerve stimulation on atrial and ventricular dynamics. Circ Res 8:1108–1122, 1960.
22. Hoffman BF, Cranefield PF: Electrophysiology of the Heart. McGraw-Hill, New York, 1960.
23. Noble D: The Initiation of the Heart Beat. Clarendon Press, Oxford, 1975.
24. Higgins CB, Vatner SF, Braunwald E: Parasympathetic control of the heart. Pharmacol Rev 25:119–155, 1973.
25. Eliakim M, Bellet S, Tawil E, Muller O: Effect of vagal stimulation and acetylcholine on the ventricle: studies in dogs with complete atrioventricular block. Circ Res 9: 1372–1379, 1961.
26. De Geest H, Levy MN, Zieske H: Carotid chemoreceptor stimulation and ventricular performance. Am J Physiol 209:564–570, 1965.
27. Daggett WM, Nugent GC, Carr PW, Powers PC, Harada Y: Influence of vagal stimulation on ventricular contractility, O_2 consumption, and coronary flow. Am J Physiol 212:8–18, 1967.
28. Randall WC, Wechsler JS, Pace JB, Szentivanyi M: Alterations in myocardial contractility during stimulation of the cardiac nerves. Am J Physiol 214:1205–1212, 1968.
29. Pace JB, Randall WC, Wechsler JS, Priola DV: Alterations in ventricular dynamics by stimulation of the cervical vagosympathetic trunk. Am J Physiol 214:1213–1218, 1968.
30. Wildenthal K, Mierzwiak DS, Wyatt HL, Mitchell JH: Influence of efferent vagal stimulation on left ventricular function in dogs. Am J Physiol 216:577–581, 1969.
31. Priola DV, Fulton RL: Positive and negative inotropic responses of the atria and ventricles to vagosympathetic stimulation in the isovolumic canine heart. Circ Res 25:265–275, 1969.
32. Randall WC, Armour A: Regional vagosympathetic control of the heart. Am J Physiol 227:444–452, 1974.
33. DeGeest H, Levy MN, Zieske H: Reflex effects of cephalic hypoxia, hypercapnia and ischemia upon ventricular contractility. Circ Res 17:349–358, 1965.
34. Levy MN, Ng M, Lipman RI, Zieske H: Vagus nerves and baroreceptor control of ventricular performance. Circ Res 18:101–106, 1966.
35. Priola DV, Spurgeon HA, Geis WP: The intrinsic innervation of the canine heart: a functional study. Circ Res 40:50–56, 1977.
36. Priola DV, Spurgeon HA: Cholinergic sensitivity of the denervated canine heart. Circ Res 41:600–605, 1977.
37. Blukoo-Allotey JA, Vincent NH, Ellis S: Interactions of acetylcholine and epinephrine on contractility, glycogen and phosphorylase activity of isolated mammalian hearts. J Pharmacol Exp Ther 170:27–36, 1969.
38. LaRaia PJ, Sonnenblick EH: Autonomic control of cardiac c-AMP. Circ Res 28:377–384, 1971.

39. Watanabe AM, Besch HR Jr: Interaction between cyclic adenosine monophosphate and cyclic guanosine monophosphate in guinea pig ventricular myocardium. Circ Res 37:309–317, 1975.
40. Bailey JC, Greenspan K, Elizari MV, Anderson GJ, Fisch C: Effects of acetylcholine on automaticity and conduction in the proximal portion of the His-Purkinje specialized conduction system of the dog. Circ Res 30:210–216, 1972.
41. Tse WW, Han J, Yoon MS: Effect of acetylcholine on automaticity of canine Purkinje fibers. Am J Physiol 230:116–119, 1976.
42. Spear JF, Moore EN: Influence of brief vagal and stellate nerve stimulation on pacemaker activity and conduction within the atrioventricular conduction system of the dog. Circ Res 32:27–41, 1973.
43. Greenspan K, Wunsch C, Fisch C: T wave of normo- and hyperkalemic canine heart: effect of vagal stimulation. Am J Physiol 208:954–958, 1965.
44. Fisch C, Knoebel SB, Feigenbaum H: The effect of acetylcholine and potassium on repolarization of the heart. J Clin Invest 43: 1769–1775, 1964.
45. Benforado JM: A depressant effect of acetylcholine on the idioventricular pacemaker of the isolated perfused rabbit heart. Bt J Pharmacol 13:415–418, 1958.
46. Kent KM, Smith ER, Redwood DR, Epstein SE: Electrical stability of acutely ischemic myocardium: influences of heart rate and vagal stimulation. Circulation 47:291–298, 1973.
47. Corr PB, Gillis RA: Role of the vagus nerves in the cardiovascular changes induced by coronary occlusion. Circulation 49:86–97, 1974.
48. Myers RW, Pearlman AS, Hyman RM, Goldstein RA, Kent KM, Goldstein RE, Epstein SE: Beneficial effects of vagal stimulation and bradycardia during experimental acute myocardial ischemia. Circulation 49:943–947, 1974.
49. Harrison LA, Harrison LH Jr, Kent KM, Epstein SE: Enhancement of electrical stability of acutely ischemic myocardium by edrophonium. Circulation 50:99–102, 1974.
50. Cohen MV: Ventricular fibrillation precipitated by carotid sinus pressure: case report and review of the literature. Am Heart J 84:681–686, 1972.
51. Cope RL: Suppressive effect of carotid sinus stimulation on premature ventricular beats in certain instances. Am J Cardiol 4:314–320, 1959.
52. Waxman MB, Wald RW: Termination of ventricular tachycardia by an increase in cardiac vagal drive. Circulation 56:385–391, 1977.
53. Hoffman BF, Siebens AA, Brooks CM: Effect of vagal stimulation on cardiac excitability. Am J Physiol 169: 377–383, 1952.
54. Prystowsky EN, Jackman WM, Rinkenberger RL, Heger JJ, Zipes DP: Effect of autonomic blockade on ventricular refractoriness and atrioventricular nodal conduction in humans: evidence supporting a direct cholinergic action on ventricular muscle refractoriness. Circ Res 49:511–518, 1981.
55. Feigl EO: Parasympathetic control of coronary blood flow in dogs. Circ Res 25:509–519, 1969.

56. Feigl EO: Reflex parasympathetic coronary vasodilation elicited from cardiac receptors in the dog. Circ Res 37: 175–182, 1975.

57. Ehinger B, Falck B, Sporrong B: Possible axonal synapses between peripheral adrenergic and cholinergic nerve terminals. Z Zellforsch Mikrosk Anat 107:508–521, 1970.

58. Sharma VK, Banerjee SP: Presynaptic muscarinic cholinergic receptors. Nature 272:276–278, 1978.

59. Jones LR, Besch HR Jr, Fleming JW, McConnaughey MM, Watanabe AM: Separation of vesicles of cardiac sarcolemma from vesicles of cardiac sarcoplasmic reticulum. J Biol Chem 254:530–539, 1979.

60. Levy MN: Sympathetic–parasympathetic interactions in the heart. Circ Res 29:437–445, 1971.

61. Shepherd JT, Lorenz RR, Tyce GM, Vanhoutte PM: Acetylcholine – inhibition of transmitter release from adrenergic nerve terminals mediated by muscarinic receptors. Fed Proc 37:191–194, 1978.

62. Muscholl E: Peripheral muscarinic control of norepinephrine release in the cardiovascular system. Am J Physiol 239:H713–H720, 1980.

63. Vanhoutte PM, Levy MN: Prejunctional cholinergic modulation of adrenergic neurotransmission in the cardiovascular system. Am J Physiol 238:H275–H281, 1980.

64. Watanabe AM, Lindemann JP, Jones LR, Besch HR Jr, Bailey JC: Biochemical mechanisms mediating neural control of the heart. In: Abboud FM, Fozzard HA, Gilmore JP, Reis DJ (eds) Disturbances in Neurogenic Control of the Circulation. Waverly Press, Inc, Baltimore, 1981, pp 189–203.

65. Loffelholz K, Muscholl E: A muscarinic inhibition of the noradrenaline release evoked by postganglionic sympathetic nerve stimulation. Naunyn Schmiedebergs Arch Pharmacol 265:1–15, 1969.

66. Loffelholz K, Muscholl E: Inhibition by parasympathetic nerve stimulation of the release of the adrenergic transmitter. Naunyn Schmiedebergs Arch Pharmacol 267:181–184, 1970.

67. Levy MN, Blattberg B: Effect of vagal stimulation on the overflow of norepinephrine into the coronary sinus during cardiac sympathetic nerve stimulation in the dog. Circ Res 38:81–85, 1976.

68. Lavallee M, de Champlain J, Nadeau RA, Yamaguchi N: Muscarinic inhibition of endogenous myocardial catecholamine liberation in the dog. Can J Physiol Pharmacol 56:642–649, 1978.

69. VanHee R, Vanhoutte PM: Cholinergic inhibition of adrenergic neurotransmission in the canine gastric artery. Gastroenterology 74:1266–1270, 1978.

70. Vanhoutte PM, Coen EP, DeRidder WJ, Verbeuren TJ: Evoked release of endogenous norepinephrine in the canine saphenous vein. Inhibition by acetylcholine. Circ Res 45:608–614, 1979.

71. Verbeuren TJ, Vanhoutte PJ: Acetylcholine inhibits potassium evoked release of ^{3}H-norepinephrine in different blood vessels of the dog. Arch Intern Pharmacodyn Ther 221:347–350, 1976.

72. Vatner SF, Rutherford JD, Ochs HR: Baroreflex and vagal mechanisms modulating left ventricular contractile responses to sympathomimetic amines in conscious dogs. Circ Res 44:195–207, 1979.

73. Hollenberg M, Carriere S, Barger AC: Biphasic action of acetylcholine on ventricular myocardium. Circ Res 26: 527–536, 1965.

74. Meester WD, Hardman HF: Blockade of the positive inotropic actions of epinephrine and theophylline by acetylcholine. J Pharmacol Exp Ther 158:241–247, 1967.

75. Dempsey PJ, Cooper T: Ventricular cholinergic receptor systems: interaction with adrenergic systems. J Pharmacol Exp Ther 167:282–290, 1969.

76. Jacob R, Miller DT, Gilmore JP: Significance of antiadrenergic effects of acetylcholine for contractility and action potential of the mammalian ventricular myocardium. Arztl Forsch 25:141–153, 1971.

77. Chamales MH, Gourley RD, Williams BJ: Effect of acetylcholine on changes in contractility, heart rate and phosphorylase activity produced by isoprenaline, salbutamol and aminophylline in the perfused guinea-pig heart. Br J Pharmacol 53:531–538, 1975.

78. Brown BS, Polson JB, Krzanowski JJ, Wiggins JR: Influence of isoproterenol and methylisobutylxanthine on the contractile and cyclic nucleotide effects of methacholine in isolated rat atria. J Pharmacol Exp Ther 212:325–332, 1980.

79. Kissling G, Reutter K, Sieber G, Nguyen-Duong H, Jacob R: Negative inotropic effects of endogenous acetylcholine on ventricular myocardium of cat and chicken. Pflugers Arch 333:35–50, 1972.

80. Sieber G, Kissling G, Miller DT, Jacob R: Indirect proof of parasympathetic nerve fibers in human ventricular myocardium. Naunyn Schmiedebergs Arch Pharmacol 276: 211–221, 1973.

81. Sadavongvivad C, Sanvarinda P, Satayavivad J: Mechanism of catecholamine antagonism in rat heart produced by pilocarpine and related drugs. Br J Pharmacol 52:97–100, 1974.

82. Grodner AS, Lahrtz HG, Pool PE, Braunwald E: Neurotransmitter control of sinoatrial pacemaker frequency in isolated rat atria and in intact rabbits. Circ Res 27:867–873, 1970.

83. Carrier GO, Bishop VS: The interaction of acetylcholine and norepinephrine on heart rate. J Pharmacol Exp Ther 180:31–37, 1972.

84. Davis LD: Effects of autonomic neurohumors on transmembrane potentials of atrial plateau fibers. Am J Physiol 229:1351–1364, 1975.

85. Bailey JC, Watanabe AM, Besch HR Jr, Lathrop DA: Acetylcholine antagonism of the electrophysiological effects of isoproterenol on canine cardiac Purkinje fibers. Circ Res 44:378–383, 1979.

86. Inui J, Imamura H: Effects of acetylcholine on calcium-dependent electrical and mechanical responses of the guinea-pig papillary muscle partially depolarized by potassium. Naunyn Schmiedebergs Arch Pharmacol 299:1–7, 1977.

87. DePalma JR: The role of acetylcholine in hydrocarbon-epinephrine arrhythmias. J Pharmacol Exp Ther 116:255–261, 1956.

88. Dresel PE, Sutter MC: Factors modifying cyclopropane-

epinephrine cardiac arrhythmias. Circ Res 9:1284–1290, 1961.

89. Vincent NH, Ellis S: Inhibitory effect of acetylcholine on glycogenolysis in the isolated guinea-pig heart. J Pharmacol Exp Ther 139:60–68, 1963.

90. Gardner RM, Allen DO: The relationship between cyclic nucleotide levels and glycogen phosphorylase activity in isolated rat hearts perfused with epinephrine and acetylcholine. J Pharmacol Exp Ther 202:346–353, 1977.

91. Watanabe Am, Hathaway DR, Besch HR Jr. Mechanism of cholinergic antagonism of the effects of isoproterenol on hearts from hyperthyroid rats. In: Kobayashi T, Sano T, Dhalla NS (eds) Recent Advances in Studies on Cardiac Structure and Metabolism. Univ Park Press, Baltimore, 1978, pp 423–429.

92. Glaviano VV, Goldberg J, Pindok MT: Acetylcholine and norepinephrine interactions on cardiac lipids and hemodynamics. Am J Physiol 228:1678–1684, 1975.

93. Samaan A: The antagonistic cardiac nerves and heart rate. J Physiol (Lond) 83:332–340, 1935.

94. Warner HR, Russell RO: Effect of combined sympathetic and vagal stimulation on heart rate in the dog. Circ Res 24:567–573, 1969.

95. Levy MN, Zieske H: Autonomic control of cardiac pacemaker activity and atrioventricular transmission. J Appl Physiol 27:465–470, 1969.

96. Wallick DW, Felder D, Levy MN: Autonomic control of pacemaker activity in the atrioventricular junction of the dog. Am J Physiol 235:H308–H313, 1978.

97. Stuesse SL, Wallick DW, Levy MN: Autonomic control of right atrial contractile strength in the dog. Am J Physiol 236:H860–H865, 1979.

98. Levy MN, Ng M, Martin P, Zieske H: Sympathetic and parasympathetic interactions upon the left ventricle of the dog. Circ Res 19:5–10, 1966.

99. Levy MN, Zieske H: Effect of enhanced contractility on the left ventricular response to vagus nerve stimulation in dogs. Circ Res 24:303–311, 1969.

100. Kolman BS, Verrier RL, Lown B: Effect of vagus nerve stimulation upon excitability of the canine ventricle. Am J Cardiol 37:1041–1045, 1976.

101. Martins JB, Zipes DP: Effects of sympathetic and vagal nerves on recovery properties of the endocardium and epicardium of the canine left ventricle. Circ Res 46:100–110, 1980.

102. Kolman BS, Verrier RL, Lown B: The effect of vagus nerve stimulation upon vulnerability of the canine ventricle: role of sympathetic–parasympathetic interactions. Circulation 52:578–585, 1975.

103. Goldstein A, Aronow L, Kalman SM: Principles of Drug Action: The Basis of Pharmacology. John Wiley and Sons, New York, 1974, pp 27–47.

104. Hoffman BB, Lefkowitz RJ: Radioligand binding studies of adrenergic receptors: new insights into molecular and physiological regulation. Ann Rev Pharmacol Toxicol 20:581–608, 1980.

105. Watanabe AM, Jones LR, Manalan AS, Besch HR Jr: Cardiac autonomic receptors: recent concepts from radiolabelled ligand binding studies. Circ Res 50:161–174, 1982.

106. Birdsall NJM, Hulme EC: Biochemical studies on muscarinic acetylcholine receptors. J Neurochem 27:7–16, 1976.

107. Ehlert FJ, Roeske WR, Yamamura HI: The nature of muscarinic receptor binding. In: Iversen, Iversen, Snyder (eds) Handbook of Pharmacology. Plenum Press, 1981.

108. Snyder SH, Chang KJ, Kuhar MJ, Yamamura HI: Biochemical identification of the mammalian muscarinic cholinergic receptor. Fed Proc 34:1915–1921, 1975.

109. Heilbronn E, Bartfai T: Muscarinic acetylcholine receptor. Prog Neurobiol 11:171–188, 1978.

110. Paton WD, Rang HP: The uptake of atropine and related drugs by intestinal smooth muscle of the guinea pig in relation to acetylcholine receptors. Proc R Soc Lond [Biol] 163B:1–44, 1965.

111. Yamamura HI, Snyder SH: Muscarinic cholinergic binding in rat brain. Proc Natl Acad Sci USA 71:1725–1729, 1974.

112. Galper JB, Klein W, Catterall WA: Muscarinic acetylcholine receptors in developing chick heart. J Biol Chem 252:8692–8699, 1977.

113. Lane MA, Sastre A, Law M, Salpeter MM: Cholinergic and adrenergic receptors on mouse cardiocytes in vitro. Dev Biol 57:254–269, 1977.

114. Cavey D, Vincent JP, Lazdunski M: The muscarinic receptor of heart cell membranes. FEBS Lett 84:110–114, 1977.

115. Fields JZ, Roeske WR, Morkin E, Yamamura HI: Cardiac muscarinic cholinergic receptors: biochemical identification and characterization. J Biol Chem 253:3251–3258, 1978.

116. Wei JW, Sulakhe PV: Regional and subcellular distribution of myocardial muscarinic cholinergic receptors. Eur J Pharmacol 52:235–238, 1978.

117. Mirro MJ, Manalan AS, Bailey JC, Watanabe AM: Anticholinergic effects of disopyramide and quinidine on guinea pig myocardium: mediation by direct muscarinic receptor blockade. Circ Res 47:855–865, 1980.

118. Galper JB, Smith TW: Properties of muscarinic acetylcholine receptors in heart cell cultures. Proc Natl Acad Sci USA 75:5831–5835, 1978.

119. Birdsall NJM, Burgen ASV, Hulme EC: The binding of agonists to brain muscarinic receptors. Mol Pharmacol 14:723–736, 1978.

120. Birdsall NJM, Burgen ASV, Hulme EC: A study of the muscarinic receptor by gel electrophoresis. Br J Pharmacol 66:337–342, 1979.

121. Ehlert FJ, Dumont Y, Roeske WR, Yamamura HI: Muscarinic receptor binding in rat brain using the agonist, [^{3}H]cis methyldioxolane. Life Sci 26:961–967, 1980.

122. Story DD, Briley MS, Langer SZ: The effects of chemical sympathectomy with 6-hydroxydopamine on alpha-adrenoceptor and muscarinic cholinoceptor binding in rat heart ventricle. Eur J Pharmacol 57:423–426, 1979

123. Yamada S, Yamamura HI, Roeske WR: Alterations in cardiac autonomic receptors following 6-hydroxydopamine treatment in rats. Mol Pharmacol 18:185–192, 1980.

124. Wei JW, Sulakhe PV: Regional and subcellular distribution of myocardial muscarinic cholinergic receptors. Eur J Pharmacol 52:235–238, 1978.

125. Hartzell HC: Distribution of muscarinic acetylcholine receptors and presynaptic nerve terminals in amphibian heart. J Cell Biol 86:6–20, 1980.

126. Laduron PM, Janssen PFM: Characterization and subcellular localization of brain muscarinic receptors labelled in vivo by [³H]dexetimide. J Neurochem 33:1223–1231, 1979.

127. Alberts P, Bartfai T: Muscarinic acetylcholine receptor from rat brain. J Biol Chem 251:1543–1547, 1976.

128. Berrie CP, Birdsall NJM, Burgen ASV, Hulme EC: Guanine nucleotides modulate muscarinic receptor binding in the heart. Biochem Biophys Res Commun 87:1000–1005, 1979.

129. Rosenberger LB, Yamamura HI, Roeske WR: Cardiac muscarinic cholinergic receptor binding is regulated by Na^+ and guanyl nucleotides. J Biol Chem 255:820–823, 1980.

130. Wei JW, Sulakhe PV: Cardiac muscarinic cholinergic receptor sites: opposing regulation by divalent cations and guanine nucleotides of receptor–agonist interaction. Eur J Pharmacol 62:345–347, 1980.

131. Galper JB, Smith TW: Agonist and guanine nucleotide modulation of muscarinic cholinergic receptors in cultured heart cells. J Biol Chem 255:9571–9579, 1980.

132. Wei JW, Sulakhe PV: Requirement for sulfhydryl groups in differential effects of magnesium ion and GTP on agonist binding of muscarinic cholinergic receptor sites in rat atrial membrane fraction. Naunyn Schmiedebergs Arch Pharmacol 314:51–59, 1980.

133. Birdsall NJM, Berrie CP, Burgen ASV, Hulme EC: Modulation of the binding properties of muscarinic receptors: evidence for receptor–effector coupling. In: Pepeu G, Kuhar MJ, Enna SJ (eds) Receptors for Neurotransmitters and Peptide Hormones. Raven Press, New York, 1980, pp 107–116.

134. Kent RS, DeLean A, Lefkowitz RJ: A quantitative analysis of beta-adrenergic receptor interactions: resolution of high and low affinity states of the receptor by computer modeling of ligand binding data. Mol Pharmacol 17:14–23, 1980.

135. Birdsall NJM, Burgen ASV, Hulme EC, Wells JW: The effects of ions on the binding of agonists and antagonists to muscarinic receptors. Br J Pharmacol 67:371–377, 1979.

136. Halvorsen SW, Nathanson NM: In vivo regulation of muscarinic acetylcholine receptor number and function in embryonic chick heart. J Biol Chem 256:7941–7948, 1981.

137. Wise BC, Shoji M, Kuo JF: Decrease or increase in muscarinic cholinergic receptor number in rats treated with methacholine or atropine. Biochem Biophys Res Commun 92:1136–1142, 1980.

138. Williams LT, Lefkowitz RJ, Watanabe AM, Hathaway DR, Besch HR Jr: Thyroid hormone regulation of beta-adrenergic receptor number. J Biol Chem 252:2787–2789, 1977.

139. Sharma VK, Banerjee SP: Muscarinic cholinergic receptors in rat heart: effects of thyroidectomy. J Biol Chem 252:7444–7446, 1977.

140. McConnaughey MM, Jones LR, Watanabe AM, Besch HR Jr, Williams LT, Lefkowitz RJ: Thyroxine and propylthiouracil effects on alpha- and beta-adrenergic receptor number, ATPase activities, and sialic acid content of rat cardiac membrane vesicles. J Cardiovasc Pharmacol 1:609–623, 1979.

141. Trautwein W: Generation and conduction of impulses in the heart as affected by drugs. Pharmacol Rev 15:277–332, 1963.

142. Michell RH: Inositol phospholipids and cell surface receptor function. Biochim Biophys Acta 415:81–147, 1975.

143. Ten Eick R, Nawrath H, McDonald TF, Trautwein W: On the mechanism of the negative inotropic effect of acetylcholine. Pflugers Arch 361:207–213, 1976.

144. Burgen ASV, Terroux KG: On the negative inotropic effect in the cat's auricle. J Physiol (Lond) 120:449–464, 1953.

145. Giles W, Tsien RW: Effects of acetylcholine on membrane currents in frog atrial muscle. J Physiol (Lond) 246:64P–66P, 1975.

146. Biegon RL, Pappano AJ: Dual mechanism for inhibition of calcium-dependent action potentials by acetylcholine in avian ventricular muscle: relationship to cyclic AMP. Circ Res 46:353–362, 1980.

147. George WJ, Polson JB, O'Toole AG, Goldberg ND: Elevation of guanosine 3,5-cyclic phosphate in rat heart after perfusion with acetylcholine. Proc Natl Acad Sci USA 66:398–403, 1970.

148. Goldberg ND, Haddox MK: Cyclic GMP metabolism and involvement in biological regulation. Ann Rev Biochem 46:823–896, 1977.

149. Kuo JF, Lee TP, Reyes PL, Walton KG, Donnelly TE Jr, Greengard P: Cyclic nucleotide-dependent protein kinases. J Biol Chem 247:16–22, 1972.

150. Lee TP, Kuo JF, Greengard P: Role of muscarinic cholinergic receptors in regulation of guanosine 3:5-cyclic monophosphate content in mammalian brain, heart muscle, and intestinal smooth muscle. Proc Natl Acad Sci USA 69:3287–3291, 1972.

151. George WJ, Wilkerson RD, Kadowitz PJ: Influence of acetylcholine on contractile force and cyclic nucleotide levels in the isolated perfused rat heart. J Pharmacol Exp Ther 184:228–235, 1973.

152. Mirro MJ, Bailey JC, Watanabe AM: Dissociation between the electrophysiological properties and total tissue cyclic guanosine monophosphate content of guinea pig atria. Circ Res 45:225–233, 1979.

153. Taniguchi T, Fujiwara M, Lee JJ, Hidaka H: Effect of acetylcholine on the norepinephrine-induced positive chronotropy and increase in cyclic nucleotides of isolated rabbit sinoatrial node. Circ Res 45:493–504, 1979.

154. McAfee DA, Whiting GJ, Siegel B: Neurotransmitter and cyclic nucleotide modulation of frog cardiac contractility. J Mol Cell Cardiol 10:705–716, 1978.

155. Linden J, Brooker G: The questionable role of cyclic guanosine 3:5-monophosphate in heart. Biochem Pharmacol 28:3351–3360, 1979.

156. Canessa de Scarnatti O, Sato M, De Robertis E: Muscarinic cholinergic stimulation of phosphatidyl inositol turnover in the CNS. Adv Exp Med Biol 83:497–503, 1977.

157. George WJ, Ignarro LJ, Paddock RJ, White L, Kadowitz PJ: Oppositional effects of acetylcholine and isoproterenol on isometric tension and cyclic nucleotide concentrations

CHAPTER 6

Alpha- and beta-adrenergic agonists and antagonists

JOHN A. OATES, DAVID ROBERTSON, ALASTAIR J. J. WOOD,
and RAYMOND L. WOOSLEY

Alpha-adrenergic agonists and antagonists

Introduction

Agonists and antagonists acting on the α-adreno-
ceptor are classified into two groups based upon
their relative potency at α_1- and α_2-receptors [1]. In
general the α_1-receptor appears to mediate vascular
smooth muscle contraction whereas the α_2-receptor
mediates inhibition of neurotransmitter release
from sympathetic neuron terminals, inhibition of
renin release from the kidney, platelet aggregation,
and central inhibition of sympathetic outflow resulting in a reduction in blood pressure. Since α_2-
agonists in high doses lead to vasoconstriction,
some vascular α_2-postsynaptic receptors probably
exist. The traditional α-agonists such as phenylephrine and methoxamine are relatively selective for
the α_1-receptor while clonidine and methylnorepi-
nephrine are relatively selective for the α_2-receptor.

α_1-agonists

Stimulation of α_1-adrenoceptors may be brought
about in at least two ways: (a) through direct receptor activation and (b) indirectly, by causing norepinephrine to be released from the postganglionic
sympathetic neuron into the synaptic cleft [2].
Norepinephrine, phenylephrine, and methoxamine
exert their major effect by direct stimulation of the
postsynaptic α-receptor whereas ephedrine, tyramine, metaraminol, amphetamine, and mephenter-
mine have significant indirect effect. The hemodynamic responses brought about by these drugs are
heterogeneous both because of interactions with re-

flexes [3] and variable direct α/β stimulation ratio.
For example, the heart rate is raised by pressor
doses of ephedrine whereas equipressor doses of
tyramine reduce heart rate [4].

A number of excellent and detailed reviews of
sympathomimetic amines are available [5–9]. To
varying degrees these agents lead to arterial and
venous constriction with attendant increased peripheral vascular resistance and central redistribution of blood volume. As a result, the heart becomes
larger. With agents such as norepinephrine, coronary blood flow may increase due to the increased
systemic pressure and the weak direct vasoconstrictor effect of α_1-agonists on coronary smooth muscle, but this rarely compensates for the associated
increase in heart work. The trigone and sphincter of
the urinary bladder are stimulated, and many patients will feel a transient urge to urinate. The contraction of the radial muscle of the iris leads to
pupillary dilatation. Pilomotor muscles are stimulated leading to a sensation of hair 'standing on
end.' Adrenergic sweating occurs, the spleen capsule contracts, and insulin secretion is inhibited.

In normal subjects sympathetic activity at rest
leads to circulating norepinephrine levels of about
250 pg/ml but plasma norepinephrine increases in
response to many stimuli [10, 11]. Usually 1–6 μg of
intravenous norepinephrine transiently yields concentrations of about 1000 pg/ml, and a rise in blood
pressure can be seen. Comparable pressor effects
are seen with phenylephrine boluses of 50–250 μg
and tyramine boluses of 1–6 mg. Caution must be
exercised in deriving dosages from the older literature [12], since contemporary preparations of some
agents appear to have more pressor effect. Norepi-

Rosen, M. R. and Hoffman, B. F. (eds.), Cardiac Therapy. ISBN 0-89838-564-4.
© 1983, Martinus Nijhoff Publishers, Boston, The Hague, Dordrecht, Lancaster. Printed in the Netherlands.

nephrine and epinephrine concentrations decline with a half life of 60–90 sec, whereas the effects of phenylephrine and tyramine last somewhat longer. There are alterations in sensitivity to pressor amines in many clinical circumstances [13]. Whereas acidosis, myxedema, and Addison's disease reduce sensitivity to these agents, hypersensitivity may be prominent in idiopathic orthostatic hypotension [14], familial dysautonomia, heart failure, scurvy, and drug therapy (guanethidine, imipramine, reserpine, monoamine oxidase inhibitors, and steroid therapy).

There are several excellent reviews of the pharmacokinetics of dopamine [15], norepinephrine and epinephrine [16, 17]. Peak plasma levels of phenylephrine following oral administration usually occur at 1 hr with plasma levels of 207 ng/ml achieved at the peak of pharmacological effect [18]. Eighty percent of the drug is excreted within 24 hr primarily as the sulfate conjugate [19].

Systemic α_1-agonists were once widely used in the treatment of shock. It is now recognized that they are seldom indicated [13] since dopamine is available. However, some authors still suggest norepinephrine for certain indications [20]. It is generally titrated toward objective evidence of clinical improvement; this often occurs at a blood pressure of 80 mmHg. Norepinephrine is conveniently administered in a concentration of 5 mg/L of 5% dextrose. Since vasoconstrictors artifactually alter sphygmomanometric pressures [21], intra-arterial blood pressure monitoring must be carried out if α-agonists are used. Extravasation of norepinephrine may cause necrosis of tissue unless the infiltration is reversed with 2 μg of phentolamine per μg of norepinephrine infiltrated.

Other uses of α-agonists include cardioversion of paroxysmal atrial tachycardia and nasal decongestion. The former can often be accomplished by minimal pressor doses of phenylephrine (100 μg), much smaller than the 500 μg doses that are commonly given. Some patients with idiopathic orthostatic hypotension are sufficiently hypersensitive to α-agonists that even ophthalmically or nasally administered phenylephrine may significantly raise blood pressure [14].

Prolonged therapy with pressor amines may lead to reduced blood volume [22]; this is also seen in pheochromocytoma [23]. Sudden withdrawal of the circulating pressor agent may lead to profound hypotension or shock. The appropriate therapy of such hypotension is volume expansion. After surgery for pheochromocytoma proper fluid management is not merely 'fluid replacement' but 'volume expansion,' as chronically contracted venous capacitance beds relax to absorb greater quantities of circulating blood.

A second complication of pressor amine therapy is myocardial necrosis. It is most likely to occur in patients receiving high doses of pressor amines for more than 24 hr. Although a typical myocardial infarction syndrome may occur, patients more commonly exhibit a diffuse myocardial injury with nonspecific ST-T wave changes on the electrocardiogram. This myocardial disease may occasionally be the dominant presentation of pheochromocytoma [24].

α_2-agonists

Two widely used antihypertensive agents act by stimulating α_2-adrenoceptors. Clonidine interacts directly as a partial agonist whereas methyldopa interacts through its metabolites α-methylnorepinephrine and α-methylepinephrine which are potent agonists at α_2-adrenoceptors in the vasomotor center of the medulla oblongata. These two agents will be considered individually although their overall clinical efficacy is similar.

Clonidine

Clonidine is a centrally acting antihypertensive agent of intermediate potency. It is the only antihypertensive drug in general use effective in microgram quantities. The drug acts as an α_2-agonist in the cardiovascular control center of the medulla oblongata, leading to reduced sympathetic outflow [25, 26]. Like α-methyldopa, clonidine reduces plasma renin activity [27].

The disposition of clonidine can be described by a two-compartment model with a rapid distribution phase of 20–30 min and a β-phase half life of 7–12 hr [28–30] following oral administration. In the 0–2 ng/ml range, the hypotensive effect parallels drug levels [30], but with large doses, giving levels greater than 10 ng/ml, resistance to the hypotensive effect may occur [31]. It has been postulated that this loss of hypotensive effect reflects stimulation of peripheral vascular α_2-receptors at the higher dosage range, thus overcoming the hypotensive effect of

146

α-mediated central reduction in sympathetic outflow. Support for this mechanism comes from the observation that patients with severe idiopathic orthostatic hypotension, in whom there is no evidence of central sympathetic outflow, not only do not show a reduction in blood pressure following clonidine but even demonstrate a marked pressor response that occasionally is of therapeutic benefit [32]. The observations suggest that a hypotensive 'window' exists above which loss of therapeutic effect occurs. Because of this, caution should be exercised if dosages greater than 1.2 mg daily are used.

Intravenous administration of clonidine may produce a brief rise in blood pressure followed by a sustained fall [33]. The transient rise is due to direct α-adrenergic stimulation in the periphery during the distribution phase. In severely hypertensive subjects this rise is infrequent and mild: a diastolic increase of about 10 mmHg was seen after the first intravenous dose in three of 19 subjects, but this was not observed in patients pretreated with a diuretic [33].

Clonidine's depressor effect usually is associated with a fall in heart rate and cardiac output [34], but renal blood flow is usually spared. In the face of reduced cardiac output, resistance is altered minimally, indicating attenuation of peripheral sympathetic reflex activity [34]. Some peripheral redistribution of blood volume occurs; this is reflected in reduced pulmonary artery wedge pressure. Exercise-induced changes in blood pressure, cardiac output, heart rate, stroke volume, and peripheral resistance are qualitatively normal but quantitatively reduced [35].

Urinary catecholamine output is reduced with clonidine [36, 37]. It is probable that the reduced sympathetic outflow reflected by catecholamine levels also contributes to the reduced plasma renin activity and hence low aldosterone level observed [27, 35, 36]. The relative importance of the sympathetic nervous system and the renin-angiotensin system in the antihypertensive effect of clonidine remains to be established.

Clonidine can provide a sustained antihypertensive effect similar to that of α-methyldopa. Tolerance is rare if concomitant diuretic therapy is given. It causes less postural hypotension than guanethidine and does not impair ejaculation. Therapy is usually begun with 0.1 mg orally twice daily [38]

with 0.1 or 0.2 mg increments at weekly intervals up to a maximum total daily dose of 1.2 mg. For more rapid blood pressure control in acute situations, oral [39] and intravenous [33] regimens have been described. Antidepressant therapy may negate the antihypertensive effect of clonidine [40].

A major problem that results from clonidine therapy is the withdrawal syndrome that occurs in some patients 24–48 hr after discontinuation of the drug [41, 42]. Nervousness, insomnia, headache, sweating, tachycardia, nausea, and premature heart beats may be seen. These are accompanied by an increase in urinary catecholamines above pretreatment levels [36, 41]. With small daily doses of clonidine, the withdrawal syndrome is rarely observed [43]. When it does occur, blood pressure can be controlled rapidly with intravenous phentolamine or reinstitution of clonidine therapy. If ectopic activity occurs during withdrawal and is unresponsive to phentolamine alone, propranolol is usually effective. Although the withdrawal syndrome associated with clonidine is nearly always mild, it has occasionally led to an erroneous diagnosis of pheochromocytoma. This differential diagnosis is made more difficult by the marginally elevated urinary catecholamine levels sometimes seen during withdrawal. In spite of all the theoretical objections to clonidine use because of its withdrawal syndrome, the published literature has not yet documented much morbidity associated with it.

Sedation and dry mouth are the most common side effects. They coincide with the initial hypotensive effect. In general they seem more severe with clonidine than with α-methyldopa, perhaps because clonidine is more rapidly effective.

Methyldopa

Methyldopa lowers blood pressure by inhibiting the output of sympathetic vasoconstrictor impulses from the brain [44]. The antihypertensive action of methyldopa was discovered during studies of its inhibition of aromatic amino acid decarboxylation in humans [45]. It soon was found that the effect of methyldopa on blood pressure is mediated by an active metabolite. In the neurons of the brain, it is metabolized to α-methylnorepinephrine and α-methylepinephrine, one or both of which act on α-receptors evoking an inhibition of the vasomotor center of the medulla [46–48]. Inhibition of the vasomotor center by the α-agonist lowers the sympathetic tone in the resistance vessels. Thus, the effects of methyldopa on the sympathetic nervous system are somewhat selectively targeted to the sympathetic neurons controlling peripheral resistance. Because this central mechanism does not totally block all sympathetic reflexes, there is greater capability to maintain some sympathetic activation in response to a decrease in blood pressure, as, for example, in the standing position or during surgical anesthesia. The stimulation of central α-receptors also results in some drug-induced sedation and diminished salivary secretion.

Methyldopa is 50% absorbed following oral administration. A large portion of the orally administered drug is metabolized by the liver: the main products appearing in the urine are free and conjugated α-methyldopa, α-methyldopamine, and their 3-O-methyl metabolites [49, 50]. Although methyldopa itself is rapidly eliminated from plasma (half-life of 2.1 hr)[51], the active metabolites are retained in neuronal stores in the brain, yielding an antihypertensive effect that persists after most of the parent drug has been eliminated. With this prolonged duration of action, twice daily doses are sufficient to maintain control of the blood pressure. There is only a modest diminution of drug effect 24 hr after the last dose [52], enabling some patients to take the drug only once daily at bedtime when the major sedative effects coincide with sleep.

Peak plasma concentrations of methyldopa occur 2–6 hr after oral administration, whereas the maximum antihypertensive effect of a single dose is not manifest for 4–8 hr.

Methyldopa produces satisfactory blood pressure control in about two-thirds of hypertensive patients who require more than a diuretic [44]. It causes considerably less orthostatic hypotension than guanethidine and ganglionic blockers. The fall in blood pressure accompanying α-methyldopa therapy is sometimes associated with a mild decrease in cardiac output in hypertensive patients [53], but it is not known if similar changes occur in those with heart failure. The fall in heart rate with methyldopa is more modest than that with propranolol.

Methyldopa reduces plasma renin activity in normotensive and hypertensive individuals, including patients with renal failure. Patients taking methyldopa have increased sensitivity to pressor amines suggestive of denervation hypersensitivity, but the relatively greater response to injected tyramine, which acts indirectly by releasing neurotransmitter, indicates that this 'hypersensitivity' is not due to reduced stores of transmitter [54].

Central nervous system side effects are sufficiently troublesome to one-third or more of patients receiving methyldopa that they would prefer an alternative antihypertensive drug. Although frank sedation usually diminishes after several days of treatment, some patients continue to experience decreased intellectual drive, drowsiness, forgetfulness, and occasionally depression. These are usually less serious than with reserpine. Failure of ejaculation is uncommon, but the psychic lassitude and depression can lead to reduced libido and functional impotence. Rarely, extrapyramidal signs have appeared. Dryness of the mouth is common, but tolerance usually develops.

Perhaps the most serious and unpredictable adverse affect is hepatotoxicity [55, 56]. The manifestations can be quite varied but may resemble viral hepatitis. Both chronic aggresive hepatitis and cholestatic jaundice have been seen, and massive hepatic necrosis and death have occurred. Since these reactions do not relate predictably to dosage or duration of therapy, they must always be kept in mind; the possibility of overlooking hepatotoxicity can be greatly diminished by measuring hepatic marker enzymes after about three weeks of therapy. Strikingly high fevers with or without associated liver disease are also reported.

Twenty percent of patients taking chronic methyldopa therapy develop a positive direct Coombs test, but only 5% will have a raised reticulocyte count and less than 1% develop hemolytic anemia. The antibody is of the IgG type [57]. Since this reaction does not occur until a patient has been taking methyldopa for about three months, it is postulated that the drug or one of its metabolites is incorporated into the developing erythocyte which is then antigenic. The Coombs test will usually, but not always, become negative within six months of withdrawal of the drug. A positive Coombs test does not mean that hepatotoxicity will develop. Hepatotoxicity may in fact occur with a persistently negative Coombs reaction. The positive Coombs test will not hinder cross-matching of blood if the blood bank is aware that the patient is taking methyldopa. Positive rheumatoid factor reactions and antinuclear antibody reactions have been reported in patients on methyldopa.

Methyldopa has a spectrum of activity similar to that of clonidine, a directly acting central α-agonist [58], but significant withdrawal symptoms are less likely to occur with methyldopa [59]. It is effective in diverse categories of hypertension [60] and its action is potentiated by diuretics [61, 62].

Compliance to a regimen of methyldopa can be assessed by a modified Watson-Schwartz test on a random urine specimen [63]. Fluorescence assays for catecholamines are interfered with by methyldopa. Assays of vanillylmandelic acid, however, are usually reliable in the presence of the drug.

α-antagonists

The principal clinical use of α-blockers is in treatment of catecholamine-dependent hypertension [64], but they have also been used in shock [65, 66], in myocardial infarction [67, 68], in pulmonary edema [69–71], and in heart failure [72].

Phenoxybenzamine

Recognition that certain ergot alkaloids could block the pressor response to epinephrine led to the systematic study of α-receptor blockade [73]. The ergot alkaloids are now known to have so many other effects that their α-blocking properties are seldom of benefit clinically [74]. Phenoxybenzamine is a useful prototype of the combined α_1- and α_2-blocker, since virtually all of its clinical effects in humans are explicable in terms of α-blockade [75], even though one metabolite is pressor in the dog [73].

Phenoxybenzamine irreversibly blocks α-receptors in smooth muscle and exocrine glands. The effect commences in hours following oral administration and disappears with a halflife of 24 hr. Thus, if a loading regimen is not employed, the maximum effect of the drug requires about a week to manifest itself. In resting supine normal subjects, blood pressure is affected little by phenoxybenzamine. However, in standing subjects, hypovolemic subjects, and subjects with excessive sympathetic activation, blood pressure is reduced significantly. Patients taking phenoxybenzamine are particularly susceptible to the hypotensive effects of nitrates and narcotics; reflex tachycardia, particularly in the upright posture, is the rule. In susceptible patients, the associated increased heart work together with re-duced (diastolic) perfusion pressure may induce or worsen angina pectoris.

Other effects of α-blockade include: (a) improvement in glucose-stimulated insulin secretion in normal subjects, (b) occasional nasal stuffiness, (c) miosis, and (d) inhibition of piloerector muscles and 'adrenergic' sweating [75]. A protective effect against certain arrhythmias has been claimed [76].

Phentolamine

The most commonly used intravenous α-blocker is phentolamine [77, 78]. Unfortunately, the effect of phentolamine is exceedingly complex, and the immediate vasodepressor effect may not be via an α-blockade [79]. In addition to α-blockade, phentolamine is known to have sympathomimetic effects, parasympathomimetic effects, histamine-like effects [80], and antiserotonin effects.

Intravenous phentolamine was formerly used as a test for pheochromocytoma. A positive test was defined as a drop in blood pressure of 35/25 mmHg following an intravenous bolus of 5 mg [64]. Because cardiovascular collapse and death have occurred, this test is now rarely done. When phentolamine is administered, it should be started with a 0.5 mg bolus with doubling of the dose every 3 min until control of blood pressure is achieved. Because phentolamine is absorbed erratically from the gastrointestinal tract, oral therapy with phenoxybenzamine (10–200 mg daily) is usually preferred.

α-Blockers are advocated in shock because inhibition of the intense reflex vasoconstriction accompanying some types of shock leads to diversion of a greater proportion of the total blood flow through channels that allow effective exchange of metabolites with tissue cells [66]. Since venoconstriction can increase transudation across capillaries, promote blood trapping in the microcirculation, and lead to plasma loss in certain models of shock, reversal of this with α-blockade would presumably increase vascular fluid volume. Unfortunately, α-blockers have not been proven to be an effective treatment for shock in humans by carefully controlled clinical trials.

Prazosin

Although it was introduced as a vasodilator [81], prazosin is now known to exert its antihypertensive effect primarily as an α-blocker [82]. However, it is unique among α-blockers in the selectivity of its action.

The classical α-adrenoreceptor blocking drugs like phentolamine and phenoxybenzamine effect dual blockade: both norepinephrine's inhibitory feedback loop (α_2) and the vasoconstrictive effect (mostly α_1) are prevented. In ligand binding studies prazosin has 5,000-fold greater affinity for the α_1- than the α_2-receptor [83]. Thus, prazosin blocks the α_1-receptor while leaving the α_2-feedback receptor unblocked [84]. Such a spectrum of inhibition should result in blood pressure lowering with relatively less norepinephrine output and hence less spillover stimulation of β-receptors.

β-receptor stimulation increases heart rate and plasma renin activity; these effects occur when patients are given classical α-blockers which induce a reflex increase in norepinephrine release. With prazosin, however, there is limited reflex release of norepinephrine; a correspondingly attenuated increase (sometime even a decrease) in heart rate and plasma renin activity [85–87] occurs.

Prazosin lowers blood pressure by reducing both peripheral vascular resistance and venous tone. The ratio of arteriolar to venous relaxation induced by oral prazosin is comparable to that induced by intravenous nitroprusside, but the duration of effect is at least 6 hr for prazosin [88].

Prazosin is almost completely absorbed following oral administration, with peak plasma levels in 2–3 hr [89, 90]. It is more than 90% protein-bound and most of it is metabolized in the liver [89].

After the first dose of prazosin, some patients feel weak and diaphoretic. In early studies syncope occurred in 13 of 934 patients [91]. This reaction typically occurs one to several hours after the institution of therapy and is most likely if the initiating dose is greater than 1 mg, if the patient maintains upright posture, and if he is sodium depleted [84]. The nature of this reaction is presumed to be postural hypotension, but why it occurs only early in the course of therapy is unclear. ECG monitoring has shown that a tachycardia suddenly gives way to bradycardia at the moment of syncope, as though a vasovagal reaction occurred. It is probably wise to keep patients supine following the first few doses of prazosin to prevent this side effect. Administration of the drug at bedtime for the first three days of therapy is one means of circumventing the syncope.

The principal use of prazosin has been in the treatment of hypertension. Its efficacy and the incidence of side effects have been roughly comparable to those of methyldopa [92, 93]. Whereas the drug has been used widely to treat mild to moderate hypertension, it is sometimes strikingly effective as an adjunct in the management of severe resistant hypertension [94]. Common side effects are dizziness, headache, and drowsiness [91]. Although *a priori* one might expect angina pectoris to be improved by prazosin, it may be worsened in some subjects even when they have mild heart failure [95].

The possibility of reduction of arteriolar resistance (afterload) and venous tone (preload) has led to the use of prazosin in treating congestive heart failure [86, 96, 97]. Preliminary data suggest that oral prazosin has hemodynamic effects similar to those of nitroprusside in this disease [88]. In patients with severe heart failure, prazosin resulted in a mean improvement in New York Heart Association class from 3.7 to 2.2 [97]. Although tolerance to the antihypertensive effect of prazosin has not generally been observed [98], there does appear to be some tolerance to the favorable effect of the drug in the chronic management of congestive heart failure [99, 100]. The role of prazosin in the management of this disease has not been established firmly.

Therapy with prazosin in an inpatient setting is usually initiated with a 0.5–1.0 mg p.o. t.i.d. regimen with stepwise increments thereafter. From the rapid absorption and 4–6 hr half life of the drug, one would anticipate a rapid onset and rapid offset of antihypertensive effect. The range of dose associated with favorable ultimate effect on blood pressure has been from 1.5 mg to greater than 40 mg daily with an average of about 12 mg daily.

Additive antihypertensive effects without unfavorable drug interactions have been found when prazosin was used in combination with diuretics, β-adrenergic blocking drugs, clonidine, methyldopa, and hydralazine [84, 101]. No deleterious effects on the clinical course of diabetes mellitus, bronchial asthma, renal failure, or gout have been reported, but the safety of the drug in children and in pregnancy remains to be established.

Other α-antagonists

Other α-blockers include tolazoline (which resembles phentolamine in the spectrum of its effects), yohimbine, and trimazosin. Trimazosin is relatively selective for the postsynaptic (α_1) receptor. Yohimbine is a relatively selective α_2-blocker which leads to activation of the sympathetic nervous system perhaps by central blockade of inhibitory α_2-adrenoceptors. Its pharmacology in humans has not been fully investigated.

Many phenothiazines and butyrophenones such as chlorpromazine and haloperidol have significant α-blocking effects in humans [73].

Labetalol is an agent with both α_1- and β-blocking properties [102]. In terms of cardiovascular effects, it appears to be more potent as a β-blocker than as an α-blocker [103]. The spectrum of activity leads to significant blood pressure reduction with less tachycardia than the usual α-blocker and less bradycardia than the usual β-blocker [104].

Beta-receptor agonists and antagonists

Beta-receptor agonists

The endogenous adrenergic agonists epinephrine and norepinephrine are both potent β-receptor stimulants. However, their hemodynamic effects are different due to epinephrine's greater potency at the β_2-receptor and norepinephrine's greater potency at the α-receptor. To minimize the unwanted alpha effects of both epinephrine and norepinephrine, relatively selective β-receptor stimulating drugs such as isoproterenol were developed. The pharmacological differences between the β-receptor agonists are due to differences in their potency at β_1- and β_2-receptors and also in their resistance to degradation by the enzyme catechol-O-methyltransferase (COMT). Because this enzyme is present in high concentrations in the liver, little of an absorbed dose of drugs which are substrates for COMT can enter the systemic circulation.

Nonselective agonists

Isoproterenol is a relatively nonselective β_1- and β_2-receptor stimulant. Its pharmacological actions can be predicted from a knowledge of the location of β_1- and β_2-receptors and the effects of their stimulation (Table 1). Stimulation of cardiac β_1-receptors causes positive chronotropic and inotropic effects. The rise in heart rate and cardiac output is further reflexly increased by the fall in peripheral resistance produced by the β_2-induced relaxation of vascular smooth muscle. This is seen particularly in skeletal muscle beds resulting in increased venous return. In addition to vascular smooth muscle, smooth muscle relaxation also occurs in the bronchi, gastrointestinal tract, and uterus. The ability to cause bronchial dilatation and to reverse airway obstruction in asthma has given isoproterenol its principal therapeutic role. More selective β_2 stimulants have, however, largely replaced isoproterenol in this area because they produce less cardiac effects at a given degree of bronchial dilatation. Isoproterenol also increases blood glucose and lipoprotein lipase concentrations resulting in a rise in free fatty acid levels.

Because isoproterenol is a potent agonist at both β_1- and β_2-receptors, its use, particularly in large or excessive doses, has been associated with cardiac toxicity. Cardiac arrhythmias are produced and may be more common under conditions of hypoxia. This has been proposed as a cause for the deaths that were associated with isoproterenol use in Australia and the United Kingdom. Isoproterenol aerosols may have been used excessively by asthmatics whose attacks were unresponsive at a time when they were somewhat hypoxic, perhaps resulting in fatal cardiac arrhythmias.

Isoproterenol is metabolized by COMT [105–107] and therefore very little enters the systemic circulation following an oral dose. However, it is highly effective in producing bronchial dilatation

Table 1. Site and effect of stimulating β_1- and β_2-receptors.

β_1-receptors		β_2-receptors	
Site	Effect of stimulation	Site	Effect of stimulation
Heart	Increased rate	Bronchi	Dilatation
	Increased contractility	Blood vessels	Dilatation
		Uterus	Relaxation
		Insulin	Increased release

when given by inhalation. Isoproterenol has also been used to increase the heart rate in severe heart block until a cardiac pacemaker can be inserted.

Selective agonists

Agents such as terbutaline, albuterol (salbutamol), fenoterol, and rimiterol are more potent agonists at β_2-receptors than at β_1-receptors. Therefore, at doses of these drugs which produce equivalent bronchial dilatation, less cardiac effects are produced than with isoproterenol [108–110]. Terbutaline, albuterol, and fenoterol do not possess the catechol nucleus and therefore are not metabolized by COMT. This means that they can reach effective levels when given orally. However, rimiterol does possess the catechol nucleus, is metabolized by COMT, and is ineffective when administered orally.

Like selective antagonists, it is important to remember that these β_2-agonists are not specific but rather they are somewhat selective for the β_2-receptor. Therefore, they usually will stimulate the β_2-receptors to produce bronchial dilatation at doses well below those which produce marked cardiac effects. Thus, although they are less likely to produce cardiac toxicity than would a nonselective β-agonist such as isoproterenol, cardiac arrhythmias do occur if a high enough dose is administered [111]. Also, there may be an additive effect on cardiac toxicity when these drugs are combined with theophylline [112].

Beta-receptor antagonists

β-receptor antagonists (β-blockers) are drugs which selectively antagonize the effects of the endogenous agents epinephrine and norepinephrine at the β-adrenergic receptor. Adrenergic receptors were subdivided by Ahlquist [113] into α- and β-receptors depending on the relative potency of antagonists of these receptors.

There are now a number of β-adrenoceptor blocking agents available, and it is likely that this number will continue to increase. All of the currently available β-blockers are competitive antagonists of the naturally occurring β-receptor agonists. There are substantial differences, however, in their pharmacokinetic properties, i.e., in the way in which they are absorbed, metabolized, and excreted. In addition, the various β-blockers currently available differ in their pharmacodynamic properties, such as their ability to block β-receptors in different tissues (selectivity), their ability to stimulate the β-receptor, and their cardiac depressant activity, as well as in their membrane-stabilizing, local anesthetic, or 'quinidine-like' activity. Rational choice of a β-blocker for an individual patient clearly depends on an understanding of the significance of these differences among the various agents.

Pharmacodynamic properties of the β-blockers

Much has been made of the differences in the actions of the various β-blockers. However, all of the β-blockers competitively inhibit the effects of both endogenous and exogenously administered catecholamines at the β-adrenergic receptors. This means that a larger concentration of agonist is required to produce an effect in the presence of the antagonist, resulting in a parallel shift to the right in the dose–response curve.

Assessment of β-blockade. The extent of β-blockade can be assessed by a variety of techniques of varying utility. All define the degree of blockade by determining the decrement in a β-receptor-mediated response (usually heart rate) to either endogenous or exogenous adrenergic agonist. The sympathetic stimulation produced by standing or exercising can be used as a stimulus for the release of the endogenous agonists epinephrine and norepinephrine. These stimuli will, in the absence of β-blockade, increase heart rate. However, the strength of the stimulus for catecholamine release varies. For example, the degree of catecholamine release following upright posture depends on the subject's previous sodium intake [114]. In addition, where the dose–response curve to β-agonists is shifted sufficiently to the right by a β-blocker (see Figure 1), a given concentration of agonist produced by a constant physiological stimulus will be insufficient to produce a rise in heart rate. A further increase in the degree of β-blockade at higher β-blocker concentrations will go undetected in this setting. This gives rise to the frequent fallacy that two β-blockers produce equal degrees of β-blockade because they both completely blocked the exercise-induced rise in heart rate.

A better approach to the measurement of the degree of β-blockade is to determine the dose of an

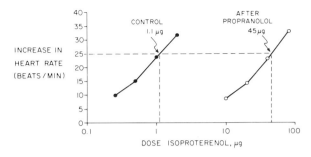

Figure 1. Increase in heart rate in response to increasing doses of isoproterenol before (●——●) and during (○——○) I.V. propranolol infusion in a normal subject.

agent such as isoproterenol which is required to produce a constant response (such as an increase in heart rate of 25 beats/min) both prior to and following the administration of a β-blocker [115]. The extent of β-blockade can then be expressed as the 'dose-ratio,' or ratio of the dose of isoproterenol required *before* β-blockade to that which is required *after* β-blockade.

Figure 1 shows the effect of increasing doses of isoproterenol on heart rate. A dose of 1.1 μg of isoproterenol was required to raise the heart rate by 25 beats/min prior to an infusion of propranolol. Following the propranolol infusion there was a more than forty-fold increase in the dose of isoproterenol required to produce the same rise in heart rate. This emphasizes a common point of confusion surrounding the effects of β-blockers. Since they are competitive antagonists of sympathetic agonists, it is always possible to overcome their effects completely, provided enough β-agonist is administered to achieve an adequate concentration at the receptor. There is therefore no such thing as complete β-blockade. One can only assess β-blockade in terms of the amount of an agonist or the strength of a stimulus required to overcome the blockade.

This technique has been used to demonstrate (Figure 2) that the dose of agonist required to raise the heart rate by a constant amount (25 beats/min) increases with advancing age, the elderly requiring around five-fold more isoproterenol than the young (Figure 2) [115]. Receptor theory would predict that following the administraton of an antagonist

$$DR - 1 = \frac{P}{K_d},$$

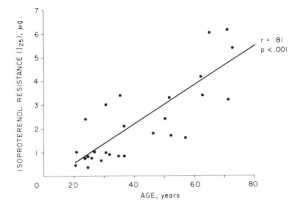

Figure 2. Relationship between age and isoproterenol resistance as measured by the dose (I_{25}) of isoproterenol required to raise the heart rate by 25 beats/min (from [115]).

where DR is the ratio of the dose of isoproterenol required to raise the heart rate by a given amount (e.g., 25 beats/min) after propranolol administration to the dose of isoproterenol required before propranolol; P is the unbound propranolol concentration in plasma, that is the concentration available for binding to receptor sites; and K_d is the apparent dissociation constant for propranolol binding to the receptor and hence is a measure of propranolol resistance, since larger values imply less effect. Following the administration of propranolol, it was found that the elderly were four to five times more resistant to propranolol than the young (Figure 3) [115].

In addition to their ability to antagonize the ef-

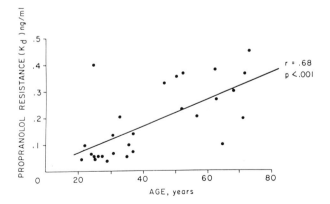

Figure 3. Relationship between age and the resistance to propranolol (K_d – see text) (from [115]).

153

fects of β-receptor agonists at the β-receptors, some of the β-blockers have additional effects that may or may not be of therapeutic importance (Table 2).

Membrane stabilizing or 'quinidine-like' activity. Early in the study of β-blocking drugs it was found that propranolol had electrophysiological properties that were not related to its antagonism of β-adrenergic receptors. Specifically, it was shown that propranolol slowed the rate of rise of the transmembrane cardiac action potential, whereas resting potential and spike duration were unchanged [116, 117]. This nonstereospecific effect is produced to an equal degree by the d- and l-isomers of propranolol [118] and has been referred to as a 'non-specific,' 'quinidine-like,' or 'direct membrane' action of propranolol. However, it is quite different from some of the actions of quinidine, and also there is no direct proof that it is due to an action on membranes. Early *in vitro* studies found that these effects on the rate of depolarization required concentrations above 300 ng/ml; 200–1,000-fold higher than usual *free* drug concentrations in patients receiving chronic therapy [119, 120]. This led many to conclude that this nonstereospecific action of propranolol does not play a role in the clinical effects of propranolol [121, 122].

However, recent studies have renewed interest in these actions by the demonstration that there are substantial differences between the rate of myocardial distribution of propranolol *in vitro* [123] and *in vivo* [24]. Propranolol accumulates more rapidly in myocardial tissue when given intravenously than when added to tissue in an *in vitro* system. Pruett et al. [123] observed electrophysiologic changes in isolated Purkinje fibers (shortening of repolarization time) that developed slowly over 2 hr of incubation with d- or l-propranolol at free drug concentrations in the range usually attained clinically. Therefore, it is likely that all prior *in vitro* studies at low concentration failed to allow adequate time for tissue accumulation of drug to occur. Similarly, early clinical electrophysiologic studies [125, 126] utilized small intravenous dosages (7–10 mg) and failed to reach plasma concentrations seen during oral therapy or to allow adequate time for tissue accumulation to occur. Likewise, a contribution of potentially active metabolites [127] would not be seen in these studies.

Whereas an increase in spontaneous cycle length

and AH conduction are effects of propranolol attributed to β-receptor blockade [128], prolongation of HV conduction and QRS widening have been described after large intravenous dosages in dogs [129] or patients [130] receiving overdosages. Slowing of HV conduction is similar to the action of local anesthetic type antiarrhythmic drugs [131] and is unlikely to be due to β-receptor blockade.

High concentrations of propranolol prolong refractoriness of isolated Purkinje tissue [117] and canine ventricular tissue *in vivo* [129]. Dawson et al. described similar effects for d-propranolol [132]. These investigators also found that the effects of d-propranolol on the AH interval could be reversed by isoproterenol but the effects on refractoriness were not influenced. Because isoproterenol shortens action potential duration, the combined effect of propranolol and isoproterenol was a significant increase in the ratio of the effective refractory period to action potential duration (ERP/APD). Theoretically, this is an antiarrhythmic action of propranolol which would be maximal during periods of adrenergic stimulation such as seen during acute myocardial infarction.

Drugs, such as bretylium [133] and amiodarone [134], which prolong cardiac repolarization, have effects similar to those of the β-adrenergic blocking drug, sotalol. Sotalol has been found to increase APD of Purkinje tissue [135], and recent studies documented the presence of this effect in patients by recording of monophasic action potential (MAP) duration using suction-electrode catheters [136]. This is likely to account for the prolongation of QT interval seen during chronic sotalol therapy. Similar effects on MAP duration have been reported after metoprolol and acebutolol administration [137, 138]. Small but statistically insignificant effects on MAP duration have been seen only after large intravenous dosages of propranolol [139]. The effects of propranolol on QT duration are not clear. Subjects with the syndrome of prolonged QT and ventricular arrhythmias have been reported to show a decreased frequency of arrhythmias without shortening of their QT duration [140], but this may be due to reversal of an underlying sympathetic imbalance in these patients. Others have reported varying effects on QT duration during propranolol therapy [139, 141–143]. It does not appear that prolongation of action potential duration by sotalol or propranolol (if it occurs clinically with this

Table 2. Pharmacodynamic properties of β-blockers.

	Potency[a]	Selectivity for β_1-receptors	Direct membrane effect[b]	Intrinsic sympathomimetic activity
Acebutolol	0.3	+	+	+
Alprenolol	0.3	0	+	+
Atenolol	1	+	0	0
Metoprolol	1	+	0	0
Nadolol	6	0	0	0
Oxprenolol	0.5–1	0	+	+
Pindolol	6	0	±	+
Propranolol	1	0	+	0
Sotalol	0.3	0	0	0
Timolol	6	0	0	0

[a] Relative to propranolol = 1.

[b] Action on cell membrane mediated directly and not via blockade at β-receptor.

drug) is due to nonstereospecific or direct membrane actions.

Selectivity. Following Ahlquist's original subdivision of adrenoceptors into two types (α and β) according to the relative potency of different sympathomimetic amines [113], almost two decades passed before these receptors were further subdivided into the so-called β_1- and β_2-receptors [144] (Table 2). Nonselective β-blockers such as propranolol act at both the β_1- and β_2-receptors. However, the so-called selective β_1-receptor antagonists, the first of which was practolol, have a relatively greater potency for the β_1-receptor than the β_2-receptor. This means that these drugs will antagonize the effects of agonists on the cardiac receptors at concentrations that have little effect on the β_2-receptors. However, with increasing concentrations of drug, the β_2-receptors will also be blocked. Considerable confusion has surrounded this area; it is important to understand that the drugs are not specific in blocking only β_1-receptors. Rather, they block these receptors at doses that are lower than those required to block β_2-receptors, conveying some degree of selectivity rather than specificity.

In patients with bronchial asthma, cardioselectivity may be a useful property, since the selective β-blockers are less likely to precipitate bronchospasm in such patients. However, it should be understood that even these selective agents may, in some patients at low doses and probably in many asthmatic patients at high doses, cause bronchial constriction [145]. Probably the ideal therapy for such patients, if a β-blocker is required, is the concurrent administration of a β_1-receptor antagonist along with a selective β_2-receptor agonist such as albuterol (salbutamol).

Another situation in which the use of a selective β-blocker may be desirable is in the treatment of diabetic patients. Nonselective β-blockers such as propranolol may delay the blood glucose recovery from hypoglycemia, whereas selective β-blockers such as metoprolol and atenolol do not [146, 147]. In addition, severe bradycardia and raised diastolic blood pressure have occurred during hypoglycemia while taking propranolol. These effects were milder with a cardioselective β-blocker [147]. Also the cardioselective β-blockers may not exaggerate the rise in blood pressure during propranolol therapy in response to sympathetic stimuli such as the cold pressor test [148]. In conclusion, therefore, cardioselectivity may be of value in some special situations, but these differences are not absolute, and antagonism of β_2-receptors does occur, particularly at higher doses.

Intrinsic sympathomimetic activity (ISA). In norepinephrine-depleted animal models, it is possible to demonstrate that some of the β-blockers (Table 2) have partial agonist activity in addition to their predominant β-antagonist properties. The maximum stimulation of the receptors that these drugs can produce is clearly much less than that with full agonists such as epinephrine or isoproterenol [149, 150]. It was suggested initially that the β-blockers which lacked ISA were more effective in the treatment of hyperthyroidism [151]. However, this has now been challenged [152, 153]. It has also been suggested that drugs with intrinsic agonist activity would be less likely to precipitate cardiac failure in patients prone to this, and that drugs with less myocardial depressant action may be safer in this regard [154]. However, it is likely that the principal reason for the precipitation of cardiac failure by β-blockers in patients already on the brink of cardiac failure is the removal of the increased sympathetic drive to the heart by β-blockade. Patients with compromised cardiac function attempt to maintain adequate cardiac output through increased sympathetic drive to the heart. Removal of this increased drive through the use of a β-blocker is likely to precipitate cardiac failure, whatever the drug's effect on the contraction of isolated cardiac tissue in vitro.

Pharmacokinetics of β-blockade

The β-blockers currently available and those that we expect to become available in the near future can be divided into two groups according to their route of elimination. Some, such as propranolol, metoprolol, and timolol, are extensively metabolized by the liver, whereas others, such as atenolol and nadolol, are excreted largely unchanged by the kidneys (Table 3); the factors controlling the excretion of the drugs in these two groups are quite different. Propranolol, the first of this group of drugs to become available, has been studied extensively partly because of its therapeutic importance but also because of its utility as a model compound.

Propranolol, metoprolol, and timolol. These drugs are almost completely absorbed following an oral dose, and peak concentrations are achieved quickly [155–160]. Food appears to enhance the systemic availability of both propranolol and metoprolol [161]. Following oral administration and absorption, the drug passes to the liver where it is exposed to the liver's drug metabolizing system. In the case of propranolol, and to a lesser extent metoprolol, the liver avidly removes the drug from the blood [162–165].

The removal of propranolol from the portal blood prior to its entry into the systemic circulation (first-pass elimination) results in a low systemic availability of the drug following oral administration, in spite of the excellent absorption [164, 165]. An additional complication is the fact that the avid removal of propranolol by the liver following oral dosing appears to be dose dependent [156, 165]. This has two important practical consequences. First, at low doses, less of the drug enters the systemic circulation than at higher doses, and, second, it is impossible to predict the disposition characteristics of the drug at steady state from a single oral dose because the bioavailability is higher during chronic oral dosing than after the first oral dose [165].

The high hepatic extraction of propranolol following oral administration, which is dependent on the liver's drug metabolizing ability, also accounts for the large difference in dosage requirements following intravenous administration (where there is no presystemic elimination) and oral administra-

Table 3. Pharmacokinetic properties of β-blockers.

	Absorption (%)	Systemic availability (%)[a]	Protein binding (%)	Half-life (hr)	Metabolism	Urinary excretion (%)[b] unchanged
Acebutolol	–	20–60	84	3–6	50-60%	40
Alprenolol	>90	15	85	2–3	Extensive	<1
Atenolol	46–62	55	<5	6–7	Minimal	85–100
Metoprolol	>95	50	12	3–4	Extensive	<5
Nadolol	15–25	20	25–30	12–24	Minimal	70
Oxprenolol	70–95	20–60	80	1.3–1.5	Extensive	2–5
Pindolol	>90	>90	46	2–5	60%	40
Propranolol	100	33	90	4–6	Extensive	<1
Sotalol	–	>60	5	5–13	Minimal	60
Timolol	>90	75	10	4–5	Extensive	13–20

[a] Dependent on both absorption and 'first-pass metabolism.'
[b] % of absorbed dose excreted unchanged in urine.

156

tion. The factors determining the clearance of propranolol, and hence steady-state levels, following oral and intravenous dosing, also are different. The oral clearance of the drug is dependent solely on the liver's drug metabolizing ability while, at steady state, the intravenous clearance is influenced mainly by liver blood flow in addition to the liver's drug metabolizing ability. Liver blood flow is much less variable between individuals than is liver drug metabolizing ability; thus, it is not surprising that the variability in propranolol concentrations is less following intravenous administration than after oral administration, when variations of up to 20-fold have been found [166, 167]. In a strictly controlled trial in which 24 normal volunteers aged 21–73 years, received 80 mg of propranolol every 8 hr in hospital, a more than ten-fold variation in plasma propranolol concentrations was found (Figure 4) [167]. As pointed out previously, the clearance following oral administration reflects the drug metabolizing ability of the liver. Since this varies widely and is affected by the patients' genetic makeup, the environment to which they have been exposed, their age, and numerous other factors [168, 169], it is not surprising that steady-state drug levels vary so widely. (Some of the factors responsible for this variation will be addressed in more detail later.)

Although most of the studies of the presystemi-

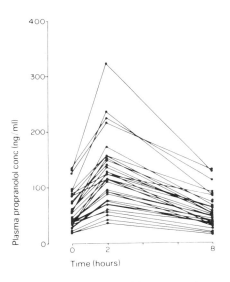

Figure 4. Variability in propranolol concentration at steady state in a group of normal hospitalized volunteers receiving 80 mg propranolol every 8 hr (from Routledge PA, Shand DG. Clin Pharmacokinet 4:73–90, 1979).

cally extracted β-blockers have used propranolol, it is likely that many of these findings can be extrapolated to the other β-blockers that are avidly removed by the liver.

Atenolol, nadolol, and sotalol. These agents are excreted mainly by the kidneys as unchanged drug [170, 171]. Thus, their elimination is impaired in renal disease, but it is not dependent on the vagaries of drug metabolism. It has therefore been suggested that the steady-state plasma levels of these drugs will be subject to much lesser interindividual variation than the highly metabolized β-blockers. Although that may well be true, it is important to note (Table 3) that both atenolol and nadolol are poorly absorbed, and although the absorption may be relatively constant [172], it is likely that variability in absorption will result in alterations in steady levels at least as large as those due to liver metabolism. One must also remember that, because of the poor absorption of atenolol and nadolol following oral administration, they, too, require lower doses intravenously than orally.

Effects of disease on the kinetics of β-blockers

Liver disease. For β-blockers such as propranolol and metoprolol and to a lesser extent timolol, all of which are extensively metabolized by the liver, liver disease might be expected to have a significant effect on plasma clearance following oral administration. In addition, the alterations in plasma proteins found in cirrhosis may alter the disposition of propranolol, which is highly bound in plasma. Because of the existence of portasystemic shunts, some of the drug coming from the gut following absorption is able to bypass the liver, resulting in a higher systemic availability of the drug.

The effect of liver disease on the kinetics of propranolol has been carefully investigated using a technique that involves the simultaneous administration of native drug orally and labeled drug intravenously [173]. This allows the measurements of all of the parameters controlling elimination including systemic availability, oral or intrinsic clearance (which, as discussed earlier, is dependent on liver drug-metabolizing ability), and systemic or intravenous clearance, which is determined at steady state by both drug-metabolizing ability (intrinsic clearance) and liver blood flow. In addition, the plasma

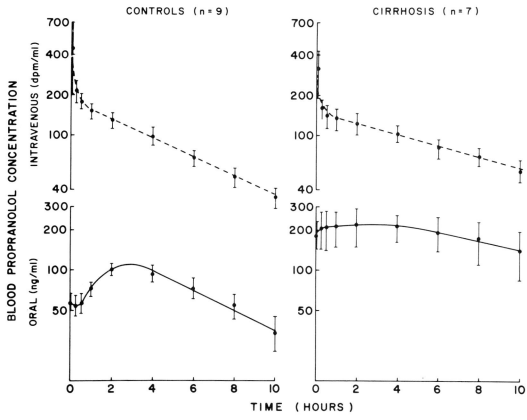

Figure 5. The concentration of unlabeled propranolol (ng/ml) in whole blood after oral administration (——) and the concentration of tritiated propranolol (dpm/ml) after intravenous administration (---) following simultaneous determination of intravenous and oral dose kinetics of propranolol at the seventh dosing interval in nine normal subjects and seven patients with cirrhosis (mean ± SEM) (from [173]).

binding of the drug was measured and used to express the drug concentrations in terms of free or unbound drug in blood. Steady-state concentrations of propranolol were markedly higher in cirrhotic patients than in controls (Figure 5). This was due to an increase in systemic availability – 38% in the control group as compared to 54% in the cirrhotic group – and a decrease in systemic clearance. Because of the increased average total steady-state concentrations in blood, coupled with an elevation in the fraction of the drug free in plasma, there was a three-fold increase in the average free drug concentration from 7.5 ng/ml to 22.3 ng/ml. It is impossible to predict accurately what the effect of liver disease will be on the steady-state levels of other β-blockers, but it is likely that drugs such as nadolol and atenolol, which are largely excreted by renal routes, will be little affected, whereas the drugs that

are highly metabolized by the liver will show changes similar to those found with propranolol. However, it should be remembered that changes in protein binding are likely to be less important for drugs such as metoprolol, which is only 12% bound in plasma.

Renal disease. It might be anticipated that β-blockers that have largely renal routes of elimination might accumulate in patients with impaired renal function; however, it is surprising that there have been suggestions that the excretion of some of the extensively metabolized drugs such as propranolol is also impaired in renal disease. Although a small proportion of timolol (13%) is eliminated unchanged in the urine, the overall clearance of timolol was not prolonged in patients with renal failure [174], and therefore no change in the oral dosage is required. However, since approximately 70% of nadolol is excreted in the urine [175], its elimination is impaired in patients with renal failure. In fact, the rate of elimination of nadolol correlated well with creatinine clearance and in patients with the most severe degree of renal failure, the half-life of nadolol was prolonged to 45 hr from the half-life of 14–20 hr in patients with normal renal function [175].

The effect of renal disease on the elimination of propranolol has been the source of some confusion with some authors [157] suggesting that the concentrations of propranolol following a single oral dose were higher in patients with renal disease, and absorption appeared to be more rapid. However, others have found impaired absorption and no change in the time-to-peak levels but did find a reduction in clearance of propranolol in patients with renal failure [176]. This area has now been clarified following a study of patients with severe renal failure, whether on hemodialysis or not yet on dialysis. No impairment of propranolol elimination, when compared to age-matched controls was found [177]. Thus, it is unlikely that any adjustment of propranolol dosage is required in patients with renal failure.

Age. It is now widely appreciated that the elderly suffer a higher incidence of adverse drug reactions than the young. This higher incidence may be due partly to alteration in their ability to eliminate drugs [178, 179].

It has been shown that following 80 mg every 8 hr, blood levels of propranolol were two-fold higher in normal subjects over the age of 35 compared to those under 35 [168] (Figure 6). In addition, when the effects of smoking were examined, it was found that smokers had significantly lower levels of propranolol throughout the dosing interval than nonsmokers (Figure 7). These changes appeared to be due to an age-related effect of smoking. The oral or intrinsic clearance of propranolol fell significantly with age only in smokers suggesting that smoking increased the ability to eliminate propranolol only in the young, the elderly being relatively resistant to this effect. Liver blood flow, on the other hand, fell significantly with age in both smokers and nonsmokers, and there appeared to be no effect of smoking on the age-related fall in liver blood flow. These changes resulted in a significant

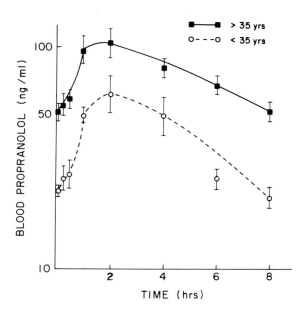

Figure 6. Steady-state blood concentrations of propranolol during the dosage intervals after oral administration of 80 mg every 8 hr in normal individuals, according to age (from [168]).

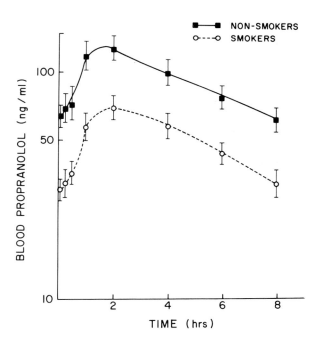

Figure 7. Steady-state blood concentrations of propranolol during the dosage intervals after oral administration of 80 mg every 8 hr in normal individuals – smokers vs nonsmokers (from [168]).

age-related fall in the systemic or intravenous clearance of propranolol in smokers alone.

Whereas propranolol is the only β-blocker whose kinetics have been studied in detail in aging, the effects of age on kinetics of some of the others can be predicted. For example, nadolol and atenolol are excreted largely by the kidneys, and as their rate of excretion is known to be closely correlated with creatinine clearance [175], which falls with advancing age, it is likely that their steady-state levels will be higher in the elderly, due to poorer renal function in this age group.

From this discussion it is clear that a number of variables affect blood levels of β-blockers. As many of the effects of β-blockers have a clear relationship to drug concentration in blood, and hence at the β-adrenergic receptor site, changes in drug concentration will alter the intensity of the drug's effect.

Adverse effects of β-blockade
Most of the adverse effects of β-blockers are due to β-blockade and, therefore, are predictable from a knowledge of their pharmacological effects. The most dramatic effects usually occur following the first dose when β-blockade quickly demonstrates the patient's dependence on adrenergic stimulation. Further doses only produce relatively (in terms of toxicity) modest increases in the degree of β-blockade. For that reason, patients thought to be particularly at risk should be given a small starting dose and observed carefully.

Bronchospasm. Blockade of β_2-receptors in the bronchi can precipitate bronchospasm in patients with asthma or obstructive airway disease. This also can occur with the relatively β_1-selective drugs; however, higher concentrations are usually required before β_2-blockade and bronchospasm are produced with the selective blockers.

Cardiac failure. The administration of β-blockers to patients with impaired cardiac reserve may precipitate cardiac failure. Although the negative inotropic actions of some of the drugs may be responsible in some cases, it is likely that most cases of β-blocker-precipitated cardiac failure are due to reversal of the increased sympathetic drive to the heart which the patients require to maintain adequate cardiac output. In such cases, reversal of this increased sympathetic drive will be produced equally effectively by all β-blockers, irrespective of their selectivity or intrinsic sympathetic activity.

Peripheral vascular disease and Raynaud's phenomena may be caused by β_2-receptor blockade. The relatively selective β-blockers would be the preferred agents in such patients, if indeed β-blockade is justified at all.

In diabetics, β-blockers can mask the usual warning signs (except sweating) of hypoglycemia which are adrenergically mediated. Increased sweating is a characteristic symptom of hypoglycemia. Though the sweat glands are innervated by the sympathetic nervous system, the neurotransmitter is acetylcholine, not norepinephrine. Therefore, it is not surprising that β-blockade does not reduce, and may increase, the degree of sweating in response to hypoglycemia. In addition to masking the symptoms of hypoglycemia, the nonselective β-blockers may worsen the physiological effects of hypoglycemia by increasing the rise in blood pressure, prolonging the period of hypoglycemia and increasing the bradycardia. Selective β_1-blockers such as metoprolol seem to produce less marked changes [147].

Bradycardia is a pharmacological manifestation of β-blockade which should only be considered an adverse effect when accompanied by signs of inadequate cardiac output. Bradycardia per se is almost never an indication for stopping or reducing the dose of β-blocker if cardiac output is maintained.

β-blocker withdrawal syndrome. There have been a number of case reports describing the development of ventricular arrhythmias, severe angina, myocardial infarction and even death soon after sudden cessation of propranolol therapy [180–185]. It was at first thought that this might occur because of the progression of the underlying cardiovascular disease during the period the patient had received β-blockade and that uncovering of this progression by withdrawal of propranolol gave rise to the exacerbation of symptoms. However, this observation cannot be the total explanation as the withdrawal syndrome has been observed in patients crossed over from propranolol to placebo during 5–6-week-long clinical trials [186].

Many of the signs such as tremulousness and tachycardia suggest a hyperadrenergic state, perhaps due to rebound increase in sensitivity to circulating catecholamines. A hypersensitivity to adrenergic agents has been shown by some [187, 188]

160

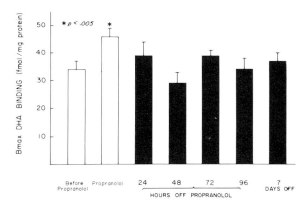

DECREASE IN LYMPHOCYTE
β-RECEPTORS IN PROPRANOLOL WITHDRAWAL

Figure 8. β-receptor density (measured by ^{3}H dihydroalprenolol (DHA) binding) on human lymphocytes following withdrawal of propranolol (from [114]).

in the period following propranolol therapy. However others, using epinephrine, have failed to confirm this [189].

The suggestion has been made that the withdrawal syndrome could be due to the increase in β-receptor number induced by propranolol persisting after the propranolol had been eliminated. One study [190] has produced data in support of this, while another [114] (Figure 8) has not. Others have suggested that the withdrawal syndrome might be due to increased levels of the active thyroid hormone triiodothyronine [191].

The existence of the withdrawal syndrome has raised several practical issues, in particular, the need to routinely withdraw propranolol before open heart surgery. Although an initial report suggested that the negative inotropic effects of the drug may last for weeks [192], this has not been substantiated [193, 194] and most agree that the drug need not be stopped before surgery. Indeed, continued treatment may be beneficial [195]. A number of studies have failed to find evidence of the withdrawal syndrome with other β-blockers. However, there is at present no evidence to suggest that this is a problem peculiar to any one β-blocker. If a β-blocker is stopped, it would seem prudent to taper the dose over a period of 4–7 days and to reinstitute therapy immediately if symptoms develop.

Indications for β-blockade

Hypertension. There is now considerable experience with the use of β-blockers in hypertensive patients, but despite this their mechanism of action remains unclear. Although the acute (intravenous) administration of propranolol produces an immediate fall in cardiac output and rate, blood pressure does not fall until later because of an initial reflex rise in the total peripheral resistance, which gradually wanes to produce a sustained fall in blood pressure [196].

A number of theories have been proposed to explain the hypotensive effect of β-blockers. It was suggested initially that the chronic reduction in cardiac output produced by long-term oral therapy resulted in resetting of the baroreceptors with a fall in blood pressure [196]. A central hypotensive action and suppression of renin secretion [197] have also been proposed as other possible mechanisms of action. It is likely that some of the confusion which still surrounds this area has resulted from the variation in dosage between studies and also because hypertension is multifactorial in its etiology.

The role of renin suppression in the hypotensive action of β-blockers, which was first suggested by Buhler et al. [197], has been clarified by Hollifield and his colleagues [198], who showed that propranolol in low dosage (160 mg/day) lowered renin levels and blood pressure of hypertensives with high and normal renin levels, but did not affect the blood pressure of the low-renin group. However, increasing the dose of propranolol, to as much as 960 mg/day in some patients, produced a fall in blood pressure even in the low-renin group and a further fall in blood pressure in the high-renin group without further reduction in renin levels. They, therefore, postulated that the hypotensive effect of propranolol in low doses is associated with suppression of renin secretion in hypertensives with high and normal renin levels whereas higher doses of propranolol lower blood pressure by a renin-independent mechanism. Others [199] have proposed a central site for the hypotensive action of propranolol. It has been shown that propranolol exerts a hypotensive effect when injected into the cerebral ventricular system of the conscious cat [200]. This effect only occurs with the l-isomer and it can be antagonized by isoprenaline.

In the treatment of hypertension, propranolol's

161

principal advantage over other agents is its lack of side effects. In particular it is not associated with postural or exercise-induced hypotension and it seldom disturbs sexual function.

A reasonable plan for treating hypertension is to start the patient on a diuretic or β-blocker and then, if control remains unsatisfactory, to add the other. A vasodilator such as hydralazine can then be added if required. The combination of hydralazine and β-blocker has been shown to be more effective than β-blocker alone [201] and to be adequate therapy for the control of severe hypertension. The combined use of a β-blocker and a vasodilator is particularly attractive because the β-blocker prevents the reflex increase in heart rate and cardiac output which would otherwise follow vasodilatation.

Angina pectoris. It was for the treatment of angina that β-blockers were developed originally [202], and their efficacy has now been shown in many clinical studies.

Angina pectoris is produced by an episode of exercise or emotional stress which increases the oxygen requirements of the left ventricle beyond the capacity of the diseased coronary arteries. β-blockade produces a dose-dependent reduction in heart rate and the arterial pressure response to exercise. This is thought to reduce the oxygen requirements of the left ventricle, and so prevent angina. Although it was suggested that the membrane stabilizing action of propranolol might account for its antianginal effect, this has not been borne out experimentally because d-propranolol has the same membrane stabilizing effect as the therapeutically active racemic mixture but has no antianginal activity [203]; other β-blockers which lack membrane stabilizing ability are potent antianginal agents.

The other mainstay of antianginal therapy is the use of nitrates, such as nitroglycerin. It is likely that their principal beneficial effect is due to peripheral vasodilation and reduction in both preload and afterload. However, this will result in a reflex increase in cardiac output and cardiac rate. These reflex changes which may increase left ventricular oxygen demands can be prevented by β-blockade so that the two drugs in combination provide complementary antianginal therapy.

Myocardial infarction. The use of β-blockade in the acute and chronic treatment of patients with myocardial infarction is an exciting but controversial area. It was suggested from studies using practolol [204] (which was subsequently withdrawn because of adverse effects) and alprenolol [205] that the number of cardiac deaths might be reduced after myocardial infarction by long-term β-blockade. This has been confirmed in a large study in which timolol or placebo was administered to patients after a myocardial infarct [206]. The death rate was reduced by 45% in the timolol-treated group. The mechanism for this beneficial effect of β-blockade following myocardial infarction is unknown. There also is evidence that β-blockers administered immediately following myocardial infarction can decrease infarct size and can prevent some patients from progressing to actual infarction perhaps by reducing myocardial oxygen demand [207].

Arrhythmias. In β-blocking concentrations, propranolol reduces sinus rate, ectopic focal activity, and conduction velocity across the A-V node. Therefore, sinus tachycardia is very responsive to β-blockade. However, it is important to determine the underlying cause for this condition before embarking on therapy. For example, reduction of the sympathetically induced tachycardia in patients with incipient cardiac failure will precipitate overt cardiac failure. On the other hand β-blockade can usefully be employed to reduce the heart rate in thyrotoxicosis without affecting the underlying thyroid status of the patient. In treating patients whose sinus tachycardia is associated with an anxiety state, β-blockade may be useful not as an anxiolytic agent but purely to interrupt the sequence of events whereby the tachycardia is contributing to the maintenance of anxiety.

Because β-blockers depress A-V conducting tissue including pathways for reentry, they are very effective in both the prophylaxis and treatment of paroxysmal supraventricular arrhythmias. Many cases of supraventricular tachycardia will revert to sinus rhythm after β-blockade. Paroxysmal atrial tachycardia, including that associated with the Wolff-Parkinson-White syndrome, can be prevented by long-term β-blockade.

Digitalis remains the drug of choice in slowing the ventricular response in atrial fibrillation. However, propranolol also depresses A-V conduction and although sinus rhythm is seldom restored, the ventricular rate may be reduced. The place of propranolol in the treatment of atrial fibrillation is probably as an adjunct to digoxin therapy. For example, if a satisfactory reduction in ventricular rate has not been obtained with digoxin, and the dosage cannot be increased due to toxicity, the synergistic effect of propranolol on the A-V conducting tissue can be used to slow the ventricular rate further.

Although it is not necessarily the drug of first choice, propranolol has been shown to be effective in nearly all types of digitalis-induced arrhythmias. However, for the reasons outlined above, the A-V block often seen in these arrhythmias may be worsened by propranolol.

The ability of propranolol to control ventricular arrhythmias in pheochromocytoma and during anesthesia results from antagonism of circulating catecholamines. Also, β-blockers have been found effective for many patients with chronic ventricular arrhythmias. However, because of less than uniform efficacy and the frequent presence of contraindications for β-blocking therapy (heart failure), β-blockers are not first-line therapy for patients with chronic ventricular arrhythmias. Yet, most studies with β-blockers have found that approximately 50% of patients have a significant reduction in ectopic frequency [208–210]. Woosley et al. [211] have evaluated a wide range of dosages of propranolol and found that 75% of 32 patients had 70–100% reduction in arrhythmia frequency (see

Figure 9). Arrhythmia suppression occurred at plasma concentrations from 12–1,100 ng/ml and at dosages from 80–640 mg/day. Because a high degree of β-blockade is usually seen at plasma concentrations from 8–200 ng/ml, these results raised the possibility that another action of propranolol may be responsible for the antiarrhythmic efficacy seen at high concentrations in approximately 40% of these patients.

However, Woosley et al. [211] also found that some patients had worsening of arrhythmia at high dosages (Figure 10), although these patients had demonstrated reduced arrhythmia frequency at lower dosages. Also, the subsequent development of suicidal depression in four subjects receiving high dosages [212] limited the usefulness of propranolol in these patients.

Propranolol has been found effective for suppressing exercise-induced arrhythmias [213] and arrhythmias seen in the first two months after myocardial infarction [214]. However, when propranolol and atenolol were given to patients with acute myocardial infarction, no significant reduction in mortality was found [215]. More importantly, the occurrence of hypotension, bradycardia, and heart failure prompted withdrawal of therapy in a large fraction of subjects receiving β-blocker therapy.

It is often assumed that the antiarrhythmic actions of drugs used to suppress ventricular arrhythmias would also reduce the incidence of sudden unexpected death in a subset of the population. Large multicenter studies have fairly conclusively

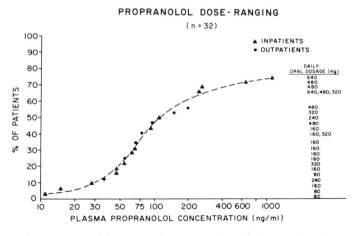

Figure 9. Relationship between plasma propranolol concentration and fraction of patients with ventricular arrhythmias, demonstrating > 70% reduction in arrhythmia frequency (from [211]).

163

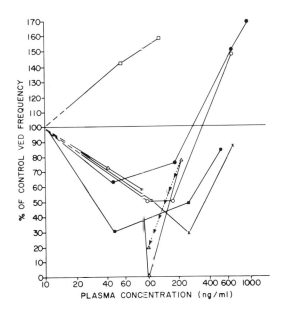

Figure 10. Plasma concentration-response curve for six patients who experienced increased arrhythmia frequency as propranolol dosage was increased. Arrows for one patient (△——△) show return of arrhythmia control after reduction in dosage: VED = ventricular ectopic depolarization (from [211]).

shown that some β-blockers, (alprenolol, practolol, and timolol) can reduce the incidence of sudden death in patients who have had a prior myocardial infarction [204–206]. A multicenter study in the United States has dosed propranolol to a fixed blood level of > 75 ng/ml and found that propranolol reduced the incidence of sudden cardiac death in patients with a prior myocardial infarction [216].

Other β-blockers have been found effective in the chronic therapy of ventricular arrhythmias [208, 209]. However, comparative studies have not been performed to determine if one β-blocker has greater efficacy in a subset of patients. Such comparisons might determine the importance of the 'direct membrane' effects of propranolol, alprenolol, and acebutolol. Also, a comparison might determine the relative importance of the lengthening of action potential duration induced by sotalol.

Hypertrophic obstructive cardiomyopathy. It has been shown that positive inotropic agents worsen the functional obstruction of ventricular outflow in this condition. There is also evidence of increased levels of catecholamines in cardiac muscle from such patients. It was natural, therefore, that propranolol would be tried in therapy, and it has been found helpful in some patients, particularly those with a high resting and exercise heart rate but without evidence of fluid retention. It has also been used to treat the cyanotic attacks associated with Tetralogy of Fallot.

Dissecting aneurysm of the aorta. The aim of therapy for this condition is to reduce blood pressure and left ventricular dp/dt. Nitroprusside, which must be given intravenously, effectively lowers blood pressure, but can produce undesirable reflex sympathetic changes which are effectively blocked by propranolol. This combination has been used successfully in treating dissecting aneurysms.

References

1. Berthelsen S, Pettinger WA: A functional basis for classification of α-adrenergic receptors. Life Sci 21:595–606, 1977.
2. Burn JH: The Autonomic Nervous System, 5th Ed. Blackwell, Oxford, 1975, pp 1–149.
3. Abboud FM et al: Reflex control of the peripheral circulation. Prog Cardiovasc Dis 18:371–403, 1976.
4. Cohn JN: Comparative cardiovascular effects of tyramine, ephedrine, and norepinephrine in man. Circ Res 16:174–182, 1965.
5. Zaimis E: Vasopressor drugs and catecholamines. Anesthesiology 29:732–762, 1968.
6. Miller JW, Lewis JE: Drugs affecting smooth muscle. Ann Rev Pharmacol 9:147–172, 1960.
7. Eckstein JW, Abboud FM: Circulating effects of sympathomimetic amines. Am Heart J 63:119–135, 1962.
8. Aviado DM: Cardiovascular effects of some commonly used pressor amines. Anesthesiology 20:71–97, 1959.
9. Szekeres L (ed): Adrenergic Activators and Inhibitors, vols I, II. Springer-Verlag, Berlin, 1981.
10. Laverty R: Catecholamines: role in health and disease. Drugs 16:418–440, 1978.
11. Robertson D et al: Comparative assessment of stimuli that release neuronal and adrenomedullary catecholamines in man. Circulation 59:637–643, 1970.
12. Keys A, Violante A: The cardiocirculatory effects in man of neosynephrine. J Clin Invest 21:1–12, 1942.
13. Nies AS: Cardiovascular disorders. II. Shock. In: Melmon KL, Morrelli HF (eds) Clinical Pharmacology: Basic Principles in Therapeutics. Macmillan, New York, 1978, pp 40–124.
14. Robertson D: Idiopathic orthostatic hypotension: contraindication to the use of ocular phenylephrine. Am J Ophthalmol 87:819–822, 1970.
15. Sandler M: Catecholamine synthesis and metabolism in man: clinical implications (with special reference to Parkinsonism). In: Blaschko H, Muscholl E (eds) Catecholamines. Springer-Verlag, Berlin, 1972, pp 845–899.

16. Holzbauer M, Sharman DF: The distribution of catecholamines in vertebrates. In: Blaschko H, Muschol E (eds) Catecholamines. Springer-Verlag, Berlin, 1972, pp 110–185.
17. Kopin IJ: Metabolic degradation of catecholamines. The relative importance of different pathways under physiological conditions and after administration of drugs. In: Blaschko H, Muscholl E (eds) Catecholamines. Springer-Verlag, Berlin, 1972, pp 270–282.
18. Bogner RL, Walsh JM: Sustained-release principle in human subjects utilizing radioactive techniques. J Pharmacol Sci 53:617–620, 1964.
19. Bruce RB, Pitts J: The determination and excretion of phenylephrine in urine. Biochem Pharmacol 17:335–337, 1968.
20. Tarazi RC: Sympathomimetic agents in the treatment of shock. Ann Intern Med 81:364–371, 1974.
21. Cohn JN: Blood pressure measurement in shock; mechanism of inaccuracy in auscultatory and palpatory methods. J Am Med Assoc 199:118–122, 1967.
22. Schmutzer KJ et al: Intravenous 1-norepinephrine as a cause of reduced blood volume. Surgery 50:452–457, 1961.
23. Manger WM, Gifford RW: Pheochromocytoma. Springer-Verlag, New York, 1977.
24. Alpert LI et al: Cardiomyopathy associated with a pheochromocytoma. Arch Pathol 93:544–549, 1972.
25. Conolly ME, Oates JA: The clinical pharmacology of antihypertensive drugs: clonidine. In: Gross F (ed) Antihypertensive Agents. Springer-Verlag, Berlin, 1977, pp 583–589.
26. Kobinger W: Pharmacologic basis of the cardiovascular actions of clonidine. In: Onesti G et al (eds) Hypertension: Mechanisms and Management. Grune and Stratton, New York, 1973, pp 369–380.
27. Weber MA et al: Renin and aldosterone suppression in the antihypertensive action of clonidine. Am J Cardiol 38:825–830, 1976.
28. Dollery CT et al: Clinical pharmacology and pharmacokinetics of clonidine. Clin Pharmacol Ther 19:11–17, 1976.
29. Keranen A et al: Pharmacokinetics and side-effects of clonidine. Eur J Clin Pharmacol 13:97–101, 1978.
30. Frisk-Holmberg M et al: Pharmacokinetics of clonidine and its relation to the hypotensive effect in patients. Br J Clin Pharmacol 6:227–232, 1978.
31. Wing LMH et al: Apparent resistance to the hypotensive effect of clonidine. Br Med J 1:136–138, 1977.
32. Robertson D et al: Clonidine raises blood pressure in idiopathic orthostatic hypotension. N Engl J Med, 1983 (in press).
33. Niarchos AP: Evaluation of intravenous clonidine in hypertensive emergencies. J Clin Pharmacol 18:220–228, 1978.
34. Onesti G et al: Antihypertensive effect of clonidine. Circ Res 28(Suppl II):53–69, 1971.
35. Muir AL et al: Circulatory effects at rest and exercise of clonidine, an imidazoline derivative with hypotensive properties. Lancet 2:181–185, 1969.
36. Hokfelt B et al: Studies on catecholamines, renin and aldosterone following Catepres in hypertensive patients. Eur J Pharmacol 10:389–397, 1970.
37. Velasco M et al: Effect of clonidine on sympathetic nervous activity in hydralazine-treated hypertensive patients. Eur J Clin Pharmacol 13:317–320, 1978.
38. Jain AK et al: Efficacy and acceptability of different dosage schedules of clonidine. Clin Pharmacol Ther 21:382–387, 1977.
39. Cohen IM, Katz MA: Oral clonidine loading for rapid control of hypertension. Clin Pharmacol Ther 24:11–15, 1978.
40. Briant RH et al: Interaction between clonidine and desipramine in man. Br Med J 1:522–523, 1973.
41. Reid JL et al: Clonidine withdrawal in hypertension: changes in blood pressure and plasma and urinary noradrenaline. Lancet 1:1171–1174, 1977.
42. Goldberg AD et al: Blood pressure and heart rate and withdrawal of antihypertensive drugs. Br Med J 1:1243–1246, 1977.
43. Whitsett TL et al: Abrupt cessation of clonidine administration: a prospective study. Am J Cardiol 41:1285–1290, 1978.
44. Oates J et al: The clinical pharmacology of antihypertensive drugs. In: Gross F (ed) Antihypertensive Agents. Springer-Verlag, Berlin, 1977, pp 571–632.
45. Oates JA et al: Decarboxylase inhibition and blood pressure reduction by α-methyl-3,4-dihydroxy-DL-phenylalanine. Science 131:1890–1891, 1960.
46. Planz G et al: Influence of the decarboxylase inhibitor benserazide on the antihypertensive effect and metabolism of alpha-methyldopa in patients with essential hypertension. Eur J Clin Pharmacol 12:429–435, 1977.
47. Heise A, Kroneberg G: Central nervous α-adrenergic receptors and the mode of action of α-methyldopa. Naunyn Schmiedebergs Arch Pharmacol 279:285–300, 1973.
48. Goldberg MR et al: Differential affinities of α-methyldopa metabolites on α_1 and α_2 receptors in rat brain. Eur J Pharmacol 69:95–99, 1981.
49. Saavedra JA et al: Plasma concentration of α-methyldopa and sulphate conjugate after oral and intravenous administration. Eur J Clin Pharmacol 8:381–386, 1975.
50. Stenbaek O et al: Pharmacokinetics of methyldopa in healthy man. Eur J Clin Pharmacol 12:117–123, 1977.
51. Barnett AJ et al: Pharmacokinetics of methyldopa: plasma levels following single intravenous, oral and multiple oral dosage in normotensive and hypertensive subjects. Clin Exp Pharmacol Physiol 4:331–339, 1977.
52. Wright JM et al: Antihypertensive effect of a single bedtime dose of methyldopa. Clin Pharmacol Ther 20:733–737, 1976.
53. Alcocer L et al: Hemodynamic and metabolic effects of methyldopa in the treatment of hypertension. Curr Ther Res 23:55–65, 1978.
54. Dollery CT et al: Hemodynamic studies with methyldopa: effect on cardiac output and response to pressor amines. Br Heart J 25:670–676, 1963.
55. Maddrey WC, Boitnott JK: Severe hepatitis from methyldopa. Gastroenterology 8:351–360, 1975.
56. Sotaniemi EA et al: Hepatic injury and drug metabolism in patients with alpha-methyldopa-induced liver damage. Eur J Clin Pharmacol 12:429–435, 1977.
57. LoBuglio AF, Jandl JH: The nature of the alpha-methyl-

dopa red-cell antibody. N Eng J Med 276:658–665, 1967.

58. Conolly ME et al: A crossover comparison of clonidine and methyldopa in hypertension. Eur J Clin Pharmacol 4:222–227, 1972.

59. Goldberg AD et al: Blood pressure and heart rate and withdrawal of antihypertensive drugs. Br Med J 1:1243–1246, 1977.

60. Leonetti G et al: Relation between the hypotensive and renin-suppressing activities of alpha methyldopa in hypertensive patients. Am J Cardiol 40:762–767, 1977.

61. McMahon FG: Efficacy of an antihypertensive agent: comparison of methyldopa and hydrocholorothiazide in combination and singly. J Am Med Assoc 231:155–158, 1975.

62. Hansen M et al: Controlled clinical study on antihypertensive treatment with a diuretic and methyldopa compared with a β-blocking agent and hydralazine. Acta Med Scand 202:385–388, 1977.

63. Pierach CA et al: Unusual Watson-Schwartz test from methyldopa. N Engl J Med 296:577–578, 1977.

64. Manger WM, Gifford RW: Pheochromocytoma. Springer-Verlag, New York, 1977, p 304–342.

65. Nickerson M, Gourzis JT: Blockade of sympathetic vasoconstriction in the treatment of shock. J Trauma 2:399–411, 1962.

66. Nickerson M: Vascular adjustments during the development of shock. Can Med Assoc J 103:853–859, 1970.

67. Riordan JF, Walters G: Effects of phenoxybenzamine in shock due to myocardial infarction. Br Med J 1:155–158, 1969.

68. Kelly DT et al: Use of phentolamine in acute myocardial infarction associated with hypertension and left ventricular failure. Circulation 47:729–735, 1973.

69. Henning RJ et al: Afterload reduction with phentolamine in patients with acute pulmonary edema. Am J Med 63:568–573, 1977.

70. Stern MA et al: Hemodynamic effects of intravenous phentolamine in low output cardiac failure: dose response relationships. Circulation 58:157–163, 1978.

71. Henning RJ, Weil MH: Effect of afterload reduction on plasma volume during acute heart failure. Am J Cardiol 42:823–827, 1978.

72. Gould LA, Reddy CVR: Oral therapy with phentolamine in chronic congestive heart failure. Chest 75:487–491, 1979.

73. Nickerson M: The pharmacology of adrenergic blockade. Pharmacol Rev 1:27–101, 1949.

74. Muller-Schweinitzer E et al: Basic pharmacological properties. In: Ergot Alkaloids and Related Compounds. Springer-Verlag, Berlin, 1978, 87–232.

75. Knapp Dr et al: Qualitative metabolic fate of phenoxybenzamine in rat, dog, and man. Drug Metab Dispos 4:164–168, 1976.

76. Williams BJ et al: The protective effect of phentolamine against cardiac arrhythmias in the rat. Eur J Pharmacol 49:7–14, 1978.

77. Richards DA et al: Circulatory and α-adrenoceptor blocking effects of phentolamine. Br J Clin Pharmacol 5:507–513, 1978.

78. Gould L, Reddy CVR: Phentolamine. Am Heart J 92:397–402, 1976.

79. Taylor S H et al: The circulatory effects of phentolamine in man with particular respect to changes in forearm blood flow. Clin Sci 28:265–284, 1965.

80. Lowry P et al: Histamine and sympathetic blockade in septic shock. Am Surg 43:12–19, 1977.

81. Hess JH et al: Antihypertensive 2-amino-4(^{3}H)-quinazolines. J Med Chem 11:130–138, 1968.

82. Davey MJ, Massingham R: A review of the biological effects of prazosin, including recent pharmacological findings. Curr Med Res Opin 4(Suppl 2):47–60, 1976.

83. U'Prichard D et al: Prazosin: differential affinities for two populations of α-noradrenergic receptor binding sites. Eur J Pharmacol 50:87–89, 1978.

84. Stokes GS, Oates HF: Prazosin: new alpha-adrenergic blocking agent in treatment of hypertension. Cardiovasc Med 2:41–57, 1978.

85. Brogden RN et al: Prazosin: a review of its pharmacological properties and therapeutic efficacy in hypertension. Drugs 14:163–197, 1977.

86. Hayes J M et al: Effect of prazosin on plasma renin activity. Med J Aust 76:562–564, 1976.

87. Massingham R, Hayden ML: A comparison of the effects of prazosin and hydralazine on blood pressure, heart rate, and plasma renin activity in conscious renal hypertensive dogs. Eur J Pharmacol 30:121–124, 1975.

88. Awan NA et al: Comparison of effects of nitroprusside and prazosin on left ventricular function and the peripheral circulation in chronic refractory congestive heart failure. Circulation 57:152–159, 1978.

89. Bateman DN et al: Prazosin, pharmacokinetics and concentration effect. Eur J Clin Pharmacol 16:177–181, 1979.

90. Rubin PC, Blaschke TF: Studies on the clinical pharmacology of prazosin. I. Cardiovascular, catecholamine and endocrine changes following a single dose. Br J Clin Pharmacol 10:23–32, 1980.

91. Pitts NE: The clinical evaluation of prazosin, a new antihypertensive agent. Postgrad Med (Nov Suppl):117–127, 1975.

92. Mroczek W et al: Prazosin in hypertension: a double-blind evaluation with methyldopa and placebo. Curr Ther Res 16:769–777, 1974.

93. Bloom DS et al: Clinical evaluation of prazosin as the sole agent for the treatment of hypertension: a double-blind crossover study with methyldopa. Curr Ther Res 18:144–150, 1975.

94. Curtis JR, Bateman FJA: Use of prazosin in management of hypertension in patients with chronic renal failure and in renal transplant recipients. Br Med J 4:432–434, 1975.

95. Charness ME et al: Exacerbation of angina pectoris by prazosin. S Med J 72:1213–1214, 1979.

96. Miller RR et al: Sustained reduction of cardiac impedance and preload in congestive heart failure with antihypertensive vasodilator prazosin. N Engl J Med 297:303–307, 1977.

97. Aronow WS et al: Effect of prazosin vs placebo on chronic left ventricular heart failure. Circulation 59:344–350, 1979.

98. Stokes GS et al: Long-term use of prazosin in combination or alone for treating hypertension. Med J Aust 2 (Suppl):13–16, 1977.

99. Packer M et al: Hemodynamic and clinical tachyphylaxis

to prazosin-mediated after-load reduction in severe chronic heart failure. Circulation 59:531–539, 1979.

100. Arnold S et al: Rapid attenuation of prazosin mediated increase in cardiac output in patients with chronic heart failure. Ann Intern Med 91:345–349, 1970.

101. Stokes GS, Weber MA: Prazosin-preliminary report and comparative studies with other antihypertensive agents. Br Med J 2:298–300, 1974.

102. Brogden RN et al: Labetalol: a review of its pharmacology and therapeutic use in hypertension. Drugs 15:251–270, 1978.

103. Richards DA, Prichard BNC: Concurrent antagonism of isoproterenol and norepinephrine after labetalol. Clin Pharmacol Ther 23:253–258, 1978.

104. Richards DA, Prichard BNC: Adrenoceptor blockade of the circulatory responses to intravenous isoproterenol. Clin Pharmacol Ther 24:264–273, 1978.

105. Gryglewski R, Vane JR: The inactivation of noradrenaline and isoprenaline in dogs. Br J Pharmacol 39:573–584, 1970.

106. Conway WD et al: Absorption and elimination profile of isoproterenol III. The metabolic fate of dl-Isoproterenol-7-^{3}H in the dog. J Pharm Sci 57:1135–1141, 1968.

107. Conolly ME et al: Metabolism of isoprenaline in dog and man. Br J Pharmacol 46:458–472, 1972.

108. Heel RC et al: Fenoterol: a review of its pharmacological properties and therapeutic efficacy in asthma. Drugs 15:3–32, 1978.

109. Pinder RM et al: Rimiterol: a review of its pharmacological properties and therapeutic efficacy in asthma. Drugs 14:81–104, 1977.

110. Hetzel MR, Clark TJH: Comparison of intravenous and aerosol salbutamol. Br Med J 919, 1976.

111. Banner AS et al: Arrhythmogenic effects of orally administered bronchodilators. Arch Intern Med 139:434–437, 1979.

112. Wilson JD et al: Has the change to beta-agonists combined with oral theophylline increased cases of fatal asthma? Lancet 1235–1237, 1981.

113. Ahlquist RP: Study of the adrenotropic receptors. Am J Physiol 153:586–589, 1948.

114. Fraser et al: Regulation of human leukocyte beta receptors by endogenous catecholamines. J Clin Invest 67:1777–1784, 1981.

115. Vestal RE et al: Reduced beta-adrenoceptor sensitivity in the elderly. Clin Pharmacol Ther 26:181–186, 1979.

116. Vaughan-Williams EM: Mode of action of beta receptor antagonists on cardiac muscle. Am J Cardiol 18:399–405, 1966.

117. Morales-Aguilera A, Vaughan-Williams EM: The effects on cardiac muscle of β-receptor antagonists in relation to their activity as local anesthetics. Br J Pharmacol 24:332–338, 1965.

118. Davis LD, Temte JV: Effects of propranolol on the transmembrane potential of ventricular muscle and Purkinje fibers of the dog. Circ Res 22:661–677, 1968.

119. Coltart DJ, Meldrum SJ: Effects of racemic propranolol, dextro-propranolol and racemic practolol on the human and canine cardiac transmembrane action potential. Arch Intern Pharmacodyn 192:188, 1971.

120. Coltart DJ, Meldrum SJ: The effect of propranolol on the human and canine transmembrane action potential. Br J Pharmacol 40:148P, 1970.

121. Prichard BNC et al: Uses of beta-adrenoceptor blocking drugs. J R Coll Phys 11:35–57, 1976.

122. Coltart DJ et al: Plasma propranolol levels associated with suppression of ventricular ectopic beats. Br Med J 1:490–491, 1971.

123. Pruett JK et al: Propranolol effects on membrane repolarization time in isolated canine Purkinje fibers: threshold tissue content and the influence of exposure time. J Pharmacol Exp Ther 215:539, 1980.

124. Kates RE, Jaillon P: A model to describe myocardial drug disposition in the dog. J Pharmacol Exp Ther 241:31–36, 1980.

125. Berkowitz ED et al: The effects of propranolol on cardiac conduction. Circulation 40:355–362, 1969.

126. Calon AH et al: The effect of propranolol on refractoriness and reentry with the His Purkinje system. Clin Res 25:211A, 1977.

127. Fitzgerald JD, O'Donnell SR: Pharmacology of 4-hydroxypropranolol, a metabolite of propranolol. Br J Pharmacol 43:222–235, 1971.

128. Seides SF et al: The electrophysiology of propranolol in man. Am Heart J 88:733, 1974.

129. Brorson L et al: Effects of concentration and steric configuration of propranolol on AV conduction and ventricular repolarization in the dog. J Cardiovasc Pharmacol 3:692–703, 1981.

130. Buiumsohn A et al: Seizures and intraventricular conduction defect in propranolol poisoning. Ann Intern Med 91:860–862, 1979.

131. Reddy CP et al: Effect of procainamide on reentry within the His Purkinje system in man. Am J Cardol 40:957–964, 1977.

132. Dawson A et al: Electrophysiological effects of high-dose propranolol in dogs: evidence in vivo for effects not mediated by the β-adrenoceptor. J Pharmacol Exp Ther, 1983 (in press).

133. Wit AL et al: Electrophysiologic effects of bretylium tosylate on single fibers of the canine specialized conducting system and ventricle. J Pharmacol Exp Ther 173:344–356, 1970.

134. Singh BN, Vaughan Williams EM: The effect of amiodarone, a new antianginal drug on cardiac muscle. Br J Pharmacol 39:657–667, 1970.

135. Vaughan Williams EM: Classification of antiarrhythmic drugs. In: Sandoe E et al (eds) Symposium on Cardiac Arrhythmias. Astra Publ, 1970, pp 449–472.

136. Edvardsson N et al: Sotalol-induced delayed ventricular repolarization in man. Eur Heart J 1:335–343, 1980.

137. Edvardsson N, Olsson SB: Effects of acute and chronic beta-receptor blockade on ventricular repolarisation in man. Br Heart J 45:628–636, 1981.

138. Amlie JP et al: Acebutolol-induced changes in refractoriness and monophastic action potential of the right ventricle of the dog heart in situ. Cardiovasc Res XII:493–496, 1978.

139. Duff HJ et al: Electrophysiologic actions of high dose propranolol independent of beta-blockade. Circulation 62(Suppl III):11, 1980.

167

140. Olley PM, Fowler RS: The surdo-cardiac syndrome and therapeutic observations. Br Heart J 32:467, 1970.

141. Raine AEG, Pickering TG: Cardiovascular and sympathetic response to exercise after long-term beta-adrenergic blockade. Br Med J 2:90–92, 1977.

142. Milne JR et al: Effect of intravenous propranolol on QT interval. Br Heart J 43:1–6, 1980.

143. Bigger JT: Braunwald E (ed) Management of Arrhythmia in Heart Disease, 1980, p 701.

144. Lands AM et al: Differentiation of receptors responsive to isoproterenol. Life Sci 6:2241–2249, 1967.

145. Decalmer PB et al: Beta-blockers and asthma. Br Heart J 40:184–189, 1978.

146. Deacon SP et al: Acebutolol, atenolol and propranolol and metabolic responses to acute hypoglycemia in diabetics. Br Med J 2:1255–1257, 1977.

147. Lager I et al: Effect of cardioselective and nonselective β-blockade on the hypoglycemic response in insuline-dependent diabetics. Lancet 1:458–462, 1979.

148. Anlauf M: Hemodynamic reactions under various stimuli before and during chronic beta-blockade. Arch Intern Pharmacodyn Ther (Suppl):76–82, 1980.

149. Kaumann AJ, Blinks JR: β-adrenoceptor blocking agents as partial agonists in isolated heart muscle: dissociation of stimulation and blockade. Arch Pharmacol (in press).

150. Kaumann AJ et al: Comparative assessment of β-adrenoceptor blocking agents as simple competitive antagonists in isolated heart muscle: similarity of inotropic and chronotropic blocking potencies against isoproterenol. Arch Pharmacol 311:219–236, 1980.

151. Turner P: β-adrenergic receptor blocking drugs in hyperthyroidism. Drugs 7:48–54, 1974.

152. Carruthers SG et al: The assessment of β-adrenoreceptor blocking drugs in hyperthyroidism. Br J Clin Pharmacol 1:93–98, 1974.

153. Nelson JK, McDevitt DG: Comparative trial of propranolol and practolol in hyperthyroidism. Br J Clin Pharmacol 2:411–418, 1975.

154. Lee RJ et al: Direct myocardial depressant effects of several β-adrenergic blocking agents in the unanesthetized atherosclerotic rabbit. Proc Soc Exp Biol Med 158:147–150, 1978.

155. Paterson JW et al: The pharmacodynamics and metabolism of propranolol in man. Pharmacol Clin 2:127–133, 1970.

156. Shand DG, Rangno RE: The disposition of propranolol. I. Elimination during oral absorption in man. Pharmacology 7:159–168, 1972.

157. Lowenthal DT et al: Pharmacokinetics of oral propranolol in chronic renal disease. Clin Pharmacol Ther 16:761–769, 1974.

158. Parsons RL et al: Absorption of propranolol and practolol in coeliac disease. Gut 17:129–143, 1976.

159. Castleden CM et al: The effect of age on plasma levels of propranolol and practolol in man. Br J Clin Pharmacol 2:303–306, 1975.

160. Tocco DJ et al: Physiological disposition and metabolism of timolol in man and laboratory animals. Drug Metab Dispos 3:361–370, 1975.

161. Melander A et al: Enhancement of the bioavailability of propranolol and metoprolol by food. Clin Pharmacol Ther 22:108–112, 1977.

162. Johnsson G et al: Combined pharmacokinetic and pharmacodynamic studies in man of the adrenergic β_1 receptor antagonist metoprolol. Acta Pharmacol Toxicol (Copenh) 36(Suppl V):31–44, 1975.

163. Shand DG et al: Plasma propranolol levels in adults, with observations in four children. Clin Pharmacol Ther 23:165–174, 1970.

164. Kornhauser DM et al: Biological determinants of propranolol disposition in man. Clin Pharmacol Ther 23:165–174, 1978.

165. Wood AJJ et al: Direct measurement of propranolol bioavailability during accumulation to steady state. Br J Clin Pharmacol 345–350, 1978.

166. Chidsey CA et al: Studies of the absorption and removal of propranolol in hypertensive patients during therapy. Circulation 52:313–318, 1975.

167. Shand DG: Individualization of propranolol therapy. Med Clin North Am 58:1063–1069, 1974.

168. Vestal RE et al: The effects of aging and cigarette smoking on propranolol's disposition in man. Clin Pharmacol Ther 26:8–15, 1979.

169. Vessel ES: Genetic and environmental factors affecting drug disposition in man. Clin Pharmacol Ther 22:659–679, 1977.

170. Dreyfuss J et al: Metabolic studies in patients with nadolol oral and intravenous administration. J Clin Pharmacol 17:300–307, 1977.

171. Conway FJ et al: Human pharmacokinetic and pharmacodynamic studies on atenolol (ICI 66082) – a new cardioselective adrenoceptor β adrenoceptor blocking drug. Br J Clin Pharmacol 3:267–272, 1976.

172. Duchin KL et al: Steady state pharmacokinetics of nadolol and therapeutic efficacy. Clin Pharmacol Ther 25:221–222, 1979.

173. Wood AJJ et al: The influence of cirrhosis on steady-state blood concentrations of unbound propranolol after oral administration. Clin Pharmacokinet 3:478–487, 1978.

174. Lowenthal DT et al: Timolol kinetics in chronic renal insufficiency. Clin Pharmacol Ther 23:606–615, 1978.

175. Herrera J et al: Elimination of nadolol by patients with renal impairment. Br J Clin Pharmacol 8(Suppl 2):227–231, 1979.

176. Thompson FD et al: Pharmacodynamics of propranolol in renal failure. Br Med J 2:434–436, 1972.

177. Bianchetti G et al: Pharmacokinetics and effects of propranolol in terminal ureamic patients and in patients undergoing regular dialysis treatment. Clin Pharmacokinet 1:373–384, 1976.

178. Wood AJJ et al: The effect of aging and cigarette smoking on the elimination of antipyrine and indocyanine green. Clin Pharmacol Ther 26:16–20, 1979.

179. Crooks J et al: Pharmacokinetics in the elderly. Clin Pharmacokinet 1:280–296, 1976.

180. Diaz RG et al: Withdrawal of propranolol and myocardial infarction. Lancet 1:1068, 1973.

181. Slome R: Withdrawal of propranolol and myocardial infarction. Lancet 1:156, 1973.

182. Alderman EL et al: Coronary artery syndrome after sud-

den propranolol withdrawal. Ann Intern Med 81:625, 1974.

183. Olsen HG et al: The propranolol withdrawal rebound phenomenon: acute and catastrophic exacerbation of symptoms and death following the abrupt cessation of large doses of propranolol in coronary artery disease. Am J Cardiol 35:162, 1975.

184. Mizgala HF, Counsell J: Acute coronary syndromes following abrupt cessation of oral propranolol therapy. Can Med Assoc J 114:1123, 1976.

185. Shand D, Wood AJJ: Propranolol withdrawal syndrome – Why? Circulation 58:202–203, 1978.

186. Miller RR et al: Propranolol withdrawal rebound phenomenon. N Engl J Med 293:1975, 1975.

187. Nattel S et al: Mechanism of propranolol withdrawal phenomena. Circulation 59:1158–1164, 1979.

188. Boudoulas H et al: Hypersensitivity to adrenergic stimulation after propranolol withdrawal in normal subjects. Ann Intern Med 87:433–436, 1977.

189. Lindenfeld J et al: Adrenergic responsiveness after abrupt propranolol withdrawal in normal subjects and in patients with angina pectoris. Circulation 62:704–711, 1980.

190. Aarons RD et al: Elevation of beta-adrenergic receptor density in human lymphocytes after propranolol administration. J Clin Invest 65:949–957, 1980.

191. Shenkman L et al: Hyperthyroidism after propranolol withdrawal. J Am Med Assoc 238:237–239, 1977.

192. Viljoen JF et al: Propranolol and cardiac surgery. J Thorac Cardiovasc Surg 64:826, 1972.

193. Faulkner SL et al: Time required for complete recovery from chronic propranolol therapy. N Engl J Med 289:607, 1973.

194. Coltart DJ et al: Investigation of the safe withdrawal period for propranolol in patients scheduled for open heart surgery. Br Heart J 37:1228, 1975.

195. Slogoff S et al: Propranolol in coronary surgery. Am Soc Anesthesiol Abstr, 1977, p 499.

196. Prichard BNC, Gillam PMS: Use of propranolol (Inderal) in treatment of hypertension. Br Med J 2:725–727, 1964.

197. Buhler FR et al: Proposed mechanisms of propranolol's antihypertensive effect in essential hypertension. Am J Cardiol 32:511–522, 1973.

198. Hollifield JW et al: Proposed mechanisms of propranolol's antihypertensive effect in essential hypertension. N Engl J Med 295:68–73, 1976.

199. Reid JL et al: Cardiovascular effects of intracerebroventricular D, L, and DL-propranolol in the conscious rabbit. J Pharmacol Exp Ther 188:394–399, 1974.

200. Day MD, Roach AG: β adrenergic receptors in the central nervous system of the cat concerned with control of arterial blood pressure and heart rate. Nature 242:30–31, 1973.

201. Hansson L et al: Treatment of hypertension with propranolol and hydralazine. Acta Med Scand 190:531–534, 1971.

202. Shanks RG: The properties of beta-adrenoceptor antagonists. Postgrad Med J 52(Suppl 4):14–20, 1976.

203. Wilson AG et al: Mechanism of action of β-adrenergic receptor blocking agents in angina pectoris: comparison of action of propranolol with dexpropranolol and practolol. Br Med J 4:399–401, 1969.

204. Green KG: Improvement in prognosis of myocardial infarction by long term beta-adrenoreceptor blockade using practolol: a multicenter international trial. Br Med J 3:735–740, 1975.

205. Wilhelmsson C et al: Reduction of sudden death after myocardial infarction by treatment with alprenolol. Lancet 2:1157–1160, 1974.

206. Norwegian Multicenter Study Group: Timolol-induced reduction in mortality and reinfarction in patients surviving acute myocardial infarction. N Engl J Med 304:801–807, 1981.

207. Lee RJ: Beta-adrenergic blockade in acute myocardial infarction. Life Sci 23:2539–2542, 1979.

208. Gibson D, Sowton E: The use of beta-adrenergic receptor blocking drugs in dysrhythmias. Prog Cardiovasc Dis 12:16, 1969.

209. de Soyza N et al: The long-term suppression of ventricular arrhythmia by oral acebutolol in patients with coronary artery disease. Am Heart J 100:631–638, 1980.

210. Naggar CZ, Alexander S: Propranolol treatment of VPBs. N Engl J Med 294:903–904, 1976.

211. Woosley RL et al: Suppression of chronic ventricular arrhythmias with propranolol. Circulation 60:819–828, 1979.

212. Petrie WW et al: Propranolol and depression. Am J Psychol 139:92–94, 1982.

213. Nixon JV et al: Efficacy of propranolol in the control of exercise-induced or augmented ventricular ectopic activity. Circulation 57:115–122, 1978.

214. Koppes GM et al: Propranolol therapy for ventricular arrhythmias 2 months after acute myocardial infarction. Am J Cardiol 46:322–328, 1980.

215. Wilcox RG et al: Randomised trial comparing propranolol with atenolol in immediate treatment of suspected myocardial infarction. Br Med J 280:885–888, 1980.

216. Goldstein S et al: Multicenter trial for secondary prevention of sudden death with propranolol. J Am Med Assoc 247:1707–1714, 1982.

CHAPTER 7

Pharmacology of the antiarrhythmic drugs

PENELOPE A. BOYDEN and ANDREW L. WIT

Antiarrhythmic drugs are compounds which influence the electrical activity of the heart and may thereby alter or abolish the abnormalities in impulse initiation and conduction which cause cardiac arrhythmias. Until the early 1960s only two drugs, quinidine and procainamide, were used widely as antiarrhythmics in the United States. During the past 15 years there has been a continuous growth in the number of agents available. In this chapter we discuss the electrophysiological bases for the action of antiarrhythmic drugs and review their pharmacological properties. The discussion will include all antiarrhythmic drugs currently approved for clinical use in the United States, as well as some of the promising agents undergoing clinical trials.

Quinidine

Quinidine is an alkaloid prepared from cinchona bark and is an optical isomer of quinine. It was originally prepared by Pasteur in 1853 for the therapy of malaria [1]. However it was not until Frey's 1918 report on the effects of cinchonine, quinine and quinidine in patients with atrial fibrillation that the efficacy of the latter drug was fully recognized and its use extended to the treatment of other cardiac arrhythmias [2].

Quinidine consists of a quinoline attached by a secondary alcohol to a quinuclidine ring (Figure 1). The secondary alcohol appears to be essential for quinidine's antiarrhythmic activity [1].

Effects on the heart and circulation

Electrophysiologic effects on cardiac cells

(A) Effects on resting membrane potential, action potential amplitude, and phase 0 upstroke velocity $(\dot{V}_{max})$. Quinidine decreases $\dot{V}_{max}$ and amplitude of phase 0 of atrial, ventricular and Purkinje fiber action potentials in a dose-dependent manner, in concentrations which do not decrease the resting membrane or maximum diastolic potential [3–8]. This effect on the upstroke of the action potential results from a direct effect of the drug to decrease the conductance of the fast Na^+ channel. Blockade of the fast Na^+ channel by quinidine is use dependent (see section on Electrophysiologic basis for antiarrhythmic drug action). It has been shown in ventricular muscle that at very slow driving rates (< 1.0 Hz) depression of $\dot{V}_{max}$ is minimal [8], while at drive rates greater than 1 Hz, $\dot{V}_{max}$ of each stimulated action potential decreases progressively until a steady-state reduction is achieved [7–9]. After steady-state reduction and during continued exposure to the drug, a period of quiescence is followed by recovery of $\dot{V}_{max}$, the degree of recovery depending on the duration of the quiescent period [7, 9]. The time constant for recovery is relatively long (in the order of seconds) and therefore it is likely that at normal heart rates a large proportion of the Na^+ channels will not recover and will remain blocked. The use-dependent block by quinidine has been explained in terms of the modulated receptor hypothesis proposed for heart by Hondeghem and Katzung [7, 10]. According to this hypothesis, during a period of activity many of the

Rosen, M. R. and Hoffman, B. F. (eds.), Cardiac Therapy. ISBN 0-89838-564-4.
© 1983, Martinus Nijhoff Publishers, Boston, The Hague, Dordrecht, Lancaster. Printed in the Netherlands.

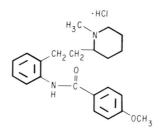

Figure 1. Chemical structures of the antiarrhythmic drugs.

antiarrhythmic drugs associate with open Na^+ channels and dissociate from inactivated or reactivated channels.

The degree of steady-state block of the Na^+ channel by quinidine is also influenced by factors other than driving rate. For example, when pH is reduced from 7.4 to 6.9, steady-state block and the reduction in $\dot{V}_{max}$ increases in Purkinje fibers and to a lesser extent in ventricular muscle [9, 11]. The time course for development of steady-state block is not influenced by the decrease in pH, but the time constant for recovery during a quiescent period is prolonged. A decrease in pH may enhance the steady-state reduction of $\dot{V}_{max}$ caused by quinidine by increasing the proportion of the drug molecule which exists in the charged form [9]. This may be the form which interacts with the receptor in the Na^+ channel to decrease Na^+ conductance. An increase in $[K^+]_0$ from 4 to 8 mM also increases the reduction in $\dot{V}_{max}$ caused by quinidine [12, 13]. This effect of K^+ most likely results from the decrease in membrane potential which usually accompanies such an increase in $[K^+]_0$. According to the modulated receptor hypothesis, there is a slower dissociation of drug from receptor at reduced membrane potentials because a greater proportion of the Na^+ channels exist in the inactivated state [10].

Quinidine also shifts the threshold potential for regenerative depolarization to less negative values. More stimulus current is therefore needed to initiate an active response from a normal level of membrane potential. The combined effects of quinidine to decrease $\dot{V}_{max}$ and increase threshold potential cause conduction velocity to slow in tissues with fast Na^+ channel-dependent upstrokes [14].

Since the blocking effect of quinidine on Na^+ conductance is enhanced at more positive membrane potentials, the drug might have a greater depressant effect on partially depolarized cardiac fibers with depressed fast response action potentials (i.e., action potentials initiated at low membrane potentials but still dependent on the fast inward Na^+ current) (see Chapter 1) [15]. Quinidine also decreases the slow inward current to a minor extent [16] and therefore may slightly decrease action potential amplitude and $\dot{V}_{max}$ of phase 0 of slow response action potentials. This is probably not a major factor in its mechanism of antiarrhythmic action, however.

(B) Effects on action potential duration and refractoriness. Quinidine prolongs the time course for repolarization, and prolongs the effective refractory period of normal atrial and ventricular muscle fibers in most animal species in which it has been studied [4–8, 17]. It also prolongs the action potential duration and refractory period of rabbit and canine Purkinje fibers [3, 11, 18, 19]. The prolongation of action potential duration results from a direct effect of quinidine to decrease the net outward membrane current at positive levels of membrane potential. This decrease in net current results mainly from a reduction of the delayed rectifier current [19]. In atrial myocardium prolongation of action potential duration might also result in part from its anticholinergic effect [20]. Curiously, quinidine shortens the duration of the sheep Purkinje fiber action potential [21]. However, there is reason to believe that in the human heart action potential duration is not shortened, since the effective refractory period of the Purkinje system is increased by the drug (see Electrophysiologic effects on the heart).

The prolongation of the effective refractory period is not entirely accounted for by the increase in action potential duration. The effective refractory period also increases because quinidine delay recovery of the Na^+ channel from inactivation [3, 6, 7, 10]. Therefore quinidine prevents the generation of new propagating action potentials until repolarization has carried membrane potential to more negative values than before drug action. When premature action potentials can be elicited they have a reduced $\dot{V}_{max}$, partly because of this delay in reactivation and partly because of a decrease in maximum inward Na^+ current that can be generated at any level of membrane potential [3].

(C) Effects on impulse initiation. Quinidine depresses normal automaticity in cardiac fibers. This effect has been demonstrated most clearly in Purkinje fibers [3] and, in high concentrations, on sinus node fibers [5]. The slowing of automatic firing results from two effects of the drug; the slope of phase 4 depolarization is decreased, and threshold potential is shifted towards 0. The decrease in phase 4 slope results from a decrease in the pacemaker current [21, 22]. Although its usual effect is to decrease the rate of automatic firing, in high (presumably toxic) concentrations quinidine may increase

the slope of phase 4 depolarization and spontaneous rate. This effect occurs only when quinidine has reduced maximum diastolic potential considerably [3].

Quinidine slightly decreases the firing rate of partially depolarized ventricular fibers by reducing the slope of phase 4 depolarization [23]. This type of automaticity is called abnormal automaticity and is probably caused by a different mechanism than normal automaticity (see Chapter 1). The effects of quinidine on other types of impulse initiation such as early and delayed afterdepolarizations have not been completely described. Preliminary data show that it increases afterdepolarization amplitude and causes triggered activity in atrial fibers exposed to norepinephrine, because it increases action potential duration [24]; this increase in duration may increase Ca^{++} influx into the cell, causing the increase in the afterdepolarization. Quinidine decreases the amplitude of afterdepolarizations caused by exposure of Purkinje fibers to toxic amounts of digitalis by decreasing the transient inward current [25].

Electrophysiologic effects on the heart

In patients without severe disease of the cardiac conducting system, therapeutic concentrations of quinidine may increase the heart rate, increase or decrease the P–R interval, and increase the QRS and QT duration [26]. These effects are the net result of direct actions of quinidine on the heart and indirect actions exerted through the autonomic nervous system. Quinidine probably attenuates the effects of the vagus on the mammalian heart [20]. It also blocks the peripheral alpha-adrenergic receptors, causing hypotension and reflex sympathetic activation [27, 28]. Both these effects may increase sinus rate and speed AV conduction. In studies on patients with cardiac transplants in whom there is persistent autonomic denervation [29] and in experimental animals with cardiac denervation [30], quinidine slows the sinus rate, increases AV nodal conduction time, prolongs His-Purkinje conduction time and the QRS and QT intervals. The atrial and ventricular effective refractory periods also increase. Thus the effects on the sinus and AV nodes reflect the influence of the autonomic nervous system, whereas in the ventricles direct effects predominate. In patients with disease of the sinus or AV nodes, quinidine may exert a more pronounced di-

rect depressant effect leading to significant slowing of the sinus rate or an increase in AV conduction time.

On the other hand, quinidine produces a dose-dependent increase in QRS and QT duration as might be expected from its direct effects on electrical activity of single cardiac cell (it depresses $\dot{V}_{max}$ and prolongs action potential duration) which predominate over any influence it may have on the ventricles through its interactions with the autonomic nervous system. The increase in the QRS duration is sometimes useful for monitoring therapy. It is generally accepted that a 25% increase in QRS duration is a cause for concern and a 50% increase should prompt a reduction in dosage [31, 32]. Such severe slowing of conduction as reflected in the prolongation of the QRS might predispose to the occurrence of reentrant ventricular arrhythmias.

Effects on circulation

When administered intravenously quinidine decreases systemic vascular resistance, causes hypotension and depresses the contractile function of the heart. The hypotension is caused to a large extent by the blockade of the alpha-adrenergic receptors [27, 28] (although a direct vasodilator effect of quinidine might also contribute [33]). Therapeutic concentrations of orally administered quinidine generally have little or no effect on left ventricular performance [34, 35]. However quinidine does have a direct depressant effect on the contractility of ventricular muscle [16, 36] which may cause an increase in left ventricular end-diastolic pressure when the blood levels are high. The direct negative inotropic effect of quinidine may also contribute to the cardiovascular depression and collapse which sometimes results from intravenous administration of the drug [31].

Pharmacokinetics

Administration, absorption, and distribution

Quinidine is most commonly administered orally because of the risk of cardiovascular depression when it is given intravenously. Several preparations are available for oral administration. Quinidine sulfate has an absorption half-time of 30 min, is 80% bioavailable and peak plasma concentrations are reached within 1–2 hr after administration. Its half-time for elimination is then 4–6 hr. The usual oral dose schedule is 300–500 mg four times a day, and this results in therapeutic plasma levels (2–6 μg/ml) which reach a steady state within 24–48 hr. A single loading dose of 600–1000 mg will also produce therapeutic plasma levels [31, 37, 38]. The range of plasma levels needed for treatment of atrial arrhythmias such as fibrillation and flutter are often higher than those required for suppression of ventricular arrhythmias. Plasma quinidine levels much above 6 μg/ml are often associated with toxicity (see below). Quinidine is also available in the form of long-acting preparations such as quinidine polygalacturonate and quinidine gluconate. These preparations need to be administered at less frequent intervals (every 12 hr) than quinidine sulfate [37, 38]. After an oral dose of quinidine gluconate the peak plasma concentration is not reached until 3–4 hr. The delay in absorption is responsible for the long duration of action. Therapeutic levels might be maintained for an 8–10-hr period after a single dose [38].

Quinidine gluconate or lactate salt is the preparation used for intramuscular administration. Absorption is often erratic and incomplete. Moreover, the injection, itself, is painful and can be associated with skeletal muscle damage as evidenced by an accompanying increase in serum creatinine kinase [37].

Eighty percent of administered quinidine rapidly binds to plasma albumin and a significant amount enters erythocytes. Quinidine also binds rapidly to the lipoprotein of cell membranes and therefore distributes rapidly to the myocardium [39, 40]. High concentrations are attained in the heart (myocardium: plasma ratios reach 10:1 or greater [40]). The volume of distribution of quinidine is 2–4 liter/kg body weight [41].

Elimination

Quinidine is eliminated both by hepatic metabolism and by renal excretion. The major fraction of biotransformation and elimination occurs in the liver (50–90%) [37]. First pass metabolism of quinidine is not great as evidenced by the 70–80% bioavailability of oral quinidine [42]. Hydroxylation of quinidine is predominantly by the mixed function oxidases [43]. The products of hepatic metabolism, 3,5-3 hydroxyquinidine and 2′ oxoquinidinone have antiarrhythmic effects in experimental animals [44,

45] and, therefore, also might be antiarrhythmic in humans. These metabolites can be present in the serum in significant concentrations, particularly in those patients on long-term quinidine therapy and might contribute to the antiarrhythmic or toxic cardiac depressant effects [45].

A small percentage of quinidine (10–30%) is cleared by the kidney, mostly via active distal tubular secretion resulting in some unmetabolized quinidine in the urine [46]. Since quinidine is a weak base, its renal excretion shows pH-dependent elimination kinetics; the more alkaline the urine, the less quinidine in the ionized form and the more back diffusion in the distal nephron. Thus, in alkaline urine there may be a decrease in quinidine excretion by the kidney [46]. However, since only a small fraction of quinidine may be excreted by the kidney, the urine pH may only significantly affect quinidine plasma levels in the presence of high drug concentrations [47].

Heart failure [48] or renal failure [45] may decrease the rate of quinidine inactivation or elimination. Some studies have reported that there is only a minimal increase in the half-time for elimination in patients with heart failure or renal insufficiency whereas in others renal clearance was reduced and plasma quinidine concentrations increased [47]. Besides an increase in plasma quinidine concentration it can be predicted that, in patients with heart or renal failure, there may be an increase in the concentrations of quinidine metabolites which also are cardioactive. Severe hepatic failure also may slow the elimination of quinidine from the plasma. However it is uncertain whether this results from a decreased ability of the liver to metabolize quinidine or the marked increase in quinidine's volume of distribution which may occur in these patients [31, 47].

Toxicity

A significant number of patients (up to one-third) suffer from toxic effects of quinidine and therefore, despite the effectiveness of the drug in the treatment of arrhythmias, toxicity can limit its usefulness [31]. Gastrointestinal distress in the form of nausea, vomiting, diarrhea, and abdominal pain, which occurs in many patients immediately upon the initiation of therapy, may require discontinuation of the drug. In some patients this may be transitory. Extracardiac effects which may occur during chronic therapy include (a) cinchonism with tinnitus, hearing loss, visual disturbances, and confusion; in severe cases there may also be headache, diplopia, photophobia, altered color perception, delirium, or psychosis; (b) anaphylactic reactions (rarely); (c) thrombocytopenia as a result of interaction of quinidine with platelets and platelet antibody, causing lysis of the platelets (after cessation of drug administration, platelet counts usually return to normal within 7–10 days); (d) hypersensitivity to quinidine which may cause fever [31, 47].

Pharmacokinetic and pharmacodynamic interactions occur between quinidine and other pharmacological agents. Moreover, electrophysiologic interaction occurs between quinidine and plasma K^+: hypokalemia may decrease the electrophysiologic effects of quinidine responsible for its antiarrhythmic action whereas hyperkalemia may potentiate the electrophysiologic effects causing cardiac toxicity [12, 13, 31].

Of recent interest is the drug interaction between quinidine and digoxin. A large percentage of patients taking maintenance doses of digoxin and having stable serum digoxin levels who then are administered quinidine show an increase in their serum digoxin levels [49, 50]. The mechanism for the increase in digoxin levels has not been completely defined. There is evidence that quinidine may displace digoxin from tissue compartments, causing a decrease in digoxin's volume of distribution in some patients. The most prominent effect of quinidine on digoxin pharmacokinetics, however, is a 40–50% reduction of the renal clearance of digoxin after quinidine administration. The mechanism is not known [50]. There are also still some questions concerning the clinical significance of the quinidine–digoxin interaction. At least part of the rise in serum digoxin levels occurs because tissue levels, including those in the heart, fall [51]. Although it has been reported that as an accompaniment of the quinidine–digoxin interaction the therapeutic effects of digoxin on myocardial contractility may be enhanced, it also has been reported that contractility may be reduced because of the reduction in myocardial digoxin [50]. This problem requires much more study. The electrophysiological effects of digoxin may also be intensified; prolongation of the P–R interval, a slowing of the ventricular response to atrial fibrillation, the occurrence of nonparoxys-

mal AV junctional tachycardia and ventricular arrhythmias have all been reported after quinidine administration to patients receiving digoxin without prior adverse effects [49, 50]. It has been proposed that these electrophysiological effects are caused by an increased action of digoxin on the autonomic nerves to the heart, because in one experimental study digoxin concentration in the brain increased after quinidine, although it decreased in other tissues [51]. Nausea and vomiting may also occur because of the interaction between quinidine and digoxin [49]. In light of this interaction, serum digoxin levels should be obtained prior to and after administration of quinidine and the clinical course and electrocardiogram of the patients carefully monitored to determine if there is either a change in the therapeutic effects or the development of toxicity [50]. At the present time, it is uncertain whether quinidine interacts with other cardiac glycosides, such as digitoxin [50].

Significant interactions occur between quinidine and drugs which alter the activity of the liver enzymes which metabolize it. Of particular importance is the influence of anticonvulsant drugs such as phenytoin and phenobarbital which increase the rate of quinidine metabolism by inducing liver enzymes [52]. Thus standard therapeutic doses of quinidine might not result in therapeutic plasma levels when given at the same time as one of these anticonvulsant drugs, and discontinuation of an anticonvulsant drug during the course of quinidine therapy might cause a precipitous rise in quinidine plasma levels.

Administration of quinidine to patients taking oral anticoagulants such as warfarin may significantly increase prothrombin time and lead to hypoprothrombinemic hemorrhage [53]. Quinidine normally decreases prothrombic activity but this is of little clinical significance. The marked increase in prothrombin time occurring when quinidine is given with an anticoagulent may result from synergistic actions on vitamin K-dependent clotting factor synthesis [54].

Quinidine can increase the intensity and duration of neuromuscular blockade caused by muscle relaxants. This could be a serious drug interaction if quinidine is administered during recovery from anesthesia [54]. This effect is caused by interaction between quinidine and acetylcholine at the neuromuscular junction.

Another type of pharmacodynamic interaction may occur between quinidine and propranolol. Propranolol may markedly decrease liver blood flow and this effect may decrease the rate of quinidine metabolism, increasing quinidine plasma levels [54].

Procainamide

The use of procainamide resulted from studies by Mautz in 1936 which showed that the local anesthetic procaine increased the threshold to electrical stimulation of ventricular myocardium [55]. Because of this effect, procaine was applied locally to the epicardium during surgical procedures which required manipulation of the heart and pericardium such as the removal of shrapnel in soldiers during World War II. Procaine, however, was a dissapointment for intravenous therapy of arrhythmias because of its rapid hydrolysis by plasma esterases, resulting in a very short duration of action, and because of its prominent toxic effects on the central nervous system. An effort to find a longer acting drug with comparable antiarrhythmic action and less central nervous toxicity resulted in the synthesis of procainamide and its application to clinical cardiac therapy [56].

Effects on the heart and circulation

Electrophysiologic effects on cardiac cells

(A) Effects on resting membrane potential, action potential amplitude and phase 0 upstroke velocity ($\dot{V}_{max}$). Procainamide has electrophysiological effects on cardiac cells which are very similar to those of quinidine. In concentrations believed to be within the therapeutic range (to 10 mg/L), it does not affect resting or maximum diastolic potential of normal cardiac fibers but does decrease these at very high concentrations (> 30 mg/L). Therapeutic concentrations of procainamide decrease $\dot{V}_{max}$ and action potential amplitude of atrial, ventricular and Purkinje fibers in the absence of an effect on resting potential, and thus probably directly block Na^+ conductance; these effects are similar to those of other drugs with local anesthetic properties [3, 57–59]. More specific information on the way in which procainamide interacts with the Na^+ channel is not available; the mechanism of action has not yet been evaluated in terms of the modulated receptor hypothesis [7]. The decrease in $\dot{V}_{max}$ caused by procainamide is enhanced by elevating the extracellular potassium concentration [12, 13, 59]. Procainamide also shifts the threshold potential to less negative values so that more stimulus current is needed to initiate an active response from a normal level of membrane potential [60]. Because of the effects on active response and threshold potential, conduction velocity usually is decreased.

The effects of procainamide on action potentials of partially depolarized or abnormal fibers have not been characterized with any degree of detail, so it is not known what its effects are on depressed fast response or slow response action potentials. However, since procainamide does depress membrane responsiveness (decreases $\dot{V}_{max}$ over a wide range of membrane potentials), it probably also decreases the upstroke velocity of depressed fast responses [58]. It does not abolish slow response action potentials in diseased human atrial myocardium [61], but it does depress conduction in such tissues.

(B) Effects on action potential duration and refractoriness. Procainamide delays repolarization and prolongs the effective refractory period of atrial and ventricular muscle fibers. It has similar effects on canine Purkinje fibers [3, 57, 58] but shortens the action potential of sheep Purkinje fibers [21]. Its effects on the human ventricular specialized conducting system resemble its effects on the canine (see below). The increase in the refractory period caused by procainamide is greater than the prolongation in action potential duration suggesting that procainamide delays the removal of inactivation of the Na^+ channel which accompanies repolarization [3, 57, 58]. The mechanism for prolongation of action potential duration is not known. In the ventricular specialized conducting system, action potential duration and effective refractory periods of Purkinje fibers are increased more in regions where they are initially short than in regions where they are long, so that the differences associated with anatomical location are reduced [58].

(C) Effects on impulse initiation. Procainamide decreases the slope of phase 4 depolarization which is associated with normal automaticity in Purkinje fibers, and slows the rate of automatic firing [3, 57,

58]. The shift in threshold potential to less negative values might also decrease the automatic firing rate because threshold potential is moved farther from maximum diastolic potential [60]. In a study on sheep Purkinje fibers, procainamide did not decrease the pacemaker current as did lidocaine and quinidine. Therefore, it was proposed that the decrease in spontaneous activity induced by procainamide may be entirely due to a reduction of Na^+ current [21].

There is very little available information on how procainamide influences other forms of impulse initiation, such as abnormal automaticity, and early or delayed afterdepolarizations. A study of normal Purkinje fibers showed that triggered activity at low membrane potentials was suppressed by procainamide [62]. Another study of diseased and depolarized human atrium having slow response action potentials found that procainamide did not decrease automaticity of these fibers [61].

Electrophysiologic effects on the heart
Procainamide's effects on the electrical activity of the heart are very similar to those of quinidine. It may increase the sinus rate in some patients through an anticholinergic action, although therapeutic doses usually do not affect sinus rate. It does not appear to have the alpha-adrenergic blocking effect of quinidine [63] so reflex sympathetic discharge is not an important factor in acceleration of rate as it is for quinidine. It also has a weak blocking effect on impulse transmission through autonomic ganglia which may influence the heart rate [63]. Procainamide may depress sinus rate in patients with sinus node disease [64]. In therapeutic amounts it usually has little effect on the P–R interval. Conduction in the atrioventricular node often is unaltered, although occasionally it may be slowed slightly [64–66]. Conduction time through the His-Purkinje system is often slightly prolonged but this slowed conduction may not be noticeable at the paper speeds usually used to record the electrocardiogram [64–66]. The relative and effective refractory periods of the AV node may be unchanged or slightly prolonged, the refractory periods of the His-Purkinje system are usually lengthened [66]. Procainamide has the potential for causing AV conduction disturbances in patients with disease of the node or ventricular conducting system although this has not been a major therapeutic problem [64].

In therapeutic concentrations procainamide prolongs the QRS duration, ventricular refractory period, and QT interval [67, 68] because of its effect on the ventricular muscle action potential; it decreases $\dot{V}_{max}$ of phase 0 to slow conduction, slightly lengthens the time course for repolarization and prolongs the time for recovery of the fast inward Na^+ current from inactivation.

Effects on the circulation
The hemodynamic effects of procainamide are dependent on the dose and route of administration. When it is given intravenously it may depress blood pressure and myocardial contractility, especially if given rapidly [67, 69, 70]. During repeated intravenous injections in doses of 100 mg, at 5-min intervals, blood pressure usually begins to decrease significantly after a total dose of 600–800 mg. Vasodilatation contributing to the decline in blood pressure may result partly from ganglionic blockade [63]. In patients whose heart or circulation is compromised, decreases in cardiac output and blood pressure may occur at lower doses. Since procainamide decreases cardiac contractility, high blood levels may be associated with an increase in left ventricular end-diastolic pressure [31, 47].

Pharmacokinetics

Administration, absorption, and distribution
Procainamide can be administered intravenously or orally. When given intravenously, a regimen utilizing intermittent injections as described by Bigger et al., is far safer than a single bolus which may have a marked depressant effect on the heart and blood pressure [31, 67, 69, 70]. The intermittent injection schedule is as follows: 100 mg of procainamide is injected over a 1-min period, and this dose is repeated every 5 min until the arrhythmia is controlled. To reduce the likelihood of cardiovascular toxicity, the total dose for intravenous injection usually is not greater than 1 g. The 5-min dosing intervals permit measurement of the blood pressure and of electrocardiographic intervals.

Arrhythmias are usually abolished when plasma procainamide concentrations reach 4–10 μg/ml. Twenty percent of this procainamide is bound to plasma proteins [71].

Procainamide equilibrates rapidly in a large apparent volume of distribution of 1.5–2.5 L/kg. This rapid equilibration causes plasma levels to fall quickly, after single intravenous injections, with a half-time of 9 min [69, 70].

After the arrhythmia is controlled by intravenous injections, antiarrhythmic plasma levels can be maintained with a constant intravenous infusion at a rate of 20–80 μg/kg/min. This infusion can be started simultaneously with the first dose to eliminate the possible decline in plasma drug levels below the minimum effective concentration which would occur if infusion were not begun until after the last I.V. injection [67, 69].

Procainamide is also administered orally in a total daily dose of 1–6 g to initiate treatment of arrhythmias which do not require immediate termination or to continue long-term treatment after intravenous administration of procainamide or another antiarrhythmic drug. Bioavailability by this route is about 80% [71, 72]. After an oral dose, peak plasma levels and antiarrhythmic effects usually are attained within 1–2 hr and, with repeated oral doses, the plasma level attains its steady-state plateau value after 24–48 hr. Procainamide is absorbed mainly from the small intestine where pH is alkaline; delayed gastric emptying thus will slow absorption and both delay the peak plasma level and decrease its magnitude [73]. Absorption of an oral dose may be poor during the first week after myocardial infarction [74]. Procainamide has a relatively short overall elimination half-life of 2.5–4 hr in patients who have normal elimination of the drug. Thus plasma levels fall rapidly after peak levels are attained with each oral dose. A 3–4 hr dosing interval may, therefore, be required to maintain therapeutic plasma levels; if oral doses are given at intervals of 6 hr, the plasma level may vary from a value less than the minimum effective concentration, just before the dose, to a toxic concentration 1 hr after the dose. In many patients undergoing oral procainamide therapy the half-time for elimination may be long; i.e., 5–8 hr, for reasons described below and a 6-hr dosing interval is sufficient to maintain therapeutic levels [31].

If a steady plasma level of procainamide has been established by constant intravenous infusion and drug administration is changed to the oral route, the first oral dose should not be given until 4 hr after termination of infusion (one elimination half-time). This allows plasma levels to fall sufficiently so that toxic levels are not reached after the first oral dose [70].

Procainamide also can be administered intramuscularly, but this route usually is employed only for patients who are unable to take oral medication. Virtually 100% of an intramuscular dose is bioavailable and peak plasma levels occur earlier than after oral administration [31].

Elimination

Procainamide is eliminated both by hepatic metabolism and renal excretion [71, 72, 75]. Between 75 and 95% of a given dose is eliminated in the urine; 30–60% appears as unchanged procainamide and the remainder as metabolites. The major metabolite in humans is N-acetylprocainamide (NAPA) which is formed through the enzymatic activity of N-acetyltransferase [31, 71, 72]. In some individuals NAPA may represent more than 50% of the total drug in the plasma. NAPA then is excreted in the urine. Two other metabolites, as yet not identified, account for an additional 8–15% of a procainamide dose [71].

NAPA has significant electrophysiological effects on cardiac fibers which are unlike those of the parent compound; moreover, NAPA is also antiarrhythmic [76, 77]. Even very high concentrations of up to 240 mg/l, do not reduce the resting potential of atrial, ventricular or Purkinje fibers and do not decrease $\dot{V}_{max}$ of phase 0. The major effect of NAPA is to prolong the action potential duration and the effective refractory period, and this may cause early afterdepolarizations and triggered activity [76]. NAPA may also accelerate automatic firing of Purkinje fibers [76]. Thus, high levels of NAPA might result in arrhythmias by enhancing impulse initiation and this may be one cause of cardiotoxicity of procainamide. Therefore in relating antiarrhythmic or toxic effects of procainamide to plasma levels, it is necessary also to evaluate NAPA plasma levels.

The rate of acetylation of procainamide varies widely among individuals [78]. The elimination half-life may be markedly prolonged in patients who are slow acetylators. Impaired renal function, such as that caused by poor renal perfusion during heart failure or shock, can also markedly prolong procainamide's elimination half-life, resulting in significant increases in plasma levels [31, 72, 79, 80]. As renal function decreases, more procainamide is metabolized by the liver and a larger fraction of administered procainamide exists in the plasma as NA-

179

PA. NAPA levels also increase when renal function is decreased because this metabolite is normally cleared by the kidney. Both elevated levels of procainamide and NAPA may cause cardiotoxicity. The volumes of distribution (V_d) can decrease in cardiac failure or shock, also causing the plasma concentration to rise [31]. The rate of excretion of procainamide and NAPA may also be influenced by the pH of the urine. Since both are weak bases, in alkaline urine more drug is present in the uncharged form and can diffuse back into the plasma from renal tubular fluid, decreasing the rate of elimination [79].

Toxicity

Procainamide may have toxic effects on the cardiovascular system, causing sinus arrest, AV block, ventricular arrhythmias, and hypotension. These effects may occur when intravenous administration of the drug is too rapid, causing high plasma or myocardial drug levels, or when plasma levels during chronic therapy are too high [31, 70]. As mentioned previously, some of these toxic effects may also be caused by accumulation of NAPA.

Procainamide also has a number of significant extracardiac effects. Gastrointestinal irritation (anorexia, nausea, vomiting) can occur during chronic oral therapy, but the incidence is less severe than with quinidine. Depression, hallucinations, psychosis, and giddiness occasionally occur from the drug's action on the central nervous system [31]. Hypersensitivity reactions are the most frequent adverse effects of oral therapy [31]. These include fever and agranulocytosis, the occurrence of which may be cause for discontinuation of therapy.

Of real importance, during chronic drug administration, is the occurrence of a syndrome resembling systemic lupus erythematosis which is seen in as many as 40% of patients receiving chronic oral therapy [81]. Common symptoms and signs include arthralgias, fever, hepatomegaly, and pleural and pulmonary pathologies. Symptomatic patients show positive tests for antinuclear factor and lupus erythematosis cells [82]. Usually symptoms disappear soon after termination of therapy but positive tests for antinuclear factor and lupus erythematosus cells revert more slowly [31]. Moreover, positive tests for antinuclear factor and/or lupus erythematosus cells often are seen in patients with no other manifestations of the lupus syndrome. It has been proposed that patients who acetylate procainamide slowly are at increased risk for the occurrence of this syndrome but definitive evidence supporting this hypothesis is lacking [78].

Disopyramide

Disopyramide is a butyramide derivative (Figure 1). It was first synthesized in 1954 and has been used widely in Europe and South America since 1963 [83]. However, it has only been approved for use in the United States since 1978.

Effects on the heart and circulation

Electrophysiologic effects on cardiac cells

(A) Effects on resting membrane potential, action potential amplitude and phase 0 upstroke velocity ($\dot{V}_{max}$). The direct effects of disopyramide on cardiac fibers resemble the effects of quinidine or procainamide. Nontoxic doses produce a concentration-dependent decrease in $\dot{V}_{max}$ and action potential amplitude in atrial, ventricular, and Purkinje fibers while resting potential is not altered [84–87]. Very high concentrations also decrease the resting potential. The effect on $\dot{V}_{max}$ becomes greater as $[K^+]_0$ is increased [88]. Associated with the decreases in action potential amplitude and $\dot{V}_{max}$ is a decrease in conduction velocity. Membrane responsiveness is also decreased so that the $\dot{V}_{max}$ of premature impulses initiated during the repolarization phase of a preceding action potential is diminished by the drug. A greater decrease in $\dot{V}_{max}$ occurs in action potentials induced at low membrane potentials than at higher membrane potentials [88]. Because of this depressant effect on $\dot{V}_{max}$ at low resting potentials, disopyramide reduces upstroke velocity of Purkinje fibers with depressed fast response action potentials surviving on the endocardial surface of infarcts [89]. Disopyramide does not decrease $\dot{V}_{max}$ or action potential amplitude of slow responses in Purkinje fibers [87].

(B) Effects on action potential duration and refractoriness. Disopyramide's direct effect results in a prolongation of the action potential duration and effective refractory period [84–87]. This effect oc-

curs in atrial, ventricular, and Purkinje fibers. The refractory period is usually prolonged to a similar extent as the duration of the action potential. In the Purkinje system action potential durations and refractory periods are prolonged more in regions where they are short than in regions where they are normally long or abnormally long because of pathology such as myocardial infarction [89]. These effects of disopyramide may be modified by its powerful anticholinergic actions [84]. This indirect effect should tend to further increase action potential duration and refractoriness in the atrium and may also influence the effects of disopyramide on the ventricle [84].

(C) Effects on impulse initiation. Disopyramide decreases the spontaneous firing rate of Purkinje fibers with normal automaticity by decreasing the rate of phase 4 depolarization [87]. Its effects on other types of impulse initiation have not yet been reported.

Electrophysiologic effects on the heart
Disopyramide has significant anticholinergic effects and these may modify its direct actions on the electrophysiology of the heart [83]. Disopyramide usually causes little change in sinus rate. However in patients pretreated with atropine, sinus rate markedly decreases, reflecting a direct depressant effect of disopyramide on phase 4 depolarization of sinus node cells [90]. When the vagus is functioning, the anticholinergic effect overcomes this direct depressant effect. The direct depressant effect can be particularly prominent in patients with sinus node disease, even in the presence of functioning vagus nerves [91, 92].

Disopyramide also has little effect on the P–R interval and does not consistently alter conduction and refractoriness in the AV node [93, 94]. The lack of effect results because the anticholinergic action nullifies the direct depressant actions of disopyramide on AV nodal conduction and refractoriness. These depressant effects become apparent when the drug is given in the presence of atropine [95]. Disopyramide consistently increases atrial refractoriness which may be the combined result of its direct electrophysiological effect and its anticholinergic effect [95]. It also increases refractoriness of accessory AV pathways [96]. Patients with AV conduction system disease may develop AV block after disopyramide administration.

His-Purkinje conduction (H–V interval of the His bundle electrogram) is not usually altered by disopyramide [93, 94] despite the experimental results showing that it decreases $\dot{V}_{max}$ of phase 0 of Purkinje fibers [86, 87, 97]. The QRS duration may be increased up to 20% because conduction in ventricular muscle is depressed. QT duration is also prolonged, reflecting the prolongation of action potential duration [93, 94]. The effective refractory period of the ventricle is also increased.

Effects on the circulation
Disopyramide can exert profound hemodynamic effects. It has a significant negative inotropic effect, the extent of which depends on the dose given, the route of administration and the status of ventricular function [98]. It can decrease left ventricular dP/dt max and ejection fraction even in patients with normal ventricular function, but these effects are more pronounced in patients with preexisting ventricular failure [99]. In patients with coronary artery disease or recent myocardial infarction left ventricular end-diastolic pressure and heart size may be increased. In some cases congestive heart failure has been precipitated [100, 101]. Disopyramide may also cause vasoconstriction of peripheral arterioles and coronary arteries, reducing blood flow [102]. Arterial pressure may increase. This may result from a direct effect on vascular smooth muscle [103].

Pharmacokinetics

Administration, absorption, and distribution
The usual oral dosage schedule for disopyramide is 150 mg, four times a day. Loading doses of 300–400 mg rapidly produce therapeutic plasma levels [31]. Nearly 90% of an oral dose is absorbed and bioavailability is high. Only a small amount of the drug is subjected to first pass hepatic metabolism [104]. The normal therapeutic plasma concentration range is 3–8 μg/ml [31] of which 30% is protein bound [105]. However, the amount of protein bound drug is proportional to the plasma concentration [106]. The apparent volume of distribution is about 1 liter/kg body weight [107].

Elimination
Disopyramide is eliminated both by hepatic metabolism (11–37%) and by renal excretion of the

unmetabolized drug (36–77%) [108]. In the liver disopyramide is N-dealkylated to form N-deisopropyldisopyramide plus other as yet uncharacterized metabolites [109]. The N-dealkylated metabolite has antiarrhythmic and anticholinergic activity [110, 111]. Drugs such as phenobarbital and phenytoin, which induce hepatic enzymes, increase the rate of disopyramide metabolism in rats [112], but this drug interaction has not been demonstrated in humans. Disopyramide metabolites are cleared by the kidney.

Unmetabolized disopyramide is also excreted by the kidney. It is filtered by the glomeruli, and the rate of renal clearance is related to the amount of drug which is free and not bound to plasma proteins. Since the fraction of disopyramide that is free increases with an increase in total drug concentration, elimination kinetics in the kidney can be nonlinear. The overall half-time for elimination of disopyramide is 6–9 hr [31].

The renal clearance of disopyramide and its metabolites is largely independent of urine pH and flow rate [113]. Nevertheless, in patients with renal insufficiency the rate of renal elimination is markedly prolonged [114]. Both disopyramide and N-deisopropyldisopyramide may accumulate in the body in this situation. There is also incomplete absorption and reduced clearance of disopyramide in patients with myocardial infarction [115–117].

Toxicity

Cardiovascular toxicity is not common in patients with relatively normal hearts. However, in patients with diseased sinus nodes or AV conducting systems or with heart failure, disopyramide can have marked adverse effects which we have already described.

Oral disopyramide generally is well tolerated; adverse gastrointestinal effects occur less frequently than with quinidine, requiring discontinuation of therapy in 10–40% of patients on chronic oral therapy. Other common adverse effects caused by the drug's anticholinergic actions are acute glaucoma and urinary retention, particularly in the elderly [31].

Lidocaine

The local anesthetic, lidocaine, was synthesized by Lofgren in 1946 as part of an effort to make an agent with a longer duration of action than procaine [118]. Lidocaine is a tertiary amine with an amide linkage to an aromatic residue (Figure 1). Southworth and associates [119] first used it as an antiarrhythmic to prevent ventricular arrhythmias in the cardiac catheterization laboratory. During the past 20 years, the drug has been widely used for the emergency treatment of ventricular arrhythmias, since it can be rapidly administered intravenously, readily attains antiarrhythmic plasma levels, and is rapidly metabolized and excreted. These characteristics are ideal for a drug used for short-term management of life-threatening ventricular arrhythmias.

Effects on the heart and circulation

(A) Effects on resting membrane potential, action potential amplitude and phase 0 upstroke velocity ($\dot{V}_{max}$). Lidocaine has no effect on resting or maximum diastolic potential of atrial, ventricular, and Purkinje fibers, and only a small depressant effect on $\dot{V}_{max}$ of phase 0 in concentrations which are within the therapeutic range (2–5 μg/ml) [120–122]. The decrease in $\dot{V}_{max}$ at these concentrations is not usually sufficient to slow conduction significantly. Above concentrations of 10 μg/ml, depression of $\dot{V}_{max}$ becomes more marked and at very high concentrations (> 30 μg/ml) resting potential is also reduced.

The effect of lidocaine on the $\dot{V}_{max}$ of phase 0 results from an interaction of the charged drug molecule with the fast Na^+ channel, thereby blocking the channel [123–125]. This effect on the Na^+ channel is influenced by the K^+ concentration in the extracellular environment [126–129], the resting membrane potential [6, 7, 129], and the rate of stimulation [7, 130]. Block of Na conductance and depression of $\dot{V}_{max}$ by lidocaine in ventricular muscle and Purkinje fibers show use-dependent characteristics [7, 131, 132]. At normal levels of resting membrane potential, a decrease in $\dot{V}_{max}$ is not apparent at slow rates of stimulation (< 1 Hz) but $\dot{V}_{max}$ decreases rapidly (over 3–5 beats) at more rapid rates of stimulation until a steady state is achieved. $\dot{V}_{max}$ will recover quickly during a subsequent quiescent period. It is believed that lidocaine interacts with the Na^+ channel when it is in an open state and dissociates from the channel most rapidly when it is in the resting state, at the time membrane potential has returned to the maximum diastolic level. Because of the rapid dissociation at the maximum diastolic potential, Na^+ conductance blockade by lidocaine at normal levels of resting membrane potential and at normal rates is not great. However, the magnitude of depression of $\dot{V}_{max}$ is increased significantly by a reduction in membrane potential because lidocaine has an increased affinity for the inactivated Na^+ channel at depolarized levels of membrane potential, and depolarization causes a larger percentage of the channels to exist in the inactivated state [7, 132]. Lidocaine's depressant effect on Na^+ conductance and $\dot{V}_{max}$ is increased by increasing $[K^+]_0$ above 4 mM [126, 127, 133] because increasing $[K^+]_0$ reduces resting membrane potential; whereas at $[K^+]_0$ levels below 4 mM lidocaine may have no noticeable effects on $\dot{V}_{max}$ [120, 121] because of the high resting membrane potential. Lidocaine's depressant effect on $\dot{V}_{max}$ also is enhanced by decreasing pH because at low pH a greater fraction of the molecule exists in the charged, active form [11, 134]. Lidocaine apparently has minimal effects on the threshold potential.

Because its effects on Na^+ conductance and $\dot{V}_{max}$ are enhanced at low membrane potentials, lidocaine markedly depresses or blocks conduction in fibers with depressed fast response action potentials [6, 133, 135]. The enhancement of lidocaine potency both by depolarization and by a decrease in pH, therefore, may cause conduction block in ischemic regions of the heart, where $[K^+]_0$ is elevated, and resting membrane potential and pH are low. Therapeutic concentrations of lidocaine do not depress the upstroke of slow response action potentials in Purkinje fibers, in high K^+, catecholamine-containing superfusate [134], but very high concentrations of lidocaine (> 30 $\mu g/ml$) will depress slow responses [136].

(B) Effects on action potential duration and refractoriness. Lidocaine shortens the action potential duration and effective refractory period of Purkinje fibers which have normal levels of membrane potential [120, 121]. The magnitude of this effect is not uniform but varies within the specialized conducting system. Lidocaine causes the greatest shortening of action potential duration in normal Purkinje fibers in which duration is the longest [137]. The available experimental data suggest that this short-

ening of duration results from an increase in net outward current in the plateau range of membrane potentials which appears not to be caused by an increase in K^+ conductance [19]. Since lidocaine fails to increase net outward current in the presence of high concentrations of TTX, it has been proposed that lidocaine's principal action is to block the inward Na^+ current that flows during the plateau through the fraction of excitatory Na^+ channels that remain open at this time [19, 21]. Lidocaine in therapeutic concentrations has no effect on action potential duration of ventricular muscle fibers and of atrial fibers [120, 122].

Although the decrease of the action potential duration caused by lidocaine in Purkinje fibers is accompanied by a shortening of the effective refractory period, the effective refractory period does not decrease as much as the action potential [120, 121]. Lidocaine delays reactivation of the fast Na channel [123–125] in ventricular muscle. The drug-associated inactivated channels behave as if the transmembrane potential is decreased by 30–40 mV and therefore recovery is slowed. As a result of lidocaine administration the earliest conducted premature responses in Purkinje fibers arise at more negative levels of membrane potential than the earliest premature impulses elicited before drug action. Under circumstances in which lidocaine does not have much depressant effect on steady-state $\dot{V}_{max}$ (such as at slow stimulation rates or at $[K^+]_0 \leqslant 4$ mM) the earliest premature responses after lidocaine may have a higher $\dot{V}_{max}$ and conduct at a more rapid velocity than the earliest responses before drug, because they arise at a higher membrane potential. Therapeutic concentrations of lidocaine have little effect on the effective refractory period of normal ventricular or atrial muscle [6, 120, 122].

Lidocaine may prolong the effective refractory period of partially depolarized ventricular muscle or Purkinje fibers with depressed fast response action potentials. The effects of the drug on action potential duration of these cells is not prominent and normally refractoriness outlasts complete repolarization [138]. Lidocaine probably increases the refractory period because it dissociates less readily from the inactivated Na^+ channel than from the resting Na^+ channel, and since a larger fraction of the Na^+ channels remain in the inactivated state in partially depolarized fibers, lidocaine effects are more pronounced than in normally polarized fibers [6, 7].

183

(C) Effects on impulse initiation. Lidocaine, in concentrations of 1–10 μg/ml, decreases the slope of spontaneous diastolic depolarization in normally polarized Purkinje fibers and slows the automatic firing rate [120, 121]. These concentrations exert no effect on automaticity of sinus node cells [122]. The decrease in slope of spontaneous diastolic depolarization in Purkinje fibers results from a decrease in pacemaker current caused by lidocaine [21]. Lidocaine only decreases very slightly the automatic firing of Purkinje and ventricular muscle fibers which occurs at low levels of membrane potential caused by long-maintained depolarizing current pulses [139–141]. However, lidocaine does stop automatic firing of Purkinje fibers at the low level of membrane potential when it can shift membrane potential to the high level by decreasing the TTX sensitive background Na^- current [142].

Lidocaine may abolish early afterdepolarizations associated with a prolonged time course of repolarization in Purkinje fibers by accelerating repolarization [62]. It does not affect delayed after depolarizations in diseased human atrial fibers [143] but does depress those afterdepolarizations caused by digitalis toxicity in Purkinje fibers [144].

Electrophysiologic effects on the heart
Lidocaine has little effect on sinus rate or on the electrophysiological properties of the atria [122]. It does not alter the action potentials of normal sinus node cells in therapeutic concentrations and, unlike other antiarrhythmic agents such as quinidine and procainamide, there appears to be little if any modification of autonomic tone by lidocaine. However lidocaine does have a depressant effect on sinus node function in some patients with sinus node disease, in whom it may cause sinus bradycardia or sinus arrest [145–148]. The diseased or abnormal sinus node therefore seems to be more sensitive than the normal node to depressant effects of this drug. Lidocaine, even in toxic concentrations, does not alter atrial conduction or the P wave but may slightly decrease the atrial effective refractory period [149].

At therapeutic plasma concentrations lidocaine has little effect on the electrocardiographic P–R interval and on the A–H interval (a measurement of AV nodal conduction) of the His bundle electrogram [150]. Usually His-Purkinje conduction (H–V interval) is not altered, consistent with the minimal effects of lidocaine on $\dot{V}_{max}$ of phase 0 of normal Purkinje fibers [120, 121]. Lidocaine has a variable effect on AV nodal refractoriness. Although pooled data indicate no effect on the AV nodal effective refractory period, in some individual cases there is significant shortening whereas in others refractoriness is slightly prolonged [151]. Lidocaine consistently shortens the effective refractory period of the His-Purkinje system as determined in studies using His bundle recordings and premature atrial stimulation [151]. This probably results from the shortening of the Purkinje fiber action potential duration by lidocaine. Despite these seemingly minor effects of lidocaine on conduction in the normal AV conducting system, instances of heart block caused by lidocaine administration have been reported in patients with an abnormal AV conducting system [151]; block may occur either in the AV node or distal to it. Therefore lidocaine may seriously impair conduction in the presence of an already diseased conducting system. Block in the diseased conducting system caused by lidocaine may be related to its enhanced depressant effect on $\dot{V}_{max}$ of Purkinje fibers with low resting potentials [133, 135, 152, 153]. Such Purkinje fibers with low resting potentials and $\dot{V}_{max}$ may be the cause of the initial conduction disturbances.

Lidocaine, even in toxic concentrations, does not affect conduction or refractoriness of normal ventricular muscle just as it does not significantly alter the ventricular muscle action potential [120, 121]. Therefore the QRS complex of the electrocardiogram is not changed [154]. However lidocaine does depress conduction in ischemic myocardium [155, 156]. Lidocaine also increases the ventricular fibrillation threshold of the ventricle [157].

Effects on the circulation
Intravenous lidocaine has not generally been associated with depressant effects on myocardial contractility or arterial blood pressure. It can depress blood pressure and contractility in patients with left ventricular function that is already depressed [158, 159].

Pharmacokinetics

Administration, absorption, and distribution
Lidocaine is usually administered intravenously because of the emergency clinical situations in which

it is used and its poor bioavailability when given orally. The effective plasma concentration is in the range of 2–5 μg/ml, although occasionally concentrations up to 8–10 μg/ml have antiarrhythmic effects without severe toxic effects [160]. About 30% of lidocaine is bound to plasma albumin. A single injection of 1–2 mg/kg body weight will achieve a therapeutic plasma concentration rapidly. If cardiac output is good, this dose initially will result in a concentration in the blood of greater than 30 μg/ml. This immediately begins to fall as the circulating drug enters and equilibrates with well-perfused tissues such as the kidneys, lungs, liver, and heart. Lidocaine also has a high affinity for fat [161]. The half-time for this initial redistribution phase is about 8 min [162, 163]. If a second dose is not given, as plasma lidocaine levels fall, the diffusion gradient from tissue to blood increases and the lidocaine which initially entered the well-perfused tissues diffuses back into the blood and is metabolized by the liver. The half-time for this second metabolic phase is approximately 108 min [162, 163]. An infusion of 20–50 μg/kg/min of lidocaine will usually maintain antiarrhythmic plasma levels for prolonged periods following a single intravenous injection.

Intramuscular lidocaine is almost completely bioavailable when administered into muscles with high blood flow such as the deltoid. This mode of administration, however, is infrequently used [31].

Only 35% of an oral dose of lidocaine is bioavailable because of the rapid first pass metabolism by the liver (50% may be cleared before the drug enters the systemic circulation) [163, 164]. Hence, oral doses as high as 250 mg do not produce therapeutic plasma levels [162]. In general, plasma levels are so unpredictable after oral administration as to contraindicate lidocaine's routine clinical use by this route.

Elimination

Most of the administered lidocaine is metabolized by the mixed function oxidases of the liver; less than 10% is excreted unmetabolized [165, 166]. Lidocaine is first de-ethylated to form N-ethyl or monethylglycylxylidide which is then cleaved to form xylidine and N-ethylglycine [167]. These metabolic products are excreted in the urine. Monethylglycylxylidide may have some antiarrhythmic properties [168], and it has been suggested that it

contributes to lidocaine's toxic effects on the central nervous system [169].

The clearance of lidocaine by the liver is very high and almost equal to hepatic blood flow [161, 164, 170–172]. Therefore any changes in blood flow markedly influence lidocaine's rate of metabolism. As might be expected for a drug so dependent on hepatic metabolism for its degradation, in instances of heart failure [173] or liver disease [174], the plasma clearance is reduced. For example, in some patients with myocardial infarction the half-life is prolonged to up to 4 hr [175]. Elderly patients who may have reduced hepatic blood flow also metabolize lidocaine more slowly than younger individuals [170]. The possibility also exists for drug interactions when lidocaine is given with another drug that alters liver blood flow. The decreased liver blood flow caused by propranolol can lead to a reduced clearance of lidocaine and increased serum levels [176]. Hence these clinical situations warrant a decrease in the rate of lidocaine infusion and total dose to avoid drug toxicity. Renal disease does not alter lidocaine elimination kinetics, but lidocaine metabolites may accumulate, causing central nervous system toxicity [174, 177]. Prolonged infusions of lidocaine can increase liver blood flow [178] and therefore can modify the clearance of lidocaine in patients [179].

Toxicity

In spite of its widespread use only a small percentage of patients receiving lidocaine show adverse reactions and usually these are relatively mild [180]. Cardiac toxicity (sinus bradycardia, AV block, depressed cardiac contractility) is relatively uncommon (see above), whereas central nervous system toxicity is the most common adverse reaction. Neurological side effects are related to the lidocaine plasma concentrations. In general a plasma concentration of around 5 μg/ml may cause dizziness, drowsiness, paresthesias, and euphoria; 10 μg/ml may cause speech disturbances, confusion, excitement, nausea, and vomiting; and higher concentrations may cause respiratory depression and seizures [181].

185

Tocainide

Removal of the two ethyl groups from the lidocaine molecule has resulted in the antiarrhythmic drug tocainide (Figure 1). Tocainide has a spectrum of antiarrhythmic efficacy similar to that of lidocaine but, unlike lidocaine, is highly effective via the oral route. This drug is now undergoing clinical investigation in the United States.

Effects on the heart and circulation

Electrophysiologic effects on cardiac cells

(A) Effects on resting membrane potential, action potential amplitude and phase 0 upstroke velocity $\dot{V}_{max}$. Tocainide and lidocaine have qualitatively the same effects on the cardiac resting and action potential. The effects of tocainide on the upstroke of the action potential are influenced by $[K^+]_0$. At low $[K^+]_0 (\leqslant 3 \text{ mM})$ even relatively high concentrations have little effect on resting membrane potential, $\dot{V}_{max}$ of phase 0 and action potential amplitude. Tocainide at therapeutic concentrations does depress $\dot{V}_{max}$ and action potential amplitude, without altering resting potential, when $[K^+]_0$ is 4 mM or greater. This depressant effect is further increased when $[K^+]_0$ itself is high enough to decrease resting membrane potential [182–184]. Although the effects of tocainide on abnormal action potentials have not been studied, because of its similarity to lidocaine, it is expected to have significant depressant effects on $\dot{V}_{max}$ of depressed fast response action potentials and little effect on slow responses.

(B) Effects on action potential duration, refractoriness, and impulse initiation. Tocainide decreases action potential duration and the effective refractory period of Purkinje fibers. It also depresses normal automatic activity of Purkinje fibers [183].

Electrophysiologic effects on the heart
Tocainide's direct electrophysiological effects resemble those of lidocaine just as its actions on cardiac transmembrane potentials are also similar to those of lidocaine. It has little or no effect on heart rate or refractory periods of the atria, AV conducting system or ventricular muscle [185, 186]. In some instances prolongation of AV nodal conduction time has been associated with termination of supra-

ventricular tachycardia but slowing of AV conduction is not a consistent drug effect. The QRS duration is not altered by tocainide but the QT interval may be slightly decreased [185]. The effects of tocainide on the function of the diseased sinus node or AV conducting system have not been described but might be expected to be similar to those of lidocaine.

Effects on the circulation
Myocardial depression does not usually occur in patients receiving oral tocainide or after intravenous infusion of tocainide, even in the presence of heart disease [187–189]. Intravenous infusion of tocainide can cause a small increase in mean arterial pressure which is probably due to an increase in systemic vascular resistance [188, 189].

Pharmacokinetics

Administration, absorption, and distribution
An oral dose of tocainide is absorbed rapidly from the stomach and peak plasma levels are attained after 30 min–4 hr. Bioavailability is nearly 100% [190], since, unlike lidocaine, there is very little metabolism during the first pass through the liver. About 50% of the drug is bound to plasma proteins [190]. The antiarrhythmic plasma levels are 6–12 μg/ml [191].

Elimination
About 50–60% of a tocainide dose is metabolized by the liver and the rest is excreted unchanged by the kidney. The half-time for elimination is 12–15 hr [190]. Tocainide is metabolized to carbamic acid and then glucuronidated [192, 193]. Animal experiments have shown dose-dependent metabolism at high drug concentrations indicating the presence of a saturable metabolic process [194]. However it is not known whether this applies to humans.

Renal excretion of tocainide and its metabolite is influenced by urine pH; in an alkaline urine, excretion is reduced [190]. There are no studies as yet on the influence of renal disease on the rate of renal elimination of the drug. The pharmacokinetics of tocainide in patients with and without acute myocardial infarction are similar, unlike that of lidocaine [195].

Toxicity

Generally, long-term studies have shown that tocainide is well tolerated and there are few adverse or toxic reactions. Patients may experience gastrointestinal side effects including nausea, anorexia, abdominal pain, constipation, and vomiting. High plasma levels (10–15 $\mu g/ml$) can exert toxic effects on the central nervous system which are similar to those of lidocaine [191]. Some data have suggested that tocainide can induce lupus-like phenomena, including antinuclear antibody titers [182], arthritis, and nonmembraneous glomerulonephritis [191].

Encainide

Encainide structurally resembles procainamide; it is 4-methoxy-2'[2-(1-methyl-2 peperidyl)-ethyl] benzanilide [196] (Figure 1). The drug is currently undergoing clinical trials in the United States [197–200] and Europe [201].

Effects on the heart and circulation

Electrophysiologic effects on cardiac cells

(A) Effects on resting membrane potential, action potential amplitude and phase 0 upstroke velocity $\dot{V}_{max}$. Encainide has no effect on the resting potential of Purkinje fibers but decreases $\dot{V}_{max}$ of phase 0 and conduction velocity [196, 202]. The membrane response curve is also depressed [202]. Similar effects are exerted on ventricular muscle cells [202]. Encainide has no effect on slow response action potentials caused by superfusing Purkinje fibers with a high $[K^+]$ superfusate containing catecholamines [202].

(B) Effects on action potential duration and refractoriness. Encainide shortens the duration of the Purkinje fiber action potential. The effective refractory period is shortened to a lesser extent [196, 202]. It has no significant effect on action potential duration of ventricular muscle.

(C) Impulse initiation. A high concentration of encainide reduces the slope of phase 4 depolarization and decreases the spontaneous rate of Purkinje fibers with high maximum diastolic potentials or of partially depolarized fibers [196]. Its effects on afterdepolarizations and triggered activity have not been described.

Electrophysiologic effects on the heart

When encainide is given intravenously, it has no effect on sinus rate or AV nodal conduction time (A–H interval on the His bundle electrogram), but the QRS, the QT intervals on the electrocardiogram, and the H–V interval on the His bundle electrogram are prolonged. Intravenous encainide has no significant effect on atrial, AV nodal or ventricular refractoriness [203, 204]. During oral encainide administration for more than 72 hr conduction in both the AV node and His-Purkinje system is slowed, and atrial and ventricular effective refractory periods are prolonged [197]. The effective refractory period of accessory atrioventricular conducting pathways is also prolonged [197]. The differences in electrophysiological effects of intravenous and oral drug may result from the occurrence of significant amounts of metabolite which have electrophysiologic effects on the heart, during oral administration (see below).

Effects on the circulation

There are no detailed studies on the effects of encainide on the circulation. One clinical report indicates that intravenous encainide in therapeutic dosages does not influence the blood pressure [204]. No effect of encainide has been detected on the mean ejection fraction of hearts in patients with cardiac disease [198].

Pharmacokinetics

After oral administration encainide is rapidly absorbed from the intestine and peak plasma levels are reached in 1.5–3 hr [199]. Encainide then undergoes a large first pass metabolism in the liver. Two of the metabolites formed, the o-demethylated and the three methoxy 4-hydroxy derivatives, both have significant electrophysiological effects on heart muscle; they decrease $\dot{V}_{max}$ and shorten the action potential duration of Purkinje fibers, and therefore the metabolites may have antiarrhythmic or toxic effects [202]. Significant plasma levels of the o-demethylated metabolite occur within 2–3 hr [198]. Although in most patients, encainide is rapidly metabolized by the liver resulting in a half-time for disposition of 0.5–4 hr, in 5–10% of patients; liver metabolism of encainide is very slow, resulting in a half-time of 7–22 hr [205]. In these patients significant amounts of the major metabolites are not formed. This inability of the liver to metabolize encainide may be determined genetically [206]. Because of the large variation in plasma levels of encainide which can occur because of different rates of liver metabolism, it is often difficult to find the correct antiarrhythmic dosage schedule.

Toxicity

Blurred vision, dizziness, and postural hypotension have been side effects noted in patients taking encainide [198, 199, 204]. Transient side effects, such as ataxia and diplopia, have been associated with a range of plasma concentrations from 135 to 570 ng/ml [198].

Mexiletine

Mexiletine is a congener of lidocaine, and it was originally developed as an anticonvulsant [207]. It is a primary amine and the ester of 2,6 dimethylphenol (Figure 1). Mexiletine was first used as an antiarrhythmic drug in 1969 and is approved for clinical use in Europe. It is undergoing clinical trials and study in the United States.

Effects on the heart and circulation

Electrophysiologic effects on cardiac cells

(A) Effects on resting membrane potential, action potential amplitude, and phase 0 upstroke velocity $\dot{V}_{max}$). Mexiletine has electrophysiological effects which are similar to those of lidocaine. It has no effect on the resting potential of atrial, ventricular and Purkinje fibers over a wide range of concentrations which most likely encompass the therapeutic range, but it decreases $\dot{V}_{max}$ of phase 0 and action potential amplitude [208–211]. The decrease in $\dot{V}_{max}$ at normal levels of resting potential is associated with a decrease in conduction velocity. Membrane responsiveness is also decreased, and, with this, conduction velocity of premature impulses is slowed. These effects of mexiletine may result

from a similar blocking action on the fast Na^+ channel as described for lidocaine.

Although the effects of mexiletine on abnormal action potentials have not been studied, because of its similarity to lidocaine, it is expected to have significant depressant effects on $\dot{V}_{max}$ of depressed fast response action potentials. It does not affect slow responses resulting from exposure of ventricular muscle to a high K^+ superfusate containing catecholamines [212].

(B) Effects on action potential duration and refractoriness. Mexiletine, like lidocaine, has almost no effect on atrial action potential duration and refractoriness [208, 209] but shortens the action potential duration and effective refractory period of Purkinje fibers [213]. The greatest amount of shortening occurs in Purkinje fibers which have the longest initial action potential durations [213]. The effective refractory period is decreased less than the action potential duration. Although the effects of mexiletine on transmembrane potentials of ventricular muscle have not been studied, it does not have any noticeable effect on the time course for repolarization of monophasic action potentials recorded from the right ventricle of human subjects. It also does not influence the effective refractory period of human ventricular muscle [214].

(C) Effects on impulse initiation. Mexiletine decreases the automatic firing rate of Purkinje fibers at normal levels of membrane potential [210, 211]. It exerts little or no effect on the slope of phase 4 depolarization but shifts the threshold voltage to less negative levels [210]. Mexiletine also suppresses normal automaticity in Purkinje fibers [210]. Digitalis-induced abnormal automaticity occurring at low levels of membrane potential and triggered activity caused by delayed afterpolarizations are both suppressed by mexiletine [210].

Electrophysiologic effects on the heart
Mexiletine does not exert effects on the heart through interactions with the autonomic nervous system [215]. When administered intravenously it has had no consistent effect on sinus rate or sinus node recovery time, even in patients with the sick sinus syndrome [216, 217]. In vitro electrophysiological studies of sinus node action potentials have also shown no effect of mexiletine [208, 209]. Mex-

188

iletine has no effect on atrial conduction or refractoriness at normal heart rates. Since it has been found to decrease the rate of phase 0 depolarization of rabbit atrial fibers it might be expected that large doses of mexiletine might depress atrial conduction [209].

The results of electrophysiological studies indicate that mexiletine may increase AV nodal conduction time on occasion [216]. Mexiletine also does not usually affect conduction in the His-Purkinje system; the H–V interval of the His bundle electrogram most often is unchanged [216]. However, instances of H–V interval prolongation by mexiletine have been reported [216]. Mexiletine consistently increases the relative and effective refractory period of the His-Purkinje system in humans, and this effect is more marked in the presence of conduction disturbances [216, 217]. This result of clinical electrophysiological studies is contrary to the effects of mexiletine on the transmembrane potentials of isolated preparations of canine cardiac Purkinje fibers: $\dot{V}_{max}$ of phase 0 is reduced [210, 211] providing the bases for prolongation in the H–V interval which sometimes occurs, but the action potential duration and the effective refractory periods of Purkinje fibers are decreased [213].

Mexiletine does not prolong the QRS duration nor does it alter the refractory period of ventricular muscle [217].

Effects on the circulation

In clinical trials, intravenous mexiletine given to patients with a history of myocardial infarction depressed cardiac contractility and caused a decrease in the mean arterial pressure [218–220]. A decrease in contractility was particularly marked in patients with depressed cardiac function. Since a major use of mexiletine may be for the prophylactic treatment of ventricular arrhythmias in patients with ischemic heart disease, its effect on cardiac function requires further examination during chronic oral administration.

Pharmacokinetics

Administration, absorption, and distribution
Mexiletine, when administered orally, is almost completely absorbed from the gastrointestinal tract [221]. Since it is almost 100% ionized at gastric pH, the major portion of absorption occurs in the small

intestine. The bioavailability of an oral dose is nearly 90%, since less than 10% is metabolized during the first pass through the liver [221]. The absorption kinetics of mexiletine are slowed in patients in whom gastric emptying is retarded [221]. This might occur in patients with acute myocardial infarction receiving atropine or morphine.

When mexiletine is given intravenously as a bolus injection, its disposition kinetics are similar to those of lidocaine. The plasma concentration falls in a biexponential manner; the initial rapid decline (half-time equals 26 min) [221] occurs as the drug in the blood rapidly equilibrates with the highly perfused tissues. The secondary decline (half-time ranges from 3 to 8 hr) [222] results from elimination by hepatic metabolism and renal excretion. The total half-life for elimination of mexiletine is about 12 hr in normal healthy subjects [223] but can increase in patients with myocardial infarction [224].

Mexiletine is highly bound to plasma proteins [225]. The therapeutic plasma concentration is 1–2 μg/ml [225].

Elimination
Approximately 92% of mexiletine in the body is metabolized by the liver, and the rest is excreted unchanged by the kidneys. Metabolism involves oxidation and reduction of the parent compound, resulting in the metabolites hydromethylmexiletine, parahydroxymexiletine, and their alcohols which are then excreted by the kidneys [225]. Reduction of hepatic blood flow or liver metabolic function, such as in patients with myocardial infarction or in elderly patients, would be expected to prolong the half-life for elimination and possibly cause toxicity. The pKas of mexiletine and its metabolites range from 7.5 to 10.5, and the renal clearance of these compounds is influenced by the urine pH; the more acidic the urine, the greater the renal clearance. Alkalinization of the urine or kidney dysfunction reduce the rate of elimination and may cause toxicity [222, 226].

Toxicity

Generally, oral mexiletine is well tolerated by patients. Gastrointestinal distress in the form of nausea, vomiting, and dyspepsia sometimes occurs.

Mexiletine rarely exerts toxic effects on the electrical activity of the heart. Sinus tachycardia, atrial

189

fibrillation, or exacerbation of existing arrhythmias have been reported in a few patients. Mexiletine can cause severe depression of cardiac contractility and blood pressure in patients with existing heart failure.

Toxic effects during chronic oral ingestion are usually manifested on the central nervous system and are related to high-plasma drug levels. The neurological effects which occur are tremor, nystagmus, confusion, diplopia, dizziness, and ataxia [227].

Phenytoin

Phenytoin, was introduced into clinical medicine as an anticonvulsant by Merritt and Putnam in 1938 [228]. Its principal use today is still for the treatment of epilepsy. The idea for its use as a cardiac antiarrhythmic drug originated in 1950 when Sidney Harris speculated that the mechanism of origin of cardiac arrhythmias due to myocardial infarction might be similar to that of epileptiform seizures [229]. It was believed that epileptic seizures were generated by the flow of current at the border between injured, necrotic brain tissue and normal tissue. A similar flow of current between injured, infarcting myocardium and adjacent normal myocardium might produce ventricular arrhythmias. Harris investigated the effects of phenytoin on arrhythmias in dogs after experimental infarction and found it to be particularly effective [229]. Subsequent studies on arrhythmias induced in animals by a variety of techniques also demonstrated that phenytoin had a significant antiarrhythmic effect [230–233]. However it was not until 1958 that phenytoin was used clinically by Leonard to successfully treat ventricular tachycardia refractory to quinidine and procainamide [234]. This result prompted a substantial investigation of the effects of phenytoin on clinical arrhythmias.

Phenytoin is structurally related to the barbiturates and shares the chemistry of that group of drugs (Figure 1). However, it does not have prominent sedative effects, since it lacks an alkyl substituent in position 5 of the hydantoin ring which is believed to be related to sedation.

Effects on the heart and circulation

Electrophysiologic effects on cardiac cells

(A) Effects on resting membrane potential, action potential amplitude and phase 0 upstroke velocity ($\dot{V}_{max}$). Phenytoin may exert several different actions on resting membrane potential, action potential amplitude and phase 0 upstroke velocity ($\dot{V}_{max}$) of atrial, ventricular and Purkinje fibers, depending on (a) the concentration of drug, (b) the [K^+] in the extracellular environment, and (c) the condition of the fibers; that is, whether resting membrane potential, action potential amplitude, and phase 0 upstroke velocity are low or within normal limits.

When the K concentration of the superfusate is at normal plasma values (4–5 mM) or slightly higher, low drug concentrations (1–3 μg/ml) do not affect resting potential and usually do not affect $\dot{V}_{max}$ of phase 0 or action potential amplitude [126, 235]. However, an increase in action potential amplitude and $\dot{V}_{max}$ in atrial fibers has been reported [235, 236]. Higher concentrations of phenytoin may decrease amplitude and $\dot{V}_{max}$ [126, 236, 237]. The membrane responsiveness curve is also shifted in a negative direction along the voltage axis, indicating a depression of $\dot{V}_{max}$ at all levels and membrane potential at which an action potential can be initiated [237]. This depressant effect is not as great as that of quinidine or procainamide. When [K^+]$_0$ is low (< 3 mM) low concentrations of phenytoin have been found to increase the resting potential, $\dot{V}_{max}$, and action potential amplitude of both atrial and Purkinje fibers, and conduction velocity is increased [238, 239]. These effects are particularly pronounced if resting potential and $\dot{V}_{max}$ are reduced by exposure of preparations to cold, mechanical trauma, or toxic concentrations of digitalis [237, 240] and usually are not seen when resting potential and $\dot{V}_{max}$ are normal. Higher concentrations of phenytoin do not generally influence resting potential or $\dot{V}_{max}$ when [K^+]$_0$ is low [238]. The mechanism by which phenytoin influences the upstroke of the action potential is not known. Phenytoin also decreases the amplitude and $\dot{V}_{max}$ of phase 0 of slow response action potentials in Purkinje fibers [237]; its direct effects on depressed fast response action potentials have not been described, but it might improve the action potential upstroke if $[K^+]_0$ is low by increasing the resting potential (see above).

(B) Effects on action potential duration and refractoriness. Concentrations of phenytoin in the therapeutic range shorten the action potential duration and effective refractory period of Purkinje fibers; the refractory period usually decreases less than action potential duration [237, 238]. The earliest premature impulses which can be initiated during repolarization arise from higher membrane potentials and therefore may have a greater $\dot{V}_{max}$ and amplitude than do the earliest premature impulses initiated prior to drug administration. As a result, at suitable concentrations of phenytoin, which do not significantly depress responsiveness but shorten action potential duration and refractoriness, early premature impulses may conduct more rapidly [238]. Phenytoin does not significantly change the action potential duration and effective refractory period of atrial fibers [239].

(C) Effects on impulse initiation. Phenytoin depresses the slope of phase 4 depolarization of Purkinje fibers with normal maximum diastolic potentials and of partially depolarized fibers and thus slows the automatic firing rate [237, 238, 241]. The increased slope of spontaneous diastolic depolarization induced by catecholamines or digitalis is also depressed by phenytoin. At low extracellular $[K^+]$ some slowing of automatic firing may also result from an increase in the maximum diastolic potential. High concentrations of phenytoin, much greater than those required to suppress Purkinje fiber automaticity, will suppress automaticity of rabbit sinus node cells [239]. Phenytoin suppresses delayed afterdepolarizations in Purkinje fibers caused by toxic amounts of digitalis [237] but its effects on early afterdepolarizations have not been studied.

Electrophysiologic effects on the heart
Phenytoin has electrophysiological actions on the heart which in some ways resemble those of lidocaine. It is not markedly depressant unless cardiac disease is present.

Phenytoin has a variable effect on sinus rate which may increase, remain unaltered, or decrease after the drug is administered. The acceleratory effect on sinus impulse initiation which has been observed in some instances after I.V. injection may

be provoked reflexly through alterations in autonomic tone resulting from hypotension or pain at the injection site [239] or may be exerted through direct effects of phenytoin on the central or autonomic nervous systems [242–244]. Although phenytoin has no direct effect on transmembrane potentials of normal sinus node fibers [239], the sinus bradycardia which may occur after drug administration in patients with sinus node disease may result from a direct depressant effect of phenytoin on the sinus node cells [239, 245]. An additional factor to be considered is the commercial solvent for phenytoin, a solution of propylene glycol and ethyl alcohol with a pH of 11 to 12 which may also depress sinus node function [246].

Phenytoin does not exert any prominent effects on the electrophysiology of the atria. No changes in the P wave of the ECG usually occur and therefore atrial conduction is probably unaltered [247]. This is consistent with the lack of effect of phenytoin on $\dot{V}_{max}$ of phase 0 of atrial action potentials [239]. Atrial refractoriness has been reported to be increased, unchanged [242, 248], or decreased [241]. Antiarrhythmic concentrations of phenytoin also have variable effects on conduction and refractoriness of the AV node. Phenytoin sometimes accelerates AV nodal conduction and reduces the AV nodal effective and functional refractory periods [233, 242, 248–250]. In experimental studies on the canine heart this improvement in AV nodal conduction is more prominent after conduction has been depressed with toxic doses of digitalis [233], but no comparable data are available from human studies. The acceleratory effect may result because of a central action of phenytoin to depress efferent vagal activity. There are no studies of the effects of phenytoin on AV nodal transmembrane potentials. Mostly it seems that phenytoin has no significant effect on AV nodal conduction or the PR interval of the electrocardiogram when the AV node is not diseased. AV nodal conduction may be depressed and progress to AV nodal block when phenytoin is given to some patients, in whom conduction is prolonged to begin with, because of a diseased AV node.

Therapeutic or toxic levels of phenytoin do not significantly slow conduction in the His-Purkinje system or ventricular muscle; there is no significant effect of the drug on the electrocardiographic QRS complex [233, 242, 248, 250, 251]. This is consistent with the observations that phenytoin does not markedly depress $\dot{V}_{\max}$ of phase 0 of the Purkinje fiber or ventricular muscle action potential [238]. Whether phenytoin has significant depressant effects on the diseased conduction system such as in patients with incomplete bundle branch block is uncertain. Phenytoin shortens the relative and effective refractory periods of the ventricular conduction system and ventricular muscle [241, 242, 252]. This effect is probably caused by the shortening of the action potential duration [238].

Effects on the circulation

As mentioned previously phenytoin may cause significant hypotension by directly vasodilating the peripheral blood vessels if an intravenous dose is administered too rapidly [229, 253]. Usually no hypotension occurs if it is given slowly or in a divided dose schedule. The propylene glycol diluent can also cause profound hypotension [246]. Intravenous phenytoin may also depress myocardial contractility and cardiac output if administered too rapidly [253–255].

Pharmacokinetics

Administration, absorption, and distribution

Phenytoin is available for intravenous or oral administration. It is not usually given intramuscularly, because absorption by this route is erratic and plasma drug levels are unpredictable. Intramuscular phenytoin is painful and also can cause tissue necrosis and sterile abscesses due to the high alkalinity of the solution [256]. The I.V. preparation usually consists of 250 mg of the sodium salt of the drug dissolved in a solution of 40% propylene glycol and 10% ethyl alcohol (pH 11–12). Sodium phenytoin is also available in capsule form for oral usage.

Bigger and associates have described a regimen for intravenous phenytoin administration which rapidly and safely results in therapeutic plasma levels [249]. Fifty to 100 mg of phenytoin is administered every 5 min until the arrhythmia is abolished, until 1,000 mg has been given, or until undesirable effects appear. This method of administration results in a stepwise increase in the plasma levels of 3–4 μg/ml after each dose and allows establishment of the minimum effective plasma level needed to abolish an arrhythmia. Once the effective antiar-

rhythmic plasma level has been achieved, supplemental doses of phenytoin are necessary to maintain it. Usually if a total dose of 1,000 mg is given over the first 24 hr, 500 mg can be given the second day to maintain plasma levels and smaller doses on subsequent days. Maintenance doses can be given intravenously or orally.

If large amounts of phenytoin are given more rapidly, therapeutic levels can be obtained much more rapidly, but the administration of the drug over a short period of time may cause significant hypotension. After a single intravenous injection of a large amount of phenytoin, plasma level decline rapidly because of distribution of the drug into peripheral tissues and therefore plasma phenytoin may fall below the therapeutic levels after 10–15 min [249, 257]. A constant I.V. infusion of phenytoin should not be given, since the high alkalinity necessary to maintain it in solution can cause intense pain and thrombosis at the infusion rate.

Phenytoin can also be administered orally. However, it is incompletely absorbed from the gastrointestinal tract, absorption is slow and there is a great deal of intersubject variation in the absorption rate. The maximum plasma level after a single oral dose is achieved only after 8–12 hr [258]. When administered without an initial loading dose, 300–500 mg/day usually results in steady-state therapeutic plasma levels in five days or more [259]. Administration of 1,000 mg orally on the first day followed by doses of 500–600 mg on the second and third days and maintenance doses of 400–500 mg/day may provide adequate control of responsive arrhythmias within 24 hr and sustained therapeutic plasma concentrations [249].

Phenytoin levels of 10–18 μg/ml are considered to be in the therapeutic range [249], although arrhythmias caused by digitalis toxicity may respond to lower plasma levels. In general, arrhythmias which do not respond to plasma concentrations of about 20 μg/ml will not be abolished by even higher drug concentrations [249]. Toxic effects (see below) occur at levels of 20 μg/ml or above. Approximately 85% of the plasma phenytoin is bound to proteins.

Elimination

Only 1–5% of the phenytoin in the body is excreted unchanged by the kidney. Inactivation of the remaining drug results from metabolism in the liver by the mixed function oxidase system; one of the phenol rings is hydroxylated resulting in the formation of 5-phenyl-5 parahydroxyphenylhydantoin (HPPH) which is conjugated with glucuronic acid or sulfate and excreted in the urine [260, 261]. Measurements of the urinary excretion of HPPH can be used as an indication of whether metabolism is occurring at a normal or reduced rate [262].

Phenytoin elimination shows first order kinetics at low plasma levels (< 5–10 μg/ml) as do other antiarrhythmic drugs such as lidocaine and procainamide. At these low concentrations the amount of drug eliminated per unit time (hydroxylated by the liver) is a fixed percentage of the total body store and the half-time for elimination is about 24 hr. Increasing the amount of drug administered results in a predictable rise in plasma concentrations and drug elimination [263]. However, unlike procainamide or lidocaine, phenytoin elimination is dose dependent [264–266]. The half-time for elimination becomes progressively longer at high plasma levels until elimination shows zero order kinetics [266]. In the dosage range where zero order kinetics of elimination occur, small increments in the daily dose of phenytoin result in large and unpredictable increases in plasma levels. This, first order kinetics may prevail during initial intravenous or oral administration. However, when administered for several days or more the fraction of drug metabolized may decrease making it difficult to predict the amount of drug in the plasma on the basis of the amount administered. These characteristics of elimination result largely from the kinetic properties of the phenytoin–liver hydroxylating enzyme system interaction. The amount of phenytoin hydroxylated increases linearly with the amount presented to the liver and is a fixed percentage of the total phenytoin until, at certain drug concentrations, the enzyme system begins to be saturated [267, 268]. Any increase in the amount of drug presented to the liver above the concentration which saturates the enzyme system does not result in an increase in the amount of drug metabolized, resulting in the zero order kinetics of elimination.

Abnormalities in plasma protein binding or metabolism may result in large deviations in plasma phenytoin levels from the expected. Since the liver is the primary site of metabolism, the state of liver function is important. Patients receiving prolonged phenytoin therapy have developed high plasma levels and signs of intoxication after infectious hepatitis or liver cirrhosis [269]. However, in many instances of liver disease clinical impairment of phenytoin metabolism is not evident, perhaps because the central area of the liver lobule, where metabolizing enzymes are located, is not critically involved [259]. The rate of liver metabolism also may be abnormally low in rare individuals with a genetic defect in the metabolizing enzyme [270] or in individuals taking other drugs which may inhibit phenytoin metabolism by the mixed function oxidase system (dicoumarol, phenylbutazone, disulfiram, phenyramidol, isoniazid, methylpenidate, chloramphenicol, and phenothiazines) [259]. Several factors may also result in accelerated phenytoin metabolism and abnormally low plasma levels. Some patients may have abnormally rapid metabolism for unknown reasons [262]. Increased activity of phenytoin metabolizing enzymes may be induced by drugs such as phenobarbital [271, 272]. Alterations in plasma protein binding of phenytoin also significantly influence the plasma drug levels. Although it is normally about 85% bound, in patients with uremia or hepatic disease protein binding may be decreased, possibly due to a decreased plasma albumin concentration as well as a qualitative change in the plasma proteins [273, 274]. As a consequence of the decreased plasma protein binding, more phenytoin may enter the tissue where it is bound to tissue proteins. The total plasma concentration of phenytoin will therefore be less than expected and tissue levels of drugs may be higher. As a result, in uremic patients therapeutic and toxic effects may occur at lower than expected plasma phenytoin levels. Phenytoin binding to proteins may also be reduced in patients receiving sulfisoxazole, phenylbutazone, and salicylic acid.

Toxicity

The toxic effects of phenytoin on the heart and circulation have already been discussed; hypotension, bradycardia, and AV block have all occurred after intravenous administration, particularly when the drug has been given rapidly or when the patients have had sinus or AV nodal disease. Toxicity occurring during long-term phenytoin therapy is most commonly manifested as central nervous system disturbances. The most prominent symptom is nystagmus which first occurs on lateral gaze, then at the 45-degree deviation from the midline, and finally on forward gaze. Other signs of toxicity are blurred vision, drowsiness, and ataxia [31].

Several nondose-related toxic reactions to phenytoin have also been observed. Gingival hyperplasia occurs in about 20% of all patients, particularly in children and young adults. Generally, this does not require withdrawal of the drug. Peripheral neuropathy and megaloblastic anemia may also occur. In some cases, the anemia is responsive to folic acid therapy [275].

Beta-adrenergic-receptor-blocking drugs

Beta-adrenergic-receptor-blocking drugs have assumed an important role in the therapy of cardiac arrhythmias. Although there are a large number of these drugs undergoing laboratory and clinical investigation, propranolol is the only one generally used for acute and chronic therapy of arrhythmias in the United States. In addition, timolol has been approved recently for prophylactic therapy in patients with prior myocardial infarction, since clinical trials have shown that timolol may prevent sudden death in these patients [276].

The beta-receptor-blocking drugs probably exert most of their antiarrhythmic effects by preventing the well-known electrophysiological effects of catecholamines on the heart [277]. A direct action on the cardiac cell membrane may also contribute to antiarrhythmic effects of some of the drugs. Some beta-receptor-blocking drugs are cardioselective whereas others are not. Cardioselective drugs mainly prevent the interaction of catecholamine with the cardiac (β_1)-adrenergic receptors and exert a much weaker blocking effect at other beta-adrenergic receptors such as those in vascular smooth muscle, bronchi, and the gastrointestinal tract (β_2-receptors). Acebutolol, atenolol, metoprolol, and practolol all are cardioselective beta-blocking agents. Oxprenolol, pindolol, sotolol, timolol, as well as propranolol are not cardioselective but block both the beta$_1$- and beta$_2$-receptors.

Although the most important property of beta-receptor-blocking drugs is to antagonize the actions of catecholamines at beta-adrenergic receptors, some of these drugs have partial beta-adrenergic agonist activity and stimulate these receptors. Beta-blocking drugs with partial agonist activity include

alprenolol, oxprenolol, pindolol, acebutolol, and practolol.

We will concentrate the majority of our discussion on propranolol, since this is the major beta-receptor-blocking drug used for antiarrhythmic therapy. Propranolol's beta-receptor-blocking properties were originally discovered by Black et al. in 1964 [278]. The blocking effect occurs because of the similarity between its chemical structure (Figure 1) and that of isoproterenol, the prototype beta-adrenergic-receptor agonist. In both compounds, the isopropyl-substituted secondary amine is similar. It is the nature of the substituents on the aromatic ring which determines whether the effects of the compound will be predominantly beta-adrenergic activation or blockade [279].

Effects on the heart and circulation

Electrophysiologic effects on cardiac cells

(A) Effects on resting membrane potential, action potential amplitude, and phase 0 upstroke velocity ($\dot{V}_{max}$). Propranolol affects the cardiac transmembrane potentials by two mechanisms of action: (a) by blocking beta-receptors, it modifies any effects that catecholamines are exerting on the resting and action potential, and (b) it exerts direct effects on the cardiac cell membrane which are independent of beta-receptor blockade and catecholamines.

Low concentrations (≤ 1 μg/ml) of propranolol which cause significant beta-receptor blockade, have no direct membrane effects; in these concentrations, propranolol does not influence the normal resting potential, action potential amplitude, or $\dot{V}_{max}$ of atrial, Purkinje, or ventricular muscle fibers [280, 281]. At concentrations which are higher than necessary for beta-blocking action (10–20 μg/ml), $\dot{V}_{max}$, action potential amplitude, the membrane responsiveness curve, and conduction in normal atrial, ventricular and Purkinje fibers are depressed [280–283]. Resting membrane potential is not altered. At these concentrations propranolol has a direct effect on fibers, reducing their Na$^+$ conductance [284, 285]. It was originally believed that the concentrations which depress the action potential upstroke are far higher than the antiarrhythmic blood levels in humans. However, more recently it has been found that the antiarrhythmic effects of propranolol may only occur in

194

some patients when plasma levels are very high [286]. Therefore, a direct membrane effect may be an important mechanism for antiarrhythmic action in some patients.

Despite the lack of effect of low propranolol concentrations on resting membrane potential and on phase 0 of the action potential described in the previous paragraph, there may be a significant effect of beta-receptor blockade on the resting and action potential under circumstances in which catecholmines are present. For example, when resting membrane potential is moderately reduced, resulting in a reduction of $\dot{V}_{max}$ and action potential amplitude, catecholamines may increase the resting membrane potential and, indirectly, $\dot{V}_{max}$. In this circumstance beta-receptor blockade might depress conduction by removing the catecholamine effect [281]. In the presence of high $[K^+]_0$, catecholamines induce slow response action potentials [287]. The upstrokes of these slow responses can be markedly depressed by beta-receptor blockade and conduction can thereby be blocked [288]. It is not known whether propranolol exerts a direct effect on $\dot{V}_{max}$ of phase 0 and conduction of slow response action potentials which are not dependent on catecholamines.

(B) Effects on action potential duration and refractoriness. In low concentrations, which have significant beta-receptor blocking effects but no direct membrane effect, propranolol does not influence repolarization or refractoriness of atrial, Purkinje, or ventricular fibers (assuming catecholamines are not exerting any significant effects on the action potential). In higher concentrations propranolol accelerates repolarization and shortens the action potential duration of Purkinje fibers through its direct membrane effect; phase 2 of repolarization is shortened more than phase 3. Repolarization of atrial and ventricular fibers also is accelerated but to a lesser extent [280, 282, 283]. The acceleration of repolarization of Purkinje fibers is most marked in areas of the ventricular conducting system where the action potential duration is the greatest [289]. At concentrations which have a direct membrane effect, propranolol shortens the effective refractory period of Purkinje fibers, but the reduction in refractory period is not as great as the reduction in action potential duration [280]. As a consequence, the earliest premature impulses which can be in-

itiated during repolarization arise from more negative membrane potentials and sometimes have a greater $\dot{V}_{max}$ than do the earliest premature impulses initiated prior to drug administration.

(C) Effects on impulse initiation. Beta-receptor blockade prevents the enhanced spontaneous diastolic depolarization caused by catecholamines in sinus node, atrial pacemaker, and Purkinje fibers. Propranolol, therefore, can slow the rate of automatic firing caused by catecholamines [281]. The direct membrane effects of propranolol also may suppress digitalis-induced spontaneous diastolic depolarization in normal Purkinje fibers [290]. The direct membrane effect of propranolol does not slow abnormal automaticity in partially depolarized Purkinje fibers, although presumably the beta-receptor blocking effects would slow abnormal automaticity when it is enhanced by catecholamines. The beta-receptor blocking capability of propranolol can decrease the amplitude of delayed afterdepolarizations and stop triggering in atrial fibers or Purkinje fibers when they are caused by catecholamines or by digitalis [291]. It is not known if the direct membrane effect of propranolol can also suppress afterdepolarizations.

Electrophysiologic effects on the heart
Clinically used doses of beta-receptor-blocking drugs probably exert most of their electrophysiological effects on the heart by blocking sympathetic influences on electrical activity. Therefore, the electrophysiological actions of beta-blocking drugs depend on the amount of autonomic activity present at the time of drug administration. If sympathetic activity and its effects on the heart are minimal, beta-blocking drugs will have little influence, whereas they will cause marked changes if sympathetic activity is high. Cardiac disease, such as myocardial infarction or failure, may result in greater sympathetic activity and therefore beta-receptor-blocking drugs may have a greater electrophysiological effect on the diseased heart rather than on the normal heart. The electrophysiological effects also may vary among different beta-blocking drugs. For example, the sympathomimetic effects of some may offset some of the effects of beta-receptor blockade. In addition, the direct membrane-depressant actions of some of the drugs also may influence electrical activity.

Propranolol and the other beta-receptor-blocking drugs attenuate the positive chronotropic effect which results from sympathetic stimulation [292]. When administered to individuals in the resting state, these drugs will also slow the sinus rate but to a lesser extent than in individuals with enhanced sympathetic activity [293–299]. Severe bradycardia occasionally results after commonly used doses of propranolol if the heart is particularly dependent on sympathetic activity to maintain an adequate rate [300]. The commonly used therapeutic concentrations of propranolol, as well as the other beta-receptor-blocking drugs, do not have direct depressant effects on normal sinus node action potentials and, thus, slowing is not caused by a direct effect. The diseased sinus node may be more sensitive to the direct depressant effects of propranolol and the possibility exists that in patients with sinus node disease some slowing may result from a direct effect. In large doses, beta-blocking drugs with direct membrane effects such as propranolol can directly cause sinus exit block or sinus arrest. Beta-blocking drugs with partial agonist activity such as acebutolol and pindolol may decrease the rate of sinus node discharge to a lesser extent than propranolol and might lessen the risk of sinus bradycardia in some patients [301–303].

Beta-receptor-blocking drugs do not significantly affect the electrophysiologic properties of the atria and do not alter the P wave unless the pacemaker site shifts as a result of sinus slowing [293, 299–305]. The beta-receptor-blocking drugs do have significant effects on the AV node; they attenuate the acceleration of conduction caused by sympathetic activation. When propranolol is given to humans in the resting state the P–R interval may not change or it may be prolonged [299, 304]. The degree of prolongation of the P–R interval depends on the intrinsic sympathetic tone. Slowing of the sinus rate also may mask the effect of beta-receptor blockade on AV conduction [299]. The increase in the P–R interval which often occurs is caused by slowing of conduction in the AV node only, and not in the His-Purkinje system [304, 306–308]. Beta-receptor blockade also increases the functional and effective refractory period of the AV node [304, 309]. The direct membrane effects of drugs such as propranolol do not usually contribute to the slowing of AV nodal conduction or the refractory period prolongation caused by therapeutic concentra-

tions, except perhaps if the node is diseased and conduction is already depressed [306]. The direct electrophysiological depressant effects of toxic amounts of propranolol may contribute to the occurrence of AV block. Beta-receptor-blocking drugs with sympathomimetic effects, such as acebutolol, pindolol, practolol, and alprenolol, may have a lesser effect on conduction and refractoriness than those drugs without an agonist action [303, 306, 310].

Beta-receptor blockade with propranolol does not slow conduction through the accessory pathway in humans with the Wolff-Parkinson-White syndrome. In one study it was also reported that the effective refractory period of the anomalous pathway was not altered [311]. However, Wellens recently has shown that beta-receptor stimulation with isoproterenol does shorten the antegrade refractory period of the accessory pathway and thus in some instances it would be expected that beta-receptor blockade could lengthen the refractory period [312].

The currently available beta-receptor-blocking drugs have no significant effects on conduction and refractoriness of the normal ventricular specialized conducting system or ventricular muscle. The H–V interval of the His bundle electrogram and the QRS duration of the electrocardiogram are not affected, since these drugs do not influence $\dot{V}_{max}$ of phase 0 of the action potential in therapeutic concentrations [281]. Even very high (toxic) concentrations do not usually depress conduction significantly in situ, although high concentrations of propranolol can decrease $\dot{V}_{max}$ in vitro [280]. Therefore, therapeutic doses of propranolol in humans do not exert a direct depressant or 'quinidine-like' effect on the heart.

Effects on the circulation
Beta-receptor-blocking drugs have important effects on cardiac output and blood pressure which are mediated largely by their effects on the heart. These hemodynamic effects are a consequence of beta-receptor blockade. Like the effects on electrical activity, the magnitude of the effects on the circulation is determined by the level of preexisting sympathetic tone. Propranolol, even in therapeutic doses, causes a reduction in cardiac output by decreasing heart rate and cardiac contractility. The decrease in contractility is manifested as a re-

duction in systolic ejection rate, and the peak rate of rise of left ventricular pressure. Peripheral resistance increases because of the compensatory sympathetic reflexes and blood flow to all tissues except the brain is reduced [313]. The decreased heart rate and contractility are especially prominent during the increased demand and sympathetic tone accompanying exercise. The decreases in end-diastolic and end-systolic ventricular size associated with exercise are also reduced. Maximum exercise tolerance is decreased in normal individuals but can be increased in patients with angina [314]. The decrease in cardiac contractility may also cause a decrease in myocardial oxygen consumption. Although the effects on hemodynamics may be well tolerated in many individuals taking propranolol therapy for arrhythmias, in some, congestive heart failure may be precipitated even by therapeutic concentrations of propranolol. This may occur in patients with preexisting heart failure in whom an adequate cardiac output is dependent on increased sympathetic tone but occasionally has occurred in patients without preexisting failure. A marked decrease in cardiac output and increase in left ventricular end-diastolic pressure may be a consequence of toxic amounts of propranolol even in patients with a normal cardiac output [315].

Propranolol also may decrease arterial blood pressure. This may result partly from the decreased cardiac output and partly from other mechanisms which as yet are poorly defined [160]. Cardiovascular collapse has occurred on occasion [316, 317].

Pharmacodynamic effects of the newer beta-blocking drugs are similar to those seen with propranolol [318–321].

Pharmacokinetics of propranolol

Administration, absorption, and distribution
Propranolol is used both for intravenous and oral therapy of arrhythmias. Although there are few studies available to relate directly plasma levels of propranolol to its antiarrhythmic effects, plasma levels which adequately block the effects of the sympathetic nervous system on the electrical activity of the heart probably will be effective against many types of arrhythmias (100–150 ng/ml after I.V. administration) [322, 323]. However, in some instances, plasma levels which are much higher than those necessary for beta-receptor blockade

must be attained before the drug is effective [286, 324].

When propranolol is administered intravenously, 0.1 mg/kg (but not exceeding a 10-mg total dose) is usually given at a rate of about 1 mg/min. This dose will result in an initial plasma level of 100–200 ng/ml [325], 90–95% of which is bound to plasma proteins [326]. After a single intravenous dose the plasma level decreases quite rapidly as a biexponential function, with an early rapid decline (half-time of about 10 min) as the drug enters the tissues, followed by a later and slower fall off with a half-time of 2–3 hr [323]. A single intravenous dose of 10 mg which produces a plasma level of 150 ng/ml may therefore decline to below 50 ng/ml within 1 hr. The sympathetic blocking effect falls off with the decline in plasma levels. The antiarrhythmic effect of a single intravenous dose of propranolol usually lasts for several hours. Maintenance of therapeutic plasma or tissue levels subsequent to I.V. propranolol administration usually is accomplished by oral administration.

When propranolol is administered orally a remarkable variability in plasma levels can occur among different patients even when they are given the same dose and complete absorption from the intestine occurs. In one study plasma levels after a single oral dose of 80 mg ranged from 30 to 200 ng/ml in five different patients [323]. This makes prediction of an exact oral dosage schedule difficult. A large quantity of the initial oral dose (70%) of propranolol is extracted immediately from the portal circulation by the liver [327]. This is due not only to metabolism but also results from binding to high affinity sites in the liver [328]. Individual differences in hepatic extraction may be at least partly responsible for the differences in plasma levels [323]. If the initial dose of oral propranolol is less than 30 mg, none of the drug may reach the systemic circulation because of almost complete hepatic extraction [328, 329]. An increase in the initial oral dose above 30 mg results in an increase in plasma levels, because more drug passes through the liver without being removed from the circulation. The high affinity hepatic binding sites are saturated by initial doses of 30 mg or more and remain saturated for up to 6 hr thereafter [328]. Therefore, a larger amount of drug reaches the systemic circulation after subsequent oral doses during the first pass of the portal blood through the liver. In the steady state about 20–50% of an oral dose is bioavailable. Since the half-time for elimination of propranolol during chronic oral therapy may range from 3–6 hr [328] oral propranolol usually is administered every 6 hr to maintain a therapeutic effect.

Elimination

Almost 95% of propranolol in the body is metabolized and very little is excreted unaltered in the urine [323, 330]. Most of the metabolism occurs in the liver where propranolol undergoes a number of degradative reactions [331, 332]. After an initial oral dose, large quantities of 4-hydroxypropranolol are formed quickly [325, 328, 333]. The quantity of 4-hydroxypropranolol formed after an initial I.V. dose is not nearly as great [333]. Apparently a high concentration of propranolol is required in the portal venous blood, as occurs after oral administration, in order for the drug to be metabolized to significant quantities of 4-hydroxypropranolol [330, 333]. Plasma levels of 4-hydroxypropranolol are insignificant by 6 hr after administration suggesting that it is further metabolized [333]. 4-hydroxypropranolol does not appear to be a major end metabolic product during periods of chronic drug administration [333].

4-hydroxypropranolol has significant pharmacologic effects. It is a beta-receptor blocker with a potency similar to propranolol, it has some sympathomimetic effects and also direct membrane actions [334]. It therefore may contribute to the antiarrhythmic effect of propranolol when it is present in the plasma in significant amounts. Other propranolol metabolites have also been identified, and many of these metabolites have pharmacological activity. α-naphthol has depressant effects on heart rate, arterial pressure, and myocardial contractility [335]; isopropylamine increases arterial pressure, heart rate, and myocardial contractile force [336], and propranolol glycol has potent anticonvulsant effects [337]. The antiarrhythmic potency of these metabolites is not yet known.

The rate of propranolol metabolism is not related linearly to plasma propranolol levels. During the course of chronic oral propranolol therapy the half-time for elimination may increase gradually by close to 50% [328]. This presumably occurs because metabolism is dose dependent and the enzyme system responsible for metabolism becomes saturated. Dosage or plasma levels at which the enzyme system is saturated completely and at which elimination occurs with zero order kinetics are not known.

Significant variations in the degree of plasma protein binding are often found between individuals, and these variations can affect the rate of propranolol metabolism [338]. Since bound propranolol is metabolized as well as free propranolol, increased plasma protein binding accelerates metabolism by reducing propranolol's volume of distribution and delivering more drug to its site of inactivation. Factors which alter hepatic blood flow also markedly affect the rate of propranolol metabolism, because the hepatic flow determines the rate of delivery of propranolol to the liver. Hepatic blood flow, reduced by congestive heart failure, may be expected to decrease the rate of propranolol metabolism. Propranolol also limits its own metabolism, since it decreases hepatic blood flow by its beta-receptor blocking effect. Liver disease also may retard the rate of propranolol metabolism. All these factors will increase propranolol plasma levels [339]. Higher propranolol plasma levels may sometimes be found in patients with chronic renal disease even though propranolol is not normally excreted by the kidneys, because renal disease may influence the extraction of propranolol by the liver [340, 341]. The metabolic products of propranolol might also accumulate in the blood and exert pharmacological effects that influence the outcome of therapy.

Pharmacokinetics of other beta-receptor-blocking drugs

Administration, absorption, distribution, and elimination

All of the other beta-blocking drugs mentioned at the beginning of this section have been effectively administered by the intravenous route. These drugs can also be given orally, since they are all well absorbed except for atenolol. Although absorption of orally administered oxprenolol and alprenolol is complete and rapid, bioavailability is low because hepatic clearance is large, as described for propranolol [342, 343]. As the dose is increased less drug is eliminated on the first pass through the hepatic circulation and thus more is available in the systemic circulation [344]. Practolol, which is eliminated largely by a renal mechanism, and pindolol, which is eliminated by both hepatic and renal mechanisms, are not extracted to any great extent by the liver during the first pass in the portal circulation and therefore bioavailability of an oral dose of these drugs is much higher than that of propranolol [345, 346].

The beta-blocking drugs show different degrees of plasma protein binding which can influence their elimination kinetics. Alprenolol is slightly bound (90%), like propranolol, facilitating metabolism by the liver [344]. Less lipophylic drugs, such as metoprolol and practolol, bind less to proteins.

Alprenolol and oxprenolol are extensively metabolized in the liver [347, 348], and the metabolites along with some unmetabolized drug are excreted by the kidneys. The beta-blocking drugs with low lipid solubility – practolol, sotolol, pindolol – are not metabolized to any great extent by the liver but, rather, are excreted by the kidney.

Toxicity

The toxic effects of beta-receptor-blocking drugs on the heart and circulation have already been mentioned. These include sinus bradycardia, sinus arrest, various degrees of AV block, ventricular failure, and hypotension. Cessation of chronic oral therapy with propranolol can also lead to a serious withdrawal syndrome characterized by exacerbation of angina pectoris, cardiac arrhythmias, as well as acute myocardial infarction [349–351]. Other adverse effects also result from blockade of beta-receptors in other organ systems. Cardioselective beta-blockers may exert fewer extracardiac toxic effects than nonselective blockers such as propranolol.

Nonselective beta-receptor blockade can cause an increase in bronchial airway resistance by blocking β_2-receptors and, in patients with asthma or chronic bronchitis, bronchospasm can result. An increase in airway resistance is less likely to occur with beta-blockers that possess partial β_2 agonist activity as well as with those that are cardioselective [352–356].

Other adverse side effects that occur with propranolol are gastrointestinal disturbances (nausea, diarrhea, gastric pain, constipation), hallucinations, dreams, and insomnia. These effects may be related to beta-adrenergic blockade.

Some of the β-blocking drugs have toxic effects that seem to be *unrelated* to β-receptor blockade.

Most importantly, patients treated with practolol, have developed a serious immune reaction, the oculomucocutaneous syndrome, that affects the skin and mucous and serous membranes [357, 358]. The syndrome is associated with a positive antinuclear factor and has led to termination of the drug's clinical use despite its effectiveness as an antiarrhythmic. In addition, there have been a few reports of this syndrome occurring in patients being treated with propranolol [359, 360] as well as oxprenolol [361, 362]. Patients being treated with practolol have also had sclerosing peritonitis [363]. These reactions are reversible after drug withdrawal.

The β-blocking drugs, tolamolol, alprenolol, practolol, and pamatolol, have all caused tumors in animals [364], yet it is unclear at this time whether this is a characteristic of all β-blocking drugs and what relationship it may have to tumor growth in humans.

Verapamil

Verapamil, which was introduced as a coronary vasodilator in 1962 by Haas and Hartfelder [365], is a synthetic derivative of papaverine (Figure 1). Although it was initially believed that verapamil was a beta-adrenergic blocking agent, subsequent studies have shown this is not the case [366, 367]. Rather, verapamil has a unique electrophysiologic action, blocking the slow inward current in cardiac fibers [368, 369]. Thus, verapamil has effects on the heart not shared by the other types of antiarrhythmic drugs.

Effects on the heart and circulation

Electrophysiologic effects on cardiac cells

(A) Effects on resting membrane potential, action potential amplitude and phase 0 upstroke velocity (V_{max}). Verapamil has no significant effect on resting potential, $\dot{V}_{max}$ of phase 0 or action potential amplitude of cardiac fibers that have normal fast response action potentials (Purkinje fibers, working atrial, and ventricular muscle fibers) [370–375]. In very high concentrations (3–10 μg/ml) a slight depression of $\dot{V}_{max}$ may occur when a racemic mixture of the drug is given, since the d-isomer has some local anesthetic effects [376]. In general, however, verapamil does not influence conduction in

199

the atria or the ventricles.

Verapamil does have a profound effect on the $\dot{V}_{max}$ of phase 0 and action potential amplitude of sinus and atrioventricular nodal cells, since these cells have slow response action potentials [372]. In the sinus node verapamil causes a decrease in action potential amplitude and $\dot{V}_{max}$, the degree of which is directly related to the drug concentration. These effects are accompanied by a small decrease in maximum diastolic potential. The depressant effects on $\dot{V}_{max}$ and action potential amplitude are less marked in the latent pacemaker cells which are found more toward the periphery of the sinus node, since some fast Na^+ current may contribute to the action potential upstrokes of these cells. The effect of verapamil on AV nodal cells also varies with their location within the node. Verapamil decreases $\dot{V}_{max}$ and action potential amplitude without altering resting potential in cells in the mid (N) and upper (AN) nodal region but has very little effect on lower nodal (NH) cells [372]. Because of these effects on nodal action potentials, verapamil slows conduction in the sinus and AV nodes.

Verapamil also depresses the phase 0 upstroke of slow response action potentials occurring under a variety of conditions. Action potential amplitude and $\dot{V}_{max}$ of slow responses in atrial, ventricular, or Purkinje fibers produced by superfusing preparations with solutions containing no Na^+ and high $[Ca^{++}]$ [371], elevated $[K^+]$ alone or with catecholamines [133], or produced by depolarizing current pulses [23] are diminished by verapamil. Drug concentrations on the order of $1–2$ $\mu g/ml$ may completely abolish excitability. The depressant effect of verapamil on action potential amplitude and $\dot{V}_{max}$ often can be reversed partly by elevating the $[Ca^{++}]$ of the superfusate [371]. Verapamil has identical depressant effects on the slow response action potentials which can be recorded from isolated preparations of diseased human atrial and ventricular myocardium [377, 378].

The effects of verapamil on slow response action potentials occur because verapamil reduces the conductance of the slow current channel through which both Ca^{++} and Na^- flow [368, 379]. Verapamil has no significant effect on fast Na^+ channel conductance. Slow channel conductance is decreased without a shift in the steady-state inactivation relationship along the voltage axis [379]. Verapamil only slightly prolongs the slow current activation

kinetics and does not affect inactivation kinetics [379]. However, it does prolong the time for recovery from inactivation [379], and this action is probably a cause for the prolongation of the effective refractory period which verapamil induces in AV nodal cells (see below).

(B) Effects on action potential duration and refractoriness. Since the slow inward current contributes to the time course of repolarization of fast response fibers, verapamil does have effects on the repolarization phase of atrial, ventricular, and Purkinje fiber action potentials. Low concentrations of verapamil (1 $\mu g/ml$) shift the plateau of Purkinje fiber action potentials to more negative levels but do not significantly alter the time for complete repolarization [370, 371, 375]. A similar effect is exerted on atrial and ventricular muscle cells [372, 373]. At these concentrations, the effective refractory period is not changed. Higher concentrations of verapamil ($5–10$ $\mu g/ml$), prolong repolarization and the effective refractory period of Purkinje fibers [370, 371]. Most of the prolongation occurs during phase 3 of the action potential. These concentrations are 5–10 times higher than the concentrations which depress or completely block slow response action potentials.

Verapamil shortens the duration of most types of slow response action potentials but prolongs the effective refractory period, because it prolongs the time course of recovery of the slow channel from inactivation as described above.

Verapamil's effects on the time course of repolarization are probably not a result of its effects on slow channel conductance alone. Verapamil also increases time independent outward (K^+) currents, an effect which should accelerate repolarization [380].

(C) Effects on impulse initiation. Verapamil decreases the spontaneous firing frequency of Purkinje fibers with normal levels of maximum diastolic potential [370]. It also has a potent depressant effect on the abnormal automaticity which can be induced experimentally in atrial, ventricular, or Purkinje fibers by reducing the level of membrane potential to around $–40$ to $–60$ mV with long depolarizing current pulses [23, 140, 371, 381] and depresses the abnormal automaticity which occurs in these fibers when they are depolarized by disease

[143, 377, 378]. Verapamil depresses and abolishes triggered activity resulting from both early [382] and delayed afterdepolarizations [144, 383] when these are induced by digitalis, K^+ free superfusates, or catecholamines. Verapamil decreases the transient inward (TI) current which causes delayed afterdepolarizations in Purkinje fibers [384]. However this may not result from a direct effect of verapamil on the conductance of the TI channel but may be a secondary effect, resulting from a decrease in slow inward current during the action potential plateau and its subsequent influence on calcium release by the sarcoplasmic reticulum [384].

Electrophysiologic effects on the heart
Intravenous verapamil may speed sinus rate, because of the reflex sympathetic discharge caused by its hypotensive effect [385]. However, verapamil directly depresses impulse initiation by sinus node fibers, because it blocks the slow inward current. Therefore, in patients receiving verapamil chronically sinus rate may be slightly decreased. If the sympathetic reflex is blocked using a beta-receptor-blocking drug, verapamil significantly slows sinus rate. It may also cause marked bradycardia in patients with diseased sinus nodes.

Verapamil has no significant effect on conduction either in the atria or ventricles, since it does not depress $\dot{V}_{max}$ of phase 0 or action potential amplitude of atrial or ventricular muscle fibers [373, 386, 387]. It does prolong the P–R interval, an effect which is not dependent on the increase in heart rate, because it occurs when heart rate is maintained constant [388]. The prolongation in the P–R interval is a result of slowed AV nodal conduction (prolonged A–H interval on the His bundle electrogram), and there is no change in His-Purkinje conduction (H–V interval) [389–392]. Verapamil also prolongs the antegrade functional and effective refractory periods of the AV node [393], probably because it slows the reactivation kinetics of the slow channel. This provides the basis for its effectiveness against reentrant AV nodal tachycardias, and for slowing the ventricular rate when there is a rapid atrial rhythm. Retrograde conduction and refractoriness do not seem to be affected as much as antegrade conduction and refractoriness. The prolongation of AV nodal conduction time and refractory periods can be reversed partially by atropine [394], but it is unlikely that any of verapam-il's actions are vagally mediated. Verapamil may cause severe depression of AV nodal conduction in patients with diseased AV nodes and prolonged P–R intervals.

Effects on the circulation
Verapamil's effects on the circulation result from the interactions between its direct effects on the heart and blood vessels and reflex effects which may increase the activity of the sympathetic nerves. The direct effects of verapamil are to depress contraction of cardiac muscle fibers [395, 396] and to relax vascular smooth muscle, because it interferes with the transarcolemmal flux of Ca^{++} necessary for excitation contraction coupling [397]. Relaxation of vascular smooth muscle caused by an intravenous injection of verapamil may initially cause a mild decrease in blood pressure. Sympathetic activity to the heart may increase, speeding heart rate. Left ventricular performance may be improved (increased ejection fraction and cardiac index), because of the positive inotropic effect of the sympathetic nervous system or the reduction in afterload caused by peripheral vasodilatation. After multiple intravenous doses of verapamil or chronic oral therapy, the decrease in blood pressure may be compensated for by the increased sympathetic discharge caused by the baroreceptor reflex [398]. Heart rate and left ventricular performance may not be altered. In patients with ischemic heart disease and angina of effort, verapamil may decrease myocardial oxygen consumption, possibly by decreasing afterload or contractility of cardiac muscle. Verapamil also has been given to patients with severely depressed left ventricular performance without further depressing contractility [399]. Nevertheless, the possibility of severe depression of the heart and blood pressure remains if verapamil is not given carefully.

Verapamil may also increase coronary blood flow by directly relaxing coronary artery smooth muscle [400]; clinical experience has shown an increase in flow in both resistance and capacitance vessels. Vasospasm of coronary arteries which may cause Prinzmetal's angina ('variant angina') may also be prevented [401].

201

Pharmacokinetics

Administration, absorption, and distribution

For the therapy of arrhythmias, most investigators report the slow intravenous administration of about 10 mg of verapamil (5–15 mg). In individuals with normal liver function this results in an initial plasma concentration of 500 ng/ml or more which begins to fall rapidly as verapamil enters the highly perfused tissues. This α phase has a half-time of 15–30 min and is followed by a second β phase of elimination, dependent on liver metabolism which has a half-time of 3–7 hr. The total half-life for elimination of an intravenous dose has been determined to range from 2 to 5 hr [398]. The plasma concentration of verapamil associated with antiarrhythmic action probably lies in the range of 150–350 ng/ml [398]. Additional data are required to determine whether therapeutic plasma concentrations are different for different types of arrhythmias. It is also possible that for some arrhythmias plasma drug levels may not correlate with antiarrhythmic effects, since verapamil has been shown to depress AV nodal conduction significantly long after plasma levels are thought to have declined. This suggests preferential uptake and binding of verapamil by the AV node [402]. Verapamil's apparent volume of distribution in subjects without liver disease is 300 liters [398].

When verapamil is given orally, greater than 90% is absorbed from the gastrointestinal tract. However, bioavailability is only 10–20% due to rapid biotransformation of verapamil in the liver during its first pass through the portal circulation [403]. Thus, dosages 10–20 times greater than those given intravenously are needed for therapeutic plasma levels to be attained. Verapamil has significant electrophysiological and hemodynamic effects within 2 hr after an oral dose, and the maximum plasma concentrations are reached within 5 hr [404].

Elimination

More than 90% of administered verapamil is metabolized by the liver. Twelve metabolites have been identified. The major metabolic process is N-dealkylation which yields a secondary amine and a primary amine. The N-methylated metabolite, norverapamil represents 6% of the metabolites excreted in the urine, whereas O-demethylated products represent 16–17% of an administered dose and are excreted as inactive conjugates [398]. Norverapamil can reach steady-state plasma concentrations which are almost equal to those of verapamil. Since norverapamil has some pharmacological activity (it has a coronary vasodilating effect which is about 20% as potent as that of verapamil), it sometimes may contribute to verapamil's antiarrhythmic action [405].

Verapamil inactivation and elimination can be impaired significantly in patients with poor liver function. Patients with hepatic cirrhosis had a mean half-time for the beta (metabolic) phase of elimination which was 476% longer than a control group in a study by Woodcock et al. [406]. Systemic plasma clearance was one-third that of controls, resulting in significantly higher plasma levels of verapamil. The increase in beta half-time in some patients was associated with an increase in the apparent volume of distribution. A diminution in hepatic blood flow correlated with the decrease in verapamil clearance. On the other hand a group of patients in an intensive care unit for treatment of trauma and septicemia showed an increased rate of verapamil elimination while being treated for associated arrhythmias [406].

Since the clearance of verapamil appears to be highly dependent on liver blood flow, it is expected that clearance would be decreased in clinical conditions in which cardiac output is low. On the other hand, a decrease in renal function, while not affecting verapamil clearance, is predicted to result in significant elevations in norverapamil levels which exert significant cardiovascular depressant effects.

Toxicity

The incidence of adverse or toxic reactions to verapamil has been low. A review of the world literature [407] indicates that about 8% of patients show toxicity. Intravenous verapamil may severely decrease blood pressure and cardiac contractility if given too rapidly but these effects usually do not occur when it is given slowly. Depression of cardiac function has occurred in patients with prior heart failure. Severe sinus bradycardia, AV block, and ventricular asystole occasionally occur, particularly in patients with disease of the sinus node and AV conducting system.

Caution has been suggested concerning concurrent use of intravenous propranolol and verapamil because of the possibility for cardiac failure and severe depression of the sinus and AV nodes. However in recent studies in which oral verapamil and propranolol have been administered at the same time for the therapy of exertional angina there have been no deleterious effects on the heart and circulation.

The adverse effects which have occurred after oral verapamil include constipation, hypotension, vertigo, dizziness, muscular weakness, and nausea.

Aprindine

Aprindine (N, N-diethyl-N′-(2-indanyl-N′-phenyl-1-3-propranediamine) is a drug with local anesthetic properties that was developed and used initially as an antiarrhythmic in Belgium [408, 409] (Figure 1). It has an aromatic residue, an intermediate chain and amino group with two attached ethyl groups and therefore has some structural similarities to the other local anesthetic antiarrhythmics, lidocaine and procainamide. Aprindine currently is used as an antiarrhythmic drug in Europe but is only available as an investigational drug in the United States.

Effects on the heart and circulation

Electrophysiologic effects on cardiac cells

(A) Effects on resting membrane potential, action potential amplitude and phase 0 upstroke velocity (V_{max}). Concentrations of aprindine which approximate the therapeutic range decrease the action potential amplitude and V_{max} of phase 0 of atrial, ventricular, and Purkinje fibers. The effects on Purkinje fibers occur at lower concentrations than on atrial and ventricular fibers [410-412]. The decrease in V_{max} is enhanced at more rapid stimulus rates, suggesting use dependent block of the Na^+ channel. Membrane responsiveness is also depressed; V_{max} of action potentials, elicited at all levels of membrane potential during repolarization of the action potential, is decreased. The decrease in V_{max} is associated with a decreased conduction velocity. Aprindine has no noticeable effect on slow response action potentials of Purkinje fibers superfused with solutions containing a high K^+ concentration and isoproterenol [410-413].

(B) Effects on action potential duration and refractoriness. Aprindine shortens Purkinje fiber action potential duration and reduces the height of the plateau. Similar effects occur in atrial and ventricular muscle at higher concentrations than in Purkinje fibers [410-412]. Aprindine decreases the effective refractory period but to a lesser extent than the shortening of action potential duration. In atrial fibers, aprindine in non-toxic concentrations does not affect either outward K^+ currents or the slow inward current [414]. Aprindine also does not increase $^{42}K^+$ efflux from myocardial fibers [410]. The shortening of action potential duration might therefore result from a decrease in inward Na^+ current during the plateau. Very high concentrations of aprindine decrease slow inward current.

(C) Effects on impulse initiation. Aprindine decreases the rate of spontaneous firing of Purkinje fibers having normal automaticity by reducing the rate of phase 4 depolarization without changing the threshold potential [410, 411]. Aprindine also suppresses automaticity which occurs at low levels of membrane potential in K^+ free superfusates, or which is induced by stretch, hypoxia, or digitalis [410, 412]. Likewise, the spontaneous firing rate of fibers superfused with sodium-free, calcium-rich solution is decreased [415, 416]. Aprindine also suppresses digitalis-induced delayed after depolarizations in Purkinje fibers [413].

Electrophysiologic effects on the heart
There is little or no interaction of aprindine with the autonomic nervous system [417, 418]. Therapeutic concentrations of the drug usually do not alter sinus rate. Whether it depresses the diseased sinus node has not been investigated. Aprindine slows conduction in the atrium and AV conducting system. Both the A–H and H–V intervals on the His bundle electrogram are prolonged [419, 420]. The atrial and AV nodal refractory periods also are lengthened [421]. The decrease in conduction in the His-Purkinje system is probably the result of a decrease in amplitude and V_{max} of phase 0 of Purkinje fiber action potentials [410, 411]. Aprindine also decreases Purkinje fiber action potential duration and effective refractory period [410-412]. Aprindine may slow conduction and cause block in accessory AV conducting pathways in patients with WPW [422]. Since aprindine also decreases V_{max} of

phase 0 of ventricular muscle fibers, it moderately prolongs the QRS complex of the electrocardiogram.

Effects on the circulation
The effects of aprindine on the heart and circulation have been investigated in individuals without heart disease. Intravenous administration of the drug results in a dose related decrease in peak left ventricular dp/dt with no significant change in left ventricular systolic or end-diastolic pressure [423]. A single oral dose of aprindine given to normal subjects also can produce a small decrease in systolic and mean aortic blood pressure [424]. The importance of the negative inotropic effect of aprindine [425, 426] in the clinical setting of poor cardiac function has not been evaluated.

Pharmacokinetics

Administration, absorption, and distribution
Orally administered aprindine is well absorbed from the gastrointestinal tract and has a high bioavailability. Therapeutic levels of the drug may be obtained within 2 hr after a 200 mg dose [427]. In patients with acute myocardial infarction therapeutic levels may not be achieved for 6–12 hr even after high oral doses, because absorption is delayed [408]. Antiarrhythmic plasma levels are believed to be in the range of 1–2 $\mu g/$ml [427, 428]. Eighty-five to 95% of aprindine in the blood is bound to plasma protein.

Elimination
Aprindine is eliminated both by hepatic metabolism (35%) and by renal excretion of the unchanged drug (65%) [427]. The half-life of elimination for oral and intravenous drug ranges from 13 to 58 hr [429]. In the liver aprindine is first hydroxylated and then N-dealkylated. The major metabolites are hydroxyaprindine and N-desethylaprindine [429]. N-desethylaprindine may have some antiarrhythmic activity but only small amounts are found in the plasma of patients on chronic oral aprindine [429]. Elimination of the drug may be delayed in patients with reduced liver function or hepatic blood flow. The metabolites and some unchanged drug are excreted in the urine and eliminated by biliary excretion [427].

Toxicity
Side effects caused by the actions of aprindine on the central nervous system may occur during chronic oral administration. In one clinical investigation slight tremor was observed in 40% of the patients [420]. Other side effects included double vision, speech disorders, dizziness, insomnia, perspiration, and psychosis, all of which were readily reversible when the dose was reduced or when therapy was stopped for a period of time. Adverse effects exerted on the cardiovascular system are not common. However, the possibility that aprindine may cause arrhythmias if given soon after myocardial infarction must still be investigated [429–432]. Also not common are adverse effects on the gastrointestinal tract.

Recently, agranulocytosis and cholestatic jaundice have developed in patients receiving aprindine therapy [433, 434]. Further studies are necessary to determine whether these adverse effects will limit the use of the drug.

Bretylium

Bretylium (Figure 1) is one of a class of drugs which inhibits responses to adrenergic nerve stimulation without impairing responses to exogenous catecholamines. It is taken up into the adrenergic nerve terminals and concentrated there. This results in an initial release of norepinephrine causing a sympathetic effect which is transient; the nerve terminals are not depleted of catecholamines. Subsequently, bretylium inhibits the release of noreprinephrine by the nerve action potential and the effect of a single dose may last 6–24 hr [435, 436]. Because of this sympatholytic action, bretylium was originally used in humans as an antihypertensive but its numerous adverse effects caused its withdrawal [437]. Subsequently, in 1966 Bacaner showed that bretylium elevated the ventricular fibrillation threshold in dogs [438], and thereafter scattered reports concerning antiarrhythmic efficacy in humans began to appear in the literature. In 1978 it was approved by the FDA for limited use in the treatment of cardiac arrhythmias.

Effects on the heart and circulation

Electrophysiologic effects on cardiac cells

(A) Effects on resting membrane potential, action potential amplitude, and phase 0 upstroke velocity ($\dot{V}_{max}$). Bretylium in concentrations up to 20 μg/ml has no *direct* effect on the resting potential, action potential amplitude, or phase 0 $\dot{V}_{max}$ of atrial, ventricular or Purkinje fibers and does not affect conduction [439–441]. Membrane responsiveness is also not influenced by this range of concentrations [439, 440]. Bretylium may exert early and transient indirect effects, however, by releasing norepinephrine from nerve fibers in close proximity to the myocardial cells [439–442]. The released norepinephrine has been shown to increase resting potential, $\dot{V}_{max}$ of phase 0 and conduction velocity in Purkinje and atrial fibers. At concentrations of 20 μg/ml and higher, action potential amplitude, overshoot, $\dot{V}_{max}$, and conduction velocity are depressed as is membrane responsiveness, but such high concentrations are probably never reached in the myocardium under clinical situations [439, 442].

(B) Effect on action potential duration and refractoriness. Bretylium prolongs the action potential duration and effective refractory period of atrial, ventricular, and Purkinje fibers in concentrations which do not depress $\dot{V}_{max}$ [439–441, 443]. This effect is unrelated to catecholamine release or depletion by bretylium, since it occurs even in catecholamine depleted hearts. The effective refractory period of ventricular muscle and Purkinje fibers is prolonged to the same extent as the action potential duration [439, 440, 443]. In general, action potential duration and refractory periods are lengthened to the greatest extent in regions of the conducting system where they are the shortest. Bretylium lengthens the action potential duration and effective refractory period of subendocardial Purkinje fibers in the noninfarcted regions of canine left ventricles with experimental myocardial infarcts; whereas it has very little effect on action potential duration and refractory periods of subendocardial Purkinje fibers surviving in the infarcted area [443]. These surviving Purkinje fibers already have long action potential durations and refractory periods. By having this preferential effect in the normal regions, premature impulses initiated in the Pur-

kinje system at the border of the infarct are less likely to cause reentry [443].

(C) Effects on impulse initiation. Bretylium transiently increases phase 4 depolarization and automatic firing rate of Purkinje fibers soon after it is administered by releasing norepinephrine from nerve terminals [439, 440]. The increase in automatic firing rate stops when norepinephrine is no longer being released and does not occur when the nerve terminals are depleted of norepinephrine or when propranolol is given prior to administration of bretylium [439, 440]. Bretylium has very little or no direct depressant effect on normal automaticity. Its effects on other types of impulse initiation are not known.

Electrophysiologic effects on the heart

The immediate effects of intravenous bretylium on the heart mostly represent the action of the norepinephrine released from sympathetic nerve terminals. Subsequently, direct effects begin to appear in combination with this sympathomimetic action, and finally the electrophysiological effects represent direct effects of bretylium combined with those of sympathetic blockade.

Bretylium causes an initial increase in the sinus rate, probably resulting from enhanced phase 4 depolarization in sinus node cells, caused by the released norepinephrine. Subsequently, sinus rate may decrease as blockade of norepinephrine release and of the tonic effect of the sympathetic nervous system on the sinus node occur [444, 445]. Bretylium prolongs the atrial effective refractory period. This effect may result from prolongation of the atrial action potential duration [444–446]. Acute administration of bretylium does not have significant effects on atrioventricular conduction in humans, although the functional refractory period of the AV node is decreased, possibly by the released catecholamines [445]. In experimental animals bretylium produces a significant slowing of AV nodal conduction which is most likely a result of its sympathetic blocking effect [446]. A similar slowing of AV nodal conduction is expected also in humans after the acute, sympathetic effects wane. Bretylium has no effect on conduction time in the ventricular specialized conduction system or in ventricular muscle; the H–V interval of the His bundle electrogram and the QRS duration of the electrocardiogram are not changed, since bretylium does not depress $\dot{V}_{max}$ of phase 0 or action potential amplitude in ventricular muscle or Purkinje fibers [444–446]. Bretylium does prolong action potential duration, sometimes markedly, thereby prolonging His Purkinje and ventricular refractory periods [444]. Bretylium also increases the ventricular fibrillation threshold. The mechanism for this antifibrillatory action is not known [437, 438, 447]. It is probably not a result only of sympathetic blockade but may result from the combined direct effect of bretylium to lengthen refractory periods and indirect effects to block norepinephrine release.

Effects on the circulation
The primary effect of bretylium is to cause a decrease in blood pressure by blocking the effects of the sympathetic nerves on the peripheral arterioles. Hypotension occurs in the supine position and is exacerbated in the upright position because the compensatory effects of the baroreceptor reflexes are blocked [437, 448]. There is no evidence that bretylium depresses contractility of the myocardium and after parenteral administration, catecholamine release may increase contractility. Detailed hemodynamic studies still are required to assess the effects of bretylium on the circulatory system of the critically ill patients to whom it is given as an antiarrhythmic agent [448].

Pharmacokinetics

Administration, absorption, and distribution
Bretylium can be administered orally, intramuscularly, or intravenously. It has been used for the emergency treatment of ventricular arrhythmias by the intramuscular or intravenous route. A common dose regimen has been initial intramuscular doses of 5–10 mg/kg, not exceeding a total of 30 mg/kg and then maintenance doses of 5 mg/kg every 6–8 hr for the control of arrhythmias. Arrhythmias which are controlled by bretylium usually begin to respond within 15–30 min after the intramuscular injection [437]. Plasma bretylium concentrations peak 30–90 min after an I.M injection. After a dose of about 5 mg/kg, plasma levels are in the vicinity of 1–1.5 μg/ml, which appear to be antiarrhythmic.

Rapid intravenous injection of 5 mg/kg of bretylium is also an effective mode of administration. An additional 10 mg/kg can be given after 15–30 min

[436]. Even after intravenous injection there may be a delay of 10–20 min before an effect on arrhythmias is seen. Although experience with chronic oral bretylium therapy for arrhythmias is limited and oral administration is not recommended [437], in some patients with arrhythmias controlled only by bretylium this type of therapy has been necessary and effective [437, 448]. The decline in plasma levels of bretylium after a single dose follows first order kinetics with a half-time for elimination of about 7–10 hr.

Elimination
Between 70% and 80% of bretylium is excreted unchanged in the urine in the first 24 hr. Thus it can be predicted that poor renal function should lead to elevated bretylium levels in the plasma [437, 448, 449].

Toxicity

The major toxic effect of bretylium on the cardiovascular system is its hypotensive effect, and this can restrict the use of the drug [31, 437]. In a small percentage of patients there may be an initial exacerbation of arrhythmias or a transient initial hypertensive effect, perhaps caused by catecholamine release from sympathetic nerve endings [450]. Nausea and vomiting also occur after intravenous administration. Painful enlargement of the parotid glands has been reported during chronic oral therapy [31].

Amiodarone

Amiodarone is an antiarrhythmic drug with a novel structure (Figure 1) and actions that are very different from the other antiarrhythmic agents. Amiodarone is a benzofuran which contains two atoms of iodine per molecule, comprising 37.2% of its molecular weight [451]. It was introduced in 1962 by Charlier et al. [452] as a coronary vasodilator and antianginal compound after extensive investigations on a group of benzofuran derivatives. In 1969 Charlier [453] first described its antiarrhythmic properties. Amiodarone currently is used as both an antianginal and antiarrhythmic in Europe and South America but is not approved in the United States.

Effects on the heart and circulation

Electrophysiologic effects on cardiac cells

(A) Effects on resting membrane potential, action potential amplitude, phase 0 upstroke velocity (V_{max}), action potential duration, and recractoriness. Amiodarone administered directly into solutions superfusing isolated cardiac tissue preparations does not have any significant effects on the resting and action potentials. Its major clinical antiarrhythmic action often occurs only after administration to patients for several weeks. Rabbits have been treated with amiodarone for comparable periods of time and their hearts studied. The atrial and ventricular fibers in preparations isolated from these hearts have normal resting potentials and V_{max} is only slightly depressed. However the action potential duration and, presumably, the effective refractory period are markedly prolonged [451]. Similarly, Purkinje fibers from animals given amiodarone for long periods of time also have prolonged action potential durations. V_{max} of phase 0 and membrane responsiveness are also reduced causing conduction to be slowed [454].

(B) Effects on impulse initiation. Amiodarone decreases the slope of phase 4 depolarization of sinus node pacemaker cells in isolated rabbit atrial preparations and slows the spontaneous firing rate [455]. This effect occurs when the drug is added directly to the tissue chamber. Amiodarone does not significantly depress phase 4 depolarization or the spontaneous firing rate of Purkinje fibers [454]. Its effects on other mechanisms of impulse initiation have not been studied.

Amiodarone may have no significant immediate and direct effects on cardiac cell membranes. It has been proposed that the effects on membrane currents responsible for the alterations in the action potential described above are a result of the drug's action on metabolism of high energy phosphate compounds which requires a long time to be established [451, 456]. The suggestion has also been made that, since chronic administration of amiodarone causes an increase in iodine in the body, amiodarone causes changes in electrical activity of the heart by altering thyroid function. Thyroidectomy, alone, in rabbits increases atrial muscle action potential duration in a similar way as amiodarone.

The change in the action potentials caused by chronic administration of amiodarone to rabbits also is prevented by administration of thyroxine [451]. Alterations in thyroid function have not always been detected in humans given amiodarone for long periods of time, although cases of both hypothyroidism and hyperthyroidism have been reported [457–461].

Electrophysiologic effects on the heart
Amiodarone has both direct and indirect effects on the heart. Its indirect effects arise from its interaction with the autonomic nervous system. It blocks the effects of sympathetic stimulation noncompetitively [461–463].

Intravenous amiodarone may increase heart rate transiently because of the cardiac actions of the alcohol and polysorbate diluent [464]. After the initial tachycardia there is slowing of sinus rate. Although inhibition of sympathetic function may contribute to this slowing, much of it is probably due to a direct action of amiodarone on sinus node cells (it suppresses spontaneous diastolic depolarization [455]), because slowing occurs even after propranolol and atropine administration. The P–R interval also is prolonged because AV nodal conduction is slowed [465–467]. Oral amiodarone also slows sinus rate and AV nodal conduction. His-Purkinje conduction may also be slowed, especially in patients with bundle branch block. Refractory periods of the atria, ventricles and AV node are prolonged as is the refractory period of accessory AV pathways [468–471].

Effects on the circulation
Amiodarone exerts many of its effects on the circulation by directly relaxing smooth muscle [462]. When administered slowly by vein it causes a decrease in peripheral resistance and an increase in coronary blood flow. Systemic vasodilatation decreases afterload, and this, in combination with the slowing of the heart rate which usually occurs, decreases cardiac work and myocardial oxygen consumption [451, 462, 472, 473]. These effects probably result in the antianginal properties of the drug. Rapid intravenous administration which results in transiently high plasma levels may cause marked hypotension, a decrease in left ventricular contractility, and an increase in left ventricular end-diastolic pressure [464]. Chronic drug administration by

the oral route does not seem to cause significant myocardial depression or hypotension [474].

Pharmacokinetics

Administration, absorption, distribution, and elimination

There is very little information on the pharmacokinetics of amiodarone and much of the information which is available is still preliminary. No observations of kinetics after intravenous administration are available in humans, but antiarrhythmic effects have been reported to occur soon after administration of 5 mg/kg indicating that plasma and tissue levels rapidly attain therapeutic concentrations of the drug. It has been advised that this dose should be administered over a 5 min period to avoid adverse effects and that the drug not be given again for at least 15 min. The antiarrhythmic effect of a single I.V. dose lasts only a short period of time. Studies on rabbits and dogs have shown that after an intravenous dose a biexponential decay of the amiodarone in the plasma occurs. The half-life of the α phase is 3–6 min and that of the beta phase is 120 min. The total volume of distribution is 1.2 L/kg. The myocardial drug concentration is 30-fold higher than plasma concentrations and declines with a similar half-time as in plasma [475].

The oral dosage schedule which has been used for the therapy of arrhythmias varies widely from 200–1,400 mg/day. After therapeutic effects are achieved the dose can be reduced to find the minimum amount which is effective. Fifty percent of an oral dose of amiodarone is bioavailable [476]. Peak plasma levels are reached 2.5–5 hr after administration and are correlated with the dose. Preliminary data have shown the half-time for elimination after a single oral dose to be quite variable ranging from less than 30 min to 3–5 hr.

The plasma levels of amiodarone which are antiarrhythmic during chronic therapy are in the range of 1–5 μg/ml. To attain this steady level may require administration of drug for several weeks, particularly if the usually recommended oral dosage schedule of 600 mg a day for one week, followed by 200–400 mg daily is used. More rapid attainment of a steady-state therapeutic level can be accomplished with an initial single loading dose of 1,400 mg or administration of 1,400 mg/day during the initial phase of therapy according to a preliminary report.

In addition to the amiodarone, the desethylamiodarone metabolite in the plasma may reach 5 μg/ml during chronic oral therapy [477]. The pharmacological properties of the metabolite are not known, and, hence, the significance of its accumulation is not understood.

After chronic oral therapy is halted, elimination of the drug is very slow explaining its long duration of antiarrhythmic action. The half-time is about 40–50 days and that of desethylamiodarone is as long. Both have been detected in the plasma as long as 12 months after discontinuation of the drug.

Toxicity

Toxic effects on the heart and circulation may occur after intravenous amiodarone, particularly if it is given too rapidly. Bradycardia, AV block, and severe hypotension have occurred as well as deaths resulting from cardiovascular collapse. Oral amiodarone may also cause AV or bundle branch block and symptomatic bradycardia in patients with preexisting conduction system abnormalities.

Amiodarone has extracardiac toxic effects. Amiodarone does not usually interfere with normal thyroid function, but the drug can alter thyroid radioiodide uptake tests and can result in high serum PBI values [478]. In a small number of patients, either hypothyroidism or hyperthroidism have been reported [458–460]. Amiodarone also causes generalized lipidosis, particularly in epithelial cells [479]. This leads to corneal microdeposits that appear as yellow-brown granules in the lower third of the cornea. Corneal deposits disappear after cessation of drug therapy and have not been reported to result in irreversible opthalmic effects. In some patients photodermatatis occurs, resulting in a blue-gray skin discoloration. Regression of this effect can take as long as two years after drug administration is stopped [454].

Recently, reports have suggested that chronic amiodarone therapy is associated with serious pulmonary fibrosis [480]. The incidence and reversibility are not known.

Ethmozin

Ethmozin (Figure 1) is a derivative of phenothiazine which has minimal central nervous system effects. It was first synthesized in Russia and developed there as an antiarrhythmic drug[481]. Clinical trials with ethmozin are currently being conducted in both the United States and USSR and the results so far suggest that it is effective against both atrial and ventricular arrhythmias [482–483].

Effects on the heart and circulation

Electrophysiologic effects on cardiac cells

(A) Effects on resting membrane potential, action potential amplitude, phase 0 upstroke velocity ($\dot{V}_{max}$), action potential duration and refractoriness. The electrophysiologic effects of ethmozin have been studied primarily on canine Purkinje fibers [484, 485]. The drug reduces $\dot{V}_{max}$ of phase 0 and action potential amplitude in a dose-dependent manner. At high concentrations (10 mg/L) ethmozin also slightly reduces the maximum diastolic potential [484]. Ethmozin has no effect on slow response action potentials in Purkinje fibers [486]. Ethmozin also decreases ventricular diastolic excitability probably by decreasing the threshold potential [486].

Ethmozin shortens the Purkinje fiber action potential duration, but the effective refractory period was not measured in these studies [484–485].

(B) Effects on impulse initiation. Ethmozin has no effect on the slope of spontaneous diastolic depolarization in Purkinje fibers. However it may decrease the spontaneous firing rate by shifting threshold potential to less negative values [484, 486]. Ethmozin does have very pronounced depressant effects on abnormal automaticity in stretched Purkinje fibers, Purkinje fibers treated with barium chloride or Purkinje fibers on the endocardial surface of one-day-old infarcts. It reduces the slope of phase 4 depolarization, causing a decrease in spontaneous rate and often totally suppresses spontaneous activity [486].

Ethmozin decreases the amplitude of delayed afterdepolarizations in Purkinje fibers on the endocardial surface of one-day-old canine infarcts [486] and in Purkinje fibers poisoned with ouabain [487].

Electrophysiologic effects on the heart
Ethmozin has no effects on sinus rate, even when injected directly into the sinus node artery in dogs

[485]. Although the drug is not usually given intravenously to humans, in studies in which it has been given intravenously to dogs, it has had no significant effects on the P–R interval or QRS duration [484]. Oral ethmozin increases the P–R interval and QRS duration slightly in humans and has no effect on the Q–T interval [483, 488, 489].

Effects on the circulation
The effects of ethmozin on the circulation have not been systematically investigated. It appears to have little or no effect on blood pressure when taken orally [482] but may cause slight hypotension when administered intravenously [484].

Pharmacokinetics

Administration, absorption, and distribution
Ethmozin is well absorbed from the stomach and small intestine and peak plasma levels occur within 60–75 min after a single oral dose [482, 483]. Oral doses of 125–500 mg produce plasma levels of 500–600 ng/ml in healthy volunteers [482]. As yet, no relationship has been established between plasma levels and antiarrhythmic effect.

The drug is almost completely metabolized but little is known concerning the site or mechanism of metabolism. The half-time for elimination in patients with normal hearts is 2–5 hr and this may be prolonged in patients with poor cardiac function [482].

Toxicity

Only mild side effects have been reported in patients receiving ethmozin [482, 483, 490, 491]. These side effects include diarrhea, dizziness, nausea, rash, and disorientation. Data from patients undergoing long-term antiarrhythmic therapy are not yet available.

Electrophysiologic basis for antiarrhytmic drug action

In Chapter 1 the electrophysiology of cardiac arrhythmias is reviewed. As explained in that chapter, cardiac arrhythmias often occur when there are certain abnormalities of the transmembrane potentials in one or another region of the heart. Ar-

Table 1. Electrophysiological mechanisms which may cause cardiac arrhythmias.

I. Arrhythmias caused by abnormal impulse generation
   A. Arrhythmias caused by automaticity
      1. Normal automaticity
      2. Abnormal automaticity
   B. Arrhythmias caused by afterdepolarizations
     (triggered arrhythmias)
      1. Early afterdepolarizations
      2. Delayed afterdepolarizations

II. Arrhythmias caused by abnormal impulse conduction
   A. Reentrant excitation

III. Simultaneous abnormalities of impulse generation
   and conduction
   A. Parasystole

---

rhythmias also can arise in cardiac cells in the absence of disease, since slow conduction, conduction block, and abnormal impulse initiation can occur in many healthy cardiac cells, such as those in the AV node. Table 1 outlines the several mechanisms thought to be responsible for the occurrence of arrhythmias [492–494]. The effects of antiarrhythmic drugs on each of these mechanisms will be discussed.

(A) Arrhythmias caused by abnormal impulse generation.

Normal Automaticity: Automaticity, the ability to initiate action potentials spontaneously is a normal property of cardiac cells in the sinus (SA) node, in some parts of the atria; in the AV valves, the atrioventricular junction, and in the Purkinje system. The normal automaticity that occurs in all these different cells results from a slow decline in membrane potential during the diastolic interval, or phase 4. The slow depolarization reflects a gradual shift in the balance between inward and outward current components in the direction of net inward (depolarizing) current. The outward current component is carried by K^+ and the inward current is carried by Na^+ and/or Ca^{+-} [495, 496]. When the spontaneous depolarization reaches threshold potential, an impulse is initiated, and, following repolarization, these events are repeated.

In the normal heart, the rate of impulse initiation due to automaticity of cells in the sinus node is sufficiently high that other potentially automatic

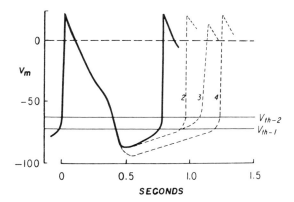

Figure 2. Mechanisms of antiarrhythmic drug action on normal automaticity. The solid line represents the time course of the change in transmembrane voltage in a Purkinje fiber that shows spontaneous diastolic depolarization. The fiber fires spontaneously when threshold voltage (V_{th-1}) is reached and the rate of firing is determined by the time it takes membrane potential to spontaneously decline from the maximum diastolic potential (MDP) to V_{th-1}. Possible mechanisms for antiarrhythmic drug effects on such an automatic rhythm are shown by action potentials 2, 3, and 4 indicated by the broken lines. Action potential 2 shows slowing of the rate caused by a decrease in the slope of phase 4 depolarization, action potential 3 shows slowing caused by a decrease in the slope of phase 4 depolarization and a positive shift in threshold potential from V_{th-1} to V_{th-2}, and action potential 4 shows a slowing caused by an increased maximum diastolic voltage and a decrease in the slope of phase 4 depolarization (reproduced from [31] with the permission of the author and the publishers).

cells are excited by propagated impulses before they can spontaneously depolarize to threshold potential. In this way the potential automaticity of other cardiac cells is suppressed [497]. A shift in the site of impulse initiation to an automatic region other than the sinus node would be expected to occur when the rate of activation of the heart by impulses from the sinus node falls considerably below the intrinsic rate of subsidiary pacemakers or when impulse initiation in a subsidiary pacemaker is enhanced, such as under the influence of the sympathetic nervous system. Thus, atrial or ventricular premature depolarizations or tachycardias may sometimes be caused by impulse initiation, caused by normal automaticity, in subsidiary pacemakers.

Antiarrhythmic drugs may sometimes exert their therapeutic effect by slowing or stopping these subsidiary or ectopic pacemakers which are generating impulses by their normal automatic mechanism (Figure 2). The use of an antiarrhythmic drug to suppress automaticity in subsidiary pacemakers should be reserved for instances when the sinus node is functioning normally or nearly normally and has been supplanted as the dominant pacemaker by enhancement of automaticity in the ectopic pacemaker. When automatic activity is depressed in the subsidiary pacemaker by the antiarrhythmic drug, the sinus node pacemaker once again can become the dominant pacemaker if it has not been depressed by the antiarrhythmic agent.

The rate at which automatic rhythms are generated by ectopic pacemakers (as well as by the sinus node) is determined by the time taken for phase 4 depolarization to carry the membrane potential to threshold, so that changes in either maximum diastolic potential, threshold potential, or the rate of spontaneous depolarization can alter the rate of automatic activity [498]. Thus, there is the potential for antiarrhythmic drugs to depress the rate of automatic activity by increasing maximum diastolic potential, by decreasing threshold potential, by slowing the rate of phase 4 depolarization (decreasing the slope), or by a combination of any or all of these actions (Figure 2).

The antiarrhythmic drugs discussed in this chapter, which suppress the initiation of impulses by normal automatic mechanisms in ectopic pacemakers, do so in concentrations which have minimal effects on the normal automaticity of the sinus node. In toxic concentrations automaticity in both sinus node and ectopic pacemakers may be suppressed.

Abnormal Automaticity: Working atrial and ventricular myocardial cells do not normally show spontaneous diastolic depolarization and do not initiate spontaneous impulses, even when they are not excited for long periods of time. However, when the resting membrane potentials of atrial or ventricular myocardial cells are experimentally reduced to less than about –60 mV, spontaneous diastolic depolarization may occur and cause repetitive impulse initiation by these fibers [499, 500]. This is called *abnormal automaticity*. A similar decrease in membrane potential of atrial and ventricular cells caused by disease also may lead to abnormal automaticity. Likewise, Purkinje fibers, which have the property of normal automaticity at normal levels of membrane potential, also show abnormal automaticity when membrane potential is reduced [501].

At the low level of membrane potential at which abnormal automaticity occurs it is likely that at least some of the ionic currents causing the automatic activity are not the same as those causing normal automatic activity. This has potential therapeutic implications since this type of automaticity may not respond to antiarrhythmic drugs in the same way as normal automaticity. In addition, because of the low level of membrane potential, the spontaneously occurring action potentials may be slow responses [501].

The rate of firing of abnormally automatic cells is determined, as for normally automatic fibers, by the time required for diastolic depolarization to carry membrane potential to threshold. Antiarrhythmic drugs might suppress arrhythmias caused by abnormal automaticity by increasing maximum diastolic potential, decreasing threshold potential or slowing the rate of phase 4 depolarization (see Figure 2). However, because of the different membrane currents involved in abnormal automaticity, it may not be suppressed by many of the drugs which suppress normal automaticity.

One major difference between normal and abnormal automaticity is the significant involvement

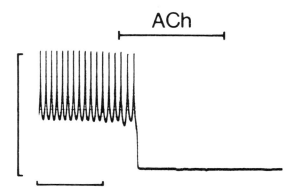

Figure 3. Abnormal automaticity in a Purkinje fiber at the low level of membrane potential. The vertical bar at the left represents 100 mV and its upper end indicates the zero potential level. The lower horizontal bar represents 10 sec. Maximum diastolic potential is about –50 mV. Acetylcholine (Ach) 10^{-5} M, was applied to the preparation for the period indicated by the horizontal bar over the record. It shifted the membrane potential from the low to the high level, probably by increasing membrane K^+ conductance. Abnormal automaticity was abolished because of this shift. Antiarrhythmic drugs which increase K^+ conductance or decrease Na^+ conductance are expected to have similar effects (reproduced from Gadsby DC, Wit AL, Cranefield PF: The effects of acetylcholine on the electrical activity of canine cardiac Purkinje fibers. Circ Res 43:29–35, 1978 with the permission of the Am Heart Assoc, Inc).

211

of slow inward current in the mechanism for spontaneous diastolic depolarization and for the action potential upstroke in abnormally automatic cells. Therefore slow channel blocking drugs may suppress impulse initiation by abnormally automatic fibers by decreasing the slope of spontaneous diastolic depolarization or by completely abolishing the upstroke of the action potential [371]. Another important means by which drugs might abolish impulse initiation by an abnormal automatic focus is to increase the level of membrane potential of the depolarized fibers. For example, normal Purkinje fibers show two quite different levels of membrane potential under appropriate experimental conditions; a high level of around –90 mV at which normal automaticity occurs and a low level at around –50 mV at which abnormal automaticity occurs. Experimentally, if membrane potential is at the low level, it can be shifted to the high level by reducing the steady state, background inward Na$^+$ current, or by increasing membrane K$^+$ conductance [142] (Figure 3). Abnormal automaticity stops when membrane potential shifts to the high level. Lidocaine has been shown to shift membrane potential from the low to the high level in Purkinje fibers [142, 502], probably because it decreases steady-state Na$^+$ currents [19]. Similar increases in membrane potential have been reported to occur after phenytoin or propranolol [502]. At the present time, most drugs have not been studied on the two stable levels of membrane potentials in Purkinje fibers, and the role of the two stable levels for causing arrhythmias has not been defined.

Abnormal automaticity might also occur as a consequence of the toxic effects of certain antiarrhythmic drugs. Toxic concentrations of quinidine and procainamide cause cardiac cells to depolarize, and automatic activity occurs at the depolarized level of membrane potential.

Early and Delayed Afterdepolarizations: Another mechanism for impulse generation in cardiac cells is that which is dependent on afterdepolarizations (see Chapter 1). The nondriven rhythmic impulses dependent on afterdepolarizations are called triggered impulses or triggered activity [503]. Early afterdepolarizations usually occur during phase 3 of repolarization of cells with high levels of maximum diastolic potential; membrane potential changes in a positive direction relative to the membrane potential expected during normal repolarization [382]

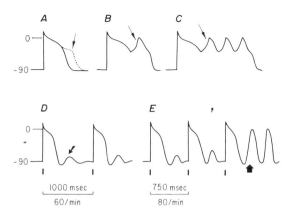

Figure 4. Triggered activity caused by early and delayed afterdepolarizations. A–C shows early afterdepolarizations in a Purkinje fiber. The normal Purkinje fiber action potential is indicated by the solid trace in A. The broken trace in A indicates the time course of the membrane potential changes during an early afterdepolarization. In B, membrane potential during the early afterdepolarization reaches threshold for the slow inward current and a second action potential occurs prior to repolarization of the first. In C, a train of triggered action potentials occurs before the fiber repolarizes. In D and E, action potentials caused by propagating impulses (indicated by vertical lines) are followed by delayed afterdepolarizations (arrow in D). In E, triggered activity caused by the afterdepolarizations occurs at the arrow (reproduced from Wit AL, Rosen MR: Cellular electrophysiology of cardiac arrhythmias. I. Arrhythmias caused by abnormal impulse generation. Mod Concepts Cardiovasc Dis 50:1–6, 1981 with permission of the publishers).

(Figure 4A). Under certain conditions membrane potential during the early afterdepolarization may reach threshold potential for reactivation of the slow inward current and a second action potential occurs prior to complete repolarization of the first (Figure 4B). The upstroke of the second action potential is caused by slow inward current since the fast Na current is inactivated at this low level of membrane potential. The second upstroke may in turn be followed by more action potentials still occurring prior to repolarization of the original initiating action potential. Because these action potentials occur at the low level of membrane potential, they may be caused by the same membrane currents responsible for abnormal automatic activity in partially depolarized fibers.

The train of triggered action potentials, if occurring at a rate more rapid than the rate at which the sinus node activates the heart, should cause a paroxysm of tachycardia. Although the exact role of triggered activity dependent on early afterdepolari-

212

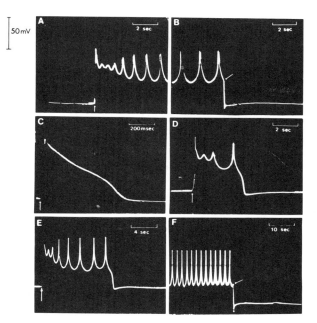

Figure 5. The effects of lidocaine on triggered activity caused by early afterdepolarizations in an isolated Purkinje fiber preparation. In panel A, the upstroke of an action potential was induced by electrical stimulus at the arrow. During repolarization slow oscillatory and triggered activity occurred which persisted for many minutes. B shows that the triggered activity had to be terminated by a hyperpolarizing current pulse applied at the arrow, which returned membrane potential to the high resting level. The fiber did not repolarize to the level by itself. After superfusion with lidocaine, shown in C, electrical stimulation induced an action potential; lidocaine caused repolarization to occur with a normal time course, and, therefore, there was no triggered activity. After lidocaine washout (D–F) early afterdepolarizations and triggered activity reappeared (reproduced from [62]).

zations in causing arrhythmias is not known, and there are little data on the effects of the antiarrhythmic drugs, certain actions of antiarrhythmic drugs can be predicted to terminate arrhythmias caused by early afterdepolarizations. First, since this type of triggered activity is so similar to abnormal automaticity, drugs which suppress abnormal automaticity, such as the slow channel blockers, can be expected to stop this kind of triggered activity. These drugs may not affect the abnormalities in repolarization but only prevent the activity occurring at the low level of membrane potential prior to complete repolarization. Second, drug actions which promote or accelerate repolarization should prevent early afterdepolarizations and triggered ac-

tivity [62] (Figure 5). Such actions may be (a) decreasing steady-state inward currents such as Na^+ and Ca^{++} currents which may retard repolarization and lead to early afterdepolarizations and (b) increasing outward K^+ currents to hasten repolarization. Lidocaine, the beta-blocker, tolamolol, and procainamide have been shown to prevent early afterdepolarizations and triggered activity in Purkinje fibers [62]; these drugs may decrease background Na^+ current [19].

Toxic effects of antiarrhythmic drugs also may cause early afterdepolarizations and triggered activity, particularly when the drugs prolong action potential duration to a large extent. N-acetylprocainamide, a metabolic product of procainamide, can cause early afterdepolarizations and triggered activity [76].

Delayed afterdepolarizations are transient or phasic depolarizations which occur after the terminal repolarization of an action potential and which are induced by that action potential (Figure 4D). If an afterdepolarization is large enough to bring the membrane potential to threshold, a nondriven (triggered) impulse arises which is also followed by an afterdepolarization. If the afterdepolarization following that triggered impulse reaches threshold, then a second triggered impulse arises and in this way a self-sustaining train of triggered action potentials may be generated. Such triggered activity caused by delayed afterdepolarizations cannot occur in the absence of an initiating action potential.

The basic mechanisms which cause delayed afterdepolarizations may be quite different from those responsible for automaticity or early afterdepolarizations. In general, the amplitude of delayed afterdepolarizations is increased by interventions which enhance calcium uptake into the cells, such as an increase in the rate of stimulation, elevation of external Ca^{++} concentration, addition of catecholamines, and application of cardiac glycosides. On the other hand, agents known to reduce Ca^{++} influx via the slow inward current channel, such as Mn^{++} and slow channel blocking drugs (D^{600}, verapamil) reduce the amplitude of delayed afterdepolarizations [504]. These results suggest that Ca^{++} is somehow involved in the genesis of these afterdepolarizations, and voltage clamp studies on the transient inward current underlying digitalis-induced delayed afterdepolarizations in Purkinje fibers have led to the conclusion that the in-

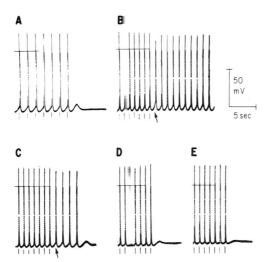

Figure 6. Effects of verapamil on delayed afterdepolarizations and triggering in atrial fibers of the canine coronary sinus. In each panel the last seven stimulated action potentials of a series of ten are shown. Panels A and B show control recordings. In A the fiber was stimulated at a cycle length of 1,100 msec. The last stimulated action potential was followed by an afterdepolarization. In B, the fiber was stimulated at a cycle length of 1,000 msec. Sustained rhythmic activity was triggered at the arrow. Panels C–E show recordings during superfusion with verapamil. The fiber is stimulated at a cycle length of 1,000 msec in all panels. At the left (C), after exposure to the drug for 10 min only a short period of sustained rhythmic activity is triggered at the arrow. In the center (D) after exposure to verapamil for 15 min, sustained rhythmic activity cannot be triggered and the last driven action potential is followed by a small afterdepolarization. In the right panel (E) after exposure to verapamil for 20 min, triggering cannot be induced and the afterdepolarization is barely noticeable (reproduced from [383] with the permission of the Am Heart Assoc, Inc).

ward current is linked in some way to a phasic release of Ca^{++} from an 'overloaded' intracellular Ca^{++} store which is probably the sarcoplasmic reticulum [384]. The effects of slow channel blockers and of variations in stimulation rate, external Ca, etc. mentioned above would then be attributable to their effects on the degree of 'loading' of that store.

Delayed afterdepolarizations and triggered activity are caused by the toxic effects of cardiac glycosides on Purkinje fibers, and some of the arrhythmias associated with digitalis toxicity may be caused by this mechanism [305]. Delayed afterdepolarizations and triggered activity have also been found to occur in atrial fibers, including those lining the coronary sinus, those in the mitral valve, and fibers from diseased human atria [504]. The

relationship between the occurrence of these delayed afterdepolarizations and atrial arrhythmias is unclear, since the studies in which afterdepolarizations have been clearly demonstrated have been on isolated, superfused preparations. Delayed afterdepolarizations and triggered activity have also been found to occur in Purkinje fibers surviving in experimental canine infarcts, raising the possibility that they might cause ischemic ventricular arrhythmias [506].

At the present time there is very little information available concerning the actions of antiarrhythmic drugs on triggered activity caused by delayed afterdepolarizations [143, 144, 237, 291, 413, 506]. For the reasons mentioned above, slow channel blocking drugs (e.g., verapamil) do prevent this sort of triggered activity [504, 144] (Figure 6). Other types of drugs also are effective. It is predicted that small increases in outward current during afterdepolarizations should diminish their amplitude and, perhaps, prevent triggered activity. Acetylcholine has this effect on atrial fibers and some antiarrhythmic drugs might exert a similar action. Drugs which decrease the inward current during afterdepolarizations should also prevent triggering. Antiarrhythmic drugs which alter the time course of the voltage change during the action potential might also indirectly influence the amplitude of delayed afterdepolarizations. Acceleration of repolarization and shortening of action potential duration may decrease the amount of calcium entering the cell, thus diminishing afterdepolarization amplitude [24]. Increases in maximum diastolic potential might also decrease afterdepolarization amplitude since the amplitude in many tissues is dependent on the level of membrane potential. Further studies must be done to determine which actions of specific antiarrhythmic drugs contribute to their effects on delayed afterdepolarizations.

(B) Arrhythmias caused by abnormal impulse conduction and reentry

Reentry occurs when a propagating impulse does not die out after complete activation of the heart but persists to reexcite it after the end of the refractory period. For this to happen, the impulse must remain somewhere in the heart while the cardiac fibers it has excited regain excitability so that the impulse can reenter and reactivate them. While

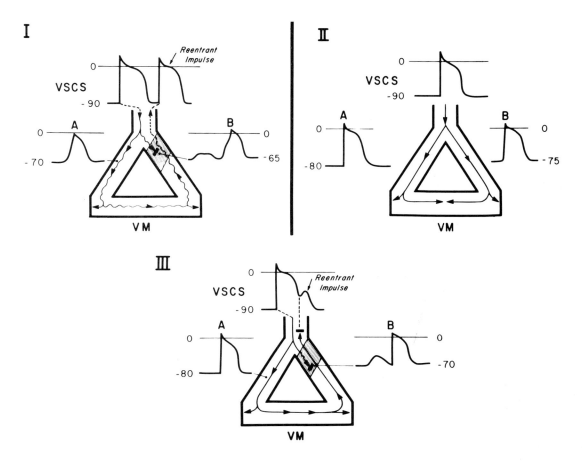

Figure 7. The Schmitt-Erlanger model for reentry and possible effects of antiarrhythmic drugs. Panel I shows reentry in a loop composed of Purkinje fiber bundles (A and B) and ventricular muscle (VM). An impulse conducts into the loop from the main bundle at the top (VSCS) prior to its bifurcation into branches A and B. The action potentials in a main bundle of the conducting system (VSCS) have a high level of membrane potential (–90 mV) and are normal. The resting and action potentials in branches A and B are depressed. Action potentials recorded from branch A arise from low membrane potentials and have a slow rate of depolarization resulting in slowed conduction through this branch as indicated by the wavy line and arrows. The Purkinje fibers near the origin of branch B (shaded area) have still lower membrane potentials and there is unidirectional conduction block in this region; there is only a low amplitude response during antegrade conduction block (1st response under B), preventing branch B from being excited. The impulse which slowly conducts through branch A and ventricular muscle can return through branch B, because of the block, and since conduction is unidirectional, an action potential with a slow upstroke is initiated in B during retrograde conduction (second action potential in trace B). The impulse which conducts retrograde in B enters the conducting system (VSCS) as the reentrant impulse. The area of unidirectional block provides the return pathway for the reentering impulse; slow conduction through the reentrant pathway (around the loop) provides the time necessary for the fibers in the VSCS to repolarize so they can be excited by the reentering impulse. Panels II and III show how reentry can be abolished if conduction is improved. As shown in II, if a drug increased membrane potential and $\dot{V}_{max}$ of phase 0 in branches A and B abolishing unidirectional block, a normal activation pattern in the peripheral loop would be restored. Speeding of conduction in the loop might abolish reentry even if unidirectional block persisted (III). Rapid conduction around the loop would result in the return of the impulse to the VSCS before fibers in this region recover excitability and conduction block of the reentering impulse would occur (reproduced from Wit AL, Rosen MR, Hoffman BF: Electrophysiological and pharmacology of cardiac arrhythmias. VIII. Cardiac effects of diphenylhydantoin B. Am Heart J 90:397–404, 1975 with permission of the publisher).

215

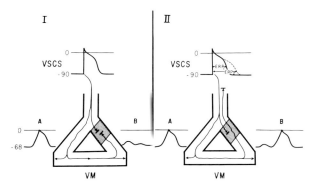

Figure 8. The Schmitt-Erlanger model for reentry and possible effects of antiarrhythmic drugs. The conduction pattern leading to reentry was shown in Panel I of Figure 7. Panel I in this figure shows the activation pattern after a drug has converted the area of unidirectional block in branch B to one of complete (bidirectional) block. The reentering impulse cannot return to reexcite the Purkinje fibers in the main bundle of the ventricular specialized conducting system (VSCS). Panel II shows the effects of a drug which prolonged the effective refractory period of fibers in the VSCS from ERP_1 to ERP_2. The pattern of impulse conduction leading to reentry is not altered, but the impulse returns to the VSCS before it has recovered excitability and, therefore, conduction of the reentering impulse is blocked.

awaiting the end of the refractory period the impulse can continue to conduct slowly through a pathway which is functionally isolated from the rest of the heart. Such a conduction pathway must provide a return route to the regions which previously have been excited and must be sufficiently long to permit propagation of the impulse during the refractory period. This reentrant pathway may be located in any region of the heart, including the sinus node, atrium, AV node, ventricular conducting system, and ventricles [507].

The role of unidirectional block and slow conduction: The exact mechanisms underlying the occurrence of reentry are described in Chapter 1. Prerequisite conditions, which usually are necessary, are transient or unidirectional block and some degree of slowed conduction. The region of block is necessary to provide the return pathway for the reentering impulse to parts of the heart that it has already excited. Reentry may occur after transient block caused by premature excitation or when there is permanent but unidirectional block (Figures 7 and 8). In addition, for reentry to occur, the site at which the impulse leaves the reentrant pathway must recover excitability by the time the impulse

conducts through this pathway and returns to reexcite regions it has already excited. If excitability has not recovered, the reentering impulse will be blocked in the refractory tissue and die out.

Antiarrhythmic drugs can stop reentrant excitation by affecting conduction and/or refractoriness in or around the reentrant circuit. They do this by altering the transmembrane action potentials of normal and abnormal cardiac fibers through their effects on inward or outward membrane currents.

One very important action of some of the drugs is to cause complete conduction block in the reentrant circuit. The area of undirectional block may be converted to an area of bidirectional block, or complete block may occur elsewhere in the circuit. In either event, conduction through the reentrant pathway is abolished. Block occurs because of the effects of the drugs on the inward current during the action potential upstroke. Drugs with local anesthetic effects interact with Na^+ channels, causing a decrease in Na^+ conductance. A model which describes this interaction is shown in Figure 9 [7, 10]. The model of use dependence proposes that the antiarrhythmic drugs can interact with membrane Na^+ channels in the resting (R), activated (A), and inactivated states (I). The drug interaction with the channel or its affinity for the channel is character-

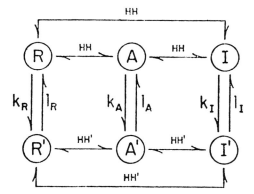

Figure 9. Schematic representation of a model of the Na^+ channel for the description of antiarrhythmic drug action (a description is in the text). R, A, and I indicate the channel in the resting, activated, and inactivated states when not occupied by drug. R', A', and I' indicate the resting, activated, and inactivated states of the drug-occupied channel. Both unoccupied and occupied channels move between states by Hodgkin-Huxley (HH) kinetics. k and l are the association and dissociation rate constants for drug interaction with the sodium channels in each of the three states: each drug has its own characteristic constants (reproduced from [10]).

ized by an association (k) and dissociation (l) rate constant which is different for each of the channel states. Thus, in the figure the R', A', and I' indicate the fraction of channels in each state which are interacting with or occupied by the drug, and this fraction is in equilibrium with unoccupied channels. Both drug-occupied and unoccupied channels cycle back and forth during an action potential between resting, activated, and inactivated states, but drug-associated channels do not conduct Na^+ ions even in the activated state. Hence, $\dot{V}_{max}$ of phase 0 and the amplitude of the action potential is reduced by the drug.

During the upstroke of the action potential some of the antiarrhythmic drugs with local anesthetic properties may interact mainly with activated channels rather than with resting or inactivated channels. A fraction of channels is occupied and blocked during each action potential upstroke, and this fraction depends on the affinity of the drug for the channel. For example, since lidocaine has a much greater affinity than quinidine for the Na^+ channel, more channels are blocked per upstroke and block develops more rapidly (after fewer upstrokes) with lidocaine than with quinidine [7]. The development of increasing block of the Na^+ channels with each successive action potential upstroke is called *use-dependent block*.

After the upstroke of the action potential both blocked and unblocked channels enter the inactivated state (I and I'). Removal of inactivation and the transition to the resting state then occurs during repolarization. The association and dissociation constants for drugs such as lidocaine and quinidine are relatively long in the inactivated state so relatively few channels block or unblock during this time. Therefore, most channels which were occupied and blocked by drug during the action potential upstroke remain occupied. During repolarization, removal of inactivation of the drug free channels and their transition to the resting state occurs normally, but removal of inactivation of the drug-associated channels is delayed. These channels behave as if the transmembrane potential is more positive than it actually is. When the drug-occupied channels do return to the resting state they unblock relatively quickly because the rate constants for dissociation and association are much smaller than during the inactivated state. Thus, there is low affinity for drug during the R–R' state.

Most of the blocking of the Na^+ channel therefore occurs during the action potential upstroke and unblocking occurs during the diastolic period between action potentials. If the heart rate is slow enough, most of the channels which are blocked during the upstroke may unblock during diastole. However, as the heart rate increases there is less time for drug-associated inactivated channels to be reactivated and enter the resting state because the time for removal of inactivation of these channels is slowed. Channels may therefore accumulate in the I' pool and remain inactivated since blocked inactivated (I' channels) only slowly unblock. The effects of the drug to depress conduction, therefore, are enhanced.

This model also suggests why some antiarrhythmic drugs exert more of a depressant effect on $\dot{V}_{max}$ of partially depolarized fibers which still have Na-dependent upstrokes (depressed fast responses) than on normal fibers (for example, see the section on Effects of lidocaine on cardiac fibers). In depolarized cells more channels exist in the I state and are probably recycled back to the R state at a much slower rate than in normally polarized cells. Since the I' to I route for unblocking is very slow, more channels are blocked by drug [7, 10, 508–510].

At the present time the precise way in which many of the different antiarrhythmic drugs interact with the Na^+ channel have not been defined. It is conceivable that some drugs may associate more rapidly with inactivated or resting channels, rather than with activated channels.

The decrease in Na^+ conductance which results from interaction of local anesthetic-type antiarrhythmic drugs with the Na^+ channel causes a decrease in conduction velocity. Because of the increased Na^+ channel blockade in depressed fast response fibers, depression of conduction is greater in reentrant pathways, where cardiac fibers are diseased, than in normal regions of the heart, and conduction block may occur, abolishing reentry. Antiarrhythmic drugs also may cause conduction block more readily in reentrant pathways during rapid arrhythmias than during sinus rhythm, since the degree of interaction between many of the antiarrhythmic drugs with local anesthetic properties and the Na^+ channel is determined to a large extent by the frequency of depolarizations (action potentials).

As described above and in Chapter 1, the slow

conduction and unidirectional block which cause reentry may also be a consequence of slow response action potentials in diseased regions of the atria or ventricles. Verapamil and other slow channel blocking drugs which decrease the slow inward current may abolish the slow response action potential and cause complete conduction block in these reentrant pathways.

Another way in which antiarrhythmic drugs may stop reentry is by increasing the effective refractory period of cardiac fibers in or around the reentrant circuit. Drugs which prolong the refractory period in the reentrant pathway may cause conduction block of reentering impulses, if these impulses arrive in the pathway prior to the recovery of excitability. Drugs which prolong refractoriness of the normal myocardium can prevent reexcitation of the heart after the impulse has traversed the reentrant circuit (Figure 8). Prolongation of the effective refractory period also might prevent the initiation of reentry by premature impulses since it may cause conduction block of these premature impulses.

The changes in refractory period caused by a drug may not be uniform throughout a given region of the heart. For example, some antiarrhythmic drugs, such as bretylium, prolong the effective refractory period of Purkinje fibers with short refractory periods to a greater extent than they prolong the refractory period of Purkinje fibers with long refractory periods. Other drugs, such as lidocaine, may, under certain circumstances, shorten the effective refractory period more in fibers with long initial refractory periods than in fibers with short initial refractory periods [43, 137]. The same sort of action might occur in atrial myocardium. Since the differences in refractory periods within a region might cause functional unidirectional block and therefore reentrant excitation, drugs which abolish these differences might prevent reentry [511].

Antiarrhythmic drugs which prolong the effective refractory period of cardiac fibers with fast response action potentials may do so by slowing the removal of inactivation of the Na^+ channels so that reactivation occurs only at higher levels of membrane potential than prior to drug action [31, 47]. Slow channel blocking drugs increase the time constant for reactivation of the slow channel in fibers with slow response action potentials, including the sinus and atrioventricular nodes [379].

The refractory period of atrial, ventricular, or Purkinje cells may also be changed by drugs which change the time course of repolarization. Repolarization results from an imbalance between maintained inward and outward membrane currents in the plateau range of membrane potentials. Inward-directed current components include a 'background' Na^+ current, flowing through incompletely inactivated Na channels, and the slow inward current, carried by both sodium and calcium ions. At least one of the outwardly directed membrane currents is likely to be a potassium current flowing in a gated channel whose permeability is both time and voltage dependent. Other contributions to outward membrane current in this potential range are expected to be made by a time-independent (background) K^+ current, by chloride influx, and by activity of the electrogenic Na^+/K^+ pump [512, 513]. Thus, drugs which decrease any of the inward currents or increase conductance for outward currents may shorten action potential duration, whereas drugs which have opposite effects may prolong action potential duration. Since recovery from inactivation of the Na current is, to a large extent, voltage dependent, these changes in action potential duration will influence the time for recovery and thus change the refractory period.

Reentry also can be abolished by improving conduction in the reentrant circuit, i.e., if the area of unidirectional block is converted to an area of normal, bidirectional conduction or if conduction velocity is increased. Converting the area of unidirectional block to an area of normal, bidirectional conduction eliminates the return pathway since this pathway is activated in the antegrade direction (Figure 7). Increasing conduction velocity results in the impulse traversing the reentrant circuit and returning to its point of origin prior to the complete recovery of excitability of cardiac cells in this region, possibly causing conduction block of reentering impulses in refractory tissue (Figure 7). Conduction of the impulse in reentrant circuits would be improved if V_{max} of depressed fast responses were increased or if slow responses in diseased areas of the heart were converted back to fast responses. Both effects might be brought about if antiarrhythmic drugs could increase the steady-state level of membrane potential in partially depolarized cells. One way in which this could occur would be for a drug to increase K^+ conductance, if conductance was low. Although it has been proposed that

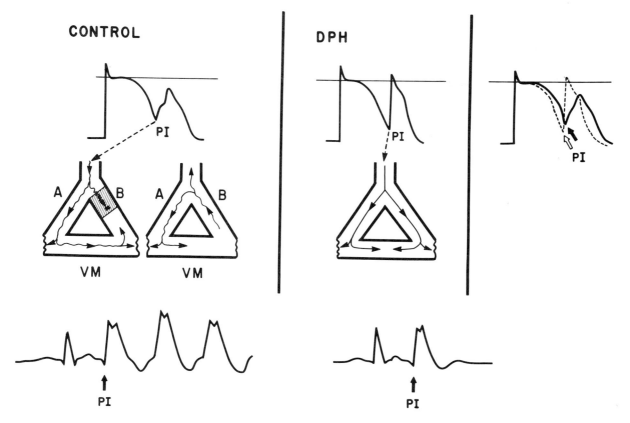

Figure 10. Mechanism by which shortening action potential duration relative to effective refractory period may abolish reentry. In the control panel (left), a premature impulse (PI) arises during the repolarization phase of a Purkinje fiber, at the end of the effective refractory period, and as a result has a very slow upstroke velocity (top). This premature impulse conducts slowly into a loop of Purkinje fiber bundles (A and B), and ventricular muscle (VM) as indicated by the arrow, blocks in the antegrade direction in branch B, and conducts slowly through branch A, VM and into B in a retrograde direction (diagram at left in control panel). The impulse continues back through B as a reentrant depolarization and then continues to conduct around the loop again (diagram at right in control panel). At the bottom, the ECG is shown; the premature impulse (PI) that causes reentry is followed by a run of ventricular tachycardia. In the center panel the proposed effects of a drug which shortens action potential duration relative to the effective refractory period is shown. Now, the earliest premature impulse arises from a higher level of membrane potential; therefore, its upstroke velocity is increased. This premature impulse conducts more rapidly and activates the Purkinje fiber muscle loop in a normal manner; there is no reentry. On the ECG at the bottom only the initial premature impulse is seen, but it is not followed by ventricular tachycardia. In the panel at the right the control action potentials (solid trace) and the action potentials after the drug (dashed trace) are superimposed. Note that the earliest premature impulse after the drug arises from a more negative membrane potential and has a more rapid rate of depolarization than the earliest premature impulse prior to administering the drug (reproduced from Wit AL, Rosen MR, Hoffman BF: Electrophysiology and pharmacology of cardiac arrhythmias. VIII. Cardiac effects of diphenylhydantoin. Am Heart J 90:397–404, 1975 with permission of the publishers).

lidocaine might have this effect, it is still a subject of controversy [31, 47]. There is no good evidence that any of the other drugs significantly increase the level of membrane potential.

Another way in which antiarrhythmic drugs might prevent reentry is to improve conduction of premature impulses. As mentioned previously, in some situations reentry might only occur when a premature impulse conducts in fibers which are relatively refractory, and thus the necessary slow conduction and block occur only because the cardiac fibers have not yet fully repolarized. Antiarrhythmic drugs which accelerate repolarization may result in premature impusles occurring at higher levels of membrane potential than prior to drug administration. Such premature impusles may conduct more rapidly after drug and reentry due to slowed conduction, and unidirectional clock of the premature impulse may be abolished (Figure 10). This might also occur when action potential duration is shortened to a greater extent than is the effective refractory period by a drug or when the effective refractory period is prolonged to a greater extent than the action potential duration [160]. Both effects may cause premature impulses to arise at higher levels of membrane potential and thus conduct more rapidly.

References

1. Moe GK, Abildskov JA: Antiarrhythmic Drugs, Inc. In: Goodman LS, Gilman A (eds) The Pharmacological Basis of Therapeutics. Macmillan Publ Co, Inc, New York, 1970, pp 709–727.

2. Frey W: Weitere Erfahrungen mit Chiniden bei absoluter Herzunregelmässigkeit. W en Klin Wochenschr 55:849–861, 1918.

3. Hoffman BF: The action of quinidine and procainamide on single fibers of dog ventricle and specialized conducting system. An Acad Bras Cienc 29:365–368, 1958.

4. Vaughan Williams EM, Szekeres L: A comparison of tests of antifibrillatory action. Br J Pharmacol 17:424–432, 1961.

5. West TC, Amory DW: Single fiber recording of the effect of quinidine at atrial pacemaker sites in the isolated right atrium of the rabbit. J Pharmacol Exp Ther 130:183–193, 1960.

6. Chen CM, Gettes LS, Katzung BG: Effects of lidocaine and quinidine on steady-state characteristics and recovery kinetics of (dv/dt) max in guinea pig ventricular myocardium. Circ Res 37:20–29, 1975

7. Hondeghem LM, Katzung BG: Test of a model of antiarrhythmic drug action: effects of quinidine and lidocaine on myocardial conduction. Circulation 61:1217–1224, 1980.

8. Johnson EA, McKinnon MG: The differential effect of quinidine and pyrilamine on the myocardial action potential at different rates of stimulation. J Pharmacol Exp Ther 120:460–468, 1957.

9. Grant AO, Trantham JL, Brown KK, Strauss HC: pH-Dependent effects of quinidine on the kinetics of dv/dt max in guinea pig ventricular myocardium. Circ Res 50:210–217, 1982.

10. Hondeghem LM, Katzung BC: Time and voltage-dependent interactions of antiarrhythmic drugs with cardiac sodium channels. Biochim Biophys Acta 474:373–398, 1977.

11. Nattel S, Elharrar V, Zipes D, Bailey JC: pH-dependent electrophysiological effects of quinidine and lidocaine on canine cardiac Purkinje fibers. Circ Res 48:55–61, 1981.

12. Dreifus LS, Azevedo IH, Watanabe Y: Electrolyte and antiarrhythmic drug action. Am Heart J 88:95–107, 1974.

13. Watanabe Y, Dreifus L, Likeff W: Electrophysiological antagonism and synergism of potassium and antiarrhythmic agents. Am J Cardio 12:702–710, 1963.

14. Hoffman BF, Rosen MR, Wit AL: Electrophysiology and pharmacology of cardiac arrhythmias VII. Cardiac effects of quinidine and procainamide. Am Heart J 90:117–122, 1975.

15. Hondeghem LM: Effects of lidocaine, phenytoin and quinidine on ischemic canine myocardium. J Electrocardiol 9:203–209, 1976.

16. Nawrath H: Action potential, membrane currents and force of contraction in mammalian heart muscle fibers treated with quinidine. J Pharmacol Exp Ther 216:176–182, 1981.

17. Vaughan Williams EM: The mode of action of quinidine on isolated rabbit atria interpreted from intracellular potential electrodes. Br J Pharmacol 13:276–287, 1958.

18. Mirro MJ, Watanabe AM, Bailey JC: Electrophysiological effects of the optical isomers of disopyramide and quinidine in the dog. Dependence on stereochemistry. Circ Res 48:867–874, 1981.

19. Colatsky T: Mechanisms of action of lidocaine and quinidine on action potential duration in rabbit cardiac Purkinje fibers: an effect on steady-state sodium currents? Circ Res 50:17–27, 1982.

20. Mirro MJ, Manalan AS, Bailey JC, Watanabe AM: Anticholinergic effects of disopyramide and quinidine on guinea pig myocardium; mediation by direct muscarinic receptor blockade. Circ Res 47:855–865, 1980.

21. Carmeliet E, Saikawa T: Shortening of the action potential and reduction of pacemaker activity by lidocaine, quinidine and procainamide in sheep cardiac Purkinje fibers: an effect on Na or K currents? Circ Res 50:257–272, 1982.

22. De Francesco D: a new interpretation of the pacemaker current in Purkinje fibers. J Physiol (Lond) 314:359–376, 1981.

23. Grant AO, Katzung BG: The effects of quinidine and verapamil on electrically induced automaticity in the ventricular myocardium of guinea pig. J Pharmacol Exp Ther 196:407–419, 1976.

24. Henning B, Wit AL: Multiple mechanisms of antiarrhythmic drug action on delayed afterdepolarizations in canine coronary sinus. Am J Cardiol 49:913, 1982 (abstract).

25. Henning B, Vereecke J, Carmeliet E, Wit AL: Block of transient inward current by TTX and local anesthetics. Circulation (Suppl II): II–356, 1982.

26. Josephson ME, Seides SF, Batsford WP, Weisfogel GM, Akhtar M, Carcacta AR, Lau SH, Damato AN: The electrophysiological effects of intramuscular quinidine on the atrioventricular conducting system in man. Am Heart J 87:55–64, 1974.

27. Roberts J, Stadter RP, Cairoli V, Modell W: Relationship between adrenergic activity and cardiac actions on quinidine. Circ Res 11:758–764, 1962.

28. Schmid PG, Nelson LD, Mark AL, Heistad DD, Abboud FM: Inhibition of adrenergic vasoconstriction by quinidine. J Pharmacol Exp Ther 188:124–134, 1974.

29. Mason JW, Winkle RA, Rider AK, Stinson EB, Harrison DC: The Electrophysiologic effects of quinidine in the transplanted human heart. J Clin Invest 59:481–489, 1977.

30. Wallace AG, Cline RE, Sealy WC, Young WG, Troyer WG: Electrophysiologic effect of quinidine: studies using chronically implanted electrodes in awake dogs with and without cardiac denervation. Circ Res 19:960–969, 1966.

31. Bigger JR Jr: Management of arrhythmias. In: Braunwald E (ed) Heart Disease: A Textbook of Cardiovascular Medicine. Saunders, Philadelphia, 1980, pp 691–743.

32. Heissenbuttel RH, Bigger JT Jr: The effect of oral quinidine on intraventricular conduction in man: correlation of plasma quinidine with changes in QRS duration. Am Heart J 80:453–462, 1970.

33. Lu G: The mechanism of the vasomotor action of quinidine. J Pharmacol Exp Ther 103:441–449, 1951.

34. Ferrer IM, Harvey RM, Wrko L, Dresdale DT, Cournand A, Richards DW Jr: Some effects of quinidine sulfate on the heart and circulation in man. Am Heart J 36:816–837, 1948.

35. Markiewicz W, Winkle RA, Binetti G, Kernoff R, Harrison DC: Normal myocardial contractile state in the presence of quinidine. Circulation 53:101–106, 1976.

36. Parmley WW, Braunwald E: Comparative myocardial depressant and antiarrhythmic properties of d-propranolol, dl propranolol and quinidine. J Pharmacol Exp Ther 158:11–21, 1967.

37. Greenblatt DJ, Pfeifer HJ, Ochs HR, Franke K, MacLaughlin DS, Smith TW, Koch-Weser J: Pharmacokinetics of quinidine in humans after intravenous, intramuscular, and oral administration. J Pharmacol Exp Ther 202:365–378, 1977.

38. Bellet S: The Clinical Disorders of the Heart Beat. Lea and Febiger, Philadelphia, 1971.

39. Conn HL Jr, Luchi RJ: Some quantitative aspects of the binding of quinidine compounds by human serum albumin. J Clin Invest 40:509–516, 1961.

40. Scherlis L, Gonzales LF, Bessman SP: Quinidine: arterial, venous, coronary sinus and myocardial concentrations. J Clin Invest 40:60–66, 1961.

41. Ueda CT, Hirschfeld DS, Scheinman MM: Disposition kinetics of quinidine. Clin Pharmacol Ther 19:30–36, 1976.

42. Ueda CT, Williamson BJ, Bzindzio BS: Absolute quinidine bioavailability. Clin Pharmcol Ther 20:260–265, 1976.

43. Palmer KH, Martin B, Baggett B, Wall ME: The metabolic fate of orally administered quinidine gluconate in humans. Biochem Pharmacol 18:1845–1860, 1969.

44. Nwangwu PU, Holcslaw TL, Small TD, Stohs SJ: A preliminary evaluation of 6'-hydroxycinchonine as an antiarrhythmic agent. Pharmacologist 19:152, 1977 (abstract).

45. Drayer DE, Lowventhal DT, Restivo KM, Schwartz A, Cook CE, Reidenberg MM: Steady-state serum levels of quinidine and active metabolites in cardiac patients with varying degrees of renal function. Clin Pharmacol Ther 24:31–39, 1978.

46. Gerhardt RD, Knouss RF, Thyrum PT, Luchi RJ, Morris JT: Quinidine excretion in aciduria and alkaluria. Ann Intern Med 71:927–933, 1969.

47. Arnsdorf MF, Hsieh Y: Antiarrhythmic agents. In: Hurst JW (ed) The Heart. McGraw Hill Inc, New York, 1978, pp 1943–1963.

48. Conrad KA, Molk BL, Chidsey CA: Pharmacokinetic studies of quinidine in patients with arrhythmias. Circulation 55:1–7, 1977.

49. Leahey EB Jr, Reiffel JA, Drusin RE, Heissenbuttel RH, Lovejoy WP, Bigger JT Jr: Interaction between quinidine and digoxin. J Am Med Assoc 240:533–534, 1978.

50. Bigger JT Jr: The quinidine–digoxin interaction. Mod Concepts Cardiovasc Dis 51:73–78, 1982.

51. Doherty JE, Straub KD, Murphey ML, de Soyza N, Bissett JK, Kane JJ: Digoxin–quinidine interaction changes in canine tissue concentration from steady state with quinidine. Am J Cardiol 45:1196–1200, 1980.

52. Data JL, Wilkinson GR, Nies AS: Interaction of quinidine with anticonvulsant drugs. N Engl J Med 294:699–702, 1976.

53. Koch-Weser J: Quinidine-induced hypoprothrombinemic hemorrhage in patients on chronic warfarin therapy. Ann Intern Med 68:511–577, 1968.

54. Shep DS, Myerberg R: Drug interactions involving antiarrhythmic drugs. In: Petrie JC (ed) Cardiovascular and Respiratory Disease Therapy. Elsevier, Amsterdam, 1980, pp 43–59.

55. Mautz FR: The reduction of cardiac irritability by the epicardial and systemic administration of drugs as a protection in cardiac surgery. J Thorac Surg 5:612–618, 1936.

56. Mark LC, Kayden HJ, Steele JM, Cooper JR, Berlin I, Rovenstein EA, Brodie BB: The physiological disposition and cardiac effects of procaine amide. J Pharmacol Exp Ther 102:5–15, 1951.

57. Rosen MR, Gelband H, Hoffman BF: Canine electrocardiographic and cardiac electrophysiologic changes induced by procainamide. Circulation 46:528–536, 1972.

58. Rosen M, Gelband H, Merker C, Hoffman B: Effects of procaine amide on the electrophysiological properties of the canine ventricular conducting system. J Pharmacol Exp Ther 185:438–446, 1973.

59. Sada H, Kojima M, Ban T: Effect of procainamide on transmembrane action potential in guinea pig papillary muscle as affected by external potassium concentration. Naunyn Schmiedebergs Arch Pharmacol 309:179–190, 1979.

60. Arnsdorf MF, Bigger JT: The effect of procaineamide on components of excitability in long mammalian cardiac Purkinje fibers. Circ Res 38:115–122, 1976.

61. Hordof A, Edie R, Malm J, Rosen M: Effects of procaineamide and verapamil on electrophysiologic properties of human atrial tissues. Pediatr Res 9:267, 1975 (abstract).

62. Arnsdorf MF: The effect of antiarrhythmic drugs on triggered sustained rhythmic activity in cardiac Purkinje fibers. J Pharmacol Exp Ther 201:689–700, 1977.

63. Schmid PG, Nelson LD, Heistad DD, Mark AL, Abboud FM: Vascular effects of procaineamide in the dog. Predominance of the inhibitory effect on ganglionic transmission. Circ Res 35:948–960, 1974.

64. Wyse DG, McAnulty JH, Stadius M, Rahimtoola SH: Electrophysiologic effects of procainamide in patients with normal and prolonged sinoatrial conduction times. Am J Cardiol 41:386, 1978 (abstract).

65. Scheinman MM, Weiss AN, Shafton E, Benowitz N, Rowland M: Electrophysiologic effects of procaine amide on patients with intraventricular conduction delay. Circulation 49:522–529, 1974.

66. Josephson ME, Carcacta AR, Riccuiti MA, Lau SH, Damato AN: Electrophysiologic properties of procainamide in man. Am J Cardiol 33:596–603, 1974.

67. Giardina EGV, Heissenbuttel RH, Bigger JT Jr: Intermittent intravenous procaineamide to treat ventricular arrhythmias. Correlation of plasma concentration with effect on arrhythmias, electrocardiogram and blood pressure. Ann Intern Med 78:183–193, 1973.

68. Giardina EGV, Bigger JT Jr: Procaine amide against reentrant ventricular arrhythmias: lengthening R–V intervals of coupled ventricular premature depolarizations as an insight into the mechanism of action of procaine amide. Circulation 48:959–970, 1973.

69. Bigger JT Jr, Giardina EGV: The pharmacology and clinical uses of lidocaine and procainamide. M Coll Va Q 9:65–71, 1973.

70. Bigger JT Jr, Heissenbuttel RH: The use of procaine amide and lidocaine in the treatment of cardiac arrhythmias. Prog Cardiovasc Dis 11:515–534, 1969.

71. Giardina EGV, Dreyfuss J, Bigger JR Jr, Shaw JM, Schreiber EC: Metabolism of procainamide in normal and cardiac subjects. Clin Pharmacol Ther 19:339–351, 1976.

72. Koch-Weser J, Klein SW: Procainamide dosage schedules, plasma concentrations and clinical effects. J Am Med Assoc 215:1454–1456, 1971.

73. Hoffman BF, Rosen MR, Wit AL: Electrophysiology and pharmacology of cardiac arrhythmias VII. Cardiac effects of quinidine and procaine amide A. Am Heart J 89:804–808, 1975.

74. Koch-Weser J, Klein SW, Foo-Canto LL, Kastor JA, DeSanctis RW: Antiarrhythmic prophylaxis with procainamide in acute myocardial infarction. N Engl J Med 281:1253–1260, 1969.

75. Dreyfuss J, Bigger JT Jr, Cohen AL, Schreiber EC: Metabolism of procainamide in rhesus monkey and man. Clin Pharmacol Ther 13:336–371, 1972.

76. Dangman KH, Hoffman BF: In vivo and in vitro antiarrhythmic and arrhythmogenic effects of N-acetylprocainamide. J Pharmacol Exp Ther 217:851–862, 1981.

77. Elison J, Strong JM, Lee WK, Atkinson AJ Jr: Antiarrhythmic potency of N-acetylprocainamide. Clin Pharmacol Ther 17:134–140, 1975.

78. Giardina EGV, Stein RM, Bigger JT Jr: The relationship between metabolism of procainamide and sulfamethazine. Circulation 55:388–394, 1977.

79. Galeazzi RL, Sheiner LB, Lock T, Benet LS: The renal elimination of procainamide. Clin Pharmacol Ther 19:55–62, 1976.

80. Gibson TP, Lowenthal DT, Nelson HA, Briggs WA: Elimination of procainamide in end stage renal failure. Clin Pharmacol Ther 17:321–329, 1975.

81. Ladd AT: Procainamide-induced lupus erythematosus. N Engl J Med 267:1357–1358, 1962.

82. Davies DM, Beedie MA, Rawlins MD: Antinuclear antibodies during procainamide treatment and drug acetylation. Br Med J 3:682–684, 1975.

83. Mokler CM, Van Arman CG: Pharmacology of a new antiarrhythmic agent α-disopropylamino α-phenyl-α-(2-pyridyl)-butyramide (SC-7031). J Pharmacol Exp Ther 136:114–124, 1962.

84. Mirro MJ, Watanabe AM, Bailey JC: Electrophysiological effects of disopyramide and quinidine on guinea pig atria

and canine cardiac Purkinje fibers. Circ Res 46:660–668, 1980.

85. Sekija A, Vaughan Williams EM: A comparison of the anti-fibrillatory actions and effects on intracellular cardiac potentials of pronetholol, disopyramide, quinidine. Br J Pharmacol 21:473–487, 1963.

86. Kus T, Sasyniuk BI: Electrophysiological actions of disopyramide phosphate on canine ventricular muscle and Purkinje fibers. Circ Res 37:844–854, 1975.

87. Danilo P Jr, Hordof AJ, Rosen MR: Effect of disopyramide on electrophysiologic properties of canine cardiac Purkinje fibers. J Pharmacol Exp Ther 201:701–710, 1977.

88. Kus T, Sasyniuk BI: The electrophysiological effects of disopyramide phosphate on canine ventricular muscle and Purkinje fibers in normal and low potassium. Can J Physiol Pharmacol 56:139–149, 1978.

89. Sasyniuk BI, Kus T: Effects of disopyramide phosphate (DP) on membrane responsiveness, conduction and refractoriness in infarcted canine ventricle. Fed Proc 35:235, 1976.

90. Chiba S, Kobayashi M, Furukawa Y: Effects of disopyramide on SA nodal pacemaker activity and contractility in the isolated blood perfused atrium of the dog. Eur J Pharmacol 57:13–19, 1979.

91. Seipel L, Breithardt G: Sinus recovery time after disopyramide phosphate. Am J Cardiol 37:1118–1119, 1976.

92. LaBarre A, Strauss HC, Scheinman MM, Evans GT, Bashore T, Tiedeman JS, Wallace AG: Electrophysiologic effects of disopyramide phosphate on sinus node function in patients with sinus node dysfunction. Circulation 59:226–235, 1979.

93. Befeler B, Castellanos A, Wells DE, Vagueiro MC, Yeh BK: Electrophysiologic effects of the antiarrhythmic agent disopyramide phosphate. Am J Cardiol 35:282–287, 1975.

94. Josephson ME, Carcacta AR, Lau SH, Gallagher JJ, Damato AN: Electrophysiological evaluation of disopyramide in man. Am Heart J 86:771–780, 1973.

95. Birkhead JS, Vaughan Williams EM: Dual effect of disopyramide on atrial and atrioventricular conduction and refractory periods. Br Heart J 39:657–660, 1977.

96. Swiryn S, Bauerfeind RA, Wyndham CRC, Dhingra RC, Palileo E, Strasberg B, Rosen KM: Effects of oral disopyramide phosphate on induction of paroxysmal supraventricular tachycardia. Circulation 64:169–175, 1981.

97. Kus T, Sasyniuk B: Disopyramide phosphate: it is just another quinidine? Can J Physiol Pharmacol 56:326–331, 1978.

98. Mathur PP: Cardiovascular effects of a newer antiarrhythmic agent – disopyramide phosphate. Am Heart J 84:764–770, 1972.

99. Marrott PK, Ruttley MST, Winterbottam JT, Muir JR: A study of the acute electrophysiologic and cardiovascular action of disopyramide in man. Eur J Cardiol 4:303–310, 1976.

100. Podrid PJ, Schoeneberger A, Lown B: Congestive heart failure caused by oral disopyramide. N Engl J Med 302:614, 1980.

101. Lawrie TDV: Comparison of newer anti-arrhythmic agents. Am Heart J 100(pt 2):990–994, 1980.

102. Kotter V, Linderer T, Schroder R: Effects of disopyramide on systemic and coronary hemodynamics and myocardial metabolism in patients with coronary artery disease: comparison with lidocaine. Am J Cardiol 46: 469–475, 1980.

103. Walsh RA, Horwitz LD: Adverse hemodynamic effects of intravenous disopyramide compared with quinidine in conscious dogs. Circulation 60:1053–1058, 1979.

104. Vismara L: Clinical studies of norpace (II). Angiology 26:132–136, 1975.

105. Chien YW, Lambert HJ, Karim A: Comparative binding of disopyramide phosphate and quinidine sulfate to human plasma proteins. J Pharmacol Sci 63:1877–1879, 1974.

106. Hinderling PH, Bres J, Garrett ER: Protein binding and erythrocyte partitioning of disopyramide and its mono-dealkylated metabolite. J Pharmacol Sci 63:1684–1690, 1974.

107. Harrison DC, Meffin PJ, Winkle RA: Clinical Pharmacokinetics of antiarrhythmic drugs. Prog Cardiovasc Dis 20: 217–242, 1977.

108. Hinderling PH, Garrett ER: Pharmacodynamics of the antiarrhythmic disopyramide in healthy humans: Correlation of the kinetics of the drug and its effects. J Pharmacokinet Biopharm 4:231–242, 1976.

109. Karim A: The pharmacokinetics of Norpace. Angiology 26:85–98, 1975.

110. Baines MW, Davies JE, Kellet DN, Munt PL: Some pharmacological effects of disopyramide and a metabolite. J Int Med Res 4:5–7, 1976.

111. Grant AM, Marshall RJ, Ankier SI: Some effects of disopyramide and its N-dealkylated metabolite on isolated nerve and cardiac muscle. Eur J Pharmacol 49:389–394, 1978.

112. Aitio ML, Aitio A: Induction of disopyramide N-dealkylation by phenobarbital and disopyramide in rat liver. Arch Intern Pharmacodyn Ther 239:16–23, 1979.

113. Hinderling PH, Garrett ER: Pharmacokinetics of the antiarrhythmic disopyramide in healthy humans. J Pharmacokinet Biopharm 4:119–229, 1976.

114. Whiting B, Elliot HL: Disopyramide in renal impairment. Lancet 2:1363, 1977.

115. Rangno RE, Wanuch W, Ogilvie RI: Correlation of disopyramide pharmacokinetics with efficacy in ventricular tachyarrhythmias. J Int Med Res 4(Supp 1):54–58, 1976.

116. Ilett K, Madsen BW, Woods JD: Disopyramide kinetics in patients with acute myocardial infarction. Clin Pharmacol Ther 26:1–7, 1979.

117. Ward JW, Kinghom CR: The pharmacokinetics of disopyramide following myocardial infarction with special reference to oral and intravenous dose regimens. J Int Med Res 4(Supp 1):49–53, 1976.

118. Lofgren N: Studies on local anesthetics. Xylocaine, A New Synthetic Drug. Ivar Haeggstroms, Stockholm, 1948 (reprinted by Marin Press, Inc, Worcester, MA).

119. Southworth JL, McKusick VA, Pierce EC, Rawson FL Jr: Ventricular fibrillation precipitated by cardiac catheterization. J Am Med Assoc 143:717–720, 1950.

120. Davis LD, Temte JV: Electrophysiological actions of lidocaine on canine ventricular muscle and Purkinje fibers. Circ Res 24:639–655, 1969.

121. Bigger JT Jr, Mandel WT: Effect of lidocaine on transmembrane potentials of ventricular muscle and Purkinje fibers. J Clin Invest 49:63–77, 1970.

122. Mandel WJ, Bigger JT Jr: Electrophysiologic effects of lidocaine on isolated canine and rabbit atrial tissues. J Pharmacol Exp Ther 178:81–93, 1971.

123. Weld FM, Bigger JT Jr: Effect of lidocaine on the early inward transient current in sheep cardiac Purkinje fibers. Circ Res 37:630–639, 1975.

124. Bean BP, Cohen CJ, Tsien RW: Lidocaine Binding to Resting and Inactivated cardiac sodium channels. Biophys J 33:208, 1981.

125. Lee KS, Hume JR, Giles W, Brown AM: Sodium current depression by lidocaine and quinidine in isolated ventricular cells. Nature 291:325–327, 1981.

126. Singh BN, Vaughan Williams EM: Effect of altering potassium concentrations on the action of lidocaine and diphenylhydantoin on rabbit atrial and ventricular muscle. Circ Res 29:286–295, 1971.

127. Obayashi K, Hayakawa H, Mandel WJ: Interrelationships between external potassium concentration and lidocaine: effects on the canine Purkinje fibers. Am Heart J 89:221–226, 1975.

128. Rosen MR, Merker C, Pippenger CE: The effects of lidocaine on the canine ECG and electrophysiologic properties of Purkinje fibers. Am Heart J 91:191–202, 1976.

129. Rosen MR, Hoffman BF, Wit AL: Electrophysiology and pharmacology of cardiac arrhythmias. V. Cardiac antiarrhythmic effects of lidocaine. Am Heart J 89:526–536, 1975.

130. Tritthart H, Fleckenstein B, Fleckenstein A: Some fundamental actions of anti-arrhythmic drugs on the excitability and contractility of single myocardial fibers. Naunyn Schmiedebergs Arch Pharmacol 269:212–219, 1971.

131. Gintant GA, Hoffman BF: Different local anesthetic characteristics of charged and uncharged forms of lidocaine and other antiarrhythmic drugs in canine cardiac Purkinje fibers. Am J Cardiol 49:1044, 1982.

132. Gintant G, Hoffman BF, Naylor RE: The influence of molecular form on the interactions of local anesthetic-type antiarrhythmic agents with canine cardiac Na^+ channel. Circ Res (in press).

133. Brennan FJ, Cranefield PF, Wit AL: Effects of lidocaine on slow response and depressed fast response action potentials of canine cardiac Purkinje fibers. J Pharmacol Exp Ther 204:312–324, 1978.

134. Grant AO, Strauss LJ, Wallace AG, Strauss HC: The influence of pH on the electrophysiological effects of lidocaine in guinea pig ventricular myocardium. Circ Res 47:542–550, 1980.

135. Lazzara R, Hope RR, El-Sherif N, Scherlag BJ: Effects of lidocaine on hypoxia and ischemic cardiac cells. Am J Cardiol 41:872–879, 1978.

136. Josephson I, Sperelakis N: Local anesthetic blockade of Ca^{+2} mediated action potentials in cardiac muscle. Eur J Pharmacol 40:201–208, 1976.

137. Wittig J, Harrison LA, Wallace AG: Electrophysiological effects of lidocaine on distal Purkinje fibers of the canine heart. Am Heart J 86:69–75, 1973.

138. Gettes LS, Reuter H: Slow recovery from inactivation of inward currents in mammalian myocardial fibers. J Physiol (Lond) 240:703–724, 1974.

223

139. Katzung BG: Drug effects on ventricular automaticity. Proc West Pharmacol Soc 17:15–18, 1974.

140. Imanishi S, McAllister RG Jr, Surawicz B: The effects of verapamil and lidocaine on the automatic depolarizations in guinea-pig ventricular myocardium. J Pharmacol Exp Ther 207:294–303, 1978.

141. Arita M, Nagamoto Y, Saikawa T: Automaticity and time dependent conduction disturbance produced in canine ventricular myocardium. Jpn Circ J 40:1408–1418, 1976.

142. Gadsby DC, Cranefield PF: Two levels of resting potential in cardiac Purkinje fibers. J Gen Physiol 70:725–746, 1977.

143. Mary-Rabine L, Hordof AJ, Danilo P Jr, Malm J, Rosen MR: Mechanisms for impulse initiation in isolated human atrial fibers. Circ Res 47:267–277, 1980.

144. Rosen MR, Danilo P: Effects of tetrodotoxin, lidocaine, verapamil and AHR-2666 on ouabain-induced delayed afterdepolarizations in canine Purkinje fibers. Circ Res 46:117–124, 1980

145. Cheng TO, Wadhwa N: Sinus standstill following intravenous lidocaine administration. J Am Med Assoc 223:790–792, 1973.

146. Lippestad CT, Forgang K: Production of sinus arrest by lignocaine. Br Med J 1:537 1971.

147. Jersaty R, Kahn A, Landry A: Sinoatrial arrest due to lidocaine in a patient receiving quinidine. Chest 61:683–684, 1972.

148. Agrawal BU, Singh RB, Vaish SK: Cardiac asystole due to lidocaine in patients with digitalis toxicity. Acta Cardiol 29:341–347, 1974.

149. Barrett PA, Laks MM, Mandel WJ, Yamaguchi I: The electrophysiologic effects of intravenous lidocaine in the WPW syndrome. Am Heart J 100:23–33, 1980.

150. Rosen KM, Lau SH, Weiss MB, Damato AN: The effect of lidocaine on atrioventricular and intraventricular conduction in man. Am J Cardiol 25:1–5, 1970.

151. Josephson ME, Carcacta AR, Lau SH, Gallagher JJ: Effects of lidocaine on refractory periods in man. Am Heart J 84:778–786, 1972.

152. Allen JD, Brennan FJ, Wit AL: Actions of lidocaine on transmembrane potentials of subendocardial Purkinje fibers surviving in infarcted canine heart. Circ Res 43:470–481, 1978.

153. Wang CM, James CA, Maxwell RA: Effects of lidocaine on the electrophysiological properties of subendocardial Purkinje fibers surviving acute myocardial infarction. J Mol Cell Cardiol 11:669–681 1979.

154. Frieden J: Antiarrhythmic drugs. VI. Lidocaine as an antiarrhythmic agent. Am Heart J 70:713–715, 1965.

155. Kupersmith J, Antman EM, Hoffman BF: In vivo electrophysiologic effects of lidocaine in canine acute myocardial infarction. Circ Res 36:84–91, 1975.

156. El-Sherif N, Scherlag BJ, Lazzara R, Hope RR: Reentrant ventricular arrhythmias in the late myocardial infarction period. IV. Mechanism of action of lidocaine. Circulation 56:395–402, 1977.

157. Gerstenbluth G, Spear JF, Moore EN: Quantitative study of the effect of lidocaine on the threshold for ventricular fibrillation in the dog. Am J Cardiol 30:242–247, 1972.

158. Grossman JI, Cooper JA, Frieden J: Cardiovascular effects of infusion of lidocaine in patients with heart disease. Am J Cardiol 24:191–197, 1969.

159. Harrison DC, Sprouse JH, Morrow AG: The antiarrhythmic properties of lidocaine and procainamide. Circulation 29:486–491, 1963.

160. Bigger JT Jr, Hoffman BF: Antiarrhythmic Drugs. In: Gilman AG, Goodman L, Gilman A (eds) The Pharmacological Basis of Therapeutics. Macmillan, New York, 1980.

161. Benowitz NL, Forsyth RP, Melmon LK, Rowland M: Lidocaine disposition kinetics in monkey and man. Clin Pharmacol Ther 16:87–98, 1974.

162. Boyes RN, Scott DB, Jebson PJ, Godman MJ, Julian DG: Pharmcokinetics of lidocaine in man. Clin Pharmacol Ther 12:105–116, 1971.

163. Rowland M, Thomson PD, Guichard A, Melmon K: Disposition kinetics of lidocaine in normal subjects. Ann NY Acad Sci 179:383–397, 1971.

164. Stenson RE, Constantino RT, Harrison DC: Interrelationship of hepatic blood flow, cardiac output and blood levels of lignocaine in man. Circulation 43:205–211, 1971.

165. Sung CV, Truant AP: The physiological disposition of lidocaine – its comparison is some respects with procaine. J Pharmacol Exp Ther 112:432–443, 1954.

166. Beckett AH, Boyes RN, Appleton PJ: The metabolism and excretion of lignocaine in man. J Pharm Pharmacol 18 (Suppl):76–81, 1966.

167. Hollunger G: On the metabolism of lidocaine. II. Biotransformation of lidocaine, hydrolysis of the amide linkage. Acta Pharmacol 17:365–373, 1960.

168. Smith ER, Duce BR: The acute antiarrhythmic and toxic effects in mice and dogs of 2-ethylamino-2'6'-acetoxylidine (L-86), a metabolite of lidocaine. J Pharmacol Exp Ther 179:580–585, 1971.

169. Blumer J, Strong JM, Atkinson AJ: The convulsant potency of lidocaine and its N-dealkylated metabolites. J Pharmacol Exp Ther 186:31–36, 1973.

170. Nation RL, Triggs EJ, Selig M: Lignocaine kinetics in cardiac patients and aged subjects. Br J Clin Pharmacol 4:439–448, 1977.

171. Perucca E, Richens A: Reduction of oral bioavailability of lignocaine by induction of first pass metabolism in epileptic patients. Br J Clin Pharmacol 8:21–31, 1979.

172. Nies AS, Shand DG, Wilkinson GR: Altered hepatic blood flow and drug disposition. Clin Pharmacokinet 1:135–155, 1976.

173. Thomson PD, Rowland M, Melmon KL: The influence of heart failure, liver disease and renal failure on disposition of lidocaine in man. Am Heart J 82:417–421, 1971.

174. Thomson PD, Melmon KL, Richardson JA, Cohn K, Steinbrunn W, Cudihee R, Rowland M: Lidocaine pharmcokinetics in advanced heart failure, liver disease and renal failure in humans. Ann Intern Med 78:499–508, 1973.

175. Prescott LF, Adjepon-Yamoah KK, Talbot RG: Impaired lignocaine metabolism in patients with myocardial infarction and cardiac failure. Br Med J 1:939–941, 1976.

176. Branch RA, Shand DG, Wilkinson GR, Nies AS: The reduction of lidocaine clearance by dl-propranolol: an example of a hemodynamic drug interaction. J Pharmacol Exp Ther 184:515–519, 1973.

177. Collinsworth KA, Strong JM, Atkinson AJ, Winkle RA, Perlroth F, Harrison DC: Pharmacokinetics and metabolism of lidocaine in patients with renal failure. Clin Pharmacol Ther 18:59–64, 1975.

224

178. Wiklund L: Human hepatic blood flow and its relation to systemic circulation during intravenous infusion of lignocaine. Acta Anaesthesiol Scand 21:148–160, 1977.

179. Le Lorier J, Latour Y, Grenon D, Caille G, Brosseau A, Solignac A, Du Mont G: The pharmcokinetics of lignocaine after prolonged intravenous infusions in man. Clin Res 28:624A, 1975.

180. Pfeifer HJ, Greenblatt DH, Koch-Weser J: Clinical use and toxicity of intravenous lidocaine. Am Heart J 92:168–173, 1976.

181. Bigger JT Jr, Heisenbuttel RH: The use of procainamide and lidocaine in the treatment of cardiac arrhythmias. In: Friedberg CK (ed) Current Status of Drug in Cardiovascular Disease. Grune and Stratton, New York, 1969, pp 125–144.

182. Investigators Brochure for Tocainide HCL. Astra Pharmaceutial Products, Inc, Jan, 1977.

183. Moore EM, Spear JF, Horowitz LN, Feldman HS, Moller RA: Electrophysiologic properties of a new anti-arrhythmic drug-tocainide. Am J Cardiol 41:703–709, 1978.

184. Oshita S, Sada H, Kojima M, Ban T: Effects of tocainide and lidocaine on the transmembrane action potentials as related to external potassium and calcium concentrations in guinea pig papillary muscles. Naunyn Schmeidebergs Arch Pharmacol 314:62–82, 1980.

185. Anderson JF, Mason JW, Winkle RA, Meffin PJ, Fowler RE, Peters F, Harrison DC: Clinical electrophysiologic effects of tocainide. Circulation 57:685–691, 1978.

186. McDevitt DG, Nies AS, Wilkinson GR, Smith RF, Woosley RL, Oates JA: Antiarrhythmic effects of a lidocaine congener, tocainide, 2-amino-2′, 6′-propionoxylidine, in man. Clin Pharmacol Ther 19:396–402, 1976.

187. Coltart DJ, Berndt TB, Kernoff R, Harrison DC: Antirrhythmic and circulatory effects of astra W36075, A new lidocaine like agent. Am J Cardiol 34:35–41, 1974.

188. Nyquist O, Forssell G, Nordlander R, Schenck-Gustafsson K: Hemodynamic and antiarrhythmic effects of tocainide in patients with acute myocardial infarction. Am Heart J 100(pt 2):1000–1005, 1980.

189. Winkle RA, Anderson JL, Peters F, Meffin PJ, Fowler RE, Harrison DC: The hemodynamic effects of intravenous tocainide in patients with heart disease. Circulation 57:787–792, 1978.

190. Lalka D, Meyer MB, Duce BR: Kinetics of oral antirrhythmic lidocaine congener tocainide. Clin Pharmacol Ther 19:757–776, 1976.

191. Winkle RA, Mason JW, Harrison DC: Tocainide of drug-resistant ventricular arrhythmias: efficacy, side effects and lidocaine responsiveness for predicting tocainide success. Am Heart J 100(pt 2):1031–1036, 1980.

192. Elvin AT, Keenagham JB, Byrnes EW, Tenthorey PA, McMaster PD, Takman BH, Lalka D, Manon CV, Baer T, Wolshin EM, Meyer MB: Conjugation of tocainide in man: evidence for a novel pathway of biotransformation for a primary amine. Pharmacologist 18:114, 1976 (abstract).

193. Elvin AT, Keenaghan JB, Byrnes EQ, Tenthorey PA, McMaster PD, Takman BH, Lalka D, Manon CV, Baer DT, Wolshin EM, Meyer MB, Ronfeld RA: Tocainide conjugation in humans: novel biotransformation pathway for a primary amine. J Pharmacol Sci 69:47–49, 1980.

194. Venkataramanan R, Axelson JE: Dose-dependent pharmcokinetics of tocainide in the rat. J Pharmacol Exp Ther 215:231–234, 1980.

195. Graffner C, Couradson T-B, Hofrendahl S, Ryden L: Tocainide kinetics after intravenous and oral administration in healthy subjects and in patients with acute myocardial infarction. Clin Pharmacol Ther 27:64–71, 1980.

196. Gibson JK, Somani P, Bassett AL: Electrophysiologic effects of encainide (MJ9067) on canine Purkinje fibers. Eur J Pharmacol 52:161–169, 1978.

197. Jackman WM, Zipes DP, Naccarelli GV, Rinkenberger RL, Heger JJ, Prystowsky EN: Electrophysiology of oral encainide. Am J Cardiol 49:1270–1279, 1982.

198. Roden DM, Reele SB, Higgins SB, Mayol RF, Gammans RE, Oates JA, Woosley RL: Total suppression of ventricular arrhythmias by encainide: pharmcokinetic and electrocardiographic characteristics. N Engl J Med 302:877–882, 1980.

199. Winkle RA, Peters F, Kates RE, Tucker C, Harrison DC: Clinical pharmacology and antiarrhythmic efficacy of encainide in patients with chronic ventricular arrhythmias. Circulation 64:290–296, 1981.

200. DiBanco R, Fletcher RD, Cohen AL, Gottdiener JS, Singh SN, Katz RJ, Mapp AF, Cockrell JL: Encainide treatment of chronic ventricular arrhythmia: a controlled prospective study. Circulation 64:IV-315, 1981.

201. Kesteloot H, Stroobandt R: Clinical experience of encainide (MJ9067): a new antiarrhythmic drug. Eur J Clin Pharmacol 16:323–329, 1979.

202. Elharrar V, Zipes DP: Effects of encainide and metabolites (MJ14030 and MJ9444) on canine cardiac Purkinje and ventricular fibers. J Pharmacol Exp Ther 220:440–447, 1982.

203. Sami M, Mason JW, Oh G, Harrison DC: Canine electrophysiology of encainide, a new anti-arrhythmic drug. Am J Cardiol 43:1149–1154, 1979.

204. Sami M, Mason JW, Peters F, Harrison DC: Clinical electrophysiologic effects of encainide, a newly developed antiarrhythmic agent. Am J Cardiol 44:526–532, 1979.

205. Carey EL Jr, Duff HJ, Roden DM, Primm RK, Oates JA, Woosley RL: Relative electrocardiographic and antirrhythmic effects of encainide and its metabolites in man. Circulation 64:IV-264, 1981.

206. Woosley RL, Roden DM, Duff HJ, Carey EL, Wood AJJ, Wilkinson GR: Co-inheritance of deficient oxidative metabolism of encainide and debrisoquine. Clin Res 29:501A, 1981.

207. Koppe HG: The development of mexiletine. Postgrad Med J 53(Suppl I):22–24, 1977.

208. Singh BN, Vaughan Williams EM: Investigations of the mode of action a new antidysrhthmic drug (Ko 1173). Br J Pharmacol 44:1–9, 1972.

209. Yamaguchi I, Singh B, Mandel W: Electrophysiological actions of mexiletine on isolated rabbit atria and canine ventricular muscle and Purkinje fiber. Cardiovasc Res 13:288–296, 1979.

210. Weld FM, Bigger JT, Swistel D, Bordiuk J, Lau YH:

Electrophysiological effects of mexiletine (Ko 1173) on ovine cardiac Purkinje fibers. J Pharmacol Exp Ther 210:222–228, 1979.

211. Iwamura N, Shimizu T, Toyoshima H, Toyama T, Yamada K: Electrophysiological actions of a new antiarrhythmic agent on isolated preparations of the canine Purkinje fiber and ventricular muscle. Cardiology 61:329–340, 1976.

212. Carmeliet E: Mechanisms of arrhythmias and of antiarrhythmic activity with special reference to mexiletine. Acta Cardiol (Suppl) 25:5–25, 1980.

213. Vaughan Williams EM: Mexiletine in isolated tissue models. Postgrad Med J (Suppl I) 53:30–34, 1977.

214. Harper RW, Olsson SB, Varnauskas E: Effect of mexiletine on monophasic action potentials recorded from the right ventricle in man. Cardiovasc Res 13:303–310, 1979.

215. Danneberg PB, Shelley JH: The pharmacology of mexiletine. Postgrad Med J 53(Suppl I):25–29, 1979.

216. Roos JC, Paalman DCA, Dunning AJ: Electrophysiological effects of mexiletine in man. Postgrad Med J 53(Suppl I): 92–94, 1977.

217. McComish M, Robinson C, Kitson D, Jewitt DE: Clinical electrophysiological effects of mexiletine. Postgrad Med J 53(Suppl I):85–91, 1977.

218. Saunamaki KI: Haemodynamic effects of a new antiarrhythmic agent, mexiletine (Ko 1173) in ischemic heart disease, Cardiovasc Res 9:738–792, 1975.

219. Pozenel H: Hemodynamic studies on mexiletine, a new antiarrhythmic agent. Postgrad Med J 53(Suppl I): 78–80, 1977.

220. Shaw TRD: The effect of mexiletine on left ventricular ejection: a comparison with lidocaine and propranolol. Postgrad Med J 53 (Suppl I):69–73, 1977.

221. Prescott LF, Pottage A, Clements JF: Absorption, distribution and elimination of mexiletine. Postgrad Med J 53(Suppl I):50–55, 1977.

222. Kiddie MA, Kaye CM, Turner P, Shaw TRD: The influence of urinary pH on the elimination of mexiletine. Br J Clin Pharmacol 1:229–232, 1974.

223. Clark RA, Julian DG, Nimmo J, Prescott LF, Talbot R: Clinical pharmacological studies of Ko 1173 – a new antiarrhythmic agent. Br J Pharmacol 47:622–623, 1973.

224. Prescott LF, Adjepon-Yamoah KK, Talbot RG: Impaired metabolism of lignocaine in patients with myocardial infarction and cardiac failure. Br Med J 1:939–941, 1976.

225. Beckett AH, Chidomere EC: The distribution, metabolism and excretion of mexiletine in man. Postgrad Med J 53(Suppl I):60–66, 1977.

226. Johnston A, Burgess CD, Warrington SJ, Wadsworth J, Hamer NAJ: The effect of spontaneous changes in urinary pH on mexiletine plasma concentrations and excretion during chronic administration to healthy volunteers. Br J Clin Pharmacol 8:349–352, 1979.

227. Talbot RG, Julian DG, Prescott LF: Long-term treatment of ventricular arrhythmias with oral mexiletine. Am Heart J 91:58–65, 1976.

228. Merrit HH, Putnam TJ: Sodium diphenylhydantoin in treatment of convulsive disorders. J Am Med Assoc 111: 1068–1073, 1938.

229. Harris AS, Kokernot RH: Effects of diphenylhydantoin sodium (dilantin sodium) and phenobarbital sodium upon

230. Mosey L, Tyler MD: The effects of diphenylhydantoin sodium (dilantin), procaine hydrochloride, procaine amide, hydrochloride and quinidine hydrochloride upon ouabain-reduced ventricular tachycardia in unanesthetized dogs. Circulation 10:65–70, 1964.

231. Coveno BG, Wright R, Charleson DA: Effectiveness of several antifibrillatory drugs in the hypothermic dog. Am J Physiol 181:54–58, 1955.

232. Scherf D, Blumenfeld S, Taner D, Yieldiz M: The effect of diphenylhydantoin (dilantin) sodium on atrial flutter and fibrillation provoked by focal application of aconitine and delphinine. Am Heart J 60:936–947, 1960.

233. Helfant RH, Scherlag BJ, Damato AN: The electrophysiological properties of diphenylhydantoin sodium as compared to procaine amide in the normal and digitalis-intoxicated heart. Circulation 36:108–118, 1967.

234. Leonard WA: The use of diphenylhydantoin (dilantin) sodium in the treatment of ventricular tachycardia. Arch Intern Med 101:714–717, 1958.

235. Jensen RA, Katzung BG: Electrophysiological actions of diphenylhydantoin on rabbit atria. Circ Res 26:17–27, 1970.

236. Katzung BG, Jensen RA: Depressant action of diphenylhydantoin on electrical and mechanical properties of isolated rabbit and dog atria: Dependence on sodium and potassium. Am Heart J 80:80–88, 1970.

237. Rosen MR, Danilo P Jr, Alonso MB, Pippenger CE: Effects of therapeutic concentrations of diphenylhydantoin on transmembrane potentials of normal and depressed Purkinje fibers. J Pharmacol Exp Ther 197:594–604, 1974.

238. Bigger JT, Strauss HC, Bassett AL, Hoffman BF: Electrophysiological effects of diphenylhydantoin on canine Purkinje fibers. Circ Res 22:221–236, 1968.

239. Strauss HC, Bigger JT, Bassett AL, Hoffman BF: Actions of diphenylhydantoin on the electrical properties of isolated rabbit and canine atria. Circ Res 23:463–477, 1968.

240. Bassett AL, Bigger JT Jr, Hoffman BF: 'Protective' action of diphenylhydantoin on canine Purkinje fibers during hypoxia. J Pharmacol Exp Ther 173:336–343, 1970.

241. Bigger JT Jr, Weinberg DI, Kovalik ATW, Harris PD, Cranefield PF, Hoffman BF: Effects of diphenylhydantoin on excitability and automaticity of canine heart. Circ Res 26:1–13, 1970.

242. Rosati RA, Alexander JA, Schaal SF, Wallace AG: Influence of diphenylhydantoin on electrophysiological properties of the canine heart. Circ Res 21:757–765, 1967.

243. Gillis RA, McClellan JR, Sauer TS, Standaert FG: Depression of cardiac sympathetic nerve activity diphenylhydantoin. J Pharmacol Exp Ther 179:599–610, 1971.

244. Evans DE, Gillis RA: Effect of diphenylhydantoin and lidocanine on cardiac arrhythmias induced by hypothalmic stimulation. J Pharmacol Exp Ther 191:506–517, 1974.

245. Unger AH, Sklaroff HJ: Fatalities following intravenous use of sodium diphenylhydantoin for cardiac arrhythmias. Report of two cases. J Am Med Assoc 200:335–336, 1967.

246. Louis S, Kutt H, McDowell F: The cardiocirculatory changes caused by intravenous dilantin and its solvent. Am Heart J 74:523–529, 1967.

247. Russell JM, Harvey SC: Effects of diphenylhydantoin on canine atria and A-V conducting system. Arch Int Pharmacodyn Ther 182:219–231, 1969.

248. Caracta AR, Damato AN, Josephson ME, Ricciutti MA, Gallagher JJ, Lau SH: Electrophysiologic properties of diphenylhydantoin. Circulation 47:1234–1241, 1973.

249. Bigger JR Jr, Schmidt DH, Kutt H: Relationship between the plasma level of diphenylhydantoin sodium and its cardiac antiarrhythmic effects. Circulation 38:363–374, 1968.

250. Damato AN, Berkowitz WD, Patton RD, Lau SH: The effect of diphenylhydantoin on atrioventricular and intraventricular conduction in man. Am Heart J 79:51–56, 1970.

251. Dhatt MS, Gomes JAC, Reddy CP, Akhtar M, Caracta AR, Lau SH, Damato AN: Effects of Phenytoin on refractoriness and conduction in the human heart. J Cardiol Pharmacol 1:3–18, 1979.

252. Bissett JK, DeSoyza NDB, Kane JJ, Murphy ML: Improved intraventricular conduction of premature beats after diphenylhydantoin. Am J Cardiol 33:493–497, 1974.

253. Mixter CG III, Moran JM, Austen WG: Cardiac and peripheral vascular effects of diphenylhydantoin sodium. Am J Cardiol 17:332–338, 1966.

254. Lieberson AD, Schumacher RR, Childress RH, Boyd DL, Williams JF Jr: Effect of diphenylhydantoin on left ventricular function in patients with heart disease. Circulation 36:692–699, 1967.

255. Puri PS: The effect of diphenylhydantoin sodium (dilantin) on myocardial contractility and hemodynamics. Am Heart J 82:62–68, 1971.

256. Wilensky AJ, Lowden JA: Inadequate serum levels after intramuscular administration of diphenylhydantoin. Neurology 23:318–324, 1973.

257. Kutt H, Winters W, Kokenge R, McDowell F: Diphenylhydantoin metabolism blood levels and toxicity. Arch Neurol 11:642–648, 1964.

258. Dill WA, Kazenko A, Wolf LA, Glazko AJ: Studies on 5, 5'-diphenylhydantoin (dilantin) in animals and man. J Pharmacol Exp Ther 118:270–279, 1956.

259. Kutt H: Biochemical and genetic factors regulating dilantin metabolism in man. Ann NY Acad Sci 179:704–722, 1971.

260. Butler TC: Metabolic conversion of 5-5-diphenylhydantoin to 5'-(phydroxyphenyl)-5 phenylhydantoin. J Pharmacol Exp Ther 119:1–11, 1957.

261. Maynert EW: The metabolic fate of diphenylhydantoin in the dog, rat and man. J Pharmacol Exp Ther 130:275–284, 1960.

262. Kutt H, Haynes J, McDowell F: Some causes of ineffectiveness of diphenylhydantoin. Arch Neurol 14:489–492, 1966.

263. Bigger JT Jr: A method for the estimation of plasma diphenylhydantoin concentration. Am Heart J 77:572–573, 1969.

264. Gerber N, Wagner JG: Explanation of dose-dependent decline of diphenylhydantoin plasma levels by fitting to the integrated form of the Michaelis-Menten equation. Res Commun Chem Pathol Pharmacol 3:455–466, 1972.

265. Arnold K, Gerber N: The rate of decline of diphenylhydantoin in human plasma. Clin Pharmacol Ther 11:121–134 1970.

266. Atkinson AJ, Shaw JJ: Pharmacokinetic study of a patient with diphenylhydantoin toxicity. Clin Pharmacol Ther 14:521–528, 1973.

267. Kutt H, Verebely K: Metabolism of diphenylhydantoin by rat liver microsomes I. Characteristics of the reaction. Biochem Pharmacol 19:675–680, 1970.

268. Gerber N, Weller WL, Lynn R, Rangno RE, Sweetman BJ, Bush MT: Study of dose-dependent metabolism of 5,5-diphenylhydantoin in the rat using new methodology for isolation and quantitation of metabolites in vivo and in vitro. J Pharmacol Exp Ther 178:567–579, 1971.

269. Kutt H, Winters W, Scherman R, McDowell F: Diphenylhydantoin and phenobarbital toxicity; the role of liver disease. Arch Neurol 11:649–656, 1964.

270. Kutt H, Wolk M, Scherman R, McDowell F: Insufficient parahydroxylation as a cause of diphenylhydantoin toxicity. Neurology 14:542–548, 1964.

271. Cucinelli SA, Conney AH, Sansur M, Burns JJ: Drug interactions in man. I. Lowering effect of phenbarbital on plasma levels of bishyoroxycoumarin (dicumarol) and diphenylhydantoin (dilantin). Clin Pharmacol Ther 6:420–429, 1965.

272. Kutt H, Haynes J, Verebely K, McDowell F: The effect of phenobarbital on plasma diphenylhydantoin level and metabolism in man and in rat liver microsomes. Neurology 19:611–616, 1969.

273. Odar-Cederhof I, Borga O: Kinetics of DPH in uraemic patients: Consequences of decreased plasma protein binding. Eur J Clin Pharmacol 7:31–37, 1974.

274. Reidenberg M, Odar-Cederlof I, Bahr Von C, Borga O, Sjogvist F: Protein binding of DPH and desmethylimipramine in plasma from patients with poor renal function. N Engl J Med 285:264–267, 1971.

275. Sparberg M: Diagnostically confusing complications of DPH therapy. Ann Intern Med 59:914–930, 1963.

276. The Norwegian Multicenter Study Group: Timolol-induced reduction in mortality and reinfarction in patients surviving acute myocardial infarction. N Engl J Med 304:801–807, 1981.

277. Wit AL, Hoffman BF, Rosen MR: Electrophysiology and pharmacology of cardiac arrhythmias. IX. Cardiac electrophysiologic effect of beta adrenergic receptor stimulation and blockade. Part A. Am Heart J 90:521–533, 1975.

278. Black JW, Crowther AF, Shanks RG, Smith LH, Dornhurst AC: A new beta-receptor antagonist. Lancet 1:1080–1081, 1964.

279. Conolly ME, Kersting F, Dollery CT: The clinical pharmacology of beta-adrenoceptor blocking drug. Prog Cardiovasc Dis 19:203–234, 1976.

280. Davis LD, Temte JV: Effects of propranolol on the transmembrane potentials of ventricular muscle and Purkinje fibers in the dog. Circ Res 22:661–677, 1968.

281. Wit AL, Hoffman BF, Rosen MR: Electrophysiology and pharmacology of cardiac arrhythmias. IX. Cardiac electrophysiologic effects of beta adrenergic receptor stimulation and blockade. Part C. Am Heart J 90:795–803, 1975.

282. Pitt WA, Cox AR: The effect of the β-adrenergic antagonist propranolol on rabbit atrial cells with the use of the ultramicroelectrode technique. Am Heart J 76:242, 1968.

283. Papp JG, Vaughan Williams SM: A comparison of the anti-arrhythmic action of ICI 50172 and (-) propranolol and their effects on intracellular cardiac action potentials and other features of cardiac function. Br J Pharmacol 36:391–398, 1969.

284. Tarr M, Luckstead EF, Jurewicz PA, Haas HG: Effect of propranolol on the fast inward sodium current in frog atrial muscle. J Pharmaco. Exp Ther 184:599–610, 1973.

285. Wu CH, Narahashi T: Mechanism of action of propranolol on squid axon membranes. J Pharmacol Exp Ther 184:155–162, 1973.

286. Woosley RL, Kornhauser D, Smith R, Reele S, Higgins SB, Nies AS, Shand DG, Oates TA: Suppression of chronic ventricular arrhythmias with propranolol. Circulation 60:819–827, 1979.

287. Carmeliet E, Vereeke J: Adrenaline and the plateau phase of the cardiac action potential. Eur J Physiol 313:300–315, 1969.

288. Pappano AJ: Calcium-dependent action potentials produced by catecholamines in guinea pig atrial muscle fibers depolarized by potassium. Circ Res 27:379–390, 1970.

289. Harrison LA, Wittig J, Wallace AG: Adrenergic influences on the distal Purkinje system of the canine heart. Circ Res 32:329–339, 1973.

290. Koerpel BJ, Davis LD: Effects of lidocaine, propranolol and sotalol on ouabain-induced changes in transmembrane potential of canine Purkinje fibers. Circ Res 30:681, 1972.

291. Hewett K, Rosen MR: β adrenergic modulation of delayed afterdepolarizations. Am J Cardiol 49:913, 1982.

292. Lucchesi BR, Whitsitt LS: The pharmacology of beta-adrenergic blocking agents. Prog Cardiovasc Dis 11:410–430, 1969.

293. Wallace AG, Troyer WG, Lesage MA, Zotti EF: Electrophysiologic effects of isoproterenol and beta blocking agents in awake dogs. Circ Res 18:140–148, 1966.

294. Epstein SE, Robinson BF, Kahler RL, Braunwald E: Effects of beta-adrenergic blockade on the cardiac response to maximal and submaximal exercise in man. J Clin Invest 44:1745–1753, 1965.

295. Sowton E: Hemodynamic changes after beta adrenergic blockade. Am J Cardiol 18:317–320, 1966.

296. Parker JO, West RO, Digiorgi S: Hemodynamic effects of propranolol in coronary heart disease. Am J Cardiol 21:11–19, 1968.

297. Dwyer EM, Wiener L, Cox JW: Effects of beta-adrenergic blockade on left ventricular hemodynamics and the electrocardium during exercise induced angina pectoris. Circulation 38:250–260, 1968.

298. Wolfson S, Gorlin R: Cardiovascular pharmacology of propranolol in man. Circulation 40:501–511, 1969.

299. Stern S, Eisenberg S: The effect of propranolol (inderal) on the electrocardiogram of normal subjects. Am Heart J 77:192–195, 1969.

300. Gibson D, Sowton E: The use of beta-adrenergic receptor blocking drugs in dysrhythmias. Prog Cardiovasc Dis 12:16–39, 1969.

301. Morgan TO, Sabto J, Anavekar SM, Louis WJ, Doyle AE: A comparison of beta adrenergic blocking drugs in the treatment of hypertension. Postgrad Med J 50:253–259, 1974.

302. Gradman AH, Winkle RA, Fitzgerald JW, Meffin PJ, Stoner J, Bell PA, Harrison DC: Suppression of premature ventricular contractions by acebutolol. Circulation 55:785–791, 1977.

303. LeClercq JF, Rosengarten MD, Kural S, Atturl P, Coumel P: Effects of intrinsic sympathetic activity of beta-blockers on SA and AV nodes in man. Eur J Cardiol 12:367–375, 1981.

304. Seides SF, Josephson ME, Batsford WP, Weisfogel GM, Lau SH, Damato AN: The electrophysiology of propranolol in man. Am Heart J 88:733–741, 1974.

305. Seipel L, Both G, Briethardt G, Gleichmann U, Loogen F: Actions of antiarrhythmic drugs on His bundle electrogram and sinus node function. Acta Cardiol (Suppl 18): 251–267, 1974.

306. Smithen CS, Balcon R, Sowton E: Use of His potentials to assess changes in atrioventricular conduction produced by a series of beta-adrenergic blocking agents. Br Heart J 33:955–961, 1971.

307. Berkowitz WD, Wit AL, Lau SH, Steiner C, Damato AN: Effects of propranolol on cardiac conduction. Circulation 40:855–862, 1969.

308. Priola DV: Effects of beta receptor stimulation and blockade on AV nodal and bundle branch conduction in the canine heart. Am J Cardiol 31:35–40, 1973.

309. Wu D, Denes P, Dhingra R, Kahn A, Rosen KM: The effects of propranolol on the induction of AV nodal reentrant paroxysmal tachycardia. Circulation 50:665–677, 1974.

310. Giudicelli JF, Lhoste F, Bossier JR: Beta-adrenergic blockade and atrioventricular conduction impairment. Eur J Pharmacol 31:216–225, 1975.

311. Rosen KM, Barwolf C, Ehsani A, Rahimtoola SH: Effects of lidocaine and propranolol on the normal and anomalous pathways in patients with preexcitation. Am J Cardiol 30:801–809, 1972.

312. Wellens H, Brugada P, Roy D, Weiss J, Bar F: Shortening of the period of the accessory pathway in the Wolff-Parkinson-White Syndrome by beta-adrenergic stimulation. Circulation 64 (Suppl IV):IV–145, 1981 (abstract).

313. Nies AS, Evans GH, Shand DG: Regional hemodynamic effects of beta-adrenergic blockade with propranolol in the unanesthetized primate. Am Heart J 85:97–102, 1973.

314. Sowton E, Smithen C, Leaver D, Barr L: Effects of practolol on exercise tolerance in patients with angina pectoris. Am J Med 51:63–70, 1971.

315. Stephen SA: Unwanted effects of propranolol. Am J Cardiol 18:463–468, 1966.

316. Vaughan Williams EM, Bagwell EE, Singh BN: Cardiospecificity of β-receptor blockade. Cardiovasc Res 7:226–240, 1973.

317. Fitzgerald JD: Perspectives in adrenergic beta-receptor blockade. Clin Pharmacol Ther 10:292–309, 1969.

318. Gibson DC: Pharmacodynamic properties of β-adrenergic receptor blocking drugs in man. Drugs 7:8–38, 1974.

319. Mason JW, Specter JM, Ingelo MB, Daughters GT, Ferris AC, Alderman EL: Haemodynamic effects of acebutolol. Br Heart J 40:29–34, 1978.

320. Robinson C, Jackson PG, Fisk C, Jewitt DE: Haemodynamic effects of atenolol in patients with coronary artery disease. Br Heart J 40:22–28, 1978.

321. Lewis CM, Brink AJ, Theron MJ, Kotze JCN: β-adrenergic blockage, hemodynamics and myocardial energy metabolism in patients with ischemic heart disease. Am J Cardiol 21:846–859, 1968.

322. Wit AL, Hoffman BF, Rosen MR: Electrophysiology and pharmacology of cardiac arrhythmias. Cardiac electrophysiologic effects of beta adrenergic receptor stimulation and blockade. Part B. Am Heart J 90:665–675, 1975.

323. Shand DG, Nuckolls EM, Oates JA: Plasma propranolol levels in adults, with observations in four children. Clin Pharmacol Ther 11:112–120, 1970.

324. Woosley RL, Shand DG, Kornhauser DM, Nies AS, Oates JA: Relation of plasma concentration and dose of propranolol to its effect on resistant ventricular arrhythmias. Clin Res 25:262A, 1977 (abstract).

325. Coltark DJ, Shand DG: Plasma propranolol levels in the quantitative assessment of β-adrenergic blockade in man. Br Med J 3:731–735, 1970.

326. Evans GH, Shand DG: Disposition of propranolol. IV. Independent variation in steady state circulating drug concentration and half-life as a result of plasma drug binding in man. Clin Pharmacol Ther 14:494–500, 1973.

327. Nies AS, Shand DG: Clinical pharmacology of propranolol. Circulation 52:6–15, 1975.

328. Evans GH, Shand DG: Disposition of propranolol. V. Drug accumulation and steady state concentration during chronic oral administration in man. Clin Pharmacol Ther 14:487–493, 1973.

329. Shand DG, Rangno RE: The disposition of propranolol. Elimination during oral absorption in man. Pharmacology 7:159–168, 1972.

330. Hayes A, Cooper RG: Studies on the absorption, distribution, and excretion of propranolol in rat, dog, and monkey. J Pharmacol Exp Ther 176:302–311, 1971.

331. Walle T, Ishizaki T, Gaffney TE: Isopropylamine, a biologically active deamination product of propranolol in dogs: identification of deuterated and unlabeled isopropylamine by gas chromatography – mass spectrometry. J Pharmacol Exp Ther 183:508–512, 1972.

332. Walle T, Gaffney TE: Propranolol metabolism in man and dog. Mass spectrometric identification of six new metabolites. J Pharmacol Exp Ther 182:83–92, 1972.

333. Cleaveland CR, Shand DG: Effect of route of administration on the relationship between beta-adrenergic blockade and plasma propranolol level. Clin Pharmacol Ther 13:181–185, 1972.

334. Fitzgerald JD, O'Donnell SR: Pharmacology of 4-hydroxypropranolol, a metabolite of propranolol. Br J Pharmacol 43:222–235, 1971.

335. Walle T, Ishizaki T, Sachens D, Privitera D, Garteiz D, Gaffney TE: Propranolol metabolism in man. Pharmacological properties of new metabolites. In: Acheson GH (ed) Abstracts of invited presentations. Fifth Int Cong Pharmacol, San Francisco, 1972, p 74.

336. Ishizaki T, Privitera PJ, Walle T, Gaffney TE: Cardiovascular actions of a new metabolite of propranolol: isopropylamine. J Pharmacol Exp Ther 189:626–632, 1974.

337. Saelens DA, Walle T, Privitera PJ, Knapp DR, Gaffney TE: Central nervous system effects and metabolic disposition of a glycol metabolite of propranolol. J Pharmacol Exp Ther 188:86–92, 1974.

338. Evans GH, Shand DG: Disposition of propranolol. VI. Independent variation in steady-state circulating drug concentrations and half-life as a result of plasma drug binding in man. Clin Pharmacol Ther 14:494–500, 1973.

339. Nies AS, Evans GH, Shand DG: The hemodynamic effects of beta adrenergic blockade on the flow-dependent hepatic clearance of propranolol. J Pharmacol Exp Ther 184:716–721, 1973.

340. Thompson F, Jaekes AM, Faulkes DM: Pharmacodynamics of propranolol in renal failure. Br Med J 2:434–436, 1972.

341. Lowenthal DT, Briggs WA, Gibson TP, Nelson H, Arksena WJ: Pharmakokinetics of oral propranolol in chronic renal disease. Clin Pharmacol Ther 16:761–769, 1974.

342. Ablad B, Ervik M, Hallgren J, Johnsson G, Solvell L: Pharmacological effects and serum levels of orally administered alprenolol in man. Eur J Clin Pharmacol 5:44–52, 1972.

343. Riess W, Rajagopalan TG, Imhof P, Schmid K, Keberle H: Metabolic studies on oxprenolol in animals and man by means of radio-tracer techniques and GLC analysis. Postgrad Med J 46(Suppl):32–39, 1970.

344. Johansson R, Regaroth CG, Sjorgren J: Absorption of alprenolol in man from tablets with different rates of release. Acta Pharm Suec 8:59–70, 1971.

345. Carruthers SG, Kelly JG, McDevitt DG, Shanks RG: Blood levels of practolol: oral and parenteral administration and their relationship to exercise heart rate. Clin Pharmacol Ther 15:497–509, 1974.

346. Gugler R, Herold W, Dengler HJ: Pharmcokinetics of pindolol in man. Eur J Clin Pharmacol 7:17–34, 1974.

347. Johnsson G, Regaroth CG: Clinical pharmcokinetics of beta-adrenoreceptor blocking drugs. Drugs II (Suppl 1): 111–121, 1976.

348. Riess W, Rajagopalan TG, Imhof P, Schmid K, Keberele H: Metabolic studies on oxprenolol in animals and man by means of radio-tracer techniques and GLC analysis. Postgrad Med J 46 (Suppl):32–39, 1970.

349. Alderman EL, Coltart DJ, Weltach GE, Harrison DC: Coronary artery syndromes after sudden propranolol withdrawal. Ann Intern Med 81:625–627, 1974.

350. Miller RR, Olson HG, Amsterdam EA, Mason DT: Propranolol withdrawal rebound phenomenon: exacerbation of coronary events after abrupt cessation of anti-anginal therapy. N Engl J Med 293:416–418, 1975.

351. Frishman WH, Christodoulou J, Weksler B, Smithen C, Killip J, Scheidt S: Abrupt propranolol withdrawal in angina pectoris: effects on platelet aggregation and exercise tolerance. Am Heart J 95:169–179, 1978.

352. Connolly CK, Batten JC: Comparison of the effect of alprenolol and propranolol on specific airway conductance in asthmatic patients. Br Med J 2:515–516, 1970.

353. Skinner C, Palmer KNV, Kerridge DF: Comparison of the effects of acebutolol and practolol in airways obstruction in asthmatics. Br J Clin Pharmacol 2:417, 1972.

354. Formgren H, Eriksson ME: Effects of practolol in combination with terbutaline in the treatment of hypertension

and arrhythmias in asthmatic patients. Scand J Resp Dis 56:217–222, 1975.

355. Skinner C, Gaddo J, Palmer KNV: Comparison of effects of metoprolol and propranolol on asthmatic airway obstruction. Br Med J 1:504, 1976.

356. Singh BN, Whitlock RML, Combes RH, Williams FH, Harris EA: Effects of cardioselective β-adrenoceptor blockade on specific airways resistance in normal subjects and in patients with bronchial asthma. Clin Pharmacol Ther 19:493–501, 1976.

357. Wright P: Untoward effect associated with practolol administration: oculomucocutaneous syndrome. Br Med J 1:595–598, 1975.

358. Felix RH, Ive FA, Dahl MGC: Cutaneous and ocular reactions to practolol. Br Med J 4:321, 1974.

359. Cubey RB, Taylor SH: Ocular reactions to propranolol and resolution on continued treatment with a different beta blocking drug. Br Med J 4:327, 1973.

360. Harty RP: Sclerosing peritonitis and propranolol. Arch Intern Med 138:1424–1426, 1978.

361. Holt PJA, Waddington E: Oculocutaneous reaction to oxprenolol. Br Med J 2:539–540, 1975.

362. Knapp MS, Gallaway HR, Clayden JR: Ocular reactions to beta blockers. Br Med J 2:562, 1975.

363. Windsor WP, Durrein F, Dyer NH: Fibrinous peritonits: a complication of practolol therapy. Br Med J 2:68, 1975.

364. Status report on beta-blockers. FDA Drug Bull 8:13, 1978.

365. Haas H, Hartfelder G: α-Isopropyl-α(N-methyl-N-homoveratryl-α-amino propyl)-3-4-dimethoxyphenyl acetonstrol, eine Substanz mit Coronäsgefäss-Eigenschaften. Arzneimittel-forsch 12:549–558, 1962.

366. Fleckenstein A, Doring HJ, Kammermaier H: Einfluss von beta-receptor Entblocker und verwandten Substanzen auf Erregung, Kontraktion und Energiestoffwechsel des Myokordifasers. Klin Wochenschr 46:343, 1968.

367. Nayler WG, McInnes I, Swann JP, Price JM, Carson V, Race D, Lowe TE: Some effects of iproveratril (isoptin) on the cardiovascular system. J Pharmacol Exp Ther 161:247, 1968.

368. Kohlhardt M, Bauer B, Krause H, Fleckenstein A: Differentiation of the transmembrane Na + Ca channels in mammalian cardiac fibers by the use of specific inhibitors. Pflugers Arch 335:309–322, 1972.

369. Tritthart H, Fleckenstein B, Fleckenstein A: Some fundamental actions of antiarrhythmic drugs on the excitability and the contractility of single myocardial fibers. Arch Pharmacol 269:212, 1971.

370. Rosen MR, Ilvento JP, Gelband H, Merker C: Effects of verapamil on electrophysiologic properties of canine Purkinje fibers. J Pharmacol Exp Ther 189:414–421, 1974.

371. Cranefield PF, Aronson RS and Wit AL: Effect of verapamil on the normal action potential and on a calcium-dependent slow response of canine Purkinje fibers. Circ Res 34:204–213, 1974.

372. Wit AL, Cranefield P: Effect of verapamil on the sinoatrial and atrioventricular nodes of the rabbit and the mechanism by which it arrests reentrant atrioventricular nodal tachycardia. Circ Res 35:413–425, 1974.

373. Singh BN, Vaughan Williams EM: A fourth class of anti-

dysrhythmic action? Effect of verapamil on ouabain toxicity, on atrial and ventricular intracellular potentials, and on other features of cardiac function. Cardiovasc Res 6:109–119, 1972.

374. Rosen MR, Wit AL, Hoffman BF: Electrophysiology and pharmacology of cardiac arrhythmias. VI Cardiac effects of verapamil. Am Heart J 89:665–673, 1975.

375. Danilo P Jr, Hordof AJ, Reder RF, Rosen MR: Effects of verapamil on electrophysiologic properties of blood superfused cardiac Purkinje fibers. J Pharmacol Exp Ther 213:222–227, 1980.

376. Bayer R, Kalusche D, Kaufmann R, Manhold R: Inotropic and electrophysiological actions of verapamil and D600 in mammalian myocardium. III. Effects of the optical isomers on transmembrane action potentials. Naunyn Schmiedebergs Arch Pharmacol 290:81–97, 1975.

377. Hordof AJ, Edie R, Malm JR, Hoffman BF, Rosen MR: Electrophysiological properties and response to pharmacologic agents of fibers from diseased human atria. Circulation 54:774–779, 1976.

378. Spear JF, Horowitz LN, Moore EN: The slow response in human ventricle. In: Zipes DP, Bailey JC, Elharrar V (eds) The Slow Inward Current and Cardiac Arrhythmias. Martinus Nijhoff, The Hague, 1980, pp 309–326.

379. Kohlhardt M, Muich Z: Studies on the inhibitory effect of verapamil on the slow inward current in mammalian ventricular myocardium. J Mol Cell Cardiol 10:1037–1052, 1978.

380. Kass RS, Tsien R: Multiple effects for calcium antagonists on plateau currents in cardiac Purkinje fibers. J Gen Physiol 66:109–119, 1972.

381. Gettes LS, Saito T: Effect of antiarrhythmic drugs on the slow inward current system. In: Zipes DP, Bailey JC, Elharrar V (eds) The Slow Inward Current and Cardiac Arrhythmias. Martinus Nijhoff, The Hague, 1980, pp 455–477.

382. Wit AL, Wiggins JR, Cranefield PF: Some effects of electrical stimulation on impulse initiation in cardiac fibers: Its relevance for the determination of the mechanism of clinical cardiac arrhythmias. In: Wellens HJJ, Lie KI, Janse M (eds) The Conduction System of the Heart: Structure, Function and Clinical Implications. Lea and Febiger, Philadelphia, 1976, p 163.

383. Wit AL, Cranefield PF: Triggered and automatic activity in the canine coronary sinus. Circ Res 41:435–445, 1977.

384. Kass R, Tsien R, Weingart R: Ionic bases of transient inward current induced by strophanthidin in cardiac Purkinje fibers. J Physiol (Lond) 281:209–226, 1978.

385. Angus JA, Richmond DR, Dhumma-Upakorn LB, Cobbin LB, Goodman AA: Cardiovascular action of verapamil in the dog with particular reference to myocardial contractility + atrioventricular conduction. Cardiovasc Res 10: 623–632, 1976.

386. Okada T: Effect of verapamil on electrical activities of SA node, ventricular muscle + Purkinje fibers in isolated rabbit hearts. Jpn Circ J 40:329–341, 1976.

387. Hirata Y, Kodama I, Iwamura N, Shimizu T, Toyama J, Yamada K: Effects of verapamil on canine Purkinje fibers and ventricular muscle fibers with particular reference to

the alternation of action potential duration after a sudden increase in driving rate. Cardiovasc Res 13:1–8, 1979.

388. Heng MK, Singh BN, Roche AHG, Norris RM, Mercer CJ: Effect of intravenous verapamil on cardiac arrhythmias and on the electrocardiogram. Am Heart J 90:487–498, 1975.

389. Neuss H, Schlepper M: Der Einfluss von Verapamil auf die atrioventrikulare Überleitung, Lokalisation des Wirkungsortes mit His Bundel Elektrogrammen. Verhandlungen der Deutschen Gesellschaft für Kreislaufforschung 37:433–438, 1971.

390. Krikler DM, Spurrell RAJ: Verapamil in the treatment of paroxysmal supraventricular tachycardia. Postgrad Med J 50:447–453, 1974.

391. Puech P: Dissection de la Conduction Sinoventriculaire pour l'étude du Verapamil injectable. Montpellier Centre Hospitalier, 1972.

392. Huisiani MH, Kvasnicka J, Ryden L, Holmberg S: Action of verapamil on sinus node, atrioventricular and intraventricular conduction. Br Heart J 35:734–737, 1973.

393. Wellens HJJ, Tan SL, Bar FWH, Düren DR, Lie KI, Dohmen HM: Effect of verapamil studied by programmed electrical stimulation of the heart in patients with paroxysmal reentrant SVT, Br Heart J 39:1058–1066, 1977.

394. Roy PR, Spurrell RAJ, Sowton E: The effect of verapamil on the cardiac conduction system in man. Postgrad Med J 50:270–275, 1974.

395. Nayler WG, Szeto J: Effect of verapamil on contractility, oxygen utilization and calcium exchange ability to mammalian heart muscle. Cardiovasc Res 6:120–128, 1972.

396. Smith HJ, Goldstein RA, Griffith JM, Kent KM, Epstein SE: Regional contractility: selective depression of ischemic myocardium by verapamil. Circulation 54:629–635, 1976.

397. Haeusler G: Differential effect of verapamil on excitation conduction coupling in smooth muscle and on excitation secretion coupling in adrenergic terminals. J Pharmacol Exp Ther 180:672–679, 1972.

398. Baky SH, Kirsten EB: Verapamil. In: Goldberg ME (ed) Pharmacological and Biochemical Properties of Drug Substances. Am Pharmaceut Assoc, Acad Pharmaceut Sci, Washington, 1981.

399. Hagemeijer F: Verapamil in the management of supraventricular tachyarrhythmias occurring after a recent myocardial infarction. Circulation 57:751–755, 1978.

400. Melville KI, Shister HE, Huq S: Iproveratril: experimental data on coronary-dilatation and anti-arrhythmic action. Can Med Assoc J 90:761–770, 1964.

401. Johnson SM, Mauritson DR, Hilles LD, Willerson JT: Verapamil in the treatment of Prinzmetals variant angina: a long term, double-blind, randomized trial. N Engl J Med 304:862–866, 1981.

402. Krikler D: Verapamil in cardiology. Eur J Cardiol 2:3–10, 1974.

403. Schomerus M, Spiegelhalder B, Stieren B, Eichelbaum M: Physiological disposition of verapamil in man. Cardiovasc Res 10:605–612, 1976.

404. Schlepper M, Thormann J, Schwarz F: The pharmacodynamics of orally taken verapamil and verapamil retard as judged by their negative dromotropic effects. Arzneim Forsch 25:1452–1455, 1975.

405. Neugebauer G: Comparative cardiovascular actions of verapamil and its major metabolites in the anesthetized dog. Cardiovasc Res 12:247–254, 1978.

406. Woodcock BG, Rietbrock I, Vohringer HF, Rietbrock N: Verapamil disposition in liver disease and intensive-care patients: kinetics clearance and apparent blood flow relationships. Clin Pharmacol Ther 29:27–34, 1981.

407. Investigator's brochure. Isoptin (verapamil hydrochloride). Knoll Pharmaceutical Co.

408. Kesteloot H: General aspects of antiarrhythmic treatment with aprindine. Acta Cardiol [Suppl] (Brux) 18:303–316, 1974.

409. Kesteloot H, Van Mieghem W, DeGeest H: Aprindine (AC 1802) a new antiarrhythmic drug. Acta Cardiol (Brux) 28:145–165, 1973.

410. Carmeliet E, Verdonck F: Effects of aprindine and lidocaine on transmembrane potentials and radioactive K efflux in different cardiac tissues. Acta Cardiol [Suppl] (Brux) 18:73–90, 1974.

411. Verdonck F, Vereecke J, Vleugels A: Electrophysiological effects of aprindine on isolated heart preparations. Eur J Pharmacol 26:338–347, 1974.

412. Steinberg MI, Greenspan K: Intracellular electrophysiological alterations in canine cardiac conducting tissue induced by aprindine and lidocaine. Cardiovasc Res 10:236–244, 1976.

413. Elharrar V, Bailey JC, Lathrop DA, Zipes DP: Effects of aprindine on slow channel action potentials and transient depolarizations in canine Purkinje fibers. J Pharmacol Exp Ther 205:410–417, 1978.

414. Gilmour RF Jr, Chikhavev VN, Jurevichus JA, Zacharov SI, Zipes DP, Rosenshtraukh LV: Effect of aprindine on transmembrane currents and contractile force in frog atria. J Pharmacol Exp Ther 217:390–396, 1981.

415. Reiser J, Freeman AR, Greenspan K: Aprindine-a calcium mediated antiarrhythmic. Fed Proc 33:476, 1974 (abstract).

416. Harker RJ, Greenspan K: Modification of calcium dependent slow responses in canine Purkinje fibers by aprindine. Fed Proc 36:946, 1977 (abstract).

417. Georges A, Hosslet A, Duvernay G: Pharmacological evaluation of aprindine (AC 1802). A new anti-arrhythmic agent. Acta Cardiol (Brux) 28:166–191, 1973.

418. Elharrar V, Foster PR, Zipes DP: Effects of aprindine HCl on cardiac tissues. J Pharmacol Exp Ther 195:201–205, 1975.

419. Seipel L, Both A, Breithardt G, Gleichmann U, Loogen F: Action of antiarrhythmic drugs on His bundle electrogram and sinus node function. Acta Cardiol [Suppl] (Brux) 18:251–267, 1974.

420. Breithardt G, Gleichmann V, Seipel L, Loogen F: Long term oral anti-arrhythmic therapy by antiarrhythmic drugs. Acta Cardiol [Suppl] (Brux) 18:341–353, 1974.

421. Schlepper M, Neuss H: Changes of refractory periods in the A-V conduction system induced by antiarrhythmic drugs. Acta Cardiol [Suppl] (Brux) 18:269–277, 1974.

422. Zipes DP, Gaum WE, Foster PR, Rosen KM, Wu D, Amat-y-Leon F, Noble RJ: Aprindine for treatment of supraventricular tachycardias. Am J Cardiol 40:586–596, 1977.

423. Piessens J, Willems J, Kesteloot H, DeGeest H: Effects of

231

aprindine on left ventricular contractility in man. Acta Cardiol [Suppl] (Brux) 15:203–216, 1971.

424. Rousseau MF, Brasseur LA, Detry JM: Hemodynamic effects of aprindine during upright exercise in normal subjects. Acta Cardiol [Suppl] (Brux) 18:195–201, 1974.

425. Remme WJ, Verdouw PD: Cardiovascular effects of aprindine, a new antiarrhythmic drug. Eur J Cardiol 314:307–313, 1975.

426. Brutsaert DL: Effects of aprindine on myocardial contractility. Acta Cardiol [Suppl] (Brux) 18:91–99, 1974.

427. Fasola AF, Carmichael R: The pharmacology and clinical evaluation of aprindine, a new antiarrhythmic agent. Acta Cardiol [Suppl] (Brux) 18:317–333, 1974.

428. Fasola AF, Noble RJ, Zipes DP: Treatment of recurrent ventricular tachycardia and fibrillation with aprindine. Am J Cardiol 39:903–909, 1977.

429. Murphy PJ: Metabolic pathways of aprindine. Acta Cardiol [Suppl] (Brux) 18:131–142, 1974.

430. Kroll DA, Lucchesi BR: Antiarrhythmic and antifibrillatory properties of aprindine. J Pharmacol Exp Ther 194:427–434, 1975.

431. Gaum WE, Elharrar V, Walker PD, Zipes DP: Influence of excitability of the ventricular fibrillation threshold in dogs. Am J Cardiol 40:929–935, 1977.

432. Elharrar V, Gaum WE, Zipes DP: Effects of drugs on conduction delay and incidence of ventricular arrhythmias induced by acute coronary occlusion in dogs. Am J Cardiol 39:544–549, 1977.

433. Leeuwen R van, Meyboom RHB: Agranulocytosis and aprindine. Lancet 2:1137, 1976.

434. Elewaut A, Van Durme JP, Goethals L, Kauffman JM, Mussche M, Elinck W, Roels H, Bogaert A, Barbier C: Aprindine-induced liver injury. Acta Gastroenterol Belg 15:236–243, 1977.

435. Boura ALA, Green AF: The actions of bretylium: adrenergic neurone blocking and other effects. Br J Pharmacol 14:536–548, 1959.

436. Boura ALA, Green AF: Adrenergic neurone blocking agents. Ann Rev Pharmacol 5:183–212, 1965.

437. Heissenbuttel RH, Bigger JT Jr: Bretylium tosylate: a newly available antiarrhythmic drug for ventricular arrhythmias. Ann Intern Med 91:229–238, 1979.

438. Bacaner MG: Bretylium tosylate for suppression of induced ventricular fibrillation. Am J Cardiol 17:528–534, 1966.

439. Bigger JR Jr, Jaffe C: The effect of bretylium tosylate on the electrophysiological properties of ventricular muscle and Purkinje fibers. Am J Cardiol 27:82–90, 1971.

440. Wit AL, Steiner C, Damato AN: Electrophysiologic effects of bretylium tosylate on single fibers of the canine specialized conducting system and ventricle. J Pharmacol Exp Ther 173:344–356, 1970.

441. Namm DH, Wang CM, El-Sayad S, Copp FC, Maxwell RA: Effect of bretylium on rat cardiac muscle: the electrophysiologic effects and its uptake and binding in normal and immunosympathectomized rat hearts. J Pharmacol Exp Ther 193:194–208, 1975.

442. Papp JG, Vaughan Williams EM: The effect of bretylium on intracellular cardiac action potentials in relation to its

antiarrhythmic and local anesthetic activity. Br J Pharmacol 37:380, 1969.

443. Cardinal R, Sasyniuk BI: Electrophysiological effects of bretylium tosylate on subendocardial Purkinje fibers from infarcted canine hearts. J Pharmacol Exp Ther 204:159–174, 1978.

444. Glassman RD, Wit AL: Electrophysiological effects of bretylium tosylate. In: Bretylium Tosylate: Current Scientific and Clinical Experience. Excerpta Medica, Amsterdam, 1979.

445. Touboul P, Porte J, Huerta F, Delahaye JP: Etude des propriétés électrophysiologiques du tosylate de bretylium chez l'homme. Arch Mal Coeur 69:503–511, 1976.

446. Waxman MB, Wallace AG: Electrophysiologic effects of bretylium tosylate on the heart. J Pharmacol Exp Ther 183:264–274, 1972.

447. Allen JD, Pantridge JF, Shanks RG: Effects of lignocaine, propranolol and bretylium on ventricular fibrillation threshold. Am J Cardiol 28:555–562, 1971.

448. Sanna G, Arcidiacono R: Chemical ventricular defibrillation of the human heart with bretylium tosylate. Am J Cardiol 32:982–987, 1973.

449. Kuntzman R, Tsai I, Chang R, Conney AH: Disposition of bretylium in man and rat. Clin Pharmacol Ther 11:829–837, 1970.

450. Bernstein JG, Koch-Weser J: Effectiveness of bretylium tosylate against refractory ventricular arrhythmias. Circulation 45:1024–1034, 1972.

451. Singh BN, Vaughan Williams EM: The effect of amiodarone, a new anti-anginal drug, on cardiac muscle. Br J Pharmacol 39: 657–667, 1970.

452. Charlier R, Deltour G, Tondeur R, Binon F: Recherches dans la série des benzofurannes. VII. Etude pharmacologique préliminaire du butyl-2-(duodo-3', 5' β-N-diethylaminoethexy-4'benzoyl)-3 benzofurane. Arch Int Pharmacodyn Ther 139:255–264, 1962.

453. Charlier R, Delaunois G, Bauthier J, Deltour G: Dans la série des benzofurannes. XL. Propriétés antiarrhythmiques d'amiodarone. Cardiologia 54:82–90, 1969.

454. Rosenbaum MB, Chiale PA, Halpern MS, Nau GJ, Przybylski J, Levi RJ, Lazzari JO, Elizari MV: Clinical efficacy of amiodarone as an antiarrhythmic agent. Am J Cardiol 38:934–944, 1976.

455. Goupil N, Lenfant J: The effects of amiodarone on the sinus node activity of the rabbit heart. Eur J Pharmacol 39:23–31, 1976.

456. Broekhuysen J, Deltour G, Gluslain M: Some biochemical effects of amiodarone. Arzneimittelforsch 19:1850–1853, 1969.

457. Grand A: Myxoedème à l'amiodarone. Coeur Med Intern 14:163–167, 1975.

458. Burger A, Dinichert D, Nicod P, Tenny M, Lemarchand-Beraud T, Vallotton MB: Effect of amiodarone on serum triiodothyronine, reverse triiodothyronine, thyroxin and thyrotropin. J Clin Invest 58:255–259, 1976.

459. Baillet J: Amiodarone et dysthyroide: colloque sur l'amiodarone. Documentation Labaz (Paris), 1977, pp 130–135.

460. Jonckheer MH, Blockx P, Kaivers R, Wyffels G: Hyperthyroidism as a possible complication of the treatment of

232

ischemic heart disease with amiodarone. Acta Cardiol 28:192–200, 1973.

461. Charlier R, Deltour G, Baudine A, Chaillet F: Pharmacology of amiodarone an antianginal drug with a new biological profile. Arzneimittelforsch 11:1408–1417, 1968.

462. Charlier R: Cardiac actions in the dog of a new antagonist of adrenergic excitation which does not produce competitive blockade of adrenoceptors. Br J Pharmacol 39:668–674, 1970.

463. Bacq AM, Blakeley AGH, Summers RJ: The effects of amiodarone, an α and β receptor antagonist, on adrenergic transmission in the cat and spleen. Biochem Pharmacol 25:1195–1199, 1976.

464. Sicart M, Besse P, Choussat A, Bricaud H: Action hémodynamique de l'amiodarone intraveineuse chez l'homme. Arch Mal Coeur 70:219–227, 1977.

465. Cabasson J, Puech P, Mellet JM, Guimond C, Bachy C, Sassine A: Analyse des effets électrophysiologiques de l'amiodarone par l'enregistrement simultane des potentiels d'action monophasiques et du faisceau de His. Arch Mal Coeur 69:691–699, 1976.

466. Touboul P, Huerta F, Porte J, Delahaye JP: Bases électrophysiologiques de l'action antiarrhythmique de l'amiodarone chez l'homme. Arch Mal Coeur 69:845–853, 1976.

467. Coulte R, Fontaine G, Franks R: Etude électrocardiologique des effets de l'amiodarone sur la conduction intracardiaque chez l'homme. Ann Cardiol Angiol (Paris) 18:543–548, 1977.

468. Rosenbaum MB, Chiale PA, Ryba D, Elizari MV: Control of tachyarrhythmias associated with Wolff-Parkinson-White syndrome by amiodarone hydrochloride. Am J Cardiol 34:215–222, 1974.

469. Wellens HJJ, Lie KI, Bar FW, Wesdorp JC, Dohmen HJ, Duren DR, Durrer D: Effect of amiodarone in the Wolf-Parkinson-White syndrome. Am J Cardiol 38:189–194, 1976.

470. Rowland E, Krikler DM: Electrophysiological assessment of amiodarone in treatment of resistant supraventricular arrhythmias. Br Heart J 44:82–90, 1980.

471. Rasmussen V, Berning J: Effect of amiodarone in the Wolff-Parkinson-White syndrome. Acta Med Scand 205:31–37, 1979.

472. Petta JM, Zaccheo VJ: Comparative profile of L 3428 and other antianginal agents on cardiac hemodynamics. J Pharmacol Exp Ther 176:328–338, 1971.

473. Cote P, Bourassa MG, Delaye J, Janin A, Froment R, David P: Effects of amiodarone on cardiac and coronary hemodynamics and on myocardial metabolism in patients with coronary artery disease. Circulation 59:1165–1172, 1979.

474. Barzin J, Freson A: Essais cliniques de l'amiodarone dans les affections coronariennes. Brux Med 49:105, 1969.

475. Kannan R, Ikeda N, Prasad K, Kay I, Ooktens M, Singh B: Plasma kinetics and myocardial disposition of intravenous amiodarone relative to its electrophysiological effects in rabbits and dogs. Circulation 64 (Suppl IV):IV–69, 1981.

476. Haffajee C, Lesko L, Canada A, Alpert JS: Clinical pharmcokinetics of amiodarone. Circulation 64 (Suppl IV):IV–263, 1981.

477. Harris L, McKenna WJ, Rowland E, Storey GCA, Krikler DM, Holt DW: Plasma amiodarone and desethyl amiodarone levels in chronic oral therapy. Circulation 64(Suppl IV):IV–263, 1981.

478. Pritchard DA, Singh BN, Hurley PJ: Effects of amiodarone on thyroid function in patients with ischemic heart disease. Br Heart J 37:856–860, 1975.

479. Bockhardt H, Drenckhahn D, Lullman-Rauch R: Amiodarone-induced lipidosis-like alterations in ocular tissues of rats. Albrecht Von Graefes Arch Klin Exp Ophthamol 207:91–96, 1978.

480. Sobol SM, Rakita L: Pneumonitis and pulmonary fibrosis associated with amiodarone treatment: a possible complication of new antiarrhythmic drug. Circulation 65:819–824, 1982.

481. Kaverina NV, Senova ZP: Ethmozin – a new preparation for treating cardiac rhythm disorders. Proc First US-USSR Symp on Sudden Death, Yalta, Oct 3–5, 1977. US Dept of HEW, PHS, NTH, DHEW Publ No 78:1470, 1978.

482. Morganroth J, Pearlman AS, Dunkman WB, Horowitz LN, Josephson ME, Michelson EL: Ethmozin: a new antiarrhythmic agent developed in the USSR. Efficacy and tolerance. Am Heart J 98:621–628, 1979.

483. Podrid PJ, Lyakishev A, Lown B, Mazur N: Ethmozin, a new antiarrhythmic drug for suppressing ventricular premature complexes. Circulation 61:450–457, 1980.

484. Danilo P Jr, Langan WB, Rosen MR, Hoffman BF: Effects of the phenothiazine analog EN 313 on ventricular arrhythmias in dogs. Eur J Pharmacol 45:127–139, 1977.

485. Ruffy R, Rozenshtraukh LV, Elharrar V, Zipes DP: Electrophysiological effects of ethmozine on canine myocardium. Cardiovasc Res 13:354–363, 1979.

486. Dangman KH, Hoffman BF: Effects of ethmozin on automatic and triggered impulse initiation in canine cardiac Purkinje fibers. J Pharmacol Exp Ther (in press).

487. Hewett K, Gessman L, Rosen MR: The effects of procaine amide, quinidine and ethmozin on ouabain-induced delayed afterdepolarizations. Eur J Pharmacol (submitted).

488. Morganroth J, Michelson EL, Klitchen JG, Dreifus LS: Ethmozin: electrophysiologic effects in man. Circulation 64(IV):263, 1981.

489. Singh SN, DiBianco R, Fletcher RD, Johnson WL, Ginsberg R: Ethmozin shown effective in reducing chronic high frequency: results of a prospective controlled trial. Am J Cardiol 49:1015, 1982.

490. Zaslovskaya RM, Skorobogatskya IF, Kolbanovskaya EY: Ethmozin therapy of patients with rhythm disturbances in heart activity. Sov Med 5:50, 1969.

491. Golochevskaya VA, Bokeriya OA: Application of ethmozin in patients with heart rhythm disturbances. In: Sivkov II, Kukes VG (eds) Questions of Pharmcotherapy of Some Cardiovascular Disease. Moscow, 1971, pp 5–7.

492. Wit AL, Rosen MR, Hoffman BF: Electrophysiology and pharmacology of cardiac arrhythmias. II. Relationship of normal and abnormal electrical activity of cardiac fibers to the genesis of arrhythmias. A. Automaticity. Am Heart J 88:515–524, 1974.

493. Wit AL, Rosen MR, Hoffman BF: Electrophysiology and

pharmacology of cardiac arrhythmias. II. Relationship of normal and abnormal electrical activity of cardiac fibers to the genesis of arrhythmias B. Reentry. Am Heart J 88:664–670, 1974.

494. Hoffman BF, Rosen MR: Cellular mechanisms for cardiac arrhythmias. Circ Res 49:1–15, 1981.

495. Vassalle M: Analysis of cardiac pacemaker potential using a 'voltage clamp' technique. Am J Physiol 210:1335–1341, 1966.

496. Noma A, Irisawa H: A time and voltage-dependent potassium current in the rabbit sino-atrial node cell. Pflugers Arch 336:251–258, 1976.

497. Vassalle M: The relationship among cardiac pacemakers. Overdrive suppression. Circ Res 41:269–277, 1977.

498. Hoffman BF, Cranefield PF: Electrophysiology of the Heart. McGraw Hill, New York, 1960.

499. Surawicz B, Imanish S: Automatic activity in depolarized guinea pig ventricular myocardium: characteristics and mechanisms. Circ Res 39:751–759, 1976.

500. Brown HF, Clark A, Noble SJ: Pacemaker current in frog atrium. Nature 235:30–31, 1972.

501. Cranefield PF: The Slow Response and Cardiac Arrhythmias. Futura Press, Mt. Kisco, 1975.

502. Arnsdorf MF, Mehlman DJ: Observations on the effects of selected antiarrhythmic drugs on mammalian cardiac Purkinje fibers with two levels of steady-state potential: influences of lidocaine, phenytoin, propranolol, disopyramide and procainamide on repolarization, action potential shape and conduction. J Pharmacol Exp Ther 207:983–991, 1978.

503. Cranefield PF: Action potentials, after potentials and arrhythmias. Circ Res 41:415–423, 1977.

504. Wit AL, Cranefield PF, Gadsby DC: Triggered activity: In: Zipes DP, Bailey JC, Elharrar V (eds) The Slow Inward Current and Cardiac Arrhythmias. Martinus Nijhoff, The Hague, 1980, pp 437–454.

505. Ferrier GR: Digitalis arrhythmias: role of oscillatory after potentials. Prog Cardiovasc Dis 19:459–474, 1977.

506. El-Sherif N, Zeiler R, Gough WB: Effects of catecholamines verapamil and tetrodotoxin on triggered automaticity in canine ischemic Purkinje fibers. Circulation 62 (pt 2): 281, 1980.

507. Wit AL, Cranefield PF: Reentrant excitation as a cause of cardiac arrhythmias. Am J Physiol 235:H1–H17, 1978.

508. Courtney KR: Mechanism of frequency-dependent inhibition of sodium currents in frog myelinated nerve by the lidocaine derivative GEA-968. J Pharmacol Exp Ther 195:225–236, 1975.

509. Hille B: Local anesthetics: hydrophilic and hydrophobic pathways for the drug-receptor reaction. J Gen Physiol 69:497–515, 1977.

510. Strichartz GR: Molecular mechanisms of nerve block by local anesthetics. Anesthesiology 45:421–441, 1976.

511. Wit AL, Rosen MR, Hoffman BF: Electrophysiology and pharmacology of cardiac arrhythmias II. Relationship of normal and abnormal electrical activity of cardiac fibers to the genesis of arrhythmias. B. Reentry, section II. Am Heart J 88:798–806, 1974.

512. Gadsby D, Cranefield PF: Electrogenic sodium extrusion in cardiac Purkinje fibers. J Gen Physiol 73:819–837, 1979.

513. Trautwein W: Membrane currents in cardiac muscle fibers. Physiol Res 53:793–835, 1973.

CHAPTER 8

Clinical use of antiarrhythmic drugs

LEONARD S. GETTES, JAMES R. FOSTER, and ROSS J. SIMPSON, Jr.

Introduction

It is axiomatic that the appropriate treatment of arrhythmias requires that each arrhythmia be correctly diagnosed. An awareness of the factors contributing to the arrhythmia, the setting of appropriate therapeutic goals, familiarity with available drugs, and documentation of efficacy are also essential elements of antiarrhythmic therapy. In this chapter, we will discuss the clinical approach to the therapy of cardiac arrhythmias by considering the general points raised above. We will discuss the specific indications, clinical pharmacology, and toxicity of the various drugs currently employed in the United States and will consider the prophylactic use of antiarrhythmic drugs in order to prevent sudden cardiac death in populations at risk.

General principles

From a practical standpoint, the decision as to whether a tachyarrhythmia with a wide QRS complex is of ventricular or supraventricular origin is the first step to appropriate therapy. This problem has been addressed by several investigators [1–5]. Most recently, Wellens et al. [5] analyzed 140 episodes of wide QRS complex tachycardia. Seventy were of ventricular origin, and 70 were of supraventricular origin. The patients with supraventricular tachycardia tended to be younger and to have less ischemic heart disease than the patients with ventricular tachycardia. A rate of less than 130/min, marked left axis deviation in the frontal plane, and a QRS duration of 140 msec were sensitive indicators of ventricular tachycardia; whereas a QRS du-

ration of 120 msec or less was a good indicator of supraventricular tachycardia. The documentation of AV dissociation was confirmed to be a valuable aid to the diagnosis of ventricular tachycardia. However, AV association, considered a useful aid in the diagnosis of supraventricular tachycardia, did not exclude ventricular tachycardia, since it was found in 33% of such episodes. Frequently, the finding of supraventricular or ventricular premature beats with QRS complexes similar to those seen during the tachycardia is also a useful diagnostic aid. If the clinical and electrocardiographic features are not adequate to separate supraventricular from ventricular tachycardia, the use of esophageal or intracardiac leads may provide the means for establishing the relationship of atrial and ventricular activation and, thus, the presence of AV dissociation or association. Carotid sinus massage and/or therapeutic trials with drugs, whose effect is largely limited to supraventricular or ventricular arrhythmias (such as verapamil or lidocaine, respectively), may also help to establish the correct diagnosis.

Once it has been determined that a tachyarrhythmia is either supraventricular or ventricular in origin, it is then important to consider the pathophysiologic and clinical factors responsible for the arrhythmia. Included in the consideration of pathophysiologic causes is a decision regarding whether the arrhythmia is due to reentry, enhanced automaticity, or triggered activity and a determination of the site of arrhythmia production, i.e., sinus node, atria, AV node, bypass tract, or ventricles. Although identification of the electrophysiologic mechanism for the arrhythmia may not contribute directly to therapeutic decisions, knowledge of the

Rosen, M. R. and Hoffman, B. F. (eds.), Cardiac Therapy. ISBN 0-89838-564-4.
© 1983, Martinus Nijhoff Publishers, Boston, The Hague, Dordrecht, Lancaster. Printed in the Netherlands.

location of a reentry circuit or the site of origin of the arrhythmia may be critical to proper therapeutic decisions.

Among the causes of tachycardias are underlying cardiac and noncardiac diseases and iatrogenic factors. For instance, mitral stenosis, Wolff-Parkinson-White syndrome, sinus node disease, and hyperthyroidism are frequent causes of supraventricular arrhythmias; whereas myocardial ischemia, congestive heart failure of any etiology, and ventricular aneurysms are frequently causes of ventricular arrhythmias. Mitral valve prolapse can be a cause of both supraventricular and ventricular arrhythmias. Among the most common iatrogenic causes are digitalis, many antiarrhythmic drugs, drug-induced hypokalemia, and cardiac surgery. The role of exercise in producing or exacerbating arrhythmias of any cause should also be evaluated. Often, such testing defines the relative role of myocardial ischemia in the genesis of the arrhythmia, contributes directly to the diagnosis of the underlying cardiac disease, assists in the choice of therapeutic agents, and provides a means of assessing drug efficacy.

The evaluation of patients with cardiac arrhythmias should include procedures designed to provide the information discussed above for assisting in the setting of therapeutic goals, to aid in the selection of agents most appropriate for meeting these goals, and to provide a means of assessing therapeutic efficacy. In addition to the history, physical examination, and routine laboratory tests, the evaluation may include echocardiography, nuclear scans, cardiac catheterization, exercise testing, ambulatory ECG monitoring, and intracardiac electrophysiologic testing. Echocardiography, nuclear scans, and cardiac catherization are employed to determine underlying cardiac diseases and to assess ventricular function. Exercise testing, ambulatory ECG monitoring, and intracardiac electrophysiologic testing are specifically aimed at gaining an understanding of the arrhythmia itself and in assessing the results of therapy. Thus, the use of these tests requires an appreciation of their sensitivity, specificity, and reproducibility.

Exercise tests

Much has been written concerning the ability of exercise testing to induce supraventricular and ventricular tachyarrhythmias and intracardiac conduction disturbances [6–12]. This literature indicates that premature beats and rhythms may occur during or after exercise in a significant percentage of patients in whom a history of symptomatic arrhythmias or findings of cardiac disease may be absent as well as in patients with documented cardiac disease. Of particular relevance to this chapter is the ability of exercise testing to provide a guide to the choice of a therapeutic agent and a means of assessing drug efficacy. These are interrelated points since both require that exercise-induced arrhythmias be reproducible. Sheps et al. [13] noted that in 13 patients subjected to two treadmill exercise tests using the Bruce protocol and separated by 45 min, the incidence of premature ventricular beats was significantly reduced in the second test as was the severity of the arrhythmia. Faris et al. [14] performed serial treadmill exercise tests at average intervals of 2.9 months on 543 state policemen. Of the 184 who had exercise-induced ventricular arrhythmias on the first test, 110 (59%) demonstrated arrhythmias on the second. Similarly, of the 211 who demonstrated arrhythmias on the second test, only 91 (43%) had arrhythmias on the first test. However, in the subgroup of subjects over age 35 with definite or suspected cardiovascular disease, 24 of 32 patients (75%) with arrhythmias on the first test had arrhythmias on the second. Ekblom et al. [15] performed repeat exercise tests within a two-week period in 38 subjects enrolled in an exercise-conditioning program. They used several exercise protocols and reported an individual reproducibility value of only 60%. However, they noted that the incidence of reproducibility increased as the number of premature beats on the first test increased. In subjects with more than ten premature beats on the first test, the chance of having a reproducibile repeat test exceeded 80%. These several studies suggest at first glance that exercise testing may not be associated with a high enough incidence of reproducibility to permit its use as a guide to antiarrhythmic therapy. However, it appears that reproducibility may be quite high in patients with cardiovascular disease and in patients with frequent ectopy. Unfortunately, there is little information on the ability of exercise testing to induce, reproducibly, ventricular tachycardia or other therapy-requiring arrhythmias. Nonetheless, Lown and co-workers [16] are quite explicit in their reliance on exercise testing as a guide to therapy in patients with malignant ventricular arrhythmias. Similarly, other investigators have used exercise testing to assess the response to therapy with a variety of antiarrhythmic drugs [17–21].

Several groups have studied the reproducibility of exercise test responses following myocardial infarction. Markiewicz et al. [22] performed serial exercise tests at two-week intervals in 46 patients from three to 11 weeks following infarction. They noted an increase in the frequency and severity of ventricular ectopic activity between the first test performed at week three and the fifth test performed at week 11, but did not comment on the reproducibility of the test in individual patients. This question was subsequently addressed in two later studies. Sami et al. [23] evaluated the reproducibility of exercise-induced ventricular arrhythmias in 155 patients in whom serial exercise tests were performed at various intervals ranging from one day to six months following myocardial infarction. They noted that the reproducibility of complex ventricular ectopy was more than 50% in virtually all pairs of tests. The highest coefficient for reproducibility was in two tests performed one to five days apart. DeBusk and Haskell (24) performed exercise tests in 200 patients three and 11 weeks following myocardial infarction. They found that ventricular ectopy occurring during a symptom-limited test at three weeks was reproducible at 11 weeks in 79% of their patients. This finding was statistically significant. Thus, in this well-defined population of patients, a reasonable degree of reproducibility can be achieved by exercise testing. However, specific information regarding reproducibility of sustained or nonsustained ventricular tachycardia in this particularly high-risk group is lacking.

Ambulatory ECG monitoring
The use of ambulatory ECG monitoring to detect arrhythmias has also resulted in an extensive bibliography [25–28]. Of particular relevance to this chapter are the studies comparing ambulatory monitoring to exercise testing and those concerned with the reproducibility of ambulatory monitoring in detecting arrhythmias. Ryan et al. [29] compared the two modes of arrhythmia detection in 100 patients with either a prior infarction or angina pectoris. Their results indicated that, whereas ambulatory

ECG monitoring revealed a higher incidence and a greater severity of arrhythmias, the data obtained by each method were complementary. Thus, of the 20 patients with couplets or at least three ventricular premature beats in a row detected by the exercise test, 15 did not demonstrate these arrhythmias during 24 hr of ambulatory monitoring. Conversely, of the 40 patients demonstrating these arrhythmias on ambulatory monitoring, 25 demonstrated lesser grades (according to the Lown classification) during or immediately after exercise.

Several groups have examined the reproducibility of the results of ambulatory monitoring [30–32]. These studies have revealed significant hour-to-hour and day-to-day variability in the frequency and severity of the arrhythmia detected. In the study of Morganroth et al. [30], 15 clinically destable patients were evaluated for three consecutive 24-hr periods. Their results demonstrated a 48% hour-to-hour variation, a 29% 8-hr variation and a 23% day-to-day variation. These investigators concluded that an 83% reduction in ventricular premature beat frequency in two 24-hr periods was needed to attribute any change in frequency to the effects of therapeutic interventions. A 65% reduction in ventricular premature beats was required if consecutive three-day periods were analyzed. In a later study [31], Michelson and Morganroth determined that a 65% decrease in the mean hourly frequency of ventricular tachycardia and a 75% reduction in frequency of couplets were required in 24-hr periods to demonstrate therapeutic efficacy. Sami et al. [32] used linear regression analysis to develop standards for assessing drug effects on serial exercise tests or 24-hr ambulatory ECG recordings. They reported that the minimum percent reduction needed to establish antiarrhythmic efficacy with a 95% confidence level was 68% for treadmill exercise and 65% for ambulatory monitoring. These studies indicate a significant variability in the frequency of ventricular extrasystoles, which precludes easy assessment of drug efficacy unless the frequency of the arrhythmia is reduced greatly.

Intracardiac electrophysiologic studies. The ability of intracardiac extrastimulus testing to induce, reproducibly, supraventricular and ventricular arrhythmias in patients with a known history of these arrhythmias is documented by an ever expanding bibliography [33–40]. For instance, Denes et al.

[35] recently studied a group of patients with the Wolff-Parkinson-White syndrome. They were able to induce tachyarrhythmias in all 20 patients with documented spontaneous arrhythmias, in eight of 12 patients with documented paroxysmal atrial fibrillation, and in five of 14 patients with paroxysmal palpitations but without documented arrhythmias. In contrast, they were able to induce arrhythmias in only one of 12 asymptomatic patients. The reported efficacy of ventricular stimulation techniques in reproducing clinically observed ventricular arrhythmias has been variable. The differences in the results can be attributed to the populations studied (children or adults, patients with ischemia or with other forms of heart disease), the site stimulated (atria, right ventricle, left ventricle), the stimulation protocol employed (single, double, or triple extrasystoles), and the characteristics of the spontaneously occurring ventricular arrhythmia (sustained, nonsustained, and exercise induced). Vandepol et al.[39] recently reported their results on 529 patients studied at the University of Pennsylvania with programmed stimulation for evaluation of documented or suspected arrhythmias. Eighty-six patients had clinically observed ventricular tachycardia. Sustained ventricular tachycardia could be induced in 52 of the 57 patients (71%) in whom this type of arrhythmia was clinically observed. Nonsustained ventricular tachycardia was observed in 18 of the 29 patients (62%) in whom this type of arrhythmia was clinically observed. Ventricular tachycardia could not be induced in 454 patients. Of these, only 14 (3%) had experienced clinically observed ventricular tachycardias. The results from other laboratories revealed reproducibility rates which range from 20% to 95%. Some investigators [41, 42] have advocated the use of isoproterenol to increase the ability to induce arrhythmias. Both supraventricular and ventricular extrastimulus testing appear to be effective means of inducing arrhythmias in susceptible patients and, thus, to provide a mechanism by which antiarrhythmic drug therapy can be designed specifically to prevent the induction of the arrhythmia [41, 43–45]. These investigators have shown that the ability to maintain therapy with drugs at concentrations found to be effective at the time of electrophysiologic testing predicts successful outpatient therapy in the majority of patients in whom the arrhythmia can be induced. However, even in the group with inducible arrhythmias, effective therapeutic regimens cannot always be found.

Setting of therapeutic goals

Were it possible to suppress all premature beats, to prevent all episodes of supraventricular or ventricular tachycardia, and to maintain sinus rhythm in patients with atrial fibrillation with drugs whose use did not carry the risk of serious and potentially life-threatening cardiac or extracardiac effects the setting of therapeutic goals would not require comment. Clearly, the goal would be to abolish whatever abnormality in cardiac rhythm was present. Unfortunately, all of the drugs in use for the treatment and/or prevention of cardiac arrhythmias are capable of causing serious, unwanted effects. For this reason, the setting of realistic therapeutic goals is critical to successful therapy. The prevention of ventricular fibrillation is the primary therapeutic goal in all patients with ventricular arrhythmias. The prevention of syncope, heart failure, or myocardial ischemia is the secondary goal in patients prone to rapid ventricular tachycardia. The prevention of the tachycardia itself is the third goal. Although the optimal therapy may result in prevention of the premature beats which initiate the ventricular tachycardia or ventricular fibrillation, the achievement of this end point often is unrealistic. If the progression of the ventricular premature beat to ventricular tachycardia cannot be suppressed without causing unacceptable, unwanted effects of the drug, then slowing of the rate of the ventricular tachycardia may be an achievable and more appropriate goal. Similarly, in patients with supraventricular tachycardias, control of the ventricular rate to prevent syncope, heart failure, and myocardial ischemia is the primary therapeutic goal. Total suppression of the arrhythmia may be the optimal result, but this end point, like the suppression of ventricular premature beats, may be unobtainable without the production of unacceptable side effects.

The setting of therapeutic goals must be individualized for each patient and then reassessed, depending on the ability to meet these goals and on the overall clinical situation. For instance, the suppression of ventricular premature beats may be the appropriate goal in the setting of an acute myocardial infarction but an inappropriate goal in a patient with no other manifestations of cardiac disease. Prevention of paroxysmal atrial fibrillation may be the appropriate goal in a patient with no other evidence of cardiac disease. However, this goal is inappropriate in a patient with atrial fibrillation and mitral valvular disease and a large left atrium.

Drugs used to treat supraventricular and ventricular tachyarrhythmias

In this section, we will discuss the various drugs according to electrophysiologic and/or clinical similarities. Thus, lidocaine, mexiletine, tocainide, and phenytoin are grouped together, as are quinidine, procainide, disopyramide, encainide, flecainide, and lorcainamide. Verapamil and the other beta-blocking drugs have different electrophysiologic effects, but share certain important clinical characteristics. Amiodarone, aprindine, and bretylium are not as easily classified and are placed in a separate category. The electrophysiologic characteristics of these drugs are detailed in Chapter 7 and have been the subject of other reviews [46–48].

Lidocaine and similar drugs (Table 1)

Lidocaine, mexiletine, and tocainide are electrophysiologically similar in that each produces a more marked effect on the steady state and recovery characteristics of the upstroke of the action potential in depressed than in normal fibers [49, 50]. Moreover, all shorten action potential duration and all are ineffective in altering slow channel-mediated responses. None lengthens the A–H or H–V intervals when they are within normal limits, and none prolongs the QRS complex. From a clinical standpoint, each is more effective in ventricular than in supraventricular arrhythmias.

Lidocaine

Indications. Lidocaine is regarded as the drug of choice for the acute treatment of serious ventricular arrhythmias in a wide variety of clinical settings, including those associated with acute myocardial infarction, general and cardiac surgery, congestive heart failure, and digitalis intoxication. Lidocaine's clinical usefulness is based on its rapid onset of action after intravenous infusion, its efficacy, the relative infrequency of severe hemodynamic or

Table 1.

	L	M	T	P
Distribution T1/2 (min)	8	6	7	?
Elimination T1/2 (hr)	1.5–2	9–12	11–23	20
Bioavailability (%)	<50	85	100	variable
Protein binding (%)	60–70	70	50	90
Route of elimination	liver	liver	liver-kidney	liver
Suggested dose				
I.V.	1.5 mg/kg	200 mg	450 mg in 30–45 min	100 mg q 5–10 min to 1,000 mg maximum
P.O.		200–400 mg q 6–8 hr	400–600 mg q 7–12 hr	300 mg/day
Therapeutic plasma levels (mcg/ml)	1.5–6	0.8–2	3–11	10–20
Common toxicity				
cardiac	rare	rare	rare	rare
extracardiac	CNS	CNS, GI	CNS, GI	CNS, hepatic

L = lidocaine
M = mexiletine
T = tocainide
P = phenytoin

electrophysiologic toxicity, and its short elimination phase half-life. Its major limitation is poor oral bioavailability which precludes its use in chronic antiarrhythmic therapy. Several recent reviews discuss in detail the clinical pharmacology and indications for lidocaine therapy [51–56].

In acute myocardial infarction, it is generally agreed that lidocaine should be administered intravenously in effective doses to patients who develop ventricular arrhythmias. However, the advisability of administering lidocaine to all patients with acute infarction, whether or not they have arrhythmias, in order to prevent primary ventricular fibrillation, remains more controversial. Only one study has tested the efficacy of intravenous 'prophylactic' lidocaine in a carefully designed, prospective fashion, using adequate doses. In this study, Lie and associates [57] found that ventricular fibrillation developed in none of 107 patients given intravenous lidocaine within 6 hr of acute infarction, but did occur in nine of 105 similar patients receiving placebo. As discussed in detail by Noneman and Rogers[58], all of the other studies of 'prophylactic' lidocaine, most of which claim no reduction in ventricular fibrillation, contain methodologic flaws that prevent reliable conclusions. Despite the methodologic difficulties, which tend to minimize possible beneficial effects of lidocaine, De Silva and associates [59] evaluated pooled data involving 1,022 patients from six of these studies [57, 60–64]. They found that 'prophylactic' lidocaine reduced the incidence of ventricular fibrillation from 5.7% (29 of 505 patients) in the control group to 3.1% (16 of 517 patients) in the treated group, a statistically significant difference. Based on these data, most authors [58, 59, 65, 66] now recommend 'prophylactic' lidocaine therapy for the first 24–36 hr in all patients suspected of having an acute myocardial infarction.

The logical extension of this conclusion is the administration of lidocaine by emergency medical personnel before and during transport to the hospital. Several studies have tested the efficacy of intramuscular lidocaine in this setting before [67] or soon after [68, 69] hospitalization for acute infarction. However, these studies also contain methodological limitations [58] which prevent definitive conclusions. For instance, the study of Lie and associates [69] failed to achieve satisfactory serum concentrations of lidocaine despite a 300-mg dose.

The low serum lidocaine levels in this study may account for a lack of a statistically significant difference in the incidence of primary ventricular fibrillation between control and treated groups. Until valid studies are performed, it seems premature to recommend the routine use of lidocaine in the prehospital phase of acute myocardial infarction.

In contrast to its high efficacy in controlling ventricular arrhythmias, lidocaine is rarely of value in treating supraventricular arrhythmias. In fact, lidocaine has been reported to increase the ventricular rate in some patients with atrial fibrillation and flutter, both in the presence of normal atrioventricular conduction [70] and in the Wolff-Parkinson-White syndrome [71].

Clinical pharmacology (Table 1 and Chapter 7). The oral bioavailability of lidocaine is only 35–40% [72, 73] due to a high presystemic clearance. Seventy percent of portal vein lidocaine is extracted and metabolized during a single pass through the liver [73, 74]. This high hepatic extraction precludes the oral use of lidocaine and makes the disposition of lidocaine very sensitive to changes in hepatic blood flow. The pharmacokinetics of intravenously administered lidocaine are described in several recent reviews [51–56]. The disposition of an intravenously administered lidocaine bolus can be described by an open two-compartment model [73, 75] and is thought to follow first-order kinetics. There is a rapid early decline in lidocaine concentration which corresponds roughly with the distribution of the drug from the central compartment, i.e., the blood volume and extracellular space, to the peripheral compartment. The half-life of this distribution phase is approximately 8–10 min and accounts for the short duration of lidocaine's antiarrhythmic effect after bolus dosing. After rapid distribution, plasma levels fall more slowly, with an elimination or beta phase half-life of 65–138 min [73, 75–79]. There is marked variability in lidocaine pharmacokinetics between normal subjects suggesting that the published calculations and computer projections of loading and maintenance doses, which are based on mean values, may be difficult to apply to an individual subject. In elderly patients without congestive heart failure, the elimination phase half-life and steady-state volume of distribution are greater than in younger subjects [79, 80]. In patients with congestive heart failure, lidocaine clearance is lower than in normals after a bolus injection, but half-life is not significantly prolonged [77]. Patients with liver disease have a lower lidocaine clearance and much longer elimination half-life than normals [77]. Lidocaine kinetics in patients with renal failure do not differ from those of normals [77].

When lidocaine is discontinued after more than 24 hr of constant rate infusion in patients with acute myocardial infarction but without congestive heart failure, the elimination phase half-life ranges from 3.2 to 7.2 hr [78, 79, 81–83], which is much longer than when calculated after bolus injection in normal subjects. Indeed, only one group of investigators reported a half-life shorter than 2-1/2 hr following a constant rate infusion [84]. A longer half-life and lower clearance of lidocaine after prolonged infusion have been demonstrated in normal subjects [76] as well as as in patients with myocardial infarction. In patients with congestive heart failure receiving prolonged infusions, lidocaine clearance is further reduced and the elimination phase half-life is further prolonged [78, 82, 83, 85].

A particularly important feature of prolonged lidocaine infusion is a progressive increase in lidocaine plasma concentration in patients with an acute myocardial infarction [78, 81, 83, 86]. This increase continues beyond the four to five half-lives usually thought to predict steady-state concentration. This may be due to an increase in alpha-1-acid glycoprotein [86, 87], the principal plasma binding protein for lidocaine [88]. These changes in protein binding in patients with acute infarction may preclude the use of total plasma lidocaine concentration as a predictor of toxicity [87] or a guide to therapy [86] since the effects of lidocaine correlate with the free rather than with the total drug concentration.

Dosage and routes of administration. Because of its poor oral bioavailability, lidocaine must be administered parenterally. The reliability of intramuscular lidocaine has not been clearly established, with three studies reporting adequate lidocaine levels after injection of 200–455 mg [89–91] but a fourth study finding subtherapeutic levels after a 300-mg injection[69]. Until this question has been resolved, lidocaine should be administered intravenously whenever possible.

Most commonly, intravenous lidocaine therapy is initiated with a single bolus. However, because of the 8-min distribution half-life, the serum concentration may fall to subtherapeutic levels in 5–15 min. Administration of the loading dose in two or more successive, smaller boluses [51, 55, 66, 92], as a rapid infusion over 10–15 min [51, 66], or by a combination of these methods [84, 93] may overcome this problem. The double bolus technique seems to offer the advantages of ease of administration, rapid attainment of adequate lidocaine concentrations, a low risk of transient toxicity, and the least possibility of a dosing error. The simplest approach is to administer slowly a 100–125-mg bolus regardless of the patient's size and to repeat the bolus at the same or a slightly reduced dose (75–100 mg) 10–15 min later. An alternative is to administer an initial intravenous bolus of 1.5 mg/kg followed by a second bolus of 1 mg/kg 10–15 min later, although there may be no need to adjust the loading dose according to body weight since the initial volume of distribution correlates poorly with weight [55, 56]. However, at the extremes of body weight, it is our practice to reduce the initial bolus to 75 mg in patients under 50 kg and to increase it to 150 mg in patients over 100 kg. Each bolus should be given over at least 1–2 min, since faster injection may produce transient neurologic toxicity.

A maintenance infusion should be started immediately after the initial bolus. Most authors recommend a maintenance infusion of 2 mg/min. The infusion rate should be reduced to 1–1.5 mg/min in patients with heart failure or liver disease and to 0.75–1.0 mg/min in patients with cardiogenic shock. Furthermore, it is reasonable to reduce the infusion rate by 25% after 24 hr because of recent data showing a lower clearance and longer half-life following a prolonged infusion, particularly in patients with acute myocardial infarction [78, 81, 82, 84, 86]. If ventricular arrhythmias occur during the first 4–6 hr of the maintenance infusion, an additional bolus of 25–50 mg should be given. If arrhythmias occur after 6–8 hr of infusion, this small bolus should be accompanied by an increase of 0.5–1.0 mg/min in the infusion rate to a maximum of 4 mg/min. It is important to realize that simply increasing the infusion rate without an additional bolus may not achieve a new steady state for 8–10 hr.

Combination therapy and interactions. Lidocaine can be used in combination with the quinidine-like drugs with little risk of additive cardiovascular toxicity. Moreover, the differences in the noncardiac side effects between these two agents will permit their combined use.

There are relatively few well-documented interactions of lidocaine with other drugs. Ochs and co-workers [76] have described a reduction in lidocaine clearance and an increase in lidocaine half-life and serum concentration during propranolol coadministration, an effect attributed to the lower cardiac output and lower hepatic blood flow caused by propranolol. In general, the high hepatic extraction of lidocaine makes its clearance very sensitive to drugs and agents that alter hepatic blood flow. Drugs that reduce hepatic blood flow might be expected to raise lidocaine serum levels, whereas those that increase hepatic blood flow might enhance lidocaine clearance and lower lidocaine serum levels. Although there is some evidence that drugs which alter hepatic microsomal activity, such as phenobarbital, halothane, isoniazid, and chloramphenicol, may affect lidocaine clearance and blood levels [94–96], this interaction is of relatively little clinical importance.

There is experimental evidence in single fibers to suspect that the effects of lidocaine may be more pronounced in the presence of hyperkalemia and less pronounced in the presence of hypokalemia, but this has not been reported in humans.

Use of blood levels. It is generally accepted that a total plasma lidocaine concentration greater than 1.5 μg/ml usually is required for a therapeutic effect, and that central nervous system toxicity occurs more frequently above a total concentration of 6.0 μg/ml. The measurement of plasma lidocaine levels may be useful clinically in the following situations: (a) when ventricular arrhythmias are not controlled by the usual doses of lidocaine; (b) when lidocaine toxicity is suspected as the cause of nonspecific neurologic signs and symptoms; (c) in patients with shock who may have a pronounced reduction in lidocaine clearance; and (d) in patients receiving infusions for more than 24 hr in whom lidocaine concentrations may rise progressively. The limited availability of a rapid lidocaine assay has contributed to the infrequent use of lidocaine levels in the routine care of critically ill patients. With the recent development of an inexpensive rapid homogeneous enzyme-linked immunoassay

(EMIT) for lidocaine [97, 98], it is possible that these obstacles will be removed and blood levels will be more extensively assayed.

However, it must be remembered that in situations of varying protein binding, such as acute myocardial infarction [86, 87], the correlation between clinical efficacy and toxicity to the total lidocaine concentration may be misleading. In these situations, the measurement of free lidocaine concentrations may prove to be more appropriate.

Toxicity and contraindications. The toxic manifestations of lidocaine are almost entirely limited to the central nervous system. These include somnolence, vertigo, disorientation, psychosis, paresthesias, muscle twitching, and, rarely, respiratory depression and seizures. These adverse effects will occur much less frequently if the lidocaine bolus is given over 1–2 min. The incidence of neurologic toxicity during prolonged infusions was shown to be only 4.1% (31 of 750 patients) in one study [99], but in six of the 31 patients, the toxic manifestations were judged to be life-threatening. Therefore, clinical vigilance is clearly indicated when prolonged lidocaine infusions are required.

Cardiovascular toxicity of lidocaine is uncommon. Several case reports attribute sinus arrest [100–103], asystole [104], and atrioventricular block [105–108] to lidocaine. In most instances, the AV block occurred in patients with bundle branch block and prior transient AV block. However, many patients with bundle branch block may experience no alteration of atrioventricular conduction [109]. Lidocaine may cause slowing of the escape rhythm associated with atrioventricular block, probably by producing exit block of the ectopic focus [110, 111]. The drug may accelerate the ventricular response to atrial fibrillation in patients with normal atrioventricular conduction [70] as well as those with the Wolff-Parkinson-White syndrome [71]. Worsening of ventricular arrhythmias might be expected with lidocaine as with any antiarrhythmic drug having direct membrane effects. However, such adverse reactions are extremely rare. Lidocaine has no important negative inotropic effect at the usual plasma concentrations, and allergic reactions to lidocaine are rare.

Although there are few absolute contradictions to lidocaine, insertion of a temporary ventricular pacemaker should be considered before lidocaine is given to patients with known advanced sinus node dysfunction or prior distal atrioventricular block. Because such patients are dependent on escape rhythms to maintain their cardiac output, lidocaine should not be given to them unless a ventricular pacemaker is in place. Finally, patients in shock may accumulate extremely high lidocaine concentrations and therefore require careful observation.

Mexiletine

Mexiletine is a recently developed drug with local anesthetic and anticonvulsant properties. It is structurally and electrophysiologically similar to lidocaine [49] but, unlike lidocaine, has a high oral bioavailability and thus can be administered orally as well as intravenously. It also differs from lidocaine in that it has a long elimination half-life. The drug has been used in Europe for several years, but remains under investigation in the United States and Canada. The antiarrhythmic properties and clinical uses of mexiletine are detailed in several recent reviews [112–115].

Indications. Studies from Europe and more recently from the United States have shown that mexiletine is effective in reducing the frequency of ventricular premature beats in patients with chronic stable heart disease [116–119], acute myocardial infarction [120, 121], and digitalis intoxication [122]. Although in one study [123] mexiletine was deemed ineffective in preventing drug-induced recurrent ventricular tachycardia, it was found to be effective in 15 of 23 similar patients in another study [124]. Mexiletine did not prevent sudden cardiac death in a long-term controlled study of patients following myocardial infarction, although it did reduce ventricular ectopy [125]. The similarity of the electrophysiologic effects of mexiletine and lidocaine would suggest that the spectrum of the drug's antiarrhythmic efficacy would parallel that of lidocaine. Like lidocaine, mexiletine to date has been found relatively ineffective in the treatment of supraventricular tachycardias. Like lidocaine, it may shorten the antegrade refractory period of the accessory pathway in patients with the Wolff-Parkinson-White syndrome [126]. Mexiletine occasionally may be effective in apparently lidocaine-resistant ventricular arrhythmias [120, 127], although lidocaine predicted the efficacy of mexiletine in one study [127]. Although these studies did not report

drug levels, it seems possible that instances of poor correlation between the efficacy of lidocaine and mexiletine may be due to noncomparable plasma levels.

Clinical pharmacology (Table 1 and Chapter 7). Mexiletine is rapidly distributed to the tissue depots following intravenous infusion. The distribution phase half-life is approximately 7 min [128, 129]. The elimination phase half-life in healthy volunteers averages approximately 11 hr after both intravenous and oral dosing [123, 128, 130]. Mexiletine is well absorbed from the gastrointestinal tract, with a bioavailability of 80–90% [129, 130].

Mexiletine is eliminated primarily by hepatic metabolism, but the hepatic extraction is relatively low. Therefore, mexiletine clearance should be relatively insensitive to changes in hepatic blood flow. This explains the observation that patients with heart failure and presumably reduced hepatic blood flow did not have significantly prolonged elimination phase half-lives [128]. Renal insufficiency does not prolong the elimination of mexiletine [131].

Dosage and route of administration. At present, intravenous mexiletine is not available in the United States. However, as a result of experience in other countries, a rapid intravenous infusion followed by several progressively slower infusions is recommended [113, 120, 128, 132]. For example, Campbell and associates [120, 128] recommended an infusion of 200 mg over 3–5 min, followed by 3 mg/min for 1 hr, and then 1.5 mg/min for 3 hr, followed by a maintenance infusion of 1 mg/min. Since many of the reported serious adverse effects have been reported after rapid intravenous infusion, it may prove safer to administer the initial 200-mg dose over 15–30 min. Side effects may also be minimized by infusing mexiletine at a rate of 10 mg/min until arrhythmia suppression or early side effects occur, to a maximum of 400–500 mg.

The oral administration of mexiletine can be initiated with a 400-mg [128, 132]–600-mg dose [121] in order to hasten the achievement of therapeutic concentrations.

The achievement of a steady-state plasma concentration requires three to four days because of the long elimination phase half-life. We have observed considerable interpatient variability in both the effective and maximum tolerated dose [124]. This is consistent with a marked interpatient variability in pharmacokinetics [128]. For this reason, and because of the low therapeutic index of mexiletine [110, 112, 118], we individualize the maintenance dose by starting with 200–250 mg every 8 hr and increasing the dose every 48–72 hr by 50–100-mg increments until the desired antiarrhythmic effect occurs or until the patient develops early signs of toxicity. These mild adverse effects often resolve when the dose is reduced by 50 mg, without loss of antiarrhythmic efficacy. We have found that some patients require and tolerate doses as large as 1,600 mg/day, usually given in four rather than three divided doses to minimize adverse effects.

Combination therapy and interactions. Several authors have reported that mexiletine may control ventricular arrhythmias when administered in combination with quinidine [124, 127, 133], procainamide [124, 133], propranolol [134], disopyramide [135], or lorcainide [136], when the individual drugs have been ineffective.

One might expect the antiarrhythmic and toxic effects of mexiletine and lidocaine to be additive. For this reason, it is our practice to decrease lidocaine infusion by 0.5–1.0 mg/min with each dose of mexiletine when mexiletine is given to patients receiving lidocaine.

Use of blood levels. Several studies agree that plasma mexiletine levels between 0.75 and 2.0 mcg/ml represent the therapeutic range and that concentrations above 2.0 mcg/ml commonly produce toxic manifestations [116, 118, 120, 128]. Measurement of mexiletine blood levels will be valuable in patients with infrequent but severe ventricular arrhythmias, in order to ensure that chronic levels equal or exceed those found to be effective during acute drug testing.

Toxicity and contraindications. Adverse effects of mexiletine are common, dose related, and reversible [113, 118, 120, 123, 124, 137]. Anorexia, nausea, epigastric discomfort, and fine tremors of the hands are the earliest symptomatic adverse effects. These symptoms are often mild and may not require a modification of the drug dosage, since the gastrointestinal effects may be minimized by the coadministration of food and antacids. At higher doses, mexiletine may produce vomiting, ataxia, diplopia,

dizziness, dysarthria, nystagmus, and confusion. A dose reduction of as little as 50 mg may result in relief of these symptoms. However, the difference between the lowest effective dose and the highest tolerated dose, i.e., the therapeutic index, is small. For this reason the lowest effective dose may produce intolerable symptoms in some patients. Thus careful attention to dose adjustment is required for each patient.

As with lidocaine, cardiovascular or life-threatening toxicity is uncommon. Hypotension, sinus arrest, sinoatrial block, and atrioventricular conduction disturbances have been observed [120, 138], but these may have occurred during rapid intravenous administration [138] and do not seem to occur with chronic therapy. A spontaneous increase in ventricular arrhythmias is rare, but does occur [120]. We have encountered two patients in whom such a response was suspected during electrophysiologic study. Although cardiac depressant effects have been observed in dogs after very large intravenous doses [139], this has not been found in humans [140–142]. No long-term toxicity from mexiletine has been recognized during published follow-up for as long as one to two years [118, 124, 137].

Tocainide

Tocainide is a structural analog of lidocaine, from which it differs in being a primary rather than a tertiary amine. It shares with mexiletine a high oral bioavailability and long half-life and is currently undergoing clinical trials in the United States. The electrophysiologic effects and pharmacologic and antiarrhythmic properties of tocainide, which resemble many of those of lidocaine and mexiletine [50], have recently been summarized by Danilo [143] and by Zipes and Troup [144].

Indications. Tocainide has been shown to reduce the frequency of ventricular premature beats in 58–100% of patients with chronic stable cardiac disease [145–151]. Tocainide may be effective in recurrent ventricular tachycardia or fibrillation refractory to other drugs [152–154] although success is not uniform. Zipes and Troup [144] found tocainide ineffective in five patients with recurrent refractory ventricular tachycardia. There are no satisfactory studies of the efficacy of intravenous or oral tocainide in acute ventricular arrhythmias, including those occurring during acute myocardial infarction. As with mexiletine, one would expect the efficacy of tocainide to parallel that of lidocaine. However, it is still uncertain whether the effect of lidocaine on a patient's arrhythmia predicts success of failure with tocainide [153–155]. As with mexiletine, it is possible that less than maximal blood levels of lidocaine [155] may explain apparent tocainide success in lidocaine-'resistant' arrhythmias. Conversely, side effects of tocainide may prevent attainment of an effective blood level. Tocainide, like lidocaine, usually is ineffective in the treatment of atrial arrhythmias. However, Waleffe et al. [156] reported that tocainide prevented AV nodal reentrant arrhythmias in one of two patients and accessory pathway reentrant arrhythmias in two of four patients.

Clinical pharmacology (Table 1 and Chapter 7). Although there is some discrepancy in the literature regarding the rapid distribution kinetics of tocainide, it appears that they are similar to those of mexiletine with a distribution phase half-life of approximately 7 min [157] and an elimination phase half-life of approximately 12–14 hr in normal subjects [157, 158]. In patients with acute myocardial infarction, both the distribution and elimination phase half-lives may be slightly prolonged [157]. The mean elimination half-life of tocainide following chronic oral dosing is similar to that reported after intravenous infusion [145, 146]. As with mexiletine, there may be considerable interpatient differences, and half-lives ranging from 11.5 to 22.8 hr have been reported [145, 146, 159]. The kinetics of tocainide have not been reported for patients with congestive heart failure or with renal or hepatic insufficiency.

Tocainide is nearly 100% bioavailable after oral administration [151, 157, 158] with no substantial first-pass effect. Approximately 40% of an intravenous or oral dose is excreted unchanged in the urine [146, 147, 157, 158, 160], and 15–30% of the remainder is conjugated in the liver to a glucuronide [160]. Lalka and associates [158] reported a 75% reduction in renal excretion of unchanged tocainide after urinary alkalinization. Differences in urinary pH might explain the large variation in renal excretion reported by Woosley and co-workers [146].

Dosage and routes of administration. The clinical use of intravenous tocainide has not been reported in detail. Single loading infusions of 450 mg over 45 min [161] or administration of 0.5–0.75 mg/kg/min over 15 min [162, 163] have been suggested. There are no published data regarding maintenance intravenous infusion rates for tocainide.

Oral dosing has been accomplished with an initial dose of 400–1,200 mg/day in two or three divided doses [145, 153, 154, 164] followed by an increase in dose every 48 hr until the desired response occurs or until adverse effects develop [145, 153, 154, 164, 165]. Most patients have been maintained on 800–2,400 mg/day in two, three, or four divided doses. It has been reported that doses over 2,400 mg/day are usually associated with side effects [152], although one study reports a daily dose as high as 3,200 mg [164].

Combination therapy and interactions. As with mexiletine, one might expect the combination of tocainide and a quinidine-like drug to be effective in some patients resistant to each drug alone. Combination therapy is mentioned in several clinical reports [152, 154, 159], but few details are provided.

Use of blood levels. Therapeutic efficacy has been reported to occur at plasma concentrations ranging from 3–19 mcg/ml [146, 154, 159]. Roden and associates [154] observed that 25% of their patients had a 60% reduction in the frequency of ventricular premature beats at plasma levels as low as 3 mcg/ml and that 25% of their patients developed adverse effects at plasma levels greater than 11 mcg/ml. As with mexiletine, plasma levels may be useful during chronic maintenance therapy to ensure that they are similar to those shown to be effective during acute drug testing.

Toxicity and contraindications. The adverse effects of tocainide resemble those of mexiletine. They are dose related and rapidly reversible [150, 152–154, 164, 165]. The most frequently occurring side effects are nausea, vomiting, anorexia, dizziness, paresthesias, tremor, confusion, and impairment of memory. In addition, allergic manifestations including skin rash, pruritis, and eosinophilia have been reported [150, 154, 165]. Rarely, tocainide may be arrhythmogenic [152, 153, 165], and one report suggests that it caused an ANA-negative immune-complex glomerulonephritis [153]. Tocainide appears to have no clinically important negative inotropic effects [162, 163, 166] and has been used in patients with congestive heart failure. The safety of tocainide in patients with preexisting disorders of sinus node function or of atrioventricular or intraventricular conduction abnormalities has not been carefully studied. The drug produced no long-term toxicity during chronic therapy for as long as three years [167].

Phenytoin

The use of phenytoin (diphenylhydantoin) as an antiarrhythmic drug received much attention during the 1960s, but relatively few investigators and clinicians now regard it as a first-line antiarrhythmic agent. There is only one detailed recent review of phenytoin as an antiarrhythmic drug [168], although a discussion of phenytoin is included in several general reviews of antiarrhythmic therapy [169–171].

Indications. Based on clinical [172–176] and animal [177–179] studies during the 1960s, phenytoin has been recommended [168, 170, 172–176] as a primary drug for the treatment of arrhythmias associated with digitalis intoxication. However, these early clinical studies were uncontrolled, tended to be descriptive rather than quantitative, often did not characterize carefully the arrhythmia being treated, and, with one exception [176], did not report serum phenytoin concentrations. Furthermore, the studies were performed before radioimmunoassay techniques were developed to measure the concentration of digitalis glycosides in the serum. Therefore, the efficacy of phenytoin in treating digitalis-induced arrhythmias remains somewhat uncertain. Nonetheless, its primary use as an antiarrhythmic drug, at present, is in the treatment of digitalis-induced atrial and ventricular tachyarrhythmias.

Despite early optimism about the efficacy of phenytoin in suppressing supraventricular and ventricular arrhythmias in the absence of digitalis intoxication [172, 174–176, 180] or preventing sudden death after myocardial infarction [181], more recent impressions have been less enthusiastic. For instance, phenytoin did not reduce death after infarction in two prospective, controlled studies [182, 183], failed to prevent recurrent ventricular tachycardia [184], was less effective than procainamide in

suppressing ventricular arrhythmias after acute myocardial infarction [185], and, in a carefully controlled recent study using a computerized Holter analysis system, did not reduce the frequency of simple or complex ventricular premature beats [186].

Clinical pharmacology (Table 1 and Chapter 7). Although estimates of phenytoin absorption are complicated by nonlinear elimination kinetics, dose-dependent absorption rates [187], and possible enterohepatic cycling [188, 189], phenytoin appears to be 70–91% bioavailable when the area under the plasma–concentration time curve after oral dosing is compared to that after intravenous administration [187, 190–192]. However, by use of a nonlinear computation method, Jusko and associates reported that phenytoin is 98% bioavailable [192]. The rate of phenytoin absorption is dose-dependent, with peak serum concentrations occurring approximately 8 hr after a single 400-mg dose but not until 32 hr after a 1,600-mg dose [187]. During chronic therapy 30 or more days may be required to achieve steady-state serum concentrations [193].

Phenytoin is nearly completely metabolized in the liver. In one study, some patients with severe hepatic disease accumulated phenytoin to high plasma levels and developed symptomatic toxicity while taking a chronic daily dose of 300 mg [194]. However, in another study the clearance of a single intravenous dose of 250 mg, which produced low serum concentrations of less than 8 mcg/ml, was not altered in the presence of viral hepatitis [195].

Phenytoin is 90–95% bound to serum proteins, principally albumin [196]. Renal failure, high serum bilirubin levels, and various drugs, including salicylates, valproic acid, sulfonylureas, and phenylbutazone, increase the free fraction of phenytoin by displacing it from protein binding sites [169, 170, 196, 197]. Lower-than-usual total phenytoin concentrations may then produce the desired therapeutic effect, and efforts to raise the total concentration into the 'therapeutic' range may result in toxicity. Many drugs, including isoniazid, coumadin, barbiturates, propoxyphene, benzodiazepines, phenothiazines, and ethyl alcohol alter hepatic metabolism of phenytoin and produce unexpectedly high or low phenytoin serum concentrations [169]. The pharmacokinetics of phenytoin differ from those of most other antiarrhythmic drugs in that its disposition is nonlinear, due to saturation of hepatic metabolic pathways [169, 170, 196]. Although it has been estimated that the half-life of phenytoin is approximately 16–22 hr [169, 191] at low serum concentrations [191], both its half-life and its clearance are highly dependent on serum level over the therapeutic range of concentrations. The nonlinearity of phenytoin kinetics may be of considerable clinical importance, since a small increase in phenytoin dose within the usual dosing range may produce a relatively large increase in serum concentration [169, 170, 196, 198]. Therefore, the dose should be increased in small increments when the concentration is near the therapeutic range in order to avoid symptomatic toxicity.

Dosage and routes of administration. Because of its long half-life, intervals of several days to a week or more are required to achieve therapeutic plasma concentrations if phenytoin therapy is started with maintenance dosing. In urgent clinical situations, therefore, a rapid intravenous loading dose is often desirable. Based on the work of Bigger and associates [176], intravenous loading with phenytoin is usually accomplished by giving 50–100 mg every 5–10 min until toxicity or the desired therapeutic effect occurs, to a maximum of 1,000 mg [169, 170]. However, on the basis of their experience with 139 patients, Cranford and associates recommend an intravenous loading dose of 18 mg/kg administered at a rate of 50 mg/min [199]. Intravenous phenytoin must be administered in a small volume of diluent having an alkaline pH (~11.7) since dilution in large volumes of fluid may result in precipitation of the drug [168, 196].

Oral loading with phenytoin also is possible. Woosley and Shand [54] suggest 300 mg initially, followed by 200 mg every 2–3 hr to a total of 900–1,100 mg. However, another study suggests that the oral loading dose may have to be larger than the intravenous loading dose, due to delayed absorption of large oral doses [187]. Several authors [53, 169, 170, 200] recommend a second smaller loading dose of 500 mg 24 hr after the initial load in order to maintain adequate plasma levels.

Intramuscular injection of phenytoin should be avoided, since it may be absorbed unreliably and erratically [201].

The usual maintenance dose of phenytoin in adults is 300–400 mg/day, usually given in divided doses although a single daily dose may be satisfactory [200, 202, 203]. After two to four weeks of maintenance therapy, it is necessary to obtain a trough plasma phenytoin level, since interpatient variability in phenytoin disposition makes prediction of the plasma level quite difficult. In general, if this concentration is less than 6 mcg/ml, the daily dose can be increased by 50–100 mg, but if the level is greater than 6 mcg/ml, a smaller daily dose increment of only 25–50 mg is desirable [204, 205]. The serum level should be checked again two to four weeks after each subsequent dose change. Several nomograms [198, 206] and graphic [204, 206, 207] techniques have been described that improve predictability of phenytoin serum levels after dose adjustments. However, even these techniques are not accurate enough [208] to obviate the need for measurement of serum phenytoin concentrations and clinical evaluation for toxicity after each dose adjustment and periodically during chronic therapy.

Combination therapy and interactions. There is little information available about the efficacy and tolerance of phenytoin when used in combination with other antiarrhythmic drugs, although such combination therapy is encountered frequently. One important interaction occurs when phenytoin and quinidine are used together, since phenytoin induces hepatic microsomal enzymes that metabolize quinidine [209]. Therefore, serum quinidine concentrations may fall if phenytoin is added or rise to toxic levels if phenytoin is discontinued at a time when quinidine concentration is in the therapeutic range. Alteration of phenytoin pharmacokinetics or serum concentration by drugs that change protein binding or hepatic metabolism of phenytoin has been discussed above. Phenytoin has been reported to decrease the diuretic effect of furosemide by impairing its absorption [210] and to cause hypotension in critically ill patients dependent on dopamine for blood pressure support [211]. This latter clinical observation was confirmed experimentally in hypotensive dogs on various pressor agents and could be explained by a systemic vasodilatory effect of phenytoin [212].

Use of blood levels. The generally accepted range of plasma phenytoin concentrations for antiarrhythmic as well as anticonvulsant efficacy is 10–20 mcg/ml [53, 54, 168, 169, 176, 196]. As discussed above, measurement of the trough concentration of phenytoin in the blood is necessary two to four weeks after starting maintenance therapy, two to four weeks after each subsequent adjustment of dose, and periodically thereafter.

Toxicity and contraindications. When administered intravenously at rates faster than 25–50 mg/min, phenytoin may cause severe cardiopulmonary toxicity, including hypotension due to systemic vasodilatation and probably depression of myocardial contractility, respiratory arrest, asystole, atrioventricular block, ventricular tachyarrhythmias, and death [50, 51, 168–171, 176, 213]. However, these complications are infrequent when the intravenous loading dose is given at a rate of 50 mg/min [199] or less. During chronic therapy, certain adverse effects are relatively predictable and correlate with plasma concentration, with nystagmus appearing at levels of 15–20 mcg/ml, ataxia above 30 mcg/ml, and lethargy or somnolence above 40 mcg/ml [213]. As reviewed recently [214], phenytoin may cause a wide variety of adverse effects not related to dose or plasma concentration, including gingival hyperplasia, coarse facial features, peripheral neuropathy, pseudolymphoma syndrome, neonatal vitamin K deficiency, hepatic injury, rickets and osteomalacia, hyperglycemia, and paradoxical seizures [158, 169, 178, 196, 214]. Dermatologic complications may consist of a mild morbilliform rash or, rarely, severe disorders such as toxic epidermal necrolysis, exfoliative dermatitis, or Stevens-Johnson syndrome [196, 214, 215]. A distinctive pattern of congenital malformations has been reported in some children of mothers treated with hydantoin anticonvulsants during pregnancy, including craniofacial abnormalities, growth deficiency, and digital hypoplasia [214, 216].

The quinidine group (Tables 2A and B)

Quinidine, procainamide, disopyramide, encainide, flecainide, and lorcainide are grouped together because of the similarities in their electrophysiological effects on single fibers and intact hearts and because of their similar clinical indications and effects. Although some of the drugs have not been studied thoroughly, the available information suggests that the drugs share with quinidine the ability to depress the rate of rise of the action potential upstroke in normal as well as depressed fibers, lengthen action potential duration, increase the refractory period out of proportion to the increase in action potential duration, and suppress spontaneous ectopic activity [46–48]. In intact hearts, the drugs tend to slow intra-atrial, His-Purkinje, and intraventricular conduction, widen the QRS complex and prolong the Q-T interval. Differences in their clinical efficacy probably are related to quantitative differences in their effects on conduction and refractoriness, in their dose–response relationships and therapeutic toxic ratios, and in their anticholinergic activity.

Quinidine

Quinidine is structurally related to quinine and is found along with quinine in the bark of the cinchona tree. This bark was first used as an antiarrhythmic agent in the mid-18th century by Jean Baptiste de Senac and was studied by Wenkebach and Frey during the early part of the twentieth century [217–219].

Indications. Acute drug testing indicates that quinidine is effective in most patients with frequent premature ventricular beats or high grade ventricular ectopy [220]. These effects can be demonstrated in patients with ectopy of acute onset following myocardial infarction and in patients with long-standing ventricular ectopy [221–225]. However, in patients with recurrent episodes of sustained ventricular tachycardia or fibrillation, the drug is less effective. Acute testing of quinidine during provocative electrophysiological testing in these patients has a success rate of 5–40%. This discrepancy between the drug's effect in the treatment of ventricular arrhythmias following a myocardial infarction or in the treatment of sporadic ectopy and of recurrent sustained ventricular tachycardia probably reflects differences in patient population and dosage of drug employed [41, 43, 133].

Quinidine has been used prophylactically to prevent recurrent sudden cardiac death in patients at high risk for this syndrome. Myerberg et al. suggested that the achievement of therapeutic blood levels of the drug resulted in a decreased mortality in patients who had suffered a prior episode of ventricular fibrillation even though ventricular ec-

Table 2A.

	Q	PA	D
Distribution T1/2 (min)	7–10	5	2
Elimination T1/2 (hr)	4–6	3–4	4–8
Bioavailability (%)	95	75–95	90
Protein binding (%)	80	15	40
Route of elimination	liver	liver-kidney	kidney
Suggested dose			
I.V.	*6–10 mg/kg over 30–45 min	50 mg/min to total 10–20 mg/kg	*0.5 mg/kg × 4 doses
P.O.	800–2,000 mg/day in divided doses	250–750 mg 3–4 hr	100–250 mg q 6 hr
Therapeutic plasma level (mcg/ml)	2–8	4–12	2–7
Common toxicity			
Cardiac	V. arrhythmia	V. arrhythmia	V. arrhythmia ↓ contractility
Extracardiac	GI, thrombocytopenia	GI, lupus	GI, urinary retention

* = not usually recommended
Q = quinidine
PA = procainamide
D = disopyramide

Table 2B.

	E	F	Lo
Distribution T1/2 (min)	?	?	18–60
Elimination T1/2 (hr)	3–5	7–26	6–13
Bioavailability (%)	40–50	95	25–50
Protein binding (%)	?	?	85
Route of elimination	liver		liver
Suggested dose			?
I.V.	?	?	
P.O.	25–100 mg q 6–8 hr	150–300 mg q 12 hr	100–150 mg q 8–12 hr
Therapeutic plasma level (mcg/ml)	variable	0.9–1.6	0.15–0.40
Common toxicity			
Cardiac	V.arrhythmia	V. arrhythmia ↓ contractility	? V. arrhythmia
Extracardiac	GI, CNS	CNS	CNS, GI

E = encainide
F = flecainide
Lo = lorcainide

topy was not necessarily suppressed [226, 227]. However, these studies have not been confirmed and the high incidence of side effects, particularly gastrointestinal, and its unproven efficacy have limited the widespread prophylactic use of quinidine (see below).

Quinidine has been used to convert atrial fibrilla-tion and flutter to normal sinus rhythm [225]. However, the practice of using progressively increasing doses of quinidine to accomplish this goal has largely been abandoned in favor of electrical cardioversion, which is considered to be more effective and less hazardous [228, 229]. Quinidine is also used to prevent recurrences of atrial fibrillation. However, there is disagreement concerning the effectiveness of the drug in this situation. For instance, Sodermark reported that quinidine reduced the recurrence rate of atrial fibrillation for at least one year following successful cardioversion in a large series of patients [229], whereas other studies have shown a less convincing success rate [230, 231]. The differences between the results of these studies may reflect differences in the patient populations under study. Patients with enlarged atria are predisposed to atrial fibrillation and quinidine may not significantly influence the recurrence rate.

Quinidine may also be used in the treatment of atrial flutter. However, its use in this setting has several limitations. Slowing of atrial conduction may result in a slower flutter rate. This, combined with a vagolytic effect that tends to shorten AV nodal refractoriness, can result in a paradoxical increase in the ventricular response. The concomitant use of digitalis is therefore necessary to increase the refractory period of the AV junction and prevent the paradoxical increase in ventricular rate.

Quinidine is effective in preventing recurrences of paroxysmal atrioventricular reentrant tachycardia in patients with and without the Wolff-Parkinson-White syndrome [232–235]. This effect may be due to the suppression of the premature atrial or ventricular beats which initiate the arrhythmia, or to changes in the refractory period of the atrioventricular junction which prevent the reentry of the premature beats. In patients with the Wolff-Parkinson-White syndrome, the drug increases refractoriness of the accessory pathway. Wellens et al. [233] noted that the magnitude of the increase in the refractory period of the accessory pathway was related to its initial refractory period. When the effective refractory period was less than 270 msec, only modest lengthening in refractoriness occurred following quinidine. When the initial refractory period was greater than 270 msec, the lengthening of the refractory period was significantly greater.

The effects of quinidine on antegrade and retrograde conduction in tachycardias using an accessory pathway appear to be independent of one another. Prolongation of the refractory period of the antegrade accessory pathway without a change in refractoriness in the retrograde pathway might widen the echo zone and facilitate the induction of reentry. In some patients, this may facilitate the spontaneous initiation of supraventricular tachycardia. Whether quinidine would prevent or potentiate the initiation and maintenance of paroxysmal supraventricular tachycardia in an individual patient with Wolff-Parkinson-White syndrome cannot be predicted without electrophysiological studies [233].

Paroxysmal supraventricular tachycardia from AV nodal reentry can also be treated effectively with quinidine. The drug has been reported to cause a major depressant effect on the retrograde fast pathway contributing to this arrhythmia and thus is highly effective in preventing recurrences of paroxysmal supraventricular tachycardia [234].

The effect of quinidine on ectopic atrial tachycardia has not been studied carefully. Some authors believe it should be beneficial because of its depressant effect on spontaneously depolarizing fibers. Current practice is to administer a drug like quinidine in order to depress the ectopic focus, in combination with digitalis, to prolong A-V nodal refractoriness in the management of these arrhythmias [34, 236].

Clinical pharmacology (Table 2A and Chapter 7). The pharmacokinetics of quinidine following an intravenous dose can be described by a two-compartment model with a distribution phase half life of approximately 7 min and an elimination phase half-life which has been reported to range from 3–4 hr to approximately 6.0 hr [237]. Quinidine is extensively metabolized in the liver and the primary metabolites have antiarrhythmic activity, which is less than 30% the activity of quinidine. Approximately 10 – 27% of quinidine is excreted unchanged in the urine, and, for most patients, quinidine elimination is affected to only a limited extent by renal insufficiency. Elderly persons may have a lower renal clearance of quinidine and the half-life of elimination of quinidine may be longer. This may partially explain the reported higher incidence of side effects from quinidine in this group of patients [238]. The drug is 80–90% protein bound [239].

Drug interactions. Quinidine metabolism is influenced by changes in hepatic microsomal function. For this reason drugs that influence microsomal enzyme activity such as the anticonvulsants may increase the rate of metabolism and thereby decrease the plasma concentration [240].

The administration of digitalis and quinidine results in another drug interaction of clinical importance. Digitalis and quinidine interact in a complex and as yet only partially understood manner. Approximately 90% of patients taking digoxin will experience an increase in the serum digoxin level when therapeutic doses of quinidine are administered [241, 242]. The magnitude of this increase is variable and depends on the dose of quinidine employed. For many patients an increase in the serum level of digoxin of approximately 50% can be expected. The time course of the interaction is rapid, beginning on the first day of quinidine therapy. A new steady-state level of digoxin is reached in approximately five days. It is thought that the quinidine displaces digoxin from tissue binding sites thereby causing a decrease in the volume of distribution of the drug and an increase in the serum digoxin levels.

It is not clear at this time whether the higher serum levels of digoxin result in a greater effect of the drug or an increase in susceptibility to toxic arrhythmias. A decrease of the ventricular response during atrial fibrillation, a further increase in the P–R interval, and the development of gastrointestinal side effects have been described as quinidine is administered to patients on fixed doses of digoxin. These symptoms have been corrected by decreasing the daily digoxin dose [243]. However, other authors have failed to show a change in the inotropic state of the heart as determined by systolic time intervals when following a similar protocol [244]. Current practice recommends that the digoxin dose be decreased by approximately 50% when quinidine is added to a patient's regimen that already includes digoxin [245].

A similar interaction between digitoxin and quinidine has not been demonstrated nor has there been an interaction of digoxin with disopyramide or procainamide [241, 242].

Dosage. A daily dose of 1.0–2.0 g/day administered in three or four divided doses is recommended. Long-acting quinidine preparations are now available, and preliminary data suggest that these preparations may be given at up to 8–12-hr intervals with maintenance of stable steady-state levels within the therapeutic range [246]. Loading dosages are generally not recommended. If it is judged necessary to achieve a therapeutic level quickly a single dose of twice the maintenance dosage can be given [53].

Quinidine can be given intravenously as an infusion of 6–10 mg/kg administered over a period of 20–45 min. However, hypotension is observed in approximately 10% of patients and for this reason the drug should be administered only in an intensive care unit or electrophysiology laboratory [247] by a physician experienced in its use.

Use of blood levels. The therapeutic level of quinidine is approximately 2–5 μg/ml. Because of intersubject variability in absorption as well as variability in the clinical response to particular plasma concentrations, clinical evaluation is necessary to regulate optimal dosing. Toxic effects are more likely to occur at higher serum concentrations [19, 53, 223, 224]. In contrast to the results reported for procainamide (see below), increasing the dosage and plasma level beyond the normal therapeutic range usually is not successful in controlling resistant ventricular ectopy [19]. Indeed, increasing the dose carries with it the risk of inducing more serious ventricular arrhythmias. Because of the risk of such arrhythmias, monitoring of plasma quinidine levels is advised in patients taking chronic oral maintenance therapy.

Toxicity. Toxic manifestations of quinidine are often serious and life threatening. They include both cardiac and extracardiac effects. The most severe cardiac manifestation is the development of a ventricular arrhythmia of the torsades de pointes type. It is thought that this arrhythmia occurs more frequently in patients with underlying heart disease who are treated concurrently with digitalis, are receiving more than 1.2 g/day of quinidine, or are hypokalemic. However, it may occur in the absence of these other risk factors. It is frequently associated with marked prolongation of the Q–T interval and may be more pronounced in patients with preexisting interventricular conduction disturbances. Potentiation of ventricular tachycardia, ventricular fibrillation and sudden cardiac death are recognized toxic manifestations of quinidine therapy [248–252].

Other cardiovascular manifestations include widening of the QRS complex, prolongation of atrioventricular conduction, sinoatrial and atrioventricular block, and hypotension [250, 253, 254]. Of the noncardiac side effects, gastrointestinal manifestations are the most common; these include anorexia, nausea, vomiting, and diarrhea. Frequently, these side effects require discontinuation of the drug [255].

Other side effects including leukopenia, thrombocytopenia, and skeletal muscle damage occur with varying frequency [256, 257].

Whether quinidine, when given in clinical doses to humans, causes significant depression of cardiac contractility is controversial. Moe et al. reported that in isolated muscle preparations large doses of quinidine resulted in a reduction of contractility [258]. Experiments in normal dogs and dog models of volume-overloaded left ventricular hypertrophy have confirmed the depressant effect on contractility of therapeutic doses of quinidine [259]. However, in normal subjects and in patients with cardiomyopathy, little adverse effect on left ventricular performance, as measured by echocardiography, can be demonstrated [260].

Procainamide
Procainamide is a local anesthetic which is similar to quinidine in electrophysiological and hemodynamic effects. Like quinidine, its anticholinergic effects contribute to its electrophysiologic activity on the atrium and the AV junction. Its electrophysiologic effects on single cells and intact hearts have been well studied [261–264].

Because of its vagolytic action, procainamide may increase the spontaneous sinus rate and speed sinoatrial and atrioventricular conduction. These effects tend to occur at lower doses. At higher doses, the drug's direct effects tend to predominate and slowing of AV conduction and prolongation of AV nodal refractoriness may occur.

Like quinidine, procainamide can induce arrhythmias, including ventricular tachycardia and fibrillation.

Indications. Procainamide is highly effective in reducing the frequency of or abolishing premature ventricular beats following acute myocardial infarction [185, 220, 265, 266]. However, like quinidine, it is less effective in reducing the frequency of sporadic premature ventricular beats in patients with and without underlying heart disease [224, 225, 267]. In the electrophysiology laboratory, procainamide has been shown to prevent or significantly modify ventricular tachycardia induced by electrical stimulation in 15–35% of studied patients [41, 43, 268, 269]. Procainamide may facilitate the induction of ventricular tachycardia in some patients [268, 269]. Because of the inability to predict whether the drug will facilitate the induction of ventricular tachycardia or prevent its occurrence, it is recommended that patients with recurrent sustained ventricular tachycardia undergo electrophysiologic studies to determine the effectiveness of the drug and the appropriate dose required to suppress the arrhythmia. Recent studies suggest that blood levels of greater than 10 mcg/ml may be required in some patients to suppress and prevent recurrent sustained ventricular tachycardia [270].

Procainamide is effective in converting atrial fibrillation to sinus rhythm in patients with normal left atrial size [271], in reducing the frequency of premature atrial beats which initiate atrial fibrillation or paroxysmal supraventricular tachycardia, and in treating ectopic atrial tachycardia and sinus and atrial echo beats [34, 272].

Procainamide also has been employed successfully to terminate episodes of paroxysmal supraventricular tachycardia both in the presence and absence of Wolff-Parkinson-White syndrome and to prevent their recurrence. It is particularly useful in the management of patients with accessory AV nodal pathways because it causes selective depression of conduction and refractoriness of the accessory pathway [232, 273]. However, as with quinidine, procainamide may potentiate recurrent supraventricular arrhythmias in some patients. For this reason, it is important that the effect of procainamide be evaluated systematically in patients with accessory AV junctional pathways and supraventricular tachycardia.

Clinical pharmacology (Table 2A and Chapter 7). Orally administered procainamide is 75–100% absorbed from the GI tract in most patients. In the range of therapeutic serum concentrations, only 15% is protein bound [53]. The distribution and elimination kinetics of procainamide can be described using a two-compartment model. The distribution half-life following an intravenous bolus is approximately 5 min. The elimination half-life averages 3.5 hr with a range of 2–5 hr [53]. The major metabolic pathway for procainamide is acetylation to the electrophysiologically active compound N-acetyl procainamide (NAPA). Approximately 50% of administered procainamide is recovered unchanged in the urine and from 7–24% is recovered as NAPA. The urinary excretion is unaffected by urinary pH [53]. The rate of procainamide acetylation in the liver parallels that of isoniazid and hydralazine. Thus, acetylation, cardiac output and glomerular filtration rate are the major determinants of the half-life of the drug [53, 274, 275].

Dosage and use of blood levels. Because of the variation in the rate of elimination of procainamide, a given dose administered orally or intravenously results in varying plasma concentrations [275–277]. This problem is further complicated by contemporary thoughts regarding the range of therapeutic plasma concentration of the drug. In early studies, a plasma concentration of 4–8 mcg/ml was reported as the therapeutic range. The occurrence of toxicity manifested by conduction and hemodynamic disturbances was reportedly most likely when the concentration exceeded 16 mcg/ml [275]. Recently, it has been suggested that the therapeutic range may be much higher [43, 270, 277, 278]. Levels in excess of 10 mcg/ml have been required to control ventricular arrhythmias in patients with acute myocardial infarction and even higher levels have been attained in treating patients with refractory ventricular tachycardias secondary to chronic ischemic heart disease. In addition, levels needed to suppress premature ventricular contractions may be different from those needed to control recurrent ventricular tachycardia [279]. In a series of 16 patients with recurrent ventricular tachycardia, drug efficacy could be correlated with a serum concentration of 13.6 ± 8.6 mcg/ml achieved during acute electrophysiologic testing [232]. Failure to maintain this blood level during chronic therapy was associated with the recurrence of ventricular tachycardia or fibrillation. For this reason and because of the drug's short and variable elimination half-life, it is important to define the blood concentration and antiarrhythmic efficacy in each patient with refractory ventricular arrhythmias.

Commonly used dosages of procainamide range from 250 to 1,000 mg every 4 hr [53]. A 'slow release' preparation of procainamide is now available and dosages of 500–2,000 mg every 6 hr can be given. Intravenous procainamide can be administered as an infusion of from 10 to 20 mg/kg over 20–45 min with constant blood pressure and electrocardiographic monitoring.

Combination therapy. There are few systematic studies of the antiarrhythmic efficacy of procainamide combined with other antiarrhythmic drugs. In theory, procainamide can be administered with other quinidine-like drugs provided the similarity of their electrophysiologic effects and their common manifestations of cardiac toxicity are recognized. However, these common manifestations may cause serious or life-threatening problems. Procainamide also can be combined with drugs having different electrophysiologic effects such as members of the lidocaine group or the beta-blocking drugs to control refractory ventricular arrhythmias [280, 281].

Toxicity. Hypotension, sinus tachycardia, ventricular tachyarrhythmias, atrioventricular block, depression of myocardial contractility, and central nervous system toxicity all have been reported during the intravenous administration of procainamide [276, 282–285]. However, Greenspan used high doses of procainamide and reported a very low incidence of toxicity with none of his patients developing hypotension, excessive Q–T lengthening or depression of infranodal conduction during acute loading with procainamide [270]. Significantly, this result is similar to that of other investigators [272, 286] who administered procainamide without adverse effects in patients with preexisting intraventricular conduction delays. Nonetheless, caution should be exercised in patients having prolonged sinoatrial conduction time or bundle branch block, as some of these patients may be affected adversely by the drug [272]. Sinus bradycardia, junctional escape rhythms, and prolongation of sinoatrial conduction time also have been reported to occur in some patients [283, 272].

Procainamide shares with the other quinidine-like drugs the ability to induce the polymorphic ventricular tachycardia termed 'torsades de pointes' [285]. This arrhythmia is probably more commonly induced by quinidine than by procainamide, perhaps because in the doses used, procainamide may cause less Q–T prolongation than quinidine.

The long-term oral usage of procainamide is limited by the development of noncardiac toxicity.

This includes gastrointestinal effects manifested by nausea, anorexia, and vomiting; and hematological effects manifested rarely by agranulocytosis [287]. However, the most significant side effect is the induction of a lupus-like syndrome with arthritis, arthralgia, rash, chest pain, fever, and pericarditis with occasional pericardial effusion and tamponade. This syndrome, which occurs in 20 to 30% of the patients receiving the drug, usually begins approximately one month after the institution of therapy, although it may be seen after a single oral dose. It can be distinguished from systemic lupus erythematosis by the absence of renal involvement and the absence of an antibody to native DNA (288). Discontinuation of the drug usually results in reversal of the syndrome; however, such resolution may take a considerable period of time and serological abnormalities may persist for years. An elevation of antinuclear antibody may be seen in over 80% of patients on long-term therapy [170, 288–289]. By itself, the presence of antibody is not an indication for discontinuation of the drug.

Kosowsky reported that 15% of patients treated with procainamide developed severe side effects early in the course of therapy which resulted in discontinuation of the drug. Eighteen to 30 months after institution of therapy, 79% of the patients had discontinued the drug [267].

N-Acetyl procainamide (NAPA). NAPA currently is undergoing clinical trials as an antiarrhythmic agent. It has a longer half-life than procainamide and was originally reported to have equal potency with procainamide [290]. Moreover, a fairly wide therapeutic margin between efficacy and toxicity was reported by Roden et al. The therapeutic concentration was reported as 14.3 mcg/ml, whereas the toxic manifestations of the drug, generally gastrointestinal, were reported to occur at 22.5 mcg/ml [291].

Other authors have not been able to fully suppress ventricular ectopic beats with NAPA. Winkle et al. reported that only two of 11 patients had a greater than 90% suppression of frequent premature beats while taking NAPA [292]. The electrophysiology of NAPA and procainamide appears to be different. NAPA prolongs atrial and ventricular refractoriness more than procainamide. Unlike procainamide, NAPA has little or no effect on His–Purkinje conduction. Several authors question the advisability of equating the antiarrhythmic efficacy of the two drugs in the treatment of ventricular arrhythmias. If a patient's therapy is changed from procainamide to NAPA, documentation of antiarrhythmic efficacy should be repeated since the response to procainamide cannot be used to predict the response to NAPA [291–294]. The observation that the lupus-like syndrome has not been reported to occur in patients treated with NAPA is important. In patients who developed the lupus-like syndrome while receiving procainamide therapy, substitution of NAPA resulted in the remission of the syndrome and preservation of antiarrhythmic efficacy [291–297]. The dosage of NAPA required to achieve blood levels associated with satisfactory control of arrhythmia ranges from 500 to 2,500 mg every 6 hr [291, 292]. N-acetyl procainamide appears to be well tolerated. Toxic manifestations including nausea, abdominal pain, nervousness, dizziness, and blurred vision may occur at higher plasma concentrations [292]. An urticarial allergic rash may also occur [291, 292].

Disopyramide
Disopyramide was developed in the 1960s and was approved for routine clinical use in the United States in the late 1970s. Although structurally different from quinidine and procainamide, its electrophysiologic effects on single fibers, intact animal models, and in humans are similar to those of, both drugs [298–300]. Disopyramide, like quinidine and procainmide, depresses the maximal rate of rise of the ventricular action potential, prolongs its duration, and suppresses automaticity. It has potent anticholinergic effects which tend to counteract the direct effects of the drug on the atrioventricular node. The drug usually causes a slight decrease in the spontaneous cycle length, a slight prolongation of atrial refractoriness, an increase in the duration of P wave, the QRS complex, and the Q–T interval, and prolongation of His-Purkinje and intraventricular conduction and refractoriness. These effects are concentration dependent. The usefulness of the drug is limited in part by its strong anticholinergic effects and by its depressant effects on cardiac contractility [298–300].

Indications. Disopyramide has been shown to suppress ventricular premature beats and recurrent sustained ventricular tachycardia in patients with and without acute myocardial ischemia or infarction[301]. Among patients suffering an acute infarction, many who do not respond to lidocaine will respond to disopyramide [302]. The long-term oral administration of the drug is capable of reducing ventricular premature beats in over 50% of tested patients [303].

Intravenous disopyramide is capable of converting ventricular tachycardia to sinus rhythm and of reducing the frequency of episodes of nonsustained venticular tachycardia [304–306]. Recent reports [305, 306] indicate that 75–85% of patients with frequent episodes of nonsustained ventricular tachycardia are controlled by intravenously administered disopyramide. Disopyramide is also effective in preventing the induction of ventricular tachycardia induced by intracardiac stimulation [304]. The favorable response to intravenously administered disopyramide during acute drug testing both with and without electrical induction of arrhythmia identifies patients likely to have a favorable response to orally administered drug [306].

Studies to test the prophylactic value of disopyramide in patients recovering from acute myocardial infarction are inconclusive. Two recent randomized placebo-controlled studies in large numbers of patients failed to document a difference in mortality or frequency of serious arrhythmias when the drug was administered in doses of 400 to 450 mg/day [307, 308]. This result contrasted with the earlier finding [301, 309] that disopyramide was of value in the prophylaxis of sudden cardiac death and life-threatening arrhythmias.

The anticholinergic effect of disopyramide can cause speeding of conduction in the AV node and acceleration of the ventricular response during atrial fibrillation [48]. However, like quinidine, disopyramide is helpful in preventing the recurrence of atrial fibrillation following conversion to sinus rhythm [310]. Intravenous disopyramide has also been used to convert atrial fibrillation to sinus rhythm [306, 311].

The drug is effective in the treatment of paroxysmal supraventricular tachycardia either in the presence or absence of the Wolff-Parkinson-White syndrome [305, 312–314]. It can slow both antegrade and retrograde conduction and prolong refractoriness in the accessory pathway. This effect makes disopyramide a useful drug in the presence of atrial fibrillation with rapid conduction through the accessory pathway.

Like procainamide and quinidine, disopyramide may affect refractoriness and conduction of the antegrade and retrograde limbs of the reentry circuit disproportionately and cause a paradoxical increase in the ease of tachycardia induction or its rate. Fortunately, this occurs only infrequently. For most patients the drug either prevents the induction of paroxysmal supraventricular tachycardia, or, failing that, significantly slows the rate of the tachycardia [314].

Clinical pharmacology (Table 2A and Chapter 7). The distribution of disopyramide can be described by the classic two-compartment model. Following intravenous administration in healthy subjects, the distribution half-life is approximately 2 min, and the elimination half-life ranges from 4 to 8 hr. The drug has almost equal hepatic and renal clearances, and like other tertiary amines, the major metabolic pathway is conversion to an N-dealkylated metabolite which has approximately 50% of the antiarrhythmic activity of the parent compound [310]. Because of these clearance pathways, the elimination half-life may be prolonged by renal insufficiency. Following myocardial infarction, an elimination half-life of up to 12 hr has been reported [53, 315].

The drug is well absorbed from the gastrointestinal tract and is protein bound in a concentration-dependent manner with approximately 40% of the drug bound at serum concentrations within the therapeutic range. Approximately 35–65% of an oral dose is recovered unchanged in the urine and from 10–35% is recovered as metabolites [315].

Dosage and blood levels. The therapeutic plasma concentration range of disopyramide is generally believed to be 2–4 mcg/ml. This level can be achieved with the oral administration of 800–1,200 mg/day in divided doses. Plasma concentrations in excess of 4 mcg/ml are associated with an increasing frequency of side effects, particularly those related to the anticholinergic effects of the drug [48, 311].

In some situations, such as following an acute myocardial infarction, blood levels greater than the usual therapeutic range may be required. Gallagher et al., in a preliminary report [316], described a small number of patients who required up to 1,600 mg/day and blood levels of from 2.5 to

7.4 mcg/ml to effectively control refractory ventricular tachycardia. These higher blood levels were well tolerated and side effects were related primarily to the drug's anticholinergic effect. These observations have been confirmed in animal models of human arrhythmias. Patterson et al. [317] demonstrated that in conscious dogs 2–4 days following a myocardial infarction, disopyramide prevented initiation of ventricular tachycardia or fibrillation only when plasma concentrations were in excess of the normal 4 mcg/ml. At the present time, the safety of maintaining these 'supratherapeutic' blood levels in patients with organic heart disease and impaired ventricular function have not been confirmed.

Intravenous disopyramide has been given as a bolus of 1–2 mg/kg administered over 10 min followed by an infusion of 0.5 to 1.0 mg/kg/hr. However, this loading scheme has been associated with a significant risk of precipitating pulmonary edema in patients with depressed ventricular function. For this reason, an alternative method has been suggested. Up to four 0.5 mg/kg boluses are given over 5 min (with at least a 5-min interval between boluses). Concurrently, a 1.0 mg/kg/hr infusion is begun which is reduced to 0.5 mg/kg/hr after 3 hr when steady-state levels are achieved. However, even with this method, there is a risk of precipitating heart failure in patients with depressed ventricular function (see below) [318]. For this reason, I.V. disopyramide administration is not recommended, particularly in patients with depressed ventricular function.

Combination therapy and drug interactions. Combined propranolol and disopyramide therapy is unwise because of their respective negative inotropic effects. An interaction of disopyramide with digoxin apparently does not occur [241].

Toxicity. Despite early hopes that disopyramide would have fewer toxic effects than quinidine, serious side effects now are known to occur following disopyramide administration. These include the precipitation of ventricular tachycardia or fibrillation and congestive heart failure. Anticholinergic side effects including dry mouth, blurred vision, nausea, constipation, and urinary retention may also be sufficiently severe to necessitate discontinuation of therapy. It is estimated that therapy

must be interrupted in approximately 10% of patients because of side effects [48].

Polymorphic ventricular tachycardia resembling the ventricular tachycardia seen after quinidine administration has been reported in some patients [220, 319, 320] (Figure 1). It can occur in the absence of hypokalemia or concomitant digitalis administration. Widening of the QRS complex by more than 25% of control values and prolongation of the Q–T interval generally are seen in association with this form of toxicity [213, 311, 321].

Hemodynamic decompensation is relatively rare in patients with normal ventricular function [48]. However, congestive heart failure may be precipitated in patients with compromised left ventricular function. Disopyramide tends to increase diastolic and mean blood pressure, decrease cardiac output, increase coronary resistance, decrease coronary artery flow, and may increase myocardial oxygen consumption. Depression of left ventricular performance is most prominent following an intravenous bolus [322–324]. The increase in total peripheral resistance and right atrial pressure and the depression of cardiac stroke index can be of such a magnitude that profound hemodynamic alterations may occur [325]. Patients with cardiomyopathy and severe left ventricular dysfunction are most prone to this type of decompensation [326].

These hemodynamic alterations also may occur during chronic oral administration. Podrid noted that over 50% of patients who had had a previous episode of congestive heart failure again manifested congestive heart failure following the addition of disopyramide to their drug regimen. Decompensation generally occurred during the initial three weeks of therapy and was reversed following discontinuation of disopyramide [327].

As indicated above, administration of smaller loading doses of intravenous disopyramide over a longer period of time has not been uniformly successful in decreasing the incidence of serious side effects [318, 328]. In our experience, low-dose, multiple bolus loading did not prevent hemodynamic deterioration. Four of our group of ten patients had compensated congestive heart failure. Of these, three developed either pulmonary edema or hypotension [318].

Disopyramide can influence sinoatrial, atrioventricular and intraventricular conduction. In normal patients, sinus node recovery time tends to shorten

Monitor Lead

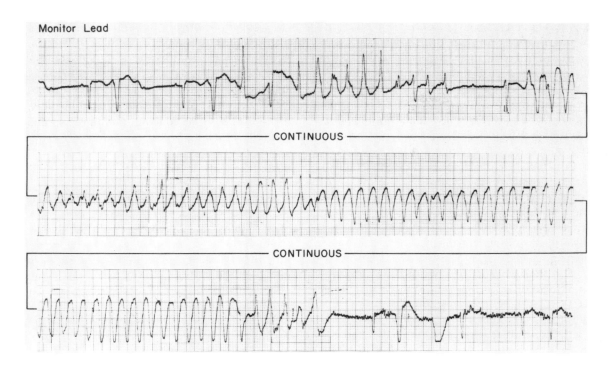

Figure 1. Polymorphic ventricular tachycardia in a patient taking disopyramide. Note the changing QRS morphology with apparent rotation of the QRS axis, the prolonged Q–T interval and AV block. This electrocardiogram is from a patient with recurrent episodes of syncope and nonsustained polymorphic ventricular tachycardia that began shortly after a physician began to administer disopyramide (600 mg/day). The patient had a long history of hypertension and was taking additional medicines including propranolol, isosorbide dinitrate, and a combination of alpha methyldopa and hydrochlorthiazide; she was not taking potassium supplements. Her serum sodium was 130 meq/L and potassium was 3.0 meq/L. Some AV conduction depression antedated her treatment with disopyramide. The arrhythmia resolved following overdrive ventricular pacing, correction of hypokalemia and discontinuation of disopyramide.

because of the drug's anticholinergic effect [329–331]. However, in patients with sinus node dysfunction, sinoatrial conduction and sinus recovery time may increase and sinoatrial block can occur [331, 332].

Disopyramide may further prolong intraventricular conduction time in patients with preexisting intraventricular conduction disturbances. However, the clinical importance of this may not be great. Desai administered disopyramide to patients with bundle branch block. Although an 18% increase in H–V interval occurred, none of the patients developed second- or third-degree AV block [333].

When disopyramide is administered to patients with atrial flutter, it may slow the atrial flutter rate and by its anticholinergic effect shorten atrioventricular nodal refractoriness and speed conduction. Thus, atrial flutter with 2:1 AV conduction may be converted to slower atrial flutter with 1:1 conduc-

tion and a resultant increase in the ventricular rate. This effect is similar to that noted with quinidine [334]. Other side effects including hypoglycemia and anaphylaxis are seen infrequently [335, 336].

In summary, disopyramide is an effective antiarrhythmic drug comparable in its antiarrhythmic efficacy to lidocaine or quinidine. It has significant anticholinergic effects and may precipitate ventricular tachyarrhythmias and sinoatrial block. Moreover, in patients with impaired ventricular function, the drug may cause congestive cardiac failure.

Encainide

Encainide may offer promise as an antiarrhythmic drug, although it is at an earlier stage of clinical testing in the United States than are mexiletine and tocainide. Its major advantages are its high therapeutic index and its efficacy, whereas its principal drawback may be its arrhythmogenic poten-

257

tial. Although there is no general review of encainide, investigators from Stanford University have recently summarized their extensive experimental and clinical experience with this drug [337].

Indications. Several studies [337–339] of small numbers of patients have shown that encainide is exceptionally effective in reducing the frequency of both single ventricular premature beats and complex ventricular arrhythmias. For example, ten of 11 patients reported by Roden and associates [338] experienced greater than 99% reduction in ventricular premature beats. Mason and Peters [340] found that encainide also was effective for at least six months in approximately half of their patients with recurrent, drug-resistant ventricular tachycardia. There are no published studies of the efficacy of encainide in converting or preventing recurrence of atrial fibrillation or flutter, although Kesteloot and Strobrandt [339] mention that intravenous encainide failed to restore sinus rhythm in two patients with atrial fibrillation. The same authors [339] also describe four patients in whom intravenous encainide abolished or reduced the frequency of atrial premature beats.

Clinical pharmacology (Table 2B and Chapter 7). The clinical pharmacology of encainide has not yet been reported in detail, although the reports of Roden and associates [338] and of Harrison and associates [337] summarize preliminary pharmacokinetic data in patients with ventricular premature beats. These authors found considerable interpatient variability in the disposition of encainide. The systemic bioavailability equaled 42 ± 24% [337], and the elimination phase half-life was 3.4 ± 1.7 hr after intravenous administration [337], 2.5 [337] to 2.7 hr [338] (range 1.9 to 3.8 hr) after single oral doses, and 3.4 hr [338] during steady-state oral dosing. Peak plasma concentrations after a single oral dose of 25 mg varied from 2.4 to 307 ng/ml [338]. Data from these [337, 338] and other [340, 341] studies suggest that an active metabolite of encainide, probably the 0-demethyl derivative, may be responsible for part of encainide's antiarrhythmic effect. This metabolite appears to have a longer elimination half-life than the parent compound. For this reason, the effects of the drug may not be fully apparent for several days after initiating therapy or changing dosage.

Dosage and routes of administration. A regimen for safe intravenous administration of encainide remains to be established, although it has been given intravenously in several studies [337, 339, 342, 343]. Based on experience in studies of its chronic efficacy [338, 340], oral encainide should be started at a dose of 25 mg every 6 hr. The dose should then be increased in increments of 5–15 mg until the desired antiarrhythmic effect is observed or adverse effects occur. However, the changes in dosing should not be made more frequently than every two to three days because of the accumulation of the active metabolite. Effective daily maintenance doses range from 100 to 250 [340] or 300 [338] mg in divided doses. The high ratio of toxic to therapeutic blood concentrations and the probable antiarrhythmic role of the more slowly eliminated 0-demethyl metabolite may permit encainide dosing at relatively convenient intervals (every 6 or 8 hr).

Combination therapy and interactions. There are no published reports describing the use of encainide in conjunction with other antiarrhythmic drugs. It would seem ill-advised, however, to combine encainide with other drugs such as quinidine, procainamide, or disopyramide that are known to prolong the QRS or Q–T intervals. Although encainide depresses cardiac pump function only slightly (see below), further studies are required to establish whether it can be used safely with negatively inotropic drugs such as beta-adrenergic and slow-channel blocking agents. If encainide's relatively low systemic bioavailability reflects a high hepatic extraction (large first-pass effect), drugs that reduce hepatic flow such as beta blockers or anesthetic agents might be expected to decrease encainide clearance and increase its concentration in the blood.

Use of blood levels. In view of the high ratio of toxic to effective encainide concentrations, the probable importance of the 0-demethyl metabolite and the wide interpatient variation in minimum effective levels measurement of encainide blood levels may be of little clinical utility except when trying to reproduce during chronic therapy drug levels found to be effective during acute drug testing. The wide range of effective concentrations, as low as 0.6 [340] and 1.3 [338] ng/ml in some patients and as high as 435 ng/ml [340] in others, makes it impractical to suggest a 'therapeutic' range of encainide concentrations.

Toxicity and contraindications. Encainide appears to be a well-tolerated antiarrhythmic drug with mean ratios between lowest toxic and therapeutic blood concentrations of 27 and 36 in two studies [337, 338]. Therefore, in most patients who respond to encainide, long-term arrhythmia control may be possible at doses that do not produce side effects. However, at high doses, encainide can produce relatively minor side effects including dizziness, ataxia, diplopia, headache, tremor, or gastrointestinal disturbance [337, 338, 340].

In contrast to the relatively minor nature of its symptomatic adverse effects, encainide may resemble currently available antiarrhythmic drugs in its potential for worsening ventricular arrhythmias. Winkle and associates [344] reported that ten of their 89 patients (11%) treated with encainide for prior sustained ventricular tachycardia and/or ventricular fibrillation appeared to develop more frequent or more malignant ventricular tachycardia after encainide. These authors [344] also reported the first occurrence of ventricular tachycardia after encainide in one of 45 patients with chronic complex ventricular ectopy, but in none of 32 normal subjects and in none of 13 patients with supraventricular arrhythmias. One preliminary report [345] suggests that arrhythmogenicity of encainide in patients with recurrent ventricular tachycardia may occur only when it lengthens the Q–T interval, although only one of the 11 patients with encainide-induced ventricular tachycardia reported by Winkle and associates [344] had marked Q–T prolongation.

Encainide probably has little clinically important negative inotropic effect. Chronic oral encainide does not alter the left ventricular ejection fraction as determined by radionuclide angiography in the resting [338] or exercise [346] state. Intravenous encainide decreases cardiac index [337, 343] and left ventricular dP/dt [343] only slightly, without altering left ventricular end diastolic pressure [337, 343] or indices of contractility [337].

Encainide produces a unique effect on the electrocardiogram in that it prolongs the QRS complex markedly but only infrequently lengthens the Q–T interval [338, 340]. The QRS prolongation, which averages 32% [340] to 44% [338] and may be as great as 90% [338] at therapeutic doses, does not appear to cause any adverse effects and may even provide a guide to the adequacy of dosing. Encainide also lengthens the P–R interval by 18% [340] to 47% [338] and the H–V interval by 31% [342]. New right bundle branch block has developed during encainide therapy [338, 340]. However, encainide-induced atrioventricular block has not been reported.

Flecainide

Flecainide is a very recently developed investigational antiarrhythmic drug that is in the early stages of clinical testing. Initial experience in humans suggests that flecainide produces nearly complete suppression of chronic ventricular premature beats in intravenous [347, 348], short-term oral [349, 350], and long-term oral [351, 352] studies. In addition, intravenous flecainide terminated sustained ventricular tachycardia in four of five patients [348] and suppressed atrial premature beats in two patients [347]. However, despite complete suppression of ventricular premature beats, two of eight patients in one chronic study continued to have recurrent ventricular tachycardia during flecainide therapy [351]. The pharmacokinetic properties of flecainide (Table 2B), which include 95% bioavailability [353], linear kinetics [348], and mean terminal elimination half-life of 14 [353] to 18 [349] hr (range 7–26 hr) are well suited for chronic oral antiarrhythmic therapy. Long-term oral dosing with 300–600 mg/day [349, 351, 352] produces arrhythmia suppression with serum concentrations of 0.4–1.6 mcg/ml [349, 351]. However, side effects at doses above 300–400 mg/day may limit the clinical use of flecainide.

Flecainide produces slight depression of left ventricular performance in experimental animals [354, 355], but two studies in humans found no decrease in echocardiographically measured left ventricular ejection fraction [349, 352], and only one report mentions worsening of congestive heart failure in a patient receiving flecainide [348]. Electrocardiographic effects of flecainide during oral dosing [349, 352] include lengthening of P–R and QRS intervals, but no significant change in sinus rate or Q–T. Symptomatic adverse effects have been relatively minor [347, 349, 352], including disequilibrium, blurred vision, abnormal taste, flushing or feeling of warmth, tinnitus, sleepiness, paresthesias, headaches, and symptomatic bradycardia, and may not require discontinuation of flecainide. Because it is highly effective and well tolerated and has desirable pharmacokinetic characteristics, flecainide appears to be a promising new investigational antiarrhythmic drug. However, further studies are needed to establish its efficacy in supraventricular and life-threatening ventricular arrhythmias, to assess the clinical importance of its possible negative inotropic effect, and to determine its arrhythmogenic potential.

Lorcainide (Table 2B)

Lorcainide has undergone pharmacokinetic and preliminary clinical studies in Europe for several years. In early trials, both intravenous [356–359] and oral [360–362] lorcainide were highly effective in reducing the frequency of simple [356–361] and complex [362] ventricular premature beats. The chronic efficacy of lorcainide in preventing recurrent ventricular tachycardia or fibrillation has not been reported. In one study, intravenous lorcainide prevented induction of ventricular tachycardia by ventricular premature stimulation [359]. However, in another similar study, lorcainide not only failed to prevent induction of ventricular tachycardia in any of the five patients tested, despite suppression of ventricular premature beats, but appeared to facilitate induction of a transient nonclinical form of ventricular tachycardia [357]. Lorcainide prolongs refractoriness of accessory pathways and may be useful in treating atrioventricular reciprocating tachycardia and atrial fibrillation in patients with Wolff-Parkinson-White syndrome [363]. There is no detailed information about the efficacy of lorcainide in treating supraventricular arrhythmias in patients who do not have Wolff-Parkinson-White syndrome.

Oral bioavailability of lorcainide varies with the size and number of doses, with less than 4% of a single 100-mg oral dose but 35–65% of a 200–300-mg dose reaching the systemic circulation [363, 364]. With multiple oral doses, bioavailability approaches 100% [363–365]. This nonlinear bioavailability suggests saturation of hepatic extraction mechanisms [363, 364]. After an intravenous bolus, the distribution half-life of lorcainide is 18–60 min [363–365], and the mean of elimination half-life is 5–8 hr (range 2.6–15.2 hr) [363–366]. Lorcainide is almost completely metabolized in the liver, largely to its N-dealkylated derivative which has a longer elimination half-life of approximately 20 hr [365–366] and some antiarrhythmic activity [366]. A lorcainide serum concentration of 0.15–0.40 mcg/ml seems to be required to suppress ventricular premature beats [365], but neither the serum level necessary to prevent recurrent ventricular tachycardia nor the level associated with adverse effects has been reported. Insomnia appears to be the most frequent symptomatic adverse effect of lorcainide and occurs in approximately 25% of patients during chronic oral therapy [358, 361, 362, 365]. Other adverse effects include diaphoresis, nightmares, a feeling of warmth, dizziness, flatulence, and gastrointestinal discomfort [358, 360–362, 365], but these are not usually severe enough to require a reduction in dose. Lorcainide causes a dose-related increase in the P–R and QRS intervals and a slight increase in the Q–T interval [366]. Its hemodynamic effects have not been reported. Winkle and associates mention two patients with lorcainide-induced ventricular tachyarrhythmias [344]. Lorcainide appears to hold promise as an antiarrhythmic drug, but its clinical value will depend on further studies of its efficacy in preventing supraventricular and life-threatening ventricular arrhythmias and of its arrhythmogenic potential.

Other drugs

We have chosen to consider propranolol, verapamil, aprindine, amiodarone, and bretylium independently, since they either exert different electrophysiologic effects or produce their antiarrhythmic effects by as yet incompletely understood mechanisms. Propranolol and verapamil are discussed as prototypes of the beta-sympathetic and slow-channel blocking agents. Although their mechanisms of action are clearly different, their antiarrhythmic effects are strikingly similar. Aprindine and amiodarone represent drugs whose electrophysiologic effects are incompletely understood, but whose efficacy in arrhythmias refractory to other agents is, on the basis of limited reports, very impressive. Although it is possible that neither drug will become available for routine use in the United States, it is not unlikely that one or both will be employed with increasing frequency in the therapy of patients whose arrhythmias prove the most difficult to treat with other agents. Bretylium is discussed because of its apparently unique place in the treatment of recurrent ventricular fibrillation.

Propranolol

Propranolol is the prototype of the class of drugs that acts by competitive blockade of the beta receptors of the sympathetic nervous system. Almost all of its antiarrhythmic effect, in particular its ability to slow sinus rate, prolong conduction and increase refractoriness of the AV node, is related to this competitive inhibition. In addition, the racemic mixture of propranolol exerts a local anesthetic or 'quinidine-like' effect which becomes manifest at drug levels approximately ten times the dosage used to induce beta adrenergic blockade. It is unlikely that this 'quinidine-like' effect contributes in a major way to the antiarrhythmic effect of propranolol [367–370].

Indications. Inappropriate sinus tachycardia may be treated with propranolol. Since the sinus rate is determined by the balance between sympathetic and parasympathetic tone, sympathetic blockade can be expected to cause depression of the sinus rate. Sinus tachycardia associated with the hyperkinetic syndrome or hyperthyroidism responds well to propranolol with improvement of symptoms and hemodynamic abnormalities [371]. The rate of the sinus tachycardia caused by other conditions will also be decreased by propranolol but care must be taken that the tachycardia is not an appropriate response to incipient congestive failure. Slowing of the heart rate in this setting may lead to serious hemodynamic deterioration [372].

Paroxysmal AV reentrant tachycardia utilizing dual AV nodal pathways or concealed or manifest accessory pathways can be effectively treated with propranolol. During acute episodes of any of these tachycardias, an intravenous bolus of propranolol causes a decrease in the rate of the tachycardia due to slowing of AV conduction. As many as 80% of these patients will convert to sinus rhythm [373].

When used alone, propranolol is less effective in preventing recurrent episodes of paroxysmal supraventricular tachycardia. Propranolol may prevent the initiation of AV junctional reentry in the electrophysiology laboratory, but, in a few patients, widening of the atrial echo zone occurs and propra-

Table 3.

	P	V	Ap	Am	B
Distribution T1/2 (min)		8–10	30–150	–	
Elimination (hr)	3–6	3–7	12–66	13–63 days	20
Bioavailability (%)	90	90	90	50	
Protein binding (%)	90–95	90	85–95		low
Route of elimination	liver	liver	liver	?	kidney
Suggested dose					
I.V.	0.15 mg/kg	0.15 mg/kg	200 mg	–	5–10 mg/kg
P.O.	20–120 mg q 6–8 hr	40–120 mg q 6–8 hr	50–100 mg q 12 hr	200–1,000 mg/day	
Therapeutic plasma					
Level	50–100 ng/ml	50–300 ng/ml	1–2 mcg/ml		–
Toxicity					
Cardiac	A-V block ↓ contractility	A-V block ↓ contractility	? ↓ contractility	? V. arrhythmia A-V block	
Extracardiac	bronchospasm, fatigue, depression	GI	GI, CNS, agranulocytosis	corneal deposits, skin discoloration, thyroid dysfunction, ? pulmonary fibrosis	hypotension GI

P   = propranolol
V   = verapamil
Ap = aprindine
Am = amiodarone
B   = bretylium

nolol may actually make the arrhythmia easier to induce. However, even in these patients, it tends to slow the rate of the tachycardia [273, 374]. In patients with accessory pathways, the beneficial effect of the drug is related to its ability to increase AV nodal refractoriness. It has little effect on conduction or refractoriness in the accessory pathway [375, 376].

Sinoatrial and intraatrial reentrant paroxysmal supraventricular tachycardias have not been studied as extensively as have AV reentrant tachycardias, and the drug's benefit in preventing these arrhythmias has not been well defined. Propranolol may be expected to decrease the ventricular response by inducing AV block during episodes of these atrial arrhythmias. Propranolol, alone or in combination with digitalis, can also be used to slow the ventricular response during ectopic atrial tachycardias [34, 377] and atrial fibrillation.

The ventricular response at rest and with exercise during atrial fibrillation can be decreased by propranolol alone or, as in common practice, in combination with digitalis [377–381]. This effect is similar but less dramatic when atrial flutter is the arrhythmia under treatment [373, 380]. Propranolol is of limited value as an aid to the conversion of atrial fibrillation and flutter to normal sinus rhythm [382], although spontaneous conversion to sinus rhythm following intravenous propranolol in postoperative patients has been reported [383].

Propranolol is effective in the management of ventricular arrhythmias associated with anesthesia, pheochromocytoma, thyrotoxicosis, and the long Q-T syndrome [348–387]. In each of these situations, prevention of beta-adrenergic stimulation is the postulated mechanism for the antiarrhythmic effect. In the long Q-T syndrome, the beneficial effect is not caused by shortening of the Q-T interval, and the mechanism of its action is not well understood [388, 389].

Exercise-induced supraventricular and ventricular arrhythmias, including exercise-induced ventricular tachycardia, are also particularly susceptible to suppression by propranolol [373, 380, 381, 390–392]. Again, prevention of beta-adrenergic stimulation is the postulated mechanism.

Digitalis-induced ventricular and supraventricular tachyarrhythmias may be beneficially affected by propranolol [369, 379, 393]. This effect is consistent with the observation that sympathetic stimu-lation can potentiate the arrhythmias of digitalis intoxication [394, 395], and that sympathectomy and drug-induced catecholamine depletion increase the dose of digitalis necessary to induce serious ventricular arrhythmias [395]. It should be noted, however, that not all of propranolol's effects are beneficial. Propranolol may convert digitalis-induced first-degree AV block to higher degrees of block and can precipitate severe sinus bradycardia or sinoatrial block [396].

Ventricular arrhythmias associated with acute myocardial infarction are less successfully treated with propranolol. Although propranolol decreases arrhythmias following coronary occlusion in experimental animals [397], it has been difficult to document a similar effect of propranolol in humans [397–399]. Recent evidence suggests that several beta-blocking drugs including propranolol may decrease the incidence of sudden cardiac death following myocardial infarction. These studies are reviewed below.

Propranolol has been advocated for the treatment of ventricular premature beats and tachycardia occurring in the setting of mitral valve prolapse [400]. However, the drug is not uniformly effective in suppressing ventricular arrhythmias in this setting. Some investigators report that only 50% of patients with mitral prolapse and frequent premature ventricular contractions have a significant reduction in ventricular ectopy following treatment with propranolol [401, 402].

Propranolol also is not generally effective in treating ventricular arrhythmias associated with other types of organic heart disease. A crossover study has shown that propranolol is not as effective as quinidine or procainamide in suppressing chronic premature beats [225]. In addition, larger doses of propranolol than are needed to induce β-adrenergic blockade may be necessary. Woosley et al., in a placebo-controlled study of efficacy in suppressing premature ventricular contractions, found a 70–100% reduction in premature beat frequency in 24 of 34 patients given propranolol 200–640 mg/day. High plasma levels of propranolol were judged necessary to control these ventricular arrhythmias [403].

Recurrent sustained ventricular tachycardia generally is not as effectively treated by propranolol as by other antiarrhythmic drugs. When studied in the electrophysiology laboratory, propranolol was successful in preventing the induction of ventricular tachycardia during acute drug testing in only a minority of patients [220, 269, 280, 404].

Thus, in most settings propranolol, when used alone, is generally ineffective in the treatment of frequent ventricular premature beats or ventricular tachycardia. Ventricular tachycardia related to exercise or ventricular ectopy associated with increased sympathetic stimulation are important exceptions to this statement.

Clinical pharmacology (Table 3 and Chapter 7). Propranolol is extensively metabolized in the liver and only a small amount of the drug is excreted unchanged in the urine. After intravenous administration, the half-life of elimination is 2.3 hr [405]. The half-life of elimination after a small oral dose is 3.2 hr [406], and, after chronic oral therapy, the half-life of elimination may be as long as 4.6 hr [405]. Plasma and cardiac tissue activity are essentially gone within 48 hr after discontinuation of therapy [407].

This difference in propranolol elimination following intravenous single oral doses and chronic oral therapy can be explained on the basis of hepatic metabolism. From 70% to 100% of a dose of propranolol is metabolized by the liver. At low portal vein concentrations as seen following a single oral dose or an intravenous dose, essentially all propranolol is metabolized. With large oral doses or during chronic administration, hepatic binding sites becomes saturated and extraction falls [53, 405].

Propranolol metabolism can be expected to be altered by changes in hepatic blood flow or by drugs or metabolic processes that interfere with the ability of the liver to metabolize the drug. Drug elimination is not significantly altered by severe renal failure [408, 409].

Some of the metabolites of propranolol are cardioactive and 4-hydroxy-propranolol has been shown to have beta-blocking activity and membrane stabilizing properties. The level of 4-hydroxy-propranolol is proportional to the serum concentration of propranolol in patients on chronic oral therapy and may be as high as 26% of the concentration of propranolol [410, 411].

Dosage and blood levels. Because of differences in hepatic blood flow and extraction rate in indi-

vidual patients, there is considerable variability in the plasma level of propranolol obtained from a given oral dose. It is impossible to predict accurately the blood concentration of drug during chronic therapy for individual patients, although the average serum concentration for patients on chronic therapy is proportional to the dosage [405]. Woosley et al. found a 5–10-fold intersubject variation in the plasma concentration of hospitalized patients taking the same dose of propranolol [403]. Blood levels are therefore very useful in the management of patients taking chronic propranolol therapy [405].

The serum level necessary to induce beta blockade may be considerably lower than that necessary for control of ventricular arrhythmias. Inhibition of exercise-induced sinus tachycardias occur at levels of approximately 50–100 ng/ml and maximal inhibition occurs in the range of 100–150 ng/ml. These levels are generally accepted as necessary for beta blockade in most patients [412]. In the treatment of ventricular arrhythmias, premature beats may be suppressed at blood levels between 40 and 320 ng/ml; however, levels as high as 1,100 ng/ml may be necessary to achieve a 70% reduction in premature ventricular beat frequency [391].

The doses normally used to achieve beta blockade for the routine control of supraventricular arrhythmias are 0.15 mg/kg intravenously given at a rate of 1 mg/min. For oral use, 80–320 mg/day are recommended, given in four equally divided doses. Larger doses of from 200–640 mg/day may be required to achieve β-adrenergic blockade or to control chronic ventricular premature beats in some patients [403].

Combination therapy. The combination of digoxin and propranolol is highly effective in slowing the ventricular response in patients with atrial fibrillation and flutter [369]. This effect may be most beneficial in patients in whom digoxin alone does not control the increase that occurs in the ventricular response to atrial fibrillation during light exercise. β-blocking drugs can minimize the inappropriate tachycardia seen even with minimal exercise [413, 414]. The combination is also effective in slowing the sinus and atrial rates in children with persistent supraventricular tachycardia [377] and can prevent recurrences of reentrant paroxysmal supraventricular tachycardia [382, 415].

Propranolol combined with an antiarrhythmic drug such as quinidine may be more effective in converting atrial fibrillation or flutter to sinus rhythm than quinidine alone. The combination has been reported to improve the success rate of electrocardioversion and in maintaining patients in sinus rhythm following cardioversion [416–418]. However, this observation is controversial, and some authors do not report any improvement in the patient's ability to maintain sinus rhythm with this combination [419].

In some circumstances, the combination of propranolol and a quinidine-like drug may be more successful in the treatment of ventricular fibrillation, frequent ventricular premature contractions, and recurrent sustained ventricular tachycardia than a 'quinidine-like' drug alone [280, 417, 420, 421].

Toxicity. The unwanted side effects of propranolol treatment are related to the induction of bronchospasm, the depression of cardiac contractility and the potential to induce sinoatrial or AV block.

The tendency of propranolol to induce bronchospasm is related to its selectivity for smooth muscle receptors of the bronchial tree which occurs at low doses and which will cause a proportionately greater effect on airway resistance than on cardiac rate. This selectivity is lost at higher doses [422]. Propranolol and other noncardiac selective β-blocking drugs increase airway resistance and can cause a deterioration of pulmonary function or precipitate acute asthma in susceptible patients [423]

Depression of cardiac contractility is also a serious complication of therapy with propranolol. This is often seen in patients with chronic congestive heart failure or in patients recovering from acute myocardial infarction who presumably have high levels of circulating catecholamines and are dependent on a relative sinus tachycardia or beta-adrenergic stimulation to maintain a satisfactory cardiac output [369, 398, 424, 425].

Whether the direct effects of propranolol on the myocardium play a role in the depression of contractility independent of the drug's beta-blocking effect is debated [426]. The effect of propranolol on rest and exercise hemodynamics in healthy males may be thought of as occurring primarily because of the alteration in heart rate rather than depression of contractility. Recent radionuclide studies suggest that the effect on rate is the dominant effect of propranolol [427]. Prolonged oral propranolol administration has little intrinsic effect on myocardial performance, and the major action is the competitive reduction of beta-adrenergic effect that is most manifest during exercise [428–430].

Conduction disturbances precipitated by propranolol also may occur. Sinoatrial and atrio-ventricular block may be precipitated, particularly if there is some degree of sinoatrial or AV conduction disturbance present initially [372, 398]. Acute conduction disturbances precipitated by propranolol generally can be ameliorated with atropine [431]. Conduction of the cardiac impulse below the level of the AV node is not affected by propranolol, and, therefore, widening of the QRS or prolongation of intraventricular conduction time is not to be expected with propranolol except in rare cases of poisoning with massive doses of the drug [368, 432].

Other side effects of propranolol administration are less frequently reported. Hypoglycemia [433], organic brain syndrome [434], exacerbation of intermittent claudication or Raynaud's phenomena [431, 435], visual hallucinations, and vivid dreams can occur [431].

Verapamil
Verapamil is the prototype of a group of drugs that inhibit the slow, calcium-dependent inward current without influencing the rapid, sodium-dependent inward current. This group of drugs currently includes nifedipine, diltiazem, and others.

Verapamil is the most effective antiarrhythmic drug of the group. It is a synthetic papaverine derivative first introduced as a peripheral and coronary artery dilator [436]. Electrophysiologic effects of verapamil include a decrease in the rate of spontaneous depolarization, maximum rate of rise of the upstroke, overshoot and duration of calcium-dependent action potentials which occur normally in the cells of the SA and AV nodes and may occur in other fibers if the fast sodium system is inactivated or blocked. Verapamil has no significant effect on the normal sodium-dependent fibers of the atria, His-Purkinje and ventricular tissues [437–442]. Verapamil does not prolong the H–V interval, the QRS complex, or Q–T interval, but, as expected from its effect on the slow inward channel, slows AV nodal conduction and prolongs the P–R interval [443, 444].

Verapamil decreases excitation–contraction coupling in smooth muscle cells and causes dilatation of the coronary and vascular bed [445]. In isolated cardiac muscle it has a negative inotropic effect and may further selectively depress regional contractility in ischemic myocardial segments [446]. When cardiac function is normal or only slightly depressed, the afterload-reducing effects caused by peripheral vasodilation tend to predominate over direct acting depressant effects and cardiac performance actually may improve [447]. However, in patients with severely depressed cardiac function contractility may be further depressed and congestive heart failure worsened [448].

Sinus rate is not altered in many patients receiving verapamil because the increase in sympathetic tone resulting from peripheral vasodilation tends to counteract the drug's intrinsic depressant effect on sinus node automaticity [449].

Indications. Verapamil is very effective in the management of many types of supraventricular tachycardia. This can be attributed to its effect on the AV node.

Intravenous verapamil causes a significant slowing of the ventricular response in almost all patients with atrial fibrillation [450], but usually does not convert atrial fibrillation to either atrial flutter or sinus rhythm [48]. Orally administered verapamil, in combination with digitalis, slows the ventricular rate more than digitalis alone. This effect is particularly impressive during exercise [451] (Figures 2 and 3). Preliminary results suggest that verapamil alone may be superior to digitalis and almost as effective as a combination of digitalis and verapamil [451].

In atrial flutter, intravenous verapamil produces a prompt reduction in the ventricular response in approximately half of the patients. Conversion to sinus rhythm or atrial fibrillation can occur [437, 450, 452–454], but, as with atrial fibrillation, conversion to sinus rhythm may be attributed to chance [455]. There is little change in the flutter rate during administration of verapamil.

A dose of 3–10 mg of intravenous verapamil has a rapid and predictable effect on sustained paroxysmal supraventricular tachycardia and over 80% of patients will convert to sinus rhythm within 5

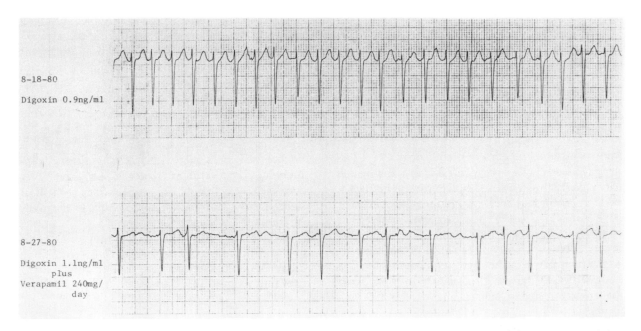

8-18-80

Digoxin 0.9ng/ml

8-27-80

Digoxin 1.1ng/ml
plus
Verapamil 240mg/
day

Figure 2. The maximum heart rate achieved in a patient taking chronic digoxin therapy (0.375 mg/day) during exercise on a treadmill for 3 min at 2 mph at 0% grade. Upper panel: The supine ventricular rate during digoxin therapy prior to the treadmill was 95 beats/min and this rate increased to a rate of 160 beats/min within 15 sec of exercise. A sustained response of 170 beats/min was achieved after 3 min of exercise. Following addition of verapamil (240 mg/day) to the regimen (lower panel), the supine ventricular response was 65 beats/min and this increased to a rate of 105 beats/min gradually over the 3 min of exercise.

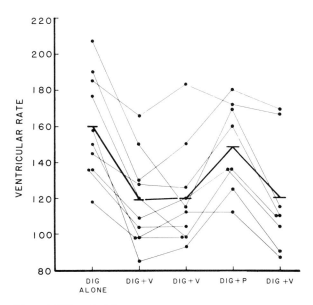

Figure 3. Effect of adding verapamil (V) to digoxin (DIG) in ten patients with atrial fibrillation. The ventricular rate represents the mean rate after three min of treadmill exercise at 2 mph and 0% grade. The first treadmill test was performed with patients taking digoxin alone (left column). Verapamil, 80 mg orally q 8 hr, was then added to the digoxin, and the treadmill test repeated one week later (second column). Subsequent treadmill tests were performed at weekly intervals while the patients were given digoxin plus verapamil, 80 mg po q 6 hr (third column), digoxin plus placebo (fourth column), and, finally, digoxin plus verapamil, 80 mg po q 6–8 hr. When verapamil was added to digoxin, the mean exercise ventricular rate decreased from 160 to 120/min. The one patient who did not experience a decrease in ventricular rate with verapamil was mildly hyperthyroid. The thin lines represent individual patient data, and the heavy line indicates the mean ventricular rate.

min of administration [443, 450, 456, 457]. The drug is effective when the reentry circuit responsible for the arrhythmia utilizes dual pathways in the AV node or AV nodal accessory pathways, concealed or manifest, [458, 459] and can be used safely in children [460, 461] as well as in adults. In clinical practice, the major advantage of intravenous verapamil over other antiarrhythmic drugs is its safe and predictable termination of sustained paroxysmal supraventricular tachycardia.

The effectiveness of orally administered verapamil in preventing recurrent episodes of paroxysmal supraventricular tachycardia has not been as well documented. Wellens et al. [459] and also Porter et al. [460] report that orally administered verapamil prevents supraventricular tachycardias in

most patients in whom intravenous verapamil is successful in preventing tachycardia induction during electrophysiologic testing.

The drug has minimal effects on the antegrade or retrograde properties of accessory AV pathways [462, 463]. In some patients, it tends to lengthen the antegrade refractory period; and in others, it may shorten the refractory period. The amount of shortening is believed to be less than that seen with digitalis [458, 459]. It is possible that verapamil, like digitalis and propranolol, may make the induction of tachycardia easier in a few patients. However, this has not been well established [459, 463]. The effect of verapamil in patients with atrial fibrillation and rapid conduction to the ventricle via an accessory pathway also has not been established, although it is likely that the drug will not decrease the ventricular response and in some patients, like digitalis [464], may accelerate it. Until the question is resolved, verapamil probably should not be administered to patients with atrial fibrillation and accessory pathway conduction.

Verapamil is not effective in the management of most ventricular arrhythmias. The drug does not generally convert ventricular tachycardia to sinus rhythm or make it more difficult to induce sustained recurrent ventricular tachycardia in the electrophysiology laboratory [269, 450]. This suggests that either slow channel-mediated responses are not important in the genesis of most ventricular arrhythmias, or that the arrhythmias are arising from a region in which perfusion is inadequate to permit effective drug concentrations from being achieved.

In single fibers, verapamil may be effective at low concentrations in decreasing the magnitude of digitalis-induced afterdepolarizations [441], and therefore verapamil may have a role in the treatment of digitalis intoxication in humans. Further testing is warranted [455].

In patients with ventricular arrhythmias associated with coronary artery spasm, verapamil may have an antiarrhythmic effect mediated by the prevention of coronary artery spasm.

Clinical pharmacology (Table 3 and Chapter 7). The onset of action of verapamil occurs within minutes of an intravenous bolus. Peak effect is seen within 10 min, and effects are still detectable after 6 hr [465]. Depression of AV nodal conduction tends to occur sooner following intravenous verapamil and to last longer than changes in vascular resistance [48].

The pharmokinetics of verapamil are complex. After an oral or intravenous dose, the initial distribution half-life is from 18 to 35 min. The slower elimination half-life is from 3 to 7 hr. Bioavailability after an oral dose ranges from 10% to 20% because of extensive first-pass metabolism by the liver. Most of the drug is metabolized by alkalinization and only 15% remains as the parent compound. The metabolites have a long half-life and their plasma concentration may exceed that of intact verapamil [466]. The metabolites are pharmacologically active, and, although they are less active than the parent compound, their high concentration contributes to the pharmacologic effect of verapamil during chronic therapy [467]. Ninety percent of the administered drug is protein-bound.

Dosage. The intravenous administration of 0.15 mg/kg over 15–60 sec is effective and safe in controlling the ventricular response to atrial fibrillation and converting paroxysmal supraventricular tachycardia to sinus rhythm. A second dose of 0.15 mg/kg administered 30 min later may be given if necessary. In atrial fibrillation, an infusion of verapamil of 0.005 mg/kg/min is suggested if the decrease in ventricular response is to be maintained. In children, the initial bolus dose is 0.1 mg/kg, repeated after 30 min if necessary. In adults, the initial oral dosage is from 40 to 80 mg administered three times per day, increased every 2–3 days to a maximum dose of 720 mg/day [48, 460].

Use of blood levels. Blood levels of verapamil are useful in predicting drug efficacy and in guiding therapy [48, 468–470]. Plasma levels of verapamil may be measured by a fluorometric assay [468] or by gas chromatography [470].

The relationship between the plasma concentration and the cardiovascular response is complex. Since active metabolites accumulate during chronic therapy, plasma concentration–response relationships during acute and chronic oral therapy may differ.

The plasma concentration–response relationship also may differ for intravenous and oral dosing. During oral therapy, a plasma concentration 2–3 times higher than during intravenous therapy may be necessary to produce the same amount of P–R

interval prolongation. This occurs because of stereo-selective presystemic elimination of the more active L isomer during passage through the liver following oral dosing [471].

Endogenous sympathetic tone also affects the plasma concentration–response relationships. In clinically stable patients with atrial fibrillation, plasma levels of 52 ± 7 ng/ml cause a decrease in the ventricular response which averages 60 beats/min. In patients with clinical evidence of congestive failure, higher doses and higher serum concentrations (95 ± 16 ng/ml) are needed to decrease the ventricular response by half as much (28 ± 11 beats/min). This difference in plasma concentration–response relationship appears to occur because of the antagonism between verapamil and catecholamines at the AV node [452].

Despite these limitations, plasma levels can be correlated with the drug's hemodynamic and electrophysiologic effects. The 'therapeutic' effect of slowing of AV conduction occurs at plasma levels which are unlikely to cause myocardial depression [469]. Plasma concentrations are correlated with the amount of P–R prolongation [471, 472], and the successful termination of supraventricular tachycardia. Serum levels of 123 ± 40 ng/ml were found necessary to successfully interrupt paroxysmal supraventricular tachycardia in most patients [456]. Some investigators believe the upper limit of the therapeutic range may be as high as 400 ng/ml [470].

The need to measure verapamil levels during long-term therapy is emphasized by the 25-fold intersubject variability in plasma concentration of patients on chronic oral therapy. This effect is probably secondary to differences in liver metabolism between patients [470]. Differences in hepatic blood flow, cardiac output, metabolic capacity of the liver, and the genetically determined pathway that verapamil follows in its metabolism may all be important in determining blood levels. Unless therapy is guided by blood levels, a proportion of patients may be undertreated because of this large intersubject variability.

Combination therapy. Prior digitalization is not a contraindication to therapy with verapamil provided there is no evidence of impaired AV conduction. In addition, verapamil may attenuate but not fully nullify the positive inotropic effect of cardiac glycosides [48]. Therefore, combination therapy with digitalis may be highly effective in certain circumstances, particularly in the management of patients with recurrent supraventricular arrhythmias. As mentioned above, this combination is very useful in preventing the rapid ventricular response to atrial fibrillation during exercise [451]. However, care must be taken in using this combination because there appears to be an interaction between digoxin and verapamil which results in an increase of digoxin blood levels of approximately 50% [473]. The mechanism for this interaction and its clinical importance have not been determined.

At present, combined verapamil and propranolol therapy are not recommended because of the potential risk of myocardial depression. Although this combination has been successfully employed in patients with chronic stable angina and apparently normal ventricular function [474], its use may be hazardous in patients with ventricular dysfunction and in patients with sinoatrial or AV conduction disturbances [475]. The combination of verapamil and other antiarrhythmic drugs has not been studied carefully.

Toxicity. Adverse reactions occur in a small percentage of patients receiving verapamil. It is estimated that adverse reactions occur in less than 10% of patients taking verapamil and that only 1% of patients have to be withdrawn from therapy. Hypotension, increased AV conduction delay, cardiac failure, and cardiac arrest can occur [441, 476, 477].

Patients with advanced left ventricular dysfunction or under concurrent treatment with propranolol may be partially prone to hemodynamic collapse or congestive failure [448]. This cardiodepressant effect in patients with congestive failure may account partially for the high incidence of hemodynamic deterioration when verapamil is used in a setting of acute myocardial infarction. In a series of 16 patients, eight with atrial fibrillation and eight with atrial flutter, one patient developed cardiogenic shock shortly after verapamil administration, and two patients had a recurrent myocardial infarction. Since patients with myocardial infarction complicated by supraventricular arrhythmias have a poor prognosis, this high percentage of complications need not necessarily be attributed to verapamil. However, until this issue is resolved, it is recommended that the drug not be used in the setting of acute myocardial infarction [478].

The effect of verapamil on patients with sinus node dysfunction is variable and not well defined. Prolongation of sinoatrial conduction and sinus node recovery times may occur [479]. Whether verapamil will depress sinoatrial conduction probably depends on whether intrinsic sinoatrial disease is present, the magnitude of the abnormality and the magnitude of the reflex increase in sympathetic tone and vagal withdrawal following the drug's depression of systemic resistance.

The effects of verapamil on AV conduction disturbances also have not been studied fully. Verapamil should be used with caution in patients with prolonged AV conduction as it may further depress conduction in these patients [443].

Verapamil's depressant effect on cardiac contractility may be reversed by intravenous calcium. The effect on AV conduction is not as readily reversible [480].

Other side effects of verapamil include constipation, vertigo, headaches, and pruritis, but they are infrequent or mild [48]. Finally, galactorrhea and hyperprolactinemia can occur during verapamil treatment [481].

Aprindine
Aprindine is available for clinical use in Europe and has been studied extensively in the United States. It appears to be effective in many patients with ventricular, atrial, and reciprocating tachyarrhythmias, but idiosyncratic neutropenia and a narrow margin between toxic and therapeutic blood levels may limit its usefulness. There are several recent reviews of the antiarrhythmic effects of aprindine [48, 144, 482, 483].

Indications. Early clinical trials in Europe suggested that aprindine reduces the frequency of ventricular premature beats in patients with stable cardiac disease [484–488] and with acute myocardial infarction [489]. More importantly, Fasola and associates found that 21 of 23 patients with recurrent ventricular tachycardia and fibrillation refractory to other agents were controlled with aprindine [490]. Strasberg and associates recently reported that nine of ten patients with very frequent ('incessant') but only four of 15 patients with infrequent ('paroxysmal') ventricular tachycardia were controlled by chronic aprindine therapy [491]. These authors [491] also found that conversion of ventricular tachycardia to sinus rhythm with intravenous aprindine predicted success of long-term oral aprindine. Patients with ventricular tachycardia associated with mitral valve prolapse may be particularly responsive to aprindine, since it prevented recurrence of ventricular tachyarrhythmia in all 17 such patients as reported by Wei and colleagues [492] and by Troup and Zipes [493].

Data on the efficacy of aprindine in patients with atrial flutter or fibrillation are limited. Several early uncontrolled observations suggest that either intravenous or oral aprindine may convert or prevent recurrence of atrial flutter and fibrillation in fewer than half of the patients treated [487, 488, 494, 495].

In nine patients with the Wolff-Parkinson-White syndrome described in detail by Zipes and associates [496], aprindine lengthened both antegrade and retrograde accessory pathway refractoriness, prevented or made more difficult the induction of tachycardia with atrial pacing techniques in five of the nine, and slowed the ventricular response to atrial flutter or fibrillation in three of these patients. In two of the patients in this study, aprindine widened the echo zone for tachycardia induction and made it more difficult to terminate the arrhythmia by pacing. Seven of these patients experienced good short-term (three to 12 months) control with aprindine, but a recent update by the same authors [483] states that long-term aprindine was ineffective in nine of their 18 patients with supraventricular tachyarrhythmias and that only four of these 18 patients continue to take aprindine. There is little information regarding the clinical usefulness of aprindine in patients with supraventricular tachycardia due to reentry within the atrioventricular node or utilizing a concealed accessory pathway.

Clinical pharmacology (Table 3 and Chapter 7). Aprindine is well absorbed after oral administration and undergoes metabolism in the liver by aromatic hydroxylation and N-dealkylation [497]. Sixty-five percent of administered aprindine and its metabolites can be recovered from the urine, with the remaining 35% excreted in the feces [498]. After single oral or intravenous doses, the disposition of aprindine in normal subjects [498, 499] and in patients with stable arrhythmias [498] can be described by a two-compartment model. The distribution phase half-life varies from 0.45 to 2.7 hr, and the

elimination phase half-life ranges from 12.5 to 66 hr with a mean of 27.9 hr [498, 499]. After multiple doses, the slow phase half-life may be considerably longer [499]. The volume of distribution exceeds total body water [499], suggesting extensive tissue binding. In the blood, aprindine is 85–95% protein bound. There are no published data on the disposition of aprindine in patients with heart failure or with renal or hepatic insufficiency, although in two patients with acute myocardial infarction, half-life was considerably longer after 60 hr than when calculated after only 12 hr of oral dosing [499].

Dosage and routes of administration. There are no detailed published data to guide recommendations for oral or intravenous dosing with aprindine. Based on considerable clinical experience, investigators at the University of Indiana [490, 496] recommend loading for several days when starting oral therapy by giving 100, 75, then 50 mg every 6 hr on the first, second, and third days, respectively, then adjusting the dose on successive days to minimize toxicity while maintaining therapeutic effect. Twice daily dosing may maintain satisfactory blood concentrations, although more frequent dosing might minimize side effects. For intravenous loading, the same authors [490, 496] recommend giving aprindine at a rate of 2 mg/min as follows: 200 mg initially, followed by 100 mg 30 min later, then 100 mg 6 hr after the start of the first 200 mg. These investigators state elsewhere [144, 483] that the antiarrhythmic effect of aprindine may not become fully manifest for several days even after initial loading.

Combination therapy and interactions. There are no detailed reports concerning the combined use of aprindine and other antiarrhythmic drugs. Fasola and associates [490] mention that aprindine plus quinidine (three patients) or propranolol (one patient) achieved a reduction in frequency of ventricular premature beats not attained with these drugs alone. These authors [490] also state that procainamide plus aprindine, at an aprindine dose producing the relatively low plasma level of 1.1 mcg/ml, produced intolerable neurologic side effects in one patient. Another report mentions three patients who developed pulmonary edema or intractable ventricular tachycardia or fibrillation while receiving both aprindine and disopyramide, but no details are provided [500]. Lidocaine and aprindine have been used together without apparent adverse interaction [144].

Use of blood levels. Fasola and associates [485, 490] found that an aprindine plasma concentration greater than 1 mcg/ml usually is necessary to reduce the frequency of ventricular premature beats [485] or to prevent recurrent ventricular tachycardia [490] and that side effects were more likely to appear above levels of 2 mcg/ml. Therefore, a 'therapeutic' range of 1–2 mcg/ml has been suggested, although our experience and that of others [490] suggest that in some cases levels greater than 2 mcg/ml may be both tolerated and required for arrhythmia control. The clinical utility of measuring aprindine concentrations in the blood remains to be established and toxicity usually is recognizable clinically.

Toxicity and contraindications. As with many other antiarrhythmic drugs, the dose or blood level of aprindine required for efficacy differs little from the dose that produces side effects. During the initial period of dose adjustment, many patients exhibit symptoms that include tremor, ataxia, vertigo, diplopia, hallucinations, nausea, and abdominal discomfort [483, 490, 491, 493]. Several reports attribute reversible abnormalities of liver function tests and mild diffuse hepatitis to aprindine [483, 501–503].

Of particular clinical importance is the occasional occurrence of reversible neutropenia [483, 504–506] or even fatal agranulocytosis [483, 504, 505] due to aprindine. Zipes and associates [483] cite a 0.6% incidence of agranulocytosis (WBC ≤ 500/ml³), with two deaths, among approximately 1,500 patients treated in the United States by 1980, with a 3% incidence of neutropenia (WBC ≤ 1,500/ml³). Weekly measurement of the white blood count is recommended during the first four months of aprindine therapy, with less frequent subsequent determinations.

Aprindine produces slight dose-dependent depression of cardiac performance in isolated papillary muscles [507], experimental animals [508–510] and humans [511]. It should be used with caution in patients with advanced left ventricular dysfunction, although there are no published reports of clinical hemodynamic deterioration due to aprindine.

Amiodarone

Originally introduced in the 1960s as an antianginal agent [512], amiodarone is now used widely in many parts of the world as an antiarrhythmic agent. As discussed in recent reviews [48, 513, 514], its very long biologic half-life and exceptional efficacy have established amiodarone as an unusually valuable antiarrhythmic agent. However, severe side effects with chronic therapy at high doses may limit its utility in some patients with serious ventricular tachyarrhythmias.

Indications. There are no rigorously controlled studies of the efficacy of either intravenous or oral amiodarone. Nevertheless, many uncontrolled series of large numbers of patients suggest that chronic oral amiodarone therapy is effective in preventing recurrent atrial flutter and fibrillation with [515–517] and without [515–519] Wolff-Parkinson-White (W-P-W) syndrome, atrioventricular reciprocating tachycardias with [515–517] and without [515, 516, 519, 520] W-P-W syndrome, including those utilizing a concealed accessory pathway [516], and ventricular tachycardia [515, 517–529], ventricular fibrillation [515, 520, 521, 523, 524, 526], and sudden cardiac death [517, 523]. In eight patients with W-P-W syndrome and a very rapid ventricular response to atrial fibrillation, amiodarone substantially lengthened both the mean and the shortest ventricular cycle length [530]. Intravenous amiodarone appears to be effective in rapidly terminating a wide spectrum of tachyarrhythmias [531–533, 535, 536].

Clinical pharmacology (Table 3 and Chapter 7). Early clinical observations [515, 536] suggested that a week or more of oral dosing might be required for arrhythmia suppression and that the duration of the antiarrhythmic [515] and electrocardiographic [536] effect of amiodarone might last as long as several weeks. Very recently, the development of a high performance liquid chromatographic assay for amiodarone has resulted in several preliminary reports of its pharmacokinetics and serum levels after oral dosing. Based on these reports, amiodarone appears to be approximately 50% bioavailable [537] and to reach peak levels of 2.8–7.7 mcg/ml after a single 800-mg oral dose [537] and 3.1–14.2 mcg/ml 5 hr after an oral dose of 1,400–1,800 mg [538]. Two to four weeks are required to

270

achieve steady-state plasma concentrations [537]. When amiodarone is discontinued after chronic therapy, its elimination half-life varies between 13 and 63 days [537–539]. Little is known about the elimination of amiodarone except that during chronic therapy in humans no amiodarone can be found in the urine [537] and the desethyl metabolite is present in plasma at concentrations approximately equal to amiodarone concentrations [539].

Dosage and routes of administration. Most studies employing intravenous amiodarone have administered approximately 5 mg/kg over several minutes [530–534]. However, hypotension and depression of atrioventricular conduction have been described after rapid, repeated injections of amiodarone. Therefore, Marcus and associates recommend that the dose not exceed 5 mg/kg, that it be given over at least 5–15 min, and that it not be repeated within 15 min [513].

Oral amiodarone therapy should be started with a period of high-dose loading if the arrhythmia requires prompt treatment, since starting treatment with maintenance doses may delay efficacy for weeks to months. Recent studies have used 1,200–2,000 mg/day in divided doses, over a period of 1–4 weeks [519, 522, 529, 542]. Even with high loading doses, ten or more days may be necessary for arrhythmia suppression [529, 542].

Based on their experience with large numbers of patients over a period of ten years, Kaski and associates recommend a maintenance amiodarone dose of at least 700 mg/day in patients with ventricular tachyarrhythmias [529]. However, more recent experience with chronic high-dose amiodarone therapy, especially in the United States, suggests that serious adverse effects often occur after 4–6 months at doses of 600 or more mg/day [534, 540]. For this reason, few if any patients should be maintained for more than a few months on amiodarone doses as high as 800 mg/day. Our current practice in patients with ventricular tachyarrhythmias is similar to that of many investigators in the United States, and consists of 600–800 mg twice daily for 7–14 days, followed by 800 mg once daily for 1–2 months. We then reduce the dose to 600 mg/day in patients with prior cardiac arrest or ventricular tachycardia, causing hemodynamic collapse, and to 300–400 mg/day in patients with more stable ventricular tachyarrhythmias. Further dose reductions are dictated by development of side effects. However, dose reduction may be accompanied by a higher risk of arrhythmia recurrence, and more experience will be necessary to determine how often dose reduction prevents side effects. Even lower maintenance doses of 200–300 mg/day are recommended for patients with supraventricular arrhythmias [529].

Combination therapy and interactions. Only two groups of investigators mention the concomitant use of amiodarone and other antiarrhythmic drugs [519, 523]. Their reports imply additive efficacy without adverse interaction when amiodarone is used in small numbers of patients in combination with quinidine, procainamide, disopyramide, phenytoin, propranolol, verapamil, aprindine, encainide, tocainide, or mexiletine. Amiodarone may cause a 20–30% increase in serum levels of quinidine, procainamide, and N-acetylprocainamide, and a reduction in the dose of these drugs may be necessary when they are used in combination with amiodarone [541]. In patients taking both amiodarone and coumadin, careful monitoring of prothrombin time and diminution of the coumadin dose may be necessary to avoid excessive anticoagulation [519, 523]. Amiodarone may cause an increase in serum digoxin concentration.

Use of blood levels. In three studies of long-term amiodarone therapy, plasma concentrations of amiodarone were 0.2–5.2 mcg/ml on 200–1,200 mg/day [539], 0.7–2.6 mcg/ml on an unstated but clinically effective dose [537], and 0.9–11.9 mcg/ml on 800–1,200 mg/day [538]. However, the relation between amiodarone levels and either efficacy or toxicity remains uncertain.

Toxicity and contraindications. After intravenous injection of 5 mg/kg over 1 min, amiodarone decreased aortic and left ventricular systolic and diastolic pressures, decreased systemic vascular resistance, and increased cardiac index, all consistent with a potent systemic vasodilating effect [543]. In another study, the same dose did not change, but 10 mg/kg depressed, indices of left ventricular contractility [544]. The combination of systemic vasodilation and depression of left ventricular function may explain the few reported cases of hypotension and cardiovascular collapse after rapid, repeated intravenous injections of amiodarone [513, 532].

There are no studies of the hemodynamic effects of chronic oral amiodarone, and no published reports attribute development or worsening of congestive heart failure to amiodarone. However, we have cared for four patients, each with left ventricular dysfunction before amiodarone (mean ejection fraction = 36%), who first developed congestive heart failure within 3-8 weeks of starting amiodarone. Until more data become available regarding the effects of amiodarone on left ventricular function, patients with ventricular dysfunction should be followed carefully during treatment with amiodarone.

Although intravenous amiodarone has produced complete atrioventricular block [532, 535], this complication has not occurred during oral therapy even in patients with preexisting bundle branch block [523, 529]. Amiodarone consistently slows the sinus rate, and symptomatic depression of sinus node function may occasionally occur [513, 515, 517, 523]. Amiodarone prolongs the electrocardiographic P–R and Q–T intervals with little effect on QRS duration [524].

Amiodarone increases protein-bound iodine, serum T4 and rT3, decreases T3 and causes no change in T3 resin uptake or thyroid stimulating hormone [536, 545]. It may produce either hyper- or hypothyroidism. A decrease in T4 and a rise in TSH may precede clinical hypothyroidism. Thyroid function tests should be followed in patients on amiodarone, especially when high doses are used.

The formation of corneal microdeposits during amiodarone therapy has received much attention. In most patients, slit-lamp examination can detect yellow-brown granular pigmentations in superficial layers of the cornea, particularly in its lower third [48, 513, 515, 518, 523, 524]. These microdeposits rarely interfere with vision and disappear after amiodarone is discontinued.

Cutaneous photosensitivity may occur in 10–17% of treated patients [515, 517]. A long-lasting bluish-gray skin discoloration occurs less commonly [48, 513, 515, 523]. Violaceous skin discoloration, especially of the forearms, may develop after chronic high-dose amiodarone.

Other side effects include gastrointestinal symptoms, constipation, proximal muscle weakness, abnormal hepatic enzymes, halo vision, tremor, ataxia, peripheral neuropathy, paresthesias, headaches, insomnia, and asthenia. In our experience, mostly with high-dose amiodarone, the most troublesome of these symptomatic side effects have been anorexia, nausea, and vomiting, which may cause marked weight loss, and a proximal myopathy involving the lower extremities. As with other antiarrhythmic drugs, amiodarone may make ventricular tachyarrhythmias faster or more frequent in some patients, especially during the first 1–2 weeks of high-dose loading.

Pulmonary toxicity is the most life-threatening complication of amiodarone therapy [523, 546]. This presents with mild dyspnea, nonproductive cough, hypoxemia, and diffuse or patchy infiltrates on chest x-ray. Although amiodarone pulmonary toxicity usually resolves when the drug is discontinued, death may occur from respiratory failure. Serial chest x-rays and clinical evaluation for pulmonary toxicity are mandatory in all patients on chronic amiodarone therapy.

Bretylium

Bretylium tosylate is a quarternary amine first introduced as an antihypertensive agent and subsequently found to have antifibrillatory activity [547, 548]. The initial effect of the drug is to release norepinephrine from adrenergic nerve endings followed by an inhibition of norepinephrine release and the prevention of epinephrine and norepinephrine uptake into the adrenergic nerve endings [549]. The drug causes electrophysiologic changes in the single cell that are unlike those caused by lidocaine, quinidine, verapamil, and similar drugs. There is no change or an increase in the maximum rate of rise of the action potential upstroke and prolongation of the action potential duration with an associated increase in refractoriness [550–552]. The latter appears to be a direct effect of bretylium. Ventricular refractoriness is also prolonged in the infarcted canine heart [553].

In the animal model, bretylium has been shown to have antifibrillatory effects in both the normal and infarcted heart [547, 553], although one group of investigators failed to find a protective effect in conscious dogs following myocardial infarction [554]. In the isolated perfused rabbit heart, bretylium did not prevent ventricular fibrillation induced by decreases in extracellular potassium or by electrical stimulation [555], suggesting that the antifibrillatory effects cited above were dependent on an intact nervous system. In isolated myocardium a positive inotropic effect has been reported [556] and is believed due in large part to catecholamine release. In humans, hemodynamic studies have shown an initial increase in heart rate and blood pressure, followed by a decrease in blood pressure and in cardiac output [556, 557]. A major problem that occurs in patients is postural hypotension.

Clinical indications. Bretylium has been used almost exclusively in the emergency management of ventricular tachycardia and fibrillation resistant to therapy with a variety of other antiarrhythmic drugs. In these life-threatening situations, the drug has been effective in approximately 60% of treated patients [558–561]. In one study, defibrillation by bretylium occurred in five of the seven patients in whom this was specifically studied [562]. This result was not duplicated in a recently reported study in which bretylium was administered to 74 patients with ventricular fibrillation persisting after an initial attempt at electrical defibrillation [563]. In all, approximately 400 patients with ventricular fibrillation or refractory life-threatening ventricular tachycardias have been treated [564]. However, there are few controlled studies in which bretylium has been used or compared to other antiarrhythmic drugs. Haynes et al. [563] found no difference between bretylium and lidocaine in the treatment of ventricular fibrillation of patients defibrillated while not in the hospital and resuscitated. Romhilt et al. [565] reported that 2–4 mg/kg of intramuscular bretylium caused a 50% or greater reduction in ectopic activity in five of the eight patients with frequent ventricular premature beats. The effectiveness of bretylium in other types of ventricular arrhythmias has not been established, and bretylium has not been tested in patients with supraventricular arrhythmias. Thus, based on a largely anecdotal, but nonetheless impressive experience, bretylium appears to be useful in the emergency management of life-threatening ventricular arrhythmias resistant to other antiarrhythmic drugs, particularly in the setting of acute myocardial infarction. Although some have suggested that bretylium be considered as a 'first line' drug in the management of such patients [564], the available information does not provide support for this recommendation, particularly since a high incidence of hypotension can be expected following intravenous administration of the drug (see below).

Clinical pharmacology (Table 3 and Chapter 7). Bretylium is poorly absorbed after oral administration and is therefore generally administered parenterally. The drug is eliminated exclusively by the kidneys with a half-life which ranges from 4.2 to 16.0 hr [46, 564, 566] when renal function is normal. Plasma protein binding is negligible. Because myocardial uptake is extensive and occurs slowly [564], pharmacological effects may persist after plasma levels approach zero.

Side effects. The most common unwanted effect of the drug is hypotension which is seen in 50–75% of treated patients [564] and may be profound enough to require therapy with fluids and vasopressors [558, 559, 564]. In these situations, hypersensitivity to infused catecholamines should be anticipated, presumably because of the impaired catecholamine uptake by the nerve endings. Other side effects include nausea and vomiting and swelling of the parotid gland, particularly after intravenous administration. A worsening of ventricular arrhythmias in the canine model has been reported in one series [554].

Dosage and blood levels. The usual dose of bretylium is 5–10 mg/kg administered intravenously or intramuscularly. In emergency situations, the drug should be administered as a 500-mg intravenous bolus. In less extreme situations, it can be administered over a 10-min period [564]. The dose may be repeated every 6–8 hr. When administered intramuscularly, the antiarrhythmic effect may be delayed by 20–60 min [564]. This lack of correlation which prevents the use of plasma levels as a guide to therapy can be explained by the extensive, but slow, uptake of the drug by the myocardium.

Drug interactions. No control studies have been performed to assess possible drug interactions in humans, although some have suggested that the antifibrillatory effects of the drug may be diminished by the prior administration of other drugs [558, 567]. Further studies are needed in this area.

Approach to specific tachyarrhythmias

In this section, we will consider the administration of the drugs in specific clinical situations. As indicated in the discussions of the individual drugs, each drug may be useful in the treatment of a variety of arrhythmias. Table 4 emphasizes that each arrhythmia may be successfully treated by several drugs. The initial choice will depend on a variety of factors including the type of arrhythmia, the urgency of the situation, the age and overall health of the patient, the cardiac status, and the familiarity of the physician with the individual drug.

In patients with ventricular fibrillation, rapid ventricular tachycardia, or poorly tolerated supraventricular tachycardia, treatment of the arrhythmia should be provided immediately using electrical cardioversion or appropriate drugs (see below). In other patients in whom the arrhythmia is not life threatening and is well tolerated, the initial approach should be the correction of predisposing or precipitating factors. This includes the correction of metabolic and electrolyte abnormalities with particular attention paid to blood gases and serum potassium. Ventricular function should be made optimal and drug toxicity should be recognized. Thereafter, the choice of the drug will depend on the therapeutic goal. In this regard, the physician should decide whether the goal is the restoration and maintenance of sinus rhythm or the slowing of the ventricular rate.

Atrial premature beats

This arrhythmia is very common and generally benign. It usually requires no therapy unless the atrial premature beats are responsible for initiating paroxysms of reentrant supraventricular tachycardias, atrial flutter, or atrial fibrillation. If the decision to treat is made, the quinidine group of drugs offers the greatest chance of success. Quinidine, procainamide, and disopyramide are all effective.

This arrhythmia rarely requires immediate suppression and, thus, the intravenous administration

Table 4.

	L	T	M	P	Q	PA	D	E	F	Lo	P	V	Ap	Am	B
APB	-	-	-	-	+	+	+	+	+	+	-	-	?	+	-
NPSVT	-	-	-	-	+	+	+	?	?	?	-	-	?	?	-
PSVT with WPW	-	±	?	-	±	±	±	?	?	±	±	±	+	+	-
PSVT without WPW	-	?	-	-	+	+	+	?	?	?	+	+	?	+	-
A flutter & fib convert	-	-	-	-	+	+	+	?	?	?	±	±	?	+	-
Slow V rate	-	-	-	-	-	-	-	?	?	?	+	+	?	?	-
VPBs	+	+	+	+	+	+	+	+	+	+	-	-	+	+	±
V Tachycardia Nonexercise induced	+	+	+	+	+	+	+	+	+	+	-	-	+	+	+
Exercise induced	±	±	±	?	±	±	±	?	?	?	+	?	?	?	?
Prevent recurrent V fib	+	+	+	+	+	+	+	?	?	?	±	-	?	+	+
Prevent SCD	+	?	?	?	±	±	±	?	?	?	+	?	?	+	?

+ = suppress or prevent
– = no effect
? = effect not reported
APB = atrial premature beat
NPSVT = nonparoxysmal supraventricular tachycardia
VPBs = ventricular premature beats
SCD = sudden cardiac death

Abbreviations for drugs as in previous tables.

of these drugs is rarely, if ever, indicated. Usually quinidine and disopyramide are preferred becaus their dosing interval is longer than that required fo procainamide.

Ectopic atrial rhythms

Ectopic atrial rhythm is a common response to sinus bradycardia or sino-atrial block. In children and young adults, it usually reflects an increase in 'vagal tone' and requires no therapy. In older patients, it frequently reflects sinus node and/or atrial disease and, in this situation, may identify the need for pacemaker implantation even though the ectopic rhythm itself causes no symptoms. Ectopic atrial tachycardia is a less common arrhythmia. It may occur in both children and adults as a manifestation of atrial disease, digitalis excess, or hypokalemia. Removal or correction of the underlying problem may suffice to eliminate the arrhythmia. Moreover, the failure to recognize problems such as digitalis excess and hypokalemia may prevent the successful employment of antiarrhythmic drugs. Therapy with the quinidine group of drugs may be attempted but is frequently unsuccessful. Drugs which increase AV nodal refractoriness such as digitalis, propranolol, and verapamil may also be used to induce AV block, provided, of course, that the arrhythmia is not a manifestation of digitalis excess. The arrhythmia rarely, if ever, requires immediate suppression, and, thus, the intravenous administration of drugs is rarely required.

Paroxysmal supraventricular tachycardia

This arrhythmia frequently requires immediate suppression. It usually is due to reentry within the AV junction and is most frequently initiated by an atrial or ventricular premature beat. When an accessory AV connection such as a Kent bundle is present, it may serve as the retrograde limb of the reentry circuit. Suppression of the arrhythmia is achieved by measures which interrupt the reentry circuit by influencing impulse conduction through the AV node or bypass pathway. Vagal maneuvers, such as carotid sinus massage, may be successful in suppressing AV nodal conduction and, thus, obviate the need for intravenous medication or electrical cardioversion. AV nodal conduction also can be suppressed by the slow-channel blocking agent, ve-

rapamil, which acts directly on the AV node and by drugs which act on the AV node via an effect on acetylcholine. These drugs include digoxin, edrophonium, and the short-acting vasopressors. Each of these drugs results in an increase in cholinergic activity, albeit via different mechanisms. Propranolol is also considered in this group since it inhibits β adrenergic effects thereby causing a 'net' increase in cholinergic activity. The nonpharmacological means of terminating this arrhythmia include atrial and ventricular pacing and direct current cardioversion.

When an anomalous AV junctional pathway forms one limb of the reentry circuit, drugs which have a direct membrane effect may be and often are effective since they often influence the electrophysiology of both the AV node and bypass tract. The goal of long-term management of these patients is twofold: (a) to prevent the recurrence of the arrhythmia and (b) to slow the rate of the arrhythmia should it recur. Often both goals can be approached with the same drugs. The drugs which act on the AV node such as digitalis, propranolol, and verapamil are often successful in preventing the recurrence of the tachycardia, although they occasionally may widen the echo zone and facilitate the induction of the tachycardia by a premature beat. If suppression of the initiating beat is required, the quinidine group of drugs is often useful. These drugs also will influence conduction and refractoriness in the AV node and in accessory pathways. Frequently, the combination of a quinidine-like drug with digitalis, propranolol, or verapamil provides effective therapy. When the arrhythmia is resistant to these therapeutic approaches, amiodarone has been found to be particularly effective.

Atrial flutter

This arrhythmia is most easily terminated by DC countershock or atrial pacing. However, it rarely requires immediate termination unless the ventricular rate is unusually rapid or unless the presence of ventricular dysfunction or coronary disease renders the patient intolerant to the ventricular response. If intravenous therapy is required, the goal of therapy should be to slow the ventricular response by increasing the degree of block at the AV node. This can be accomplished most readily by the intravenous administration of verapamil, digitalis, or propranolol. It is important to recognize that slowing the ventricular response to atrial flutter with digitalis may be more difficult to achieve and require more drug than slowing the ventricular response in atrial fibrillation. Pharmacological cardioversion may often occur after the administration of these agents. However, more frequently atrial flutter persists. In this situation, the AV block should be maintained with the oral administration of the above drugs, again recognizing the need for digitalis doses greater than those usually required in atrial fibrillation, and a quinidine-like drug added. Quinidine has been most frequently used in this situation, although there is no evidence to suggest that procainamide or disopyramide would be more or less effective. These drugs generally slow the rate of atrial flutter and this effect, when combined with a possible shortening of the AV nodal refractory period mediated via the anticholinergic effect, may result in one-to-one AV conduction and a paradoxical speeding of the ventricular rate. This effect is prevented by the prior administration of digitalis, propranolol, or verapamil and forms the basis for combined therapy. Quinidine should be administered in increasing doses starting at 200–300 mg q 6 hr. It is the authors' policy to turn to electrical cardioversion if quinidine doses in excess of 400 mg q 6 hr are required. Maintenance therapy with digoxin and quinidine is usually required following cardioversion.

Atrial fibrillation

The choice of therapy for this arrhythmia clearly depends on whether the goal is to restore sinus rhythm, to prevent recurrences once sinus rhythm has been restored, or to control the ventricular rate. Frequently the goal is determined by the likelihood of maintaining sinus rhythm. Younger patients without underlying cardiac disease in whom atrial fibrillation is idiopathic (lone atrial fibrillation) or occurs as the result of thyrotoxicosis can have their arrhythmia converted most easily to sinus rhythm, particularly after the correction of underlying problems. Conversion to sinus rhythm is least likely in elderly patients and in patients with enlarged atria. The search for underlying or precipitating factors may disclose sinus node disease, congestive heart failure, mitral stenosis, or mitral valve prolapse;

or less frequently, constrictive pericarditis, thyrotoxicosis, or atrial septal defects. An additional consideration in determining appropriate therapy is the presence or absence of AV nodal bypass tracts. The primary goal of therapy in atrial fibrillation should be the control of ventricular rate regardless of the decision concerning the restoration and maintenance of sinus rhythm. Rapid, although temporary, rate control often can be accomplished by intravenously administered verapamil, propranolol, or digoxin, although digoxin will not act as rapidly as the other two agents.

Each of these drugs acts by prolonging refractoriness and slowing conduction in the AV node. Thus, none may be effective in the patient with W-P-W who is conducting over the bypass tract with a resultant rate of $>$ 200 beats/min. Indeed, in this situation, therapy with digoxin, and perhaps verapamil, is contraindicated because of the possibility of shortening the refractory period in the bypass tract, increasing the ventricular rate and increasing the likelihood of the development of ventricular fibrillation. In this situation, immediate electrical defibrillation is the treatment of choice although intravenously administered procainamide may also slow the ventricular response. In patients with known W-P-W but in whom most of the ventricular responses are conducted via the AV node, we consider propranolol to be the drug of choice for slowing the ventricular rate.

Once the immediate therapeutic goal of slowing the ventricular response has been met, the decision must be made regarding restoration of sinus rhythm. As with atrial flutter, conversion to sinus rhythm can be accomplished with the quinidine group of drugs or with electrical current. Following the restoration of sinus rhythm, the patient is usually maintained on one of the quinidine-like drugs and digoxin. Quinidine is used to prevent the recurrence of atrial fibrillation and digoxin is given to control the ventricular response should it recur.

The long-term management of the patient with persistent atrial fibrillation traditionally has been accomplished by digoxin. However, it is important to remember that reasonable control of the resting ventricular response does not guarantee adequate control of the ventricular rate during exercise. The combination of digoxin and propranolol [413, 414], digoxin and verapamil [451] (Figure 2) or perhaps even verapamil alone provides better rate control of the exercise response. Figure 3 shows our experience in a group of patients treated with digoxin and then with a combination of digoxin and verapamil. This result is similar to the experience of Klein et al.[451].

Ventricular premature beats

In general, ventricular premature beats, like atrial premature beats, are not an indication for antiarrhythmic drug therapy. Although frequent ventricular premature beats are regarded as a risk factor for subsequent coronary events including sudden cardiac death [171, 568–572], there is no evidence to suggest that suppression of the premature beats confirms protection against such occurrences. Moreover, Myerberg et al.[226, 279] have suggested that protection from sudden death in patients who have experienced a prior episode of ventricular fibrillation can occur even though the ventricular premature beats are not suppressed. Thus, it rarely is necessary to treat ventricular ectopy with the following exceptions: (a) patients with an acute myocardial infarction in whom treatment with lidocaine is indicated to prevent ventricular fibrillation, (b) patients in whom the ventricular ectopy is the result of digitalis excess or hypokalemia and in whom cessation of digitalis and/or the correction of hypokalemia not only abolishes the ectopy but, more importantly, prevents the subsequent development of more serious ventricular arrhythmias, and (c) patients who are unusually sensitive to the symptoms associated with the ventricular ectopy. In this last situation, the drugs in the quinidine group and the analogs of lidocaine which can be administered orally such as mexiletine and tocainide have been found to be approximately equally effective. Frequently in an individual patient, the drugs of one group may be more or less effective than the drugs in the other. Although the intravenous administration of these drugs is not essential, an argument can be made for using intravenous therapy to establish efficacy and to determine the plasma level required for suppression.

Ventricular tachycardia

Sustained, rapid ventricular tachycardia should be regarded as a life-threatening emergency requiring immediate therapy. However, the appropriate therapy must be individualized. If indeed the arrhythmia is life-threatening, intravenous lidocaine is indicated and, if unsuccessful, should be followed by electrical cardioversion. If the arrhythmia recurs, rapid ventricular pacing following cardioversion should be considered. This modality is particularly useful when a bradyarrhythmia underlies the tachycardia or when the tachycardia can be attributed reasonably to quinidine, disopyramide, or procainamide excess. Administration of potassium should be considered if hypokalemia alone or in the presence of digitalis excess is the responsible factor. If the quinidine group can be excluded as contributing to the arrhythmia, the combination of intravenously administered procainamide and lidocaine may be successful when either alone fails.

As mentioned throughout the preceding sections of the chapter, recurrent ventricular tachycardia is best managed on the basis of electrophysiologic or exercise testing. It is our practice to attempt to prevent the tachycardias induced by electrical testing using a quinidine-type drug, usually procainamide, in doses adequate to produce the blood levels achieved in the electrophysiology laboratory. If procainamide fails, our second drug is usually one of the lidocaine group, either mexiletine or tocainide, particularly if lidocaine is found to be effective in the laboratory. If necessary, we will employ the combination of mexiletine and quinidine or procainamide. If this fails, we will use amiodarone. At the same time, we attempt to achieve optimal ventricular performance with pre- and after-load reducing agents if they are clinically indicated.

Exercise-induced tachycardias generally are treated initially with propranolol or other beta-blocking agents. If the arrhythmia is both electrically and exercise induced, we usually choose the drug or combination of drugs which prevents both types of tachycardia. If the various drugs, given alone or in combination, fail to prevent recurrences of the arrhythmia, we may accept slowing of the rate of the tachycardia as an alternative goal. However, it should be emphasized that this goal is accepted only when we are unable to prevent the induction of the arrhythmia. We have no fixed policy regarding therapy for short bursts of ventricular tachycardia, i.e., those characterized by three or four beat runs, and therapy is adjusted to the individual case and to the results of the various testing procedures. We are, however, reluctant to initiate therapy empirically, particularly with a quinidine-type drug, because of its known ability to induce more serious and potentially life-threatening arrhythmias.

Ventricular fibrillation

The treatment of ventricular fibrillation requires immediate electrical cardioversion in concert with the administration of drugs capable of preventing its recurrence. The drug of choice in this situation is lidocaine administered as one or two boluses followed by a constant infusion. If ventricular fibrillation recurs after instituting lidocaine therapy, then a variety of options may be exercised depending on the factors thought to be important in the genesis of the arrhythmia. These include (a) increasing the dose of lidocaine until CNS toxicity occurs, (b) adding a second drug such as procainamide, bretylium, or propranolol, and (c) ventricular pacing.

When ventricular fibrillation occurs, and particularly if it recurs, the role of digitalis, antiarrhythmic drugs, hypoxia, acidosis, and electrolyte abnormalities, particularly hypokalemia should be determined and abnormalities corrected as rapidly as possible. We have found the combination of rapid ventricular pacing and lidocaine to be particularly useful when the recurrent ventricular fibrillation is due to quinidine, procainamide, or disopyramide. Occasionally, bretylium is particularly useful in patients with recurrent ventricular fibrillation associated with acute ischemia. As indicated above, hypotension should be anticipated when bretylium is used.

The subsequent management of ventricular fibrillation depends on the etiology of the arrhythmia. If ventricular fibrillation occurs in the setting of an acute myocardial infarction, no other evaluation usually is required. However, if ventricular fibrillation occurs in the absence of an acute myocardial infarction, intracardiac stimulation techniques are often indicated in order to determine the most appropriate therapy.

Prevention of sudden cardiac death

Lown has labeled sudden cardiac death as 'the major challenge confronting contemporary cardiology' [573]. In discussing this topic, we have chosen to categorize the patients at risk, since the approach and the results of therapy may differ depending upon the underlying cardiac problem.

The first group includes those who have sustained an episode of ventricular fibrillation from which they have been resuscitated. The second includes those with documented ventricular tachycardias and the third includes those who have recovered from an acute myocardial infarction.

The studies of Cobb et al. [574, 575] have clearly shown that patients surviving an episode of sudden cardiac death, usually from ventricular fibrillation, are at high risk for sudden death, particularly if they do not sustain an acute myocardial infarction and if they have findings of congestive heart failure. In this group of patients, three approaches have been considered. These include: (a) evaluation for coronary disease and coronary artery bypass where appropriate, (b) institution of drug therapy based on the results of provocative testing, and (c) empirical therapy without provocative testing.

The first approach acknowledges the fact that as many as 75% of patients suffering an episode of sudden cardiac death have coronary disease and, in the absence of an acute myocardial infarction, are at high risk (30%) for sustaining a recurrent episode of ventricular fibrillation within one year [575]. Although no control studies have been performed to determine the effect of coronary artery bypass surgery on subsequent mortality in this group of high risk patients, current practice includes a thorough evaluation for coronary disease including exercise testing and, if necessary, coronary angiography, and a decision regarding coronary artery bypass surgery based on the findings. Clearly needed are studies designed to determine the role of coronary surgery in the treatment of patients surviving an episode of sudden cardiac death who may not have the more classical indications for bypass surgery.

The second approach to this group of patients is exemplified by the report of Ruskin et al. [133]. They used intracardiac provocative stimulation techniques in 31 patients who survived an episode of sudden cardiac death not associated with an acute infarction. They were able to induce ventricular arrhythmias in 25 (81%) of these patients. In 19 patients, complete suppression was obtained using single or double drug therapy and none died during the mean follow-up period of 15 months. In the remaining six patients, the induced arrhythmia could not be suppressed in the laboratory. Of these, three died suddenly within the follow-up period.

Ventricular tachycardia could not be induced in the laboratory in six patients and none of these died within the follow-up period. However, this should not be interpreted to indicate that noninducibility identifies patients who are not at risk. It is also of interest that ventricular arrhythmias could not be induced in two of the three patients who received coronary bypass grafts. Thus, this study suggests that sudden cardiac death can be prevented by pharmacological therapy as determined by the results of provocative intracardiac stimulation. It is possible that the reproducible induction of ventricular arrhythmias during exercise in some patients who have sustained an episode of sudden cardiac death may provide an alternative to intracardiac stimulation as a means of determining effective therapy. A similar approach has been utilized by Lown and his colleagues in patients with ventricular tachycardia [16]. However, this has not yet been proven to be effective in this group of patients.

The third approach is exemplified by the studies of Myerberg and co-workers [226, 279]. These investigators administered procainamide or quinidine in doses adequate to provide a plasma concentration within the commonly accepted therapeutic range to a group of patients who survived an episode of sudden cardiac death and reported a one-year mortality of 6%. They also noted that the administered dose did not necessarily suppress ventricular ectopy as recorded on the standard ECG and during ambulatory monitoring. However, these provocative reports must be interpreted with caution since the number of patients was small and the study did not contain a control group. Moreover, the concept that the attainment of a predetermined plasma level of a quinidine-like drug provides protection against recurrent ventricular fibrillation is somewhat contrary to the experience of other groups. This difference is made more significant by the knowledge of the quinidine group's ability to cause life-threatening ventricular arrhythmias. For these reasons, confirmation of these results is required.

The approach to the second group of patients, that is, those with documented episodes of recurrent tachycardia, has been discussed above and need not be repeated here other than to stress the need to document drug efficacy whenever possible. This is best accomplished by electrical testing or by exercise tests. However, there are three situations in which documentation of drug efficacy may not be possible: (a) when the arrhythmia cannot be induced by electrical testing, (b) when the arrhythmia cannot be suppressed by any of the tested drugs, administered singly or in combination, and (c) when amiodarone is administered.

There are no clearcut guidelines for the management of patients in whom arrhythmias cannot be induced in the laboratory. It is our practice to administer procainamide as the initial drug to this group of patients if the need to treat has been established. We administer the drug at the time of electrical testing to establish that the drug does not facilitate arrhythmia induction and will then attempt to reproduce, by oral dosing, the plasma level present at the time of electrical testing. If procainamide facilitates arrhythmia induction, we use mexiletine, again performing electrical testing after the steady-state plasma level is achieved by oral dosing.

When arrhythmia induction cannot be prevented by the administered drugs, we usually choose that drug or combination of drugs that makes the induction more difficult as determined by the number of premature beats or the ventricular pacing rate required to induce the arrhythmia, or by selecting the drug that slows the rate of the induced tachycardia by the greatest amount.

In patients treated with amiodarone, clinical suppression has occurred in spite of the ability to induce the arrhythmia [523]. As a result, the documentation of effectiveness must be determined empirically.

The third group of patients includes those who have survived an acute myocardial infarction. Two approaches to therapy can be considered in this group of patients. One is the identification of high risk patients and the second is prophylactic treatment of the entire group.

It is clear that high risk patients can be identified by a variety of indicators including ventricular function, the presence of ventricular ectopy and arrhythmias, the results of exercise testing, the status of the coronary circulation, and the presence of delayed electrical activity as recorded by an electrode catheter [576] or by high frequency surface electrocardiogram [577]. However, the ability to prevent subsequent sudden death in these high risk patients by pharmacological interventions has not been established. Green et al. reported that the induction of a spontaneous ventricular response

Table 5.

Drug [Ref.]	Dose mg/day	Onset of therapy following MI	Duration of therapy months	No. of patients		Total cardiac deaths		Sudden cardiac deaths		Reinfarction	
				Control	Treated	Control (%)	Treated (%)	Control	Treated	Control	Treated
Alprenolol [580]	400	immediate	12	39	38	3 (7.7)	3 (7.9)	1	2	4	4
Alprenolol [581]	400	at discharge	24	116	114	14 (12.1)	7 (6.1)	11	3	18	16
Alprenolol [582]	400	at discharge	24	93	69	11 (11.8)	5 (7.2)	9	1*	15	4*
Practolol [583, 584]	400	1–4 weeks	12	1,514	1,524	73 (7.8)	47* (3.1)	58	41	89	69
Timolol [585]	20	1–4 weeks	12–33	939	945	113 (12.0)	58* (6.1)	95	47*	141	88*
Metoprolol [586]	200	immediate	3	697	698	62 (8.9)	40 (5.7)				
Propranolol [587]	120	8.5 days	3–9	365	355	18 (4.9)	19 (5.3)	NR		14	15
Propranolol [588]	120	immediate	12	129	132	10 (7.8)	5 (3.8)	NR		NR	
Propranolol [589]	180–240	13.8 days	30	1,916	1,921	171 (8.9)	127 (6.6)	89	64	NR	
Total β blockers				5,808	5,496	475 (8.1)	311 (5.7)	263	161	281	196
Sulfinpyrazone [594, 595]			16	783	775	62 (7.9)	43 (5.5)	37	22	NR	

* = Statistically significant

NR = Not reported

induced by a single atrial extrastimulus provided a means of identifying the subset of patients at high risk following myocardial infarction [578]. They based their conclusions on the results of studies of 50 patients with refractory ventricular arrhythmias, 48 survivors of a recent myocardial infarction and 12 normal subjects. They also reported that in a separate group of 23 patients with refractory ventricular tachycardia, suppression of the repetitive ventricular response by aprindine in 20 patients was associated with long-term suppression of the arrhythmia [579]. Whether the use of this technique following acute myocardial infarction will prove preferable to other methods of identifying patients at risk for sudden death and gain widespread acceptance cannot be stated at this time since confirmatory studies from other laboratories are lacking.

The prevention of sudden cardiac death following myocardial infarction has been attempted with a variety of antiarrhythmic drugs administered prophylactically including quinidine, procainamide, and phenytoin. These studies, recently reviewed by Bigger et al. [171] and Warnowicz and Denes (220) were limited by a high incidence of side effects and largely failed to show a statistically significant improvement in survival in the treated patients. Recent trials, primarily in Europe with several beta blockers [580–588] and most recently with propranolol in the United States [589], suggest that the routine administration of these drugs may exert a protective effect (Table 5). More than 10,000 patients have been enrolled in the nine studies shown in Table 5. Not included are the acute propranolol studies of the 1960s [590–593] which, with the exception of the original study by Snow [590], failed to show a difference in mortality within 28 days of acute infarction. The results of the sulfinpyrazone study [594] also suggest that this drug may prevent sudden death. It is worth noting that, in most of these studies, the exclusions from entry prevented many of the patients at high risk for sudden death from being included in the treatment groups. Clearly, the challenge of the future is to develop interventions which will be appropriate for the high risk patients as well as for those in whom the risk is lower.

Conclusion

In this chapter, we have attempted to review the clinical pharmacology, indications and contraindications of those drugs currently available or in clinical trials for the treatment and prevention of cardiac arrhythmias. We have outlined our general approach to the patient with serious cardiac arrhythmias and our approach to the therapy of specific rhythm disturbances. The ever increasing number of antiarrhythmic drugs is likely to render this chapter incomplete in the near future. It also is probable that the future will see the more rigorous standardization of various test procedures. It is our bias, however, that the general approach, aimed as it is at providing specific means of determining the pathogenesis of the arrhythmia and the sensitivity of the arrhythmia to the various drugs and of determining drug efficacy, will remain essentially the same and that the cataloging of the various drugs according to their lidocaine-, quinidine-, verpamil-, or propranolol-like characteristics will facilitate an appreciation of their therapeutic efficacy, their side effects and their ability to potentiate as well as to treat cardiac arrhythmias.

Acknowledgment

Some of the studies reported in this chapter were supported by National Institutes of Health grant no. HL-23624 and no. HL-26484.

References

1. Pick A, Langendorf R: Differentiation of supraventricular and ventricular tachycardias. Prog Cardiovasc Dis 2: 391–407, 1960.
2. Kistin AD: Problems in the differentiation of ventricular arrhythmias from supraventricular arrhythmia with abnormal QRS. Prog Cardiovasc Dis 9:1, 1966.
3. Marriott HJL, Sandler JA: Criteria, old and new, for differentiating between ectopic ventricular beats and aberrant ventricular conduction in the presence of atrial fibrillation. Prog Cardiovasc Dis 9:18, 1966.
4. Massumi RA, Tawakkol AA, Kistin AD: Re-evaluation of electrocardiographic and bedside criteria for diagnosis of ventricular tachycardia. Circulation 36:628, 1967.
5. Wellens HJJ, Bar FWHM, Lie KI: The value of the electrocardiogram in the differential diagnosis of a tachycardia with a widened QRS complex. Am J Med 64:27–33, 1978.

6. McHenry PL, Fisch C, Jordan JW, Corya BR: Cardiac arrhythmias observed during maximal treadmill exercise testing in clinically normal men. Am J Cardiol 29:331–336, 1972.

7. Blackburn H, Taylor HL, Hamrell B, Buskirk E, Nicholas WC, Thorsen RD: Premature ventricular complexes induced by stress testing: their frequency and response to physical conditioning. Am J Cardiol 31:441–449, 1973.

8. Frolicher VF, Thomas MM, Pillow C, Lancaster MC: Epidemiologic study of asymptomatic men screened by maximal treadmill testing for latent coronary artery disease. Am J Cardiol 34:770–776, 1974.

9. Jelinek MV, Lown B: Exercise stress testing for exposure of cardiac arrhythmias. Prog Cardiovasc Dis 16:497–522, 1974.

10. DeMaria AN, Vera Z, Amsterdam EA, Mason DT, Massumi R: Disturbances of cardiac rhythm and conduction induced by exercise: diagnostic, prognostic and therapeutic implications. Am J Cardiol 33:732–736, 1974.

11. McHenry PL, Morris SN, Kavalier M, Jordan JW: Comparative study of exercise-induced ventricular arrhythmias in normal subjects and patients with documented coronary artery disease. Am J Cardiol 37:609–616, 1976.

12. Goldschlager N, Cohn K, Goldschlager A: Exercise-related ventricular arrhythmias. Cardiovasc Dis 48:67–71, 1979.

13. Sheps DS, Ernst JC, Briese FR, Lopez LV, Conde CA, Castellanos A, Myerburg RJ: Decreased frequency of exercise-induced ventricular ectopic activity in the second of two consecutive treadmill tests. Circulation 55:892–895, 1977.

14. Faris JV, McHenry PL, Jordan JW, Morris SN: Prevalence and reproducibility of exercise-induced ventricular arrhythmias during maximal exercise testing in normal men. Am J Cardiol 37:617–622, 1976.

15. Ekblom B, Hartley LH, Day WC: Occurrence and reproducibility of exercise-induced ventricular ectopy in normal subjects. Am J Cardiol 43:35–40, 1979.

16. Lown B, Graboys TB: Management of patients with malignant ventricular arrhythmias. Am J Cardiol 39:910–918, 1977.

17. Gey GO, Levy RH, Fisher L, Pettet G, Bruce RA: Plasma concentration of procainamide and prevalence of exertional arrhythmias. Ann Intern Med 80:718–722, 1974.

18. Gettes LS, Surawicz B: Long-term prevention of paroxysmal arrhythmias with propranolol therapy. Am J Med Sci 254:257–265, 1967.

19. Gey GO, Levy RH, Pettet G, Fisher L: Quinidine plasma concentration and exertional arrhythmia. Am Heart J 90:19–24, 1975.

20. Talbot S, Kilpatrick D, Krikler D, Oakley CM: Ventricular tachycardia due to cardiac ischaemia: assessment by exercise electrocardiography. Br Med J 2:733–736, 1978.

21. LeWinter MM, Engler RL, Karliner JS: Tocainide therapy for treatment of ventricular arrhythmias: assessment with ambulatory electrocardiographic monitoring and treadmill exercise. Am J Cardiol 45:1045–1052, 1980.

22. Markiewicz W, Houston N, DeBusk RG: Exercise testing soon after myocardial infarction. Circulation 56:26–31, 1977.

23. Sami M, Kraemer H, DeBusk RF: Reproducibility of exercise-induced ventricular arrhythmia after myocardial infarction. Am J Cardiol 43:724–730, 1979.

24. DeBusk RF, Haskell W: Symptom-limited vs heart-rate-limited exercise testing soon after myocardial infarction. Circulation 61:738–743, 1980.

25. Hinkle LE, Carver ST, Stevens M: The frequency of asymptomatic disturbances of cardiac rhythm and conduction in middle-aged men. Am J Cardiol 24:629–650, 1969.

26. Bleifer SB, Bleifer DJ, Hansmann DR, Sheppard JJ, Darpman HL: Diagnosis of occult arrhythmias by Holter electrocardiography. Prog Cardiovasc Dis 16:569–599, 1974.

27. Harrison DC, Fitzgerald JW, Winkle RA: Ambulatory electrocardiography for diagnosis and treatment of cardiac arrhythmias. N Engl J Med 294:373–380, 1976.

28. Winkle RA: Ambulatory electrocardiography. Mod Concepts Cardiovasc Dis 49:7–12, 1980.

29. Ryan M, Lown B, Horn H: Comparison of ventricular ectopic activity during 24-hour monitoring and exercise testing in patients with coronary heart disease. N Engl J Med 292:224–229, 1975.

30. Morganroth J, Michelson EL, Horowitz LN, Josephson ME, Pearlman AS, Dunkman WB: Limitations of routine long-term electrocardiographic monitoring to assess ventricular ectopic frequency. Circulation 58:408–414, 1978.

31. Michelson EL, Morganroth J: Spontaneous variability of complex ventricular arrhythmias detected by long-term electrocardiographic recording. Circulation 61:690–695, 1980.

32. Sami M, Kraemer H, Harrison DC, Houston N, Shimasaki C, DeBusk RF: A new method for evaluating antiarrhythmic drug efficacy. Circulation 62:1172–1179, 1980.

33. Bigger JT Jr, Goldreyer BN: The mechanism of supraventricular tachycardia. Circulation 42:673–688, 1970.

34. Josephson ME, Kastor JA: Supraventricular tachycardia: mechanisms and management. Ann Intern Med 87:346–358, 1977.

35. Denes P, Wu D, Amat-y-Leon F, Dhingra R, Wyndham C, Kehoe R, Ayres BF, Rosen KM: Paroxysmal supraventricular tachycardia induction in patients with Wolff-Parkinson-White syndrome. Ann Intern Med 90:153–157, 1979.

36. Wellens HJ, Schuilenburg RM, Durrer D: Electrical stimulation of the heart in patients with ventricular tachycardia. Circulation 46:216–226, 1972.

37. Denes P, Wu D, Dhingra RC, Amat-y-Leon F, Wyndham C, Mautner RK, Rosen KM: Electrophysiological studies in patients with chronic recurrent ventricular tachycardia. Circulation 54:229–236, 1976.

38. Josephson ME, Horowitz LN: Electrophysiologic approach to therapy of recurrent sustained ventricular tachycardia. Am J Cardiol 43:631–642, 1979.

39. Vandepol CJ, Farshidi A, Spielman SR, Greenspan AM, Horowitz LN, Josephson ME: Incidence and clinical significance of induced ventricular tachycardia. Am J Cardiol 45:725–731, 1980.

40. Wellens HJJ, Duren DR, Lie KI: Observations on mechanisms of ventricular tachycardia in man. Circulation 54:237–244, 1976.

41. Mason JW, Winkle RA: Electrode-catheter arrhythmia

induction in the selection and assessment of antiarrhythmic drug therapy in recurrent ventricular tachycardia. Circulation 58:971–985, 1978.

42. Reddy CP, Gettes LS: Use of isoproterenol as an aid to electric induction of chronic recurrent ventricular tachycardia. Am J Cardiol 44:705–713, 1979.

43. Horowitz LN, Josephson ME, Farshidi A, Spielman SR, Michelson EL, Greenspan AM: Recurrent sustained ventricular tachycardia. 3. Role of the electrophysiologic study in selection of antiarrhythmic regimens. Circulation 58: 986–997, 1978.

44. Wellens HJJ: Value and limitations of programmed electrical stimulation of the heart in the study and treatment of tachycardias. Circulation 57:845–853, 1978.

45. Mason JW, Winkle RA: Accuracy of the ventricular tachycardia induction study for predicting long-term efficacy and inefficacy of antiarrhythmic drugs. N Engl J Med 103: 1073–1077, 1980.

46. Bigger JT Jr, Hoffman BF: Antiarrhythmic drugs. In: Gilman AG, Goodman LS, Gilman A (eds) The Pharmacological Basis of Therapeutics. Macmillan, New York, 1980, pp 761–792.

47. Gettes LS, McAllister R, Chen C-M: Electropharmacology and clinical pharmacology of antiarrhythmic drugs. In: Eliot RS, Wolf GL, Forker AD (eds), Cardiac Emergencies. Futura Publ, New York, 1977, pp 245–282.

48. Singh BN, Collett JT, Chew CYC: New perspectives in the pharmacologic therapy of cardiac arrhythmias. Prog Cardiovasc Dis 22:243–301, 1980.

49. Sada H, Tan T, Oshita S: Effects of mexiletine on transmembrane action potentials as affected by external potassium concentration and by rate of stimulation in guinea-pig papillary muscles. Clin Exp Pharmacol Physiol 7: 583–593, 1980.

50. Oshita S, Sada H, Kojima M, Ban T: Effects of tocainide and lidocaine on the transmembrane action potentials as related to external potassium and calcium concentrations in guinea-pig papillary muscles. Arch Pharmacol 314: 67–82, 1980.

51. Greenblatt DJ, Balognini V, Koch-Weser J, Harmatz JS: Pharmacokinetic approach to the clinical use of lidocaine intravenously. J Am Med Assoc 236: 273–277, 1976.

52. Collingsworth KA, Kalman SM, Harrison DC: The clinical pharmacology of lidocaine as an antiarrhythmic drug. Circulation 50:1217–1230, 1974.

53. Harrison DC, Meffin PJ, Winkle RA: Clinical pharmacokinetics of antiarrhythmic drugs. Prog Cardiovasc Dis 20:217–242, 1977.

54. Woosley RL, Shand DG: Pharmacokinetics of antiarrhythmic drugs. Am J Cardiol 41:986–995, 1978.

55. Bernowitz NL, Meister W: Clinical pharmacokinetics of lidocaine. Clin Pharmacokinet 3:177–201, 1978.

56. Rodman JH: Lidocaine. In: Evans WE, Schentag JJ, Jusko WJ (eds), Applied Pharmacokinetics: Principles of Therapeutic Drug Monitoring. Applied Therapeutics, San Francisco, 1980, pp 350–391.

57. Lie KF, Wellens HJ, Van Capelle FJ, Durrer D: Lidocaine in the prevention of primary ventricular fibrillation: a double-blind randomized study of 212 consecutive patients. N Engl J Med 291:1324–1326, 1974.

58. Noneman JW, Rogers JF: Lidocaine prophylaxis in acute myocardial infarction. Medicine 57:501–515, 1978.

59. DeSilva RA, Hennekins CH, Lown B, Casscells W: Lignocaine prophylaxis in acute myocardial infarction: an evaluation of randomized trials. Lancet 2:855–858, 1981.

60. Bleifeld W, Merx W, Heinrich KW, Effert S: Controlled trial of prophylactic treatment with lidocaine in acute myocardial infarction. Eur J Clin Pharmacol 6:119–126, 1973.

61. Bennett MA, Wilner JM, Pentecost BL: Controlled trial of lignocaine in prophylaxis of ventricular arrhythmias complicating myocardial infarction. Lancet 2:909–911, 1970.

62. Mogensen I: Ventricular tachyarrhythmias and lignocaine prophylaxis in acute myocardial infarction. Acta Med Scand [Suppl] 513:1–80, 1970.

63. O'Brien KP, Taylor PM, Corxson RS: Prophylactic lignocaine in hospitalized patients with acute myocardial infarction. Med J Aust 2 (Suppl):36–37, 1973.

64. Church G, Biern R: Prophylactic lidocaine in acute myocardial infarction. Circulation 45–46 (Suppl II):II–139, 1972 (abstract).

65. Ribner HS, Isaacs ES, Frishman WH: Lidocaine prophylaxis against ventricular fibrillation in acute myocardial infarction. Prog Cardiovasc Dis 21:287–313, 1979.

66. Harrison DC: Should lidocaine be administered routinely to all patients after acute myocardial infarction? Circulation 58:581–584, 1978.

67. Valentine PA, Frew JL, Mashford ML, Sloman JG: Lidocaine in the prevention of sudden death in the pre-hospital phase of acute infarction. N Engl J Med 291:1327–1331, 1974.

68. Sandler G, Dey N, Amonkar J: Prophylactic intramuscular lidocaine in myocardial infarction. Curr Ther Res 20:563–571, 1976.

69. Lie KL, Liem KL, Louridtz WJ, Janse MH, Willebrands AF, Durrer D: Efficacy of lidocaine in preventing primary ventricular fibrillation within 1 hour after a 300 mg intramuscular injection: a double-blind, randomized study of 300 hospitalized patients with acute myocardial infarction. Am J Cardiol 42:486–488, 1978.

70. Danahy DT, Aronow WS: Lidocaine-induced cardiac rate changes in atrial fibrillation and atrial flutter. Am Heart J 95:474–482, 1978.

71. Akhtar M, Gilbert CJ, Shenasa M: Effect of lidocaine on atrioventricular response via the accessory pathway in patients with Wolff-Parkinson-White syndrome. Circulation 63:435–551, 1981.

72. Huet PM, Lelorier J, Pomier G, Marleau D: Bioavailability of lidocaine in normal volunteers and cirrhotic patients. Gastroenterology 75:969, 1978 (abstract).

73. Boyes RN, Scott DB, Jebson PJ, Godman MJ, Julian DG: Pharmacokinetics of lidocaine in man. Clin Pharmacol Ther 12:105–116, 1971.

74. Stenson RE, Constantine RT, Harrison DC: Interrelationships of hepatic blood flow, cardiac output and blood levels of lidocaine in man. Circulation 43:205–211, 1971.

75. Rowland M, Thomson PD, Uiuchard A, Melmon RL: Disposition kinetics of lidocaine in normal subjects. Ann NY Acad Sci 179: 383–398, 1971.

76. Ochs HR, Carstens G, Greenblatt DJ: Reduction in lidocaine clearance during continuous infusion and by coad-

ministration of propranolol. N Engl J Med 303:373–377, 1980.

77. Thomson PD, Melmon KE, Richardson JA, Cohn K, Steinbrunn W, Cudihee R, Rowland M: Lidocaine pharmacokinetics in advanced heart failure, liver disease and renal failure in humans. Ann Intern Med 78:499–508, 1973.

78. Bax NDS, Tucker GT, Woods HF: Lignocaine and indocyanine green kinetics in patients following myocardial infarction. Br J Clin Pharmacol 10: 353–361, 1980.

79. Nation R, Triggs EJ, Selig M: Lignocaine kinetics in cardiac patients and aged subjects. Br J Clin Pharmacol 4:439–448, 1977.

80. Cusack B, Kelly JG, Lavan J, Neol J, O'Malley K: Pharmacokinetics of lignocaine in the elderly. Br J Clin Pharmacol 9:293P–294P, 1980 (abstract).

81. LeLorier J, Grenon D, Latour Y, Caille G, Dumont G, Brosseau A, Solignac A: Pharmacokinetics of lidocaine after prolonged intravenous infusions in uncomplicated myocardial infarctions. Ann Intern Med 87:700–702, 1977.

82. Prescott LF, Adjepon-Yamoah KK, Talbet RG: Impaired lidocaine metabolism in patients with myocardial infarction and cardiac failure. Br Med J 1:939–941, 1976.

83. Sawyer DR, Ludden TM, Crawford MH: Continuous infusion of lidocaine in patients with cardiac arrhythmias: unpredictability of plasma concentrations. Arch Intern Med 141:43–45, 1981.

84. Aps C, Bell JA, Jenkins BS, Poole-Wilson PA, Reynolds F: Logical approach to lignocaine therapy. Br Med J 1:13–15, 1975.

85. Zito RA, Reid PR: Lidocaine kinetics predicted by indocyanine green clearance. N Engl J Med 298:1160–1163, 1978.

86. Routledge PA, Stargel WW, Wagner GS, Shand DG: Increased alpha-1-acid glycoprotein and lidocaine disposition in myocardial infarction. Ann Intern Med 93:701–704, 1980.

87. Pieper JA, Wyman MG, Goldreyer BN, Cannon DS, Slaughter RL, Lalka D: Lidocaine toxicity: effects of total vs free lidocaine concentrations. Circulation 62 (Suppl III):III-181, 1980 (abstract).

88. Piafsky KM, Knoppert D: Binding of local anesthetics to alpha-1-acid glycoprotein. Clin Res 26:836A, 1978 (abstract).

89. Zener JC, Kerber RE, Spivack AP, Harrison DC: Blood lidocaine levels and kinetics following high dose intramuscular administration. Circulation 47:984–988, 1973.

90. Cohen LS, Rosenthal JE, Horner DW Jr, Atkins JM, Matthews OA, Sarnoff SJ: Plasma levels of lidocaine after intramuscular administration. Am J Cardiol 29:520–523, 1972.

91. Ryden L, Wasir H, Conradsson TB, Olsson B: Blood levels of lignocaine after intramuscular administration to patients with proven or suspected acute myocardial infarction. Br Heart J 34:1012–1017, 1972.

92. Wyman MG, Lalka D, Hammersmith L, Cannon DS, Goldreyer BN: Multiple bolus technique for lidocaine administration during the first hours of an acute myocardial infarction. Am J Cardiol 41:313–317, 1978.

93. Stargel WW, Shand DG, Routledge PA, Barchowsky A, Wagner GS: Clinical comparison of rapid infusion and

94. DiFazio LA, Brown RB: Lidocaine metabolism in normal and phenobarbitol pre-treated dogs. Anesthesiology 36: 238–243, 1972.

95. Heinonen J: Influence of some drugs on toxicity and rate of metabolism of lidocaine and mepivacaine. Ann Med Exp Biol Fenn 44 (Suppl III):1–43, 1966.

96. Heinonen J, Takki S, Jarho L: Plasma lidocaine levels in patients treated with potential inducers of microsomal enzymes. Acta Anaesthesiol Scand 14:89–95, 1970.

97. Pape BE, Whiting R, Parker KM, Mitra R: Enzyme immunoassay and gas–liquid chromatography compared for determination of lidocaine in serum. Clin Chem 24: 2020–2022, 1978.

98. Buckman K, Claiborne K, de Guzman M, Walberg CB, Haywood LJ: Lidocaine efficacy and toxicity assessed by a new, rapid method. Clin Pharmacol Ther 28:177–181, 1980.

99 Pfeifer HJ, Greenblatt, DJ Koch-Weser J: Clinical use and toxicity of intravenous lidocaine. Am Heart J 92:168–173, 1976.

100. Lippestad CT, Forfang K: Production of sinus arrest by lignocaine. Br Med J 1:537, 1971.

101. Cheng TO, Wadwha K: Sinus standstill following intravenous lidocaine administration. J Am Med Assoc 223: 790–792, 1973.

102. Levy S, Balansard P, Bouteau JM, Gerard R: L'arrêt sinusal: complication grave de la lidocaine intraveineuse Arch Mal Coeur 68:1069–1073, 1975.

103. Klein HO, Jutrin I, Kaplinsky E: Cerebral and cardiac toxicity of a small dose of lignocaine. Br Heart J 37: 775–778, 1975.

104. Manyari-Ortega DE, Brennan FJ: Lidocaine-induced cardiac asystole. Chest 74:227–229, 1978.

105. Lichstein E, Chadda KD, Gupta PK: Atrioventricular block with lidocaine therapy. Am J Cardiol 31:277–281, 1973.

106. Josephson ME, Caracta AR, Lau SH, Gallagher JJ, Damato AN: Effects of lidocaine on refractory periods in man. Am Heart J 84:778–786, 1972.

107. Gianelly RE, von der Groeben JO, Spivack AP, Harrison DC: Effects of lidocaine on ventricular arrhythmias in patients with coronary heart disease. N Engl J Med 277:1215–1219, 1967.

108. Gupta PK, Lichstein E, Chadda KD: Lidocaine-induced heart block in patients with bundle branch block. Am J Cardiol 33:487–492, 1974.

109. Kunkel F, Rowland M, Scheinman MM: The electrophysiologic effects of lidocaine in patients with intraventricular conduction defects. Circulation 49:894–899, 1974.

110. Aravandakshan V, Kuo CS, Gettes LS: Effect of lidocaine on escape rate in patients with complete atrial ventricular block. Am J Cardiol 40:177–183, 1977.

111. Kuo CS, Reddy CP: Effect of lidocaine on escape rates in patients with complete atrioventricular block: B. Proximal His bundle block. Am J Cardiol 47:1315–1320, 1981.

112. Leahy EB Jr, Bigger JT: Mexiletine: a new antiarrhythmic drug. Ann Intern Med 92:427–429, 1980.

113. Chew CYC, Collett J, Singh BN: Mexiletine: A review of

its pharmacological properties and therapeutic efficacy in arrhythmias. Drugs 17:161–181, 1979.

114. Kulbertus HE: Clinical antiarrhythmic efficacy of mexiletine: a review. Acta Cardiol Suppl 25: 111–120, 1980.

115. Danilo P Jr: Mexiletine. Am Heart J 97:399–403, 1979.

116. Jewitt D, McComish M, Jackson G: Ambulatory monitoring in the controlled assessment of antiarrhythmic drug therapy. Postgrad Med J 5 (Suppl 7):67–71, 1976.

117. VanDurme JP, Bogaert M, Weyne T, Pannier R: Comparison of the antidysrhythmic efficacy of mexiletine, isocainide and placebo. Circulation 55–56(Suppl III):III–176, 1977 (abstract).

118. Talbot RG, Julian DG, Prescott LF: Long term treatment of ventricular arrhythmias with oral mexiletine. Am Heart J 91: 58–65, 1976.

119. Abinader EG, Cooper M: Mexiletine: use in control of chronic drug resistant ventricular arrhythmias. J Am Med Assoc 242:337–339, 1979.

120. Campbell NPS, Pantridge JF, Adgey AAJ: Mexiletine in the management of ventricular dysrhythmias. Eur J Cardiol 6:245–258, 1977.

121. Campbell RWF, Achuff SC, Pottage A, Murray A, Prescott LF, Julian DG: Mexiletine in the prophylaxis of ventricular arrhythmias during acute myocardial infarction. J Cardiovasc Pharmacol 1:43–52, 1979.

122. Talbot RG, Clark RA, Nimmo J, Nielsson JMM, Julian DG, Prescott LF: Treatment of ventricular arrhythmias with mexiletine (Ko 1173). Lancet 2:399–404, 1973.

123. Heger JJ, Nattel S, Rinkenberger RL, Zipes DP: Mexiletine therapy in 15 patients with drug-resistant ventricular tachycardia. Am J Cardiol 45:627–632, 1980.

124. Friedman IM, Simpson RJ, Foster JR, Gettes LS: Mexiletine: an effective drug in preventing refractory recurrent ventricular tachycardias. Circulation 62 (Suppl III): III–154, 1980 (abstract).

125. Chamberlain DA, Julian DG, Boyle DM, Jewitt DE, Campbell RWF, Shanks RG: Oral mexiletine in high-risk patients after myocardial infarction. Lancet 2:1324–1327, 1980.

126. McComish M, Robinson C, Kitson D, Jewitt D: Clinical electrophysiologic effect of mexiletine. Postgrad Med J 53 (Suppl I): 85–91, 1977.

127. Duff HJ, Roden DM, Primm K, Carey EL, Oates JA, Woosley RL: Mexiletine for resistant ventricular tachycardia: comparison with lidocaine and enhancement of efficacy by combination with quinidine. Am J Cardiol 47: 438, 1981 (abstract).

128. Campbell NPS, Kelly JG, Adgey AAJ, Shanks RG: The clinical pharmacology of mexiletine. Br J Clin Pharmacol 6:103–108, 1978.

129. Campbell NPS, Kelly JG, Adgey AAJ, Shanks RG: Mexiletine in normal volunteers. Br J Clin Pharmacol 6: 372–373, 1978.

130. Prescott LF, Clements JA, Pottage A: Absorption, distribution and elimination of mexiletine. Postgrad Med J 53 (Suppl I):50–55, 1977.

131. Baudinet G, Henrard L, Quinaux N, el Allaf D, De Laudsheere C, Carlier J, Dresse A: Pharmacokinetics of mexiletine in renal insufficiency. Acta Cardiol Suppl XXV: 55–65, 1980.

132. Bogaert M: Adaptation of the dose of mexiletine according to pharmacokinetic data. Acta Cardiol Suppl XXV:67–73, 1980.

133. Ruskin JN, DiMarco JP, Garan H: Out-of-hospital cardiac arrest: Electrophysiologic observations and selection of long-term antiarrhythmic therapy. N Engl J Med 303: 607–613, 1980.

134. Leahey EB, Heissenbuttel RJ, Bigger JT: Combined mexiletine and propranolol for resistant ventricular arrhythmias. Circulation 62 (Suppl III) III–181, 1980 (abstract).

135. Breithardt G, Seipel L, Abendroth RR: Comparative crossover study of the effects of disopyramide and mexiletine on stimulus-induced ventricular tachycardia. Circulation 62 (Suppl III):III–153, 1980 (abstract).

136. Meinertz T, Kasper W, Kersting F, Bechtold H, Jahnchen E, Lollgen H, Just H: Comparison of the antiarrhythmic activity of mexiletine and lorcainide on refractory ventricular arrhythmias. Circulation 62 (Suppl III):III–184, 1980 (abstract).

137. Stavenow L, Hanson A, Johansson BW: Mexiletine in treatment of ventricular arrhythmias: a long-term follow-up. Acta Med Scand 205:411–415, 1979.

138. Paalman ACA, Roos JC, Siebelink J, Dunning AJ: Development of a dosage scheme for simultaneous intravenous and oral administration of mexiletine. Postgrad Med J 53 (Suppl I):128–132, 1977.

139. Carlier J: Hemodynamic, electrocardiographic and toxic effects of the intravenous administration of increasing doses of mexiletine in the dog: comparison with similar effects produced by other antiarrhythmics. Acta Cardiol Suppl XXV:81–100, 1980.

140. Campbell NPS, Zaidi SA, Adgey AAJ, Patterson GC, Pantridge JF: Observations on haemodynamic effects of mexiletine. Br Heart J 41:182–186, 1979.

141. Renard M, De Hemptinne J, Gillet JM, Bernard R: Hemodynamic effects of parenteral and oral mexiletine. Acta Cardiol Suppl XXV:75–80, 1980.

142. Henrard L, Carlier J: Hemodynamic effects of an intravenous injection of mexiletine in patients hospitalized in intensive care units. Acta Cardiol Suppl XXV:101–107, 1980.

143. Danilo P: Tocainide. Am Heart J 97:259–262, 1979.

144. Zipes DP, Troup PJ: New antiarrhythmic agents. Am J Cardiol 41:1005–1024, 1978.

145. Winkle RA, Meffin PJ, Fitzgerald JW, Harrison DC: Clinical efficacy and pharmacokinetics of a new orally effective antiarrhythmic, tocainide. Circulation 54:884–889, 1976.

146. Woosley RL, McDevitt DG, Nies AS, Smith RF, Wilkinson GR, Oates JA: Suppression of ventricular ectopic depolarizations by tocainide. Circulation 56:980–984, 1977.

147. Ryan W, Engler R, LeWinter M, Karliner JS: Efficacy of a new oral agent (tocainide) in the acute treatment of refractory ventricular arrhythmias. Am J Cardiol 43:285–291, 1979.

148. Engler R, Ryan W, LeWinter M, Bluestein H, Kerliner JS: Assessment of long-term antiarrhythmic therapy: studies on the long-term efficacy and toxicity of tocainide. Am J Cardiol 43: 612–618, 1979.

149. Kuck KH, Hanrath P, Lubda J, Mathey D, Bleifeld W.: Die antiarrhythmische Wirkung von tocainid bei ventricu-

laren Herzrhythmusstörungen. Dtsch Med Wochenschr 104: 1701–1705, 1979.

150. Sonnhag C: Efficacy and tolerance of tocainide during acute and long-term treatment of chronic ventricular arrhythmias. Eur J Clin Pharmacol 18: 301–310, 1980.

151. McDevitt DG, Nies AS, Wilkinson GR, Smith RF, Woosley RL, Oates JA: Antiarrhythmic effects of a lidocaine congener, tocainide, 2-amino-2',6'-propionoxylidide in man. Clin Pharmacol Ther 19:396–402, 1976.

152. Maloney JD, Nissen RG, McColgan JM: Open clinical studies at a referral center: chronic maintenance tocainide therapy in patients with recurrent sustained ventricular tachycardia refractory to conventional antiarrhythmic agents. Am Heart J 100:1023–1030, 1980.

153. Winkle RA, Mason JW, Harrison DC: Tocainide for drug-resistant ventricular arrhythmias: efficacy, side effects and lidocaine responsiveness for predicting tocainide success. Am Heart J 100:1031–1036, 1980.

154. Roden DM, Reele SB, Higgins SB, Carr RK, Smith RF, Oates JA, Woosley RL: Tocainide therapy for refractory ventricular arrhythmias. Am Heart J 100:15–22, 1980.

155. Koransky A, Kehoe R, Sherman M, Tommaso C, Myers S, Lesch M: Comparative effects of tocainide and lidocaine on sustained ventricular tachycardia. Circulation 64 (Suppl IV): IV–38, 1981 (abstract).

156. Waleffe A, Bruninx R, Mary-Rabine L, Kulbertus HE: Effects of tocainide studied with programmed electrical stimulation of the heart in patients with reentrant tachyarrhythmias. Am J Cardiol 43:292–299, 1979.

157. Graffner C, Conradson T, Hofvendahl S, Ryden L: Tocainide kinetics after intravenous and oral administration in healthy subjects and in patients with acute myocardial infarction. Clin Pharmacol Ther 27: 64–71, 1980.

158. Lalka D, Meyer MB, Duce BR, Elvin AT: Kinetics of the oral lidocaine congener, tocainide. Clin Pharmacol Ther 19: 757–766, 1976.

159. Winkle RA, Meffin PJ, Harrison DC: Long-term tocainide therapy for ventricular arrhythmias. Circulation 57: 1008–1016, 1978.

160. Elvin AT, Keenaghan JB, Byrnes EW, Tenthorey PA, MCMaster PD, Takman BH, Lalka D, Manion CV, Baer DT, Wolshin EM, Meyer MB, Ronfeld RA: Conjugation of tocainide in man: a novel pathway of biotransformation for a primary amine. J Pharmacol Sci 69: 47–49, 1980.

161. Swedberg K, Pehrson J, Ryden L: Electrocardiographic and hemodynamic effects of tocainide (W-36095) in man. Eur J Clin Pharmacol 14:15–19, 1978.

162. Nyquist O, Forssel G, Norlander R, Schenck-Gustafsson K: Hemodynamic and antiarrhythmic effects of tocainide in patients with acute myocardial infarction. Am Heart J 100:1000–1005, 1980.

163. Winkle RA, Anderson JL, Peters F, Meffin PJ, Fowles RE, Harrison DC: The hemodynamic effects of intravenous tocainide in patients with heart disease. Circulation 57:787–792, 1978.

164. Haffajee CJ, Alpert JS, Dalen JE: Tocainide for refractory ventricular arrhythmias of myocardial infarction. Am Heart J 100: 1013–1016, 1980.

165. Horn H, Hadidian Z., Johnson JL, Vassallo HG, Williams JH, Young MD: Safety evaluation of tocainide in the American Emergency Use Program. Am Heart J 100: 1037–1040, 1980.

166. Ryan WF, Karliner JS: Effects of tocainide on left ventricular performance at rest and during acute alterations in heart rate and systemic arterial pressure: an echocardiographic study. Br Heart J 41:175–181, 1979.

167. Young MD, Hadidian Z, Horn HR, Johnson JL, Vassallo HG: Treatment of ventricular arrhythmias with oral tocainide. Am Heart J 100:1041–1045, 1980.

168. Atkinson AJ, Davison R: Diphenylhydantoin as an antiarrhythmic drug. Ann Rev Med 25:99–113, 1974.

169. Winkle RA, Glantz SA, Harrison DC: Pharmacologic therapy of ventricular arrhythmias. Am J Cardiol 36: 629–650, 1975.

170. Anderson JL, Harrison DC, Meffin PJ, Winkle RA: Antiarrhythmic drugs: clinical pharmacology and therapeutic uses. Drugs 15:271–309, 1978.

171. Bigger JT, Dresdale RJ, Heissenbussel RH, Weld FM, Wit AL: Ventricular arrhythmias in ischemic heart disease: mechanism, prevalence, significance and management. Prog Cardiovasc Dis 19:255–300, 1979.

172. Karliner JS: Intravenous diphenylhydantoin sodium (dilantin) in cardiac arrhythmias. Dis Chest 51:256–269, 1967.

173. Rosen M, Lisak R, Rubin IL: Diphenylhydantoin in cardiac arrhythmias. Am J Cardiol 20:674–678, 1967.

174. Conn RD: Diphenylhydantoin sodium in cardiac arrhythmias. N Engl J Med 272:277–282, 1965.

175. Mercer EN, Osborne JA: The current status of diphenylhydantoin in heart disease. Ann Intern Med 67:1084–1107, 1967.

176. Bigger JT Jr, Schmidt DH, Kutt H: Relationship between the plasma level of diphenylhydantoin sodium and its cardiac antiarrhythmic effects. Circulation 38: 363–374, 1968.

177. Mosey L, Tyler MD: The effect of diphenylhydantoin sodium (dilantin), procaine hydrochloride, procaine amide hydrochloride, and quinidine hydrochloride upon ouabain-induced ventricular tachycardia in unanesthetized dogs. Circulation 10:65–70, 1954.

178. Helfant RH, Scherlag BJ, Damato AN: Protection from digitalis toxicity with the prophylactic use of diphenylhydantoin sodium. Circulation 36:119–124, 1967.

179. Lang TW, Bernstein H, Barbieri F, Gold H, Corday E: Digitalis toxicity: treatment with diphenylhydantoin. Arch Intern Med 116:573–580, 1965.

180. Eddy JD, Singh SP: Treatment of cardiac arrhythmias with phenytoin. Br Med J 4:270–273, 1969.

181. Vajda FJE, Prineas RJ, Lovell RRH, Sloman JG: The possible effect of long-term high plasma levels of phenytoin on mortality after acute myocardial infarction. Eur J Clin Pharmacol 5:138–144, 1973.

182. Collaborative group: Phenytoin after recovery from myocardial infarction. Lancet 2:1055–1057, 1971.

183. Peter T, Ross D, Duffield A, Luxton M, Harper R, Hunt D, Sloman G: Effect on survival after myocardial infarction of long-term treatment with phenytoin. Br Heart J 40:1356–1360, 1978.

184. Stone N, Klein MD, Lown B: Diphenylhydantoin in the prevention of recurring ventricular tachycardia. Circulation 43:420–427, 1971.

185. Karlsson E: Procainamide and phenytoin: comparative

studies of their antiarrhythmic effects at apparent therapeutic plasma levels. Br Heart J 37:731–740, 1975.

186. Krone RJ, Miller JP, Kleiger RE, Clark KW, Oliver GC: The effectiveness of antiarrhythmic agents on early-cycle premature ventricular complexes. Circulation 63:664–669, 1981.

187. Jung D, Powell JR, Walson P, Perrier D: Effect of dose on phenytoin absorption. Clin Pharmacol Ther 28:479–485, 1980.

188. Glazko AJ: Diphenylhydantoin. Pharmacology 8:163–177, 1972.

189. Albert KS, Sakmar E, Hallmark MR, Weidler DJ, Wagner JG: Bioavailability of diphenylhydantoin. Clin Pharmacol Ther 16:727–735, 1974.

190. Lund L, Alvan G, Berlin A, Alexanderson B: Pharmacokinetics of single and multiple doses of phenytoin in man. Eur J Clin Pharmacol 7:81–86, 1974.

191. Gugler R, Manion CV, Azarnoff DL: Phenytoin: pharmacokinetics and bioavailability. Clin Pharmacol Ther 19:135–142, 1976.

192. Jusko WJ, Koup JR, Alvan G: Nonlinear assessment of phenytoin bioavailability. J Pharmacokinet Biopharm 4:327–336, 1976.

193. Ludden TM, Allen JP, Schneider LW, Stavchansky SA: Rate of phenytoin accumulation in man: a simulation study. J Pharmacokinet Biopharm 6:399–415, 1978.

194. Kutt H, Winters W, Scherman R, McDowell F: Diphenylhydantoin and phenobarbital toxicity: the role of liver disease. Arch Neurol 11:649–656, 1964.

195. Blaschke TF, Meffin PJ, Melmon KL, Rowland M: Influence of acute viral hepatitis on phenytoin kinetics and protein binding. Clin Pharmacol Ther 17:685–691, 1975.

196. Olanow CW, Finn AL: Phenytoin: pharmacokinetics and clinical therapeutics. Neurosurgery 8:112–117, 1981.

197. Olanow CW, Finn AL, Prussak C: The effects of salicylate on the pharmacokinetics of phenytoin. Neurology 31:341–342, 1981.

198. Richens A, Dunlop A: Serum phenytoin levels in management of epilepsy. Lancet 2:247–248, 1975.

199. Cranford RE, Leppik IE, Patrick B, Anderson CB, Kostick B: Intravenous phenytoin: clinical and pharmacokinetic aspects. Neurology 28:874–880, 1978.

200. Buchanan RA, Kinkel AW, Goulet JR, Smith TC: The metabolism of diphenylhydantoin (dilantin) following once-daily administration. Neurology 22:126–130, 1972.

201. Kostenbauder HB, Rapp RP, McGovern JP, Foster TS, Perrier DG, Blacker HM, Hulon WC, Kinkel AW: Bioavailability and single-dose pharmacokinetics: intramuscular phenytoin. Clin Pharmacol Ther 18:449–456, 1975.

202. Strandjord RE, Johanessen SI: One daily dose of diphenylhydantoin for patients with epilepsy. Epilepsia 15:317–327, 1974.

203. Cocks DA, Critchley EMR, Hayward HW, Owen V, Mawer GE, Woodcock BG: Control of epilepsy with a single daily dose of phenytoin sodium. Br J Clin Pharmacol 2:449–453, 1975.

204. Mawer GE, Mullen PW, Rodgers M: Phenytoin dose adjustment in epileptic patients. Br J Clin Pharmacol 1:163–168, 1974.

205. Ludden TM, Allen JP, Valutsky WA, Vicuna AV, Nappi JM, Hoffman SF, Wallace JE, Lalka D, McNay JL: Individualization of phenytoin dosage regimens. Clin Pharmacol Ther 21:287–293, 1977.

206. Martin E, Tozer TN, Sheiner LB, Riegelman S: The clinical pharmacokinetics of phenytoin. J Pharmacokinet Biopharm 5: 579–596, 1977.

207. Mullen PW: Optimal phenytoin therapy: a new technique for individualizing dosage. Clin Pharmacol Ther 23:228–232, 1978.

208. Vozeh S, Koelz A, Martin E, Magun H, Scollo-Lavizzari G, Follath F: Predictability of phenytoin serum levels by nomograms and clinicians. Eur Neurol 0:345–352, 1980.

209. Data JL, Wilkinson GR, Nies AS: Interaction of quinidine with anticonvulsant drugs. N Engl J Med 294:699–702, 1976.

210. Fine A, Henderson IS, Morgan DR: Malabsorption of frusemide caused by phenytoin. Br Med J 2:1061–1062, 1977.

211. Bivins BA, Rapp RP, Griffen WO Jr, Blouin R, Bustrack J: Dopamine–phenytoin interaction: a cause of hypotension in the critically ill. Arch Surg 113:245–249, 1978.

212. Tibbs PA, Bivens BA, Rapp RP, Young AB, Griffon WO Jr, Haack DG: Phenytoin-induced hypotension in animals receiving sympathomimetic pressor support. J Surg Res 29:338–347, 1980.

213. Kutt H, Winters W, Kokenge R, McDowell F: Diphenylhydantoin metabolism, blood levels and toxicity. Arch Neurol 11:642–648, 1964.

214. Kutt H, Schoman GE: Phenytoin: relevant side effects. In: Glaser GH, Penry JK, Woodbury DM (eds) Antiepileptic Drugs: Mechanism of Action. Raven Press, New York, 1980.

215. Levantine A, Almeyda J: Cutaneous reactions to anticonvulsants. Br J Dermatol 87:646–649, 1972.

216. Hanson JW, Smith DW: The fetal hydantoin syndrome. J Pediatr 87:285–290, 1975.

217. Willius FA, Keys TE: A remarkably early reference to the use of cinchona in cardiac arrhythmia. In: Staff Meetings of the Mayo Clinic XCIV, 1942, pp 294–296.

218. Wenckebach KF: Die unregelmässige Herztätigkeit und ihre klinische Bedeutung. Engelmann W, Leipzig, 1914.

219. Frey W: Weitere Erfahrungen mit chinidin bei absoluter Herzunregelmässigkeit. Wien Klin Wochenschr 55:849–853, 1918.

220. Warnowicz MA, Denes P: Chronic ventricular arrhythmias: comparative drug effectiveness and toxicity. Prog Cardiovasc Dis 23:225–236, 1980.

221. Bloomfield SS, Romhilt DW, Chou T, Fowler NO: Natural history of cardiac arrhythmias and their prevention with quinidine in patients with acute coronary insufficiency. Circulation 47:967–973, 1973.

222. Bloomfield SS, Romhilt DW, Chou T, Fowler NO: Quinidine for prophylaxis of arrhythmias in acute myocardial infarction. N Engl J Med 285:979–986, 1971.

223. Gaughan CE, Lown B, Lanigan J, Voukydis P, Besser HW: Acute oral testing for determining antiarrhythmia drug efficacy. Am J Cardiol 38:677–684, 1976.

224. Jelinek MV, Lohrbauer L, Lown B: Antiarrhythmic drug therapy for sporadic ventricular ectopic arrhythmias. Circulation 49:659–666, 1974.

225. Winkle RA, Gradman AH, Fitzgerald JW, Bell PA: Antiarrhythmic drug effect assessed from ventricular arrhythmia reduction in the ambulatory electrocardiogram and treadmill test: comparison of propranolol, procainamide and quinidine. Am J Cardiol 42:473–480, 1978.

226. Myerburg RJ, Conde C, Sheps DS, Appel RA, Kiem I, Sung RJ, Castellanos A: Antiarrhythmic drug therapy in survivors of prehospital cardiac arrest: comparison of effects on chronic ventricular arrhythmias and recurrent cardiac arrest. Circulation 59:855–863, 1979.

227. Kletzkin M: Antiarrhythmic therapy: quinidine gluconate vs procainamide. Circulation 61: 214, 1980.

228. Cramer G: Early and late results of conversion of atrial fibrillation with quinidine: a clinical and hemodynamic study. Acta Med Scand [Suppl] 490:5–96, 1968.

229. Sodermark T, Edhag O, Sjogren A, Jonsson B, Olsson A, Oro L, Danielsson M, Rosenhamer G, Wallin H: Effect of quinidine on maintaining sinus rhythm after conversion of atrial fibrillation or flutter: a multicentre study from Stockholm. Br Heart J 37:486–492, 1975.

230. Hillestad L, Bjerkelund C, Dale J, Maltau J, Storstein O: Quinidine in maintenance of sinus rhythm after electroconversion of chronic atrial fibrillation: a controlled clinical study. Br Heart J 33:518–521, 1971.

231. Waris E, Kreus K, Salokannel J: Factors influencing persistence of sinus rhythm after DC shock treatment of atrial fibrillation. Acta Med Scand 189:161–166, 1971.

232. Wellens HJJ, Durrer D: Effect of procaine amide, quinidine, and ajmaline in the Wolff-Parkinson-White syndrome. Circulation 50:114–120, 1974.

233. Wellens HJJ, Bar FW, Dassen WRM, Brugada P, Vanagt EJ, Farre J: Effect of drugs in the Wolff-Parkinson-White syndrome: importance of initial length of effective refractory period of the accessory pathway. Am J Cardiol 46:665–669, 1980.

234. Wu D, Hung J, Kuo C, Hsu K, Shieh W: Effects of quinidine on atrioventricular nodal reentrant paroxysmal tachycardia. Circulation 64:823–831, 1981.

235. Hoffman BF, Rosen MR, Wit AL: Appraisal and reappraisal of cardiac therapy: electrophysiology and pharmacology of cardiac arrhythmias. VII. Cardiac effects of quinidine and procaine amide. Part A. Am Heart J 89:804–840, 1975.

236. Gillette PC, Garson A: Electrophysiologic and pharmacologic characteristics of automatic ectopic atrial tachycardia. Circulation 56:571–579, 1977.

237. Ueda CT, Hirschfeld DS, Scheinman MM, Rowland M, Williamson BJ, Dzindzio BS: Disposition kinetics of quinidine. Clin Pharmacol Ther 19:30–36, 1975.

238. Ochs HR, Greenblatt DJ, Woo E, Smith TW: Reduced quinidine clearance in elderly persons. Am J Cardiol 42:481–485, 1978.

239. Conn HL, Luchi RJ: Some quantitative aspects of the binding of quinidine and related quinoline compounds by human serum albumin. J Clin Invest 40: 509–516, 1961.

240. Data JL, Wilkinson GR, Nies AS: Interaction of quinidine with anticonvulsant drugs. N Engl J Med 294:699–702, 1976.

241. Doering W: Quinidine–digoxin interaction: pharmacokinetics, underlying mechanism and clinical implications. N Engl J Med 301:400–404, 1979.

242. Leahey EB, Reiffel JA, Drusin RE, Heissenbuttel RH, Lovejoy WP, Bigger JT: Interaction between quinidine and digoxin. J Am Med Assoc 240: 533–534, 1978.

243. Leahey EB, Reiffel JA, Heissenbuttel RH, Drusin RE, Lovejoy WP, Bigger JT: Enhanced cardiac effect of digoxin during quinidine treatment. Arch Intern Med 139: 519–521, 1979.

244. Hirsh PD, Weiner HJ, North RL: Further insights into digoxin–quinidine interaction: lack of correlation between serum digoxin concentration and inotropic state of the heart. Am J Cardiol 46:863–867, 1980.

245. Bigger JT: The quinidine–digoxin interaction: what do we know about it? N Engl J Med 301: 779–781, 1979.

246. Ochs HR, Greenblatt DJ, Woo E, Franke K, Pfeifer HJ, Smith TW: Single and multiple dose pharmacokinetics of oral quinidine sulfate and gluconate. Am J Cardiol 41: 770–777, 1978.

247. Hirschfeld DS, Ueda CT, Rowland M, Scheinman MM: Clinical and electrophysiological effects of intravenous quinidine in man. Br Heart J 39:309–316, 1977.

248. Anderson JL, Mason JW: Successful treatment of overdrive pacing of recurrent quinidine syncope due to ventricular tachycardia. Am J Med 64:715–718, 1978.

249. Koster RW, Wellens HJJ: Quinidine-induced ventricular flutter and fibrillation without digitalis therapy. Am J Cardiol 38:519–523, 1976.

250. Luchi RJ: Intoxication with quinidine. Chest 73:129–131, 1978.

251. Reynolds EW, Vander Ark CR: Quinidine syncope and the delayed repolarization syndromes. Mod Concepts Cardiovasc Dis 45:117–122, 1976.

252. Selzer A, Wray HW: Quinidine syncope: paroxysmal ventricular fibrillation occurring during treatment of chronic atrial arrhythmias. Circulation 30:17–26, 1964.

253. Grayzel J, Angeles J: Sino-atrial block in man provoked by quinidine. J Electrocardiol 5:289–294, 1972.

254. Mason JW, Winkle RA, Rider AK, Stinson EB, Harrison DC: The electrophysiologic effects of quinidine in the transplanted human heart. J Clin Invest 59:481–489, 1977.

255. Cohen IS, Jick H, Cohen SI: Adverse reactions to quinidine in hospitalized patients: findings based on data from the Boston Collaborative Drug Surveillance Program. Prog Cardiovasc Dis 20:151–163, 1977.

256. Nair MRS, Duvernoy WFC, Leichtman DA: Severe leukopenia and thrombocytopenia secondary to quinidine. Clin Cardiol 4: 247–257, 1981.

257. Yagiela JA, Benoit PW: Skeletal-muscle damage from quinidine N Engl J Med 301:437, 1979.

258. Moe GK, Abildskow JA: Antiarrhythmic drugs. In: Goodman LS, Gilman AG (eds) The Pharmacological Basis of Therapeutics. Macmillan, New York, 1970, pp 709–727.

259. Engler RL, Le Winter MM, Karliner JS: Depressant effects of quinidine gluconate on left ventricular function in conscious dogs with and without volume overload. Circulation 60:828–835, 1979.

260. Crawford MH, White DH, O'Rourke RA, Amon KW: Effects of oral quinidine on left ventricular performance in normal subjects and patients with congestive cardiomy-

opathy. Am J Cardiol 44:714–718, 1979.

261. Arnsdorf MF, Bigger JT: The effect of procaine amide on components of excitability in long mammalian cardiac Purkinje fibers. Circ Res 38:115–122, 1976.

262. Kastor JA, Josephson ME, Guss SB, Horowitz LN: Human ventricular refractoriness: II. Effects of procainamide. Circulation 56:462–467, 1977.

263. Woske H, Belford J, Fastier FN, Brooks CM: The effect of procaine amide on excitability, refractoriness and conduction in the mammalian heart. J Pharmacol Exp Ther 107:134–140, 1953.

264. Michelson EL, Spear JF, Moore EN: Effects of procainamide on strength–interval relations in normal and chronically infarcted canine myocardium. Am J Cardiol 47:1223–1232, 1981.

265. Kayden HJ, Brodie BB, Steele JM: Procaine amide: a review. Circulation 15:118–126, 1957.

266. Koch-Weser J, Klein SW, Foo-Canto LL, Kastor JA, DeSanctis RW: Antiarrhythmic prophylaxis with procainamide in acute myocardial infarction. N Engl J Med 281:1253–1260, 1969.

267. Kosowsky BD, Taylor J, Lown B, Ritchie RF: Long-term use of procaine amide following acute myocardial infarction. Circulation 47:1204–1210, 1973.

268. Engel TR, Meister SG, Luch JC: Modification of ventricular tachycardia by procainamide in patients with coronary artery disease. Am J Cardiol 46:1033–1038, 1980.

269. Wellens HJJ, Bar FWHM, Lie KI, Duren DR, Dohmen HJ: Effect of procainamide, propranolol and verapamil on mechanism of tachycardia in patients with chronic recurrent ventricular tachycardia. Am J Cardiol 40:579–585, 1977.

270. Greenspan AM, Horowitz LN, Spielman SR, Josephson ME: Large dose procainamide therapy for ventricular tachyarrhythmia. Am J Cardiol 46:453–462, 1980.

271. Halpern SW, Ellrodt G, Singh BN, Mandel WJ: Efficacy of intravenous procainamide infusion in converting atrial fibrillation to sinus rhythm: relation to left atrial size. Br Heart J 44:589–595, 1980.

272. Wyse DG, McAnulty JH, Rahimtoola SH: Influence of plasma drug level and the presence of conduction disease on the electrophysiologic effects of procainamide. Am J Cardiol 43:619–626, 1979.

273. Wyndham CR, Meeran MK, Wu D, Rosen KM: Recent insights into paroxysmal supraventricular tachycardia – An integrated approach to disgnosis and therapy. Aust N Z J Med 7:212–231, 1977.

274. Koch-Weser J: Pharmacokinetics of procainamide in man. Ann NY Acad Sci 179:370–382, 1971.

275. Koch-Weser J, Klein SW: Procainamide dosage schedules, plasma concentrations, and clinical effects. J Am Med Assoc 215:1454–1460, 1971.

276. Lima JJ, Goldfarb AL, Conti DR, Golden LH, Bascomb BL, Benedetti GM, Jusko WJ: Safety and efficacy of procainamide infusions. Am J Cardiol 43:98–105, 1979.

277. Mattiasson I, Hanson A, Johansson BW: Massive doses of procainamide for ventricular tachyarrhythmias due to myocardial infarction. Acta Med Scand 204:27–34, 1978.

278. Embree LJ, Levine SA: Ventricular tachycardia: a case requiring massive amounts of procaine amide (pronestyl) for reversion. Ann Intern Med 50:222–231, 1959.

279. Myerburg RJ, Kessler KM, Kiem I, Pefkaros KC, Conde CA, Cooper D, Castellanos A: Relationship between plasma levels of procainamide, suppression of premature ventricular complexes and prevention of recurrent ventricular tachycardia. Circulation 64:280–290, 1981.

280. Fisher JD, Cohen HL, Mehra R, Altschuler H, Escher DJW, Furman S: Cardiac pacing and pacemakers. II. Serial electrophysiologic-pharmacologic testing for control of recurrent tachyarrhythmias. Am Heart J 93:658–668, 1977.

281. Winkle RA, Alderman EL, Fitzgerald JW, Harrison DC: Treatment of recurrent symptomatic ventricular tachycardia. Ann Intern Med 85:1–7, 1976.

282. Berry K, Garlett, EL, Bellet S, Gefter WI: Use of pronestyl in the treatment of ectopic rhythms–treatment of ninety-eight episodes in seventy-eight patients. Am J Med 11:431–441, 1951.

283. Epstein MA: Ventricular standstill during the intravenous procaine amide treatment of ventricular tachycardia. Am Heart J 45:898–908, 1953.

284. Stearns NS, Callahan EJ III, Ellis LB: Value and hazards of intravenous procaine amide ("pronestyl") therapy. J Am Med Assoc 148:360–364, 1952.

285. Strasberg B, Sclarovsky S, Erdberg A, Duffy CE, Lam W, Swiryn S, Agmon J, Rosen KM: Procainamide-induced polymorphous ventricular tachycardia. Am J Cardiol 47:1309–1314, 1981.

286. Scheinman MM, Weiss AN, Shafton E, Benowitz N, Rowland M: Electrophysiologic effects of procaine amide in patients with intraventricular conduction delay. Circulation 49:522–529, 1974.

287. Konttinen YP, Tuominen L: Reversible procainamide-induced agranulocytosis twice in one patient. Lancet 2:925, 1971.

288. Blomgren SE, Condemi JJ, Vaughan JH: Procainamide-induced lupus erythematosus: clinical and laboratory observations. Am J Med 52: 338–348, 1972.

289. Anderson RJ, Genton E: Procainamide-induced pericardial effusion. Am Heart J 83:798–800, 1972.

290. Elson J, Strong JM, Lee W, Atkinson AJ: Antiarrhythmic potency of n-acetylprocainamide. Clin Pharmacol Ther 17:134–140, 1975.

291. Roden DM, Reele SB, Higgins SB, Wilkinson GR, Smith RF, Oates JA, Woosley RL: Antiarrhythmic efficacy, pharmacokinetics and safety of n-acetylprocainamide in human subjects: comparison with procainamide. Am J Cardiol 46:463–468, 1980.

292. Winkle RA, Jaillon P, Kates RE, Peters F: Clinical pharmacology and antiarrhythmic efficacy of n-acetylprocainamide. Am J Cardiol 47:123–130, 1981.

293. Jaillon P, Rubenson D, Peters F, Mason JW, Winkle RA: Electrophysiologic effects of n-acetylprocainamide in human beings. Am J Cardiol 47:1134–1140, 1981.

294. Jaillon P, Winkle RA: Electrophysiologic comparative study of procainamide and n-acetylprocainamide in anesthetized dogs: concentration–response relationships. Circulation 60:1385–1394, 1979.

295. Ahmad S: Procainamide, NAPA and systemic lupus (Letter to the Editor). Circulation 61:865, 1980.

296. Stec GP, Lertora JJL, Atkinson AJ, Nevin MJ, Kushner W, Jones C, Schmid FR, Askenazi J: Remission of procainamide-induced lupus erythematosus with n-acetylprocainamide therapy. Ann Intern Med 90:799–801, 1979.

297. Winkle RA, Jaillon P: Procainamide, NAPA and systemic lupus. Circulation 61:865–866, 1980.

298. Mokler CM, Van Arman CG: Pharmacology of a new antiarrhythmic agent, γ-diisopropyl-amino-α-phenyl-α-(2-Pyridyl)-butyramide (SC-7031). J Pharmacol Exp Ther 136:114–124, 1962.

299. Kus T, Sasyniuk BI: Electrophysiological actions of disopyramide phosphate on canine ventricular muscle and Purkinje fibers. Circ Res 37:844–854, 1975.

300. Yu PN: Disopyramide phosphate (norpace): a new antiarrhythmic drug. Circulation 59:236–237, 1979.

301. Jennings G, Jones MBS, Besterman EMM, Model DG, Turner PP, Kidner PH: Oral disopyramide in prophylaxis of arrhythmias following myocardial infarction. Lancet 10:51–54, 1976.

302. Sbarbaro JA, Rawling DA, Fozzard HA: Suppression of ventricular arrhythmias with intravenous disopyramide and lidocaine: efficacy comparison in a randomized trial. Am J Cardiol 44:513–520, 1979.

303. Vismara LA, Mason DT, Amsterdam EA: Disopyramide phosphate: clinical efficacy of a new oral antiarrhythmic drug. Clin Pharmacol Ther 16:330–335, 1974.

304. Benditt DG, Pritchett ELC, Wallace AG, Gallagher JJ: Recurrent ventricular tachycardia in man: evaluation of disopyramide therapy by intracardiac electrical stimulation. Eur J Cardiol 9/4:255–276, 1971.

305. Deano DA, Wu D, Mautner RK, Sherman RH, Ehsani AE, Rosen KM: The antiarrhythmic efficacy of intravenous therapy with disopyramide phosphate. Chest 71:597–606, 1977.

306. Vismara LA, Vera Z, Miller RR, Mason DT: Efficacy of disopyramide phosphate in the treatment of refractory ventricular tachycardia. Am J Cardiol 39:1027–1034, 1977.

307. Nicholls DP, Haybyrne T, Barnes PC: Intravenous and oral disopyramide after myocardial infarction. Lancet 2:936–938, 1980.

308. Wilcox, RG, Hampton JR, Rowley JM, Mitchell JRA, Roland JM, Banks DC: Randomized placebo-controlled trial comparing oxprenolol with disopyramide phosphate in immediate treatment of suspected myocardial infarction. Lancet 2:765, 1980.

309. Zainal N, Griffiths JW, Carmichael DJS, Besterman EMM, Kidner PH, Gillham AD, Summers GD: Oral disopyramide for the prevention of arrhythmias in patients with acute myocardial infarction admitted to open wards. Lancet 2:887–889, 1977.

310. Hartel G, Louhija A, Konttinen A: Disopyramide in the prevention of recurrence of atrial fibrillation after electroconversion. Clin Pharmacol Ther 15:551–555, 1974.

311. Niarchos AP: Disopyramide: serum level and arrhythmia conversion. Am Heart J 92:57–64, 1976.

312. Bennett DH: Disopyramide in patients with the Wolff-Parkinson-White syndrome and atrial fibrillation. Chest 74:624–628, 1978.

313. Spurrell RAJ, Thorburn CW, Camm J, Sowton E, Deuchar DC: Effects of disopyramide on electrophysiological properties of specialized conduction system in man and on accessory atrioventricular pathway in Wolff-Parkinson-White syndrome. Br Heart J 37:861–867, 1975.

314. Swiryn S, Bauernfeind RA, Wyndham RC, Dhingra RC, Palileo E, Strasberg B, Rosen KM: Effects of oral disopyramide phosphate on induction of paroxysmal supraventricular tachycardia. Circulation 64:169–175, 1981.

315. Cunningham JL, Shen DD, Shudo I, Azarnoff DL: The effects of urine pH and plasma protein binding on the renal clearance of disopyramide. Clin Pharmacokinet 2:373–383, 1977.

316. Gallagher JJ, Pritchett ELC, Benditt DG, Wallace AG: High dose disopyramide phosphate: an effective treatment for refractory ventricular tachycardia. Circulation 55 (Suppl III):225, 1977.

317. Patterson E, Gibson JK, Lucchesi BR: Electrophysiologic effects of disopyramide phosphate on reentrant ventricular arrhythmia in conscious dogs after myocardial infarction. Am J Cardiol 46:792–799, 1980.

318. Simpson RJ, Foster JR, Benge C, Gettes LS: Safety of multiple bolus loading in intravenous disopyramide. Am Heart J (in press).

319. Dhurandhar RW, Nademanee K, Goldman AM: Ventricular tachycardia-flutter associated with disopyramide therapy: a report of three cases. Heart Lung 7:783–787, 1978.

320. Frieden J: Quinidine effects due to disopyramide. N Engl J Med 298: 975, 1978.

321. Meltzer RS, Robert EW, McMorrow M, Martin RP: Atypical ventricular tachycardia as a manifestation of disopyramide toxicity. Am J Cardiol 42:1049–1053, 1978.

322. Kotter V, Linderer T, Schroder R: Effects of disopyramide on systemic and coronary hemodynamics and myocardial metabolism in patients with coronary artery disease: comparison with lidocaine. Am J Cardiol 46:469–475, 1980.

323. Walsh RA, Horwitz LD: Adverse hemodynamic effects of intravenous disopyramide compared with quinidine in conscious dogs. Circulation 60:1053–1058, 1979.

324. Kinney EL, Field EH, Salmon MP, Zelis R: Cardiac arrhythmias associated with disopyramide. N Engl J Med 302:1146, 1980.

325. Leach AJ, Brown JE, Armstrong PW: Cardiac depression by intravenous disopyramide in patients with left ventricular dysfunction. Am J Med 68:839–844, 1980.

326. Hulting J, Rosenhamer G: Hemodynamic and electrocardiographic effects of disopyramide in patients with ventricular arrhythmia. Acta Med Scand 199:41–51, 1976.

327. Podrid PJ, Schoeneberger A, Lown B: Congestive heart failure caused by oral disopyramide. N Engl J Med 302:614–617, 1980.

328. Reddy CP, Benes J: Efficacy and safety of a new intravenous dosage regimen of disopyramide in treating patients with ventricular arrhythmia. Circulation 64 (Suppl):IV-265, 1981 (abstract).

329. Befeler B, Castellanos A,. Wells DE, Vagueiro MC, Yeh BK: Electrophysiologic effects of the antiarrhythmic agent disopyramide phosphate. Am J Cardiol 35:282–287, 1975.

330. Ross D, Vohra J, Cole P, Hunt D, Sloman G: Electrophysiology of disopyramide in man. Aust NZ J Med 8: 377–383, 1978.

331. Seipel L, Breithardt G: Sinus recovery time after disopyramide phosphate. Am J Cardiol 37:1118. 1976.

332. LaBarre A, Strauss HC, Scheinman MM, Evans GT, Bashore T, Tiedeman JS, Wallace AG: Electrophysiologic effects of disopyramide phosphate on sinus node function in patients with sinus node dysfunction. Circulation 59:226–235, 1979.

333. Desai JM, Scheinman M, Peters RW, O'Young J: Electrophysiological effects of disopyramide in patients with bundle branch block. Circulation 59:215–225, 1979.

334. Robertson CE, Miller HC: Extreme tachycardia complicating the use of disopyramide in atrial flutter. Br Heart J 44:602–603, 1980.

335. Porterfield JG, Antman EM, Lown B: Respiratory difficulty after use of disopyramide. N Engl J Med 303:584, 1980.

336. Goldberg IJ, Brown LK, Rayfield EJ: Disopyramide (Norpace®)-induced hypoglycemia. Am J Med 69:463–466, 1980.

337. Harrison DC, Winkle R, Sami M, Mason J: Encainide: a new and potent antiarrhythmic agent. Am Heart J 100:1046–1054, 1980.

338. Roden DM, Reele SB, Higgins SB, Mayol RF, Gammans RE, Oates JA, Woosley RL: Total suppression of ventricular arrhythmias by encainide. N Engl J Med 302:877–882, 1980.

339. Kesteloot H, Stroobaudt R: Clinical experience of encainide (MJ 9067): a new anti-arrhythmic drug. Eur J Clin Pharmacol 16:323–326, 1979.

340. Mason JW, Peters FA: Antiarrhythmic efficacy of encainide in patients with refractory recurrent ventricular tachycardia. Circulation 63:670–675, 1981.

341. Roden DM, Duff HJ, Wang T, Woosley RL: Contribution of a metabolite to the ECG and antiarrhythmic actions of encainide. Circulation 62 (Suppl III):III–141, 1980 (abstract).

342. Sami M, Mason JW, Peters F, Harrison DC: Electrophysiologic effects of encainide, a new antiarrhythmic drug. Am J Cardiol 44:526–532, 1979.

343. Metcalfe JM, Daly KM, Atkinson L, Monaghan M, Jewitt DE: Dose-related hemodynamic effects of intravenous encainide. Am J Cardiol 47:483, 1981 (abstract).

344. Winkle RA, Mason JW, Griffin JC, Ross D: Malignant ventricular tachyarrhythmias associated with use of encainide. Am Heart J 102: 857–864, 1981.

345. Bren GB, Varghese PJ, Katz RJ, Ross AM: Arrhythmogenicity of encainide: the role of QT interval. Am J Cardiol 47:498, 1981 (abstract).

346. DiBianco R, Gottdiener JS, Fletcher RD, Single S, Katz RJ, Sauerbrunn B: Effects of encainide on left ventricular function: assessment with treadmill exercise and radionuclide ventriculography. Circulation 62 (Suppl III):III–182, 1980.

347. Somani P: Antiarrhythmic effects of flecainide. Clin Pharmacol Ther 27:464–470, 1980.

348. Campbell RWF, Henderson A, Bryson LG, Reid DS, Sheridan DJ, Rawlins MD, Julian DG: Intravenous flecainide – Pharmacokinetics and efficacy. Circulation 64 (Suppl IV): IV–265, 1981 (abstract).

349. Anderson JL, Stewart JR, Perry BA, Van Hamersveld DD, Johnson TA, Conard GJ, Chang SF, Kvam DC, Pitt B: Oral flecainide acetate for the treatment of ventricular arrhythmias. N Engl J Med 305: 473–477, 1981.

350. Morrison H, Haugland JM, Granrud G, Asinger RW, Mikell FL, Krejci J: Flecainide acetate, a new antiarrhythmic agent: dose-ranging and efficacy study. Am J Cardiol 47:482, 1981 (abstract).

351. Van Hamersveld DD, Stewart JR, Johnson TA, Anderson JL: Oral flecainide acetate for long-term treatment of ventricular arrhythmias in man. Circulation 64 (Suppl IV): IV–316, 1981 (abstract).

352. Granrud G, Krejci J, Coyne T, Hodges M: Sustained elimination of ventricular arrhythmias during chronic flecainide dosing. Circulation 64 (Suppl IV):IV–316, 1981 (abstract).

353. Conrad GJ, Carlson GL, Frost JW, Ober RE: Human plasme pharmacokinetics of flecainide acetate (R-818), a new antiarrhythmic, following single oral and intravenous doses. Clin Pharmacol Ther 25:218, 1979 (abstract).

354. Verdouw PD, Deckers JW, Conard GJ: Antiarrhythmic and hemodynamic actions of flecainide acetate (R-818) in the ischemic porcine heart. J Cardiovasc Pharmacol 1:473–486, 1979.

355. Welter AN, Schmid JR, Kvam DC: Cardiovascular profile of R-818, a new antiarrhythmic. Fed Proc 36:1003, 1977 (abstract).

356. Klotz U, Muller-Seydlitz PM, Heimburg P: Lorcainide infusion in the treatment of ventricular premature beats. Eur J Clin Pharmacol 16:1–6, 1979.

357. Sung RJ, Somani P: Discordant antiarrhythmic effects of intravenous lorcainide on ventricular premature beats and ventricular tachycardia. Circulation 64 (Suppl IV): IV–37, 1981 (abstract).

358. Kesteloot H, Stroobandt R: Clinical experience with lorcainide (R 15889), a new antiarrhythmic drug. Arch Intern Pharmacodyn 230:225–234, 1977.

359. Somberg JC, Willens H, Camilleri W, Maguire W, Miura DS: Effect of lorcainide on suppressing ventricular tachycardia induced by programmed stimulation. Circulation 64 (Suppl IV):IV–37, 1981 (abstract).

360. Cocco G, Strozzi C: Initial clinical experience of lorcainide (Rol3–1042), a new antiarrhythmic agent. Eur J Clin Pharmacol 14:105–109, 1978.

361. Meinertz T, Kasper W, Kersting F, Bechtold H, Jahnchen E, Lollgen H, Just H: Comparison of the antiarrhythmic activity of mexiletine and lorcainide on refractory ventricular arrhythmias. Circulation 62 (Suppl III):III–184, 1980 (abstract).

362. Morganroth J, Dreifus LS, Michelson EL, Sawin HW: Efficacy and tolerance of lorcainide. Circulation 62 (Suppl III): III–180, 1980 (abstract).

363. Klotz U, Muller-Seydlitz P, Heimburg P: Pharmacokinetics of lorcainide in man: a new antiarrhythmic agent. Clin Pharmacokinet 3:407–418, 1978.

364. Jahnchen E, Bechtold H, Kasper W, Kersting F, Just H, Heykants J: Lorcainide: I. Saturable presystemic elimination. Clin Pharmacol Ther 26: 187–195, 1979.

365. Klotz U, Muller-Seydlitz P, Heimburg P: Disposition and antiarrhythmic effect of lorcainide. Int J Clin Pharmacol Biopharm 17:152–158, 1979.

366. Meinertz T, Kasper W, Kersting F, Just H, Bechtold H, Jahnchen E: Lorcainide: II. plasma concentration–effect relationship. Clin Pharmaco Ther 26:196–204, 1979.

367. Davis LD, Temte JV: Effects of propranolol on the transmembrane potentials of ventricular muscle and Purkinje fibers of the dog. Circ Res 22:661–677, 1968.

368. Berkowitz WD, Wit AL, Lau LH, Steiner C, Damato AN: The effects of propranolol on cardiac conduction. Circulation 40:855–862, 1969.

369. Gettes LS: Beta adrenergic blocking drugs in the treatment of cardiac arrhythmias. Cardiovasc Clin 2:211–237, 1970.

370. Lucchesi BR, Whitsitt LSm Stickney JL: Antiarrhythmic effects of beta adrenergic blocking agents. Ann NY Acad Sci 139:940–951, 1967.

371. Gorlin R: The hyperkinetic heart syndrome. J Am Med Assoc 182:823–829, 1962.

372. Schamroth L: Immediate effects of intravenous propranolol on various cardiac arrhythmias. Am J Cardiol 18:438–443, 1966.

373. Gibson D, Sowton E: The use of beta-adrenergic receptor blocking drugs in dysrhythmias. Prog Cardiovasc Dis 12:16–39, 1969.

374. Wu D, Denes P, Dhingra E, Khan A, Rosen KM: The effects of propranolol on induction of A-V nodal reentrant paroxysmal tachycardia. Circulation 50:665–677, 1974.

375. Denes P, Cummings JM, Simpson R, Wu D, Amat-Y-Leon F, Dhingra R, Rosen KM: Effects of propranolol on anomalous pathway refractoriness and circus movement tachycardias in patients with preexcitation. Am J Cardiol 41:1061–1067, 1978.

376. Rosen KM, Barwolf C, Ehsani A, Rahimtoola SH: Effects of lidocaine and propranolol on the normal and anomalous pathways in patients with preexcitation. Am J Cardiol 30:801–809, 1972.

377. Walters L, Gettes LS, Noonan JA, Surawicz B: Long-term management of chronic tachycardias of childhood with orally administered propranolol. Am J Cardiol 21:119, 1968 (abstract).

378. Brown RW, Goble AJ: Effect of propranolol on exercise tolerance of patients with atrial fibrillation. Br Med J 2:279–280, 1969.

379. Luria MH, Adelson EI, Miller AJ: Acute and chronic effects of an adrenergic beta-receptor blocking agent (propranolol) in treatment of cardiac arrhythmias. Circulation 34:767–773, 1966.

380. Sloman G, Stannard M: Beta-adrenergic blockade and cardiac arrhythmias. Br Med J 4:508–512, 1967.

381. Stock JPP: Beta adrenergic blocking drugs in the clinical management of cardiac arrhythmias. Am J Cardiol 18:444–449, 1966.

382. Arnsdorf MF: Electrophysiologic properties of antidysrhythmic drugs as a rationa basis for therapy. Med Clin North Am 60:213–232, 1976

383. Wolfson S, Herman MV, Sullivan JM, Gorlin R: Conversion of atrial fibrillation and flutter by propranolol. Br Heart J 29:305–309, 1967.

384. Davis LD, Temte JV, Murphy QR: Epinephrine – cyclopropane effects on Purkinje fibers. Anesthesiology 30:369–377. 1969.

385. Katz RL, Epstein RA: The interaction of anesthetic agents and adrenergic drugs to produce cardiac arrhythmias. Anesthesiology 29:763–784, 1968.

386. Krasnow N, Barbarosh H: Clinical experiences with beta-adrenergic blocking agents. Anesthesiology 29:814–827, 1968.

387. Prichard BNC, Ross EJ: Use of propranolol in conjunction with alpha receptor blocking drugs in pheochromocytoma. Am J Cardiol 18:394–398, 1966.

388. Garza LA, Vick RL, Nora JJ, McNamara DG: Heritable Q-T prolongation without deafness. Circulation 41:39–48, 1970.

389. Olley PM, Fowler RS: The surdo-cardiac syndrome and therapeutic observations. Br Heart J 32:467–471, 1970.

390. Gettes LS, Surawicz B: Long-term prevention of paroxysmal arrhythmias with propranolol therapy. Am J Med Sci 254:257–265, 1967.

391. Nixon JV, Pennington W, Ritter W, Shapiro W: Efficacy of propranolol in the control of exercise-induced or augmented ventricular ectopic activity. Circulation 57:115–122, 1978.

392. Taylor RR, Halliday EJ: Beta-adrenergic blockade in the treatment of exercise-induced paroxysmal ventricular tachycardia. Circulation 32:778–781, 1965.

393. Turner JRB: Propranolol in the treatment of digitalis-induced and digitalis-resistant tachycardias. Am J Cardiol 18:450–457, 1966.

394. Becker DJ, Nonkin PM, Bennett LD, Kimball SG, Sternberg MS, Wasserman F: Effect of isoproterenol in digitalis cardiotoxicity. Am J Cardiol 10:242–247, 1962.

395. Roberts J, Ito R, Reilly J, Cairoli VJ: Influence of reserpine and βTM 10 on digitalis-induced ventricular arrhythmia. Circ Res 13:149–158, 1963.

396. Greene R, Oliver LC: Sensitivity to propranolol after digoxin intoxication. Br Med J 4:413–414, 1968.

397. Kupersmith J, Shiang H, Litwak RS, Herman MV: Electrophysiological and antiarrhythmic effects of propranolol in canine acute myocardial ischemia. Circ Res 38:302–307, 1976.

398. Stephen SA: Propranolol in acute myocardial infarction: a multicentre trial. Lancet 31:1435–1437, 1966.

399. Lemberg L, Castellanos A, Arcebal AG: The use of propranolol in arrhythmias complicating acute myocardial infarction. Am Heart J 80:479–487, 1970.

400. Shand DG: Drug therapy: propranolol. N Engl J Med 293:280–285, 1975.

401. Naggar CZ, Alexander S: Propranolol treatment of VPB's. N Engl J Med 294:903–904, 1976.

402. Winkle RA, Lopes MG, Goodman DJ, Fitzgerald JW, Schroeder JS, Harrison DC: Propranolol for patients with mitral valve prolapse. Am Heart J 93:422–427, 1977.

403. Woosley RL, Kornhauser D, Smith R, Reele S, Higgins SB, Nies AS, Shand DG, Oates JA: Suppression of chronic ventricular arrhythmias with propranolol. Circulation 60:819–827, 1979.

404. Horowitz LN, Josephson ME, Kastor JA: Intracardiac electrophysiologic studies as a method for the optimization of drug therapy in chronic ventricular arrhythmia. Prog Cardiovasc Dis 23:81–98, 1980.

405. Evans GH, Shand DG: Disposition of propranolol: V. Drug accumulation and steady-state concentrations during

chronic oral administration in man. Clin Pharmacol Ther 14:487–493, 1973.

406. Shand DG, Nuckolls EM, Oates JA: Plasma propranolol levels in adults with observations in four children. Clin Pharmacol Ther 11:112–120, 1969.

407. Faulkner SL, Hopkins JT, Boerth RC, Young JL, Jellett LB, Nies AS, Bender HW, Shand DG: Time required for complete recovery from chronic propranolol therapy. N Engl J Med 289:607–609, 1973.

408. Lowenthal DT, Briggs WA, Gibson TP, Nelson H, Cirksena WJ: Pharmacokinetics of propranolol in chronic renal disease. Clin Pharmacol Ther 16:761–769, 1974.

409. Thompson FD, Joekes AM, Foulkes DM: Pharmacodynamics of propranolol in renal failure. Br Med J 2:434–436, 1972.

410. Fitzgerald JD, O'Donnell S, Austin M: Pharmacology of 4-hydroxypropranolol, a metabolite of propranolol. Br J Pharmacol 43:222–235, 1971.

411. Walle T, Gaffney TE: Propranolol metabolism in man and dog: mass spectrometric identification of six new metabolites. J Pharmacol Exp Ther 182:83–92, 1972.

412. Coltart DJ, Shand DG: Plasma propranolol levels in the quantitative assessment of β-adrenergic blockade in man. Br Med J 3:731–734, 1970.

413. David D, Di Segni E, Klein HO, Kaplinsky E: Inefficacy of digitalis in the control of heart rate in patients with chronic atrial fibrillation. Chest 71:592–596, 1977.
nergic blocking agent. Am J Cardiol 44:1378–1382, 1979.

414. Yahalom J, Klein H, Kaplinsky E: Beta-adrenergic blockade as adjunctive oral therapy in patients with chronic atrial fibrillation. Chest 71:592–596, 1977.

415. Gettes LS, Yoshonis KF: Rapidly recurring supraventricular tachycardia: a manifestation of reciprocating tachycardia and an indication for propranolol therapy. Circulation 41:689–700, 1970.

416. Stern S: Conversion of chronic atrial fibrillation to sinus rhythm with combined propranolol and quinidine treatment. Am Heart J 74:170–172, 1967.

417. Stern S: Treatment and prevention of cardiac arrhythmias with propranolol and quinidine. Br Heart J 33:522–525, 1971.

418. Visioli O, Bertaccini G: Combined propranolol and quinidine treatment in cardiac arrhythmias. Am Heart J 75:719, 1968.

419. Hillestad L, Storstein O: Conversion of chronic atrial fibrillation to sinus rhythm with combined propranolol and quinidine treatment. Am Heart J 77:137–139, 1969.

420. Korte DW, Nash CB: Ventricular electrophysiology of quinidine–propranolol combinations in the dog heart. J Pharmacol Exp Ther 197:452–457, 1976.

421. Ikram H, Nixon PGF: Propranolol in myocardial infarction. Lancet 19:1134, 1966.

422. Williams EMV, Bagwell EE, Singh BN: Cardiospecificity of β-receptor blockade: a comparison of the relative potencies on cardiac and peripheral vascular β-adrenoceptors of propranolol, of practolol and its ortho-substituted isomer, and of oxprenolol and its para-substituted isomer. Cardiovasc Res 7:226–240, 1973.

423. McNeill RS, Ingram CG: Effect of propranolol on ventilatory function. Am J Cardiol 18:473–475, 1966.

424. Chidsey CA, Braunwald E, Morrow AG: Catecholamine excretion and cardiac stores of norepinephrine in congestive heart failure. Am J Med 39:442–451, 1965.

425. Vogel JHK, Chidsey CA: Cardiac adrenergic activity in experimental heart failure assessed with beta receptor blockade. Am J Cardiol 24:198–208, 1969.

426. Parmley WW, Braunwald E: Comparative myocardial depressant and anti-arrhythmic properties of d-propranolol, dl-propranolol and quinidine. J Pharmacol Exp Ther 158:11–21, 1967.

427. Port S, Cobb FR, Jones RH: Effects of propranolol on left ventricular function in normal men. Circulation 61:358–366, 1980.

428. Crawford MH, Lindenfeld J, O'Rourke RA: Effects of oral propranolol on left ventricular size and performance during exercise and acute pressure loading. Circulation 61:549–554, 1980.

429. Parker JO, West RO, Di Giorgi S: Hemodynamic effects of propranolol in coronary heart disease. Am J Cardiol 21:11–19, 1968.

430. Wolfson S, Gorlin R: Cardiovascular pharmacology of propranolol in man. Circulation 40:501–511, 1969.

431. Conolly ME, Kersting F, Dollery CT: The clinical pharmacology of beta-adrenoceptor-blocking drugs. Prog Cardiovasc Dis 19:203–234, 1976.

432. Buiumsohn A, Eisenberg ES, Jacob H, Rosen N, Bock J, Frishman WH: Seizures and intraventricular conduction defect in propranolol poisoning: a report of two cases. Ann Intern Med 91:860–862, 1979.

433. Kotler MN, Berman L, Rubenstein AH: Hypoglycaemia precipitated by pronanolol. Lancet 24:1389–1390, 1966.

434. Kurland ML: Organic brain syndrome with propranolol. N Engl J Med 300:366, 1979.

435. Frohlich ED, Tarazi RC, Dustan HP: Peripheral arterial insufficiency: a complication of beta-adrenergic blocking therapy. J Am Med Assoc 208:2471–2472, 1969.

436. Sandler G, Clayton GA, Thornicroft SG: Clinical evaluation of verapamil in angina pectoris. Br Med J 3:224–227, 1968.

437. Antman EM, Stone PH, Muller JE, Braunwald E: Calcium channel blocking agents in the treatment of cardiovascular disorders. Part I: basic and clinical electrophysiologic effects. Ann Intern Med 93:875–885, 1980.

438. Chen CM, Gettes LS: Effects of verapamil on rapid Na channel-dependent action potentials of K^+-depolarized ventricular fibers. J Pharmacol Exp Ther 290:415–421, 1979.

439. Gettes LS, Saito T: Effect of antiarrhythmic drugs on the slow inward current system. In: Zipes DP, Bailey JC, Elharrar V (eds) The Slow Inward Current and Cardiac Arrhythmias. Martinus Nijhoff, The Hague, 1980, pp 455–477.

440. Nayler WG, Szeto J, Berry D: Effect of verapamil on contractility, oxygen utilization, and calcium exchangeability in mammalian heart muscle. Cardiovasc Res 6:120–128, 1972.

441. Rosen MR, Wit AL, Hoffman BF: Electrophysiology and pharmacology of cardiac arrhythmias. VI. Cardiac effects of verapamil. Am Heart J 89:665–673, 1975.

442. Saito S, Chen CM, Buchanan J, Gettes LS, Lynch MR:

293

Steady state and time-dependent slowing of conduction in canine hearts – Effects of potassium and lidocaine. Circ Res 42:246–254, 1978.

443. Henry PD: Comparative pharmacology of calcium antagonists: nifedipine, verapamil and diltiazem. Am J Cardiol 46:1047–1058, 1980.

444. Husaini MH, Kvasnicka J, Ryden L, Holmberg S: Action of verapamil on sinus node, atrioventricular, and intraventricular conduction. Br Heart J 35:734–737, 1973.

445. Haeusler G: Differential effect of verapamil on excitation-contraction coupling in smooth muscle and on excitation-secretion coupling in adrenergic nerve terminals. J Pharmacol Exp Ther 180:672–682, 1972.

446. Smith HJ, Goldstein RA, Griffith JM, Kent KM, Epstein SE: Regional contractility: selective depression of ischemic myocardium by verapamil. Circulation 45:629–635, 1976.

447. Ferlinz J, Easthope JL, Aronow WS: Effects of verapamil on myocardial performance in coronary disease. Circulation 59:313–319, 1979.

448. Chew CYC, Hecht HS, Collett JT, McAllister RG, Singh BN: Influence of severity of ventricular dysfunction on hemodynamic responses to intravenously administered verapamil in ischemic heart disease. Am J Cardiol 47:917–922, 1981.

449. Singh SN, Roche AHG: Effects of intravenous verapamil on hemodynamics in patients with heart disease. Am Heart J 94:593–599, 1977.

450. Schamroth L, Krikler DM, Garrett C: Immediate effects of intravenous verapamil in cardiac arrhythmias. Br Med J 1:660–662, 1972.

451. Klein HO, Pauzner H, Segni ED, David D, Kaplinsky E: The beneficial effects of verapamil in chronic atrial fibrillation. Arch Intern Med 139:747–749, 1979.

452. Dominic J, McAllister RG Jr, Kuo CS, Reddy CP, Surawicz B: Verapamil plasma levels and ventricular rate response in patients with atrial fibrillation and flutter. Clin Pharmacol Ther 26:710–714, 1979.

453. Heng MK, Singh BN, Roche AHG, Norris RM, Mercer CJ: Effects of intravenous verapamil on cardiac arrhythmias and on the electrocardiogram. Am Heart J 90:487–498, 1975.

454. Stone PH, Antman EM, Muller JE, Braunwald E: Calcium channel blocking agents in the treatment of cardiovascular disorders. Part II. Hemodynamic effects and clinical applications. Ann Intern Med 93:836–904, 1980.

455. Lazzara R, Scherlag B: Treatment of arrhythmias by blocking slow current. Ann Intern Med 93:919–921, 1980.

456. Sung RJ, Elser B, McAllister RG Jr: Intravenous verapamil for termination of re-entrant supraventricular tachycardias: intracardiac studies correlated with plasma verapamil concentrations. Ann Intern Med 93:682–689, 1980.

457. Singh BN, Ellrodt G, Peter CT: Verapamil: a review of its pharmacological properties and therapeutic use. Drugs 15:169–197, 1978.

458. Spurrell RAJ, Krikler DM, Sowton E: Concealed bypasses of the atrioventricular node in patients with paroxysmal supraventricular tachycardia revealed by intracardiac electrical stimulation and verapamil. Am J Cardiol 33:590–595, 1974.

459. Wellens HJJ, Tan SL, Bar FWH, Curen DR, Lie KI, Dohmen HM: Effect of verapamil studied by programmed electrical stimulation of the heart in patients with paroxysmal re-entrant supraventricular tachycardia. Br Heart J 39:1058–1066, 1977.

460. Porter, CJ, Gillette PC, Garson A, Hesslein PS, Karpawich PP, McNamara DG: Effects of verapamil on supraventricular tachycardia in children. Am J Cardiol 48:487–491, 1981.

461. Soler-Soler J, Sagrista-Sauleda J, Cabrera A, Sauleda-Pares J, Iglesias-Berengue J, Permanyer-Miralda G, Roca-Llop J: Effect of verapamil in infants with paroxysmal supraventricular tachycardia. Circulation 59: 876–879, 1979.

462. Matsuyama E, Konishi T, Okazaki H, Matsuda H, Kawai C: Effects of verapamil on accessory pathway properties and induction of circus movement tachycardia in patients with the Wolff-Parkinson-White syndrome. J Cardiovasc Pharmacol 3:11–24, 1981.

463. Spurrell RAJ, Krikler DM, Sowton E: Effects of verapamil on electrophysiological properties of anomalous atrioventricular connexion in Wolff-Parkinson-White syndrome. Br Heart J 36:256–264, 1974.

464. Sellers TD, Bashore TM, Gallagher JJ: Digitalis in the pre-excitation syndrome: analysis during atrial fibrillation. Circulation 56:260–267, 1977.

465. Opie LH: Drugs and the heart. III. Calcium antagonists. Lancet 1:806–809, 1980.

466. Schomerus M, Spiegelhalder B, Stieren B, Eichelbaum M: Physiological disposition of verapamil in man. Cardiovasc Res 10:605–612, 1976.

467. Eichelbaum M, Ende M, Remberg G, Schomerus M, Dengler HJ: The metabolism of DL-[^{14}C]verapamil in man. Drug Metab Dispos 7:145–148, 1979.

468. McAllister RG, Howell SM: Fluorometric assay of verapamil in biological fluids and tissues. J Pharm Sci 65:431–432, 1976.

469. Mangiardi LM, Hariman RJ, McAllister RG Jr, Bhargava V, Surawicz B, Shabetai R: Electrophysiologic and hemodynamic effects of verapamil. Circulation 57:366–372, 1978.

470. Woodcock BG, Hopf R, Kaltenbach M: Verapamil and norverapamil plasma concentrations during long-term therapy in patients with hypertrophic obstructive cardiomyopathy. J Cardiovasc Pharmacol 2:17–23, 1980.

471. Eichelbaum M, Birkel P, Grube E, Gutgemann U, Somogyi A: Effects of verapamil on P–R intervals in relation to verapamil plasma levels following single I.V. and oral administration and during chronic treatment. Klin Wochenschr 58:919–925, 1980.

472. Koike Y, Shimamura K, Shudo I, Saito H: Pharmacokinetics of verapamil in man. Res Commun Chem Pathol Pharmacol 24:37–47, 1979.

473. Klein HO, Lang R, Segni ED, Kaplinsky E: Verapamil-digoxin interaction. N Engl J Med 303:160, 1980.

474. Leon MB, Rosing DR, Bonow RO, Lipson LC, Epstein SE: Clinical efficacy of verapamil alone and combined with propranolol in treating patients with chronic stable angina pectoris. Am J Cardiol 48:131–139, 1981.

475. Urthaler F, James TN: Experimental studies on the pathogenesis of asystole after verapamil in the dog. Am J Cardiol

44:651–656, 1979.

476. Abinader EG, Berger A: Verapamil and PSVT. Circulation 60:1198–1199, 1979.

477. Benaim ME: Asystole after verapamil. Br Med J 2: 169–170, 1972.

478. Hagemeijer F: Verapamil in the management of supraventricular tachyarrhythmias occurring after a recent myocardial infarction. Circulation 57:751–755, 1978.

479. Grendahl H, Miller M, Sivertssen E: Registration of sinus node recovery time in patients with sinus rhythm and in patients with dysrhythmias. Acta Med Scand 197: 403–408, 1975.

480. Hariman RJ, Mangiardi LM, McAllister RG Jr, Surawicz B, Shabetai R, Kishida H: Reversal of the cardiovascular effects of verapamil by calcium and sodium: differences between electrophysiologic and hemodynamic responses. Circulation 59:797–804, 1979.

481. Gluskin LE, Strasberg B, Shah JH: Verapamil-induced hyperprolactinemia and galactorrhea. Ann Intern Med 95:66–67, 1981.

482. Danilo P: Aprindine. Am Heart J 97:119–124, 1979.

483. Zipes DP, Elharrar V, Gilmour RF, Heger JJ, Prystowsky EN: Studies with aprindine. Am Heart J 100:1055–1062, 1980.

484. Kesteloot H, Van Mieghem W, De Geest H: Aprindine (AC 1802), a new anti-arrhythmic drug. Acta Cardiol 28:145–165, 1974.

485. Fasola AF, Carmichael R: The pharmacology and clinical evaluation of aprindine, a new antiarrhythmic agent. Acta Cardiol Suppl 18:317–333, 1974.

486. Van Durme JP, Rousseau M, Mbuyamba P: Treatment of chronic ventricular dysrhythmias with a new drug: aprindine (AC 1802). Acta Cardiol Suppl 18:335–340, 1974.

487. Breithardt G, Gleichmann U, Seipel L, Loogen F: Long-term oral antiarrhythmic therapy with aprindine (AC 1802). Acta Cardiol Suppl 18:341–353, 1974.

488. Besse P, Giraudel JL, Grosgogeat Y, Haiat R, Puech P, Saulnier JP: Traitement des troubles du rhythme par l'aprindine. Acta Cardiol Suppl 18:389–407, 1974.

489. Hagemeijer F, Janse C, Hugenholtz PG: Efficacité antiarythmique de l'aprindine à la phase aiguë de l'infarctus du myocarde. Acta Cardiol Suppl 18:409–421, 1974.

490. Fasola AF, Noble RJ, Zipes DP: Treatment of recurrent ventricular tachycardia and fibrillation with aprindine. Am J Cardiol 39:903–909, 1977.

491. Strasberg B, Palileo E, Prechel D, Bauernfeind R, Swiryn S, Wyndham CR, Dhingra R, Kehoe R, Rosen KM: Ventricular tachycardia: prediction of response to oral aprindine with intravenous aprindine. Am J Cardiol 47: 676–682, 1981.

492. Wei JY, Bulkley BH, Schaeffer AH, Greene HL, Reid PR: Mitral valve prolapse syndrome and recurrent ventricular tachyarrhythmias. Ann Intern Med 89:6–9, 1978.

493. Troup PJ, Zipes DP: Aprindine treatment of recurrent ventricular tachycardia in patients with mitral valve prolapse. Am Heart J 97:322–328, 1981.

494. Bollen G, Enderle J: Preliminary experience in the treatment of cardiac arrhythmias with aprindine. Acta Cardiol Suppl 18:355–360, 1974.

495. Palma-Gamiz JL, Boedo C, Lopez-Pujol FJ, de Uria JS: Etude clinique d'un nouvel anti-arhythmique: aprindine. Acta Cardiol Suppl 18:361–368, 1974.

496. Zipes DP, Gaum WE, Foster PR, Rosen KM, Wu D, Amat-Y-Leon F, Noble RJ: Aprindine for treatment of supraventricular tachycardia with particular application to Wolff-Parkinson-White syndrome. Am J Cardiol 40:586–596, 1977.

497. Murphy PJ: Metabolic pathways of aprindine. Acta Cardiol Suppl 18:131–142, 1974.

498. Fasola AF, Carmichael R: The pharmacology and clinical evaluation of aprindine, a new antiarrhythmic agent. Acta Cardiol Suppl 18: 317–335, 1974.

499. Delcroix C, Martin L, Van Durme JP, Kesteloot H, Hagemeijer F, Mbuyamba P, Deblecker M: Model for exchange kinetics of aprindine in man after single and multiple doses. Acta Cardiol Suppl 18:177–194, 1974.

500. Rosenberg P, Fisher J, Furman S, Scheuer J: Unexpected disopyramide toxicity. Circulation 60 (Suppl II):II-183, 1979 (abstract).

501. Brandes J-W, Schmitz-Moormann PS, Lehmann F-G, Martini GA: Gelbsucht nach aprindin: eine hepatitisähnliche Arzneimittelschädigung. Dtsch Med Wochenschr 101:111–113, 1976.

502. Elewaut A, Van Durme JP, Goethals L, Kauffman JM, Mussche M, Elinck W, Roels H, Bogaert M, Barbier F: Aprindine-induced liver injury. Acta Gastroenterol Belg 40:236–243, 1977.

503. Herlong HF, Reid PR, Boitnott JK, Maddrey WC: Aprindine hepatitis. Ann Intern Med 89:359–361, 1978.

504. van Leeuwen R, Meyboom RHB: Agranulocytosis and aprindine (letter). Lancet 2:1137, 1976.

505. van Leeuwen R: Agranulocytose tijdens het gebruik van aprindine. Ned Tijdschr Geneeskd 120:1549–1550, 1976.

506. Baedeker W, Rastetter J: Agranulozytose nach Aprindin-behandlung. Münch Med Wochenschr 119:1047–1048, 1977.

507. Brutsaert PL: Effects of aprindine on myocardial contractility. Acta Cardiol Suppl 18:91–99, 1974.

508. Gerin M, Gerin Y, Duvernay G, Georges A: Effects of aprindine (AC1802) on cardiac function in conscious dogs. Acta Cardiol Suppl 18:143–162,, 1974.

509. Mertens HM, Neuhaus KL: Investigation on the cardiovascular effects of aprindine. Acta Cardiol Suppl 18: 163–169, 1974.

510. Remme WJ, Verdouw PD: Cardiovascular effects of aprindine, a new antiarrhythmic drug. Eur J Cardiol 3:307–313, 1975.

511. Piessens J, Willems J, Kesteloot H, de Geest H: Effects of aprindine on left ventricular contractility in man. Acta Cardiol Suppl 18:203–216, 1974.

512. Vastesaeger M, Gillot P, Rasson G: Etude clinique d'une nouvelle médication anti-angoreuse. Acta Cardiol 22: 483–500, 1967.

513. Marcus FI, Fontaine GH, Frank R, Grosgogeat Y: Clinical pharmacology and therapeutic applications of the antiarrhythmic agent, amiodarone. Am Heart J 101:480–493, 1981.

514. Dreifus LS, Ogawa S: Quality of the ideal antiarrhythmic drug. Am J Cardiol 39:466–468, 1977.

515. Rosenbaum MB, Chiale PA, Halpern MS, Nau GJ, Przy-

bylski J, Levi RJ, Lazzari JR, Elizari MV: Clinical efficacy of amiodarone as an antiarrhythmic agent. Am J Cardiol 38:934–944, 1976.

516. Rowland E, Krikler DM: Electrophysiological assessment of amiodarone in treatment of resistant supraventricular arrhythmias. Br Heart J 44:82–90, 1980.

517. Ward DE, Camm AJ, Spurrell RAJ: Clinical antiarrhythmic effects of amiodarone in patients with resistant paroxysmal tachycardias. Br Heart J 44:91–95, 1980.

518. Wheeler PJ, Puritz R, Ingram DV, Chamberlain DA: Amiodarone in the treatment of refractory supraventricular and ventricular arrhythmias. Postgrad Med J 55:1–9, 1979.

519. Podrid PJ, Lown B: Amiodarone therapy in symptomatic sustained refractory atrial and ventricular tachyarrhythmias. Am Heart J 101:374–379, 1981.

520. Leak D, Eydt JN: Control of refractory arrhythmias with amiodarone. Arch Intern Med 139:425–428, 1979.

521. Troup PJ, Zipes DP: Amiodarone in patients with drug resistant ventricular tachyarrhythmias. Clin Res 26:655A, 1978 (abstract).

522. Groh, WC, Kastor JA, Josephson ME, Horowitz LN: Amiodarone: an effective drug for refractory ventricular tachycardia. Circulation 62 (Suppl III):III–152, 1980 (abstract).

523. Heger JJ, Prystowsky EN, Rinkenberger RL, Jackman WM, Naccarelli G, Zipes DP: Amiodarone – clinical efficacy and electrophysiology during long-term therapy for recurrent ventricular tachycardia or ventricular fibrillation. N Engl J Med 305:539–545, 1981.

524. Nademanee K, Hendrickson JA, Cannom DS, Goldreyer BN, Singh BN: Control of refractory life-threatening ventricular tachyarrhythmias by amiodarone. Am Heart J 101:759–768, 1981.

525. Edwards AC, Shenasa M, Curry PVL, Sowton E: Amiodarone in management of chronic refractory ventricular tachycardia. Br Heart J 42:236, 1979 (abstract).

526. Nademanee K, Cannom D, Hendrickson J, Goldreyer B, Singh B: Recurrent sudden arrhythmic cardiac deaths prevented by amiodarone: efficacy predictable by the initial suppression of ventricular tachyarrhythmias. Circulation 64 (Suppl IV):IV–36, 1981 (abstract).

527. Peter T, Hamer A, Weiss D, Mandel W: Sudden death survivors: experience with long-term empiric therapy with amiderone. Circulation 64 (Suppl IV):IV–36, 1981 (abstract).

528. Morady F, Scheinman M, Hess D: Amiodarone in the management of patients with malignant ventricular arrhythmias. Circulation 64 (Suppl IV):IV–36, 1981 (abstract).

529. Kaski JC, Girotti LA, Messutti H, Rutitzky B, Rosenbaum MB: Long-term management of sustained, recurrent, symptomatic ventricular tachycardia with amiodarone. Circulation 64:273–279, 1981.

530. Rowland E, McKenna W, Holt D, Harris L, Krikler D: Control of the ventricular response with oral amiodarone in patients with rapidly conducted atrial fibrillation complicating the Wolff-Parkinson-White syndrome. Circulation 64 (Suppl IV):IV–317, 1981 (abstract).

531. Benaim R, Denizeau J-P, Melon J, Domengie B, Kolsky H, Chapelle M, Chiche P: Les effets antiarhythmiques de l'amiodarone injectable: à propos de 100 cas. Arch Mal Coeur 69:513–522, 1976.

532. Benaim R, Uzan C: Les effets antiarhythmiques de l'amiodarone injectable: à propos de 153 cas. Rev Med 19:1959, 1978.

533. Waleffe A, Bruninx P, Kulbertus HE: Effects of amiodarone studied by programmed electrical stimulation of the heart in patients with paroxysmal re-entrant supraventricular tachycardia. J Electrocardiol 11:253–260, 1978.

534. Rotmensch HH, Belhassen B, Ferguson RK: Amiodarone-benefits and risks in perspective. Am Heart J 104:1117–1119, 1982.

535. Gomes J, Kang P, Behl A, Lyons J, El-Sherif N: Intravenous amiodarone: a potent and effective drug for atrioventricular nodal reentrant paroxysmal tachycardia. Circulation 64 (Suppl IV):IV–317, 1981 (abstract).

536. Pritchard DA, Singh BN, Hurley PJ: Effects of amiodarone on thyroid function in patients with ischaemic heart disease. Br Heart J 37:856–860, 1975.

537. Haffajee C, Lesko L, Canada A, Alpert JS: Clinical pharmacokinetics of amiodarone. Circulation 64 (Suppl IV): IV–263, 1981 (abstract).

538. Kannan R, Nademanee K, Hendrickson JA, Rostami HJ, Singh BN: Amiodarone kinetics after oral doses. Clin Pharmacol Ther 31:438–444, 1982.

539. Harris L, McKenna WJ, Rowland E, Storey GCA, Kvikier DM, Holt DW: Plasma amiodarone and desethyl amiodarone levels in chronic oral therapy. Circulation 64 (Suppl IV): IV–263, 1981 (abstract).

540. Harris L, McKenna WJ, Rowland E, Holt DW, Storey GCA, Krikler DM: Side effects of long-term amiodarone therapy. Circulation 67:45–51, 1983.

541. Saal AK, Werner JA, Gross BW, Gorham JR, Graham EL, Sears GK, Greene HL: Interaction of amiodarone with quinidine and procainamide. Circulation (Suppl II):II–224, 1982 (abstract).

542. Rakita L, Sobol SM: Amiodarone treatment for refractory arrhythmias: dose-ranging and importance of high initial dosage. Circulation 64 (Suppl IV):IV–263, 1981.

543. Cote P, Bourassa MG, Delaye J, Janin A, Froment R, David P: Effects of amiodarone on cardiac and coronary hemodynamimics and on myocardial metabolism in patients with coronary artery disease. Circulation 59:1165–1172, 1979.

544. Sicart M, Besse P, Choussat A, Bricaud H: Action hémodynamique de l'amiodarone intra-veineuse chez l'homme. Arch Mal Coeur 70:219–227, 1977.

545. Nademanee K, Melmed S, Hendrickson J, Reed AW, Hershman JM, Singh BN: Role of serum T4 and reversed T3 in monitoring antiarrhythmic efficacy and toxicity of amiodarone in resistant arrhythmias. Am J Cardiol 47:482, 1981 (abstract).

546. Marchlinski FE, Gansler TS, Waxman HL, Josephson ME: Amiodarone pulmonary toxicity. Ann Intern Med 97:839–845, 1982.

547. Bacaner MB: Bretylium tosylate for suppression of induced ventricular fibrillation. Am J Cardiol 17:528–534, 1966.

548. Bacaner MB: Treatment of ventricular fibrillation and oth-

er acute arrhythmias with bretylium tosylate. Am J Cardiol 21:530–543, 1968.

549. Boura ALA, Green AF: The actions of bretylium: adrenergic neurone blocking and other effects. Br J Pharmacol 14:536–548, 1959.

550. Wit AL, Steiner C, Damato AN: Electrophysiologic effects of bretylium on single fibers of the canine specialized conducting system and ventricle. J Pharmacol Exp Ther 173:344–356, 1970.

551. Bigger JT Jr, Jaffe CC: The effect of bretylium tosylate on the electrophysiologic properties of ventricular muscle and Purkinje fibers. Am J Cardiol 27:82–92, 1971.

552. Cardinal R, Sasynink BI: Electrophysiologic effects of bretylium tosylate on subendocardial Purkinje fibers from infarcted canine hearts. J Pharmacol Exp Ther 204:159–174, 1978.

553. Patterson E, Gibson JK, Lucchesi BR: Prevention of chronic canine ventricular tachyarrhythmias with bretylium tosylate. Circulation 64:1045–1050, 1981.

554. Allen JD, Zaidi SA, Shanks RG, Pentridge JF: The effects of bretylium on experimental cardiac dysrhythmias. Am J Cardiol 29:641–649, 1972.

555. Aravindakshan V, Gettes LS: effects of bretylium and lidocaine on ventricular fibrillation in the isolated rabbit heart. Cardiovasc Res 9:19–28, 1975.

556. Chatterjee K, Mandel WJ, Vyden JK, Parmley WW, Forrester JS: Cardiovascular effects of bretylium tosylate in acute myocardial infarction. J Am Med Assoc 223:757–760, 1973.

557. Taylor SH, Donald KW: The circulatory effects of bretylium in man. Br Heart J 22:588–590, 1960.

558. Bernstein JG, Koch-Weser J: Effectiveness of bretylium tosylate against refractory ventricular arrhythmias. Circulation 45:1024–1034, 1972.

559. Cohen HC, Gozo EG, Langendorf R, Kaplan BM, Chan A, Pick A, Glick G: Response of resistant ventricular tachycardia to bretylium: relation to site of ectopic focus and location of myocardial disease. Circulation 47:331–340, 1973.

560. Djiramdjar RW, Teasdale SJ, Mahon WA: Bretylium tosylate in the management of refractory ventricular fibrillation. Can Med Assoc J 105:161–166, 1971.

561. Day HW, Bacaner M: Use of bretylium tosylate in the management of acute myocardial infarction. Am J Cardiol 27:177–189, 1971.

562. Sanna G, Arcidiacono R: Chemical ventricular defibrillation of the human heart with bretylium tosylate. Am J Cardiol 32:982–987, 1973.

563. Haynes RE, Chinn TL, Copass MK, Cobb LA: Comparison of bretylium tosylate and lidocaine in management of out of hospital ventricular fibrillation: a randomized clinical trial. Am J Cardiol 48:353–360, 1981.

564. Koch-Weser J: Drug therapy: bretylium. N Engl J Med 300:473–477, 1979.

565. Romhilt DW, Bloomfield SS, Lipicky RJ, Welch RM, Fowler O: Evaluation of bretylium tosylate for the treatment of premature ventricular contractions. Circulation 45:800–807, 1972.

566. Anderson JT, Patterson, Wagner JG, Stewart JR, Belm HL, Lucchesi BR: Oral and intravenous bretylium disposi-

tion. Clin Pharmacol Ther 28:468–476, 1980.

567. Bacaner MB: Quantitative comparison of bretylium with other antifibrillatory drugs. Am J Cardiol 21:504–512, 1968.

568. The Coronary Drug Project Research Group: Prognostic importance of premature beats following myocardial infarction: experience in the Coronary Drug Project. J Am Med Assoc 223:1116–1124, 1973.

569. Kotler MN, Tabatznik B, Mower MM, Tominaga S: Prognostic significance of ventricular ectopic beats with respect to sudden death in the late postinfarction period. Circulation 47:959–966, 1973.

570. Hinkle LE, Carver ST, Argyros DC: The prognostic significance of ventricular premature contractions in healthy people and in people with coronary heart disease. Acta Cardiol (Suppl 18):5–53, 1974.

571. Ruberman W, Weinblatt E, Goldberg JD, Frank CW, Shapiro S: Ventricular premature beats and mortality after myocardial infarction. N Engl J Med 297:750–757, 1977.

572. Moss AJ: Clinical significance of ventricular arrhythmias in patients with and without coronary artery disease. Prog Cardiovasc Dis 23:33–52, 1980.

573. Lown B: Sudden cardiac death: the major challenge confronting contemporary cardiology. Am J Cardiol 43:313–328, 1979.

574. Cobb LA, Werner JA, Trobaugh GB: Sudden cardiac death. I. A decade's experience with out-of-hospital resuscitation. Mod Concepts Cardiovasc Dis 49:31–36, 1980.

575. Cobb LA, Werner JA, Trobaugh GB: Sudden cardiac death. II. Outcome of resuscitation management, and future directions. Mod Concepts Cardiovasc Dis 49:37–42, 1980.

576. Josephson ME, Horowitz LN, Farshidi A: Continuous local electrical activity: a mechanism of recurrent ventricular tachycardia. Circulation 57:659–665, 1978.

577. Simson MB: Use of signals in the terminal QRS complex to identify patients with ventricular tachycardia after myocardial infarction. Circulation 64:235–242, 1981.

578. Greene HL, Reid PR, Schaeffer AH: The repetitive ventricular response in man: a predictor of sudden death. N Engl J Med 299:729–734, 1978.

579. Schaeffer AH, Greene HL, Reid PR: Suppression of the repetitive ventricular response: an index of long-term antiarrhythmic effectiveness of aprindine for ventricular tachycardia in man. Am J Cardiol 42:1007–1012, 1978.

580. Reynolds JL, Whitlock RML: Effects of a beta-adrenergic receptor blocker in myocardial infarction treated for one year from onset. Br Heart J 34:252–259, 1972.

581. Wilhelmsson C, Vedin JA, Wilhelmsen L, Tibblin G, Werko L: Reduction of sudden deaths after myocardial infarction by treatment with alprenolol: preliminary results. Lancet 2:1157–1160, 1974.

582. Andersen MP, Bechsgaard P, Frederiksen J: Effect of alprenolol on mortality among patients with definite or suspected acute myocardial infarction: preliminary results. Lancet 2:865–868, 1979.

583. Multicentre International Study: Improvement in prognosis of myocardial infarction by long-term beta-adrenoreceptor blockade using practolol: a multicentre international study. Br Med J 3:735–740, 1975.

584. Multicentre International Study: Reduction in mortality with long-term beta-adrenoceptor blockade: a multicentre international study. Br Med J 2:49–51, 1977.

585. The Norwegian Multicenter Study Group. Timolol-induced reduction in mortality and reinfarction in patients surviving acute myocardial infarction. N Engl J Med 304:801–807, 1981.

586. Hjalmarson A, Herlitz J, Malek I, Ryden L, Vedin A, Waldenstrom A, Wedel H, Elmfeldt D, Holmberg S, Nyberg G, Swedberg K, Waagstein F, Waldenstrom J, Wilhelmsen L, Wilhelmsson C: Effect on mortality of metoprolol in acute myocardial infarction: a double-blind randomised trial. Lancet 2:823–826, 1981.

587. Baber NS, Wainwright ED, Howitt G: Multicentre postinfarction trial of propranolol in 49 hospitals in the United Kingdom, Italy and Yugoslavia. Br Heart J 44:96–100, 1980.

588. Wilcox RG, Roland JM, Banks DC, Hampton JR, Mitchall JRA: Randomised trial comparing propranolol with atenolol in immediate treatment of suspected myocardial infarction. Br Med J 2:885–888, 1980.

589. β-Blocker Heart Attack Trial Research Group: A randomized trial of propranolol in patients with acute myocardial infarction. I. Mortality results. J Am Med Assoc 247:1707–1714, 1982.

590. Snow PJD, Manc MD: Effect of propranolol in myocardial infarction. Lancet II:551–553, 1965.

591. Balcon R, Jewitt DE, Davies JPH, Oram S: A controlled trial of propranolol in acute myocardial infarction. Lancet II:917–920, 1966.

592. A Multicentre Trial: Propranolol in acute myocardial infarction. Lancet II:1435–1438, 1966.

593. Norris RM, Caughey DE, Scott PJ: Trial of propranolol in acute myocardial infarction. Br Med J 2:398–400, 1968.

594. The Anturane Reinfarction Trial Research Group: Sulfinpyrazone in the prevention of sudden death after myocardial infarction. N Engl J Med 302:250–256, 1980.

CHAPTER 9

Cardiac pacing: role in diagnosis and treatment of disorders of cardiac rhythm and conduction

ALBERT L. WALDO

Introduction

Cardiac pacing is the application of external electrical stimuli to the heart. Because cardiac tissue is excitable, external electrical stimuli delivered to the heart will evoke a propagated response provided the stimulus is of appropriate strength and duration and is delivered during a period when the cardiac tissue is capable of responding. External stimuli can be applied epicardially or endocardially to any of the cardiac chambers or, under special circumstances, to the His bundle or bundle branches via a suitable electrode placed temporarily or permanently. The heart also can be paced from electrodes placed in the correct position in the esophagus, or even from the anterior chest wall [1, 2]. This chapter will deal with the application of cardiac pacing for the diagnosis and treatment of abnormalities of cardiac rhythm and conduction.

Modes and methods of cardiac pacing

Unipolar and bipolar pacing

In the unipolar pacing mode, one electrode is in contact with the tissue of the cardiac chamber one wishes to pace, and serves as the cathode. The other (indifferent) electrode is distant from that chamber, generally on or near the body surface (skin or subcutaneous tissue) and serves as the anode. In the bipolar pacing mode, both electrodes are in contact with the cardiac chamber one wishes to pace. When a catheter electrode is placed endocardially to pace the heart, the distal electrode serves as the cathode.

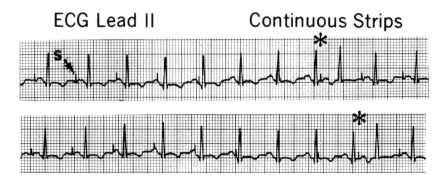

Figure 1. ECG lead II recorded during a spontaneous sinus tachycardia at a rate of about 112 beats/min with a competitive rhythm being caused by asynchronous atrial pacing at a rate of 105 beats/min. The first two beats in the top trace are paced atrial beats. Beginning with the third beat, atrial capture is lost as the faster sinus tachycardia becomes manifest. Note that the stimulus artifact (S) marches through successive P waves and QRS complexes so the pacing stimulus again finds the atria excitable and produces a premature beat (asterisk) which is conducted to the ventricles. There then follows a brief period of atrial capture until, with the third beat of the bottom trace, the faster sinus tachycardia again becomes manifest and the cycle repeats itself (from [3] with permission).

Rosen, M. R. and Hoffman, B. F. (eds.), Cardiac Therapy. ISBN 0-89838-564-4.

Asynchronous pacing

In this type of pacing, the pacing rate is fixed and is totally uninfluenced by any spontaneous beats that may occur. Thus, a pacemaker used in this mode will fire regardless of the spontaneous heart rate or rhythm. As a result, competitive rhythms may occur (Figure 1). During such rhythms, the pacemaker stimulus may fall during the vulnerable period of a previous spontaneous beat. Thus, asynchronous atrial pacing may precipitate atrial fibrillation but, more importantly, asynchronous ventricular pacing may precipitate a life-threatening ventricular arrhythmia such as ventricular fibrillation. In addition, during competitive rhythms caused by asynchronous pacing, the external stimuli in effect produce premature beats which may precipitate rhythms such as ventricular tachycardia or paroxysmal atrial tachycardia in patients with a predisposition to these arrhythmias. Therefore, except for attempts to interrupt or precipitate ventricular arrhythmias, the asynchronous pacing mode is used primarily for temporary atrial pacing and rarely is used for ventricular pacing, even in the presence of complete A-V block.

Demand pacing

In this type of pacing, the pacing rate is fixed, but the pacemaker will fire only when a spontaneous beat fails to occur during a preset interval. Spontaneous beats are identified by the pacemaker by using the pacing electrodes to sense the cardiac signal (electrogram). Thus, when a spontaneous beat occurs, it will be sensed by the pacemaker which will automatically reset its pacing cycle. Therefore, when sensing properly, demand mode pacing should not produce competitive rhythms. More importantly, it should eliminate the possibility of inadvertent precipitation of serious arrhythmias such as ventricular fibrillation. In practice, however, the pacemaker occasionally may fail to sense one or more spontaneous beats for any number of reasons, and thereby, in effect, may become an asynchronous pacemaker with all its attendant problems. Conversely, the pacemaker may be inhibited inappropriately for any number of reasons (e.g., it may sense muscle movement inappropriately, it may sense atrial activation, or it may sense the T wave inappropriately), resulting in failure of the pacemaker to fire at the preset interval, occasionally with disastrous consequences.

Coordinated atrioventricular pacing (A-V sequential pacing)

With this type of pacing, a stimulus is delivered to the ventricles at a preset interval following atrial activation. Atrial activation may be spontaneous, may result from atrial asynchronous pacing, or may result from atrial demand mode pacing. Ventricular activation may result from asynchronous pacing or from demand mode pacing. Clearly, there are many possible combinations. A-V sequential pacing can be used to treat bradyarrhythmias, particularly when the atrial contribution to cardiac output is critical or clinically important. Also, coordinated A-V pacing modes that utilize atrial sensing have the unique and potentially important advantage of permitting the intrinsic sinus or atrial rate to determine the ventricular rate. However, in such instances, the pacemaker must have a built-in capability for rate-related A-V block so that the development of a spontaneous supraventricular tachycardia such as atrial flutter does not result in an excessively rapid ventricular rate resulting from a 1:1 A-V response. In addition, use of these types of pacemakers in the treatment (interruption or suppression or both) of several tachyarrhythmias is developing rapidly.

Underdrive pacing

This type of cardiac pacing consists of applying stimuli to the heart at a rate slower than the spontaneous rate of the cardiac chamber being paced. In effect, it is the introduction of premature beats at random intervals following a spontaneous beat. This technique may be used in an effort to initiate or terminate some nonautomatic cardiac arrhythmias, primarily paroxysmal atrial tachycardia (both the intra A-V nodal reentrant type and the A-V bypass pathway type) and ventricular tachycardia.

Overdrive pacing

This type of cardiac pacing consists of applying stimuli to the heart at a rate faster than the spontaneous rate of the chamber being paced. This technique may be used to initiate or interrupt nonautomatic cardiac arrhythmias (paroxysmal atrial tachycardia, ventricular tachycardia, atrial flutter, ectopic atrial tachycardia), to suppress cardiac arrhythmias, to treat bradyarrhythmias, to test sinus node function, and to assess A-V conduction.

Paired- and coupled-pacing

Paired-pacing is a technique in which the atria or ventricles are paced asynchronously at a fixed rate, and, following each paced beat, a premature stimulus is delivered at a fixed preset interval. Coupled-pacing is a technique in which the basic atrial or ventricular rhythm is spontaneous, and, following each sensed spontaneous beat, a premature stimulus is delivered to the atria (atrial coupled-pacing) or ventricles (ventricular coupled-pacing) at a fixed preset interval.

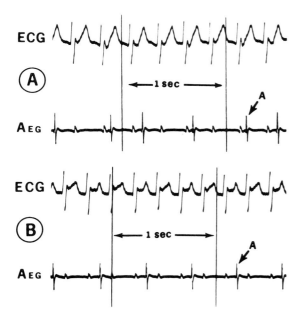

Figure 2. Panels A and B both illustrate an ECG recorded simultaneously with a bipolar atrial electrogram (AEG) from a four-month-old patient in the immediate postoperative period following a Mustard procedure for correction of transposition of the great vessels. Panel A demonstrates an A-V junctional tachycardia at a rate of 220 beats/min with variable retrograde conduction to the atria. Panel B, recorded 19 min following the rhythm shown in Panel A, demonstrates that the A-V junctional tachycardia has increased to 285 beats/min with 2:1 retrograde conduction to the atria now present. This was associated with a mean aortic pressure of 40 mmHg and anuria. This arrhythmia was refractory to standard modes of therapy: A = atrial electrogram (from [5] with permission).

Ventricular paired-pacing may be used to treat refractory A-V junctional tachycardia or ventricular tachycardia either by interrupting the rhythm if it is reentrant or suppressing it if it is automatic [3, 5–7]. When used selectively and with proper indications, ventricular paired-pacing offers highly effective treatment and, in fact, may be life-saving. An example of the effect of ventricular paired-pacing on a patient whose arrhythmia had resulted in hemodynamic decompensation (Figure 2) is shown in Figure 3. A clinical role for atrial paired- or coupled-pacing or ventricular paired-pacing in the treatment of cardiac arrhythmias has not been clearly demonstrated.

Ventricular paired-pacing must be used carefully to avoid precipitation of ventricular fibrillation. However, methods have been outlined which, if followed properly, make precipitation of ventricular fibrillation highly unlikely [3–7]. The following is a summary of these methods: (a) Probably most important, the duration and strength of the delivered stimuli must not be excessive. They are best limited to a stimulus duration of 2 msec or less and a stimulus strength that does not exceed twice the diastolic threshold. (b) The electrode(s) used to deliver the stimuli should be in sustained, firm contact with the myocardium. (c) As with any form of cardiac pacing, care must be taken to prevent the inadvertent delivery of ground loop currents to the heart. This is best accomplished by using a battery-powered pacemaker or connecting the electrodes to an isolation device. (d) The manner of induction of ventricular paired-pacing to control tachyarrhythmia probably is performed best as follows: Using an appropriate stimulator, the S_1–S_2 interval, i.e., the interval from the basic driving stimulus (S_1) to the premature stimulus (S_2), should be set at an interval which is somewhat shorter than the cycle length of the spontaneous ventricular rate, and the S_1–S_1 interval, i.e., the interval of the basic driving stimulus (S_1), should be set at twice the S_1–S_2 interval. This will produce a regular paced rhythm which is just faster than the spontaneous ventricular rate. After the paired-pulse stimulator has been connected to the electrodes and pacing has been initiated, the stimulus strength should be increased gradually until constant ventricular capture is obtained. The S_1–S_2 interval then is shortened gradually until the S_2 produces an electrical response (QRS complex) for which there is no effective mechanical response

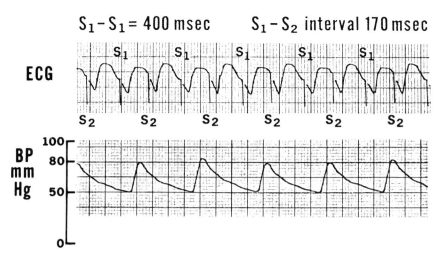

$S_1 - S_1 = 400\text{ msec}$ $S_1 - S_2$ interval 170 msec

ECG

S_1 S_1 S_1 S_1 S_1

S_2 S_2 S_2 S_2 S_2 S_2

BP
mm
Hg

100
80
50

0

Figure 3. These traces are recorded from the same patient as in Figure 2, and demonstrate ventricular paired-pacing initiated to control the rapid ventricular rate in this patient. The top panel demonstrates an ECG recorded during ventricular paired-pacing at an S_1–S_1 interval of 400 msec and an S_1–S_2 of 170 msec. The bottom trace demonstrates the blood pressure recorded from a catheter in the femoral artery. These traces were monitored simultaneously and were recorded sequentially. Note that there is only one pressure pulse in the bottom trace for every two QRS complexes in the top trace. Thus, despite the fact that the ventricles were being paced at a rate of 300 beats/min, because each deliberately induced premature ventricular beat (S_2) failed to eject blood from the ventricles, the effective ventricular rate was 150 beats/min, a rate considerably less than the spontaneous rate. Using this pacing technique, the mean aortic pressure quickly rose to 60–65 mmHg and normal urine output resumed (from [5] with permission).

(Figure 3). The mechanical response is monitored best by recording the arterial pulse pressure directly using standard techniques (Figure 3). (e) An ECG should be monitored continuously during the ventricular paired-pacing, and preferably, simultaneously with an arterial pulse pressure.

The following is an example of the technique of paired-pacing: If the spontaneous rate is 150 beats/min (cycle length 400 msec), the S_1–S_2 interval should be set for a rate which is about 160 beats/min (cycle length 375 msec). The S_1–S_1 interval should be set at a rate of 80 beats/min (cycle length 750 msec). The S_1–S_2 interval then should be shortened until the S_2 impulse produces an electrical event (QRS complex) without an effective mechanical response. Thus, the pacing rate will remain 160 beats/min, but the rate of mechanically effective beats will be only 80/min.

Introduction of premature beats at selected intervals

Following a train of spontaneous or paced beats, a single premature beat may be introduced at selected intervals following the last beat of the train in order to study excitability and refractoriness of cardiac tissues and to assess sinus node function. Introduc-

tion of premature beats following a train of spontaneous or paced beats also may be used to initiate nonautomatic cardiac arrhythmias (ventricular tachycardia, paroxysmal atrial tachycardia, atrial fibrillation, atrial flutter, ectopic atrial tachycardia, ventricular fibrillation), either during electrophysiological evaluation or during studies of the efficacy of antiarrhythmic drug therapy [8, 9]. In these circumstances, premature beats are introduced at selected intervals singly or as doublets or triplets following the last beat of the train. This technique also may be used to interrupt ventricular tachycardia or paroxysmal atrial tachycardia [3, 7]. It is largely ineffective when used to interrupt atrial flutter and totally ineffective as treatment of atrial or ventricular fibrillation [3, 7, 10–13].

Programmed cardiac pacing

This form of pacing combines introduction of premature beats at selected intervals (section above) and overdrive pacing (section above) in an effort to precipitate and/or characterize and/or interrupt tachycardias [8, 9]. It also is used to assess efficacy of treatment modalities of tachycardias, e.g., to assess the efficacy of drug therapy, cardiac surgical therapy, or pacemaker therapy.

302

Programmed cardiac pacing usually is performed during cardiac catheterization, but also may be performed using temporarily placed epicardial wire electrodes. The technique most commonly employs electrode catheters inserted using standard pervenous techniques (percutaneous insertion via a femoral vein, a subclavian vein, an external jugular vein, or insertion via a brachial or antecubital vein cutdown) and placed in selected portions of the heart. The electrode catheters are used for pacing and/or recording from selected sites, the standard sites being the high right atrium, the coronary sinus, the His bundle, and the right ventricle. In addition, depending on the indication, catheters may be placed at other regions of the right atrium and also may be placed in the proximal right pulmonary artery to record from the region of Bachmann's bundle [14-17]. Catheters also may be placed intraarterially via standard techniques (percutaneous insertion via a femoral artery or, rarely, insertion via a brachial artery cutdown) when left ventricular pacing and/or recording is required.

Standard studies include assessment of sinus node function, A-V conduction, and atrial and ventricular refractoriness. However, the procedure is carried out most frequently to identify, characterize, and/or interrupt an underlying tachyarrhythmia and/or to assess efficacy of antiarrhythmic therapy, be it drug, pacemaker, or surgical therapy. Each study usually is tailored to the known or suspected underlying abnormality. Nevertheless, a standard routine would be to introduce premature atrial beats to explore atrial diastole after a train of at least eight spontaneous beats in order to determine atrial refractoriness (both functional and effective refractory periods), and to determine the nature of A-V nodal conduction and refractoriness (both functional and effective refractory periods). Ventricular functional and effective refractory periods also would be determined by introducing ventricular beats to explore ventricular diastole after a train of at least eight spontaneous beats. These procedures then would be repeated following a train of at least eight paced atrial and/or ventricular beats during pacing at one or two rates faster than the spontaneous rate. These pacing rates are usually at least 100-120 beats/min. Depending on the purpose of the study, these pacing procedures may be performed at several sites, e.g., from the high right atrium and coronary sinus, or from the right ventricular outflow tract, right ventricular apex, and left ventricle. When programmed cardiac pacing is performed to precipitate or to characterize a tachyarrhythmia, and/or to assess the efficacy of antiarrhythmic therapy, these pacing procedures usually involve introduction of single, double, or triple premature beats as well as bursts of rapid pacing from selected sites. A more detailed discussion of these and other pacing procedures used in the diagnosis, characterization, and treatment of abnormalities of rhythm and conduction is found elsewhere in this chapter.

Patient safety

Whenever temporary cardiac pacing is initiated, the presence of a physician is required, particularly when the heart is paced at rapid rates or when a deliberate attempt to precipitate a tachyarrhythmia is made. Also, it is recommended that, whenever possible, a battery-powered pacemaker be used, as it avoids the necessity of using an electrical isolation device between the electrodes and the pacemaker. Similarly, all electrode catheters in contact with the heart and used for recording of electrograms should be isolated electrically to prevent inadvertent delivery of current (microshock hazard) to the heart which might cause ventricular fibrillation. At least one body surface ECG lead, preferably lead II or V_1, should be recorded when pacing is initiated. Should continuous cardiac pacing be required on a temporary basis, the rhythm should be monitored constantly and direct ECG print-out capabilities should be readily available. When these techniques are used, and particularly in the case of acutely ill patients, the capability for cardiopulmonary resuscitation, including DC cardioversion, should be available.

Cardiac pacing in the determination of mechanisms responsible for arrhythmias

Automaticity

Cells which are capable of initiating impulses through the process of spontaneous self-excitation are said to be automatic, and this property of self-excitation has been called automaticity [18]. It is important to stress here that the clinical pacing techniques used to identify automatic rhythms are based on observations made about so-called 'normal' automaticity (for a further discussion, see Chapter 1). Normal automaticity is a property thought to be limited to the specialized tissues of the heart. Although the sinus node is the normal pacemaker of the heart, other normal pacemaker sites are located in the atrial internodal pathways, portions of the A-V node and the His-Purkinje system [18, 19]. More recently, cells capable of demonstrating automatic activity have been demonstrated in the anterior leaflet of the mitral valve, the septal leaflet of the tricuspid valve, and the coronary sinus of canine hearts [20–22]; and the anterior mitral valve leaflet of human hearts [23].

Rhythms which are due to normal automaticity can be neither initiated nor terminated by cardiac pacing, but do demonstrate characteristic responses to cardiac pacing, as will be discussed shortly. In Chapter 1 of this volume, mechanisms responsible for abnormal pacemaker function are described. There is an important difference in the response to pacing of normal and abnormal automatic mechanisms in that the latter are less readily overdrive suppressed than the former. Although it is likely that some arrhythmias resulting from abnormal automaticity can be overdrive suppressed clinically, at present, the clinical applicability of the former is far better known and will now be described.

Overdrive suppression and warm up
All normal automatic cardiac pacemakers demonstrate the phenomemon of overdrive suppression [24]. In the presence of normal conduction, the fastest pacemaker (usually the sinus node) will determine the heart rate, and the spread of activation from that pacemaker will depolarize the rest of the cardiac cells, including latent pacemaker cells. This fastest or dominant pacemaker does not merely depolarize subsidiary pacemakers before they can attain threshold and fire, but actually suppresses them. Any normally automatic focus that is depolarized by the spread of activation from a faster pacemaker, whether the latter is a spontaneous pacemaker or an external battery-operated pacemaker, will not immediately recover to its intrinsic rate following abrupt cessation of pacing from the faster pacemaker, but will do so with some delay. This phenomenon has been termed overdrive suppression [24].

In considering the differential diagnosis of a tachyarrhythmia, the use of pacing techniques to induce overdrive suppression may be important in establishing the presence of a rhythm resulting from a normal automatic mechanism (and, possibly, from an abnormal automatic mechanism). For instance, if one paces the heart (either atria or ventricles) at a rate faster than the intrinsic rate of an automatic rhythm, then following abrupt cessation of pacing, one should see a pause longer than the intrinsic cycle length of the automatic rhythm (overdrive suppression) before the spontaneous pacemaker resumes firing. Then, over the next several beats, the pacemaker rate will increase, i.e., warm-up, until the pacemaker returns to its previous spontaneous rate. In some instances, particularly in the presence of sinus tachycardia, the rate may briefly exceed the previous spontaneous rate [24].

These principles of overdrive suppression and warm-up of such automatic fibers have important practical implications. For instance, if the ventricles are being paced because a patient has A-V block, or if the atria are being paced because a patient had sinus bradycardia, and one wishes to determine the underlying spontaneous rhythm, one should not simply turn off the pacemaker because overdrive suppression of the spontaneous pacemaker may result in prolonged asystole with all its attendant hazards. It is worth noting that a spontaneous equivalent to overdrive suppression occurs in patients with the sick sinus syndrome whenever a tachycardia stops abruptly (Figure 4) and is often the cause of syncope associated with the tachycardia-bradycardia syndrome. Therefore, regardless of the cardiac chamber being paced, the

Continuous

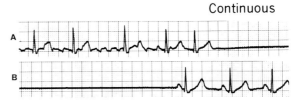

Figure 4. Panels A and B are continuous monitor ECG traces and demonstrate spontaneous termination of atrial fibrillation followed by an asystolic period of just over 5 sec before sinus rhythm becomes manifest. The asystolic period suggests sinus node dysfunction as well as dysfunction of the A-V junctional pacemaker, both of which are common manifestations of the sick sinus syndrome (from [3] with permission).

pacing rate should be slowed gradually and the pacing stopped only when the spontaneous rhythm reappears or when the lowest clinically acceptable rate of the pacemaker (usually 50 beats/min) has been achieved. There are occasions when abrupt termination of cardiac pacing is appropriate or indicated, such as in assessment of sinus node function. However, if one elects to terminate pacing abruptly, one should be prepared to reinitiate the pacing promptly should the overdrive suppression result in prolonged asystole or should the rate of the spontaneous rhythm be inadequate.

Finally, the phenomenon of overdrive suppression of a spontaneous pacemaker must be distinguished from overdrive suppression of a focus that is protected by entrance block. In this instance, the impulses produced in overdrive pacing cannot enter and depolarize or interrupt the rhythm generated by the protected focus. Therefore, with cessation of overdrive pacing the rhythm generated by the protected focus will reappear promptly (unless there is some exit block from the focus) and there should not be any period of warm up.

Reset of the dominant pacemaker

If a premature beat depolarizes the spontaneous pacemaker before the latter reaches threshold and fires, the pacemaker will be reset, i.e., its cycle will resume following repolarization. This characteristic of automatic tissue has been used in the clinical assessment of sinus node function. However, it should be noted that the demonstration of reset of a rhythm by a premature beat does not per se identify the rhythm as being due to automaticity, because reset of reentrant rhythms by premature beats also occurs [25]. For a more complete discussion of reset of a pacemaker, see below the section on the introduction of premature atrial beats and overdrive atrial pacing to evaluate sinoattrial conduction time.

Inability to initiate or terminate with pacing techniques

A characteristic of normal automatic rhythms is that they typically are neither initiated nor terminated with any pacing techniques [8]. However, they can be influenced by pacing techniques, to wit: introduction of premature atrial beats may reset an automatic rhythm, and pacing at rates faster than the automatic rhythm may result temporarily in

overdrive suppression of that rhythm. We must emphasize, however, that the inability to initiate or terminate an arrhythmia with pacing techniques (i.e., introduction of premature beats or overdrive pacing) does not necessarily mean the rhythm in question is automatic. For instance, it is possible that premature beats may not influence or may only reset a reentrant rhythm [25] and that overdrive pacing of a reentrant rhythm may fail to interrupt the arrhythmia (see following discussion of transient entrainment) [6, 7, 26–31].

Reentry

Ability to initiate and terminate with pacing techniques

A characteristic of reentrant rhythms is that usually they can be initiated and/or terminated reproducibly with cardiac pacing techniques [8, 32]. The principle involved in initiation of the arrhythmia is that impulses are introduced in such a way that slow conduction and unidirectional block, the requisites for reentrant rhythms, become operative in a potentially reentrant circuit so that an arrhythmia will occur. This appears to occur because the introduc-

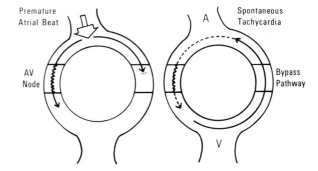

Figure 5. Diagrammatic representation of the onset of an A-V bypass pathway-type paroxysmal atrial tachycardia. In the left diagram, a premature atrial beat (large arrow) is introduced. The wavefront from this beat is blocked in an antegrade direction in the A-V bypass pathway but is conducted slowly (serpentine line) through the A-V node (as expected because it is a premature beat) to the ventricles. In the right diagram, when the wavefront from this beat which is now activating the ventricles reaches the A-V bypass pathway, it is conducted in a retrograde direction to reactivate the atria. The impulse then is conducted again through the A-V node and a reentry or circus movement tachycardia has been precipitated. Thus, unidirectional block in the A-V bypass pathway and slow conduction in the A-V node permit the initiation of a reentry or circus movement tachycardia: A = atria; V = ventricles.

tion of one, two, or three premature impulses or even rapid pacing may result in the wavefront from the pacing impulse being blocked from propagating in one pathway while being conducted slowly in another pathway such that circus movement of excitation occurs (Figure 5).

Although reentrant rhythms can, in most instances, be initiated with cardiac pacing techniques, it should be emphasized that neither spontaneous nor induced premature beats nor rapid pacing always will initiate reentrant rhythms in patients who, in fact, have a predisposition to or known occurrence of these arrhythmias. Thus, the fact that an arrhythmia is not initiated by pacing techniques does not mean per se that the arrhythmia is not reentrant. In the same vein, the fact that an arrhythmia is not interrupted by pacing techniques does not mean it is not reentrant per se. This is because the ability to terminate reentrant rhythms with cardiac pacing requires that the pacing impulse enter the reentrant loop in such a fashion that block of both the antidromic (opposite direction as the wavefront of the spontaneous tachycadia) and orthodromic

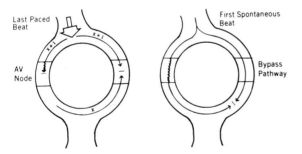

Figure 6. Diagrammatic representation of the same A-V bypass pathway-type paroxysmal atrial tachycardia in Figure 5 interrupted with overdrive pacing from the high right atrium. The large arrow in the left diagram indicates the last pacing impulse from the high right atrium entering into the reentry loop, whereupon it is conducted orthodromically (X + 1) and antidromically (X + 1). Antegrade block of the antidromic wavefront from the pacing impulse (X + 1) and retrograde block of the orthodromic wavefront from the previous beat (X) occur in the A-V bypass pathway, and antegrade block of the orthodromic wavefront (X + 1) of the pacing impulse occurs in the A-V node. Thus, when the pacing is stopped, the reentry or circus movement tachycardia has been interrupted because there is no wavefront still traveling in the reentry loop. The right diagram shows the first spontaneous beat following cessation of pacing. It is a sinus beat in which normal conduction occurs to the ventricles via the A-V node and also via the accessory A-V bypass pathway (the Wolff-Parkinson-White syndrome). The serpentine lines indicate slow conduction.

(same direction as the wavefront of the spontaneous tachycardia) wavefronts of the pacing impulse occur in the reentry loop (Figure 6), and this is not always accomplished. Thus, ostensibly reentrant rhythms such as atrial fibrillation and ventricular fibrillation cannot be interrupted, likely due in part to the presence of multiple and continuously changing reentry loops which characterize these arrhythmias.

However, it also is possible that there may be reentrant rhythms with a single and constant reentry loop, perhaps such as Type II atrial flutter (i.e., the very rapid form of atrial flutter), which cannot be interrupted with pacing techniques. For instance, if the mechanism of a reentrant rhythm is of the leading circle type (i.e., circus movement without an anatomical obstacle as described in Chapter 1) [32] in which the reentry loop consists of the head of excitability chasing the tail of the refractoriness, there is no excitable gap. The wavefront from the pacing impulse may be unable to enter such a reentry loop. In addition, it is possible that a reentrant rhythm with an excitable gap is protected by entrance block into the loop. Such a reentry loop would then be protected from interruption by overdrive pacing. Furthermore, it is possible that the pacing site may be so far from the reentry loop that the combination of conduction time from the pacing site to the reentry loop and refractoriness of the tissue being paced make it impossible for the pacing impulse to enter the reentry loop [8]. Under these conditions, it is impossible for overdrive pacing to interrupt the arrhythmia [28, 32].

Finally, because an arrhythmia can be initiated and/or terminated by pacing techniques does not make the arrhythmia reentrant per se. This is because rhythms that utilize the mechanism of triggered activity also can be initiated and terminated with cardiac pacing [33–37]. Therefore, it would seem that specific identification of reentrant arrhythmias on the basis of cardiac pacing techniques is not yet possible. However, it has recently been suggested that if one can demonstrate transient entrainment (see below) and subsequent interruption of an arrhythmia with overdrive pacing, the arrhythmia can be caused only by a reentrant mechanism [30].

Transient entrainment
Transient entrainment occurs when overdrive pac-

306

ing of a tachycardia results in an increase in the rate of firing of the cardiac chamber being paced to the overdrive pacing rate. On abrupt cessation of pacing or slowing of the pacing rate below the intrinsic rate of the tachycardia, there is resumption of the intrinsic rate of the tachycardia [27, 30]. Transient entrainment was first described when studying overdrive pacing to interrupt atrial flutter [26]. Until that time, it had been thought that atrial flutter could not always be interrupted by overdrive pacing, and that overdrive pacing was therefore a relatively ineffective treatment mode for management of atrial flutter [38]. However, it was demonstrated that atrial flutter always could be interrupted by overdrive atrial pacing provided pacing was performed at a critically rapid rate [26]. Overdrive pacing of atrial flutter at rates short of the critically rapid rate simply entrained the atrial flutter transiently without interrupting it [26, 39]. Other rhythms such as ventricular tachycardia [27, 40], A-V bypass pathway-type paroxysmal atrial tachycardia [30], ectopic atrial tachycardia [31], and A-V

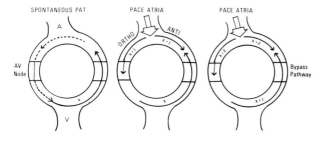

Figure 7. The left diagram is a representation of the reentry loop during spontaneous A-V bypass pathway-type paroxysmal atrial tachycardia. X represents the orthodromic wavefront of the reentrant rhythm. The middle diagram is a representation of the introduction of the first pacing impulse (X + 1) during overdrive pacing from the high right atrium during the paroxysmal atrial tachycardia. The large arrow indicates the pacing impulse entering into the reentry loop, whereupon it is conducted orthodromically (ortho) and antidromically (anti). The antidromic wavefront from the pacing impulse (X + 1) collides with the orthodromic wavefront of the previous spontaneous beat (X). The right diagram is a representation of the introduction of the second pacing impulse (X + 2) during overdrive pacing from the high right atrium during the paroxysmal atrial tachycardia. The large arrow again indicates the pacing impulse entering into the reentry loop, whereupon it is conducted orthodromically and antidromically. This next antidromic wavefront (X + 2) collides with the orthodromic wavefront of the previous paced beat (X + 1). The arrows indicate the direction of spread of the impulse, and the serpentine line indicates slow conduction in the A-V node: A = atria; V = ventricles (from [30] with permission).

nodal reentrant tachycardia also demonstrate transient entrainment.

The importance of transient entrainment and subsequent interruption of tachyarrhythmias, apart from its practical significance (see section below on cardiac pacing in the treatment of tachyarrhythmias) stems from recent studies [28–31] which suggest that their demonstration means that the mechanism of the tachyarrhythmia is reentry. Data from these studies indicate that transient entrainment is explained by early entrance of each wavefront from the pacing impulse into the reentry loop in both the antidromic and orthodromic directions (e.g., see Figure 7). The antidromic wavefront of each pacing impulse repeatedly collides with the orthodromic wavefront of the previous beat, extinguishing the tachycardia, but the orthodromic wavefront of each pacing impulse reinitiates the tachycardia, with resultant increase in the tachycardia rate to the pacing rate. Interruption of the tachycardia occurs when both the antidromic and orthodromic wavefronts of the same pacing impulse are blocked (Figure 6) [30].

Based on these observations, it has been postulated that if one can demonstrate transient entrainment and subsequent interruption of an arrhythmia, the rhythm must be due to reentry [28–31]. However, this hypothesis must be carefully qualified in order to distinguish transient entrainment and subsequent interruption of a reentrant rhythm from either overdrive suppression of a rhythm generated by a protected focus (i.e., a focus protected by entrance block) or from a triggered rhythm. It is our opinion at present that if any of the following criteria are demonstrated during overdrive pacing of a tachyarrhythmia, the underlying mechanism of the arrythmia is reentry: (a) Prior to the interruption of a tachyarrhythmia with overdrive pacing, if one can demonstrate constant fusion beats during a period of transient entrainment of the tachycardia *except* during the last entrained beat or, if during a period of transient entrainment of the tachycardia at two or more different pacing rates, one can demonstrate constant fusion beats at each of the two different pacing rates, but different degrees of fusion (progressive fusion) at the different rates, we believe the mechanism must be reentry; (b) Associated with the interruption of a tachyarrhythmia with overdrive pacing, if one can demonstrate block localized to a site which then is acti-

307

vated by the next pacing impulse coming from a different direction and with a shorter conduction time than before the localized block occurred, then the underlying mechanism of the arrhythmia must be reentry. The basis for these criteria and a further discussion of them are presented in reference 30.

Unfortunately, transient entrainment and interruption of a tachyarrhythmia can occur without the demonstration of any of the above criteria [30]. Therefore, if overdrive pacing of a tachyarrhythmia fails to demonstrate any of the above, it may be impossible to distinguish between a reentrant mechanism, a triggered mechanism, or a protected focus. And, if overdrive pacing is performed without successful interruption of the arrhythmia, and neither of the first two criteria is met, one must add an automatic mechanism to the list of indistinguishable mechanisms.

Triggered activity

As summarized recently [33], rhythms clearly demonstrating triggered activity have been shown only in vitro and in experimental animals. Although it is entirely likely that these arrythmias have a clinical counterpart, none has been identified beyond doubt, let alone studied in vivo with clinical pacing techniques. Therefore, the responses of these rhythms to cardiac pacing only can be extrapolated from the in vitro data. As indicated above, these rhythms can be initiated and terminated either by premature beats introduced at appropriate intervals or by rapid pacing [33–37]. Thus, on this basis alone, these rhythms cannot be distinguished from reentrant rhythms. However, a few differentiating points between the two have been suggested [33, 41, 42]. If an inverse relationship exists between the premature beat which initiates the tachycardia and the first beat of the tachycardia, such as exist in A-V nodal reentrant rhythms (in which there is an inverse relationship between the P–R interval and the subsequent R–P interval), it is quite unlikely that the arrhythmia is due to triggered activity. This is because no such observations have been made in studies of the in vitro model. In addition, if a single premature beat introduced during a tachyarrhythmia results in sustained shortening of the cycle length of the tachycardia, the arrhythmia is likely to be due to triggered activity. Responses to cardiac pacing that can identify this mechanism when pres-

ent clinically and distinguish it from a reentrant or, in fact, any other type of arrhythmia clearly are important, but unfortunately at this time have not been characterized. Nevertheless, recent in vitro studies of overdrive pacing of triggered rhythms have demonstrated some unique responses [37]. The most noteworthy of these is acceleration of the rhythm in response to overdrive pacing.

Cardiac pacing in the treatment of tachyarrhythmias

Introduction

Virtually all the techniques that will be described are temporary pacing techniques. However, it is important to note that these techniques now are being applied using implanted pacemaker systems for chronic treatment of recurrent tachyarrhythmias. Although modalities are available for treating tachyarrhythmias, clinical circumstances in which temporary pacing should be considered include situations in which: (a) rhythms continue to recur with only short intervals between each episode (e.g., ventricular tachycardia or paroxysmal atrial tachycardia); (b) prior antiarrhythmic drug treatment has been ineffective (e.g., classical atrial flutter); (c) DC cardioversion may be hazardous (e.g., because of prior digitalis therapy, or in the face of chronic obstructive pulmonary disease); (d) it is anticipated that prolonged bradycardia or asystole may follow DC cardioversion or interruption of the arrhythmia by drug therapy (e.g., as in the tachycardia-bradycardia syndrome); (e) the previous drug history is unknown; (f) electrodes to pace the heart are readily available (e.g., in patients following open heart surgery in whom temporarily placed epicardial wire electrodes are available or during cardiac catheterization); (g) a Swan-Ganz catheter with atrial or ventricular electrodes is in place; and (h) demonstration of the efficacy of cardiac pacing is necessary prior to placement of a permanent pacemaker system to treat that arrhythmia [7]. In most instances in which temporary pacing is used to treat tachyarrhythmias, it is used in concert with or followed by administration of appropriate antiarrhythmic drugs.

Atrial fibrillation

Atrial fibrillation cannot be treated with presently

available cardiac pacing techniques. However, when atrial fibrillation is associated with a relatively slow ventricular response rate, or when atrial fibrillation is present in the face of complete A-V block and a slow A-V junctional escape rhythm, temporary ventricular pacing at an appropriate rate can be and usually should be initiated. A permanent ventricular pacing system may be indicated subsequently, depending on the etiology of the problem.

Atrial flutter

Classical (Type I) atrial flutter, i.e., a regular atrial rhythm with a range of rates from about 230–340 or 350 beats/min [43, 44], always can be interrupted with rapid atrial pacing [3, 6, 7, 26, 28, 29, 43, 44]. This treatment mode is the therapy of choice in patients following open heart surgery who have

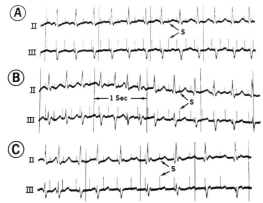

Figure 8. Panels A, B, and C are continuous traces of ECG leads II and III during the period of overdrive pacing of Type I atrial flutter in a patient whose spontaneous atrial rate was 294 beats/ min (cycle length of 204 msec). In this patient, overdrive atrial pacing was initiated at a cycle length of 194 msec, and then the ramp pacing technique (in which the pacing rate is gradually increased until the atrial complexes become positive, and then is decreased) was used. As the pacing cycle length was decreased from 171 to 157 msec (panel A), the atrial complexes became positive in both leads II and III. The atrial pacing cycle length then was increased, i.e., the pacing rate was decreased (panels B and C). Note that as the pacing cycle length became longer than that of the spontaneous atrial flutter (end of panel B), the atrial complexes remained positive. As the atrial pacing cycle length was further increased (panel C), the atrial flutter did not recur. In fact, atrial capture was maintained as the pacing cycle length was increased to 545 msec, a pacing rate of 110 beats/min (not shown). Thus, using the ramp atrial pacing technique, the atrial flutter was initially transiently entrained and finally interrupted by rapid pacing: S = stimulus artifact. Time lines are at 1-sec intervals (modified after [26] with permission).

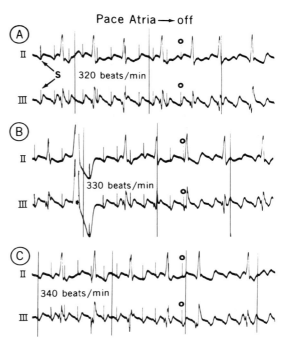

Pace Atria → off

Figure 9. ECG leads II and III recorded simultaneously at the termination of 30 sec of atrial pacing at 320 beats/min (panel A), 330 beats/min (panel B), and 340 beats/min (panel C) in a patient whose spontaneous atrial flutter rate was 300 beats/min. In each instance, following termination of atrial pacing (circle), the atrial flutter rate, which had increased to the atrial pacing rate, promptly returned to its previous spontaneous rate. Note that despite the fact that the atria were being paced from a pair of atrial electrodes placed in the region of the sinus node, the morphology of the atrial complexes during the rapid atrial pacing was essentially unchanged from that of the spontaneous atrial flutter. Thus, this figure illustrates three examples of transient entrainment of Type I atrial flutter without its interruption by rapid pacing: S = stimulus artifact. Time lines are at 1-sec intervals (from [3] with permission).

temporary atrial wire electrodes in place, and is quite useful, and even may be the therapy of choice in other clinical circumstances. The very rapid (Type II) atrial flutter, i.e., atrial flutter with a regular atrial rhythm and rates greater than 340– 350 beats/min [43, 44], to date has not been interrupted with rapid atrial pacing [3, 6, 7, 43, 44]. In fact, it was the inability to interrupt this more rapid rhythm with overdrive pacing techniques which first suggested that Type II atrial flutter was a distinctly different rhythm from Type I atrial flutter.

Either the ramp technique (defined in Figure 8) or the constant pacing rate technique (Figures 9 and 10) can be used effectively to treat Type I atrial

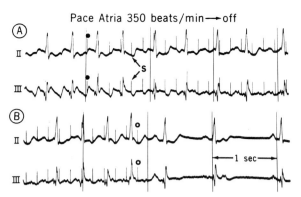

Pace Atria 350 beats/min → off

Figure 10. ECG leads II and III recorded from the same patient as in Figure 9. Panels A and B are not continuous traces. The dot in panel A marks the onset of atrial pacing at 350 beats/min. Note that in short order, the morphology of the atrial complex changes dramatically such that by the end of the trace in panel A, the atrial complexes are positive in both leads II and III. Panel B shows the termination of 30 sec of atrial pacing at 350 beats/min (circle). Note that with abrupt termination of the overdrive atrial pacing, sinus rhythm appears: S = stimulus artifact. Time lines are at 1-sec intervals (from [3] with permission).

flutter. With either technique, bipolar atrial pacing from the high right atrium is recommended while the ECG is recorded continuously. With either technique, a sufficiently rapid overdrive atrial pacing rate must be achieved that the atrial complexes in lead II, which previously had been negative, become frankly positive (Figures 14 and 16). The successful overdrive pacing rate for interuption of Type I atrial flutter is approximately 120–135% of the spontaneous rate [3, 44]. The development of positive atrial complexes during high right atrial pacing of atrial flutter indicates that the overdrive pacing rate is no longer transiently entraining the atrial flutter, but rather that the atrial flutter has been successfully interrupted [3, 6, 7, 26]. Therefore, when the atrial complexes in ECG lead II become positive, the atrial pacing can be abruptly terminated (Figure 10) or the pacing rate can be quickly slowed (Figure 8) to maintain control of the atrial rhythm.

It should be noted that, depending on the pacing site, one might not see the development of positive atrial complexes in lead II associated with interruption of the arrhythmia. Thus, if one paces from the mid or low right atrium, or from the coronary sinus or inferior left atrium, one could not use the hallmark of change in the configuration of the atrial complexes of ECG lead II as an index of successful interruption of the atrial flutter. Thus, one would not want to use a ramp technique but rather would use a constant pacing rate technique and simply observe whether or not, following each pacing sequence, the atrial flutter had been interrupted. Similarly, when pacing from the right atrial appendage, one may achieve clearly positive atrial complexes in ECG lead II, yet only transiently entrain rather than interrupt the atrial flutter. This appears to be explained by a considerable degree of fusion when pacing from this site that, resulting in clearly positive atrial complexes on occasion during the period of transient entrainment. Parenthetically, this suggests that the right atrial appendage pacing site is more distant from the reentry loop than sites closer to the sinus node. In any event, should this occur, one must simply increase the atrial pacing rate until the atrial flutter is interrupted.

Regardless of what pacing technique is used, sometimes pacing at rates over 400 beats/min may be required to interrupt Type I atrial flutter, and, in a small percentage of patients, rapid atrial pacing will precipitate atrial fibrillation despite careful application of the technique [3, 6, 7, 41]. This usually occurs in patients in whom the atrial pacing rate required to interrupt the atrial flutter is 35% greater than the spontaneous atrial flutter rate. The atrial fibrillation precipitated by rapid atrial pacing is very often transient, lasting seconds to minutes before spontaneously converting to sinus rhythm. In a small percentage of cases, the atrial fibrillation so precipitated may persist. Nevertheless, it is almost always a more desirable rhythm than atrial flutter, since the ventricular response rate to atrial fibrillation is usually slower and usually can be controlled easily with digitalis or other agents, such as beta blockers and calcium antagonists, which depress A-V conduction.

Despite the successful interruption of atrial flutter, it may recur in short order, either because it is precipitated by the occurrence of premature atrial beats during sinus rhythm, or because atrial fibrillation spontaneously reverts to atrial flutter. If the atrial flutter recurs two or more times following successful interruption with rapid atrial pacing and is associated with a rapid ventricular response, rapid atrial pacing at a rate of 450 beats/min may be initiated and maintained so that atrial fibrillation will be precipitated and sustained [3, 6, 7, 45]. In almost all instances, this will permit effective con-

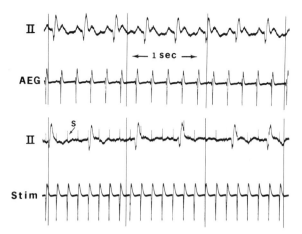

Figure 11. The top panel demonstrates ECG lead II recorded simultaneously with a bipolar atrial electrogram (AEG) during Type I atrial flutter at a rate of 320 beats/min with 2:1 A-V conduction, producing a ventricular rate of 160 beats/min. In this post-open-heart surgical patient, the atrial flutter was interrupted successfully on several occasions with overdrive atrial pacing. However, the atrial flutter recurred each time. Therefore, as shown in the bottom panel, continuous rapid atrial pacing at 450 beats/min was initiated. Pacing at this rate precipitated and sustained atrial fibrillation and was associated with a slowing of the ventricular rate to about 120 beats/min. Digoxin was then administered to slow the ventricular rate still further. Continuous rapid atrial pacing to sustain atrial fibrillation for control of ventricular rate was required for 26 hr in this patient while antiarrhythmic drug therapy (digoxin and quinidine) was administered. After rapid atrial pacing was terminated, atrial fibrillation was present but was transient, spontaneously converting to sinus rhythm within several minutes: S = stimulus artifact. Time lines are at 1-sec intervals (modified after [45] with permission).

trol of the ventricular response (Figure 11). Should additional slowing of the ventricular rate be desirable, digitalis, and, if necessary, either propranolol or verapamil also can be administered. Continuous rapid atrial pacing should then be continued as long as necessary along with the administration of appropriate antiarrhythmic therapy such as quinidine or procainamide. When rapid atrial pacing is used for a prolonged period, if the electrodes are not fixed epicardially or endocardially, great care must be taken to ensure a stable position for the electrode(s) used in pacing.

As indicated earlier, the more rapid type of atrial flutter, i.e., Type II atrial flutter, has not been interrupted successfully with rapid atrial pacing from sites high in the right atrium [3, 6, 7, 43]. Because of an overlap between the upper range of rates of Type I and lower range of rates of Type II atrial flutter, a

trial of rapid atrial pacing sometimes may be necessary to distinguish between the two.

Paroxysmal atrial tachycardia

Paroxysmal atrial tachycardia is probably the simplest tachyarrhythmia to interrupt with cardiac pacing. There are several acceptable methods of cardiac pacing to interrupt this arrhythmia. The simplest method is to pace the atria at a rate somewhat faster than the spontaneous rate. After achieving capture of the atria, the pacing can be terminated abruptly or the pacing rate may be slowed to a predetermined rate (Figure 12). However, because paroxysmal atrial tachycardia, be it due to A-V nodal reentry or A-V bypass reentry, can be transiently entrained, overdrive pacing to interrupt this arrhythmia may require pacing at rates 20–50 beats/min faster than the spontaneous rate of the tachycardia [3, 6, 7, 30].

Paroxysmal atrial tachycardia often can be interrupted with an appropriately timed premature atrial beat. Therefore, one simply can initiate atrial pacing at a rate considerably slower than that of the spontaneous rhythm, e.g., 100 beats/min. One of the pacing stimuli ultimately will produce an atrial beat at an appropriate interval after a spontaneous beat such that it will interrupt the tachyarrhythmia (Figure 13). One can also introduce premature atrial beats at selected intervals following a train of spontaneous beats during the tachycardia and interrupt the arrhythmia in that fashion. Because paroxysmal atrial tachycardia may be transiently entrained, it is possible that the introduction of a premature beat may simply transiently entrain the rhythm for one beat, i.e., it will fail to produce the necessary block in the reentry loop to interrupt the arrhythmia. Should that occur, it usually is possible to interrupt the rhythm by introducing two premature beats at appropriately timed intervals (Figure 14).

In some patients, the paroxysmal atrial tachycardia may be recurrent despite successful interruption with the pacing techniques described above. In these instances, it usually is desirable to suppress this arrhythmia to maintain a clinically acceptable ventricular rate [3, 6, 7, 45]. On occasion, atrial pacing at rates between 90–110 beats/min may successfully suppress the inciting premature atrial or ventricular beats and therefore permit suppression

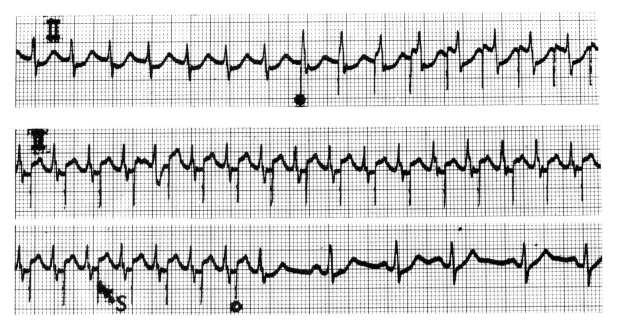

Figure 12. The top trace shows ECG lead II recorded during an episode of paroxysmal atrial tachycardia at a rate of 150 beats/min. Beginning with the eighth beat in this trace, rapid atrial pacing at a rate of 165 beats/min was initiated (dot). In the middle trace, which begins 12 sec after the last beat of the top trace, atrial capture with 1:1 A-V conduction is demonstrated clearly. In the bottom trace, which is continuous with the middle trace, sinus rhythm appears when atrial pacing is terminated abruptly (circle): S = stimulus artifact (from [6] with permission).

Continuous Strips

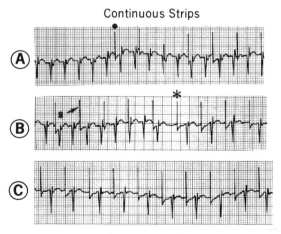

Figure 13. Panels A, B, and C are continuous traces of ECG lead II. Panel A shows the onset of atrial pacing (dot) at a rate of 110 beats/min during an episode of paroxysmal atrial tachycardia at a rate of 195 beats/min. The asynchronous atrial pacing results in the random introduction of premature atrial beats, one of which ultimately interrupts the tachycardia (panel B). There then follows a paced atrial rhythm at a rate of 110 beats/min (panels B and C). The asterisk denotes the first beat of the paced atrial rhythm. Note that the third and sixth beats during the paced atrial rhythm are premature atrial beats which are conducted to the ventricles: S = stimulus artifact (from [3] with permission).

of recurrent paroxysmal atrial tachycardia. Should this be unsuccessful (Figure 15), an alternative therapeutic modality is continuous rapid atrial pacing at rates sufficiently rapid to ensure 2:1 A-V conduction. This type of pacing should provide effective suppression of the recurrent paroxysmal atrial tachycardia and will also provide an acceptable ventricular response rate (Figure 16). During the period of continuous rapid atrial pacing, antiarrhythmic drug therapy should be administered to permit termination of the continuous rapid pacing. Some patients may require programmed cardiac pacing studies in concert with serial drug testing before a successful therapeutic regimen is found. Also, some patients may require either cardiac surgery or implantation of a permanent pacing system to provide satisfactory control of the arrhythmia.

Ectopic nonparoxysmal atrial tachycardia

This is an ectopic rhythm that presumably is initiated somewhere in the atria. This rhythm generally is associated with a variable degree of A-V block, although when the atrial rate is relatively slow (e.g., 140–150 beats/min), 1:1 A-V conduction may be

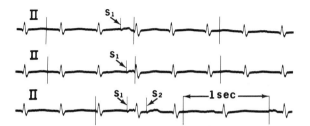

Figure 14. All three panels show ECG lead II recorded during an episode of paroxysmal atrial tachycardia. Following a train of eight spontaneous atrial beats, either a single premature atrial beat (upper two panels) or two premature atrial beats (lower panel) are introduced at selected intervals. In each of these traces, only the last three spontaneous beats of a train of eight beats are shown prior to introducing a premature beat (S). In the upper panel, a premature atrial beat (S_1) was introduced 220 msec following the last spontaneous beat of an eight-beat train. Atrial capture was obtained, and, although the tachycardia was reset (note that the interval between the fourth and fifth beats is shorter than the other intervals during the paroxysmal atrial tachycardia), the paroxysmal atrial tachycardia was not interrupted. In the middle panel, the premature atrial beat (S_1) was introduced 280 msec following the train of eight spontaneous atrial beats. Although atrial capture was obtained, the paroxysmal atrial tachycardia was not influenced by the introduction of the premature atrial beat. In the lower panel, two premature atrial beats were introduced, the first (S_1) 280 msec following the train of eight spontaneous atrial beats and the second (S_2) 220 msec following the first (S_1) premature atrial beat, with atrial capture being obtained each time. Note that the paroxysmal atrial tachycardia was interrupted with return to spontaneous sinus rhythm. In the upper two panels, the tachycardia was transiently entrained for one beat. In the lower panel, the tachycardia was interrupted, undoubtedly because block of both the antidromic and orthodromic wavefronts of the second premature atrial beat occurred. Time lines are at 1-sec intervals (modified after [6] with permission).

present. The mechanism of this rhythm is uncertain. Because some forms of this arrhythmia can be entrained transiently and ultimately interrupted by overdrive atrial pacing, it seems reasonable to suggest that some forms of this rhythm are due to reentry [3, 6, 7, 31]. In addition, some forms are likely due to automaticity and conceivably even to triggered activity, the latter being suggested if only because one of the well-described associations of this arrhythmia is with digitalis toxicity. However, this rhythm also is seen frequently in patients with chronic lung disease and on occasion in patients following open heart surgery. It should be emphasized that, in most settings, this arrhythmia usually is not associated with digitalis toxicity.

When this rhythm is associated with 2:1 A-V

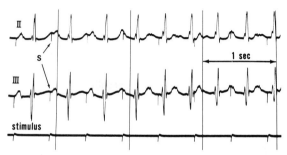

Figure 15. ECG leads II and III recorded simultaneously with stimulus artifact during atrial pacing at a rate of 120 beats/min in a patient who had recurrent paroxysmal atrial tachycardia following open heart surgery. In this patient, atrial pacing at a rate of 180 beats/min had successfully interrupted the paroxysmal atrial tachycardia. However, with cessation of the rapid pacing, the rhythm returned to sinus rhythm with frequent premature atrial beats which reprecipitated the paroxysmal atrial tachycardia. Atrial pacing at rates of 100, 110, and 120 beats/min failed to suppress the premature beats. This figure illustrates a premature beat (fourth beat) precipitating another episode of paroxysmal atrial tachycardia which was not interrupted by continuous atrial pacing at 120 beats/min: S = stimulus artifact. Time lines are at 1-sec intervals (from [45] with permission).

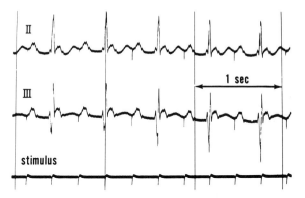

Figure 16. ECG leads II and III recorded simultaneously with a stimulus artifact from the same patient as in Figure 15 during continuous atrial pacing at a rate of 210 beats/min. Pacing at this rate produced 2:1 A-V conduction and a clinically acceptable ventricular rate (105 beats/min). It also resulted in complete suppression of the premature atrial beats and therefore prevented recurrence of the paroxysmal atrial tachycardia. During the period of continuous rapid atrial pacing, digitalis and procainamide were administered. After about 20 hr of continuous rapid atrial pacing, cessation of the pacing resulted in return of normal sinus rhythm. Earlier termination of rapid atrial pacing was associated with reprecipitation of the paroxysmal atrial tachycardia: S = stimulus artifact. Time lines are at 1-sec intervals (from [45] with permission).

313

conduction, it may not require any therapeutic intervention apart from the cessation of digitalis therapy, should digitalis toxicity be suspected. However, should the degree of A-V block diminish or should the rate of the atrial tachycardia slow, the ventricular response rate may increase, producing undesirably rapid ventricular rates. In addition, it may be desirable for other reasons to obtain a normal sinus rhythm. Therefore, interruption or control of this rhythm usually is desirable.

Some ectopic nonparoxysmal atrial tachycardias such as those resulting from digitalis toxicity have not been successfully interrupted with presently available pacing techniques. Alternatively, the form of ectopic atrial tachycardia that we believe to be due to reentry can always be interrupted with over-

drive pacing techniques [3, 6, 7, 31]. Because this form of ectopic atrial tachycardia will demonstrate transient entrainment during overdrive pacing, a critically rapid pacing rate (usually 120–130% of the spontaneous atrial rate) must be achieved to interrupt the arrhythmia (Figure 17). Should precipitation of atrial fibrillation be considered undesirable, atrial pacing at rates above 300–350 beats/min probably should be avoided.

When an ectopic atrial tachycardia cannot be terminated by pacing, pacing the atria still may be desirable to slow the ventricular rate. In patients in whom the spontaneous atrial rate is slow enough (e.g., 150–170 beats/min) that either 1:1 or variable A-V conduction occurs and is associated with a clinically unacceptable rapid ventricular rate, the

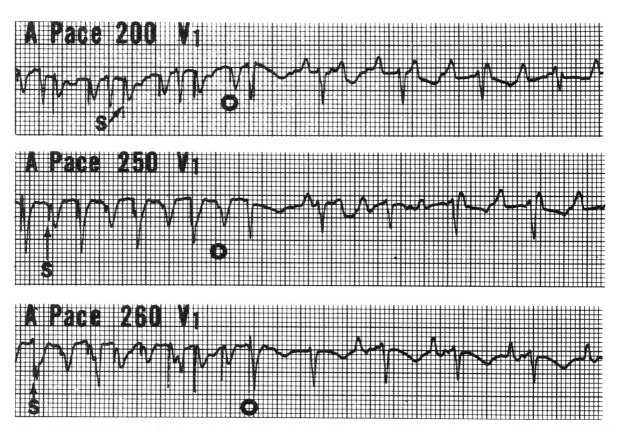

Figure 17. ECG lead V_1 recorded at the termination of 40 sec of atrial pacing at rates of 200 beats/min (top trace), 250 beats/min (middle trace), and 260 beats/min (bottom trace), in a patient who had an ectopic atrial tachycardia at a rate of 180 beats/min with 2:1 A-V conduction. In each trace, the circle marks the last paced atrial beat. The ectopic atrial tachycardia has not been interrupted by atrial pacing at rates of 200 (top trace) 210, 220, 230, 240, and 250 (middle trace) beats/min. However, atrial pacing at 260 beats/min (bottom trace) interrupted the ectopic atrial tachycardia, with development of sinus rhythm following abrupt cessation of atrial pacing (bottom trace): S = stimulus artifact (from [3] with permission).

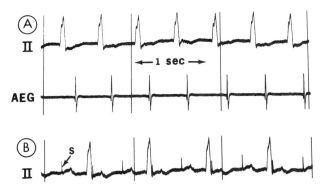

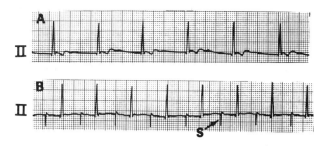

Figure 18. Panel A shows ECG lead II recorded simultaneously with a bipolar atrial electrogram (AEG) demonstrating an ectopic atrial tachycardia at a rate of 135 beats/min with 1:1 A-V conduction in a patient following open heart surgery. Overdrive atrial pacing suppressed the arrhythmia, but with cessation of pacing, the tachycardia promptly returned. Antiarrhythmic drug therapy also failed to interrupt the arrhythmia. Therefore, continuous rapid atrial pacing at a rate of 180 beats/min was initiated. As shown in panel B, this produced 2:1 A-V conduction with a clinically satisfactory ventricular rate of 90 beats/min: S = stimulus artifact. Time lines are at 1-sec intervals (from [6] with permission).

Figure 19. ECG lead II. Panel A demonstrates a spontaneous A-V junctional rhythm at a rate of 65 beats/min with retrograde A-V conduction. Panel B demonstrates that with atrial pacing at a rate of 90 beats/min in the same patient, 1:1 antegrade A-V conduction is obtained: S = stimulus artifact (from [3] with permission).

ventricular rate can be controlled by pacing the atria at rates between 180–230 beats/min to achieve 2:1 A-V conduction with ventricular rates between 90–115 beats/min (Figure 18) [3, 6, 7, 45].

Nonparoxysmal A-V junctional tachycardia

This presumably automatic rhythm cannot be interrupted by rapid atrial pacing. However, the rhythm always can be overdriven by atrial pacing at rates somewhat faster than the spontaneous rate provided the arrhythmia is not associated with a significant degree of A-V block. When a rate faster than the A-V junctional rate is desirable or when the atrial contribution to cardiac output is desirable, simple initiation of atrial pacing often is a successful form of treatment (Figure 19). If this arrhythmia is associated with a degree of A-V block such that overdrive atrial pacing will not suppress the arrhythmia, sequential atrioventricular pacing provides an alternative for effective pacing therapy.

On occasion, the ectopic pacemaker in the A-V junction may be so enhanced that it will produce an extremely rapid rate that is incompatible with a satisfactory clinical course (as was shown in Figure 2). In addition, it may be sufficiently rapid that neither the usual atrial or ventricular pacing tech-

niques nor antiarrhythmic drug therapy can successfully treat this rhythm. In such instances, ventricular paired-pacing may be required [5, 7] (refer to Figure 3). When ventricular paired-pacing is used to provide a reasonable and effective rate of ventricular contraction during an automatic A-V junctional tachycardia, the paired-pacing very likely will have to be continued for many hours while the factors that have enhanced the automaticity of the A-V junction either subside spontaneously or subside in association with drug therapy.

Sinus tachycardia

Because sinus tachycardia may be associated with very rapid ventricular rates, it may be desirable to slow it. Unfortunately, use of cardiac pacing to accomplish this has been rather disappointing. Rapid atrial pacing at rates faster than the spontaneous sinus rate can always overdrive the atria, but, of course, cannot interrupt the arrhythmia because sinus tachycardia results from enhancement of a normal pacemaker, i.e., it is an automatic rhythm. Attempts have been made to overdrive sinus tachycardia by rapid atrial pacing in an effort to produce 2:1 A-V conduction and thus decrease the ventricular rate by increasing the atrial rate. Unfortunately, this technique is rarely successful because in all instances, the factors that generate the sinus tachycardia also enhance A-V conduction. The result is an inability to produce 2:1 A-V conduction at atrial pacing rates that will result in a clinically acceptable ventricular response rate. It has been suggested that the use of digitalis with or without a beta blocker or verapamil therapy may be

315

helpful in these instances. During rapid atrial pacing, these drugs may produce acceptable A-V block such that rapid atrial pacing can be used to overdrive the sinus rate and slow the ventricular response. Unfortunately, there is no published experience in this regard. There are a few reports demonstrating that either coupled or paired atrial pacing is capable of slowing the ventricular rate, but this has been performed only when the sinus rate was 105 beats/min or less [46, 47]. This limited experience does not permit an assessment of the efficacy of this technique in the treatment of more rapid sinus tachycardias.

Ventricular tachycardia

The reentrant form of this arrhythmia usually is amenable to treatment with cardiac pacing techniques. However, depending on the clinical circumstances, either intravenous drug therapy (lidocaine or procainamide) or DC cardioversion initially may be the treatment of choice. If a diagnosis of torsades de pointes is made, any drugs that prolong the Q–T interval such as quinidine, procainamide, disopyramide, phenothiazines, or tricyclic antidepressants should be terminated [48]. In addition, depending on the clinical circumstances, treatment that shortens the Q–T interval may be indicated. This includes use of drugs such as lidocaine, phenytoin, propranolol, or a catecholamine, and use of atrial (or rarely ventricular) pacing at relatively fast rates (up to 120–130 beats/min) [3, 7]. If either the serum potassium or magnesium is low, the abnormality should be corrected.

Several pacing techniques have been described for the successful interruption of ventricular tachycardia. These include introduction of premature ventricular beats, either randomly (underdrive pacing) or at selected intervals; overdrive ventricular pacing; overdrive atrial pacing (provided 1:1 A-V conduction is possible at the appropriately fast atrial rate); ventricular paired-pacing; and so-called ventricular burst pacing [3, 7, 8, 49]. At the outset, it should be emphasized that, although all these techniques are remarkably safe when used properly, one should be prepared to treat ventricular fibrillation.

Overdrive ventricular pacing to interrupt ventricular tachycardia provides an effective mode of treatment. Recent studies have suggested that, much as with atrial flutter, paroxysmal atrial tachycardia, and ectopic tachycardia, it may be necessary to pace the ventricles at a rate considerably faster than the spontaneous rate in order to interrupt ventricular tachycardia [3, 7, 27, 50, 51]. Pacing at rates which are faster than the spontaneous rate of the tachycardia but slower than a critically rapid rate may merely transiently entrain the tachycardia without interrupting it.

Based on previous studies of the successful interruption of Type I atrial flutter, it is currently suggested that ventricular pacing at rates 35% faster than the spontaneous ventricular tachycardia rates may be hazardous in terms of the danger of precipitating ventricular fibrillation. Therefore, ventricular pacing at rates 35% greater than the spontaneous rate probably should be avoided. The duration of pacing will vary from 2–30 sec, largely determined by the hemodynamic status of the patient and the effects of the pacing rate on hemodynamic status. It is unclear whether these admonitions apply to atrial pacing of ventricular tachycardia, although it is likely that A-V block will prevent 1:1 A-V conduction of very rapid atrial rates.

The technique of ventricular burst pacing as described by Fisher et al. [49] also may provide a clinically useful technique for interruption of ventricular tachycardia. With this technique, ventricular pacing at a rate 40–50 beats/min faster than the spontaneous rate is applied to the ventricles for periods of 5–7 capture beats. Following cessation of pacing, if the ventricular tachycardia persists, pacing at the same rate is performed for 10–12 capture beats. Following cessation of pacing, if ventricular tachycardia still persists, the pacing rate is increased in increments of 25 beats/min and the pacing is repeated, first to obtain 5–7 capture beats and then, if necessary, to obtain 10–12 capture beats. This technique has proven highly effective, particularly in otherwise resistant ventricular tachycardia. It also is useful to note that ventricular tachycardia may be interrupted successfully by ventricular paired-pacing. The technique is applied in exactly the same manner as described previously in this chapter, and the same admonitions also apply.

When overdrive ventricular pacing techniques are used to interrupt ventricular tachycardia, a more rapid ventricular tachycardia may be precipitated [3, 7, 27, 49]. This rhythm may be transient, with a subsequent return to the previous spontaneous rate; it may be stable and amenable to

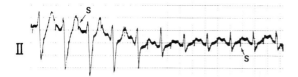

Ventricular Tachycardia - 150 beats/min
Atrial Pacing - 160 beats/min

Figure 20. ECG lead II demonstrating a ventricular tachycardia at 150 beats/min during atrial pacing at 160 beats/min. Note the progressive fusion at the fourth, fifth, and sixth QRS complexes following which complete atrial capture of the ventricles is established: S = stimulus artifact (from Waldo et al., Ala J Med Sci 11:120–128, 1974 with permission).

further overdrive pacing; or it may be associated with a clinically unacceptable state, requiring prompt DC cardioversion.

In some instances, ventricular tachycardia may not be interrupted by overdrive pacing for any of several reasons; e.g., the arrhythmia may be automatic, the site generating the tachycardia may be protected by entrance block, or the pacing rate required to interrupt the tachycardia may be such that development of ventricular fibrillation is a concern. In such instances, continuous atrial pacing at a rate faster than that of the tachycardia may produce a more satisfactory rhythm if 1:1 A-V conduction is possible and the rate produced is acceptable (Figure 20). Alternatively, continuous ventricular paired-pacing may be used to suppress such a ventricular tachycardia. Either of these pacing techniques may be used temporarily until other forms of therapy (e.g., antiarrhythmic drugs or cardiac surgery) permit resolution of the problem.

Once ventricular tachycardia has been interrupted by any method and the spontaneous heart rate is relatively slow, atrial or ventricular pacing may be desirable. Such pacing at rates faster than the sinus rate, either alone or in association with drug therapy, may be associated with significant or complete suppression of the premature ventricular beats which were responsible for initiating the tachycardia (Figure 21).

Ventricular fibrillation

Ventricular fibrillation is not amenable to treatment with cardiac pacing techniques. Defibrillation is the appropriate therapy here.

Continuous ECG Strips

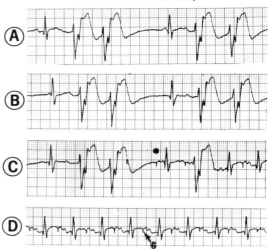

Figure 21. Panels A, B, C, and D are continuous recordings of a monitor ECG lead. Note that two premature atrial beats follow each sinus beat in a trigeminal pattern (panels A, B, and C). With the onset of atrial pacing at a rate of 100 beats/min, atrial capture is obtained (dot in panel C). This increase in the atrial rate is associated with 1:1 A-V conduction and results in complete suppression of premature ventricular beats (panel D): S = stimulus artifact (from [3] with permission).

Cardiac pacing in the treatment of bradyarrhythmias

Introduction

The use of temporary and permanent pacing techniques is well established for the treatment of various forms of bradycardia. Bradycardia, of course, may be due to many abnormalities: sinus node dysfunction with sinus bradycardia; sinus node exit block; sinus node dysfunction with a slow ectopic atrial rhythm; sinus rhythm with any form of second-degree A-V block; third-degree A-V block; or atrial bigeminy with nonconducted premature atrial beats. In addition, other A-V conduction abnormalities such as first-degree A-V block, bundle branch block, and A-V dissociation also may require treatment.

Sick sinus syndrome

The sick sinus syndrome refers to dysfunction of the sinus node with its attendant clinical signs and symptoms [52]. Sinus node dysfunction may be manifest as: (a) sinus bradycardia, i.e., a sinus rate less than 60 beats/min; (b) periods of sinus arrest or sinus node exit block, most often accompanied by failure of an escape rhythm to appear in a clinically satisfactory manner during the resulting pause in sinus rhythm; (c) failure of sinus rhythm to resume following termination (spontaneous or induced) of any supraventricular arrhythmia (Figure 4). This syndrome is frequently associated with abnormalities of A-V conduction and/or the A-V junctional escape pacemaker. In fact, the latter ultimately is responsible for the clinical symptoms of dizziness, lightheadedness, or frank syncope which result from ventricular asystole during periods of sinus arrest or sinus node exit block and which make this arrhythmia potentially life threatening.

Sinus bradycardia is infrequently a life-threatening arrhythmia except when associated with dizziness, lightheadedness, fatigue, syncope, or precipitation of either angina pectoris or congestive heart failure. Emergency treatment, when necessary, usually is placement of a temporary ventricular demand mode pacemaker to provide a satisfactory rate until the underlying cause of the arrhythmia is identified and appropriate long-term therapy is initiated. Occasionally, temporary atrial or A-V sequential pacing may be indicated.

When patients with the sick sinus syndrome develop a paroxysmal supraventricular tachycardia (e.g., atrial fibrillation, atrial flutter, paroxysmal atrial tachycardia), treatment with a demand mode ventricular pacemaker (initially a temporary system and subsequently a permanent system) is necessary. This will provide a satisfactory minimal rate, thereby preventing prolonged periods of ventricular asystole with its attendant hazards (Figure 22). This will also permit administration of appropriate medication to suppress or prevent the paroxysmal tachycardia despite the fact that the medication might adversely affect sinus node function.

Until recently, the primary mode of treatment of

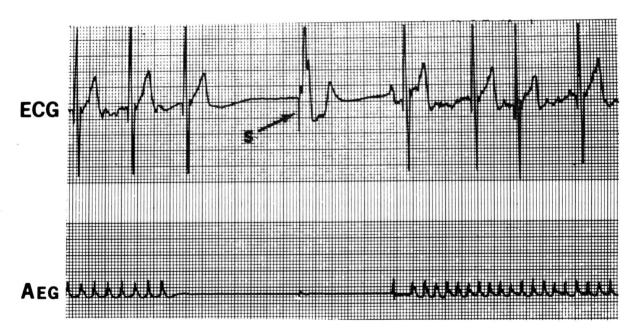

Figure 22. Monitor ECG lead recorded simultaneously with a bipolar atrial electrogram from a patient with sick sinus syndrome. The patient developed paroxysms of supraventricular tachycardia which terminated spontaneously and were associated with prolonged periods of asystole. Therefore, this patient's temporary epicardial ventricular wire electrodes were attached to a ventricular pacemaker set in the demand pacing mode to provide a rate floor of 40 beats/min. This figure illustrates the spontaneous termination of an episode of atrial flutter (probably Type II) in this patient which is followed by an almost 3-sec period of atrial asystole. Note, however, than when the ventricular asystolic period exceeds the preset interval of the pacemaker, it delivers a stimulus (S) which captures the ventricles (from [3] with permission).

the sick sinus syndrome was placement of a ventricular pacemaker, virtually always in the demand mode and often with an adjustable rate (i.e., programmable). However, with the advent of sophisticated coordinated atrioventricular pacemakers, the opportunity exists to provide the patient with a normal A-V contraction sequence, and thereby with all the attendant advantages of the atrial contribution to cardiac output. In fact, some of the systems that recently have become available not only pace the atria, but also sense the atrial rate, so that if it is adequate (i.e., not too slow), the spontaneous atrial rate governs the ventricular rate. Such pacemakers also have an automatic A-V block, so that, if the atrial rate becomes too fast, e.g., as in atrial flutter, the ventricles will respond with a clinically acceptable rate.

A-V block

Third-degree (complete) A-V block

The development of third-degree A-V block is virtually always a life-threatening arrhythmia, either overtly or potentially and, therefore, virtually always requires prompt treatment. Usually, the treatment of choice is temporary demand mode ventricular pacing at an appropriate rate, followed by placement of an appropriate permanent pacemaker system (ventricular or A-V sequential pacemaker). Prior to placement of a temporary ventricular pacemaker system, if the spontaneous ventricular rate is so slow that it is life threatening, therapy with intravenous isoproterenol (1–4 mcg/min) and/or atropine (1–2 mg) usually will increase the ventricular rate satisfactorily.

Second-degree A-V block

Second-degree A-V block with significant ventricular bradycardia is treated in a manner similar to that described for third-degree A-V block. However, the ultimate placement of a permanent ventricular pacemaker will be determined by the underlying cause of the second-degree A-V block. For instance, if due to digitalis toxicity or toxic effects of therapy with a beta-blocking agent, only a temporary pacemaker may be necessary. Mobitz Type I second-degree A-V block, i.e., Wenckebach periodicity (progressive P–R interval lengthening preceding a dropped beat), rarely requires emergency treatment, and – unless due to a lesion in the A-V

conduction system distal to the A-V node (infrequent) – infrequently requires placement of either a temporary or permanent ventricular pacemaker [53]. Mobitz Type II second-degree A-V block (constant P–R interval with a sudden and unexpected dropped beat), however, is most often due to a lesion distal to the A-V node, and, because of the natural history of such a lesion, placement of a permanent ventricular pacemaker system is almost always indicated whenever this diagnosis is established [53, 54]. Occasionally, electrophysiological studies, including atrial pacing and His bundle electrogram recordings, must be performed to establish the location of the block and determine whether or not there is an indication for placement of a permanent ventricular pacemaker system.

1:1 A-V conduction with bundle branch block and abnormal axis deviation

Whether or not patients with 1:1 A-V conduction in the presence of various degrees of A-V block (P–R interval prolongation and/or bundle branch block with or without abnormal axis deviation, i.e., including the so-called hemiblocks or bifascicular blocks) are at an increased risk for sudden death (presumably because of the abrupt development of third-degree A-V block with an inadequate ventricular rhythm) is an important and somewhat controversial question, particularly for patients who have had a myocardial infarction.

Patients who have not had an acute myocardial infarction. Prospective studies [55–58] have demonstrated that in this group of patients the incidence of progression to spontaneous third-degree A-V block is quite low at about 4–5%, (20 of 452 patients in one study [55]). Furthermore, as summarized recently [59], attempts to identify factors that might predict who is at risk for development of advanced A-V block and sudden death have, for the most part, not proven useful. However, a breakdown of the subgroup of patients into smaller subsets seems useful.

i) Patients without symptoms related to advanced A-V block: There is general agreement that for patients in this group, without symptoms possibly related to advanced A-V block, a prophylactic ventricular pacemaker system need not be used, although such patients should be followed carefully. Although the problem of sudden death in this group of patients is yet to be solved, the data from the prospective studies suggest it most commonly results from ischemic heart disease with ventricular tachyarrhythmia and not from advanced A-V block. However, the data from one group [60] suggest that asymptomatic patients over 70 years of age with a bundle branch block pattern and abnormal axis deviation (so-called bifascicular block) associated with marked prolongation of the H–V interval beyond 70 msec (the normal range is 35–55 msec [61]) represent a subgroup at increased risk of sudden death, presumably due to development of advanced A-V block. A more recent study has suggested that if the H–V interval is greater than 100 msec, this small subset of patients is at extremely high risk for development of complete heart block and sudden death, and, therefore, placement of a ventricular pacing system is required [62].

ii) Patients with symptoms possibly related to advanced A-V block: Symptomatic patients, i.e., primarily those with syncope, require careful evaluation. The causes of syncope in this group of patients include intermittent A-V block, sinoatrial block, ventricular tachycardia, central nervous system disease, postural hypotension (often due to drug therapy), paroxysmal supraventricular arrhythmias (atrial fibrillation, atrial flutter, ectopic atrial tachycardia, paroxysmal atrial tachycardia) with rapid ventricular response rates, aortic stenosis, hypertrophic cardiomyopathy, and idiopathic vasovagal mechanisms. Most of these causes of syncope clearly will not be helped by prophylactic placement of a pacemaker. Therefore, this group of patients needs careful evaluation, including a thorough history and physical examination, prolonged ECG monitoring, and often electrophysiologic studies during cardiac catheterization in addition to other appropriate noncardiologic laboratory investigation. If paroxysmal A-V block or bradycardia can be demonstrated as the cause, or if no cause for the syncope can be demonstrated, prophylactic cardiac pacing appears to be indicated [60].

iii) Value of His bundle recordings: This discussion is presented in such a way as to avoid almost completely the controversy of the significance of H–V interval prolongation associated with various forms of A-V conduction abnormalities in the presence of 1:1 A-V conduction. In particular, the significance of H–V interval prolongation as a predictor of the development of third-degree A-V block remains controversial. Two prospective studies [58, 63–65] clearly indicate that it has no predictive value and data from three other groups [56, 60, 66] indicate that it does, at least in symptomatic patients. Perhaps the middle ground is found in the much longer follow-up studies by Dhingra and co-workers [67] of their earlier studies of patients with 1:1 A-V conduction in the presence of so-called bifascicular block. The longer follow-up studies now demonstrate that the development of third-degree A-V block is eight times more frequent in patients with a prolonged (greater than 55 msec) H–V interval (15 of 319 patients, for a 4.5% incidence) than in patients with a normal H–V interval (19 of 198 patients, for a 0.6% incidence). Despite this significant difference in incidence, Dhingra and associates initially did not recommend placement of permanent ventricular pacemaker systems in the group having H–V interval prolongation because the incidence of development of complete heart block was so low. In one of their most recent reports [67], they appear to have modified their approach because there is no question from their data that the cumulative seven-year incidence of development of complete heart block was 3% in patients with normal H–V intervals and 12% of patients with prolonged H–V intervals (p < 0.01). Furthermore, the seven-year cumulative cardiovascular mortality was 32% in patients with normal H–V intervals and 57% in patients with prolonged H–V intervals (p < 0.005). However, the difference in mortality between these two groups was almost certainly related to the marked difference in the incidence and severity of organic heart disease in patients with prolonged H–V intervals as opposed to those with normal H–V intervals.

Two recent observations do appear to be predictive for the development of advanced A-V block: (a) the development of paroxysmal A-V block as a result of block distal to the His bundle recording site produced during rapid atrial pacing in the presence of normal A-V conduction time [59]; and (b) H–V intervals greater than 100 msec [62]. Thus, when performing electrophysiological studies, these important subgroups of A-V conduction block should be carefully sought and evaluated.

In summary, the available data make it difficult to be dogmatic about indications for prophylactic placement of a ventricular pacemaker in the presence of 1:1 A-V conduction associated with the various forms of A-V conduction abnormalities. In the absence of symptoms, we believe the data suggest that prophylactic pacemaker placement in the presence of 1:1 A-V conduction is indicated infrequently. In the presence of symptoms, the data suggest that the best approach is careful evaluation of the symptoms, with placement of a ventricular pacemaker system when it is clearly indicated or when an etiology cannot be demonstrated and the symptoms reasonably can be explained by advanced A-V block.

Patients who have had an acute myocardial infarction. The role of cardiac pacing in acute myocardial infarction still is being debated, but there are enough data to provide a few noncontroversial guidelines. The development of Mobitz Type II second-degree A-V block, unexpected third-degree A-V block, or third-degree A-V block which develops following antecedent Mobitz Type II A-V block now are generally accepted indications for placement of a temporary ventricular pacemaker and, later, a permanent ventricular pacemaker [68-70]. Also, the development of Mobitz Type I second-degree A-V block in association with an anterior myocardial infarction is an indication for placement of a temporary, followed by a permanent, ventricular pacemaker [68, 69]. The development of Mobitz Type I A-V block or third-degree A-V block following antecedent Mobitz Type I A-V block in the absence of an anterior infarction (i.e., in the presence of a posterior infarction) often necessitates temporary ventricular pacing, particularly if the ventricular rate is unsatisfactory or unstable or is associated with bradycardia-related ventricular arrhythmias, but rarely will require placement of a permanent ventricular pacemaker [69, 70]. The development of right bundle branch block with either abnormal left axis deviation or right axis deviation (so-called bifasicular block) is an indication for placement of a temporary ventricular pacemaker, but unless there is subsequent evolution of high degree A-V block, it is not at present thought to be an indication for placement of a permanent ventricular pacemaker [68-70]. Parenthetically, during acute myocardial infarction and in the period following the acute myocardial infarction, bradycardia-related arrhythmias have the same indication for placement of a permanent pacemaker system as in the absence of myocardial infarction.

The role of His bundle recording in determining which patients in this group are at risk for the development of permanent advanced A-V block is unclear. However, one group [70] has shown that prolongation of the H-V interval in patients with an anteroseptal myocardial infarction and abnormal axis deviation (i.e., so-called bifascicular block) is highly predictive for the development of third-degree A-V block. This group has also demonstrated that, for patients with an inferior myocardial infarction who temporarily develop third-degree A-V block, the His bundle recording will localize the block either to the A-V node or to an infranodal site, the implications being different for an infranodal locus of the block (permanent ventricular pacemaker system implantation indicated) than for an A-V nodal locus of the block (temporary ventricular pacemaker as needed).

Finally, it is important to emphasize that in patients thought to be at increased risk for development of advanced A-V block following an acute myocardial infarction, sudden death still may occur despite the placement of a permanent ventricular pacemaker. This is because these patients often have other serious myocardial problems (significant congestive heart failure, ventricular arrhythmias, etc.) for which ventricular pacing is inadequate therapy [68, 69].

First-degree A-V block
First-degree A-V block generally is diagnosed from the standard ECG when the P-R interval is prolonged (>0.20 sec in adults). When P-R interval prolongation is due to delayed conduction of the impulse from the sinus node to the A-V node, so-called internodal conduction delay [71], the presence of the prolonged P-R interval usually is of no clinical consequence. The more usual causes of a prolonged P-R interval (i.e., first-degree A-V block) are abnormal conduction in the A-V node, in the His bundle, and/or in the bundle branches. When first-degree A-V block becomes manifest for the first time and is not drug-related, depending on the clinical circumstances, it may be advisable to utilize a temporary ventricular pacemaker system to provide a minimum rate of about 60 beats/min until either the problem is resolved, or until it is clear that such pacing is not necessary. Then, if A-V conduction fails such that first-degree A-V block

progresses to second- or third-degree block and the ventricles are not activated at least once per second by a spontaneous rhythm, the ventricular pacemaker will discharge automatically, preventing potentially serious consequences.

When first-degree A-V block is present, it may prevent effective use of atrial pacing to treat other rhythm disturbances. This is because the atrial pacing rate required to suppress the arrhythmia may result in second-degree A-V block. For example, a patient may have a sinus bradycardia at 50 beats/min with first-degree A-V block. Because of the presence of underlying first-degree A-V block, atrial pacing at an appropriate rate, e.g., 70 beats/min, may produce second-degree A-V block making the ventricular response rate clinically inadequate. In such instances, either ventricular pacing in a demand mode or coordinated A-V pacing would provide effective therapy.

Atrioventricular (A-V dissociation)
In this A-V conduction abnormality, the atria and ventricles each are governed by separate rhythms, the ventricular rate is faster than the atrial rate, and there is unidirectional retrograde A-V block. Thus, in this type of A-V block an ectopic rhythm, most commonly from an A-V junctional pacemaker, activates the ventricles at a rate exceeding that of the rhythm (usually a sinus rhythm) which governs atrial activation. The presence of retrograde A-V block prevents 1:1 retrograde conduction to the atria of the faster rhythm governing ventricular activation. This arrhythmia is common following open heart surgical repair of various forms of congenital heart lesions, particularly when there has been manipulation of the A-V junction resulting in enhanced A-V junctional automaticity. This rhythm also may be a manifestation of digitalis toxicity or acute myocardial infarction. If, in the presence of functional A-V dissociation, the cardiac index is too low or clinically unacceptable, atrial pacing at a rate somewhat faster than the A-V junctional rate should be initiated. Since retrograde but not antegrade A-V conduction block usually is the rule for this arrhythmia, simply pacing the atria at a rate faster than the A-V junctional rate should achieve 1:1 antegrade A-V conduction. The cardiac index should increase, often substantially, as the atrial contribution to cardiac output is accomplished. Rarely, the lesion which has resulted in the A-V

junctional rhythm also produces a degree of antegrade A-V block such that pacing the atria at a rate faster than the A-V junctional rate will not permit 1:1 antegrade A-V conduction. Furthermore, 1:1 A-V conduction during atrial pacing may result in substantial first-degree A-V block resulting in minimal improvement of cardiac output. In these instances, coordinated A-V pacing alone or in combination with drug therapy (phenytoin, atropine or atropine-like agents, or catecholamines) to improve A-V conduction may be desirable.

Cardiac pacing in the diagnosis of abnormalities of rhythm and conduction

Introduction

The use of cardiac pacing for the diagnosis of various abnormalities of rhythm and conduction is now well established as an important clinical technique. Most of these pacing techniques are applied during cardiac catheterization in which one or more electrode catheters are introduced pervenously using standard techniques and placed in selected regions of the heart (the high right atrium, the coronary sinus, the His bundle recording position along the posterior leaflet of the tricuspid valve, and the right ventricle) [9] for purposes of pacing the heart and/or recording local electrograms. In addition, it is not uncommon to place an electrode catheter selectively in the left ventricle (primarily for studies of ventricular tachycardia), and in the right pulmonary artery to record from the superior left atrium [14–17]. Cardiac pacing and/or recording also can be performed using stainless steel wire electrodes temporarily placed epicardially on the atria and ventricles at the time of open heart surgery [3, 5, 7]. Also, through the use of newly developed, programmable pacemaker systems, permanently placed epicardial or endocardial electrodes also may be used to study abnormalities of rhythm and conduction.

Assessment of sinus node function

Overdrive atrial pacing for the assessment of sinus node recovery time
Because sinus rhythm results from an automatic mechanism, atrial pacing at rates faster than the

intrinsic rate of the sinus node should suppress the sinus node pacemaker. Therefore, following abrupt termination of atrial pacing, the first sinus beat should appear after an interval which is longer than the sinus cycle length prior to the onset of pacing, i.e., abrupt termination of pacing should result in a period of overdrive suppression. The latter is then followed by a period during which the sinus cycle length shortens until it returns to its prepacing interval. This period is variable in duration, and frequently includes a period during which the sinus cycle length transiently becomes shorter than its prepacing cycle length [24]. These responses have been applied clinically in a studied fashion to assess sinus node function [72–75].

Atrial pacing should be performed in the absence of all cardioactive drugs or any medications known to affect sinus node function or autonomic tone. The atria should be paced at selected rates generally beginning 10–20 beats/min faster than the spontaneous sinus rate. Pacing is continued for at least 15 sec and sometimes for as long as 2 min. The duration of pacing is only important in the assessment of sinus node function if prolonged pacing at a rapid rate causes hypotension with a resultant reflex increase in sympathetic tone, or if the pacing period is too short (less than 15 sec) [76]. Therefore, the atria are generally paced for periods of 15–30 sec followed by abrupt cessation of pacing. This pacing procedure is repeated, increasing the rate by

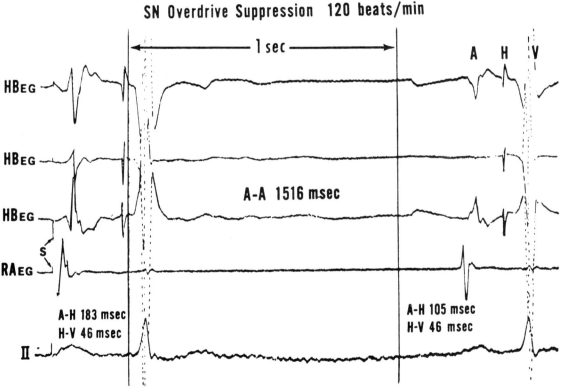

Figure 23. This record was recorded from a patient during a study of sinus node function using the technique of overdrive suppression. A tripolar electrode catheter was used to record electrograms from the region of the His bundle. Using a simple junction box, each of the electrodes was connected to the other such that three bipolar electrograms were recorded. The fourth trace represents a bipolar atrial electrogram recorded from the mid-portion of the right atrium. The fifth trace is ECG lead II. The first beat in this figure is the last beat of 30 sec of atrial pacing at a rate of 120 beats/min. The subsequent beat is the first spontaneous sinus beat which follows the abrupt termination of the atrial pacing. The sinus escape interval, in this instance measured from the atrial electrogram recorded during the last paced atrial beat to the atrial electrogram recorded during the first spontaneous sinus beat, was 1,516 msec. In this patient, the cycle length during the spontaneous rhythm was 1,245 msec. Thus, the corrected sinus node recovery time is normal at 271 msec. This sinus escape interval represents 126% of the basic sinus cycle length, also normal (from Waldo et al. Ala J Med Sci 11:120–128, 1974 with permission).

increments of 10–20 beats/min as the clinical state will permit until a rate of at least 130 beats/min and preferably 170 beats/min has been reached. Between each period of pacing, an interval of at least 60 sec should be allowed to elapse.

Sinus node recovery time (SNRT) is determined for each pacing period by measuring the interval from the last paced atrial beat to the first spontaneous sinus beat (Figure 23). This interval is then corrected (CSNRT) for rate by subtracting the spontaneous sinus cycle length (SCL) which was present prior to pacing from the actual sinus node recovery time: CSNRT = SNRT – SCL. Values that exceed 525 msec are considered abnormal and values between 450–525 msec may also be abnormal [74]. Additionally, the corrected sinus node recovery time may be expressed as a percentage of the sinus cycle length: $\text{CSNRT} = \dfrac{\text{SNRT}}{\text{SCL}} \times 100$ in which case values greater than 130% are considered abnormal [72].

In some patients with sinus node dysfunction, the abnormal response following termination of overdrive pacing is manifest by a so-called secondary

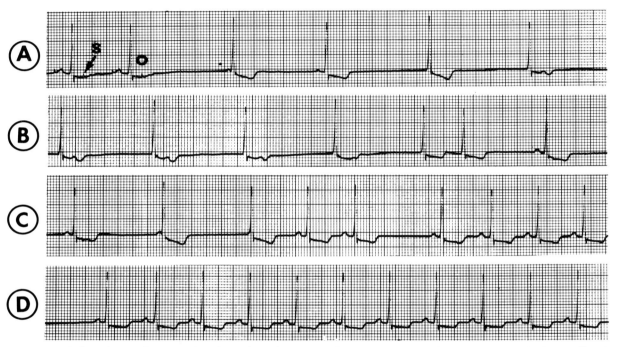

Figure 24. This figure is taken from a portion of an atrial pacing study performed because the patient's spontaneous rhythm manifested occasional periods of asystole which were as long as three seconds. During the atrial pacing study, pacing at rates at or above 120 beats/min resulted in 2:1 A-V conduction (abnormal). Panels A through D are continuous traces of ECG lead I following the the abrupt termination (circle) of 30 sec of atrial pacing at a rate of 150 beats/min. The interval from the last paced atrial beat to the first spontaneous atrial beat (sinus node recovery time) is about 1,130 msec. Because the spontaneous sinus rate was 93 beats/min (645 msec), the corrected sinus node recovery time is 485 msec and is probably abnormal. However, the subsequent so-called secondary pauses are clearly abnormal and document the presence of sinus node dysfunction. Note that the interval between the first and second spontaneous sinus beat is somewhat longer than the interval between the last paced atrial beat and the first spontaneous beat. With the slowing of the sinus rate, the patient develops a spontaneous A-V junctional rhythm at a rate of about 47 beats/min (panels A and B) with A-V dissociation. The latter is present as evidenced by the appearance of sinus P waves which progressively march through the QRS complex, S–T segment, and T wave of subsequent A-V junctional beats (panels A and B) until with the sixth QRS complex in panel B, an atrial capture beat occurs. The second and third QRS complexes in panel C represent A-V junctional escape beats, following which, despite two subsequent pauses (panels C and D), sinus rhythm resumes at its prior rate of 93 beats/min. Note that the P–P intervals in panel B and the first portion, i.e., the first three P waves, in panel C are twice the spontaneous sinus cycle length (panel D). Thus, the apparent sinus bradycardia (panels A, B, and C) and sinus pauses (panels C and D) may result from sinus node exit block. In fact, the apparent sinus node exit block makes evaluation of sinus node recovery time problematical. In sum, the atrial pacing study in this patient demonstrated both sinus node dysfunction and A-V conduction abnormalities, both manifestations of the sick sinus syndrome: S = stimulus artifact (from [3] with permission).

pause (Figure 24). In these patients, the first spontaneous beat may have a normal corrected sinus node recovery time, but subsequent sinus beats may then display abnormally prolonged cycle lengths [77]. In fact, these secondary pauses may be so marked that a sinus rhythm does not become evident for many beats (Figure 24).

Introduction of premature atrial beats and overdrive atrial pacing to evaluate sinoatrial conduction time

Sinoatrial conduction time is the time required for the sinus impulse to exit from the sinus node and initiate atrial excitation. A prolonged sinoatrial

conduction time may be associated with the sick sinus syndrome. The current established method for measuring sinoatrial conduction time is indirect and, therefore, of limited accuracy [78, 79]. The recording of sinus node electrograms may be more satisfactory. The current method uses a spontaneous or induced premature atrial beat during which there is sinus node reset [80]. The interval that follows the premature atrial beat is assumed to include the time for conduction of the premature atrial beat into the sinus node and the basic sinus cycle length. It also assumes there has been no overdrive suppression. Figure 25 shows the various types of responses of the sinus node to premature

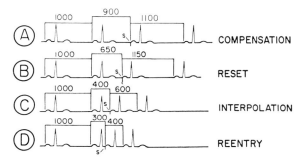

Figure 25. Responses of the sinus node to premature atrial beats. In this example, the premature atrial beats are induced by pacing stimuli (S) introduced at selected intervals during a regular sinus rhythm whose cycle length is 1,000 msec. Panel A shows an example of a *compensatory pause* in response to a late premature atrial beat, in this instance introduced at a coupling interval of 900 msec. The premature atrial beat is so late that it does not enter and depolarize the sinus node, but it does prevent the next sinus beat from capturing the atria. However, because the sinus node keeps firing at its basic cycle length of 1,000 msec, the subsequent sinus beat occurs at its expected time, in this instance 1,100 msec after the premature atrial beat, or two sinus cycles from the sinus beat which preceded the premature atrial beat (900 msec + 1,100 msec = 2,000 msec, i.e., two sinus cycle lengths). Panel B shows an example of *sinus node reset* following a premature atrial beat, in this instance introduced at a coupling interval of 650 msec. The sinus beat which follows the premature atrial beat occurs following an interval of 1,150 msec. Had the premature atrial beat not interfered in any way with the sinus cycle, the sinus beat which follows the premature atrial beat should have occurred at an interval of 1,350 msec, i.e., after a compensatory pause (650 msec + 1,350 msec = 2,000 msec). Note, however, that the two intervals add up to less than two sinus cycles (650 msec + 1,150 msec = 1,800 msec), indicating that the premature atrial beat entered and depolarized the sinus node and caused it to reset its cycle. The result is that the next spontaneous sinus beat occurs earlier than its normally expected time. These intervals can also be used to assess *sinoatrial con-

duction time,* assuming that when the premature atrial beat resets the sinus pacemaker, it does not also produce any overdrive suppression of the sinus pacemaker. When the regular sinus cycle length (1,000 msec) is subtracted from the interval from the premature atrial beat to the subsequent sinus beat (1,150 msec), the difference (150 msec) reflects the total time it takes the premature atrial beat to enter the sinus node and reset the sinus pacemaker, and the subsequent sinus beat to exit the sinus node and excite the atria. Assuming conduction time into the sinus node is identical to conduction time out of the sinus node, one can determine the sinoatrial conduction time simply by dividing the above difference by two. In this example, the sinoatrial conduction time is 75 msec

$$\frac{1,150 \text{ msec} - 1,000 \text{ msec}}{2} = 75 \text{ msec}$$

The range of normal sinoatrial conduction time in humans is uncertain, but the upper limit of normal may be as high as 120 msec. Panel C shows an example of *interpolation* of an early premature atrial beat, in this instance introduced at a coupling interval of 400 msec. The sinus beat which follows the premature atrial beat occurs very early, only 600 msec after the premature atrial beat. The two intervals add up to a normal spontaneous sinus cycle (400 msec + 600 msec = 1,000 msec), indicating that the premature atrial beat neither entered and depolarized the sinus node nor affected exit of the sinus impulse from the sinus node. Thus, the premature atrial beat was interpolated between two normal sinus beats. Panel D shows an example of *sinus node reentry* produced by a very early premature atrial beat, in this instance introduced at a coupling interval of 300 msec. The premature atrial beat is followed after 400 msec by a spontaneous beat with a normal P wave. The two intervals add up to less than a normal spontaneous sinus cycle (300 msec + 400 msec = 700 msec). Therefore, the beat following the premature atrial beat could not have been a spontaneous pacemaker-induced sinus beat. In fact, it represents a sinus node reentrant beat which presumably uses the perinodal fibers as an important part of the reentry circuit (modified after Jordan et al. In: Bonke FIM (ed) The Sinus Node, Structure, Functional and Clinical Relevance. Martinus Nijhoff, The Hague, 1978, p 11 with permission).

atrial beats and the figure legend explains the calculation of the sinoatrial conduction time. The upper limits of normal sinoatrial conduction time calculated using this technique are uncertain, estimates ranging from 80–120 msec.

Another method of calculating sinoatrial conduction time has been proposed by Narula et al. [81] and may prove to be the most useful. This technique uses overdrive atrial pacing for a train of eight beats at a rate of 10 beats/min faster than the patient's spontaneous sinus rate. The interval from the last paced beat to the first spontaneous sinus beat reflected by the atrial electrogram recorded at the pacing site is considered to be the total time for retrograde and antegrade conduction time. At this pacing rate, the sinus node pacemaker does not appear to be suppressed detectably, if at all, and no apparent shift in the pacemaker site has been appreciated following cessation of pacing, both limitations of other techniques of assessing sinoatrial conduction time. Furthermore, the technique offers the advantage of ease of application of the pacing technique and ease of measurement of the data.

Limitations

Unfortunately, studies of sinus node recovery time and sinoatrial conduction time when used to assess sinus node function may yield normal results despite the clinically demonstrable presence of sinus node dysfunction. In addition, when these studies do yield an abnormal result, it usually is in patients who already have demonstrated evidence of significant sinus node dysfunction spontaneously, as in 24-hr Holter monitor recordings. Thus, it is reasonable to state that these techniques are of limited clinical utility. However, when they reveal abnormalities not otherwise apparent, they are helpful. In addition, these techniques are still being refined, particularly in association with the administration of autonomic blocking agents [82], such that there is the promise that they will have greater sensitivity and specificity in the near future. The use of the recently described technique of recording extracellular sinus node electrograms [83–85] still requires evaluation.

Finally, it should be stressed that, for all studies that use atrial pacing to assess sinus node function, the role of the perinodal fibers is very important and not well understood. It is clear that the perinodal fibers act in a manner analogous to the way in which the A-V node acts, i.e., they manifest a marked delay in recovery of excitability following repolarization and also serve as a site of normal conduction delay or block propagation of ectopic impulses into the sinus node [86]. Thus, this tissue normally functions to limit depolarization of the sinus node, and if this tissue is in itself abnormal, it is unclear how this might affect the response to various pacing techniques.

Assessment of A-V conduction

There is a limited role for cardiac pacing in the assessment of A-V conduction. As indicated elsewhere in this chapter, the development of A-V block in which a beat is blocked distal to the His bundle recording site (i.e., each atrial beat is conducted through the A-V node to the His bundle, but block of one a more of these beats then occurs in the specialized A-V conduction system, presumably in the distal His bundle or at the bifurcation of the left and right bundle branches) is an indication of serious A-V conduction disease and appears to be an indication for placement of a permanent ventricular pacemaker [59].

There are times when it may be difficult to distinguish first-degree A-V block on the basis of an A-V conduction abnormality or on the basis of an internodal abnormality (i.e., prolonged conduction time between the sinus node and the A-V node). In such circumstances, atrial pacing may be quite useful. If the prolonged P–R interval is due to internodal conduction delay, then atrial pacing at progressively faster rates should affect A-V conduction in a normal fashion. Thus, A-V nodal Wenckebach periodicity should develop at the expected range of pacing rates, the lower limit of which is about 130 beats/min in adults. However, if the prolonged P–R interval is due to A-V nodal disease, A-V nodal Wenckebach periodicity and even 2:1 A-V conduction will develop at relatively slow atrial pacing rates.

Deliberate precipitation of arrhythmias to establish arrhythmia diagnosis, to characterize the arrhythmias, and to establish efficacy of various therapeutic interventions

Pacing studies to establish arrhythmia diagnosis

Overdrive atrial pacing. On occasion, simple overdrive atrial pacing at selected rates may be very useful in establishing the diagnosis of an arrhythmia that is only suspected. For instance, for the patient in whom the Wolff-Parkinson-White syndrome is suspected but not demonstrated, this technique may be effective. It is well known that the diagnostic electrocardiographic manifestations of the Wolff-Parkinson-White syndrome, i.e., a short P–R interval (<0.12 sec) associated with a delta wave in the QRS complex, are not always present and the only clinical indication of the presence of Wolff-Parkinson-White syndrome may be a history of recurrent tachyarrhythmia. Cardiac electrophysiological studies that use atrial pacing may establish the diagnosis. The technique takes advantage of the normal prolongation of A-V nodal conduction time that occurs during overdrive atrial pacing when the atrial pacing rate is increased [87].

In the occasional patient in whom the Wolff-Parkinson-White syndrome is suspected, and in whom a delta wave is not present in the ECG during sinus rhythm, the following methods can be employed. An electrode catheter is placed in the His bundle recording position, and a His bundle electrogram and as many ECG leads as possible are recorded simultaneously during the spontaneous sinus rhythm. The atria then are paced, usually via another electrode catheter introduced into the right atrium. Atrial capture is obtained at a rate just faster than the spontaneous rate. The atrial pacing rate then is increased by increments of 5–10 beats/min until either a delta wave is recorded in the ECG, or a manifestation of second degree A-V block is achieved. Since A-V nodal conduction time will prolong progressively with increasing rate, the A–H interval will progressively increase as the atrial pac-

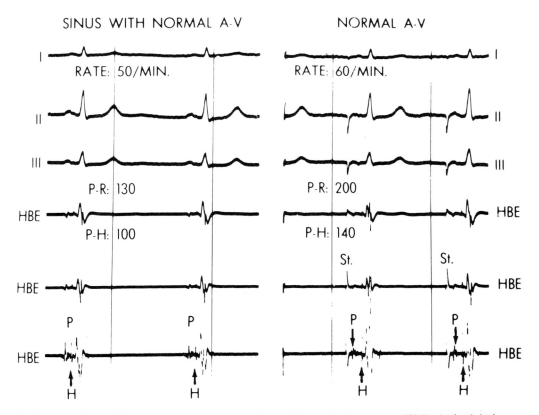

Figure 26. ECG leads I, II, and III recorded simultaneously with the His bundle electrogram (HBE) obtained during spontaneous bradycardia at a rate of 50 beats/min (left panel) and during atrial pacing at a rate of 60 beats/min (right panel). Note that no delta wave is apparent in the ECG leads in either panel. Note also that the P–R interval prolongs from 130 to 200 msec simply on increasing the rate by 10 beats/min with atrial pacing. Note also that the P–H interval prolongs, reflecting an increase in A-V nodal conduction time: P = P wave; H = His bundle deflection; St = stimulus artifact. Time lines are at 1-sec intervals. All intervals are expressed in msec (from Castellanos et al. Circulation 41:399–411, 1970 with permission).

327

ing rate is increased. This usually will permit more and more of the ventricles to be activated via the A-V bypass pathway, thereby eliciting the clear or clearer appearance of a delta wave in the ECG (Figures 26 and 27). It should be noted that recording the His bundle electrogram is not always necessary for this technique, although it is desirable.

Overdrive atrial pacing also may be useful in establishing the diagnosis of paroxysmal atrial tachycardia, whether of the intra A-V nodal or the A-V bypass pathway reentrant type. Although this is not the most common way to precipitate paroxysmal atrial tachycardia, it certainly is one of the effective ways of doing this, particularly when the only pacemaker available is one capable only of pacing asynchronously at constant cycle lengths. More often, techniques that employ introduction of premature atrial and/or ventricular beats alone or in pairs during a complete cardiac electrophysiological study (programmed cardiac pacing) provide more information for characterization of the various components of the reentrant pathway.

Overdrive atrial pacing at very rapid rates, in the range of 240–340 beats/min, on occasion may be useful in attempts to precipitate atrial flutter in patients who are suspected of having this arrhythmia, but in whom it has not been documented. Unfortunately, the specificity and sensitivity of this test to induce atrial flutter are not known. Also, as indicated earlier, overdrive atrial pacing may be required to distinguish Type I from Type II atrial flutter when the atrial rate is in the range of 340–360 beats/min [3, 7, 43]. Finally, it is not clear what role, if any, overdrive atrial pacing plays in estab-

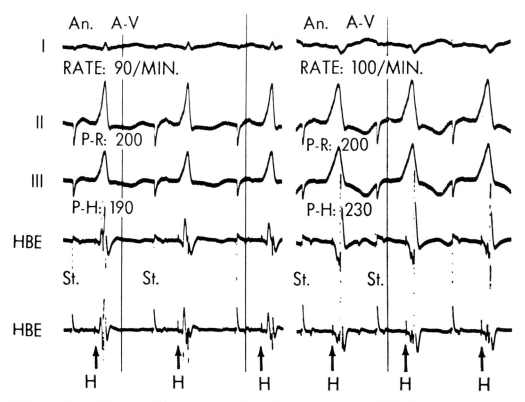

Figure 27. ECG leads I, II, and III recorded simultaneously with the His bundle electrogram (HBE) in the same patient as in Figure 26 during atrial pacing at a rate of 90 beats/min (left panel) and 100 beats/min (right panel). Despite the fact that the P–R interval remained 200 msec, note that the P–H interval prolonged with each increase in the pacing rate. Note the appearance of the delta wave in both panels, the delta wave being more prominent in the right panel than the left panel. Thus, as A-V nodal conduction time prolonged, as evidenced by prolongation of the P–H interval, antegrade conduction over an accessory A-V bypass pathway became apparent, and was more apparent at the faster pacing rate. In fact, in the right panel, the His bundle deflections appear after the onset of the QRS complex, i.e., after the onset of ventricular activation: H = His bundle deflection; St = stimulus artifact; An. A-V = anomalous A-V conduction. Time lines are at 1-sec intervals. All intervals are in msec (from Castellanos et al. Circulation 41:399–411, 1970 with permission).

lishing the diagnosis of rhythms suspected to be sinus node reentry, ectopic atrial tachycardia, or atrial fibrillation.

Introduction of premature atrial beats. This technique is useful primarily in efforts to precipitate paroxysmal atrial tachycardia. As discussed earlier, this technique is employed during programmed cardiac pacing studies and involves introduction of premature atrial beats at selected intervals from selected atrial sites (usually the high right atrium and/or coronary sinus, although other sites may also be selected) in an effort to precipitate a tachyarrhythmia. The technique usually is quite effective in provoking a tachyarrhythmia in patients whose underlying arrhythmia is paroxysmal atrial tachycardia, whether it is the A-V nodal reentrant type or the type using an A-V bypass pathway (Figure 5). Also, the introduction of premature atrial beats should precipitate sinus node reentrant rhythms in patients in whom this is the underlying tachyarrhythmia, although this rhythm is quite difficult to diagnose with confidence [88]. It should be emphasized that premature atrial beats can precipitate ventricular tachycardia [89, 90], and one must always be aware of this possibility.

Premature atrial beats may be used to induce atrial flutter, but most studies suggest that it is quite difficult to precipitate atrial flutter in this manner in patients in whom this is the underlying tachyarrhythmia [10–13]. The role of induced premature atrial beats in patients whose underlying disease may be one form of ectopic atrial tachycardia or atrial fibrillation is unclear.

Overdrive ventricular pacing. Overdrive ventricular pacing is a technique that can be used in an attempt to precipitate ventricular tachycardia and usually is part of a programmed cardiac pacing study. Pacing is performed in bursts beginning at rates of 10–20 beats/min faster than the spontaneous rate. The pacing stimulus strength is usually twice diastolic threshold. The duration of the pacing bursts largely depends on the pacing rate, the hemodynamic status of the patient and the laboratory performing the study. Usually, pacing lasts no longer than 10–20 beats at each rate, and may be as short as 5–10 beats at the very rapid pacing rates. The upper limit of pacing rates is somewhat controversial, although most now suggest that pacing

should be performed until either ventricular tachycardia is precipitated, or 2:1 ventricular capture at twice diastolic threshold is obtained. The pacing usually is initiated in the right ventricle. When pacing from the initial site in the right ventricle does not start a ventricular tachycardia, it is recommended that pacing be performed from several additional sites. If pacing still does not evoke ventricular tachycardia, and ventricular tachycardia still is suspected as the underlying tachyarrhythmia, it is recommended that the pacing procedures be repeated with the electrode in the left ventricle.

It should be recognized that, on occasion, particularly in patients who have an A-V bypass pathway (manifest or concealed), rapid ventricular pacing may produce paroxysmal atrial tachycardia. This serves to underscore the need in virtually all instances to perform diagnostic studies during cardiac catheterization employing formal programmed cardiac pacing.

Introduction of ventricular premature beats. This technique is used primarily in attempts to precipitate ventricular tachycardia. Premature ventricular beats at twice stimulus threshold are introduced to scan ventricular diastole during a spontaneous sinus rhythm, during atrial pacing at selected rates and during right and, if necessary, left ventricular pacing at selected rates. In each instance, the premature beat or beats are introduced following a train of at least eight paced beats at a constant cycle length or a train of eight spontaneous beats. When ventricular tachycardia is not precipitated by single premature ventricular beats that have scanned the diastolic interval until the effective refractory period has been reached, a second premature beat and, if necessary, a third premature ventricular beat also should be introduced at selected intervals scanning diastole once again. When a second premature ventricular beat is to be introduced, the first premature beat should be delivered at a constant interval just longer (5–20 msec) than its effective refractory period at that site. When three premature beats are to be delivered, the first and the second premature beats should be introduced at constant cycle lengths just longer (5–20 msec) than the cycle length for the effective refractory period of each of those beats at that pacing site. When neither introduction of premature ventricular beats nor rapid ventricular pacing precipitates ventricular tachycardia in patients

329

in whom this rhythm is suspected, the pacing site should be changed and the study repeated. If pacing from at least two sites (usually the apex and outflow tract) in the right ventricle does not produce the arrhythmia, the pacing should be repeated from the left ventricle.

It is important to note that introduction of premature ventricular beats also may precipitate paroxysmal atrial tachycardia, particularly in patients with an A-V bypass pathway. Often a single premature ventricular beat will produce such an arrhythmia, but it is not at all uncommon that two premature ventricular beats are required to precipitate the arrhythmia. In fact, in patients in whom the A-V bypass pathway type of paroxysmal atrial tachycardia is suspected and in whom premature atrial beats at selected intervals have failed to precipitate the tachycardia, the introduction of premature ventricular beats at selected intervals, either alone or in pairs, is indicated in an effort to precipitate the tachyarrhythmia.

Pacing studies to characterize known arrhythmias

Introduction. In some patients, particularly those with tachyarrhythmias resistant to empirical drug therapy, it is useful and often imperative to study the tachycardia and its response to drugs using invasive electrophysiological techniques. When this clinical situation occurs, the standard techniques of clinical cardiac electrophysiological studies described above should be used to study the mode of initiation and termination of the tachycardia and the sequence of atrial activation during the tachycardia. This should permit several questions to be answered: (a) What is the mechanism of the tachycardia (within the limitations previously discussed); (b) What is the site or region of origin of the tachycardia, and, if the tachycardia is reentrant, what are the components and characteristics of the reentry loop; (c) What are effective treatment modes?

Paroxysmal atrial tachycardia. This arrhythmia generally is acknowledged to be reentrant, due either to intra A-V nodal reentry, or reentry via a pathway in which antegrade A-V conduction occurs over the A-V node-His-Purkinje system, and retrograde A-V conduction occurs via an A-V bypass pathway (manifest, as in the Wolff-Parkinson-White syndrome, or concealed, as in the presence of

an A-V bypass pathway that only can conduct in a retrograde direction). A standard study includes programmed cardiac pacing of both the atria and ventricles to characterize: (a) the onset of the arrhythmia; (b) the width of the window for precipitation of the arrhythmia; (c) the sequence of atrial activation during the arrhythmia; (d) the nature of A-V nodal conduction at the onset of the arrhythmia; (e) the ability to preexcite the atria with a premature ventricular beat delivered after antegrade His bundle activation but before antegrade ventricular activation (i.e., a premature ventricular beat delivered during the H–V interval). These studies should differentiate the A-V nodal from the A-V bypass pathway type of paroxysmal atrial tachycardia.

The following criteria suggest that the paroxysmal atrial tachycardia circuit includes ventriculo-atrial activation via an A-V bypass pathway (manifest or concealed) [8, 25, 91]: (a) eccentric retrograde atrial activation (Figure 28); (b) early atrial activation following a premature ventricular beat delivered during the refractory period of the His bundle, i.e., during the H–V interval, with the atrial activation demonstrating the same relative sequence as during the spontaneous tachycardia; (c) slowing of the tachycardia rate and development of a longer retrograde V-A conduction time with the development of a bundle branch block (indicating that the A-V bypass pathway is on the same side as the 'blocked' bundle branch); (d) prolongation of the H–A interval with prolongation of the H–V interval. A very short V–A interval (<60 msec) and the sudden increase in the A–H interval following introduction of a premature beat which finally initiates the tachycardia are criteria for establishing the tachyarrhythmia as being of the A-V nodal reentrant type [92]. On occasion, the distinction between these two mechanisms can be very difficult.

Ventricular tachycardia. Through the use of programmed cardiac pacing [93], one can determine: (a) whether and how easily the arrhythmia can be started (i.e., following single, double, or triple premature ventricular beats or with rapid ventricular pacing); (b) what is the rate of the tachycardia, and how stable is it once it occurs; (c) what is the response of the tachycardia to overdrive or underdrive atrial or ventricular pacing or to introduction

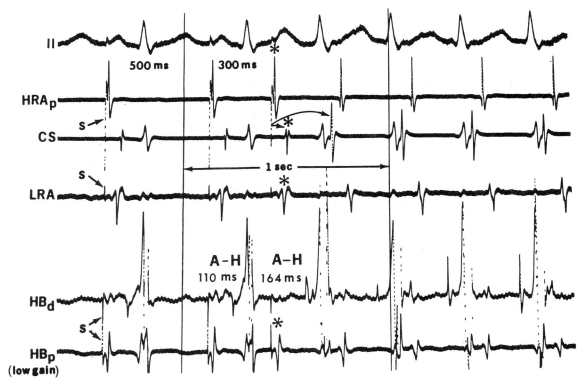

Figure 28. ECG lead II recorded simultaneously with bipolar electrograms from the proximal pair of the electrode catheter placed in the high right atrium (HRA$_p$), the coronary sinus (CS), the low lateral right atrium (LRA), the distal pair (HB$_d$) and proximal pair (HB$_p$) of electrodes of the tripolar catheter placed in the His bundle position in the same patient as in Figure 5. The first two beats in this figure are the last two beats of a train of eight paced atrial beats at a cycle length of 500 msec. The atria are being paced from the distal pair of the high right atrial catheter electrode. The third beat is a premature atrial beat introduced at an interval (S$_1$–S$_2$ interval) of 300 msec following the previous beat. This premature atrial beat then precipitates paroxysmal atrial tachycardia. The asterisks indicate capture at each atrial recording site which results from the premature atrial stimulus. However, as indicated by the arrows in the coronary sinus recording site, the premature atrial stimulus results in activation of this site twice. Initially, the coronary sinus site is activated in the normal direction by the pacing-induced premature atrial beat (asterisk). However, this premature atrial beat is conducted through the A-V node with delay, as evidenced by prolongation of the A–H interval from 110 msec during the train of eight paced atrial beats to 164 msec with the premature atrial beat. The orthodromic wavefront of the premature atrial beat continues down the His-Purkinje system to activate the ventricles. Because the delay in A-V nodal conduction permits recovery of excitability of the A-V bypass pathway and the atria, the orthodromic wavefront of the premature atrial beat continues from the ventricles over the A-V bypass pathway, resulting in retrograde activation of the atria. The first atrial site activated is the coronary sinus site, indicating an ectopic locus of retrograde atrial activation, and documenting the presence of a left sided A-V bypass pathway: S = stimulus artifact; H = His bundle electrogram. Time lines are at 1-sec intervals.

of premature ventricular beats (alone or in pairs) delivered at selected intervals. All these factors are important in guiding therapy and in the subsequent assessment of the efficacy of that therapy. The techniques utilized to characterize the nature of the arrhythmia are as described earlier.

Wolff-Parkinson-White syndrome. Several aspects of pacing in the study of this syndrome have already been discussed. Perhaps the most important is identification of patients with this syndrome who are

high at risk for the development of life-threatening arrhythmias. The reason arrhythmias may be life threatening in these patients is related primarily to the actual or potential ability of the A-V bypass pathway to conduct impulses rapidly from the atria to the ventricles during supraventricular arrhythmias such as atrial fibrillation, atrial flutter, or ectopic atrial tachycardia (Figure 29).

The most common arrhythmia in patients with this syndrome is paroxysmal atrial tachycardia, followed in frequency by atrial fibrillation and ven-

ECG Monitor Strip

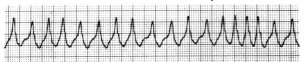

Figure 29. ECG lead recorded from a patient with Type A Wolff-Parkinson-White syndrome during an episode of atrial fibrillation. Note that QRS complexes are all wide, but the ventricular rate is very rapid (about 200 beats/min), and that there are cycle lengths as short as 200 msec (from Schwartz et al. In: Rackley CE (ed) Critical Care Cardiology. F. A. Davis, New York, 1981, pp 25–48 with permission).

tricular fibrillation [94, 95]. Atrial fibrillation resulted in ventricular fibrillation in 28% of the cases in one series [95]. Ventricular fibrillation may present as the first and only manifestation of this syndrome or follow atrial fibrillation with a rapid ventricular response, especially with the injudicious use of digitalis to control the ventricular response to atrial fibrillation. Therefore, it becomes very important to determine the effective refractory period of the A-V bypass pathway at the time of cardiac electrophysiological study and to pace the atria rapidly, even to atrial fibrillation, to determine the nature of antegrade A-V conduction over this pathway. This should demonstrate or predict who is at risk for the development of clinically unacceptable ventricular response rates to atrial fibrillation, atrial flutter, and ectopic atrial tachycardia [96]. Appropriate therapy would critically depend on this demonstration.

Other arrhythmias. It is often difficult to characterize other arrhythmias using the various pacing techniques because their initiation by these techniques is unpredictable at best. Rhythms such as atrial fibrillation, atrial flutter, and ectopic atrial tachycardia fall into this category. However, some arrhythmias, especially ectopic automatic atrial tachycardias may be identified and characterized by programmed cardiac pacing studies.

Pacing studies in the evaluation of antiarrhythmic therapy

Programmed cardiac pacing seems particularly useful in determining the efficacy of antiarrhythmic therapy and is becoming a standard way to test the efficacy of drug therapy, surgical therapy, and pacemaker therapy of cardiac arrhythmias [97, 98]. Once the characteristics of an arrhythmia have been

established and, in particular, once it is known that the arrhythmia can be initiated predictably with various pacing techniques, the effects of the therapeutic intervention in preventing precipitation of the arrhythmia by pacing can be studied systematically. This is particularly valuable in patients in whom the arrhythmia had previously been treated empirically, but in whom treatment has been unsuccessful. There are now numerous studies which suggest, particularly in patients with life-threatening ventricular arrhythmias, that this form of evaluation often provides the best means of assessing efficacy of most antiarrhythmic agents [97–99]. Thus, although administration of a standard drug such as quinidine may ostensibly suppress spontaneous premature ventricular beats, programmed cardiac pacing studies may demonstrate that the patient still is at risk for ventricular tachycardia and changes in the therapeutic regimen may be required. However, this does not seem to be true in all circumstances, the most obvious being the administration of a new drug, amiodarone, an agent that is still investigational in the United States. This drug seems to be highly effective clinically in the treatment of ventricular tachycardia in a large number of patients (who are often resistant to other antiarrhythmic drugs), yet when these patients are tested with various pacing techniques, the arrhythmia still can be precipitated. Thus, it is clear we have more to learn about these techniques. Nevertheless, for drugs such as quinidine, procainamide, disopyramide, phenytoin, and, in fact, most of the antiarrhythmic agents now under investigation, it appears that the ability to precipitate a tachycardia such as ventricular tachycardia or paroxysmal atrial tachycardia in a patient receiving these drugs indicates that the patient remains at risk to develop the arrhythmia spontaneously. Thus, this form of pacing seems highly important in determining efficacy of drug treatment. For both the above examples, i.e., ventricular tachycardia and A-V bypass pathway-type paroxysmal atrial tachycardia, and, in fact, for recalcitrant A-V nodal reentrant tachycardia, surgical techniques and pacing techniques may be required to treat these arrhythmias should drug therapy fail.

With the advent of surgical techniques to treat cardiac arrhythmias (see Chapter 10) such as ventricular tachycardia, paroxysmal atrial tachycardia, and the Wolff-Parkinson-White syndrome, once again, the efficacy of the treatment should be tested postoperatively with programmed cardiac pacing. Finally, the new so-called 'antitachycardia' pacemaker systems now under development and undergoing clinical trials afford yet another indication for pacing studies to evaluate therapeutic efficacy. In these instances, the tachycardia is deliberately provoked after the pacemaker system has been placed to ensure effectiveness of the therapy even though this has been demonstrated by a prior study using an equivalent temporary pacemaker system [7].

Conclusion

The applications of cardiac pacing to the understanding, diagnosis, and treatment of disorders of rhythm and conduction are myriad. Clearly, pacing is one of the important tools for providing improved patient care and for understanding the basis for rhythm disturbances.

Acknowledgment

This project was supported in part by USPHS NHLBI Program Project Grant HL 11310 and SCOR on Ischemic Heart Disease Grant 1P17HL17667 and by a Grant-in-Aid from the American Heart Association. Work performed in part during Dr. Waldo's tenure as the Otto G. Storm Established Investigator of the American Heart Association.

References

1. Zoll PM: The resuscitation of the heart in ventricular standstill by external electrical stimulation. N Engl J Med 247: 768–771, 1952.
2. Gallagher JJ, Smith WM, Kerr CR, Kasell J, Cook L, Reiter M, Sterba R, Harte M: Esophageal pacing: a diagnostic and therapeutic tool. Circulation 65:336–341, 1982.
3. Waldo AL, MacLean WAH: Diagnosis and Treatment of Cardiac Arrhythmias Following Open Heart Surgery. Emphasis on the Use of Atrial and Ventricular Epicardial Wire Electrodes. Futura Publ, Mt. Kisco, NY, 1980.
4. Maloney JD, Medina-Ravell V, Pieretti OH, Portillo B, Maduro C, Castellanos A, Berkovits B: Follow up assessment of dual-demand, dual chamber DVI-DVO pacing for automatic conversion, control and prevention of refractory paroxysmal supraventricular tachycardia. PACE 4:A–57,

5. Waldo AL, Krongrad E, Kupersmith J, Levine OR, Bowman FO Jr, Hoffman BF: Ventricular paired-pacing to control rapid ventricular heart rate following open heart surgery: observations on ectopic automaticity: report of a case in a four-month-old patient. Circulation 53:176–181, 1976.
6. Cooper TB, MacLean WAH, Waldo AL: Overdrive pacing for supraventricular tachycardia. A review of theoretical implications and therapeutic techniques. PACE 1:196–221, 1978.
7. Waldo AL, Wells JL Jr, Cooper TB, MacLean WAH: Temporary cardiac pacing. Applications and techniques in the treatment of cardiac arrhythmias. Prog Cardiovsc Dis 23:451–473, 1981.
8. Wellens HJJ: Value and limitations of programmed electrical stimulation of the heart in the study and treatment of tachycardias. Circulation 57:845–853, 1978.
9. Josephson ME, Seides SF: Clinical Cardiac Electrophysiology. Techniques and Interpretations. Lea and Febiger, Philadelphia, 1979.
10. Haft JI: Treatment of arrhythmias by intracardiac electrical stimulation. Prog Cardiovasc Dis 16:531–568, 1974.
11. Wellens HJJ: Electrical Stimulation of the Heart in the Study and Treatment of Tachycardia. Univ Park Press, Baltimore, 1971.
12. MacLean WAH, Karp RB, Kouchoukos NT, James TN, Waldo AL: Uniformly successful interruption of atrial flutter with rapid atrial pacing in 100 patients. Circulation 54:II–167, 1976 (abstract).
13. Watson RM, Josephson ME: Atrial flutter. Electrophysiological substrates and modes of initiation and termination. Am J Cardiol 45:732–741, 1980.
14. Puech P: L'Activité Électrique Auriculaire Normale et Pathologique. Masson and Cie, Paris 1956.
15. Amat-y-Leon F, Prakash D, Miller RH, Dhingra RC, Rosen K: A new approach for indirect recording of anterior left atrial activation in man. Am Heart J 93:408–410, 1977.
16. Ogawa S, Dreifus LS, Kitchen JG III, Shenoy PN, Osmick MJ: Catheter recordings of Bachmann's bundle activation from the right pulmonary artery: a new technique for mapping and study of supraventricular tachycardias. Am J Cardiol 41:1089–1096, 1978.
17. Cooper TB, Hageman GR, James TN, Waldo AL: Neural effects on sinus rate and A-V conduction produced by electrical stimulation from a transvenous electrode catheter in the canine right pulmonary artery. Circ Res 46:48–57, 1980.
18. Hoffman BF, Cranefield PF: The physiologic basis of cardiac arrhythmias. Am J Med 37: 670–684, 1964.
19. Cranefield PF, Wit AL, Hoffman BF: Genesis of cardiac arrhythmias. Circulation 47:190–201, 1973.
20. Wit AL, Fenoglio JJ Jr, Wagner BM, Bassett AL: Electrophysiological properties in the cardiac muscle in the anterior mitral valve leaflet and the adjacent atrium in the dog. Possible implications for the genesis of atrial dysrhythmias. Circ Res 32:731–745, 1973.
21. Bassett AL, Fenoglio JJ Jr, Wit AL, Myerburg RJ, Gelband H: Electrophysiologic and ultrastructural characteristics of the canine tricuspid valve. Am J Physiol 230:1366–1373, 1976.
22. Wit AL, Cranefield PF: Triggered and automatic activity in

the canine coronary sinus. Circ Res 41:435–445, 1977.

23. Wit AL, Fenoglio JJ Jr, Hordof AJ, Reemtsma K: Ultra-structure and transmembrane potentials of cardiac muscle in the human anterior mitral valve leaflet. Circulation 59: 1284–1292, 1979.

24. Vasalle M: The relationship among cardiac pacemakers. Overdrive suppression. Circ Res 41:269–277, 1977.

25. Barold SS, Coumel P: Mechanisms of the atrioventricular junctional tachycardia. Role of reentry and concealed accessory bypass tracts. Am J Cardiol 39:97–106, 1977.

26. Waldo AL, MacLean WAH, Karp RB, Kouchoukos NT, James TN: Entrainment and interruption of atrial flutter with atrial pacing: studies in man following open heart surgery. Circulation 56:737–745, 1977.

27. MacLean WAH, Plumb VJ, Waldo AL: Transient entrainment and interruption of ventricular tachycardia. PACE 4:358–366, 1981.

28. Plumb VJ, MacLean WAH, Cooper TB, James TN, Waldo AL: Atrial events during entrainment and interruption of atrial flutter by rapid atrial pacing. Circulation 60:II-64, 1979 (abstract).

29. Plumb VJ, James TN, Waldo AL: Evidence that atrial flutter is due to a circus movement with an excitable gap. Circulation 62:III-46, 1980 (abstract).

30. Waldo AL, Plumb VJ, Arciniegas JG, James TN: Transient entrainment and interruption of A-V bypass pathway type paroxysmal atrial tachycardia. A model for understanding and identifying reentrant arrhythmias. Circulation 67:73–83, 1983.

31. Henthorn RW, Plumb VJ, Arciniegas JG, Waldo AL: Entrainment of 'ectopic atrial tachycardia': evidence for re-entry. Am J Cardiol 49:920, 1982 (abstract).

32. Allessie MA, Bonke FIM, Schopman FJG: Circus movement in rabbit atrial muscle as a mechanism of tachycardia. III. The 'leading circle' concept: a new model of circus movement in cardiac tissue without the involvement of an anatomical obstacle. Circ Res 41:9–18, 1977.

33. Rosen MR, Reder RF: Does triggered activity have a role in the genesis of cardiac arrhythmias? Ann Intern Med 94: 794–801, 1981.

34. Cranefield PF: The Conduction of the Cardiac Impulse. Futura Publ, Mt. Kisco, NY, 1975.

35. Cranefield PF: Action potentials, afterpotentials, and arrhythmias. Circ Res 41:415–423, 1977.

36. Wit AL, Cranefield PF: Triggered activity in cardiac muscle fibers of the simian mitral valve. Circ Res 38:85–89, 1976.

37. Wit AL, Cranefield PF, Gadsby DC: Electrogenic sodium extrusion can stop triggered activity in the canine coronary sinus. Circ Res 49:1029–1042, 1981.

38. Rosen KM, Sinno MZ, Gunnar RM, Ruhimtoola SH: Failure of rapid atrial pacing in the conversion of atrial flutter. Am J Cardiol 29:524–528, 1972.

39. Inoue H, Matsuo H, Takayunagi K, Murao S: Clinical and experimental studies of the effects of atrial extrastimulation and rapid pacing on atrial flutter cycle. Evidence for macro-reentry with an excitable gap. Am J Cardiol 48:623–631, 1981.

40. Fisher JD, Kim SG, Furman S, Matos JA: Role of implantable pacemakers in control of recurrent ventricular tachycardia. Am J Cardiol 49:194–206, 1982.

41. Wellens HJJ, Brugada P, Vanagt EJDM, Ross DL, Barr FW: New studies with triggered automaticity. In: Harrison DC (ed) Cardiac Arrhythmias. A Decade of Progress. GK Hall Med Publ, Boston, 1981, pp 601–612.

42. Zipes DP: A defense of triggered automaticity. In Harrison DC (ed) Cardiac Arrhythmias. A Decade of Progress. GK Hall Med Publ, Boston, 1981, pp 591–599.

43. Wells JL Jr, MacLean WAH, James TN, Waldo AL: Characterization of atrial flutter. Studies in man after open heart surgery using fixed atrial electrodes. Circulation 60:665–673, 1979.

44. Waldo AL, Wells JL Jr, Plumb VJ, Cooper TB, MacLean WAH: Characterization of atrial flutter – studies in patients following open heart surgery. In: Narula OS (ed) Cardiac Arrhythmias. Mechanism, Diagnosis, Management. Williams and Wilkins, Baltimore, 1979, pp 256–271.

45. Waldo AL, MacLean WAH, Karp RB, Kouchoukos NT, James TN: Continuous rapid atrial pacing to control recurrent or sustained supraventricular tachycardias following open heart surgery. Circulation 54:245–250, 1976.

46. Langendorf R, Pick A: Observations on the clinical use of paired electrical stimulation of the heart. Bull NY Acad Med 41:535–540, 1965.

47. Lister JW, Damato AN, Kosowsky BD, Lau SH, Stein E: The hemodynamic effect of slowing the heart rate by paired or coupled stimulation of the atria. Am Heart J 73:362–368, 1967.

48. Krikler DM, Curry PVL: Torsade de pointes, an atypical ventricular tachycardia. Br Heart J 38:117–120, 1976.

49. Fisher JD, Mehra R, Furman S: Termination of ventricular tachycardia with bursts of ventricular pacing. Am J Cardiol 41: 94–102, 1978.

50. Wellens HJJ, Duren DR, Lie KI: Observations on mechanisms of ventricular tachycardia in man. Circulation 54: 237–244, 1976.

51. MacLean WAH, Cooper TB, James TN, Waldo AL: Entrainment and interruption of ventricular tachycardia by rapid atrial pacing in man. Clin Res 27:771A, 1979 (abstract).

52. Ferrer MI: The Sick Sinus Syndrome. Futura Publ, Mt. Kisco, NY, 1974.

53. Narula OS: Atrioventricular block. In: Narula OS (ed) Cardiac Arrhythmias. Electrophysiology, Diagnosis and Management, Williams and Wilkins, Baltimore, 1979, pp 85–110.

54. Langendorf R, Pick A: Atrioventricular block, Type II (Mobitz): its nature and clinical significance. Circulation 38: 819–821, 1968.

55. Dhingra RC, Wyndham C, Amat-y-Leon F, Denes P, Wu D, Sridhar S, Bustin AG, Rosen KM: Incidence and site of atrioventricular block in patients with chronic bifascicular block. Circulation 59:238–246, 1979.

56. Scheinman MM, Peters RW, Modin G, Brennan M, Mies C, O'Young J: Prognostic value of infranodal conduction time in patients with chronic bundle branch block. Circulation 56:240–244, 1977.

57. Kulbertus HE, de Leval-Rutten F, Du Bois M, Petit JM: Prognostic significance of left anterior hemiblock with right bundle branch block in mass screening. Am J Cardiol 41:385, 1978 (abstract).

58. McAnulty JH, Rahimtoola SH, Murphy ES, Kauffman S,

Ritzmann LW, Kanarek P, DeMots H: A prospective study of sudden death 'high-risk' bundle-branch block. N Engl J Med 299:209–215, 1978.

59. Dhingra RC, Wyndham C, Bauernfeind R, Swiryn S, Deedwania PC, Smith T, Denes P, Rosen KM: Significance of block distal to the His bundle induced by atrial pacing in patients with chronic bifascicular block. Circulation 60: 1455–1464, 1979.

60. Narula OS: Intraventricular conduction defects: current concepts and clinical significance. In: Narula OS (ed) Cardiac Arrhythmias. Electrophysiology, Diagnosis, and Management, Williams and Wilkins, Baltimore, 1979, pp 114–139.

61. Kupersmith J, Krongrad E, Waldo AL: Conduction intervals and conduction velocity in the human cardiac conduction system: studies during openheart surgery. Circulation 47:776–785, 1973.

62. Scheinman M, Peters R, Sauve MJ, Desai J, Cogan J, Wohl B: Graded influence of the H-V interval on the incidence of spontaneous infranodal block. Circulation 64:IV–144, 1981 (abstract).

63. Denes P, Dhingra RC, Wu D, Chuquimia R, Amat-y-Leon F, Wyndham C, Rosen KM: H-V interval in patients with bifascicular (right bundle branch block and left anterior hemiblock). Clinical, electrocardiographic, and electrophysiologic correlations. Am J Cardiol 35:23–29, 1975.

64. Dhingra RC, Denes P, Wu D, Chuquimia R, Amat-y-Leon F, Wyndham C, Rosen KM: Chronic right bundle branch block and left posterior hemiblock. Clinical, electrophysiologic and prognostic observations. Am J Cardiol 36:867–872, 1975.

65. Dhingra RC, Denes P, Wu D, Wyndham CR, Amat-y-Leon F, Towne WD, Rosen KM: Prospective observations in patients with chronic bundle branch block and marked H-V prolongation. Circulation 53:600–609, 1976.

66. Altschuler H, Fisher JD, Furman S: Significance of isolated H-V interval prolongation in symptomatic patients without documented heart block. Am Heart J 97:19–26, 1979.

67. Dhingra RC, Palileo E, Strasberg B, Swiryn S, Bauernfein RA, Wyndham CRC, Rosen KM: Significance of the HV interval in 517 patients with chronic bifascicular block. Circulation 64:1265–1271, 1981.

68. Atkins JM, Leshen SJ, Blomqvist G, Mullins CB: Ventricular conduction blocks and sudden death in acute myocardial infarction: potential indications for pacing. N Engl J Med 288:281–284, 1973.

69. Hindman MC, Wagner GS, JaRo M, Atkins JM, Scheinmann MM, DeSanctis RW, Hutter AH Jr, Yeatman L, Rubenfire M, Pujura C, Rubin M, Morris JJ: The clinical significance of bundle branch block complicating acute myocardial infarction. 2. Indications for temporary and permanent pacemaker insertion. Circulation 58:689–699, 1978.

70. Lie KI, Durrer D: Conduction disturbances in acute myocardial infarction. In: Narula OS (ed) Cardiac Arrhythmias. Electrophysiology, Diagnosis, and Management, Williams and Wilkins, Baltimore, 1979, pp 140–163.

71. Waldo AL, Kaiser GA, Bowman FO Jr, Malm JR: Etiology of prolongation of the P-R interval in patients with an endocardial cushion defect: further observations on internodal conduction and the polarity of retrograde P wave. Circulation 48:19–27, 1973.

72. Mandel W, Hayakawa H., Danzig R, Marcus HS: Evaluation of sino-atrial node function in man by overdrive suppression. Circulation 44:59–66, 1971.

73. Mandel WJ, Hayakawa H, Allen HN, Danzig R, Kermaier AI: Assessment of sinus node function in patients with the sick sinus syndrome. Circulation 46:761–769, 1972.

74. Narula OS, Samet P, Javier, RP: Significance of sinus-node recovery time. Circulation 45:140–158, 1972.

75. Strauss HC, Bigger JT Jr, Saroff AL, Giardina EV: Electrophysiologic evaluation of sinus node function in patients with sinus node dysfunction. Circulation 53:763–776, 1976.

76. Jordan J, Yamaguchi I, Mandel WJ, McCullen AE: Comparative effects of overdrive on sinus and subsidiary pacemaker function. Am Heart J 93:367–374, 1977.

77. Benditt DG, Strauss HC, Scheinman MM, Behard VF, Wallace AG: Analysis of secondary pauses following termination of rapid atrial pacing in man. Circulation 54:436–441, 1976.

78. Breithardt G, Seipel L, Loogen E: Sinus node recovery time in calculated sinoatrial conduction in normal subjects and patients with sinus node dysfunction. Circulation 56:43–50, 1977.

79. Miller HC, Strauss HC: Measurement of sinoatrial conduction time by premature atrial stimulation in the rabit. Circ Res 35:935–947, 1974.

80. Strauss HC, Saroff AL, Bigger JT Jr, Giardina EV: Premature atrial stimulation as a key to the understanding of sinoatrial conduction in man. Presentation of data and critical review of the literature. Circulation 47:86–93, 1973.

81. Narula OS, Shantha N, Vasquez M, Towne WD, Linhart JW: A new method for measurement of sinoatrial conduction time. Circulation 58:706–714, 1978.

82. Jose AD, Collison D: The normal range in determinants of the intrinsic heart rate in man. Cardiovasc Res 4:160–167, 1970.

83. Cramer M, Siegal M, Bigger JT Jr, Hoffman BF: Characteristics of extracellular potentials recorded from the sinoatrial pacemaker of the rabbit. Circ Res 41:292–300, 1977.

84. Hariman J, Krongrad H, Boxer RA, Weiss MB, Steeg CN, Hoffman BF: Method for recording electrical activity of the sinoatrial node and automatic atrial foci during cardiac catheterization in human subjects. Am J Cardiol 45:775–781, 1980.

85. Reiffel JA, Gang E, Gliklich J, Weiss MB, Davis JC, Patton JN, Bigger JT Jr: The human sinus node electrogram: a transvenous catheter technique and a comparison of directly measured and indirectly estimated sinoatrial conduction time in adults. Circulation 62:1324–1334, 1980.

86. Strauss HC, Bigger JT Jr: Electrophysiological properties of the rabbit's sinatrial perinodal fibers. Circ Res 37:490–506, 1972.

87. Lister JW, Stein E, Kosowsky BD, Lau SH, Damato AN: Atrioventricular conduction in man. Effect of rate, exercise, isoproterenol, and atropine on the P-R interval. Am J Cardiol 16:516–523, 1965.

88. Waldo AL, Cooper TB, MacLean WAH: Editorial: need for additional criteria for the diagnosis of sinus node reentrant tachycardias. J Electrocardiol 10:103–104, 1977.

89. Myerburg RJ, Sung RJ, Gerstenblith G, Mallon SM, Castellanos A, Lazzara R: Ventricular ectopic activity after premature atrial beats in acute myocardial infarction. Br Heart J 39:1033–1037, 1977.

90. Wellens, HJJ, Bar FW, Farre J, Ross DL, Weiner I, Vanagt EJ: Initiation and termination of ventricular tachycardia by supraventricular stimuli. Incidence and electrophysiologic determinants as observed during programmed stimulation of the heart. Am J Cardiol 46:576–582, 1980.

91. Josephson ME: Paroxysmal supraventricular tachycardia. An electrophysiological approach. Am J Cardiol 41:1123–1126, 1978.

92. Gallagher JJ, Smith WM, Kasell J, Smith WM, Grant AO, Benson DW Jr: Use of the esophageal lead in the diagnosis of mechanisms of reciprocating supraventricular tachycardia. PACE 3:440–451, 1980.

93. Josephson ME, Horowitz LN: Electrophysiologic approach to therapy of recurrent sustained ventricular tachycardia. Am J Cardiol 43:631–642, 1979.

94. Sherf L, Neufeld HN: Preexcitation Syndrome. Facts and Theories. Yorke Med Books, New York, 1978.

95. Gallagher JJ, Sealy WC, Pritchett ELC, Kasell J, Wallace AG: Wolff-Parkinson-White syndrome: experience with 83 patients. In: Kelly DT (ed) Advances in the Management of Arrhythmias. Telectronics, Pty, Ltd, New South Wales, Australia, 1978, pp 47–72.

96. Wellens HJJ, Durrer D: Wolff-Parkinson-White syndrome and atrial fibrillation. Relations between refractory period, accessory pathway, and ventricular rate during atrial fibrillation. Am J Cardiol 34:777–782, 1974.

97. Horowitz LN, Josephson ME, Kastor JA: Intracardiac electrophysiologic studies as a method for the optimization of drug therapy in chronic ventricular arrhythmia. Prog Cardiovasc Dis 23:81–98, 1980.

98. Fisher JD, Cohen HL, Mehra R, Altschuler H, Escher DJW, Furman S: Cardiac pacing and pacemakers. II. Serial electrophysiologic – pharmacologic testing for control of recurrent tachyarrhythmias. Am Heart J 93:658–668, 1977.

99. Ruskin JN, DiMarco JP, Garan H: Out-of-hospital cardiac arrest. Electrophysiologic observations and selection of long-term antiarrhythmic therapy. N Engl J Med 303:607–613, 1980.

CHAPTER 10

Surgical therapy of arrhythmias

MARK E. JOSEPHSON* and ALDEN H. HARKEN

Paroxysmal tachyarrhythmias, both supraventricular and ventricular, remain a difficult therapeutic
challenge to the physician. Despite the availability
of a multitude of antiarrhythmic agents and the
development of novel pacing techniques, in a significant number of patients these therapeutic modalities either are ineffective or induce unacceptable
side-effects. In such patients, surgery provides an
alternative method for treating disabling and/or
life-threatening arrhythmias.

The rationale for surgical intervention is the assumption that the mechanism for the tachyarrhythmia can be identified and/or its site of origin
or pathway can be localized to specific regions of
the heart. Such site(s) might then be removed,
transsected, excluded, or otherwise altered either to
prevent the occurrence of the arrhythmia or to eliminate its disabling consequences. The evolution of
such surgical techniques has been accomplished by
advances in the use of programmed stimulation of
the heart and activation mapping techniques in
both the clinical electrophysiology laboratory and
the operating room.

In the following pages we will review the surgical
procedures for the therapy of supraventricular tachycardias, particularly those associated with the
Wolff-Parkinson-White syndrome, and ventricular
tachycardias. Future directions for the surgical
treatment of other arrhythmias will also be discussed.

* Recipient of Research Career Development Award #K04
HL00361, National Heart, Lung, and Blood Institute, Bethesda,
Maryland. Dr. Josephson is the Robinette Foundation Associate
Professor of Medicine (Cardiovascular Diseases).

Surgery for tachycardias associated with the Wolff-Parkinson-White syndrome

Tachycardias associated with the Wolff-Parkinson-
White syndrome are well suited to surgical therapy
since both the electrophysiologic mechanisms and
anatomic substrate of these arrhythmias are well
characterized. The concept of circus movement tachycardias associated with an accessory pathway
began with the observations of Kent [1, 2] in the late
nineteenth and early twentieth centuries and the
insight of Mines in 1913 and 1914 [3, 4]. Scattered
case reports of probable examples of the Wolff-
Parkinson-White syndrome appeared over the next
15 years [5-7]; but it was not until the classic paper
by Wolff, Parkinson, and White in 1930 [8] that
the association of tachycardias, in apparently
normal subjects who had short P-R intervals, and a
bundle branch block-like pattern on their electro-
cardiograms was reported. Over the next 50 years
the anatomic and electrophysiologic basis of this
syndrome became established. The initial descrip-
tions of an atrioventricular muscle bundle associated with the Wolff-Parkinson-White syndrome
were made by Wood, Wolferth, and Geckeler [9] in
the United States and by Öhnell [10] in Europe.
Further corroboration of their data has demonstrated that the Wolff-Parkinson-White syndrome
results from the presence of accessory atrioventricular connections which usually course on the epicardial surface of the annulus fibrosis of the atrioventricular rings [11-13]. In a majority of cases,
the tissue of which the atrioventricular bypass tract
is composed appears similar to working myocardium [11-13]. These connections generally arise as

Rosen, M. R. and Hoffman, B. F. (eds.), Cardiac Therapy. ISBN 0-89838-564-4.
© 1983, Martinus Nijhoff Publishers, Boston, The Hague, Dordrecht, Lancaster. Printed in the Netherlands.

a single trunk in the atrium and enter the ventricular myocardium in several ramifying branches over an area of a few millimeters; frequently there is patchy fibrosis at the ventricular insertion sites [11–13]. The pathways usually are not visible or palpable and usually are 5–10 mm in length. On occasion several tracts can be present. In fact, from the surgical experience at Duke University, it is believed that the atrial muscle of the coronary sinus also may serve as a source of atrioventricular connections; in this instance they are somewhat remote from the mitral annulus [14, 15].

Localization of the pathways in the intact human heart became feasible with the development of epicardial mapping, as described by Durrer and Ross in 1967 [16]. They performed epicardial mapping during cardiac surgery and were able to demonstrate the presence of ventricular preexcitation at the right lateral base of the heart in a patient with the Wolff-Parkinson-White syndrome. Similar observations were made by Burchell and associates [17] who were unable to divide the accessory pathway. In 1968 a patient with intractable arrhythmias associated with the Wolff-Parkinson-White syndrome underwent successful surgery at Duke University Medical Center [18, 19]. Epicardial mapping had localized the site of preexcitation to the right lateral base of the heart, and Dr. Will Sealy successfully divided the pathway using an external dissection to the right lateral base of the heart. The patient has remained free of tachycardia since that time. This successful surgical procedure marked the beginning of a new frontier of cardiac surgery for arrhythmias based upon electrophysiologic guidance. Since that time there have been many reports of surgical attempts to divide or modify accessory pathways associated with the Wolff-Parkinson-White syndrome [14, 15, 20–31]. In general, all current approaches to the surgical therapy of tachycardias associated with the Wolff-Parkinson-White syndrome rely on both preoperative and intraoperative mapping studies, as initially described at Duke University. Most of the modifications used throughout the world have evolved through the efforts of Dr. Sealy and his colleagues [14, 22, 26, 27, 29–31]. As a consequence, most of the preoperative and intraoperative mapping techniques and surgical interventions described in this chapter will be a review of their work.

Classifications of atrioventricular accessory pathways

Originally, accessory pathways were divided into either left-sided (type A Wolff-Parkinson-White syndrome) or right-sided (type B Wolff-Parkinson-White syndrome) [32]. However, from anatomic, electrocardiographic, vectorcardiographic, and activation mapping data, it has become clear that bypass tracts can occur at multiple sites almost anywhere around the mitral and tricuspid annuli [11–14, 28–30, 33–37]. Although electrocardiographic or electrophysiologic analysis of the direction of the delta wave can divide bypass tracts into approximately eight areas, [14, 28, 33, 34, 37] for purposes of surgery, we believe the classification used by Sealy and his colleagues is most appropriate [14]. They divide accessory pathways into four groups: right parietal (free wall), left parietal, anterior septal, and posterior septal (Figure 1). Such a classification has been derived from their surgical experience as well as the anatomic studies by McAlpine [38]. Two important but frequently unrecognized facts which are clearly pointed out by McAlpine are: (a) the atria and ventricles appose each other and are separated by the annulus fibrosis around their entire circumference *except* at the point at which the left atrium is attached to the aortic ring; at this point there is no continuity of atrium and ventricle; and (b) the left atrium *and* part of the right atrium straddle the superior process of the left ventricle which lies in the crux of the heart [38]. These findings suggest that it is possible to have atrioventricular connections along any part of the mitral or tricuspid annulus except that point at which the mitral valve and left atrium are attached to the aortic ring. Since no portion of the left ventricle is continuous with the left atrium at the area of aorto-mitral continuity, no accessory pathways should be expected in that region. This assumption has been confirmed by the surgical experience at Duke [29].

Left free wall pathways are those that begin anteriorly at the left fibrous trigone and extend posteriorly to the posterior-superior process of the left ventricle [14, 15] (Figure 1). This part of the left ventricle links the annulus fibrosis to the posterior portion of the muscular ventricular septum. These left free wall bypass tracts may be further sub-divided into anterior, lateral, and posterior sections

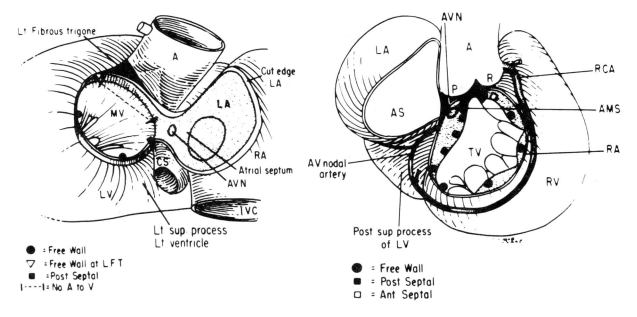

Figure 1. Sites of atrioventricular bypass tracts. Left-sided pathways are shown on the left and right-sided pathways on the right: A = aorta; AMS = atrial extension of membranous septum; AS = atrial septum; AVN = A-V node; AVNA = A-V nodal artery; CS = coronary sinus; IVC = inferior vena cava; LA = left atrium; LFT = left fibrous trigone; MV = mitral valve; P = posterior sinus of valsalva; R = right sinus of valsalva; RA = right atrium; TV = tricuspid valve (from [14], with permission of C V Mosby Co).

[15]. Posterior free wall pathways can arise from the muscular wall of the coronary sinus which is part of the left atrium. Moreover, since there is overlap of the right atrium and the posterior-superior process of the left ventricle, it is possible that bypass tracts can arise from the right atrial free wall and enter the posterior-superior process of the left ventricle. Right free wall accessory pathways cross the atrioventricular groove in proximity to parietal portions of the tricuspid annulus (see Figure 1) with its most anterior point being adjacent to the area at which the right coronary artery enters the atrioventricular sulcus [14].

Septal pathways are divided into anterior and posterior locations [14, 27]. The atrial extension of the membranous septum divides the two. This dividing point is related anatomically to the right fibrous trigone and is a region in which the normal atrioventricular conducting system is located. Since the posterior-superior process of the left ventricle can receive bypass fibers from either the right or left atrium, the original classification into types A and B [32] is clearly an oversimplification that can lead to erroneous conclusions and surgical failures. This critical area, the posterior septum, is anatomically

the most complex and provides the most difficult surgical approach.

Preoperative electrophysiologic examination

The preoperative electrophysiologic study is necessary to: (a) confirm the diagnosis of preexcitation due to an atrioventricular bypass tract, (b) demonstrate that the bypass tract is involved in producing the arrhythmia for which surgery is contemplated, (c) determine whether or not additional bypass tracts are present, and (d) select appropriate patients for surgery. Originally the indications for surgery were circus movement, supraventricular tachycardia refractory to all antiarrhythmic agents and atrial flutter or fibrillation with life-threatening ventricular responses. As surgical techniques have improved, these indications have been extended to include young adults with supraventricular tachycardia that would require long-term medication and the presence of the Wolff-Parkinson-White syndrome in patients undergoing cardiac surgery for other reasons. The electrophysiologic methods used for the preoperative evaluation include: (a) programmed stimulation for diagnosis of preexci-

339

tation and assessment of the functional capacity of the bypass tract as well as for identifying the mode of induction of arrhythmias and (b) endocardial atrial mapping and multiple-site atrial pacing to localize the atrial and ventricular sites of insertion of the bypass tract. These methods have been reviewed in detail elsewhere [35, 37, 39-43]. Localization of the bypass tract requires atrial mapping during ventricular pacing or, more importantly, during induced or spontaneous circus movement tachycardia. An atrial insertion in the inferior or lateral left atrium typically can be localized by mapping through the coronary sinus. The superior left atrium can be mapped via the pulmonary artery or through a patent foramen ovale. Right atrial mapping is carried out with a catheter moved along the A-V ring. Although special catheters have been developed to accomplish mapping of the tricuspid ring [44], a standard catheter with an exaggerated

curve at the tip probably is sufficient.

The ventricular insertion is less easily located by catheter mapping due to the technical difficulties of ventricular mapping. Thus, ventricular mapping is not widely used during sinus rhythm. However, mapping the inflow tract of the right ventricle is possible, and a left ventricular electrogram can be recorded from the coronary sinus. In general, catheter localization of the atrial insertion is more precise than localization of the ventricular site of insertion. An example of the ability to localize both the atrial and ventricular sites of insertion by catheter mapping is shown in Figure 2.

The preoperative study is performed in the catheterization laboratory, and the investigator can take several hours to complete the study. The preoperative study, therefore, has none of the potential limitations of intraoperative mapping, i.e., the effects of anesthesia and cardiopulmonary bypass on the

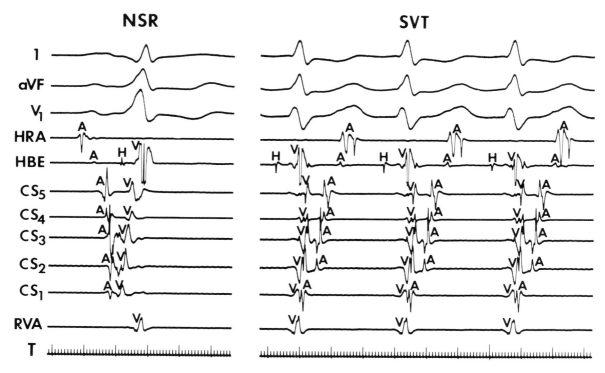

Figure 2. Determination of location of bypass tract by ventricular activation in sinus rhythm and atrial activation during supraventricular tachycardia. Both panels are arranged from top to bottom. ECG leads I, aVF, and V_1 and intracardiac recordings from the high right atrium (HRA), His bundle (HBE), distal to proximal coronary sinus (CS_1-CS_5 respectively) and right ventricular apex (RVA). The map during sinus rhythm (NSR) is on the left panel and during supraventricular, tachycardia (SVT), on the right. During NSR the earliest ventricular activation is the posterolateral left ventricle recorded from CS_1. This coincides with the delta wave, thus localizing the ventricular insertion of the bypass tract. During SVT, retrograde atrial activation is also earliest in CS_1. Therefore both the atrial and ventricular insertions are at the posterolateral left atrium and ventricle: T = 10- and 100-ms time lines.

function of the bypass tract as well as inadvertent trauma to the bypass tract. Although catheter mapping is a less precise technique than intraoperative mapping, it can serve as a guide to the surgeon in cae of intraoperative complications that prohibit adequate localization of the bypass tract at the time of surgery.

Intraoperative mapping

The purpose of intraoperative mapping is to determine more precisely than is possible with catheterization techniques the atrial and ventricular insertions of the accessory pathway. The intraoperative map can confirm the catheter map and also can allow more precise estimation of the presence of other bypass tracts. A thorough preoperative study complements the intraoperative map in the following ways: it can serve as a useful guide to the surgeon, and it also may be the only information available if the bypass tract ceases to function in the operating room due to inadvertent trauma or because an unexpected intraoperative event precludes mapping. Most mapping performed in the operating room is epicardial. The techniques used are those initially employed by Durrer and Roos [16].

Mapping is performed with a standard stick or ring probe electrode connected to amplifiers capable of recording unipolar and bipolar signals; two reference electrograms and three ECG leads also are recorded. Although on-line data acquisition is possible using an interval counter, the earliest sites of activation, either on the ventricle or atrium, can be determined readily by eye. A complete ventricular map as well as a more limited map of the atria just around the A-V rings usually is obtained. The information obtained can demonstrate multiple sites of preexcitation. Knowledge of the normal activation sequence of the ventricles is required to determine whether or not multiple bypasses are operative during sinus rhythm. On occasion a second bypass tract can be obscured by excessive preexcitation over another tract [35–37]. This may be diagnosed by demonstrating abnormal early epicardial activation at two sites along the A-V groove. On occasion, atrial pacing at different atrial sites can be useful in making both pathways more readily recognized.

Reference electrograms are recorded from the atrium and the ventricle near the A-V ring at the area at which the bypass tract is expected on the basis of ECG, vectorcardiographic, and/or electrophysiologic data. Both unipolar and bipolar recordings provide useful information [36, 45, 46]. The bipolar recordings provide a more discrete spike for accurate measurement of the time of local excitation. However, the epicardium sometimes may be some distance from bypass tracts which may lie within the fat pad of the atrioventricular sulcus. In such instances bipolar recordings may be inadequate and unipolar recordings more helpful. Analysis of the timing and morphology of unipolar electrograms is very useful. A QS or rS usually is present at the site closest to the bypass tract.

Leads for recording the reference electrograms usually are sutured into the atrium and ventricle to provide a stable sharp deflection in relation to which all other signals are timed. These reference electrograms are required because we are unable to determine accurately the onset of the delta wave which frequently is distorted when the chest is opened and the heart displaced. The site of ventricular insertion of the bypass tract is determined by mapping the regions of the ventricle near the A-V sulcus during either sinus rhythm or atrial pacing. The site of the ventricular end of the bypass tract is most readily determined when preexcitation is brought out by atrial pacing; this is easiest when the pacing catheter is placed close to the presumed atrial site of the bypass tract. In some instances no evidence of antegrade preexcitation can be determined since the bypass tract can conduct only in a retrograde fashion. In such instances only the atrial insertion site can be determined. In these patients (concealed bypass tracts) and those with the typical Wolff-Parkinson-White syndrome, the site of atrial insertion can be determined by mapping the atrium in the area of the atrioventricular ring during ventricular pacing or induced supraventricular tachycardia. When bypass tracts are located on parietal portions of the ventricles, the earliest ventricular activation precedes the onset of the delta wave [36, 45, 46], whereas, if a septal bypass tract is present, the earliest activity recorded by epicardial mapping follows the onset of the delta wave (Figure 3) [36, 45, 46].

In the experience of investigators at Duke [14, 29, 30, 35–37], as well as that of Iwa and colleagues [26, 28], approximately 10% of patients have had multiple pathways, necessitating repeat studies fol-

341

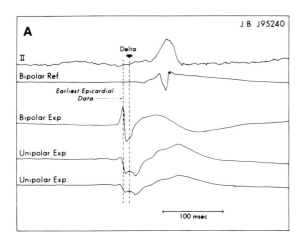
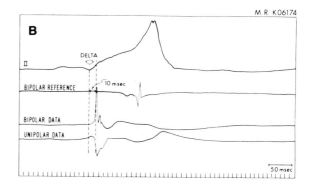

Figure 3. Epicardial activation during preexcitation via free wall (A) and septal (B) bypass tracts. In panels A and B, during sinus rhythm lead II is shown along with bipolar and unipolar epicardial electrograms and a bipolar reference electrogram. With a free wall bypass tract (A), the rapid components of both unipolar and bipolar electrograms from the area of earliest epicardial ventricular excitation precede the onset of the delta wave (dark arrow) noted on the ECG. When the bypass tract is located septally (B), the rapid components of the unipolar and bipolar electrograms recorded from the earliest area of epicardial ventricular excitation follow the onset of the delta wave observed on the surface ECG (arrow) (from [45], with the permission of Lea and Febiger).

lowing surgery. In addition, approximately 13% of their patients have had bypass tracts that conducted only retrogradely [29, 37]; thus, only the atrial site of insertion could be determined. Mapping has been especially difficult during atrial fibrillation and has required that the reference electrode be placed on the ventricle near the site at which the tract is suspected. The recording of both unipolar (QS) and bipolar electrograms is important in this situation and care should be taken to measure the earliest complexes. It is important to recognize that mechanically induced ventricular premature depolarizations that occur during mapping may be early. Thus, reproducibility of the mapping data is required to distinguish inadvertent mechanically induced complexes from the reproducible early activation at the site of the bypass tract.

There are several limitations to epicardial mapping. As noted above, the trauma secondary to stretch caused by lifting of the heart or retraction can incapacitate the bypass tract temporarily. Another important problem is related to the angle at which the atrium joins the ventricle. If the angle is sharp, the bypass tract can be at some distance from the atrial and/or ventricular sites suggested by epicardial mapping. The disparity is greatest when the angle of atrioventricular insertion is greatest and the bypass tract extends obliquely from one chamber to another. Another problem results from the presence of fat in the A-V sulcus; if this is excessive, it can prevent precise determination of the location of the bypass tract by prohibiting direct recording over the annulus. The effects of extensive fat plus the abnormal angulation of atrium and ventricle at the A-V ring can be minimized by endocardial mapping [14, 29]. This is accomplished more easily on the right side of the heart, since the right atrium can be entered readily and endocardial mapping around the tricuspid ring accomplished without difficulty. Both entering and mapping the left atrium are more difficult because of this chamber's more posterior position. Epicardial mapping is also of limited value in the case of septal bypass tracts [14, 35–37, 45, 46]. In such instances, endocardial mapping of the atrium, specifically on the right atrium, is required during a tachycardia to localize adequately the origin of the bypass tract.

In addition to standard electrode mapping of the accessory pathway, investigators at Duke have used a cryothermal probe [47]. This technique, which is applicable only to those pathways that are quite near the epicardium, is based on the ability of local cooling to 0 °C to suppress temporarily the function of the bypass tract. However, only a small fraction of bypass tracts appears to be located at or near the epicardium where they can be cooled reversibly by this technique [29]. In such cases, permanent ablation of the bypass tract can be accomplished by freezing the area that was reversibly incapacitated by cooling to 0°C. Permanent ablation is accomplished by cooling the site to –60°C [47].

Specific surgical procedures for ablating atrioventricular bypass tracts

Depending on the site of the bypass tract and the clinical status of the patient, the surgical approach may be a direct attack on the bypass tract itself, either by transsection or cryosurgery, or may be indirect with disruption of the normal atrioventricular conduction system by cryosurgery, transsection, cautery, or ligature. For the most part, the indirect approaches are reserved for cases in which the direct approach fails to obliterate the bypass tract or for patients in whom prolonged bypass time would incur excessive risk. Moreover, ligation, cautery, and/or incision in the region of the A-V nodal–His bundle structure are associated with potential risks of tricuspid insufficiency, atrial and/or ventricular septal defects, and distortion of the sinuses of Valsalva which might result in aneurysms or fistulae. Following any of the direct procedures, epicardial mapping is again performed during normal sinus rhythm and atrial and ventricular pacing to ascertain whether the bypass tract and His bundle are functioning.

The first successful procedure was performed by Dr. Will Sealy at Duke University, who disarticulated the right atrium from the free wall of the right ventricle using an epicardial approach [18, 19]. The disarticulating incision was made on the ventricular side of the annulus. With more experience it became apparent that right ventricular free wall bypass tracts, although the easiest to sever, were the least common. Since most bypass tracts requiring surgical intervention appeared to be localized to the left free wall and/or the septum [14, 29], an epicardial approach could not be utilized because: (a) epicardial mapping was inadequate for the septal bypass tracts and (b) inadequate hemostasis could result if the posterior left atrial epicardium were incised. The evolution of these procedures has established that the primary approach for all bypass tracts should be incision from the atrial *endocardium* just above the annulus, with variations depending upon the site; i.e., right free wall, septal, or left free wall [22]. These variations in procedure are necessary because bypass tracts in the posterior septum may run from the right atrium to the superior process of the left ventricle through the pyramidal space and because bypass tracts can be present at varying distances from the annulus to the epicardium within the fat pad of the A-V sulcus. Presently, the operation always is performed via a median sternotomy which gives the best exposure, particularly if multiple pathways are involved. Subtle differences in procedures depending on the site of the bypass tract will be described below based on the techniques currently used by Sealy and co-workers [14, 15, 27, 29, 30].

Surgical approach to right free wall bypass tracts
Parietal right side pathways are easy to localize and divide, since their location is most accessible. Unfortunately, these bypass tracts are encountered least commonly in those patients who require surgery. Since exposure is so good, the concern for adequate hemostasis following an epicardial incision is not warranted. As a result, cardiopulmonary bypass time can be decreased by using both an epicardial and endocardial approach. The technique of dividing a free wall right side pathway is shown in Figure 4. Dissection is begun externally at the site at which the epicardial reflection moves from the atrium over the fat pad in the A-V sulcus at the atrial site demonstrated to be activated earliest during supraventricular tachycardia. The epicardium is divided at this juncture and a dissection is begun along the atrial wall to the tricuspid annulus. The right coronary artery is protected during this dissection by pulling the fat pad inferiorly. Once the annulus is reached, dissection is begun along the superior surface of the right ventricle up to, but not through, the epicardium while retracting the coronary vessels superiorly. Following this dissection, a right atriotomy is performed and an endocardial incision is made through the entire wall of the atrium opposite to the dissected area and just above the annulus beginning at the point of earliest excitation during the tachycardia and extending 1–1.5 cm on either side. Closure of the endocardium, the right atriotomy and epicardium then is accomplished. The total cardiopulmonary bypass time for this procedure as performed at Duke University is approximately 40–60 min [29, 31]. Once the heart

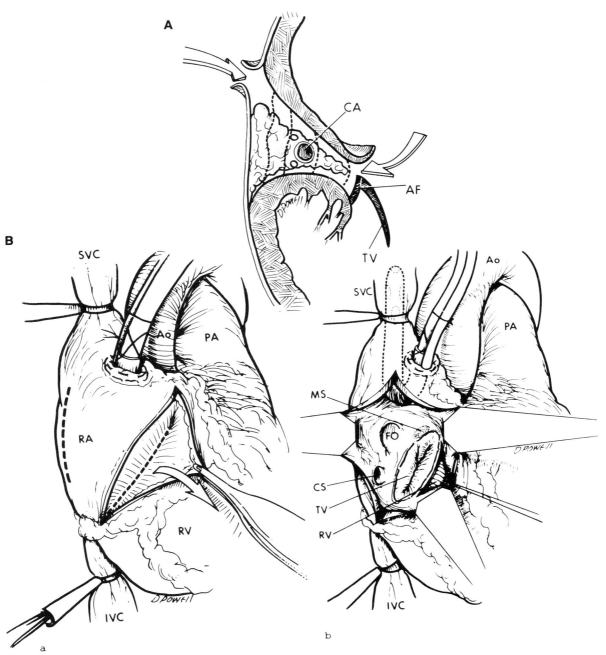

Figure 4. The surgical approach to right free wall bypass tracts. The possible locations of atrioventricular bypass tracts as they cross the A-V sulcus fat pad in the right free wall are demonstrated in panel A (CA = coronary artery, AF = annulus fibrosis, TV = tricuspid valve). The arrows demonstrate epicardial and endocardial approaches to the dissection. In panel B, the surgical methods for interrupting right free wall bypass tracts are shown. The procedure is begun by an incision through the epicardial attachment to the right atrium at the site of earliest atrial excitation during ventricular pacing or supraventricular tachycardia. The fat and coronary vessels are deflected downward (a) as shown by the arrow. Following an atriotomy (vertical broken lines on the left), the tricuspid valve is exposed (right, b) and an incision just above the annulus on the endocardial side is made exposing the right ventricle from which the remainder of the fat pad is dissected. See text for further explanation: AO = aorta; CS = coronary sinus; FO = fossa ovale; IVC = inferior vena cava; MS = membranous septum: PA = pulmonary artery; RA = right atrium; RV = right ventricle; SVC = superior vena cava; TV = tricuspid valve (from [14], with permission of C V Mosby Co).

344

has been rewarmed, the entire epicardial mapping study during sinus rhythm and atrial and ventricular pacing is repeated. Lack of ventricular preexcitation during atrial pacing and a normal retrograde atrial activation sequence during ventricular pacing, as well as pacing-induced antegrade and retrograde Wenckebach periodicity strongly suggest that the bypass tract has been ablated.

Surgical approach for left free wall pathways
Left free wall pathways are those most commonly associated with arrhythmias requiring surgical intervention [14, 15, 29]. Although the endocardial approach to these pathways is similar to that for right free wall pathways, anatomic considerations prohibit a simultaneous epicardial approach due to inability to control bleeding adequately following surgery and an increased risk of injuring cardiac vessels which lie posteriorly in the fat pad of A-V sulcus. As a result, once epicardial mapping has identified the atrial and ventricular insertions of the bypass tract, a suture ligature or needle is passed through the atrium at the area of earliest excitation to crudely mark where the endocardial incision should begin [14, 15, 29]. This marker is necessary since the mitral annulus is somewhat distant from the epicardium due to the number of vessels in the A-V sulcus fat pad, the thickness of the left ventricle, and the relatively small area of the mitral annulus. The initial incision is made in the left atrium at the level of the inter-atrial groove. If there is concern that epicardial mapping has not adequately identified the site of the bypass tract, endocardial mapping along the atrial side of the mitral annulus can be accomplished with the patient supported by cardiopulmonary bypass and with the left ventricle vented. Once the bypass tract has been localized adequately, an incision is made just above the mitral annulus at that site and extended for 1–2 cm on either side. Since bypass tracts can exist anywhere in the A-V sulcus fat pad from the annulus to the epicardium (including the wall of the coronary sinus), extensive dissection through the fat in the A-V sulcus is required (Figure 5). Initially, the dissection is carried out inferiorly along the ventricle until the epicardial attachment to the ventricle is reached. The dissection is repeated along the atrial surface with care being taken not to enter the coronary sinus or damage the coronary arteries. The epicardium is left intact to minimize bleeding postopera-

tively. The endocardial incision and atriotomy then are closed and the patient rewarmed. Once warming has occurred, epicardial mapping and stimulation are repeated to ascertain whether or not the bypass tract has been ablated.

Surgical approach to anterior septal bypass tracts
Right anterior septal pathways are those just anterior to the atrial extension of the membranous septum extending approximately 1.5–2 cm to the region opposite the site at which the right coronary artery dips into the A-V groove [14, 27, 29]. Thus, these pathways are just anterior to the His bundle. On the ventricular side these pathways insert at the base of the right ventricular outflow tract near the crista supraventricularis. Experience at Duke suggests that the earliest epicardial ventricular excitation usually occurs over the outflow tract at some distance from the annulus, with epicardial activation following the onset of the delta wave [14, 27, 29]. In some instances, epicardial breakthrough can suggest that the pathway is on the free wall (parietal) part of the right ventricle. Two facts suggest this is not the case: (a) The earliest ventricular activation occurs after the onset of the delta wave, whereas in parietal pathways earliest epicardial activation typically precedes the onset of the delta wave, and (b) endocardial mapping of the atrium during supraventricular tachycardia or ventricular pacing demonstrates earliest activity at the anterior septum adjacent to the region of the His bundle. In fact, at times these tracts can insert to within a millimeter of the His bundle.

The surgical approach to these pathways begins following the atriotomy which has been performed to permit endocardial atrial mapping. The initial incision begins at the anterior edge of the atrial extension of the membranous septum and extends to the free wall of the right ventricle (Figure 6). The dissection is then carried out over the atrial extension of the fat pad to the epicardium and then over the right ventricle. In contrast to surgery for right free wall pathways, the epicardium is usually left intact. The right coronary artery usually is clearly visible in this region and can be protected readily. It is critical to begin the incision of the A-V ring anterior to the atrial extension of the membranous septum since heart block can be induced if the incision is begun more posteriorly. On occasion, however, it is impossible to avoid injuring the His

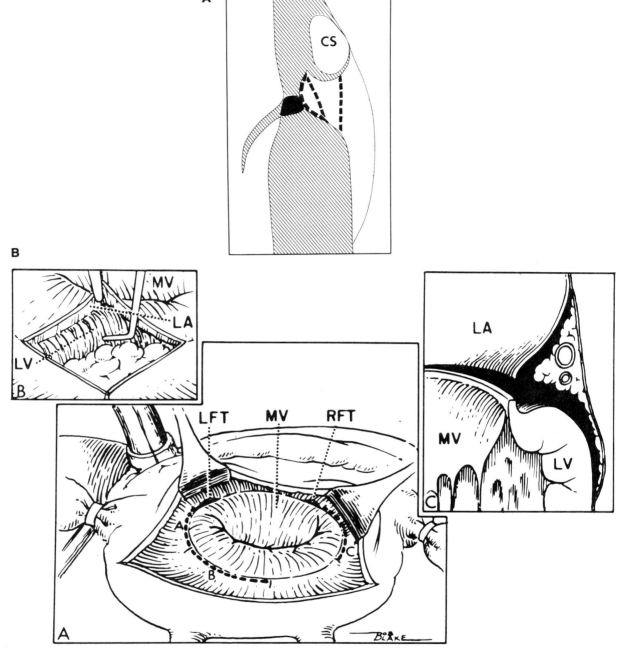

Figure 5. Surgical approach to left free wall atrial ventricular bypass tracts. On the top (A) is a schema of the left atrium, left ventricle, and mitral valve with bypass tract locations shown by broken lines running between the atrium and the ventricle, including the wall of the coronary sinus (CS). On the bottom in the three panels (A, B, C) is shown the surgical method used to transect left parietal bypass tracts. Following a left atriotomy through the interatrial groove, an incision is made above the mitral annulus. This incision can be anywhere from the anterior margin of the left fibrous trigone (LFT) opposite the free wall of the left ventricle. The fat is separated from the left ventricle (LV) and left atrium (LA) using a nerve hook. The separation of fat from both the left atrium and left ventricle and incision over the mitral valve (MV) is shown in C. An incision adjacent to the right fibrous trigone (RFT) will allow entrance to the pyramidal space to approach to septal pathways (see text and Figure 8) (from [14, 15], with permission of C V Mosby Co).

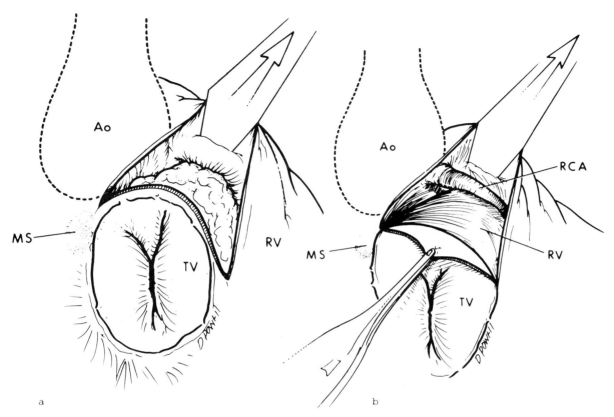

Figure 6. Surgical approach to anteroseptal bypass tracts. Following right atriotomy an incision is made above the tricuspid annulus extending from the atrial extension of the membranous septum anteriorly opposite the parietal portion of the right ventricle. This exposes the right coronary artery which is retracted. The fat pad in the A-V sulcus is dissected and separated from the atrium and ventricle. The epicardium is left intact: Ao = aorta; MS = muscular septum; RV = right ventricle; RCA = right coronary artery; TV = tricuspid valve (from [27], with permission of C V Mosby Co).

bundle, and, in fact, in certain instances the bypass tract inserts through the His bundle region in the right fibrous trigone. Total cardiopulmonary bypass time is 40–60 min [29].

Surgical approach to posterior septal bypass tracts
Posterior septal bypass tracts have been the most difficult to ablate surgically because of the complex anatomy of the crux of the heart. As noted earlier, both the right and left atrium overlie the superior-posterior process of the left ventricle; it may not be possible to distinguish right- and left-sided pathways by presently available mapping techniques when these pathways are located in the region of the crux. This region, the pyramidal space which was initially described by Koch in 1922 [48] and later by Anderson and Becker [12] and McAlpine [38], is

bounded anteriorly by the right fibrous trigone, posteriorly by the epicardium, inferiorly by the interventricular septum and the posterior-superior process of the left ventricle, and superiorly and laterally by both atria.

Localization of septal bypass tracts is contingent upon: (a) the earliest epicardial activation being in the region of the crux and occurring after the onset of surface delta wave and (b) right atrial endocardial mapping showing earliest activation usually at the os of the coronary sinus. The approach to posterior septal bypass tracts is depicted in Figure 7 [14, 27]. After atriotomy and endocardial mapping to identify the earliest activity during supraventricular tachycardia, the His bundle and atrial extension of the membranous septum are identified. The right atrial wall then is incised above the tricuspid annulus

347

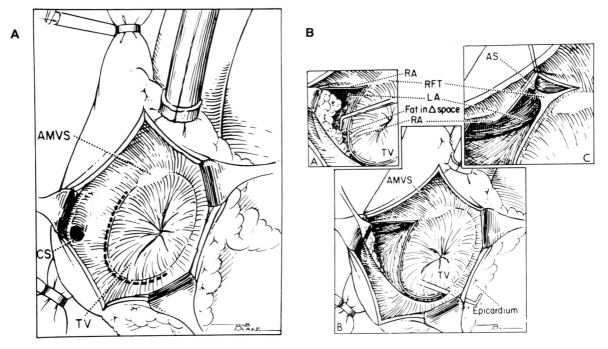

Figure 7. Surgical approach to posteroseptal pathways. Following a right atriotomy an incision is made above the tricuspid annulus beginning just posterior to the atrial extension of the membranous septum (AMVS, Figure 7A). This is continued posteriorly and laterally to include the free wall (Figure 7A). This incision exposes the pyramidal space (Figure 7B – panel A) in which a nerve hook is shown separating the fat pad from the posterior/superior process of the left ventricle. The dissection is carried through to the superior aspect of the space, i.e., the base of the right and left atrium (Figure 7B – B and C). See text for further explanation: AS = atrial septum; RFT = right fibrous trigone; RA = right atrium; LA = left atrium; TV = tricuspid valve; CS = coronary sinus.

beginning just posterior to the point at which the atrial extension of the membranous septum is located. This usually is approximately 1 cm anterior to the coronary sinus. The incision is continued posteriorly under the region of the coronary sinus to extend at least a centimeter onto the parietal wall. As demonstrated in Figure 7, this exposes the pyramidal space. Initially, dissection with a nerve hook is carried out inferiorly to separate the fat from the muscular ventricular septum and the posterior-superior process of the left ventricle. The dissection is then carried superiorly along the right and left atrial walls up to the epicardium and along the coronary sinus as it crosses the space and joins the right atrium. Knowledge of the complex anatomy of this area is necessary to adequately dissect the entire region. The A-V node–His bundle axis can be preserved only if the dissection does not extend into the region of the atrial septum.

After adequate dissection of the pyramidal space, the incision is closed and the heart rewarmed. If stimulation demonstrates that the bypass tract has not been ablated, the left atrium must be entered and incision of the mitral annulus in the region of the pyramidal space must be accomplished with further dissection originating from the incision over the mitral annulus. Great care must be taken to dissect along the wall of the coronary sinus since bypass tracts have been identified as extending from the muscular wall of the coronary sinus to the ventricles.

As noted above, bypass tracts may exist within or in close proximity to the His bundle, and in these instances ablation of the bypass tract invariably has resulted in the development of heart block.

Cryosurgical ablation of bypass tracts

Cryosurgical ablation of bypass tracts initially was described by Gallagher et al. [47]. There are two roles for cryosurgery in management of arrhythmias associated with the Wolff-Parkinson-White syndrome. The first indication occurs when the bypass tract lies close to the epicardium. As previously noted, in such instances local cooling to 0° C at the site of the bypass tract results in temporary and reversible cessation of function of the bypass tract. Demonstration that cooling blocks the bypass tract suggests that permanent freezing would ablate it. The one limitation of this technique is that the pressure exerted by the cryoprobe may damage the bypass tract and not the cooling per se, thereby falsely suggesting localization to the superficial epicardium. Even if the bypass tract is epicardial, it can be cooled to –60° C only if coronary vessels are not adjacent to the region of cooling. Obviously, if the region were contiguous to the coronary artery, damage to that vessel might occur. The cryosurgical approach to bypass tracts is therefore limited to the few epicardially localized tracts which are not adjacent to coronary vessels.

A second indication for cryosurgery arises if the bypass tract is localized to the region of the A-V bundle in the right fibrous trigone. In such instances, the cryosurgical approach is a safe and effective alternative to local incision as a means to interrupt the bypass tract.

To date, the Duke group has reported the use of cryothermia on free wall bypass tracts in 16 cases of preexcitation [29, 47]. In 12, transient cessation of bypass tract function was produced by local cooling to 0° C. Of these 12 cases, in three, permanent cooling was not attempted due to proximity of the tract to a coronary artery; in five, attempts to cryoablate the lesion permanently failed; permanent ablation was successful in the remaining four patients. Thus, the cryosurgical approach to free wall bypass tracts was only successful in 25% (4/16) of the cases in which it was attempted. In two additional cases, cryosurgery ablated bypass tracts traversing the tricuspid annulus near the septum. Others also have used cryosurgery successfully to treat arrhythmias utilizing A-V bypass tracts [49]. Although cryothermia offers a means for directly ablating the atrioventricular bypass tract, direct surgical dissection of these accessory pathways remains the most effective method.

Indirect approaches for bypass tracts – indications and methods of division of the His bundle

The indirect approach to the management of circus

movement tachycardia in the Wolff-Parkinson-White syndrome involves ablation of the His bundle [29, 50, 51]. Such a method is successful because the normal atrioventricular conducting system forms one limb of the macro-reentrant circuit operative in this tachycardia. Such surgery is not applicable to patients in whom the presenting arrhythmia is atrial fibrillation associated with a rapid ventricular response over the accessory pathway. Although the primary objective in the surgical treatment of arrhythmias associated with the Wolff-Parkinson-White syndrome should be the ablation of the bypass tract, in some instances it is more appropriate to ablate the His bundle. One such indication is the presence of severe cardiac dysfunction, particularly when associated with a septal bypass tract in which the operative risk would be too high if a direct approach were used. In such instances, ablation of the A-V nodal–His bundle axis by cryothermia may be the method of choice. Freezing the His bundle creates heart block with a junctional escape pacemaker [47, 52–54]. Permanent ventricular pacing is needed as a back-up in case both the bypass tract and His bundle escape rhythm cease to function. Other methods of destroying the His bundle which have been used in the management of circus movement tachycardia include surgical ligation, direct transsection, and cautery [54, 55]. The one limitation of cryosurgery appears to be atrial hypertrophy which may prevent the cryothermal injury from extending deep enough to damage the His bundle permanently [29, 53, 55]. An alternative explanation for failure to ablate the His bundle might be an eccentrically located A-V conducting system. However, this should be identified prior to any surgical attempt to destroy it.

Results of surgery for arrhythmias using atrioventricular bypass tracts

Surgical therapy for arrhythmias associated with the Wolff-Parkinson-White syndrome has evolved over a period of 13 years. Although many centers have operated on a few patients, the group at Duke University has the most experience. The results of their series at various stages have been published in detail [14, 15, 19, 22, 27, 29, 30]. Only Iwa and his colleagues [25, 26, 28] have acquired a significantly large experience (in excess of 20 patients) over the

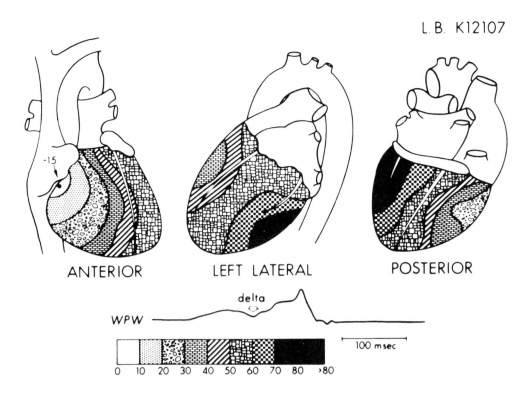

L.B. K12107

ANTERIOR   LEFT LATERAL   POSTERIOR

WPW

delta

100 msec

0 10 20 30 40 50 60 70 80 >80

EARLY AREA

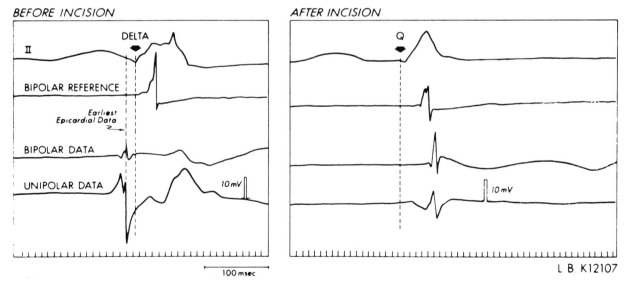

BEFORE INCISION

AFTER INCISION

II

DELTA

Q

BIPOLAR REFERENCE

Earliest
Epicardial Data

BIPOLAR DATA

UNIPOLAR DATA

10 mV

10 mV

100 msec

L.B. K12107

Figure 8. Surgery in a patient with a right free wall bypass tract. In the top panel (A), the epicardial map during sinus rhythm is shown along with a surface ECG lead. The epicardial map demonstrates epicardial breakthrough at the lateral free wall of the right ventricle. Early epicardial activation is noted 15 msec prior to the onset of the delta wave seen on the surface ECG (arrow). In panel B below epicardial activation at this site is shown in analog records before and after incision. On the left side of panel B, the bipolar and unipolar electrograms are recorded prior to the onset of the delta wave. Following surgery the delta wave is no longer present and is replaced by a normal Q wave (arrow), and the bipolar and unipolar electrograms follow the onset of the QRS by approximately 55 msec (from [45], with permission of Lea and Febiger).

350

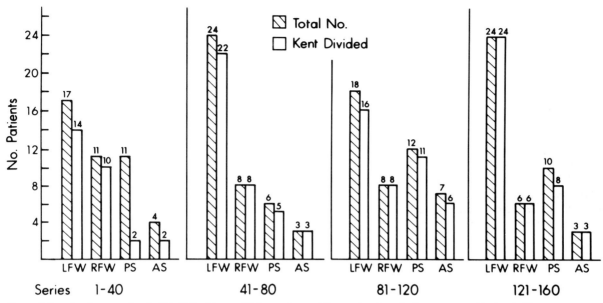

RESULTS OF SURGERY ON 172 KENT BUNDLES IN 160 PATIENTS

Figure 9. Results of surgery for the Wolff-Parkinson-White syndrome. The results of surgical attempts at ablating A-V bypass tracts as a function of time are shown in groups of 40: LFW = left free wall; RFW = right free wall; PS = posterior septal; AS = anteroseptal (kindly supplied by J J Gallagher).

Table 1. 190 patients with Kent bundles operated upon for arrhythmias.

Age (years)	No. of patients	Female	Male
0–10	8	3	5
11–20	53	11	42
21–30	50	21	29
31+	79	35	44
Total	190	70	120

Table 2. Unusual findings (190 patients).

Two pathways	15
Three pathways	4
Retrograde function only	24
Antegrade function only	3

Table 3. Results of surgery for interruption of 206 pathways in 190 patients.

	No. of pathways	No. divided
Left free wall	93	85
Right free wall	39	37
Posterior septal	53	41
Anterior septal	21	18
Total	206	181

Table 4. Mortality (patient series 1 to 190).

		No. of patients
Deaths pt. series 1 to 40		
Cardiomyopathy	2	
Operative failure	1	3
Deaths pt. series 41 to 120		
Pancreatitis	1	
Respiratory insufficiency	1	2
Deaths pt. series 121 to 190		0
Total		5

years, and their results parallel those of the Duke group. Presently both centers use similar techniques, with the major surgical goal being to disarticulate the atrium from the ventricle using an endocardial approach just above the annulus of the A-V rings. When surgery is successful evidence of preexcitation and the ability to develop atrioventricular reentry are permanently lost (Figures 8 and 9). The most recent reports from Duke University include data for 190 patients with 206 bypass tracts (Tables 1–4 kindly supplied by Dr. Will Sealy, unpublished data). One hundred and twenty of the 190 patients were male, reflecting the typical male preponderance of surgical candidates, and ranged in age from childhood to adulthood. Interestingly, slightly more than 50% of the patients with potentially lethal arrhythmias operated upon at Duke University were 10-30 years old (Dr. Will Sealy, personal communication). Among these patients, approximately 75% were operated on for circus movement tachycardias and 25% for proven or potentially life-threatening arrhythmias. As noted earlier, the indications for surgery have been expanded to include not only drug-refractory arrhythmias but also young patients with symptomatic arrhythmias requiring drug therapy or patients with arrhythmias who undergo cardiac surgery for other reasons. As in all investigators' experience, approximately half of the bypass tracts operated upon are left free wall bypass tracts [29]. Of note, 10-15% of patients operated on by Sealy's and Iwa's groups had multiple bypass tracts; in such cases surgery is more complicated and in some instances several surgical attempts are required [14, 26, 28-30, 35-37].

With the increased use of clinical electrophysiologic techniques, there has been an increased awareness of concealed bypass tracts, i.e., those which only conduct in a retrograde fashion [43, 56-59]. These bypass tracts are identical in structure to those which result in overt preexcitation. There have been 24 patients with concealed bypass tracts in the Duke series (Dr. Will Sealy, personal communication), and it is expected that a larger percentage will appear as a result of the increased use of the clinical electrophysiologic laboratory in the diagnosis and treatment of arrhythmias.

With the evolution of more specific surgical approaches, the use of cardioplegia, and increasing experience, surgical results improve with time [14, 26-29, 31, 35]. An example of the changing success rate, particularly with posteroseptal bypass tracts, is shown in Figure 9 [31]. These data suggest that, with improving techniques, successful ablation of atrioventricular bypass tracts can be accomplished in 90% of cases. In the remaining patients, multiple operations, including His bundle ablation and/or the addition of drugs, can be used to prevent recurrences of arrhythmias.

Summary

From its initial description, both clinically and pathologically, it became apparent that the Wolff-Parkinson-White syndrome was an ideal model for surgical therapy. In this model a clear understanding of both the electrophysiologic and anatomic basis for the arrhythmias being treated was obtained, and electrophysiologically directed surgery was developed. Much of the knowledge gained in the surgical management of the Wolff-Parkinson-White syndrome has been the basis for surgical approaches to the other arrhythmias discussed in this chapter.

Surgery for supraventricular tachyarrhythmias unrelated to bypass tracts

A variety of supraventricular tachyarrhythmias can produce disabling and, on occasion, life-threatening symptoms. Although the exact mechanism for each of these arrhythmias has not been established in humans, they generally can be divided into: (a) reentrant tachycardias localized most commonly to the A-V node and less often to the atrium or region of the sinus node, (b) automatic atrial tachycardias, and (c) atrial flutter and/or fibrillation with a rapid ventricular response. In a small number of patients, the arrhythmia cannot be prevented and/or the ventricular rate controlled by pharmacologic means. In selected patients surgery may remain the only therapeutic option. Unlike patients in whom a bypass tract provides an anatomic substrate for the arrhythmia which can be directly attacked surgically, a well-defined anatomic substrate for these arrhythmias has not been established. Therefore, for the most part, indirect surgical methods are utilized for their control. In the majority of patients, surgery is directed at decreasing an inappropriately rapid ventricular response. The techniques used and the specific indications are described below.

His bundle ablation

Atrial flutter/fibrillation with a rapid ventricular response is the most common supraventricular arrhythmia, with the exception of preexcitation, for which surgery is undertaken [54]. In most instances rapid A-V nodal conduction is responsible for the rapid ventricular rate [37, 43, 60, 61]. In rare cases of flutter with a 1:1 ventricular response or atrial fibrillation with a rapid ventricular response, an atrio-His bypass tract is present [62, 63]. These two mechanisms for accelerated A-V conduction can be distinguished by analyzing the response of the atrioventricular conducting system to programmed atrial stimulation and rapid atrial pacing. In patients with an atrio-His bypass tract, no A-H prolongation is produced by either perturbation, whereas blunted A-V nodal conduction is observed in patients in whom accelerated A-V nodal conduction is present on a functional basis. Specific criteria used for the diagnosis of accelerated A-V conduction include an A–H interval ≤ 60 msec, a blunted A–H response to pacing; i.e., less than 100 msec change from a sinus rhythm to the fastest paced rate at which 1:1 A-V conduction occurs, and a 1:1 ventricular response during pacing at cycle lengths ≤300 msec. Furthermore, the ability to modify the response to stimulation by drugs which can alter autonomic tone (e.g., digitalis or propranolol), or those which act relatively selectively on nodal tissue (e.g., verapamil) also may be used to distinguish functional accelerated A-V nodal conduction from an atrio-His bypass tract.

Other arrhythmias for which His bundle ablation has been used include atrial tachycardias (reentrant or automatic) and A-V nodal reentry [29, 37, 53, 54, 64–66]. These arrhythmias do not produce life-threatening ventricular responses but can produce paroxysmal syncope or may be incessant and induce heart failure. In patients with A-V nodal reentrant supraventricular tachycardia, attempts to ablate the His bundle may produce damage to the A-V node which forms a functional substrate for the arrhythmia. In this way, a surgical procedure may have a direct effect on the arrhythmia. The anatomy of the A-V node–His bundle region has been described in detail [11–13, 67] and localization of the proximal His bundle can be attained readily by endocardial mapping.

A variety of surgical procedures that produce A-V block have been evaluated in animals. Sealy et al. [54, 66] were convinced that division of the atrial septum at its insertion into the right fibrous trigone was necessary to interrupt conduction reliably at the A-V nodal–His bundle junction. They previously had demonstrated experimentally and clinically

that ligature and electrocautery were unreliable and potentially hazardous techniques [55].

Based on anatomic knowledge of the area, a direct surgical approach was developed by the Duke group (Figure 10) [54, 66]. Once the His bundle is identified, an incision is made through the right atrium beneath the coronary sinus. This provides entry into the pyramidal space just above the muscular ventricular septum. From this region the posterior aspect of the atrial septum at its insertion into the right fibrous trigone can be identified. The incision then is extended across the superior aspect of the right fibrous trigone separating it completely from the atrial septum and dividing the His bundle. On occasion this procedure may result in entry into the left atrium, but this can be corrected readily by suture.

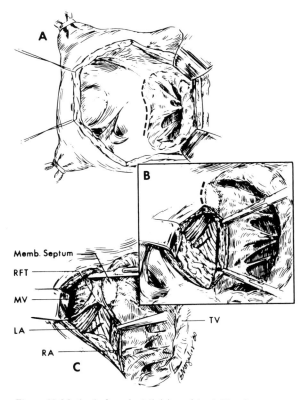

Figure 10. Method of surgical division of the A-V node-penetrating His bundle junction. Following atriotomy, an incision is made just above the atrial extension of the membranous septum and extended posteriorly allowing entrance to the pyramidal space (A, B). In C, the atrial septum has been separated from the right fibrous trigone (RFT). The anterior extension of the atrial septum is shown with the right and left atrial walls (RA, LA) entering it (from [66], with permission of C V Mosby Co).

353

At the same time that the Duke group developed its surgical approach, Harrison et al. [52] demonstrated that cryosurgery could be used to produce a similar result without complication. Cryothermia has become more popular in recent years due to the discrete injury which can be produced and which is not associated with the complications potentially caused by other procedures – i.e., tricuspid valve dysfunction, trauma to the sinus of Valsalva, or creation of a septal defect (Figure 11).

The cryothermal apparatus allows regulation of flow of nitrous oxide through the tip of a cryoprobe. The expansion of the gas at the tip results in cooling by the Joule-Thompson effect. With cooling to –60° to –65° C, there is permanent cryoinjury which usually has smooth borders and a sharp demarcation from the normal myocardium [68, 69]. The size and shape of this cryolesion can be altered by variations in the procedure. Increasing the surface area of the probe in contact with the myocardium, increasing the duration of cooling, decreasing probe temperatures, and refreezing the tissue all increase cryothermal injury. Cryothermal injury,

unlike electrocautery, incision and surgical ligatures, does not damage fibrous structures.

Once the most proximal His bundle electrogram is recorded with a probe, cryothermia to 0° C is applied to assess whether or not A-V block occurs. If A-V block occurs, the temperature can be reduced to –60° to 65° C resulting in permanent A-V block. Two or more additional freezing procedures over adjacent atrial septum superiorly, anteriorly, and posteriorly to the initial cryolesion are also performed. As noted above, since cryoinjury does not cause necrosis of the supporting fibrous tissue, sloughing of that tissue will not occur. The major problem with cryosurgery is the lack of control over the depth of penetration.

Results of His bundle ablation

Although the creation of A-V block was used sporadically to treat supraventricular arrhythmias associated with the Wolff-Parkinson-White syndrome prior to 1975 [29, 50, 51], Sealy was the first to evaluate in a critical manner the various methods

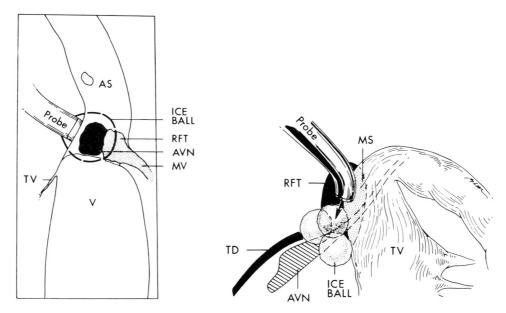

Figure 11. Cryosurgical approach to the junction of the A-V node and penetrating His bundle. Panel A on the left is a cross-section of the septal area at a level just posterior to the junction of A-V node (AVN) and penetrating His bundle. The cryoprobe is positioned on the right atrium at the level of the right fibrous trigone (RFT). The circular broken line shows the extent of the cryolesion. In another view, looking down at the septum from the superior lateral right atrium, one can see the production of three ice ball lesions by the cryoprobe at the region of the A-V node–His bundle junction, which lies at the right fibrous trigone. The tendon of Todaro (TD) extends to this junction and can be used as a landmark for it: MV = mitral valve; TV = tricuspid valve; MS = membranous septum; AS = atrial septum; V = ventricle (from [66], with permission of C V Mosby Co).

by which His bundle ablation could be accomplished and their relative effectiveness and complication rates in the management of other supraventricular arrhythmias [54, 55, 66]. The use of cryothermal A-V block first was reported by Harrison et al. in 1977 [52]. The first large series was reported by Klein et al. in 1980 [53]; this has recently been updated by Sealy and co-workers [66]. In the vast majority of these cases the arrhythmia for which surgery was undertaken was atrial fibrillation with a rapid ventricular response, although approximately one-fourth of the patients had arrhythmias without accelerated A-V conduction.

The results of four series using cryothermia or surgery are shown in Table 5. Of the 45 patients, cryosurgery was used in 30. Thirty-seven of 45 patients undergoing either cryosurgery or surgical division of the A-V junction had A-V block with a His bundle escape rhythm produced by the procedure. Moreover, in three patients with return of A-V function there was no recurrence of the arrhythmia which in each case had been A-V nodal reentry. There was only one operative death in the entire series, which occurred during the surgical approach to the A-V junction.

The escape rhythm in all studies has been a His bundle rhythm. Gonzalez et al. [70] and Klein et al. [53] evaluated the functional status of the escape pacemaker by analyzing the spontaneous rhythm, the His bundle recovery time, and the response of the escape pacemaker to exercise and/or isoproterenol, atropine, and lidocaine. The escape pacemaker had a mean cycle length of 1,244 msec at seven to ten days [53], and when analyzed at three to four months, both series showed similar escape cycle lengths of approximately 1,450 msec (mean rate of 38-45 beats/min) [53, 70]. Neither exercise nor atropine affected the escape rhythm; however, in Klein's series isoproterenol produced a dose-dependent increase in the rate of the escape rhythm which however never exceeded that of the permanent pacemaker [53]. In Gonzalez's series, lidocaine had no effect on the escape rhythm in all, except with one patient in whom the His escape rhythm and recovery time were increased [70]. The major difference in the two studies was in the analysis of the His bundle recovery time. Gonzalez et al. [70] found marked variability in His bundle recovery time with significant prolongation of this measurement, which in one patient was 8.4 sec. Klein et al. [53], on the other hand, found minimal suppression of His bundle recovery time. The differences between the two groups may have been due to the fact that Klein's patients were studied seven to ten days following surgery, whereas Gonzalez's were studied three months or more following surgery. In addition, the paced cycle length of the overdrive rhythm may have been faster in the series by Gonzalez. Finally, it is possible that the effect on His bundle recovery time was dependent on the surgical

Table 5. Indirect surgical treatment of supraventricular arrhythmias.

Author	No. of patients	Arrhythmias		Methods (patients)	AVB	Arrhythmic control
Sealy et al. [53, 54, 66]	27	AF/AFl	17	Cryosurgery (25)	22	25*
		AVNRT	5	Incision & other (2)	2	
		IART	2			
		AAT	3			
Gonzalez et al. [70]	9	AF	9	Incision (9)	7[†]	8**
Baird and Uther [64]	4	AVNRT	4	Incision (4)	2	4***
Camm et al. [49]	5	AF	4	Cryosurgery (5)	4	5**
		IART	1			

*   One patient with intact A-V conduction but AVNRT cured.
**   One patient had persistent but impaired A-V conduction that allowed control of ventricular response during AF.
***   Two patients with return of A-V conduction but control of AVNRT.
[†]   – one operative death

AF   – atrial fibrillation
AFl   – atrial flutter
AAT   – automatic atrial tachycardia

AVB   – atrioventricular block
AVNRT – A-V nodal reentrant tachycardia
IART   – intraatrial reentrant tachycardia

approach used – cryosurgery was used in Klein's patients and surgical division of the A-V junction in Gonzalez's series.

Thus, in the majority of supraventricular arrhythmias refractory to medications or associated with unacceptable ventricular responses, an indirect approach – His bundle ablation – offers a reasonable therapeutic alternative. In most instances A-V block can be produced and the arrhythmia controlled. This procedure may be performed by either cryothermal injury or by surgical incision which must extend to the superior aspect of the right fibrous trigone separating it from the atrial septum. Both these methods have been employed successfully with a reasonable morbidity and mortality.

Left atrial isolation – a new indirect method for the management of supraventricular arrhythmias

Although the creation of A-V block by His bundle ablation is an effective method for treating a variety of supraventricular arrhythmias, it necessitates a permanent ventricular pacemaker. The concept of atrial isolation as a method for treating atrial arrhythmias evolved from the pioneering work of Guiraudon et al. [71] who have developed an isolation procedure in the management of ventricular tachycardia (see below). Sealy and Seaber have studied the effects of exclusion of various components of the atria to assess the effects on exclusion of these atrial sites on escape atrial rhythms [72]. More recently, Williams et al. [73] developed a technique of left atrial isolation which has potential applications for the management of left atrial tachycardias and atrial fibrillation which is initiated in the left atrium. Williams et al. [73] studied ten adult dogs in which they were able to isolate the left atrium from the right atrium electrically while maintaining normal A-V conduction. These canine studies suggest that there are no adverse hemodynamic consequences associated with loss of synchronous left atrial contraction. More experimental studies in animals with preexistent abnormalities of ventricular function are necessary before the safety of this procedure is established for patients. However, left atrial isolation does appear to have theoretical advantages over His bundle ablation for the management of left atrial tachyarrhythmias.

Direct approaches to the management of supraventricular tachyarrhythmias

With the experience developed with intraoperative mapping techniques, it is possible to attack focal atrial tachycardias directly. A directed local disc excision of the area might cure the arrhythmia and preserve atrioventricular conduction. Obviously, the ability to accomplish this requires that the tachycardia be present in the operating room so that an adequate localization can be obtained by mapping techniques. Such tachycardias must therefore either be inducible in the operating room or be persistent. The experience with such directed surgical ablative procedures on atrial tachycardias is small. Coumel et al. [74] initially described a cure of a focal atrial tachycardia located at the junction of the right superior pulmonary vein with the left atrium. Wyndham et al. [75] recently described the surgical cure of a focal paroxysmal atrial tachycardia which was well studied in both the catheterization laboratory and intraoperatively. The arrhythmia could be initiated and terminated reproducibly by programmed stimulation, and catheter endocardial mapping localized the earliest activity to the posterolateral rim of the right atrial appendage. Intraoperative mapping confirmed this site of early activity and the appendage was excised, resulting in cure of the arrhythmia. In vitro electrophysiologic studies were performed on the surgical specimen, and these revealed the presence of triggered activity; however, the rate of the triggered rhythm, even in the presence of epinephrine, never exceeded 80 beats/min, whereas the clinical tachycardia averaged 140 beats/min. Whether or not the rhythm in vivo was a direct counterpart of that shown by in vitro investigation could not be established.

We have had the opportunity to operate on an incessant atrial tachycardia in a 26-year-old patient. Unlike the patients in the two prior studies, our patient had a rhythm that was neither induced nor terminated by programmed stimulation but could be reset by premature stimuli and showed overdrive suppression followed by warm-up. Digoxin, propranolol, quinidine, disopyramide, and procainamide failed to terminate the arrhythmia. Catheter endocardial mapping localized the area of early activity to the posterior lip of the fossa ovalis. The patient was discharged on digoxin and propranolol to control her ventricular response, but this proved ineffective and she returned six months later for surgery. At that time a repeat catheter map was identical to the one obtained six months earlier and localized the origin to the posterior lip of the fossa ovalis. When the patient was taken to the operating room, the tachycardia was not present. With the infusion of catecholamines, frequent ectopic impulses were observed and mapped. In addition, the P waves induced by pacing various regions of the atria, including the region of the fossa ovalis, were compared to those of the tachycardia. Both the pace-mapping procedure and mapping of the catecholamine-initiated rhythms localized the earliest activity to the lip of the fossa ovalis, as predicted by the catheter map. A 1.5×2 cm wedge of atrial tissue was resected and the patient has been free of tachycardias for the past two years. Histological examination of the tissue revealed a mesenchymal tumor at the border of the lip of the fossa ovalis. In vitro electrophysiologic studies revealed a catecholamine-induced automatic rhythm with a very long cycle length (2,000 msec) which was abolished by verapamil. The significance of these in vitro findings remains unclear.

Thus, with advances in mapping techniques both in the catheterization laboratory and intraoperatively, it is possible to excise local regions of the atrium from which focal arrhythmias arise. This more limited and direct attack on atrial arrhythmias clearly provides the most desirable postoperative result in terms of mechanical and electrical atrioventricular function.

Surgical therapy of ventricular tachyarrhythmias

The surgical management of malignant ventricular arrhythmias has evolved over the past 25 years. The surgical techniques employed in the management of these arrhythmias have as their goal either an alteration of the electrophysiologic milieu which predisposes to the arrhythmia or ablation or isolation of the tissue responsible for the arrhythmia. A variety of surgical techniques has been proposed to accomplish this goal including coronary artery bypass grafting, aneurysmectomy with or without coronary artery bypass grafting, simple ventriculotomy, encircling endocardial ventriculotomy, cryosurgery, and subendocardial resection. Although each of these procedures claims efficacy for managing

such arrhythmias, evaluation of efficacy has been extremely difficult, particularly in surgical series conducted prior to 1975. A number of reasons account for this: (a) the definition of life-threatening arrhythmia varied from study to study and included isolated or complex ventricular ectopic activity, nonsustained ventricular tachycardia, sustained ventricular tachycardia, and ventricular fibrillation; (b) the electrophysiologic characterization and clinical setting of the arrhythmias was poorly described; (c) the extent to which pharmacologic therapy was used preoperatively varied; (d) the hemodynamic status and coronary anatomy of the patients was not described uniformly and, as a result, patients with and without coronary artery disease in various states of cardiac decompensation were included in the same groups; (e) preoperative and postoperative evaluation of the arrhythmia as well as the follow-up (both the method of follow-up and the definition of success) were incomplete; and (f) there was selective reporting of cases. Therefore, not unexpectedly, the reported efficacy of such procedures varied from 10% to 100%. Among the factors which never can be controlled, even if the same procedure is utilized, are interinstitutional differences in surgical technique, methods of myocardial preservation, and anesthesia.

The development of clinical electrophysiology has led to the ability to characterize and treat arrhythmias. With the tools of programmed stimulation and catheter as well as intraoperative mapping, our ability to select appropriate pharmacologic and/or surgical therapy for individual patients has been improved. Importantly, the electrophysiologist now serves as a link to the surgeon in helping develop new procedures to treat specific arrhythmias. As a result, a systematic approach to the electrophysiologic investigation and subsequent surgical therapy for ventricular arrhythmias have become possible. In this section particular emphasis will be placed on the surgical therapy of arrhythmias which have been characterized electrophysiologically and clinicopathologically. These include: (a) ventricular tachycardia/fibrillation related to acute ischemia and/or infarction and (b) sustained ventricular tachycardia with and without associated coronary artery disease.

Surgery for ventricular arrhythmias associated with acute ischemia or infarction

Several groups of patients fall into this category. They include those with recurrent episodes of ventricular fibrillation, exercise-induced ventricular tachycardia or fibrillation, ventricular tachycardia or fibrillation associated with angina pectoris, and recurrent ventricular tachycardia/fibrillation associated with acute myocardial infarction. Since myocardial ischemia predisposes to the development of ventricular fibrillation, restoration of coronary blood flow to ischemic myocardium might be expected to correct the physiologic abnormality responsible for the electrophysiologic derangement [76]. Thus, several reports attest to the role of coronary revascularization for the management of recurrent ventricular tachycardia/fibrillation associated with acute and *reversible* ischemia [77–82]. In these patients, who invariably have advanced obstructive coronary artery disease but reasonably good ventricular function, the malignant arrhythmias are associated with episodes of severe angina or exercise. The use of coronary revascularization in patients surviving an episode of unexpected cardiac arrest in the absence of myocardial infarction also has been suggested [83–85]. Whereas these procedures appear promising, it must be recognized that they represent a small number of case reports from various centers. Thus, although the procedure undoubtedly can be successful, a larger prospective series is required to evaluate efficacy more carefully. Clearly, revascularization alone for arrhythmias unassociated with ischemia is without significant benefit (vide infra).

Patients with recurrent ventricular tachycardia/fibrillation associated with acute myocardial infarction have severe cardiac dysfunction. Most commonly this results from a large anterior infarction with the development of a ventricular aneurysm. Medical management of these patients is difficult [86, 87]. Unlike the patients with reversible ischemia described above, these patients have irreversibly damaged myocardium which places abnormal wall stresses on the surviving muscle and is associated with local cellular electrophysiologic derangements which predispose to arrhythmias. In such cases, revascularization must be accompanied by aneurysmectomy or infarctectomy. The initial results of Mundth et al. [88] showed a high operative mortality rate ($3/7 = 42\%$) with surgical survivors having excellent long-term results. Recently, more aggressive approaches have included early intervention with intraaortic counterpulsation prior to surgery [89, 90]. Use of counterpulsation was associated with resolution of the arrhythmia in 12 of 22 patients (55%) and with improvement of the arrhythmias in seven of the 22 patients (31%) [90]. The association of decreasing arrhythmias with improvement of left ventricular function supports the rationale for resection and revascularization to improve both ventricular function and coronary perfusion. These procedures have shown good long-term results in survivors even though antiarrhythmic agents have been employed in many patients to control asymptomatic ventricular ectopy (the need for antiarrhythmic therapy here is unclear) (Table 6).

Whether or not electrophysiologic evaluation pre- and/or intraoperatively will permit more di-

Table 6. Results of coronary revascularization and myocardial resection for recurrent ventricular tachycardia/fibrillation with acute myocardial infarction.

Authors	No. of patients	Operative deaths	Late deaths	Arrhythmias controlled*	Follow-up months
Mundth et al. [88]	7	3	0	3	3–24
Yashar et al. [82]	11	0	2	9	3–57
Tabry et al. [83]	23	6	1	15	4–32
Waldo et al. [86]	16	5	1	10	8–39
Walker et al. [89]	5	0	0	5	12–96
Hanson et al. [90]	15	8	0	7	9–92
Bar et al. [87]	10	2	0	8	2–21
Total	87	24 (28%)	5	57 (64%)	

* This number includes patients who are controlled postoperatively with or without drugs.

rected and successful therapy (vide infra) is not yet established. Unpublished observations from our laboratory suggest that many of the patients with ventricular tachycardia which rapidly degenerates to ventricular fibrillation can have their arrhythmia initiated reproducibly by programmed stimulation. The additional use of antiarrhythmic agents frequently slows the rate of the arrhythmia, allowing a stable and uniform QRS morphology to be present, thereby facilitating the mapping of the arrhythmia.

Surgery for recurrent sustained ventricular tachycardia

Recurrent sustained ventricular tachycardia is a well-known complication of chronic ischemic heart disease. It is a major cause of postinfarction morbidity and is frequently the initiating arrhythmia in sudden cardiac death [91]. The most common anatomic substrate for recurrent sustained ventricular tachycardia is prior myocardial infarction associated with left ventricular wall motion abnormalities, in particular, left ventricular aneurysms [91]. Less commonly, sustained ventricular tachycardia is unassociated with prior infarction. This latter group is heterogeneous, including patients with right ventricular dysplasia, cardiomyopathies, valvular heart disease, congenital heart disease, and idiopathic ventricular tachycardia. In view of the fact that coronary artery disease, in particular, myocardial infarction complicated by a left ventricular aneurysm, is the most common substrate for this arrhythmia, it is not surprising that the first surgical approach to the management of this arrhythmia was simple ventricular aneurysmectomy [92]. Since this initial attempt, a variety of surgical procedures have been employed to deal with this arrhythmia, specifically in the setting of coronary artery disease. It is impossible to evaluate these procedures adequately, since this series is composed of patients with a variety of different anatomic substrates and arrhythmias and with an inadequate preoperative and postoperative assessment of the arrhythmia and the result of surgery. By far the most commonly employed procedure has been aneurysmectomy with or without bypass grafting [93–103]. Although it is clear that this procedure may provide effective therapy in some cases, it is nonetheless unpredictable. Coronary revascularization alone appears to be without effect on this arrhythmia which is not related to episodes of myocardial ischemia [100]. In our own studies comparing matched patients with identical arrhythmias (i.e., recurrent sustained ventricular tachycardia), aneurysmectomy with or without bypass grafting was a failure with a higher operative mortality and recurrence of ventricular tachycardia than reported in the literature. The success rate was less than 30% [104].

With the advent of invasive electrophysiologic investigation as well as the knowledge gained in experimental models, a greater understanding of the mechanisms of ventricular tachycardia was obtained [105–113]. Two major mechanisms are thought to be operative in sustained ventricular tachycardia: (a) enhanced automaticity and (b) reentry. For practical purposes, the ability to initiate and terminate the tachycardia by programmed premature stimulation has been considered highly suggestive of reentry. Findings which further support reentry as the mechanism of sustained ventricular tachycardia include: (a) the association of initiation and maintenance of the arrhythmia with fragmented electrical activity spanning diastole; (b) an inverse relationship (of the coupling interval of the stimulus (S_1–S_2) that initiates the tachycardia to the interval from that initiating stimulus to the onset of the tachycardia); and (c) the ability of drugs such as procainamide to slow and/or abolish the tachycardia and failure of verapamil to affect the tachycardia [105–109]. These findings are incompatible with triggered activity. A schema of the proposed mechanism of ventricular tachycardia associated with coronary artery disease is shown in Figure 12.

The results of catheter and intraoperative mapping of ventricular tachycardia associated with coronary artery disease suggest that the reentrant circuit is located near the endocardium [107, 108, 114–116]. This information explains why simple aneurysmectomy failed to ablate the arrhythmia in patients with coronary artery disease. With standard aneurysmectomy a cuff of tissue is left at the edge of the aneurysm as a sewing ring, and, in addition, the septum is never resected even if it is clearly infarcted. Since experimental data and data from the laboratory indicated that in the presence of coronary artery disease the 'border zone' is where these arrhythmias arise [107–109, 113–116], standard aneurysmectomy would necessarily be insufficient.

359

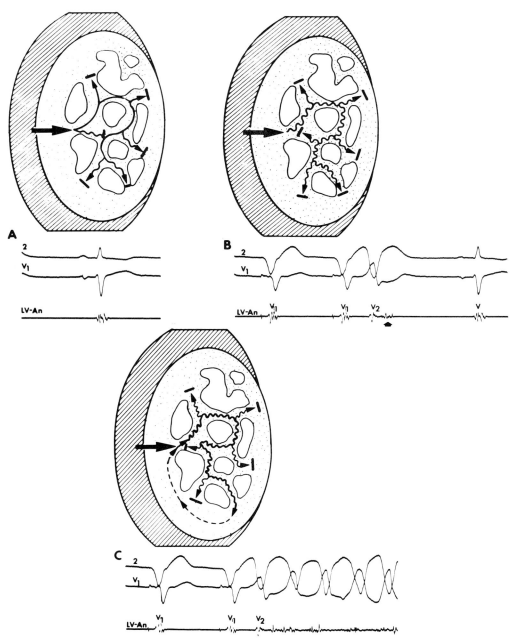

Figure 12. Schema of the mechanism of ventricular tachycardia associated with coronary artery disease. On the left-hand side of the figure, a portion of the left ventricle is shown with normal muscle shown in oblique lines and ischemically damaged muscle in the stippled area. Islands of dead tissue are represented by the empty spaces enclosed within the ischemic area. An electrocardiogram and an electrogram from this area which represents the border of an infarct at the left ventricular aneurysm (LV-An) is shown below each of the panels. In the top panel, during sinus rhythm the cardiac impulse enters the ischemically injured area and conducts slowly but cannot exit since the surrounding area is refractory. The slow conduction is shown by fractionated electrogram in the LV-An recording (panel A). In panel B, during ventricular pacing (V_1) a premature ventricular stimulus (V_2) is delivered which results in marked slowing of impulse propagation through this damaged area. This is associated with more marked fractionation of the electrogram in the LV-An. In panel C, a slightly more premature impulse is introduced during ventricular pacing and conduction of the impulse is slow enough to allow recovery of the surrounding tissue. Reentry occurs resulting in ventricular tachycardia. Note that the fractionated electrogram in the LV-An extends through diastole becoming continuous before and between complexes of the tachycardia.

360

In patients with sustained ventricular tachycardia unrelated to coronary artery disease, programmed stimulation has for the most part demonstrated that the arrhythmias are inducible in a manner similar to tachycardias associated with coronary artery disease [105, 106, 117–121]. Delayed fractionated electrograms have been recorded from patients with right ventricular dysplasia [117–121] and ventricular tachycardia and may represent a marker for reentry, since these electrograms are thought to represent slow conduction, one of the requirements for reentry. Thus, preoperative electrophysiologic evaluation is important for patients undergoing surgery for ventricular tachycardia. It is important to demonstrate that the arrhythmia can be initiated and terminated reproducibly, and, if possible, catheter mapping should be performed to give the surgeon an idea of sites involved in the initiation or propagation of the arrhythmia. This is important for two reasons: (a) if the arrhythmia is inducible in the catheterization laboratory, it is almost always inducible in the operating room, where it can be mapped in more detail; (b) if intraoperative mapping cannot be undertaken for one of a variety of reasons, the preoperative catheter map may be useful in directing the surgical intervention. Of note is the fact that surgery for tachycardias that cannot be initiated in the laboratory is usually unsuccessful [120, 121]. This is true particularly for tachycardias not associated with coronary artery disease, but we believe it applicable also to patients with coronary artery disease. A description of the preoperative and intraoperative mapping procedures is provided below.

Method of catheter endocardial mapping

The purpose of catheter endocardial mapping is to provide information that can help guide the surgical procedure undertaken to ablate the arrhythmia. Catheter endocardial mapping usually is performed in patients in whom the tachycardia is induced by programmed stimulation but can also be used in patients with automatic ventricular tachycardia which is present at the time of the electrophysiologic study but which may not be present at the time of the operation [107, 108, 114]. In addition to giving the surgeon an operative guide, the results of catheter mapping may be the only information on which to base surgery in patients with ventricular tachy-

cardias which are not inducible intraoperatively either prior to and/or following aneurysmectomy and in patients with automatic ventricular tachycardias which are not present at the time of surgery.

To obtain adequate activation maps, multiple electrode catheters are inserted percutaneously or by cutdown and positioned at the atrioventricular junction at the His bundle recording site, the right atrium, the coronary sinus, and the right ventricular apex. These electrodes provide reference electrograms to which the activation data can be compared. They also provide anatomic reference points to the septum (catheter at the right ventricular apex) and posterobasal (coronary sinus catheter) portions of the heart. The mapping catheters are introduced into the venous and arterial systems and positioned in the right and left ventricles. To obtain adequate maps, fluoroscopy in multiple planes is required to identify the catheter position.

A variety of catheters can be used for mapping. We have used interelectrode distances of 1.5 mm– 1 cm without observing any marked differences in activation times; therefore, standard bipolar woven dacron catheters or the new USCI catheter with a 5-mm interelectrode distance can be used. Recordings are made from 15 to 20 sites during sinus rhythm and during the tachycardia. A schema of the mapping sites is depicted in Figure 13. These represent segments of the heart approximately 5–10 cm² in area. When aneurysms are present, one should attempt to record from several sites within

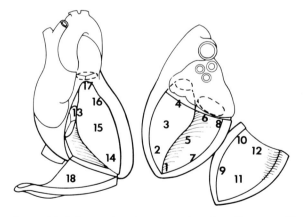

Figure 13. Schema of catheter mapping sites. There are 18 general areas in both the right and left ventricles which are mapped. The left ventricle has 12 sites. These numbered sites represent areas of 5–10 cm² within the ventricles (from [114], with permission of Yorke Publ Co).

361

and on the lateral borders of the aneurysm. We usually use bipolar recordings filtered at 30–500 Hz and a 1-mV calibration signal [107, 108, 114]. Unipolar recordings have been used during the tachycardia but do not appear to be helpful. Each position must be verified in multiple planes and several complexes must be recorded before moving to the next site. We are currently able to localize the pathway of the tachycardia to an area as small as 4 cm^2.

Very low amplitude signals are often recorded from apical aneurysms containing mural thrombus. Similar low amplitude electrograms, however, have been recorded intraoperatively in nine of these patients following removal of the clot [14]. Thus, although interference with recordings may occur because of the clot, we do not believe this is a serious problem. In sinus rhythm and during the tachycardia, in addition to measuring activation times, a qualitative description of the electrogram is recorded. This is particularly important during sinus rhythm where fractionated, split, or late electrograms may have therapeutic importance [114].

To map ventricular tachycardia, the arrhythmia must be present at the time of the procedure, whether spontaneous or induced by programmed stimulation. In addition, the patient must be hemodynamically stable for a long enough time during the tachycardia to permit completion of the map. Although the vast majority of tachycardias can be initiated, 20–30% may be too rapid to map (unpublished observations). In such instances, the rate of the tachycardias may be slowed by antiarrhythmic therapy in order to better define electrical systole and diastole and/or to ensure hemodynamic stability, both of which facilitate the acquisition of mapping data. The presence of the antiarrhythmic drug does not alter the sequence of activation [114]. All stable and morphologically distinct tachycardias should be mapped. Of note, is that, in patients with constantly changing ventricular complexes, the administration of an antiarrhythmic agent may produce a rhythm having a uniform morphology [122]. Depending on the skill and the experience of the catheterizer, construction of a map may take from 25 to 60 min. Obviously, more time is required if multiple QRS morphologies are present. In contrast to the operating room where bypass time is a critical factor, the catheterization laboratory offers a more stable situation in which mapping can take place over a period of several hours without significant complications. If necessary, several catheterizations can be performed.

When a tachycardia is initiated its so-called 'site of origin' is determined by locating the earliest discrete or fragmented electrogram. The presence of a presystolic fragmented electrogram strongly suggests that activity is being recorded from a part of a reentrant circuit [107, 108, 114, 123]. It is not always possible to record holodiastolic activity since such recordings are dependent on the spatial relation of the reentrant circuit to the recording electrodes. Although continuous electrical activity throughout the cardiac cycle occasionally can be recorded and related to initiation and maintenance of the tachycardia, this is uncommon [108]. More often than not, only presystolic activity (i.e., nonholodiastolic activity preceding the QRS) can be recorded. Occasionally broad, fractionated electrograms recorded during rapid heart rate may simulate continuous activity. Such apparent 'continuous activity' should be distinguished from fractionated continuous activity which is required for initiation and maintenance of the tachycardia. This may be accomplished by (a) slowing the tachycardia with drugs to allow separation of systole and diastole or (b) applying local pressure or cryothermia. Termination of the tachycardia by these techniques suggests the continuous electrical activity represented electrical events associated with the reentrant circuit. Proof of reentry would require detailed mapping to demonstrate the reentrant pathway, and technical limitations make this an improbable task to accomplish.

We have been able to map 96 tachycardias in 75 patients with coronary artery disease and 18 morphologically distinct tachycardias in 14 patients without coronary disease [114]. All of the tachycardias in patients with coronary disease arose from the left ventricle or the septum regardless of QRS morphology. In all but three cases, electrical activity could be recorded prior to the onset of the QRS. An example of catheter maps of ventricular tachycardias from a patient with coronary artery disease is shown in Figures 14 and 15. In patients without coronary artery disease, the tachycardias may originate in either the right or the left ventricle. An example of a catheter map of a tachycardia originating in the right ventricle from a patient with right ventricular dysplasia is shown in Figure 16.

362

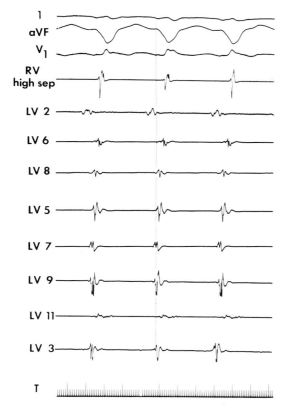

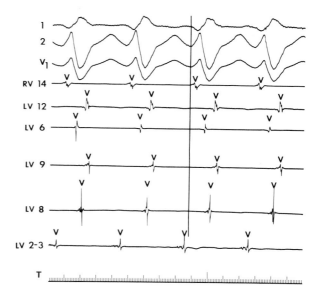

Figure 14. Catheter endocardial map of ventricular tachycardia with a right bundle branch block pattern. From top to bottom are leads I, aVF, V_1, and electrograms from the right ventricular high septum and multiple left ventricular (LV) sites. The earliest recorded activity can be seen at site 2 in the left ventricle. The electrogram at this site begins 55 msec before the onset of the QRS of the tachycardia (dotted line).

Figure 15. Catheter endocardial map of ventricular tachycardia of left bundle branch block morphology. From top to bottom are leads I, 2 and V_1 and electrograms from the right ventricular apex (site 14) and multiple left ventricular sites. The earliest recorded activity can be seen at the junction of sites 2 and 3 in the left ventricle where activity precedes the onset of the QRS by 70 msec with a rapid deflection at 30 msec prior to the onset of the QRS.

The role of mapping during sinus rhythm in patients with ventricular tachycardia is not yet established. However, we have evaluated the possibility of localizing the origin of ventricular tachycardia by analyzing the timing and duration of local ventricular electrograms during sinus rhythm. Although the data are preliminary, it appears that patients with recurrent sustained ventricular tachycardia associated with coronary artery disease have more marked fractionation of electrograms than do normals or other patients with coronary artery disease, infarction and/or aneurysms who do not have ventricular tachycardia [124]. In the majority of instances, the electrogram of longest duration was recorded close to the region at which the earliest activity was recorded by mapping during the tachycardia [125]. Such fractionated activity was observed in all patients in whom continuous activity was associated with initiation and maintenance of the tachycardia [108, 114, 125] (Figure 17). The role of these fractionated and delayed endocardial electrograms in the genesis and localization of ventricular tachycardia remains to be defined both in patients with and those without coronary artery disease.

The ability to perform intraoperative mapping does not detract from the value of catheter mapping. Preoperative catheter mapping is particularly valuable for the following reasons: (a) In some patients a previously inducible tachycardia is no longer inducible in the operating room for a variety of reasons, (b) the tachycardia is automatic in mechanism and is not present at the time of surgery, (c) in some patients not all morphological forms of the tachycardia can be induced or mapped intraoperatively, and (d) it may not be possible to conduct intraoperative endocardial mapping because of physical impediments such as mural thrombosis,

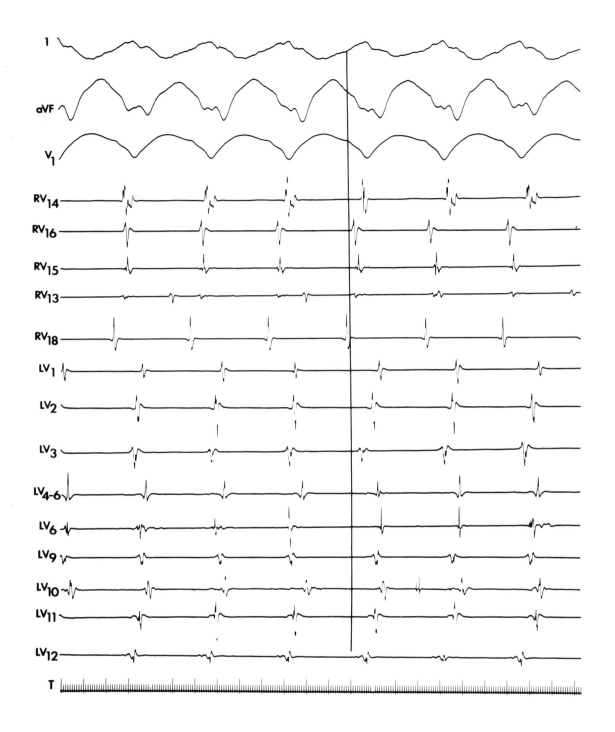

Figure 16. Catheter endocardial map during ventricular tachycardia in a patient with right ventricular dysplasia. Leads I, aVF, and V₁ are shown with local electrograms from multiple right and left ventricular sites. The earliest activity recorded during this tachycardia appeared in the anterior wall of the right ventricle (site 18). This site had markedly abnormal contraction on right ventricular angiography.

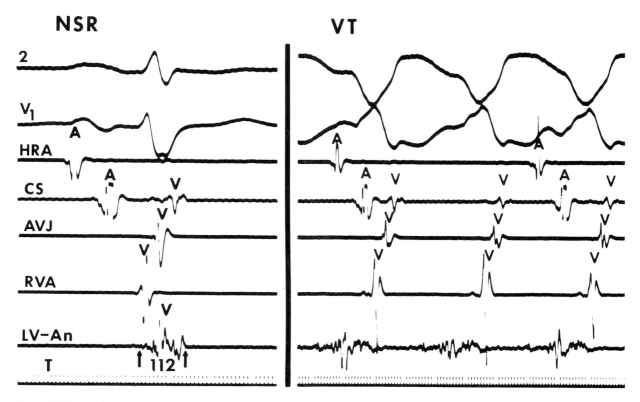

Figure 17. Correlation of electrograms during sinus rhythm and ventricular tachycardia in a patient with coronary artery disease. From top to bottom in both panels are leads 2, V$_1$ and electrograms from the high right atrium (HRA), coronary sinus (CS), atrioventricular junction (AVJ), right ventricular apex (RVA), and the border of the left ventricular aneurysm (LV-An). In sinus rhythm on the left, in the LV-An a broad fractionated electrogram is noted with a duration exceeding that of the QRS. On the right during ventricular tachycardia, the same site demonstrates markedly fractionated activity that spans diastole with the major deflection just preceding the onset of the QRS. See text for further discussion (from [108], with permission of the Am Heart Assoc, Inc).

etc. Although the potential role of catheter mapping during sinus rhythm is not yet established, it may be useful in patients in whom the tachycardia rapidly degenerates to ventricular fibrillation. We believe, therefore, that it is important to perform preoperative endocardial mapping to provide data which can be used to plan surgical ablation, although preoperative endocardial mapping should not replace the more detailed intraoperative map. Our experience suggests that it is a reasonable alternative when intraoperative studies cannot be performed.

Intraoperative mapping of ventricular tachycardia

Intraoperative mapping in patients with ventricular tachycardia uses procedures similar to those employed for intraoperative mapping of the Wolff-

Parkinson-White syndrome [36]. Mapping of ventricular tachycardia is carried out using hand-held or fingertip ring electrodes with two or three electrodes having an interelectrode distance of 1–2 mm. The electrodes are connected to a junction box and either unipolar or bipolar signals can be recorded. In most instances bipolar recordings are used since they record more local electrical activity. Unipolar electrograms may be used in conjunction with the bipolar electrogram and may be of value in analyzing the wavefront of activation. The electrograms recorded from the roving or mapping electrode are displayed with one or two reference electrodes obtained by either fixed electrodes sewn to selected portions of the heart, stainless steel plunge electrodes, and/or catheter electrodes which are positioned preoperatively. We prefer two reference electrodes since the variability of the surface electrocardiogram during surgery may result either from changing activation patterns or changing cardiac position. The reference electrograms as well as the electrograms recorded from the mapping probe are displayed with two or three simultaneous ECG leads. We usually use leads 1, aVF, and either V_5, V_6, V_{5R}, or V_{6R}, and set filters at 40–500 Hz. Usually a 1-mV calibration signal is used to measure the amplitudes of the recorded electrograms. The epicardial recording sites usually are identified by a grid dividing the epicardial surface of the heart into approximately 50 segments. The grid used at the University of Pennsylvania (Figure 18) has 54 standards sites but allows for mapping in half-sites both vertically and horizontally. The timing of the electrograms is measured using one of the reference electrograms and later its relationship to the onset of the QRS is established. The measurements can be made by computerized techniques and epicardial maps constructed [117–121, 126, 127]; however, if stable tachycardias are present, the site of earliest activation can be identified visually and measured manually in a short period of time [116].

Mapping is performed first during sinus rhythm in order to identify abnormal electrograms (low amplitude, fractionated, split, and late potentials) which may reflect slow conduction and therefore a potential substrate for reentry (Figure 19) [116–121, 128]. The tachycardia is induced by programmed stimulation and the map repeated to obtain the earliest site of epicardial activation. More than one epicardial breakthrough site may be present. If more than one morphologically distinct ventricular tachycardia is present, epicardial activation studies

should be obtained for each of the different morphologies. It is critical to maintain the patients at normothermia or slightly hyperthemic, since it may not be possible to initiate a sustained tachycardia reproducibly unless the perfusing solutions are maintained at these temperatures (unpublished observations). Cooling of the heart frequently either prevents initiation of the tachycardia or produces immediate fibrillation.

Once epicardial mapping of the tachycardia is completed, the aneurysm and/or infarction can be opened and/or resected. In many instances, the tachycardia will continue despite this procedure and endocardial mapping can be undertaken. Initially we map the endocardium around the cut edge of the aneurysm in clockwise fashion with an ever increasing radius: usually 40–60 endocardial sites are mapped. If the tachycardia ceases following ventriculotomy and/or resection, in our experience, it almost always can be reinitiated. Failure to reinitiate the tachycardia can occur and does not necessarily mean the reentrant circuit has been interrupted. Stretch of the myocardium can render the circuit temporarily unable to sustain reentry. In addition to endocardial maps of the tachycardia, it may be desirable to perform endocardial mapping during sinus rhythm. This procedure, which has been employed by Waldo et al. [128], is used to localize abnormal electrograms suggesting slow conduction. Once the epicardial and endocardial activation sequences are mapped, the surgical procedure can be undertaken. Mapping usually requires 30–75 min of cardiopulmonary bypass time, and this is a limiting factor in patients who have multiple morphologies of ventricular tachycardia.

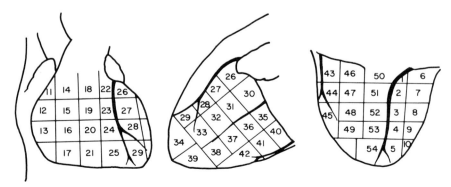

Figure 18. Scheme of epicardial mapping sites. The heart is shown in the anterior, left lateral, and inferior views. Fifty-four predetermined sites are demonstrated as a guide to the surgeon (from [115], with permission of the Am Heart Assoc, Inc).

epicardial, transmural, and endocardial mapping is required in order to evaluate more properly the mechanism of the arrhythmia as well as the optimal surgical therapy.

Results of intraoperative mapping in patients with ventricular tachycardia associated with coronary artery disease

The early experience of Fontaine et al. [117, 119–121], Wittig and Boineau [139], and Moran et al. [101], as well as experimental data [134] emphasized that epicardial recording may not adequately localize the site of origin of ventricular tachycardias associated with coronary artery disease. In fact, epicardial mapping studies during tachycardia frequently revealed one or more epicardial breakthrough sites which always followed the onset of the surface QRS during the tachycardia [101, 116, 120, 135, 136], suggesting that the epicardium was not the source of the arrhythmia. Support of a subendocardial origin of the arrhythmia has been suggested by catheter mapping techniques [107, 108, 114], intraoperative endocardial mapping [115, 116, 129], and pathologic data [137].

Late potentials have not been as consistent a finding in patients with myocardial infarction as they are in patients with arrhythmogenic right ventricular dysplasia. Fontaine et al. [117, 119] found late potentials in six of 19 patients with ventricular tachycardia associated with coronary artery disease, and in only two of these cases was there a correlation with the earliest epicardial breakthrough. In the remaining patients, the data have been described as uninterpretable but were not presented. The group at the University of Pennsylvania [116, 138, 139] have found epicardial late potentials in eight of 60 patients, in four of whom they appeared related to the site of origin or the tachycardia which always arose from the underlying endocardium on the free wall of the left ventricle. In the remaining four patients in whom there was no correlation, the site of origin of the tachycardia was on the left side of the interventricular septum. On the other hand, Waldo et al. [128, 140] have reported fractionated epicardial and endocardial electrograms in 20 of 21 patients with ventricular arrhythmias (17 of whom had sustained ventricular tachycardia), but recorded delayed potentials in 12 of the 21 patients. This group believes such fractionation and late potentials are specific for patients with arrhythmias but have not correlated these findings with the results of mapping of ventricular tachycardia. It is the authors' opinion that fractionated electrograms and delayed potentials can occur in areas of prior infarction and may be unrelated to the tachycardia. The demonstration that such activity is correlated with the area of earliest activity of the tachycardia is required to support the relationship of late potentials to arrhythmogenic sites. In the absence of such data, extrapolation of the finding of fractionated electrograms and/or late potentials during sinus rhythm to the site of origin of ventricular tachycardia cannot be made.

Mapping during ventricular tachycardia associated with coronary artery disease has been reported primarily by the group at the University of Pennsylvania [116, 138, 139]. Their studies are the only ones that report both epicardial and endocardial activation in this group of patients. Although there have been other isolated reports of epicardial maps in such patients [101, 129, 135], all of which demonstrated rather late epicardial breakthrough, these have not analyzed epicardial and endocardial mapping during ventricular tachycardia. Mason et al. recently have reported intraoperative mapping data on 60 patients with ventricular tachycardia associated with coronary artery disease [133]. Ninety-five morphologically distinct ventricular tachycardias in the 60 patients were studied. Thirty-one of the patients had more than one morphologically distinct tachycardia. Although complete epicardial and endocardial activation maps were obtained in at least one morphologically distinct tachycardia in almost all patients, such data were not obtainable during each morphologically distinct tachycardia for a variety of reasons, including mural thrombus, degeneration of the rhythm to ventricular fibrillation, failure to initiate the arrhythmia, prolonged bypass time, or intraoperative complications. As observed by others [101, 127, 129, 135], epicardial activation typically began after the onset of the QRS. In one patient, epicardial breakthrough occurred at the onset of the QRS and in the remaining patients, epicardial breakthrough appeared 10–76 msec following the onset of the QRS. In tachycardias with a right bundle branch block morphology, epicardial breakthrough always was on the left ventricle, whereas in those tachycardias with left bundle branch morphology epicardial breakthrough was usually on the right ventricle adjacent to the interventricular groove. In patients with ventricular aneurysms, low amplitude, fractionated, or no activity was recorded over parts of the aneurysm during the tachycardia. Such fractionated and/or low amplitude potentials have been described by others over aneurysms and in border zones [117, 120, 128].

Detailed analysis of endocardial activation during ventricular tachycardia has revealed that endocardial activity always can be recorded prior to epicardial activation (14–85 msec) and that activity could be recorded prior to the onset of the QRS during the tachycardia (Figure 20). This closely corresponded to what Josephson et al. reported during catheter endocardial mapping [107, 108, 114, 115]. Continuous activation spanning the cardiac cycle in a sequential fashion was observed

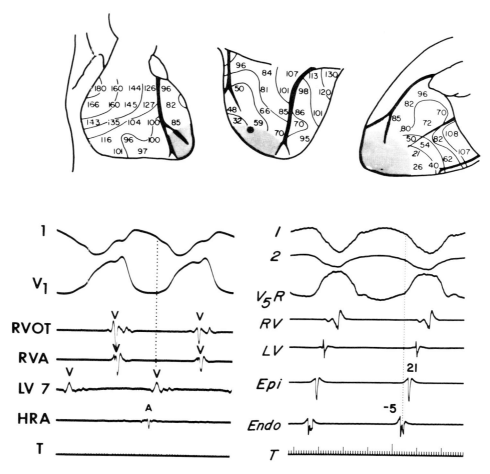

Figure 20. Relationship of epicardial to endocardial activation during ventricular tachycardia. An isochronic epicardial map is shown on top in the anterior, inferior, and lateral views. The stippled area represents the aneurysm. Earliest epicardial breakthrough can be seen 21 msec after the onset of the QRS at the anterior lateral border of the aneurysm. The earliest activation recorded was on the endocardium on the inferior apical border of the aneurysm (dark circle in inferior view of heart). On the bottom of the figure are analog records. On the left is a catheter map in which recordings from the right ventricular outflow tract (RVOT), right ventricular apex (RVA), the high right atrium (HRA), and left ventricular (LV) site 7 are shown. LV site 7 was the earliest site of activity, the onset of which preceded the onset of the QRS during the tachycardia. Site 7 is at the inferior lateral apex of the heart at the site found to be the earliest activated during intraoperative mapping. The earliest epicardial and endocardial activation noted intraoperatively is shown in the lower right-hand panel. Leads 1, 2, and V_5 are shown with reference electrograms from the right ventricle (RV) and left ventricle (LV). Earliest epicardial (epi) activation was noted 21 msec following the onset of the QRS while earliest endocardial (endo) activation was 5 msec preceding the QRS. The endocardial activation times, both intraoperatively and preoperatively, were nearly identical.

during three tachycardias and was interpreted as recording of a reentrant circuit (Figure 21). In one-third of the patients discrete systolic and diastolic activity bridging the cardiac cycle could be recorded at the same or adjacent sites, again suggesting recording from different limbs of a reentrant circuit. In this group of patients there were regions in which electrograms recorded presystolic activity which continued into systole; digital pressure at these sites frequently terminated the arrhythmia. In 25 of the 31 patients with multiple morphologically distinct tachycardias, the earliest activity during

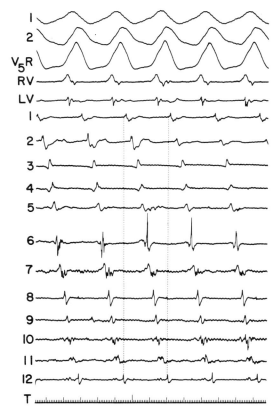

Figure 21. Endocardial map during ventricular tachycardia. Leads 1, 2, and V_5 are shown with reference electrograms from the right ventricle and left ventricle (RV, LV). Numbers 1 through 12 represent clock positions around the border of the left ventricular aneurysm. It can be seen that activity spans the cardiac cycle and is continuous around the border of the aneurysm. Each electrogram remained in fixed relationship to the preceding one. Digital pressure at several sites reproduced the terminated tachycardia. Demonstration of a continuum of activity suggested recording of the reentrant circuit. See text for further discussion (from [116], with permission of the Am Heart Assoc, Inc).

each tachycardia was recorded within 3 cm, suggesting that the different morphologies represented different exit points from a reentrant circuit with subsequently different ventricular activation patterns. In six patients, however, there appeared to be two widely disparate areas of origin.

There was no correlation of epicardial break-through and earliest site of endocardial activation when the tachycardias originated on the septum. In such cases, epicardial breakthrough always appeared along the interventricular groove in either the right or left ventricle, and this location was 3–8 cm away from the site of earliest recorded endocardial activity. When the tachycardia arose on the free wall of the left ventricle, the earliest epicardial and endocardial activation were correlated (within 2 cm) in half the patients, whereas in the remaining patients epicardial breakthrough and endocardial area of origin were disparate. These data are similar to those of Wittig and Boineau [129] and Moran et al. [101] and stress the limitations of epicardial mapping in patients with coronary artery disease.

Surgical procedures for ventricular tachycardia

Although many surgical procedures have been employed to treat various ventricular arrhythmias, only those procedures based on an understanding of the underlying pathophysiology of arrhythmias will be described. By and large, ventricular tachycardias which can be surgically ablated are reentrant in nature or at least can be initiated reproducibly and evaluated. In rare cases an incessant automatic tachycardia can be present at surgery and activation studies can be useful as a guide to its therapy.

Although routine aneurysmectomy with or without bypass grafting has been the most commonly employed surgical intervention for the management of ventricular tachycardia associated with chronic ischemic heart disease [93–103], it will not be further discussed due to the inherent limitations of the procedure described earlier. Clearly, this procedure, which has its unequivocal successes, is out of date as a procedure to ablate ventricular tachycardia. The data which have relegated standard aneurysmectomy to the 'outdated' classification include: (a) standard aneurysmectomy routinely leaves in place the border zone which is a source of

371

the reentry phenomenon and (b) standard aneurysmectomy has no effect on tachycardias originating in the septum. Standard aneurysmectomy can work only if a suture modifies a border zone or if the resection or suturing interrupts the reentrant circuit.

Another procedure that will not be discussed at length is sympathectomy, particularly left cervical stellectomy, for the management of patients with ventricular tachycardia resulting from the long QT syndrome [141–143]. Left stellectomy was initially performed by Moss and McDonald [141] in order to decrease the QT interval. Although shortening of the QT interval was initially the goal of such surgery, it was apparent that stellectomy could increase fibrillation thresholds regardless of its effect on the QT interval [142]. Moreover, propranolol, which is the initial therapy of choice, is also successful without necessarily shortening the QT interval. Propranolol therapy is, however, associated with a 6% failure rate, and its sudden discontinuation can lead to syncope and/or sudden death [142]. The exact number of patients who have undergone left stellectomy for the management of this disorder is unknown but is probably less than 30. Twenty patients were reported by Schwartz, all of whom are alive and without syncope [142]. Of note, more than half still have a prolonged QT interval [142]. The side effects of the procedure and the incidence of maintained drug therapy were not discussed. Thus, the exact role of stellectomy in the management of the long QT syndrome remains to be defined.

The surgical procedures which are currently used to treat ventricular tachycardia include simple transmural ventriculotomy, encircling endocardial ventriculotomy, radical myocardial resection, cryosurgery, or subendocardial resection. Combinations of these procedures may be employed in addition to concomitant resection of dysplastic right ventricle, aneurysms, and/or coronary bypass grafting. All the procedures except encircling endocardial ventriculotomy [71, 120, 121] require some form of guidance by activation mapping.

Simple transmural ventriculotomy

Simple transmural ventriculotomy guided by epicardial mapping has its major role in the management of recurrent sustained ventricular tachycardia in the absence of coronary artery disease [117–121,

127]. Transmural ventriculotomy was always employed at sites of epicardial breakthrough during ventricular tachycardia. In many instances these workers used multiple ventriculotomies which could be 4–5 cm in length. In addition to the ventriculotomy at the site of epicardial breakthrough, Guiraudon, Fontaine and colleagues [117–121] have performed ventriculotomy in areas of late potentials (i.e., those exhibiting the postexcitation phenomenon) or excision if these potentials are located in thin-walled dysplastic right ventricles. Somewhat inconsistent was their decision not to perform ventriculotomy or other surgical procedures in areas of postexcitation if such areas were found in macroscopically normal parts of the heart [119]. Similar procedures have been described by Spurrell et al. [127] and Waldo and Kirklin [128].

Fontaine and Guiraudon and colleagues from Paris have the greatest experience using this technique. Of 19 patients with ventricular tachycardia in the absence of coronary artery disease, these workers attempted to ablate the arrhythmia using simple transmural ventriculotomy with or without excision in 16 [120, 121]. In the three remaining patients, excision alone (two) or plication (one) was used to treat the arrhythmia. (In the two cases with excision alone, endocardial encircling ventriculotomy may also have been employed.) Twelve of the 16 patients treated with a simple transmural ventriculotomy, including all nine with arrhythmogenic right ventricular dysplasia, were cured by the procedure. The four failures included one with idiopathic left ventricular tachycardia who presented with at least seven areas of epicardial breakthrough all of which could not be included in the ventriculotomy. This patient died postoperatively on the fifth day due to ventricular tachycardia and low cardiac output. There was a second operative death related to low output failure in a patient with Uhl's anomaly. In the remaining three patients in whom ventriculotomy did not ablate the arrhythmia, no late potentials were found during epicardial mapping and the tachycardias could not be initiated by programmed stimulation and were therefore considered to be automatic in nature. Since the rationale for the procedure was the interruption of large reentrant loops, Fontaine and Guiraudon and colleagues [119–121] now recommend that such surgery only be undertaken in patients with inducible arrhythmias. The hallmarks of the studies of their patients were late potentials recorded during sinus rhythm by epicardial mapping and the ability to determine accurately the sites of epicardial breakthrough. Although the sites of late potentials and early epicardial breakthrough were not always identical (vide supra), such potentials were consistent findings in the successfully treated patients.

Attempts to extrapolate the use of ventriculotomy to patients with tachycardias associated with coronary artery disease have not been successful. Fontaine et al. operated on 13 patients with ventricular tachycardia associated with prior myocardial infarction [117]. They attempted to use epicardial mapping to guide the site of ventriculotomy. In 11 of the 13 the epicardial mapping data were considered uninterpretable, since multiple epicardial breakthrough sites and absence of late potentials prevented them from selecting appropriate sites at which the ventriculotomy was to be made. In the only two cases in whom the data were considered to be interpretable (i.e., late potentials adjacent to the site of breakthrough) ventriculotomy was performed. Even so, only one of these operations was a success. The inability to localize adequately the origin of ventricular tachycardia by epicardial mapping has been corroborated by experimental studies and clinical experience [101, 115, 116, 129, 134–136]. Moreover, late potentials, which commonly are observed in patients with tachycardias not associated with coronary artery disease, are, according to most investigators, infrequently present in patients with coronary artery disease [116, 119, 121, 138, 139]. Spurrell et al. [127], however, successfully treated ventricular tachycardia in a patient by using multiple ventriculotomies. The extensive surgical interventions employed in his patient, however, were followed by hemodynamic decompensation. Thus, simple transmural ventriculotomy in the management of ventricular tachycardia associated with coronary artery disease appears to be of limited use, and probably should be reserved for patients with ventricular tachycardias unassociated with coronary artery disease. The patients to whom this procedure appears to be most successfully applied are those with arrhythmogenic right ventricular dysplasia.

Encircling endocardial ventriculotomy

Guiraudon et al. [71, 120, 121, 144] have developed a new surgical approach to the management of ventricular tachycardia associated with coronary artery disease. Based on their surgical data which demonstrated that the most severe ischemic lesions in myocardial infarction are subendocardial and extend beyond the limits of apparent epicardial damage and that experimental animal and human data suggesting that the areas responsible for ventricular tachycardia are located at the subendocardial junction of ischemic and normal tissue [106–110, 113, 116], these workers believed a circular ventriculotomy performed outside the limits of this subendocardial border zone would interrupt and/or isolate the reentrant circuit from the remainder of the myocardium. Thus, the encircling endocardial ventriculotomy was designed to exclude all the abnormal myocardium, through which slow conduction must occur as a requisite for reentrant activity, from electrical continuity with the remaining normal myocardium. With this procedure, spontaneous ventricular premature depolarizations could not initiate reentry since the area of slow conduction was isolated from the normal myocardium. Even if reentry were to occur, the tachycardia would not be able to exit from the area to the remaining myocardium.

The procedure is carried out following entrance to the ventricular cavity by standard ventriculotomy through the aneurysm or infarction. A nearby transmural ventriculotomy is then performed with a perpendicular incision around the visible border of endocardial fibrosis, sparing the epicardium and coronary arteries (Figure 22). When the septum is involved, the procedure must virtually disarticulate the septum from the remaining ventricle. The ventriculotomy is then repaired with running sutures buttressed with teflon strips or pledgets.

Guiraudon et al. have operated on 23 patients using this technique [144]. The site of infarction was anterior in 13 patients, septal in two patients, and posterior in eight patients [144]. There were two operative deaths, both in patients with low ejection fractions (EF = 25%). Four of the survivors had recurrent episodes of ventricular tachycardia, two of whom have been treated successfully pharmacologically. There have been two late nonarrhythmic deaths in a follow-up ranging from one to 55 months.

Waldo and colleagues also have utilized a complete or modified encircling endocardial ventricu-

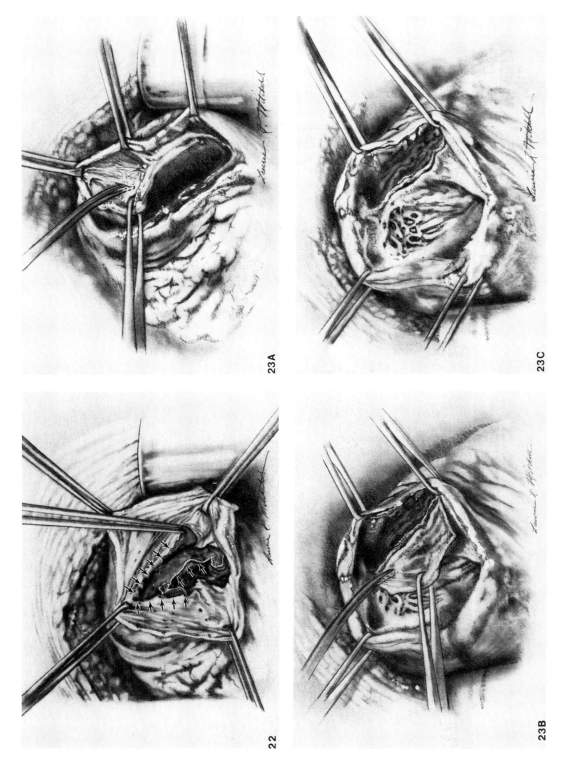

22

23A

23B

23C

Figure 22. Encircling endocardial ventriculotomy. A sketch of an encircling endocardial ventriculotomy is shown with the arrows delineating the perpendicular incision at the border of the endocardial scar. *Figure 23.* Subendocardial resection. Panels A through C demonstrate sequence of subendocardial resection from the septal border of an aneurysm. At the top (A) the endocardium is undermined by scissors. A 1–3-mm thick sheet of endocardium is undermined (panel B). Following subendocardial resection the septum is left denuded (C) (adapted from [136] and [150]).

374

lotomy guided by sinus rhythm epicardial and endocardial mapping in 16 patients [128, 140]. Three of the seven patients in whom a complete encircling endocardial ventriculotomy was performed died of low cardiac output; two of these patients had ventricular tachycardia. There was one late sudden death (probably due to recurrent ventricular tachycardia) and another death from sepsis. Of the 11 remaining patients, all are alive without evidence of recurrent tachycardia with a follow-up of one to 54 months. Eight of these patients are on antiarrhythmic agents, one for ventricular tachycardia. Cox (J. R. Cox, personal communication), Mason (J. W. Mason, personal communication) and Engel [145] report hemodynamic impairment in patients undergoing encircling endocardial ventriculotomy. Ungerleider et al. [146] have demonstrated that the procedure causes an ischemic insult to the viable myocardial tissue overlying the subendocardial scar. Thus, the viable tissue between the limits of subendocardial fibrosis and the epicardial extension of the infarction is placed in jeopardy by this procedure. Guiraudon and co-workers [120, 121, 144], as well as Waldo [128], Mason (J. W. Mason, personal communication), and Cox (J. R. Cox, personal communication) no longer recommend performing encircling endocardial ventriculotomy in patients in whom significant myocardial dysfunction is present preoperatively.

Encircling endocardial ventriculotomy offers a new approach to management of ventricular tachycardias which appears quite successful in selected patients. The advantages of the procedure are chiefly that neither the induction of the tachycardia nor mapping are really required intraoperatively since the incision is guided by visual delineation of the border of subendocardial fibrosis in normal tissue. Therefore, it theoretically can be applied widely since sophisticated equipment and experienced electrophysiologists are not necessary. The procedure does have limitations. A major concern is the effect of the procedure on ventricular function. Hemodynamic evaluation of this procedure has not been undertaken prospectively, and the exact role of this procedure in the management of ventricular tachycardia depends upon its ability to prevent tachycardias and preserve ventricular function. Unfortunately, low cardiac outputs and low ejection fractions are the rule in patients with ventricular tachycardia associated with coronary artery dis-

ease. Thus, the hemodynamic effects of this procedure must be established prior to establishing its role in the management of these arrhythmias.

Another potential limitation is the requirement for septal disarticulation to deal with arrhythmias arising in the septum, a fairly frequent finding. Moreover, certain structures may pose difficulty in performing a ventriculotomy – for example, the base of the papillary muscle may be composed of several trunks matted closely to the ventricular wall, a condition which would make encircling this area difficult if not impossible. Finally, the effects of sutures on thrombus formation and/or endocarditis have not been commented upon.

Radical myocardial resection

Although standard aneurysmectomy has not proven to be effective routinely in the management of ventricular tachycardia, the group from the Mayo Clinic has suggested that radical surgical resection of abnormal myocardium might be effective [147]. This group reported a series of 13 patients with recurrent ventricular tachycardia. They used epicardial mapping to delineate epicardial breakthrough sites and concluded that these breakthrough sites were relevant if they occurred within the first 25–30 msec of the tachycardia. Using mapping as a guide, aneurysmectomy was done including the entire scar and normal muscle in the area showing epicardial breakthrough. This extensive excision included the rim of tissue around the aneurysm which usually is left in place. In addition, in five of the patients a portion of the interventricular septum was removed. There were two operative deaths, one with recurrence of the ventricular tachycardia. Of the 11 survivors, there has been one recurrence of ventricular tachycardia. Several of the survivors, however, are maintained on antiarrhythmic therapy for reasons that are unclear. Detailed electrophysiologic studies were not performed postoperatively to assess the efficacy of the procedure. All survivors were said to improve hemodynamically over a mean follow-up of 19 months (range 2–40 months), although no specific data have been given.

Whether or not radical resection will offer any advantages over less extensive surgical ablation remains to be seen (vide infra, subendocardial resection). As a result of the nature of the radical resection, normal myocardium must necrose due to placement of sutures through it. This myocardial necrosis could impair hemodynamic function. Another potential complication of extensive excision is reduction of the cavity size of the left ventricle, further decreasing cardiac output. Finally, resection of significant portions of the septum necessitates replacement of the septum with a patch. This procedure markedly increases cardiopulmonary bypass time, increasing the hematologic complications caused by prolonged 'pump-time.' Thus, although radical resection can ablate the tachycardia, it seems that an inordinate amount of tissue is removed which may result in compromise of ventricular function. More experience is necessary to evaluate this technique.

Cryosurgery for ventricular tachycardia

With the development of cryosurgical techniques to ablate the His bundle [52, 53], the use of cryoablation to treat ventricular tachycardia has been explored [49, 130, 148]. In addition, cryothermia has been used as a method for localizing critical areas of the reentrant circuit in a manner similar to that used to identify bypass tracts. Transient abolition of the tachycardia by cryothermia suggests that the region cooled was a critical component of the tachycardia circuit [49, 130]. Cryothermia has been shown to produce predictable lesions in the myocardium as first described by Haas [149]. The cryolesion has smooth borders and is sharply demarcated from normal myocardium [52, 68, 149]. The scar is firm and does not disrupt anatomic continuity of adjacent myocardium. Moreover, the size and shape of the lesion can be controlled by adjusting the surface area of the probe in contact with the myocardium, increasing the duration of cooling, decreasing the probe temperatures and the use of multiple cryothermal applications. A disadvantage of the standard flat probe is that the depth of the cryothermal lesion varies and the lesion may not be transmural. However, if the cryothermal probe is used in an area that is already thinned by infarction, multiple applications of cryothermia should produce a homogeneous lesion. In addition, a trocar probe may be used to freeze at deeper sites.

Klein et al. [69] have evaluated the electrophysiologic effects of cryothermal injury on the myocardium. They analyzed electrophysiologic character-

istics of the site of the cryothermal injury as well as adjacent sites using multipolar transmural electrograms. Initially, transmural myocardial damage was produced as evidenced by QS complexes over the lesions. By four weeks some of the epicardial complexes had small R waves. The deeper areas near the subendocardium showed evidence of survival of Purkinje fibers. Overall, there were decreased R wave voltages and reduced slopes of the intrinsicoid deflection of the unipolar electrograms, which are consistent with loss of the outer layers of the myocardium. The electrophysiologic abnormalities were discrete with a sharp transition between the scar produced by the cryothermal injury and normal muscle. This sharp transition also was noted in pathologic studies. Of interest was the fact that all animals studied demonstrated spontaneous ventricular premature depolarizations of various frequencies, all of which appeared to arise at the border of the cryothermal lesion, usually near the subendocardium. Two dogs actually demonstrated ventricular tachycardia with characteristics similar to those of accelerated ventricular tachycardia. However, nearly all the ventricular irritability disappeared by the end of the first week. Thus, the technique appears safe and effective in the production of discrete myocardial lesions.

There has been a limited experience in the use of cryothermal damage to treat ventricular tachycardia. The first application of cryothermal injury in the treatment of a ventricular tachycardia was reported by Gallagher et al. [130] in a patient in whom an automatic ventricular tachycardia associated with scleroderma was ablated. This tachycardia, whose origin was identified in the right ventricle, was transiently terminated by temporary cooling and permanently terminated with cryothermal application at –60 °C for 3 min. Of note, however, was the recurrence of ventricular tachycardia with a different morphology but originating from the right ventricle eight months later. This may have reflected inadequate cryothermal damage. Camm et al. [48, 148] also have employed cryosurgery in the treatment of ventricular tachycardia. Cryothermal mapping was performed in a manner analogous to that of Gallagher et al. [130] in which the effects of temporary cooling on the tachycardia were assessed. Termination of the tachycardia upon temporary cooling suggested that the site that was cooled was a critical component of the tachycardia circuit. That site was then cryoablated. Camm used these techniques in two patients [49, 148]. In one, epicardial mapping could not be used to delineate the tachycardia which ultimately was shown to arise from the septum. In the second patient, cryothermal damage at the earliest epicardial breakthrough at the edge of an aneurysm terminated the tachycardia. Cryothermia was applied multiple times in adjacent regions so that the extent of the cryolesion, although not described, must have been several cm^2. Mason et al. have used cryosurgery in three patients with good results (J. W. Mason, personal communication).

Whereas cryothermia appears promising, it does require some form of mapping. It has theoretical advantages in that it can be used to locate the tachycardia as well as abolish it. Since the fibrous stroma is not affected by cryothermia, the major structural substrate of the patient's heart remains intact. The major limitation will be the size of the probe and the tissue interface. Lesions of only a limited size can be produced with one application and several applications must be used. Endocardial mapping and application of cryothermia may improve the efficacy of this procedure. Further work is necessary to establish the exact role of cryosurgery in the management of ventricular tachycardia, but we believe that it may play an important role, particularly in conjunction with subendocardial resection.

Subendocardial resection for ventricular tachycardia

With the advent of invasive electrophysiologic investigations, a greater understanding of the mechanisms of ventricular tachycardia was obtained. These data suggested that ventricular tachycardia associated with chronic coronary artery disease was due to reentry and that the reentrant circuit was located near the endocardium [105–109, 114–116]. Based on these data, we developed the technique of subendocardial resection to treat ventricular tachycardia associated with coronary artery disease [136, 150]. With this procedure the subendocardium in the region of earliest recorded activity determined by intraoperative and/or catheter mapping (see above) is undermined and resected (10–15 cm^2) (Figure 23).

Sixty consecutive patients with medically refrac-

tory recurrent sustained ventricular tachycardia associated with prior myocardial infarction underwent subendocardial resection at the hospital of the University of Pennsylvania [138]. All patients had failed at least two standard antiarrhythmic agents (range 2–6 drugs) during serial electrophysiologic studies. In ten patients experimental antiarrhythmic agents also failed to prevent initiation of the tachycardia by programmed ventricular stimulation.

Fifty-eight of the 60 patients underwent catheter endocardial mapping as described above. In all patients operated on, electrical activity preceding the onset of the QRS could be recorded from the area of infarction and/or border of left ventricular aneurysm.

All patients underwent complete angiographic and hemodynamic catheterization. All patients had coronary artery disease, most with multivessel disease (mean 2.0 vessels with ≥50% obstruction). The mean cardiac index was 2.7 l/min/m^2, mean ejection fraction was 27% and mean left ventricular end-diastolic pressure was 17.5 mmHg. Fifty-two patients had left ventricular aneurysms; two had had prior aneurysmectomy for recurrent ventricular tachycardia. Eight patients had infarctions without aneurysms; in each of these the infarction was inferior in location.

Surgical results
Subendocardial resection was accomplished in 60 patients with ventricular tachycardia associated with coronary artery disease, 52 of whom had concomitant aneurysmectomies. Forty patients also received coronary artery bypass grafts with an average of 1.6 grafts per patient. There were five deaths within 30 days. Three patients died from pump failure in the first week; two of these had suffered a myocardial infarction within a week prior to surgery. One patient had an acute infarction on the eighth postoperative day and died in electrical-mechanical dissociation. Both bypass grafts were widely patent and infarction was assumed to be secondary to spasm. The remaining death occurred in a patient in whom ventricular tachycardia arose in the posterior papillary muscle; thus, only partial subendocardial resection could be accomplished. Ventricular tachycardia was inducible by programmed stimulation two weeks postoperatively (none occurred spontaneously) and the

patient was treated with disopyramide to control his inducible arrythmia. Two days after initiating therapy, he developed acute cardiogenic shock and died. At the time of death he was in sinus rhythm. There was no evidence of myocardial infarction, and death was attributed to disopyramide-induced cardiac dysfunction.

The remaining 55 patients underwent programmed ventricular stimulation ten to 28 days postoperatively. The study included single and double, and on occasion, triple ventricular extrastimuli from the right and, when necessary, from the left ventricle. In 42 patients no ventricular tachycardia was inducible (group 1), and they were discharged on no medication. Ventricular tachycardia was inducible in the remaining 13 patients (group 2), in three of whom ventricular tachycardia occurred spontaneously prior to electrophysiologic study. Each underwent serial electrophysiologic studies to assess drug therapy. In five patients ventricular tachycardia was no longer inducible on antiarrhythmic agents, in eight patients ventricular tachycardia was still inducible, although in most patients it was both more difficult to induce and slower in rate than prior to antiarrhythmic therapy. All group 2 patients were discharged with prescriptions for these drugs which made the tachycardia either noninducible or more difficult to induce.

Forty-nine patients underwent cardiac catheterization prior to discharge; the preliminary results of these studies have been reported [138, 151]. As noted above, 52 patients had aneurysmectomies and the remaining patients had ventriculotomy and endocardial resection alone. Sixty-three coronary bypass grafts were placed in 40 patients. In the patients studied all but two grafts were patent (96%). In the patients with aneurysmectomy, the mean ejection fraction rose from 27% to 39% (p < 0.0005), and mean left ventricular end-diastolic pressure decreased from 17 to 12 mmHg (p < 0.001), while cardiac index was unchanged. No thrombus was observed nor was there any evidence of ventricular septal defect at the time of left ventricular angiography.

Follow-up
Of the 55 surviving patients, 42 (group 1) were discharged with no antiarrhythmic agent for prevention of ventricular tachycardia. The 13 group 2 patients were discharged on antiarrhythmic agents.

On follow-up of two to 41 months, there have been nine late deaths: six in group 1 and three in group 2 (Table 7). Four have been due to progressive heart failure, two have been due to myocardial infarction, one due to pneumonia, one due to rupture of a mycotic aneurysm of the pulmonary artery, and one due to cardiac rupture. The site of cardiac rupture was at an area of recent ischemia adjacent to the ventricular suture line. The area of endocardial resection, which was on the septum, was intact and coated with an endothelial fibroblastic layer without evidence of thrombosis. There have been two recurrences in group 1, both of which were controlled with antiarrhythmic agents. There have been two recurrences in group 2 which were controlled by increasing the dose of medication. No other patients have required hospitalization for arrhythmias. Half of the surviving patients have complex ventricular ectopic activity but remain asymptomatic and untreated. An actuarial predicted survival curve demonstrates 62% at 40 months (Figure 24). Mason and colleagues (J. W. Mason, personal comunication) have observed similar successes in a smaller number of patients.

Values and limitations of subendocardial resection
The advantages of subendocadial resection are related to the fact that surgery is directed to the area or areas responsible for the arrhythmia. As a result, the resection is limited and only involves the subendocardial border of the aneurysm or infarct. This allows the surgeon to utilize the cuff or fibrous rim of the aneurysm to close the aneurysmectomy. This

Table 7. Endocardial resection for VT (follow-up 55 patients).

Noninducible (42 patients)	Inducible (13 patients)	
	Antiarrhythmic agents	
	Noninducible (5 patients)	Inducible (8 patients)
2 Recurrences	0 Recurrences	2 Recurrences

Late deaths 9 (1.5–31 mos)

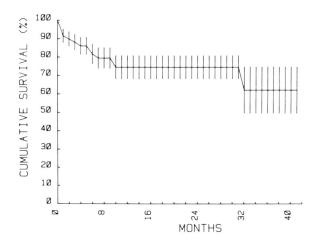

Figure 24. Life table analysis of results of subendocardial resection for ventricular tachycardia. A 60% 40-month predicted survival is expected following subendocardial resection for recurrent sustained ventricular tachycardia. Vertical bars represent 1 standard error (from [138], with permission of the NY Acad Sci).

technique also allows the surgeon to abolish tachycardias arising on the septum without either disarticulating or removing large parts of the septum. The hemodynamic results of limited resection are gratifying in that the ejection fraction is improved and left ventricular end-diastolic pressure reduced in the majority of cases [138, 151].

The major limitations of the technique are related to the requirement that the tachycardia be inducible so that it can be mapped intraoperatively, or at least preoperatively. Intraoperative inducibility is affected by cardiac temperature, anesthetic agents, and other miscellaneous pharmacologic and metabolic factors. Moreover, it may not be possible to map all the morphologies of the tachycardia completely because of other factors such as: (a) failure to induce the arrhythmia following aneurysmectomy, (b) failure to induce all clinical morphologies during both epicardial and endocardial mapping, (c) rapid degeneration of the tachycardia to ventricular fibrillation, (d) inability to distinguish early from late areas due to too rapid a tachycardia, (e) inability to map the endocardium due to large mural thrombi, and (f) unexpected surgical complications which prohibit detailed mapping. We have been able to obviate most of these problems by maintaining normothermia, using multiple stimu-

lation techniques from both ventricles, using antiarrhythmics (e.g., procainamide) to slow the rate of very rapid tachycardias and/or prevent their degeneration to ventricular fibrillation, and to rely on the preoperative catheter map for morphologic forms which can neither be induced nor completely mapped intraoperatively.

Another limitation of this procedure is inability to resect the base of papillary muscle should the tachycardia arise there. Although limited resection can be accomplished, other techniques (e.g., cryosurgery) probably will be required to ablate such arrhythmias uniformly. Activation mapping usually takes 30–60 min of normothermic cardiopulmonary bypass. Although this might potentially influence surgical mortality and morbidity, we have not found this to be the case. Our data demonstrate a mortality comparable to that of aneurysmectomy and bypass grafting for heart failure [104]. Despite these limitations, most of which we have been able to deal with, subendocardial resection appears to be a very promising surgical approach for the treatment of ventricular tachycardia.

Conclusion

Recent advances in our understanding of the pathophysiology of ventricular tachycardia have led to the development of new surgical approaches for the management of this arrhythmia. These electrophysiologically based approaches to arrhythmia surgery offer great promise for the treatment of ventricular tachycardia; however, several questions remain:

1. Are preoperative and/or intraoperative mapping required? In patients with ventricular tachycardia not associated with coronary artery disease there is general agreement that mapping is necessary to guide the surgical procedure. The lack of, or poorly understood, pathologic substrate necessitates mapping. However, if ventricular tachycardia is associated with coronary artery disease, a nondirected surgical approach, encircling endocardial ventriculotomy, is available. If one uses this technique, neither pre- nor postoperative mapping is required, although Waldo et al. [128] suggest that mapping is useful when a limited encircling endocardial ventriculotomy is contemplated. If a nondirected approach is used, a greater amount of

Table 8. Surgery for recurrent ventricular tachycardia associated with coronary artery disease.

Author	No. of patients	Procedure*		Operative mortality	Follow-up** (months)	Patients on drugs	Late recurrences
Fontaine, Guiraudon et al. [71, 120, 121, 144]	23	EEV		2 (9%)	1–55	4	2
Mason et al. (personal communication)	40	SER	(24)	9 (20%)	1–24	11	1
		SER & TMV	(1)		(9.4)		
		SER & EEV	(4)				
		EEV	(6)				
		TMV	(2)				
		CRYO	(2)				
		CRYO & SER	(1)				
Waldo et al. [128, 140]	16	EEV		3 (19%)	1–54	8	2
		EEV					
Allen et al. [147]	13	RMR		2 (15%)	2–40	? several	1
Josephson et al. [131, 136, 138, 139, 150]	60	SER		5 (8%)	2–42 (20)	13	4

* Number of patients with each procedure in parentheses.
** Mean follow-up in parentheses if available.

CRYO – cryosurgery
EEV – encircling endocardial ventriculotomy
RMR – radical myocardial resection

SER – subendocardial resection
TMV – transmural ventriculotomy

tissue must be resected and/or excluded, leaving less functioning myocardium. This is consistent with reports of severe hemodynamic impairment by this procedure with large aneurysms and/or infarctions and low ejection fractions [120, 121, 128, 144, 145]. Of the mapping-directed procedures, radical aneurysmectomy can also theoretically produce hemodynamic compromise.

We believe that the less tissue resected, the better the patient. This can be accomplished only if mapping procedures are used to guide surgery.

2. Which procedure produces the most satisfactory hemodynamic result? As noted above, encircling ventriculotomy and radical aneurysmectomy can be associated with significant alterations of ventricular function. The hemodynamic effects of subendocardial resection have been studied in detail [138, 151]. This procedure has produced no significant detrimental hemodynamic effects and has actually resulted in improved ejection fraction. However, one patient experienced rupture of the heart. On autopsy, however, this was associated with a recent ischemic event and unrelated to the septal endocardial resection [136]. The hemodynamic effects of other procedures have not been documented. Thus, in patients with ventricular tachycardia associated with coronary artery disease, subendocardial resection appears to be hemody-namically least detrimental.

3. Is anticoagulation required? This question has not been addressed. No anticoagulation has been reported to be routinely used with any procedure. The University of Pennsylvania experience, including repeat catheterizations and pathologic studies of two late deaths, have revealed no thrombus formation. No embolic events have been reported with any procedure; therefore, it appears that anticoagulation is not necessary.

These approaches have improved the success of surgery in the treatment of ventricular tachycardia. The results of several series are summarized in Table 8.

Clinical, experimental, and human electrophysiologic investigation have given us remarkable insights into the mechanisms of supraventricular and ventricular tachycardias. This information has allowed the development of new surgical procedures to treat arrhythmias. Such procedures have been a major advance in the therapy of medically refractory arrhythmias.

Acknowledgment

This project was supported in part by grants #1 R01 HL24278 and #1 R01 HL22315 from the National

Heart, Lung, and Blood Institute, Bethesda, Maryland; grants from the American Heart Association, Southeastern Pennsylvania Chapter, Philadelphia, PA; and the Fannie E. Ripple Foundation, Morristown, NJ.

References

1. Kent AFS: Researches on the structure and function of the mammalian heart. J Physiol 14:233–254, 1893.
2. Kent AFS: Observations of the auriculo–ventricular junction of the mammalian heart. Q J Exp Physiol 7:193–195, 1913.
3. Mines GR: On dynamic equilibrium in the heart. J Physiol 46:349–383, 1913.
4. Mines GR: On circulation excitations in heart muscles and their possible relation to tachycardia and fibrillation. Trans R Soc Can Sec 4:43–53, 1914.
5. Wilson FN: A case in which the vagus influenced the form of the ventricular complex of the electrocardiogram. Arch Intern Med 16:1008–1027, 1915.
6. Wedd AM: Paroxysmal tachycardia with reference to nomotopic tachycardia and the role of the extrinsic cardiac nerves. Arch Intern Med 27:571–590, 1921.
7. Hamburger WW: Bundle branch block. Four cases of intraventricular block showing some interesting and unusual clinical features. Med Clin North Am 13:343–362, 1929.
8. Wolff L, Parkinson J, White PD: Bundle-branch block with short P–R intervals in healthy young people prone to paroxysmal tachycardia. Am Heart J 5:685–704, 1930.
9. Wood FC, Wolferth CC, Geckeler GD: Histological demonstration of accessory muscular connections between auricle and ventricle in a case of short P–R interval and prolonged QRS complexes. Am Heart J 25:454–462, 1943.
10. Öhnell RF: Preexcitation a cardiac abnormality. Acta Med Scand 152:1–167, 1944.
11. Becker AE, Anderson RH, Durrer D, Wellens HJJ: The anatomical substrates of Wolff-Parkinson-White syndrome. A clinicopathologic correlation in seven patients. Circulation 57:870–879, 1978.
12. Becker AE, Anderson RH: Anatomic substrates of ventricular preexcitation. In: Bircks W, Loogen F, Schulte HD, Seipel L (eds) Medical and Surgical Management of Tachyarrhyhthmias. Springer-Verlag, Berlin, 1980, pp 81–93.
13. Anderson RH, Becker AE: Stanley Kent and accessory atrioventricular connections. J Thorac Cardiovasc Surg 81:649–658, 1981.
14. Sealy WC, Gallagher JJ, Pritchett EL: The surgical anatomy of Kent bundles based on electrophysiological mapping and surgical exploration. J Thorac Cardiovasc Surg 76:804–815, 1978.
15. Sealy WC, Gallagher JJ: Surgical treatment of left free wall accessory pathways of atrioventricular conduction of the Kent type. J Thorac Cardiovasc Surg 81:698–706, 1981.
16. Durrer D, Roos JP: Epicardial excitation of the ventricles in a patient with Wolff-Parkinson-White syndrome type B. Circulation 35:15–21, 1967.
17. Burchell HB, Fry RL, Anderson MW, McGoon DC: Atrioventricular and ventriculo-atrial excitation in Wolff-Parkinson-White syndrome type B. Temporary ablation at surgery. Circulation 36:663–672, 1967.
18. Cobb FR, Blumenschein SD, Sealy WC, Boineau JP, Wagner GS, Wallace AG: Successful surgical interruption of the bundle of Kent in a patient with Wolff-Parkinson-White syndrome. Circulation 38:1018–1029, 1968.
19. Sealy WC, Hattler BG, Blumenschein SD, Cobb FR: Surgical treatment of Wolff-Parkinson-White syndrome. Ann Thorac Surg 8:1–10, 1969.
20. Iwa T, Kazui T, Sugii S, Wada J: Surgical treatment of Wolff-Parkinson-White syndrome. Jpn J Thorac Surg 23:513–517, 1970.
21. Sealy WC, Boineau JP, Wallace AG: The identification and division of the bundle of Kent for premature ventricular excitation and supraventricular tachycardia. Surgery 68:1009–1017, 1970.
22. Sealy WC, Gallagher JJ, Wallace AG: The surgical treatment of Wolff-Parkinson-White syndrome: evolution of improved methods of identification and interruption of the Kent bundle. Ann Thorac Surg 22:443–457, 1976.
23. Boineau JP, Moore EN: Evidence for propagation of activation across an accessory atrioventricular connection in types A and B pre-excitation. Circulation 41:375–397, 1970.
24. Sealy WC, Gallagher JJ, Pritchett ELC, Wallace AG: Surgical treatment of tachyarrhythmias in patients with both an Ebstein anomaly and a Kent bundle. J Thorac Cardiovasc Surg 75: 847–853, 1978.
25. Iwa T: Surgery of supraventricular tachycardia. I. Operative treatment of Wolff-Parkinson-White syndrome. Nippon Jukankiyaku Shi 42:287–293, 1978.
26. Iwa T, Magara T, Watanabe Y, Kawasuji M, Misaki T: Interruptions of multiple accessory conduction pathways in the Wolff-Parkinson-White syndrome. Ann Thorac Surg 30:313–325, 1980.
27. Sealy WC, Gallagher JJ: The surgical approach to the septal area of the heart based on experiences with 45 patients with Kent bundles. J Thorac Cardiovasc Surg 79:542–551, 1980.
28. Iwa T, Kawasuji M, Misaki T, Iwase T, and Magara T: Localization and interruption of accessory conduction pathway in the Wolff-Parkinson-White syndrome. J Thorac Cardiovasc Surg 80:271–279, 1980.
29. Gallagher JJ, Sealy WC, Kasell JH: Intraoperative localization and division of accessory pathways associated with the Wolff-Parkinson-White syndrome. In: Bircks W, Loogen, F, Schulte HD, Seipel L (eds) Medical and Surgical Management of Tachyarrhythmias. Springer-Verlag, Berlin, 1980, pp 114–137.
30. Sealy WC, Gallagher JJ: Surgical problems with multiple accessory pathways of atrioventricular conduction. J Thorac Cardiovasc Surg 81:707–712, 1981.
31. Gallagher JJ, Sealy WC, Kasell JH: Epicardial mapping and surgical treatment of preexcitation syndrome (in press).
32. Rosenbaum FF, Hecht HH, Wilson FN, Johnston FD: Potential variations of the thorax and the esophagus in anomalous atrioventricular excitation W.P.W. syndrome. Am Heart J 29:281–326, 1945.

33. Boineau JP, Moore EN, Spear JF, Sealy WC: Basis on static and dynamic electrocardiographic variations in Wolff-Parkinson-White syndrome: anatomic and electrophysiologic observations in right and left preexcitation. Am J Cardiol 32:32–45, 1973.

34. Tonkin AM, Wagner GS, Gallagher JJ, Cope GD, Kasell J, Wallace AG: Initial forces of ventricular depolarization in the Wolff-Parkinson-White syndrome: analysis based upon localization of the accessory pathway by epicardial mapping. Circulation 52:1030–1036, 1975.

35. Gallagher JJ, Gilbert M, Svenson RH, Sealy WC, Kasell J, Wallace AG: Wolff-Parkinson-White syndrome. The problem, evaluation, and surgical correction. Circulation 51:767–785, 1975.

36. Gallagher JJ, Kasell J, Sealy WC, Pritchett EL, Wallace AG: Epicardial mapping in the Wolff-Parkinson-White syndrome. Circulation 57:854–866, 1978.

37. Gallagher JJ, Pritchett EL, Sealy WC, Kasell J, Wallace AG: The preexcitation syndromes. Prog Cardiovasc Dis 20:285–327, 1978.

38. McAlpine WA: Heart and Coronary Arteries. Springer, New York-Heidelberg-Berlin, 1975, pp 12–18, 68–73, 87–92.

39. Wellens HJJ, Schuilenberg RM, Durrer D: Electrical stimulation of the heart in patients with the Wolff-Parkinson-White syndrome type A. Circulation 43:99–114, 1971.

40. Coumel P, Waynberger M, Fabiato A, Slama R, Aiqueperse J, Bouvrain Y: Wolff-Parkinson-White syndrome. Problems in evaluation of multiple accessory pathways and surgical therapy. Circulation 40:1216–1230, 1972.

41. Svenson RH, Miller HC, Gallagher JJ, Wallace AG: Electrophysiological evaluation of the Wolff-Parkinson-White syndrome. Problems in assessing antegrade and retrograde conduction over the accessory pathway. Circulation 52:552–562, 1975.

42. Wellens HJJ, Farré J, Bär FW: Wolff-Parkinson-White syndrome: value and limitations of programmed electrical stimulation. In: Narula OS (ed) Cardiac Arrhythmias. Electrophysiology, Diagnosis and Management. Williams and Wilkins, Baltimore, 1979, pp 589–617.

43. Josephson ME, Seides SF: Clinical Cardiac Electrophysiology. Techniques and Interpretations. Lea and Febiger, Philadelphia, 1979, pp 211–245.

44. Gallagher JJ, Pritchett ELC, Benditt DG, Tonkin AM, Campbell RWF, Dugan FA, Bashore TM, Tower A, Wallace AG: New catheter techniques for analysis of the sequence of retrograde atrial activation in man. Eur J Cardiol 6:1–14, 1977.

45. Wallace AG, Sealy WC, Gallagher JJ, Kasell J: Ventricular excitation in the Wolff-Parkinson-White syndrome. In: Wellens HJJ, Lie KI, Janse MJ (eds) The Conduction System of the Heart. Lea and Febiger, Philadelphia, 1976, pp 613–630.

46. Durrer D, Janse MJ, van Dam RT, van Capelle FJL, Moulijn A, Meyne NG: Electrophysiologic observations during cardiac surgery of patients with Wolff-Parkinson-White syndrome. In: Bircks W, Loogen F, Schulte HD, Seipel L (eds) Medical and Surgery Management of Tachyarrhythmias. Springer-Verlag, Berlin, 1980, pp 106–113.

47. Gallagher JJ, Sealy WC, Kasell J, Millar R, Campbell RWF, Harrison L, Pritchett ELC, Wallace AG: Cryosurgical ablation of accessory atrioventricular connections: a new technique for correction of the preexcitation syndrome. Circulation 55:471–479, 1977.

48. Koch W: Der functionelle Bau des menschlichen Herzens. Urban und Schwarzenberg, Berlin, 1922, p 92.

49. Camm J, Ward DE, Spurrell RA, Rees GM: Cryothermal mapping and cryoablation in the treatment of refractory cardiac arrhythmias. Circulation 62:67–74, 1980.

50. Dreifus LS, Nichols H, Dryden M, Watanabe Y, Truex R: Control of recurrent tachycardia of Wolff-Parkinson-White syndrome by surgical ligature of the A-V bundle. Circulation 38:1030–1036, 1968.

51. Edmonds JH, Ellison RG, Crews TL: Surgically induced atrioventricular block as treatment for recurrent atrial tachycardia in Wolff-Parkinson-White syndrome. Circulation 39:I-105–111, 1969.

52. Harrison L, Gallagher JJ, Kasell J, Anderson RW, Mikat E, Hackel DB, Wallace AG: Cryosurgical ablation of the AV node–His bundle a new method for producing A-V block. Circulation 55:463–470.

53. Klein GJ, Sealy WC, Pritchett ELC, Harrison L, Hackel DB, Davis D, Kasell J, Wallace AG, Gallagher JJ: Cryosurgical ablation of the atrioventricular node–His bundle: long-term follow-up and properties of the junctional pacemaker. Circulation 61:8–15, 1980.

54. Sealy WC, Anderson RW, Gallagher JJ: Surgical treatment of supraventricular tachyarrhythmias. J Thorac Cardiovasc Surg 73:511–522, 1977.

55. Sealy WC, Hackel DB, Seaber AV: A study of methods for surgical interruption of the His bundle. J Thorac Cardiovasc Surg 73:424–430, 1977.

56. Coumel P, Attuel P: Reciprocating tachycardia in overt and latent re-excitation. Eur J Cardiol 1:423–436, 1974.

57. Farshidi A, Josephson ME, Horowitz LN: Electrophysiologic characteristics of concealed bypass tracts: clinical and electrocardiographic correlates. Am J Cardiol 41:1052–1060, 1978.

58. Sung RJ, Gelband H, Castellanos A, Aranda JM, Myerburg RJ: Clinical and electrophysiologic observations in patients with concealed atrioventricular bypass tracts. Am J Cardiol 40:839–847, 1977.

59. Tonkin AM, Gallagher JJ, Svenson RH, Wallace AG, Sealy WC: Anterograde block in accessory pathways with retrograde conduction in reciprocating tachycardia. Eur J Cardiol 3:143–152, 1975.

60. Caracta AR, Damato AN, Gallagher JJ, Josephson ME, Varghese PJ, Lau SH, Westura EE: Electrophysiologic studies in the syndrome of short P-R interval, normal QRS complex. Am J Cardiol 31:245–253, 1973.

61. Iannone L: Electrophysiology of atrial pacing in patients with short P-R, normal QRS complex. Am Heart J 89:74–78, 1975.

62. Brechenmacher C, Laham J, Iris L, Gerbaux A, Lenégre J: Etude histologique des voies anormales de conduction dans un syndrome de Wolff-Parkinson-White et dans un syndrome de Lown-Ganong-Levine. Arch Mal Coeur 67:507–519.

63. Brechenmacher C: Atrio-His bypass tracts. Br Heart J

37:853–855, 1975.

64. Baird DK, Uther JB: Surgical management of supraventricular tachycardia. In: Kelly DT (ed) Advances in the Management of Arrhythmias.Telectronics Pty Ltd, Lane Cove, Australia, 1978, pp 150–161.

65. Pritchett ELC, Anderson RW, Benditt DG, Kasell J, Harrison L, Wallace AG, Sealy WC, Gallagher JJ: Reentry within the atrioventricular node: surgical cure with preservation of atrioventricular conduction. Circulation 60: 440–446, 1979.

66. Sealy WC, Gallagher JJ, Kasell J: His bundle interruptions for control of inappropriate ventricular responses to atrial arrhythmias. Ann Thorac Surg (in press).

67. Becker AE, Anderson RH: Morphology of the human atrioventricular junctional area. In: Wellens HJJ, Lie KI, Janse MJ (eds) The Conduction System of the Heart. Lea and Febiger, Philadelphia, 1976, pp 263–286.

68. Mikat EM, Hackel DB, Harrison L, Gallagher JJ, Wallace AG: Reaction of the myocardium and coronary arteries to cryosurgery. Lab Invest 37:632–641, 1977.

69. Klein GJ, Harrison L, Ideker RF, Smith WM, Kasell J, Wallace AG, Gallagher JJ: Reaction of the myocardium to cryosurgery: electrophysiology and arrhythmogenic potential. Circulation 59: 364–372, 1979.

70. Gonzalez R, Scheinman M, Thomas A, Desai J, Peters R, Dzindzio B: Electrophysiologic characterization of surgically induced His bundle rhythm in man. PACE 4:152–162, 1981.

71. Guiraudon G, Fontaine G, Frank R, Escande G, Etievent P, Cabrol C: Encircling endocardial ventriculotomy: a new surgical treatment for life-threatening ventricular tachycardias resistant to medical treatment following myocardial infarction. Ann Thorac Surg 26:438–444, 1978.

72. Sealy WC, Seaber AV: Surgical isolation of the atrial septum from the atria. Identification of an atrial septum pacemaker. J Thorac Cardiovasc Surg 80:742–749, 1980.

73. Williams JM, Ungerleider RM, Lofland GK, Cox JL, Sabiston DC Jr: Left atrial isolation. New technique for the treatment of supraventricular arrhythmias. J Thorac Cardiovasc Surg 80:373–380, 1980.

74. Coumel PH, Aigueperse J, Perrault MA, Fantoni A, Slama R, Bouvrain Y: Repérage et tentative d'exérèse chirurgical d'un foyer ectopique auriculaire gauche avec tachycardie rebelle. Evolution favorable. Ann Cardiol Angeiol (Paris) 22:189–199, 1973.

75. Wyndham CRC, Arnsdorf MF, Levitsky S, et al: Successful surgical excision of focal paroxysmal atrial tachycardia. Observations in vivo and in vitro. Circulation 62:1365–1372, 1980.

76. Dixon ME, Trank JW, Dobell ARC: Ventricular fibrillation threshold: variation with coronary flow and its value in assessing experimental myocardial revascularization. J Thorac Cardiovasc Surg 47:620–627, 1964.

77. White M, Hershey JE: Multiple transmyocardial puncture revascularization in refractory ventricular fibrillation due to myocardial ischemia. Ann Thorac Surg 6:557–563, 1968.

78. Lambert CJ, Adam M, Geisler GF, Verzosa E, Nazarian M, Mitchel BF: Emergency myocardial revascularization for impending infarctions and arrhythmia. J Thorac Cardiovasc Surg 62:522–528, 1971.

79. Hutchinson JE, Kemp HG, Schwarz MJ: Emergency treatment of cardiac arrest in CHD with coronary artery bypass graft. J Am Med Assoc 216:1645, 1971.

80. Cline RE, Armstrong RG, Stanford W: Successful myocardial revascularization after ventricular fibrillation induced by treadmill exercise. J Thorac Cardiovasc Surg 65:802–805, 1973.

81. Bryson AL, Parisi AF, Schechter E, Wolfson S: Life-threatening ventricular arrhythmias induced by exercise. Cessation after coronary bypass surgery. Am J Cardiol 32: 995–997, 1973.

82. Yashar J, Yashar JJ, Witoszka M, Kitzes DL, Simeone FA: The treatment of patients with recurrent ventricular fibrillation. Am J Surg 133:453–457, 1977.

83. Tabry IF, Geha AS, Hammond GL, Baue AE: Effect of surgery on ventricular tachyarrhythmias associated with coronary arterial occlusive disease. Circulation 58:I 166–170, 1978.

84. Nordstrom LA, Lillehei JP, Adicoff A, Sako Y, Gobe FL: Coronary artery surgery for recurrent ventricular arrhythmias in patients with variant angina. Am Heart J 89: 236–241, 1975.

85. Myerburg RJ, Gharramani A, Mallon SM, Castellanas A Jr, Kaiser G: Coronary revascularization in patients surviving unexpected ventricular fibrillation. Circulation 52:III 219–222, 1975.

86. Wald RW, Waxman MB, Corey PN, Gunstensen J, Goldman BS: Management of intractable ventricular tachyarrhythmias after myocardial infarction. Am J Cardiol 44:329–338, 1979.

87. Bar FW, Lie KI, Wellens HJJ: Surgical treatment of ventricular tachyarrhythmias complicating acute myocardial infarction. Circulation 54:II–37, 1976 (abstract).

88. Mundth ED, Buckley MJ, DeSanctis RW, Daggett W, Austen WG: Surgical treatment of ventricular irritability. J Thorac Cardiovasc Surg 66:943–951, 1973.

89. Walker WE, Stoney WS, Alford WC, Burrus GR, Glassford DM, Thomas CS: Results of surgical management of acute left ventricular aneurysms. Circulation 62:I 75–78, 1980.

90. Hanson EC, Levine FH, Kay HR, et al: Control of postinfarction ventricular irritability with the intraaortic balloon pump. Circulation 62:I 130–137, 1980.

91. Josephson ME, Horowitz LN, Spielman SR, Greenspan AM: Electrophysiologic and hemodynamic studies in patients resuscitated from cardiac arrest. Am J Cardiol 46:948–955, 1980.

92. Couch OA: Cardiac aneurysm with ventricular tachycardia and subsequent excision of aneurysm. Circulation 20: 251–253, 1959.

93. Magidson O: Resection of postmyocardial infarction ventricular aneurysms for cardiac arrhythmias. Dis Chest 56:211–218, 1969.

94. Ritter ER: Intractable ventricular tachycardia due to ventricular aneurysm with surgical cure. Ann Intern Med 71:1155–1157, 1969.

95. Hunt D, Sloman G, Westlake G: Ventricular aneurysmectomy for recurrent tachycardia. Br Heart J 31:264–266, 1969.

96. Thind GS, Blakemore WS, Zinnsser HF: Ventricular aneu-

rysmectomy for the treatment of recurrent ventricular tachyarrhythmia. Am J Cardiol 27:690–694, 1971.

97. Kenaan G, Mendez A A, Zubiate P, Gray P, Kay JH: Surgery for ventricular tachycardia unresponsive to medical treatment. Chest 64:574–578, 1973.

98. Graham AF, Miller DC, Stinson EB, Daily PO, Fogarty TJ, Harrison DC: Surgical treatment of refractory life-threatening ventricular tachycardia. Am J Cardiol 32: 909–912, 1973.

99. Liotta D, Ferrari H, Pisano A, Pujadas G, Oliveri R, Donato O: Medically uncontrollable recurrent ventricular tachyarrhythmia in association with ventricular aneurysm. Am J Cardiol 33:693–694, 1974.

100. Ricks WB, Winkle RA, Shymway NE, Harrison DC: Surgical management of life-threatening ventricular arrhythmias in patients with coronary artery disease. Circulation 56:38–42, 1977.

101. Moran JM, Talano JV, Euler D, Moran JF, Montoya A, Pifarre R: Refractory ventricular arrhythmia. The role of intraoperative electrophysiological study. Surgery 82:809–815, 1977.

102. Sami M, Chaitman BR, Bourassa MG, Charpin D, Chabot M: Long-term follow-up of aneurysmectomy for recurrent ventricular tachycardia or fibrillation. Am Heart J 96: 303–308, 1978.

103. Buda AJ, Stinson EB, Harrison DC: Surgery for life-threatening ventricular tachyarrhythmias. Am J Cardiol 44:1171–1177, 1979.

104. Harken AH, Horowitz LN, Josephson ME: Comparison of standard aneurysmectomy and aneurysmectomy with directed endocardial resection for the treatment of recurrent sustained ventricular tachycardia. J Thorac Cardiovasc Surg 80:527–534, 1980.

105. Wellens HJJ, Duren DR, Lie KI: Observations on mechanism of ventricular tachycardia in man. Circulation 54: 237–244, 1976.

106. Josephson ME, Horowitz LN, Farshidi A, Kastor JA: Recurrent sustained ventricular tachycardia. 1. Mechanisms. Circulation 57:431–439, 1978.

107. Josephson ME, Horowitz LN, Farshidi A, Spear JF, Kastor JA, Moore EN: Recurrent sustained ventricular tachycardia. 2. Endocardial mapping. Circulation 57:440–447, 1978.

108. Josephson ME, Horowitz LN, Farshidi A: Continuous local electrical activity: a mechanism of recurrent ventricular tachycardia. Circulation 57:659–665, 1978.

109. Josephson ME, Horowitz LN, Farshidi A, Spielman SR, Michelson EL, Greenspan AM: Sustained ventricular tachycardia: evidence for protected localized reentry. Am J Cardiol 42:416–424, 1978.

110. Karagueuzian H, Fenoglio JJ, Weiss MB, Wit AL: Protracted ventricular tachycardia induced by premature stimulation of the canine heart after coronary occlusion and reperfusion. Circ Res 44:833–846, 1979.

111. El-Sherif N, Scherlag BJ, Lazzarra R, Hope RR: Reentrant ventricular arrhythmias in the late myocardial infarction period. 1. Conduction characteristics in the infarction zone. Circulation 55:686–702, 1977.

112. El-Sherif N, Hope RR, Scherlag BJ, Lazzara R: Reentrant ventricular arrhythmias in the late myocardial infarction period. 2. Pattern of initiation and termination of reentry. Circulation 55:702–719, 1977.

113. Michelson EL, Spear JF, Moore EN: Electrophysiologic and anatomic correlates of sustained ventricular tachyarrhythmias in a mode of chronic myocardial infarction. Am J Cardiol 45:583–590, 1980.

114. Josephson ME, Horowitz LN, Spielman SR, Waxman HL, Greenspan AM: The role of catheter mapping in the preoperative evaluation of ventricular tachycardia. Am J Cardiol 49:207–220, 1982.

115. Josephson ME, Horowitz LN, Spielman SR, Greenspan AM, Vandepol C, Harken AH: Comparison of endocardial catheter mapping with intraoperative mapping of ventricular tachycardia. Circulation 61:395–404, 1980.

116. Horowitz LN, Josephson ME, Harken AH: Epicardial and endocardial activation during sustained ventricular tachycardia in man. Circulation 61:1227–1238, 1980.

117. Fontaine G, Guiraudon G, Frank R, et al: Stimulation studies and epicardial mapping in ventricular tachycardia. Study of mechanisms and selection for surgery. In: Kulbertus HE (ed) Re-entrant Arrhythmias: Mechanisms and Treatment. Univ Park Press, Baltimore, 1977, pp 334–350.

118. Fontaine G, Guiraudon G, Frank R, Coutte R, Dragodanne C: Epicardial mapping and surgical treatment in six cases of resistant ventricular tachycardia not related to coronary artery disease. In: Wellens HJJ, Lie KI, Janse MJ (eds) The Conduction System of the Heart. Lea and Febiger, Philadelphia, 1976, pp 545–563.

119. Fontaine G, Guiraudon G, Frank R, Fillette F, Tonet J, Grosgogeat Y: Correlations between latest delayed potentials in sinus rhythm and earliest activation during chronic ventricular tachycardia. In: Bircks W, Loogen F, Schulte HD, Seipel L (eds) Medical and Surgical Management of Tachyarrhythmias. Springer-Verlag, Berlin, 1980, pp 138–154.

120. Guiraudon G, Fontaine G, Frank R, Pavie A, Grosgogeat Y, Cabrol C: Is the reentry concept a guide to the surgical treatment of chronic ventricular tachycardia? In: Bircks W, Loogen F, Schulte HD, Seipel L (eds) Medical and Surgical Management of Tachyarrhythmias. Springer-Verlag, Berlin, 1980, pp 155–172.

121. Fontaine G, Guiraudon G, Frank R, Carbrol C, Grosgogeat Y: The surgical management of ventricular tachycardia. Herz 4:276–284, 1979.

122. Horowitz LN, Greenspan AM, Spielman SR, Josephson ME: Torsades de pointes. Electrophysiologic studies in patients without transient pharmacologic or metabolic abnormalities. Circulation 63:1120–1128, 1981.

123. Josephson ME, Horowitz LN, Farshidi A, Spielman SR, Michelson EL, Greenspan AM: Recurrent sustained ventricular tachycardia. 4. Pleomorphism. Circulation 59: 459–468, 1979.

124. Spielman SR, Untereker WJ, Horowitz LN, Greenspan AM, Simson MB, Kastor JA, Josephson ME: Fragmented electrical activity. Relationship to ventricular tachycardia. Am J Cardiol 47:448, 1981 (abstract).

125. Spielman SR, Horowitz LN, Greenspan AM, Untereker WJ, Simson MB, Kastor JA, Josephson ME: Activation mapping in sinus rhythm in patients with ventricular tachycardia. Relationship to cycle length and site of origin.

Am J Cardiol 47:497, 1981 (abstract).

126. Ideker RE, Smith WM, Wallace AG, Kasell J, Harrison LA, Klein GJ, Kinicki RE, Gallagher JJ: A computerized method for the rapid display of ventricular activation during the intraoperative study of arrhythmias. Circulation 59:449–458, 1979.

127. Spurrell RAJ, Sowton E, Deuchar DC: Ventricular tachycardia in 4 patients evaluated by programmed electrical stimulation of heart and treated in 2 patients by surgical division of anterior radiation of left bundle branch. Br Heart J 35:1014–1025, 1973.

128. Waldo AL, Arciniegas JG, Klein H; Surgical treatment of life-threatening ventricular arrhythmias. The role of intraoperative mapping and consideration of the presently available surgical techniques. Prog Cardiovasc Dis 23: 247–264, 1981.

129. Wittig JH, Boineau JP: Surgical treatment of ventricular arrhythmias using epicardial, transmural and endocardial mapping. Ann Thorac Surg 20:117–124, 1975.

130. Gallagher JJ, Anderson RW, Kasell J, Rice JR, Pritchett ELC, Gault JH, Harrison L, Wallace AG: Cryoablation of drug-resistant ventricular tachycardia in a patient with a variant of scleroderma. Circulation 57:190–197, 1978.

131. Horowitz LN, Harken AH, Kastor JA, Josephson ME: Ventricular resection guided by epicardial and endocardial mapping for treatment of recurrent ventricular tachycardia. N Engl J Med 302:589–593, 1980.

132. Harken AH, Horowitz LN, Josephson ME: Surgical correction of recurrent sustained ventricular tachycardia following complete repair of tetralogy of Fallot. J Thorac Cardiovasc Surg 80: 779–781, 1980.

133. Mason JW, Stinson EB, Derby G, Griffin JC, Winkle RA, Ross DL, Oyer PE, Harrison DC: Advantages of activation sequence mapping in the treatment of ventricular tachycardia. In: Harrison DC, Winkle RA, Mason JW (eds) Symposium on Cardiac Arrhythmias – A Decade of Progress 1980. G K Hall, San Bernadino, CA, 1981.

134. Spielman SR, Michelson EL, Horowitz LN, Spear JF, Moore EN: The limitations of epicadial mapping as a guide to the surgical therapy of ventricular tachycardia. Circulation 57:666–670, 1978.

135. Gallagher JJ, Oldham HN, Wallace AG, Peter RH, Kasell J: Ventricular aneurysm with ventricular tachycardia. Report of a case with epicardial mapping and successful resection. Am J Cardiol 35:696–700, 1975.

136. Josephson ME, Harken AH, Horowitz LN: Endocardial excision. A new surgical technique for the treatment of recurrent ventricular tachycardia. Circulation 60:1430–1439, 1979.

137. Fenoglio JJ Jr, Albala A, Silva FG, Friedman PL, Wit AL: Structural basis of ventricular arrhythmias in human myocardial infarction. A hypothesis. Human Pathol 7:547–563, 1976.

138. Josephson ME, Horowitz LN, Harken AH: Surgery for recurrent sustained ventricular tachycardia associated with coronary artery disease: the role of subendocardial resection. Ann NY Acad Sci (in press).

139. Horowitz LN, Harken AH, Josephson ME: Electrophysiologically directed ventricular resection for recurrent sustained ventricular tachycardia. The University of Pennsylvania experience 1977–80. In: Harrison DC, Winkle RA, Mason JW (eds) Symposium on Cardiac Arrhythmias – A Decade of Progress 1980. G K Hall, San Bernadino, CA, 1981.

140. Arciniegas JG, Klein, J, Karp RB, Kouchoukos NT, James TN, Kirklin JW, Waldo AL: Surgical treatment of life-threatening ventricular tachyarrhythmias. Circulation 62:III–42, 1980 (abstract).

141. Moss AJ, McDonald J: Unilateral cervico-thoracic sympathetic gangliomectomy for the treatment of the long Q-T interval syndrome. N Engl J Med 285:903–904, 1971.

142. Schwartz PJ. The long QT syndrome. In: Kulbertus HE, Wellens HJJ (eds) Sudden Death. Martinus Nijhoff, The Hague, 1980, pp 358–378.

143. Sealy WC, Oldham HN: Surgical treatment of malignant ventricular arrhythmias by sympathectomy, coronary artery grafts and heart wall resection. In: Kelly DT (ed) Advances in the Management of Arrhythmias. Teletronics Pty Ltd, Lane Cove, Australia, 1978, pp 218–224.

144. Guiraudon G, Fontaine G, Frank R, Gorsgogeat Y, Cabrol C: Encircling endocardial ventriculotomy. Late follow-up results. Circulation 62:III–320, 1980 (abstract).

145. Engle TR: Endocardial surgery for ventricular tachycardia. The inside story. Ann Intern Med 94:402–404, 1981.

146. Ungerleider RM, Stanley TE, Williams JM, Lofland GK, Cox JL: Physiologic effects of encircling endocardial ventriculotomy (EEV) for refractory ischemic ventricular tachycardia. Circulation 62:III–61, 1980 (abstract).

147. Allen WB, Maloney JD, Hartzler GO, Holmes DR Jr, Puga FJ: Resection of ventricular aneurysm modified by electrophysiologic assessment in patients with intractable ventricular tachycardia and left ventricule aneurysm. Am J Cardiol 45:417, 1980 (abstract).

148. Camm J, Ward DE, Cory-Pearce R, Rees GM, Spurrell RAJ: The successful cryosurgical treatment of paroxysmal ventricular tachycardia. Chest 75:621–624, 1979.

149. Hass GM, Taylor CB: A quantitative hypothermal method for the production of local injury of tissue. Arch Pathol 45:563–580, 1948.

150. Harken AH, Josephson ME, Horowitz LN: Surgical endocardial resection for the treatment of malignant ventricular tachycardia. Ann Surg 190:456–460, 1979.

151. Josephson ME, Horowitz LN, Harken AH, Kastor JA: Hemodynamic and electrocardiographic changes produced by endocardial resection and aneurysmectomy for ventricular tachycardia. Circulation 62:III–320, 1980 (abstract).

385

CHAPTER 11

The pharmacology of cardiac glycosides

BRIAN F. HOFFMAN

Introduction

The first systematic description of the use of digitalis was provided in 1785 by William Withering in his book *An Account of the Foxglove and Some of its Medical Uses: With Practical Remarks on Dropsy and Other Diseases.* Since that time digitalis has been used to treat a variety of illnesses including most forms of edema. In more recent times digitalis was used first to treat atrial fibrillation and then it was used to treat what we would now accept as heart failure. There have been a great many studies on the pharmacology of digitalis, but in spite of this it still is a frequent subject for investigation and there probably is much we still need to learn about its actions and mechanisms of action.

Digitalis is the term used to describe the cardiac glycosides that are obtained from a number of plants including *digitalis purpurea* and *digitalis lanata*. The cardiac glycosides consist of an aglycone or genin, which is responsible for the main pharmacologic actions, and one to four sugar molecules which modify solubility and potency. At present two preparations are used to the almost complete exclusion of others: digoxin and digitoxin. Ouabain or G-strophanthin is a glycoside employed quite frequently in experiments on animals and differs from digoxin and digitoxin only in terms of kinetic parameters.

General indications

Digitalis has two primary uses; it has for many years been the most important drug employed to treat heart failure and, until the advent of the beta-adrenergic-blocking drugs and verapamil, digitalis was the only drug consistently effective in controlling ventricular rate during rapid atrial rhythms. Recently systemic arterial and venous vasodilators have been found effective in a number of types of heart failure, either alone or in conjunction with digitalis, and new positive inotropic agents such as amrinone have appeared. Nevertheless, it seems likely that digitalis will continue to be the drug prescribed most often for chronic heart failure and for chronic or recurrent atrial fibrillation and flutter. A detailed description of the indications for use of digitalis to treat failure is presented in Chapter 14, and its use to treat arrhythmias is covered in Chapter 8; here we will provide only some general considerations about indications and use.

Heart failure

Digitalis usually will improve cardiac performance when there is failure of either the right or left ventricle or both, and, although arrhythmias may modify the response of the heart to digitalis, the presence of most arrhythmias usually is not a contraindication to its use. From what is known concerning its mechanism of action (see below), it is obvious that digitalis can exert a positive inotropic effect on both the failed and normal myocardium; this suggests that digitalis might be employed to prevent or slow the development of failure and cardiomegaly in patients with heart disease. There are no convincing data showing the effectiveness of prophylactic administration of digitalis (in part because of the difficulty in designing a reasonable experiment), but it

Rosen, M. R. and Hoffman, B. F. (eds.), Cardiac Therapy. ISBN 0-89838-564-4.
© 1983, Martinus Nijhoff Publishers, Boston, The Hague, Dordrecht, Lancaster. Printed in the Netherlands.

seems likely that if digitalis increases the work capacity of the stressed heart, the progression of heart failure may be less rapid.

In general digitalis is likely to be effective in improving mechanical function if the heart has not been too severely damaged and if an increase in end-diastolic pressure and volume have occurred as a compensation for inadequate pump function. If heart failure results from the direct effect of some agent that depresses myocardial metabolism or contractility, such as severe thiamin deficiency or the action of toxins, digitalis will be of little value. Digitalis typically is not consistently effective in treating heart failure caused by thyrotoxicosis or chronic severe hypoxia. If there has been severe structural damage to the ventricles, as in cardiomyopathy, and in the presence of acute inflammatory responses, such as in rheumatic fever or infectious myocarditis, the response to digitalis usually is limited. Finally, when the cause of failure is an obstructive lesion that severely limits forward flow from the ventricles, digitalis cannot be expected to cause significant improvement and in the case of obstructive forms of cardiomyopathy may actually increase the hindrance to ejection.

In general the treatment of heart failure must be based on an understanding of the cause or causes of the abnormality and the possible and reasonable changes that might improve the circulation. Thus if failure results from systemic arterial hypertension, it would be unreasonable to use digitalis without reducing arterial pressure and often, if pressure can be controlled adequately, left ventricular performance will be adequate without digitalization. If an increase in circulating blood volume with or without edema accompanies heart failure, diuretics which bring about the loss of sodium and water will alleviate some of the symptoms and will increase the benefits to be derived from digitalization. Similarly, if data on the hemodynamic status of the patient indicate that a reduction in afterload, preload, or both can be expected to improve the adequacy of cardiac function, agents that accomplish these changes should be employed either separately or in addition to digitalis. It seems reasonable to assume that, if the heart has been weakened from any cause and that the resultant cardiac failure reflects its inability to perform the needed work, a lessening of work requirement by reduction in afterload will help. If the ventricles are greatly overdis-

tended and thus are placed in an unfavorable position with respect to the Laplace relationship, such that excessive wall tension is needed to generate a reasonable intraventricular pressure during systole, a reduction in preload may help. Nevertheless, an estimate of what reasonably can be accomplished still is essential. If the ventricles have been so weakened by disease that they generate reasonable force only from the optimum end-diastolic pressure and length, too great a reduction in preload may cause marked and severe deterioration in cardiac performance. A similar effect might be expected if, for any reason, the distensibility of the ventricles is markedly reduced; once again an excessive reduction in filling pressure with diuretics or vasodilators would impair performance.

Arrhythmias

Traditionally, digitalis has been used to reduce excessively rapid ventricular rates in patients with atrial fibrillation or to prevent the occurrence of rapid ventricular rates in patients likely to experience episodes of atrial fibrillation, flutter, or tachycardia. Digitalis acts in this case mainly by increasing the effective refractory period of the A-V node so that only a limited proportion of rapidly recurring atrial impulses can be conducted to the ventricles. This effect is due primarily to a vagomimetic indirect action. If digitalis is ineffective in this regard beta-adrenergic-blocking drugs or verapamil can be employed in place of or in conjunction with digitalis. Many paroxysmal supraventricular tachycardias can be determinated by digitalis through its ability to increase vagal activity. Digitalis can be employed to slow the ventricular rate in patients with atrial flutter and may convert flutter to fibrillation. Finally, in some patients with anomalous A-V conduction paths, digitalis can be used to control arrhythmias.

Pharmacodynamics

There was some confusion about the primary action by which digitalis improves the circulation in patients with heart failure from the time of Withering until relatively recently [1]. In part this resulted from an inadequate understanding of the pathophysiology of heart failure and in part from an inability to discriminate among the several causes of edema. At present there is general agreement that the beneficial effects of digitalis in heart failure result primarily from an ability to increase directly the capacity of the heart to develop active tension and do work. This is called the direct positive inotropic effect of digitalis. Undoubtedly digitalis causes a number of other changes which may contribute to the relief of heart failure, such as a decrease in sinus rate and modification of autonomic reflexes, but the direct effect on contraction is of paramount importance. This is not surprising since heart failure occurs when the work required of the heart exceeds the heart's capacity to do work.

Direct effects on mechanical activity

The direct positive inotropic effect of digitalis can be demonstrated most clearly by studies on isolated preparations of cardiac muscle. With such preparations variables that influence contraction such as rate, end-diastolic fiber length, and load can be controlled. Also the effects of other factors that modify contraction, such as autonomic neurotransmitters, can be blocked with appropriate drugs. Typically, studies are conducted on fine trabecula in which diffusion is not limited. Measurements can be made during both isometric and isotonic contractions.

During isometric contractions suitable concentrations of digitalis increase both the rate at which force is developed and also the peak force developed at any end-diastolic fiber length (Figure 1).

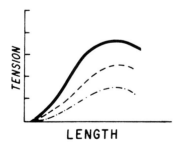

LENGTH

Figure 1. Diagrammatic representation of the length–tension relationship for isolated cardiac muscle contracting under isometric conditions and showing the peak force developed as resting length is increased from slack length to a length greater than optimal. The lower curve represents control data and the interrupted and solid curves show the effects of half-maximal and maximal doses of ouabain, respectively.

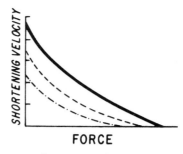

FORCE

Figure 2. Diagrammatic representation of the relationship between maximum shortening velocity and load for isolated cardiac muscle contracting under isometric conditions. The lowest trace shows control data and the interrupted and solid traces show contractile responses after exposure to half-maximal and maximal concentrations of ouabain, respectively.

The time-to-peak force and duration of contraction are not modified greatly. During isotonic contractions digitalis causes an increase in the velocity of shortening at all loads between the minimum and the maximum that can be lifted (Figure 2). As for isometric contractions this effect is present over a wide range of end-diastolic fiber lengths. For both modes of contraction the increment in force or shortening velocity, relative to the control, is greater if the preparation has 'failed,' i.e., if contraction has become impaired prior to exposure to digitalis. The effects are similar for right and left ventricular and for atrial muscle.

Admittedly, neither the isometric nor the isotonic contraction of an isolated preparation of cardiac muscle mimics the contraction of the left ventricle in situ. Nevertheless, the data obtained from these experiments can be transformed [2] so as to be somewhat more relevant (Figure 3). The data for

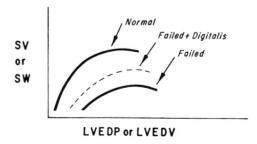

LVEDP or LVEDV

Figure 3. Diagrammatic representation of the relationship between stroke volume or stroke work and left ventricular end-diastolic pressure (LVEDP) or volume (LVEDV) for an isolated supported heart. Note that digitalis increases the work capacity of the failed ventricle at all values of LVEDP or LVEDV.

389

isotonic contractions show that digitalis can be expected to increase ejection velocity and decrease the ejection period. The data also show that the left ventricle will be able to eject against a given aortic pressure from a shorter end-diastolic fiber length.

Mechanism of the positive inotropic effect
The mechanism by which digitalis exerts its direct positive inotropic effect remained a mystery for many years. Because of some similarities between the effects of digitalis and those of an elevated extracellular calcium concentration ($[Ca^{2+}]_o$) and because of the central role of calcium in causing contraction and relaxation, many studies attempted to attribute the inotropic effect of digitalis to an increase in intracellular calcium stores [3]. The evidence for this, and an explanation of how the change is brought about, can be summarized briefly, but first the regulation of intracellular cation concentrations in heart fibers must be explained.

In mammalian hearts calcium ions (Ca^{2+}) enter the fibers as slow inward current (i_{si}) during the plateau of the transmembrane action potential. This calcium is not sufficient to cause contraction; rather, it triggers the release of a larger amount of Ca^{2+} from the sarcoplasmic reticulum (SR). This is the calcium that causes contraction [4, 5]. The reuptake of Ca^{2+} by the SR terminates contraction and permits relaxation. At steady state the calcium that enters the fibers during each action potential must be eliminated from the fibers to prevent a continuing buildup of calcium content. Calcium is eliminated in exchange for sodium [6, 7]; this mechanism is a form of exchange diffusion and the net flux of Na^+ and Ca^{2+} depends on the concentrations of Na^{2+} and Ca^{2+} inside and outside the sarcolemma and perhaps also on transmembrane potentials. An active transport system that carries a significant amount of Ca^{2+} out across the sarcolemma only recently has been demonstrated for the heart [8].

The intracellular concentration of Na^+ ($[Na^+]_i$) is the crucial variable in controlling the removal of Ca^{2+} from the heart fibers. If $[Na^+]_i$ increases, the efflux of Na^+ will increase and more calcium will be brought into the cell or less calcium will be removed from it. The steady-state value of $[Na^+]_i$ is controlled by active extrusion of Na^+ by means of the so-called sodium–potassium pump. This active transport system is an integral part of a specific membrane Na^+, K^+-ATPase and exchanges intracellular Na^+ for extracellular K^+ in a ratio of 3:2 [9]. Digitalis binds to the ATPase and decreases the activity of the pump [10–13]. As a result $[Na^+]_i$ increases and $[K^+]_i$ decreases. The elevated $[Na^+]_i$ causes an increase in calcium content via the Na^+--Ca^{2+} exchange mechanism; the elevated $[Ca^{2+}]_i$ in turn causes the increase in contraction.

The binding of tritiated digoxin to the Na^+, K^+-ATPase from calf heart has been studied to provide further information on the nature of the binding and the nature of inhibition of the drug-bound enzyme [14]. The results suggest that the drug binds to the phosphorylated conformation of the enzyme and that inhibition results from the stability of the drug-enzyme complex. In other studies an estimate has been made of the fraction of drug-bound ATPase sites in cat myocardium, and this fraction was found to correlate well with the magnitude of the inotropic effect [15].

The evidence for this mechanism for the direct positive inotropic action of digitalis is quite convincing. It has been shown that the uptake of rubidium by the in situ mammalian heart is depressed in a dose-dependent manner by digoxin [16] and that both the inotropic effect and toxic effects of digoxin are related to the magnitude of inhibition of the ATPase. Here Rb^+ substitutes for K^+ and the decreased Rb^+ uptake results from depression of active transport by the pump. In studies on isolated cardiac tissues it has been shown that digitalis directly inhibits the active transport of Na^+ and K^+ and that this effect is associated with an increase in $[Na^+]_i$, a decrease in $[K^+]_i$, and an increase in $[Ca^{2+}]_i$ [17–23]. Finally, other interventions that depress the active transport of Na^+ cause changes in $[Na^+]_i$, $[Ca^{2+}]_i$, and in contractility similar to those seen with digitalis [24–26].

Studies with intracellular sodium-sensitive electrodes have directly demonstrated that after exposure to dihydro-ouabain, there was a strong correlation between the increase in intracellular sodium activity and the increase in contractile force [21]. In similar experiments using voltage clamp it has been shown that when the Na^+–K^+ pump is inhibited by a reduction in $[K^+]_o$, there is a rise in intracellular Na^+ activity and an increase in twitch and tonic tension. Further, when the pump is reactivated by addition of Rb^+ to the superfusate, intracellular Na^+ activity and tension both decline [25, 26].

Several studies have suggested that very low concentrations of digitalis substances may stimulate rather than inhibit the Na^+, K^+-ATPase; recent investigations on enzyme purified from cat heart have failed to support this conjecture and have shown only inhibition at concentrations from 10^{-10} to 10^{-7} M [27]. Partially confirmatory results were obtained by studying the effects of very low concentrations of ouabain on isolated cardiac tissues from several species [28]. The relationship between pump inhibition and positive inotropy also has been examined in a study which used Rb^+ to inhibit the active transport of Na^+ and assessed the inotropic effect by measuring transmembrane potentials and contraction of isolated guinea pig atrium and ventricle [29]. For the ventricle it was shown that low concentrations of Rb^+ transiently decreased developed force and action potential duration. This finding may merely reflect the fact that Rb^+ can activate the pump, at least in the K^+-free solutions [30].

The observation that low concentrations of digitalis may increase contractile force but not significantly increase intracellular sodium activity has been examined by use of a computer simulation and the assumptions (a) that Na^+ entering the fiber during the action potential upstroke accumulates near the sarcolemma and (b) that the net increment in intracellular Na^+ is pumped out before the next action potential. Under these conditions, one could assume that the partial inhibition of active transport caused by low concentrations of ouabain would increase the time required for Na^+ to be extruded (and thus augment Na^+ for Ca^{2+} exchange) without increasing measured sodium activity in the myoplasm [31].

Although the evidence supporting the idea that the positive inotropic action of digitalis is caused by inhibition of sodium transport, recent evidence has been obtained for rat ventricle [32] showing that ouabain binding to a high affinity site exerts a positive inotropic effect and that this site is not related to the Na^+, K^+-ATPase. Other studies question the causal relationship between enzyme inhibition and positive inotropy. Studies on the Na^+, K^+-ATPase from rabbit heart showed a temporal correlation between the extent of inhibition and positive inotropy; in dogs, however, this relationship was not demonstrated [33]. The question of how digitalis increases contractile force also has been posed in terms of correlation between the

rate of onset of the positive inotropic effect in different cardiac chambers and both the ATPase concentration and capacity for cation transport of those chambers. No clear correlations were found [34].

The effects of intracellular and extracellular application of digoxin on bovine ventricular myocardium [35] have been compared. Extracellular but not intracellular application resulted in a positive inotropic effect that could be prevented or reversed by digoxin antibody. This finding substantiates the concept that digitalis binds to the ATPase from the outer surface of the membrane.

Effects on slow inward current
It has been suspected for some time that, because the Ca^{2+} for excitation–contraction coupling is delivered by the slow inward current, digitalis might directly or indirectly modify the slow inward channels and thus augment i_{si}. Although some evidence for a direct interaction of digitalis with slow channels has been obtained [36], recent careful studies using voltage clamp and intracellular Ca^{2+}-sensitive electrodes have provided strong evidence that digitalis causes an *indirect* increase in i_{si} [37]. The change results from the inhibition of the Na^+, K^+-pump, the decrease in active Na^+ extrusion and the consequent increase in $[Ca^{2+}]_i$. This increase in $[Ca^{2+}]_i$ acts to augment the conductance of the slow inward channels and increase inward (calcium) current. It has been suggested that this is a mechanism by which a modest inhibition of the pump can result in a fairly significant increase in $[Ca^{2+}]_i$ [38] and also a mechanism that provides a phasic increase in $[Ca^{2+}]_i$ during systole. Interestingly, other evidence suggests that increase in $[Ca^{2+}]_i$ promotes the inactivation of slow inward channels [38]; this effect might assist in decreasing the risk of toxicity due to an increase in $[Ca^{2+}]_i$.

Direct effects on mechanical activity of the isolated heart

The direct positive inotropic effect of digitalis can be demonstrated in studies on the isolated, supported heart or heart–lung preparation. These preparations offer advantages for studying the direct effects of digitalis because heart rate, end-diastolic intraventricular pressure, and aortic pressure can be controlled. This control eliminates the pos-

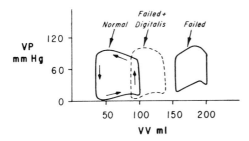

Figure 4. Diagrammatic representation of the pressure–volume loop for the left ventricle under control conditions, after failure associated with a marked increase in left ventricular diastolic volume and pressure and after action of a maximal dose of digitalis: VP = left ventricular pressure; VV = left ventricular volume.

sibility that a change in mechanical performance of the ventricle results from the inotropic effects of alterations in rate, fiber length, or afterload. In studies on isolated hearts it has been shown that digitalis increases the maximum rate of development of intraventricular pressure, decreases the duration of isovolumic contraction and the ejection period, increases ejection velocity and peak systolic pressure, and decreases the duration of systole. Usually, stroke volume increases and end-diastolic volume decreases. If the study is conducted on a failed heart; that is, one in which a high end-diastolic pressure is required for development of an adequate stroke volume and systolic pressure, the ability of digitalis to improve cardiac function can be demonstrated clearly. The decrease in end-systolic volume, with constant filling during diastole, results in a decrease in end-diastolic pressure and volume. In spite of the resulting decrease in fiber length, the positive inotropic effect of digitalis causes a sufficiently strong contraction to achieve adequate emptying during systole. This effect is shown graphically in Figure 4. The manner in which digitalis improves the function of the failed human heart is described in Chapter 14.

Direct effects on electrical activity

Digitalis exerts both direct and indirect effects on the electrical activity of cardiac cells, and, to some extent, the changes in electrical activity caused by digitalis differ for different types of cardiac cells. The most extensive studies on this problem have employed cardiac Purkinje fibers because they are best suited to studies by voltage clamp techniques.

In addition, it is important to remember that the effects of digitalis on normal fibers may differ from those exerted on fibers which have been modified by disease or the actions of other drugs.

Purkinje fibers

The changes in the transmembrane potentials of Purkinje fibers are dependent on the concentration of digitalis; for the most part different preparations of digitalis exert similar effects [39–43]. If the drug concentration is low and the stimulus rate low, digitalis causes a modest initial increase in the action potential duration; this increase is not seen at rapid rates. Subsequently, action potential duration decreases, largely as a result of a decrease in the duration of the plateau. Typically, there is no reduction in the maximum rate of depolarization during phase 0 ($\dot{V}_{max}$) and no decrease in action potential amplitude. These effects may be the changes that represent the action of a 'therapeutic' concentration of digitalis; unfortunately, most studies have employed concentrations sufficiently high to result in clear toxic effects after a suitable time. With such concentrations there are additional changes in the transmembrane potentials. Maximum diastolic potential is decreased and, if $[K^+]_o$ is normal or low, the slope of phase 4 depolarization appears to increase. Associated with the increase in phase 4 depolarization, there may be a decrease in $\dot{V}_{max}$. The apparent increase in the slope of phase 4 may be the result of an automatic mechanism or of the occurrence of delayed afterdepolarizations (DAD) [44–46]. DADs usually appear as a damped oscillation; their amplitude is a function of the cycle length, and at rapid rates the first or second DAD can attain threshold and elicit a premature response. Because the premature response follows a short cycle, it gives rise to a larger DAD, and thus a train of impulses can be initiated. The relationships between DAD amplitude and rate are complex [47] and are discussed elsewhere (Chapter 1). Finally, at very high concentrations of digitalis there seems to be a direct depression of fast inward channels due to a shift of the inactivation curve and a significant decrease in $\dot{V}_{max}$ [40]. This usually is accompanied by a further reduction in MDP or resting potential.

The effect of digitalis on the electrical activity of Purkinje fibers need be discussed both in terms of the mechanisms probably responsible for the observed changes and also in relation to changes in activity of the *in situ* heart. Clearly, some of the effects noted for isolated fibers seem to result from a stronger toxic effect than would occur during administration of digitalis to patients. For example, in humans digitalis typically does not directly increase QRS duration and thus a marked depression of fast inward current would not seem a likely effect of therapeutic doses of digitalis in patients. If huge doses of digitalis are ingested in attempts at suicide, QRS duration may increase but this probably results from K^+ loss from muscle and an increase in serum K^+ concentration.

The increase in action potential duration observed at low drug concentrations and slow rates of stimulation might reflect a change in passive electrical properties of the membrane [40], but more likely results from the effect of digitalis on the Na^+, K^+-pump. A decrease in Na^+ extrusion will diminish the transient increase in pump current that follows each action potential upstroke, and this will delay repolarization somewhat. The decrease in electrogenic pumping of Na^+ also will tend to slightly decrease MDP and increase the slope of phase 4 depolarization. The shortening of the action potential seen with higher drug concentrations and higher rates of stimulation may result from the increase in $[Ca^{2+}]_i$ that results from depressed Na^+ extrusion described above. There is convincing evidence that an elevated $[Ca^{2+}]_i$ can increase the conductance of some K^+ channels and augment outward current [48]. This increase in outward current would decrease plateau duration and shorten the action potential. All of these postulated effects would be influenced to some extent by the simultaneous changes in $[Na^+]_i$ and $[K^+]_i$ which result from depression of the pump. The reduction in $[K^+]_i$ has been demonstrated directly and would tend to decrease resting potential or MDP; the increase in $[Na^+]_i$ has been demonstrated directly with Na-sensitive intracellular electrodes and, because it would decrease the driving force for inward Na^+ current, would be expected to diminish slightly both V_{max} and action potential amplitude. The alteration in intracellular Na^+ and K^+ concentrations also might have effects on the conductance of other transmembrane channels. Finally, to the extent that an increae in $[Ca^{2+}]_i$ increases slow channel conductance (see above) this change will counteract the decrease in action potential duration.

Uncertainly about the exact causes of the observed changes in transmembrane potentials of isolated Purkinje fibers is enhanced because, at least for canine and ungulate hearts, the extracellular spaces immediately adjacent to rather large areas of the sarcolemma are narrow and concentrations of ions in these spaces tend not to be in equilibrium with the bulk phase [49, 50]. The narrow extracellular clefts between Purkinje cells make interpretation of voltage-clamp experiments difficult and also introduce uncertainties in estimates of extracellular ion concentrations during rest and activity. Typically, during the action potential the concentration of K^+ in the clefts increases and the more rapid the rate, the greater the increase [50–52]. If digitalis decreases pump function and decreases the rate of transport of K^+ back into the fiber, the change in $[K^+]_o$ would be augmented and more so at higher rates. However, the transport of Na^+ and K^+ by the pump is a function of both $[Na^+]_i$ and $[K^+]_o$, and thus the increase in cleft $[K^+]$ might reduce the extent to which a given concentration of digitalis depressed the pump. Recent data show also that $[Ca^{2+}]_o$ decreases during the action potential and $[Na^+]_o$ may undergo a similar change. Thus the manner in which digitalis modifies cellular electrical activity is indeed complex, such that interactions among the factors that are modified by primary effects of digitalis modulate the net changes in electrical activity.

Production of delayed afterdepolarizations. It is interesting that, although the causes of many of the effects of digitalis on the Purkinje fiber action potential are uncertain, the basis for digitalis-induced delayed afterdepolarizations (DADs) seems reasonably clear. DADs can result from many interventions other than the action of digitalis, including the action of catecholamines, increases extracellular $[Ca^{2+}]$, or intracellular $[Na^+]$ and changes in the pattern of relaxation [53–55]. In each case the significant change appears to be an increase in $[Ca^{2+}]_i$. This is thought to 'overload' the storage mechanisms for Ca^{2+} in the sarcotubular system so that, during each cycle of electrical and mechanical activity, after relaxation and reuptake of Ca^{2+} by the SR, there is an oscillatory release and reuptake of Ca^{2+} by that structure. This has been shown by a variety of techniques perhaps the most convincing of which is the association of an aftercontraction with the DAD. The secondary release of Ca^{2+} is

393

thought to initiate a transient inward current, carried mainly by Na^+, and this current causes the DAD. This common mechanism for DAD would explain the ease with which a variety of pharmacological agents abolish the abnormal oscillation in transmembrane potential. Local anesthetic antiarrhythmic drugs, by decreasing the net entry of Na^+ during each action potential and decreasing background inward Na^+ current, would lead to a decrease in $[Ca^{2+}]_i$ as would drugs that act directly on slow inward channels to diminish i_{si}.

Other aspects of digitalis action. In experiments on isolated preparations of cardiac muscle, it has been shown that extremely toxic concentrations of digitalis, by elevating intracellular calcium concentration [56], cause partial uncoupling of cells at the nexuses [57]. This uncoupling increases the resistance to current flow between fibers and decreases both the safety factor for conduction and conduction velocity. It is not likely that this effect is a frequent result of the clinical exhibition of digitalis; nevertheless, if digitalis acts on abnormal cells that either have an increased permeability to Ca^{2+} or a decreased ability for Ca^{2+} extrusion, the mechanism might become operative.

It has been shown clearly that the intensity of effect of a given concentration of digitalis can be modified by the condition of the fiber. Thus, the development of toxic effects is more rapid if the rate of stimulation is high [39]; this would be expected in terms of the mechanisms of action since with a higher rate the pump is required to effect more net transport of Na^+ and K^+ per unit time. The intensity of effect also is a function of $[K^+]_o$ and $[Ca^{2+}]_o$. Again these relationships seem reasonable. An increase in $[K^+]_o$ would decrease the intensity of digitalis effect because the capacity of the pump to transport Na^+ and K^+ is, within limits, a function of the value of $[K^+]_o$. Also, there is evidence that the binding of digitalis to the pump is a function of $[K^+]_o$ [58] so that an elevated potassium concentration decreases binding and inhibition. Indeed, there is some evidence that the number of pump sites in the membrane also may be controlled in part by $[K^+]_o$ [59]. The effects of changes in $[Ca^{2+}]_o$ also can be explained. The net uptake of Ca^{2+} by a fiber on which digitalis has acted is a function of $[Ca^{2+}]_o$ because of the nature of the Na^+–Ca^{2+} exchange mechanism. Also, with an increase in $[Ca^{2+}]_o$, slow

inward current would be augmented and Ca^{2+} loading increased. Finally, there is evidence that $[Ca^{2+}]_o$ may directly inhibit the Na–K pump [60].

Other types of cardiac fibers
The direct effects of digitalis on other types of cardiac fibers are not prominent at low, and presumably therapeutic, concentrations. Digitalis, by its direct effect, causes slowing and then acceleration of spontaneous action potential generation in the sinus node [61, 62], but most of the clinically important effects on sinus rhythm are indirect. Very high concentrations of digitalis depress both impulse generation and conduction in the node. In the case of the A-V node clearly toxic concentrations of digitalis can cause a decrease in MDP, a decrease in action potential amplitude and slowing of conduction and block. These changes are associated with an increase in the duration of the effective refractory period. As for the sinus node, most of the usual effects of digitalis on the A-V node are due to the indirect effects mentioned subsequently. Specialized atrial fibers, or atrial plateau fibers [63], respond to digitalis in much the same manner as do Purkinje fibers and under the influence of digitalis can develop both increased automaticity and DAD [64]. Electrical activity of atrial and ventricular muscle fibers also changes under the influence of digitalis. In both fiber types there will be changes in action potential duration like those described for Purkinje fibers; in the case of ventricular fibers the plateau is abbreviated and the slope of phase 3 decreased. These changes in ventricular repolarization seem to be the cause of the changes in the S–T segment and T wave noted in the ECG. Ventricular fibers are less sensitive to a given concentration of digitalis than are Purkinje fibers in that changes in transmembrane potentials are less marked and develop less rapidly [38]. Digitalis does not cause phase 4 depolarization to appear in ordinary atrial or ventricular muscle fibers, but it can cause these fibers to develop DAD [65].

Digitalis has been shown to have clear effects on fibers in the canine coronary sinus which typically develop DAD even in the absence of glycoside effect [66]. This action might tend to enhance triggered coronary sinus arrhythmias in the following way. When DAD cause a tachyarrhythmia the resulting stimulation of the electrogenic pump usually terminates the rapid rhythm by increasing outward current and hyperpolarizing the fibers [67]. If the pump is depressed by digitalis this effect will be decreased or absent and the arrhythmia will persist.

Indirect effects on electrical activity

Many of the effects of digitalis on the heart and circulation result from the ability of digitalis to modify the autonomic control of the cardiovascular system. This modification results from direct effects of digitalis on blood vessels, the central nervous system, autonomic neural structures, and from alterations in reflex activity. The changes in reflex activity are caused both by the direct effects and also the digitalis-induced changes in the contraction of the heart and in the circulation. Indeed, there is strong evidence that indirect, autonomically mediated actions are important in the genesis of digitalis-induced arrhythmias [68, 69].

The widespread effects of digitalis on excitable tissues should be expected in light of the major mechanism of action of this drug. Since digitalis binds to and depresses active transport by the membrane Na, K-ATPase, it is reasonable to expect that digitalis will exert direct effects on all excitable cells that depend on this transport mechanism to maintain normal transmembrane concentration gradients of ions. Thus digitalis should be expected to modify the function of all neural elements and smooth muscle cells. One recent study [70] has shown that there is a significant uptake of digoxin by peripheral autonomic nerves in the dog and that the uptake by sympathetic ganglia is particularly marked. In addition, as noted during severe digitalis poisoning, the Na^+, K^+-pump in skeletal muscle also is influenced strongly with release of K^+ into the circulation.

There is no doubt that digitalis influences the activity of both parasympathetic and sympathetic nervous systems. The magnitude and nature of the influence is a function of the dose of digitalis and the state of the heart and circulation. Other agents such as angiotension II also are involved in the net adjustment of the circulation to the effects of digitalis and may be of some importance in determining the effects of digitalis in patients with heart failure.

Modification of parasympathetic activity
In normal experimental mammals, and probably also in humans, digitalis increases efferent vagal activity. This increase results from actions of digitalis at multiple sites. At each site the primary effect appears to be an inhibition of the membrane Na^+, K^+-ATPase. Evidence is convincing that digitalis exerts effects on baroreceptors, synapses in the afferent and efferent limbs of autonomic reflex paths, and on peripheral muscarinic receptors.

The effects of digitalis on arterial baroreceptors have been studied in a number of preparations. Digitalis increases the sensitivity of the reflex so that afferent signals are augmented [71]. As a result there is an increase in vagal and a decrease in sympathetic efferent activity. The change in sensitivity of the baroreceptors probably results from the ability of digitalis to inhibit partially the active transport of Na^+ and K^+ in the afferent nerve terminals [72, 73]. Digitalis also acts in the central vagal nuclei and the nodose ganglia [74] to augment efferent signals. Other studies have shown that digitalis alters the electrical excitability of efferent vagal fibers and impulse transmission in autonomic ganglia [75]. Finally, there is evidence that digitalis may increase the sensitivity of cardiac fibers to the actions of acetylcholine [76].

The net effect of the augmented vagal activity on the normal heart and circulation has been evaluated carefully in experimental animals and to some extent in humans. Sinus rate typically decreases. This change is not prominent in normal humans at rest but in dogs the augmented vagal effect is sufficient to decrease the maximum sinus rate achieved during exercise [77]. In the presence of heart failure with sinus tachycardia in humans, digitalis causes a significant slowing; in this case a decrease in sympathetic activity results from improvement in the circulation and contributes strongly to the net effect.

Acetylcholine modifies impulse generation in the sinus node by increasing the potassium conductance of specific sarcolemmal channels [78]. Because of the increase in K^+ conductance and augmented outward current the maximum diastolic potential is increased and the rate of slow depolarization during phase 4 is diminished. Both changes tend to decrease sinus rate. Very intensive vagal activity, or quite high concentrations of acetylcholine, also can decrease the amplitude of the SA nodal action potential and slow or block conduction of impulses from the node to the atrium [79–81]. The decrease in action potential amplitude may in part reflect an ability of acetylcholine to decrease i_{si} [82], but the predominant effect of acetylcholine is brought about through the increased K^+ conductance. The impaired conduction probably results from both the changes in the action potential and the increased K^+ conductance which diminishes net excitatory currents and decreases the space constant. Recent studies on both isolated [80] and in situ [81] canine hearts have shown that when vagal stimulation causes asystole, the absence of activity may be the result either of arrest of sinus impulse generation or complete block of sinoatrial conduction. Digitalis markedly augments these ef-

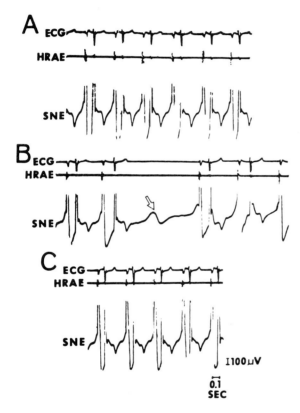

Figure 5. Records of sinus node electrograms from a conscious chronically instrumented dog (SNE) recorded simultaneously with an electrocardiogram (ECG) and high right atrial electrogram (HRAE). Sinus node electrograms are recorded through a unipolar electrode and with polarity reversed from electrocardiographic convention (negative deflections upward). The records in A are recorded under control conditions, those in B after intravenous administration of ouabain, 15 μg/kg, and C after intravenous administration of atropine, 2 mg. Note that after ouabain the sinus electrogram shows prolongation of the sinoatrial conduction. The arrow points to a sinus potential that is not followed by atrial excitation.

fects of the vagus on sinus node function (Figure 5).

The augmented vagal activity due to digitalis also has clear effects on the speed of impulse conduction through the A-V node and on the effective refractory period for A-V transmission. The mechanism of action here is like that described for the sinus node. Acetylcholine augments K^+ conductance, and this increases resting potential and maximum diastolic potential and diminishes the amplitude of the action potential [83]. These effects are prominent in the upper node (AN and N regions) but not in the lower node (NH region) [84].

Modification of sympathetic activity
Data from many types of experiments show that alterations in activity of the sympathetic nervous system contribute to both the therapeutic and toxic effects of digitalis on the heart; alterations in sympathetic neural activity also contribute to the effects of digitalis on vascular smooth muscle. The effects probably are dose-related and may differ among different tissues.

In relation to cardiac electrical activity the following seems reasonably well established. Digitalization, through sensitization of the baroreceptor reflexes, causes some decrease in efferent sympathetic activity and this decrease contributes to the decrease in sinus rate and prolongation of A-V conduction and refractoriness. For both tissues there is evidence that high doses of digitalis also may decrease the sensitivity of the effectors to norepinephrine [85, 86], but the applicability of this finding to the clinical actions of digitalis is unclear. For digitalis to significantly increase the automaticity of isolated Purkinje fibers, the presence of catecholamines is essential [87]; also, acute sympathectomy [88] and chronic cardiac denervation [89] change the response of the heart to toxic doses of digitalis. With removal of the influence of the sympathetic nervous system, lethal doses of digitalis do not cause ventricular arrhythmias; instead there is progressive bradycardia and asystole. The interactions between digitalis and norepinephrine may be rather complex. There is some evidence that digitalis increases the net release of catecholamines from sympathetic nerve terminals, either by causing some depolarization of the terminals or by blocking reuptake [90] or both; this effect would augment both automatic rhythms and triggered rhythms caused by delayed afterdepolarizations.

The interactions of digitalis with the central nervous system, and the resulting modifications of efferent sympathetic activity, are numerous and complex and have been reviewed recently [68, 69]. There is strong evidence that the occurrence of toxic arrhythmias depends in part on enhanced efferent sympathetic signals to the heart [68, 69, 71, 91]. The augmented sympathetic activity may result from effects both directly on the autonomic nervous system and from actions on the central nervous system. It has been shown in experiments on cats that transection of the spinal cord at the C-1 level increases the dose of ouabain needed to cause ventricular tachycardia and also the myocardial content of ouabain at the onset of tachycardia [92]. Also, although arrhythmias can be produced in dogs with highly polar glycosides that do not gain general access to the central nervous system [93] during digitalis intoxication, there is significant accumulation of digitalis in the region of the area postrema. Data from the same studies suggest that digitalis probably gains access to the crucial CNS structures through the choroid plexus. Digitalis also modifies the activity of autonomic afferents in the heart. For example, local application of acetyl-strophathidin causes sensitization of receptors and initiates afferent signals in the vagus that markedly decrease renal sympathetic activity [94].

In summary, digitalis alters activity in the sympathetic nervous system in several ways, and these alterations probably are important to the toxic effects of the glycosides. It seems quite clear that, in the absence of effects of norepinephrine on the heart, toxic tachyarrhythmias are not likely and tolerance of toxic amounts of glycoside is enhanced. With respect to the function of the S-A and A-V nodes it seems as though modification of sympathetic effects probably makes some contributions to the overall response to digitalis, but the major indirect action is exerted through the vagus.

Effects on electrical activity of the heart

The effects of digitalis on the electrical activity of the *in situ* heart depend on the dose, or better total body store, of glycoside, on the physiological state of the heart and circulation, and on such other factors as serum electrolyte balance, the presence of noncardiac disease, and the concurrent administration of other drugs. Much of the data available

comes from studies on experimental animals, and it is not always correct to assume that there will be quantitative correspondence between these data and findings for the human with heart failure or atrial arrhythmias. In spite of these complicating factors most of the effects can be predicted with reasonable accuracy.

Effects on excitability and conduction

Data from experiments on the canine heart indicate that digitalis has a biphasic effect on electrical excitability; unfortunately, these findings are not correlated with data for serum concentrations [95]. Low doses of digitalis are reported to increase excitability and higher doses to decrease it in both the atrium and ventricle. The increase in excitability might well reflect depression of the Na^+, K^+-pump and a resulting decrease in both outward (repolarizing) current and resting potential or a slight increase in K^+ concentration just outside the sarcolemma. This also would shift resting potential towards the threshold potential and increase excitability. The subsequent decrease in excitability might result from sufficient depolarization to partially inactive fast inward channels, from a shift in the voltage-dependence of fast channels [40] or other factors. Since digitalis typically does not increase QRS duration in humans, it seems likely that therapeutic concentrations probably do not cause a significant decrease in electrical excitability of specialized or ventricular fibers. Several studies have shown that atrial and Purkinje fibers are more sensitive to digitalis than are fibers from the ventricles [96, 97]. The indirect effects of digitalis also may be involved in causing changes in electrical excitability. For the atria, the enhanced vagal effect would be expected to increase resting potential and thereby increase the requirement for stimulus strength. The magnitude of the effect of changes in sympathetic activity is difficult to predict.

Effects of digitalis on conduction of the impulse in different parts of the heart are well documented. In dogs, digitalis, through its ability to enhance vagal activity, causes some depression of impulse conduction from the sinus pacemaker to the atrium; this action seems to be less prominent in humans [98]. In the atrium several factors influence conduction. The depolarization resulting from the direct effect of digitalis would be antagonized by the action of acetylcholine; the net effect on transmembrane potential and thus on conduction would depend on the balance between these two actions. It does not seem likely that with usual therapeutic or even toxic concentrations of digitalis in humans there will be marked impairment of conduction even though digitalis has been reported to cause broadening of the P wave. The most important effect of digitalis on conduction is exerted at the A-V node where both the direct effect and indirect effects – enhanced vagal and reduced sympathetic activity – act to depress impulse propagation. This depression occurs in the AN and N regions of the node and not in the NH region or His bundle. This slowing of impulse propagation in the A-V node appears as an increase in the A–H interval of the His bundle electrogram and as an increase in P–R interval of the ECG; the prolongation of refractoriness in the node, discussed elsewhere, is the primary cause of the higher degree of heart block. In the case of the canine heart it has been shown that lower concentrations of digitalis are needed to impair conduction in the His-Purkinje system than in ventricular muscle [99, 100], but for the human heart this action usually is not demonstrable.

Effects of digitalis on refractoriness
Digitalis will influence refractoriness both by its direct and indirect actions. Also, to the extent that digitalis changes heart rate it will also modify the duration of refractoriness. The net effects can be estimated only by assessing the importance of the individual factors.

For the atria the major effect of digitalis in low concentrations is to decrease the duration of the effective refractory period through the action of acetylcholine to shorten the action potential. With higher levels of digitalis the direct action will tend to increase the duration of refractoriness and this effect will be enhanced if atropine is used to block the vagal action. Changes in the duration of refractoriness of human hearts, including the atria of transplanted hearts, are not marked [101, 102]. The most important effect on refractoriness is that exerted on the A-V node [103, 104]; here again the direct action, the indirect actions, and the changes in heart rate interact to cause the net change. The enhanced vagal action and the direct effect of digitalis increase the effective refractory period of the A-V node, and the change is most prominent in AN and N regions. To the extent that there is a decrease in

the liberation or effect of norepinephrine this will further prolong refractoriness. It is this increase in duration of effective refractoriness that is primarily responsible for the slowing of ventricular rate during atrial tachyarrhythmias. In atrial fibrillation a large proportion of the impulses generated in the atria block in the node because of repetitive concealed conduction. Under the influence of digitalis the net atrial rate during fibrillation usually increases because the duration of the atrial action potential is shortened. This increase in atrial rate also makes a direct contribution to the increased block in the A-V node.

Special consideration should be given to the effects of digitalis on refractoriness of the different parts of the conduction path in patients who have anomalous A-V bypass tracts. The usual effects will be exerted at the A-V node; if the bypass tract conducts only in the retrograde direction the increase in A-V conduction time may be sufficient to increase the likelihood of reentry to the atria over the anomalous tract. In humans data for effects of digitalis on refractoriness of atrial muscle are conflicting with both decreases and no change reported [103, 104]. The important finding is that digitalis can *decrease* the effective refractory period of the bypass tract and thus increase the maximum rate at which atrial impulses will be transmitted to the ventricles. In the extreme case ventricular activation during atrial fibrillation may be so rapid as to cause ventricular fibrillation.

Refractoriness of Purkinje and ventricular fibers is influenced to a small extent by direct actions of acetylcholine and probably to a greater extent by the effects of norepinephrine on both β- and α-receptors (see Chapter 6). Also, acetylcholine acts on presynaptic sympathetic terminals to decrease the liberation of transmitter. The possibilities for various net effects of the indirect actions of digitalis thus are great. In the few studies that report direct measurements in humans, changes in refractoriness of Purkinje fibers have not been great, but a decrease in the effective refractory period of the ventricles has been seen [105]. For this reason the possibility for reentry involving the ventricles and Purkinje system is increased.

Effects in patients with sinus node disease
Since digitalis, by its direct and vagal actions, depresses both impulse generation in the sinus pace-

maker cells and impulse transmission from the sinus node to the atrium, one would expect digitalis to cause serious problems in most patients with sinus node disease or the sick sinus syndrome. In dogs it has been shown that digitalis consistently enhances vagal effects on the node and increases the likelihood of sinus node reentry [106]. In humans, on the other hand, digoxin does not consistently decrease sinus rate in the absence of heart failure and decreases, not increases, corrected sinus node recovery time [107, 108]. In spite of these data there have been reports of severe depression of pacemaker function with sinus node disease [109], and so caution should be exercised if digitalis is to be used to treat patients with sinus node dysfunction.

Effects on the electrocardiogram

Digitalis causes minor but reasonably consistent changes in the electrocardiogram. The P–R interval will be prolonged, and with high levels of digitalis or in the presence of preexisting depression of A-V conduction there may be higher degrees of heart block. The S–T segment and T wave usually change with a decrease in T amplitude and displacement of the S–T segment opposite to the major QRS direction. In some cases the T-wave will invert. The Q–T interval typically is shortened somewhat but the QRS complex is not increased in duration as a result of the direct effects of digitalis. Obviously, with the occurrence of arrhythmias due to digitalis intoxication other changes in the ECG will be present. Also, in patients with the Wolff-Parkinson-White syndrome the degree of QRS deformation by the delta wave often will increase as a result of slowing of A-V nodal transmission.

Effects on systemic and coronary vessels

Typically, in animals, digitalis causes constriction of arterioles and an increase in systemic vascular resistance. This effect is counterbalanced in part by reflex activation of baroreceptors since their denervation results in a further increase in resistance. Digitalis also causes constriction of veins; except for hepatic veins in dogs this effect probably is weak since there usually is no important decrease in venous return.

Studies on the effects of ouabain and acetylstrophanthidin on the vascular resistance of the per-

fused gracilis muscle during hypotension showed a consistent vasodilation brought about through a cholinergic mechanism; in normotensive animals the same drugs caused vasconstriction that was abolished by α-receptor blockade [110]. These studies demonstrate the importance of the level of sympathetic activity in determining the vascular response to glycosides. In intact spontaneously hypertensive rats it has been shown that digitoxin reduces systemic arterial pressure, whereas in rats with sinoaortic denervation it increases pressure. These findings emphasize the importance of the effect of digitalis to sensitize afferent terminals [111].

Other recent studies on cerebral, mensenteric, renal, and femoral artery strips from dogs and monkeys suggest that for cerebral arteries the digitalis-induced contraction results mainly from inhibition of the Na^+, K^+-pump and a resulting increase in intracellular calcium. For the other vessels the contraction induced by ouabain could be abolished by α-adrenergic blockade and thus appeared to result from release of norepinephrine from intravascular nerve terminals [112].

Digitalis also causes constriction of coronary arteries. Presumably this results from a direct effect to increase inward Ca^{2+} current [113]. The net effect on the coronary circulation, however, may not reflect this action. Studies in humans [114] have shown no significant change in coronary flow in normal subjects after intravenous administration of stophanthus glycosides, and data from studies on dogs [115] indicate that digitalis may increase perfusion of ischemic segments of the ventricle after coronary occlusion. In addition, if digitalis causes changes in heart work or heart rate these factors will strongly influence coronary tone as will any significant alteration in sympathetic nerve traffic to the heart. One would hope that, when administered to treat failure, the decrease in ventricular volume (and wall tension) and the decrease in heart rate would tend to cause an improvement in the ratio between flow capacity and actual need.

Effects of digitalis on the cardiovascular system

The effects of digitalis on cardiac function and on the pulmonary and systemic circulations depend on the dose of digitalis, the initial condition of the heart and circulation, and the capacity of the heart to develop increased force from a reduced end-diastolic pressure and volume. Thus digitalis would bring about different changes in the circulation when given to patients with atrial fibrillation and heart failure. In general, however, certain predictions can be made in terms of data derived from experiments on animals and observations made on humans. The observations deal with the direct effects of digitalis on cardiac and vascular muscle, the indirect effects that result from interactions with neural structures, and the secondary changes, as in blood volume, that result from improvement in the circulation.

Effects on the normal heart and circulation

If a full dose of digitalis is administered to a normal dog there will be consistent changes in cardiac activity and in systemic pressure and flow [116, 117]. All indices of ventricular contractility increase, but the changes are not large; typically, systolic and mean arterial pressures increase. The increase in force of ventricular contraction does not depend on activation of adrenergic receptors or on a change in end-diastolic fiber length. There usually is an increase in stroke volume and a decrease in aortic flow or cardiac output. There is a modest decrease in heart rate that largely can be abolished by prior denervation of the carotid and aortic baroreceptors. If heart rate is kept constant by pacing, the decrease in cardiac output is less marked or absent. Thus, the major direct effect on the heart is to increase the force of contraction. The increase in systemic arterial pressure clearly results from vasoconstriction since flow is decreased or unchanged. The increase in arterial resistance is augmented by baroreceptor denervation showing that the primary effect of digitalis is to constrict arterioles and the effect of this on pressure is modulated by the autonomic nervous system. Digitalis also acts on the veins to cause constriction; the effect probably is more prominent in the dog than in humans. In any case, since there is no significant decrease in the end-diastolic heart size, the venous constriction is not sufficient to limit cardiac filling. When digitalis is studied in exercising dogs it can be shown that the bradycardia caused by digitalis diminishes the maximum work capacity, and this effect can be abolished by atropine; similarly, the inotropic effect of digitalis is not additive with that of the catecholamines liberated during exercise [77]. In normal humans the effects are like those described for the dog [118–121]. Dig-

italis causes some increase in systemic arterial resistance and pressure and exerts a clear positive inotropic effect. Cardiac slowing is not prominent [122, 123], and cardiac output is unchanged or slightly diminished.

Effects in the presence of heart failure

The changes in the circulation that occur when digitalis is administered to patients with heart failure are described in detail in Chapter 14. A brief summary of the major components will be given here. In failure, usually there will be an increase in end-diastolic heart size and pressures, corresponding increases in pulmonary venous or systemic venous pressures, and often an increase in intravascular and extravascular volume. If failure compromises the circulation, most often the activity of the sympathetic nervous system will be augmented and circulating levels of catecholamines increased. One consequence of this will be an increase in sinus rate. With modest failure cardiac output will be normal when the subject is at rest, but with more severe failure output will be diminished. Hepatic and renal blood flow may be decreased markedly. When digitalis is given, the primary effect is the direct positive inotropic action. Because of an increase in the capacity of the ventricles to develop force, ejection is more complete, end-diastolic volume and pressure decrease, and the relationship between wall tension and intraventricular pressure improves. With improved ejection, heart rate can decrease without compromising cardiac output. With improvement in the circulation, sympathetic activity decreases and this contributes to a decrease in systemic vascular resistance and heart rate. The diminished afterload and lower heart rate both contribute to the improved stroke volume. With improvement in the circulation, renal function changes and there is elimination of salt and water and a decrease in intravascular volume and venous and capillary pressure. The increase in renal perfusion may result, in part, from a direct effect of digitalis on autonomic fibers to the heart. Local application of digitalis to the canine heart causes a marked reduction in renal sympathetic nerve activity [94].

An additional indirect means by which digitalis can improve ventricular function in patients with coronary artery disease is brought about as follows. The decrease in rate and the decrease in wall tension both permit an increase in coronary flow and cause a decrease in requirement for flow. Thus, in patients in whom myocardial perfusion is inadequate during failure, the changes caused by digitalis may improve the relationship between myocardial requirement and flow.

Pharmacokinetics

A detailed description of the clinical administration of digitalis is provided in Chapter 14. Here we will summarize information on absorption, distribution, elimination, and dosage of digoxin and digitoxin. Although other preparations are available, these two are the most widely used and are suitable for most, if not all, situations. Table 1 presents most of the essential data.

Absorption

Both digoxin and digitoxin are adequately absorbed after oral administration. Absorption of digoxin is more variable than for digitoxin, and bioavailability also varies more for the former preparation. It generally is advisable to become familiar with one commercial product and use it whenever possible.

The fraction of the dose of digoxin absorbed after oral administration is a function of the type of preparation employed. Absorption is almost com-

Table 1. Clinical pharmacology of digoxin and digitoxin.

	Digoxin	Digitoxin
Average digitalizing dose		
Oral	1.0–2.5 mg	0.8–1.2 mg
I.V.	0.5–2.0 mg	0.8–1.2 mg
Average daily maintenance		
Oral	0.125–0.75 mg (0.375)	0.05–0.2 mg (0.10)
I.V.	0.25 mg	0.10 mg
Onset of action		
Oral	1.5–4 hr[a]	3–4 hr
I.V.	5–30 min	30–120 min
Maximum effect		
Oral	4–6 hr	6–12 hr
I.V.	1.5–3.0 hr	4–8 hr
GI absorption	$\leqslant$ 40–90%[b] (75%)	90–100%
Plasma protein binding	20%	97%
Apparent volume of distribution	1000 liters	100 liters
Distribution half-time	1–3 hr	Unknown
Final disposition half-time		
Normal renal function	1.00–2.00 days	3–6 days
Anephric	4.5 days	3–5 days
Route of elimination	Renal excretion of unchanged drug; small amount of hepatic metabolism	Hepatic degradation of molecule; renal excretion of metabolites
Effect of enzyme induction	No significant effect	Moderate to large effect
Enterohepatic circulation	Small	Large
Percent of dose excreted as unchanged drug	70–90%	10–30%
'Therapeutic' plasma concentration	0.5–2.0 ng/ml (1.2 ng/ml)	10–50 ng/ml (25 ng/ml)

[a] Dependent on relation of dose to meal, gastric emptying time, type of preparation.
[b] About 90% of an alcohol elixir is absorbed from a normal GI tract.

401

plete when digoxin is administered in an alcoholic vehicle (90% or more) and usually approximates 75% with highly bioavailable tablets. For some preparations, however, absorption may be as low as 40%. The differences in bioavailability result mainly from differences in rate and extent of dissolution among tablets from different sources [124–127]. Absorption of digoxin also is modified by the presence of food in the gastrointestinal tract, by abnormalities of gastric emptying, and by malabsorption syndromes. Some antibiotics such as neomycin retard absorption as do steroid-binding resins. It has been shown that in approximately 10% of patients there is substantial conversion of digoxin to cardioinactive products by enteric organisms. During the administration of a constant daily dose of digoxin to such patients the simultaneous administration of erythromycin or a tetracycline can increase the serum concentration of digoxin as much as two-fold [128].

After oral administration plasma levels of digoxin typically peak in 2–3 hr and the maximum effect is attained in 4–6 hr. With chronic oral administration the plateau plasma level is attained in about one week; this is expected for a drug for which the $t_{1/2e}$ is between 1–2 days. Obviously, if elimination of digoxin is retarded both peak plasma levels resulting from a given dose and also the time required to attain a plateau level will be altered.

Absorption of digitoxin after oral administration is almost complete in nearly all patients [90–99%], and significant problems with bioavailability have not been reported. Absorption will be influenced by most of the factors mentioned in relation to digoxin. Because the $t_{1/2e}$ for digitoxin is long, the time required to reach a steady plasma level is quite long (Table 1), as is the time required for the plasma level to fall if a toxic concentration has been attained.

Distribution

The volume of distribution for both digoxin and digitoxin is quite large and thus a reasonably long interval is required for distribution and equilibration with all body compartments. Distribution is slowed in the presence of heart failure. Digitoxin is more extensively bound to plasma protein (97%) than is digoxin (20%), and thus the apparent volume of distribution for digitoxin is smaller than for digoxin and the therapeutic plasma levels are considerably higher. Both glycosides are distributed to almost all body tissues including red cells, skeletal muscle, and heart. At equilibrium the concentration in cardiac muscle is 15–30 times the plasma concentration. Binding to heart and skeletal muscle is decreased when serum potassium is elevated. Recently it has been reported that potassium depletion decreases the number of digitalis binding sites in skeletal muscle [59]. Other studies have demonstrated a considerable accumulation of ^{3}H-digoxin in some parts of the central nervous system (area postrema) and in the neurohypophysis and superior cervical ganglia [129].

For both digoxin and digitoxin the peak inotropic effect lags behind attainment of the peak plasma level and maximum inotropic effect may not be attained until 1 hr after the cardiac level attains its maximum value. This may result from the time required for pump inhibition to result in a significant change in intracellular calcium. In the heart the functionally significant uptake of glycosides is that bound to the Na^+, K^+-ATPase.

Elimination

Digoxin and digitoxin differ in terms of the primary route of elimination. Digoxin is eliminated mainly by the kidney through glomerular filtration and tubular secretion, whereas digitoxin is eliminated mainly by hepatic metabolism. Digoxin is reabsorbed from renal tubular fluid, and thus the rate of elimination will be decreased with significant decreases in the rate of flow of tubular fluid. Some patients form an inactive metabolite of digoxin, 2-hydroxydigoxin, and in such patients a therapeutic effect may be difficult to attain. A very few patients form antibodies to digoxin which prevent its therapeutic effect.

The half-time for elimination of digoxin is strongly dependent on renal function and usually the elimination correlates closely with the endogenous creatinine clearance or the blood urea nitrogen level. Vasodilator therapy [130] and interventions that modify renal perfusion pressure thus will change the rate of elimination of digoxin [131]. Hepatic disease does not significantly influence the elimination rate of either digoxin or digitoxin. There is an enteroheptic circulation of digitoxin but only a small fraction of the drug is eliminated unchanged in the intestine.

Dosages

Since digitalis is used most often either to alleviate heart failure or to control ventricular rate during a persistent atrial arrhythmia, usually it is necessary both to establish and to maintain a therapeutic plasma and cardiac level of glycoside. In most patients the desired effect can be achieved with sufficient speed by oral administration. If there is no urgency the maintenance dose can be given daily and for digoxin the peak effect will develop in 3–7 days; with digitoxin the interval will be 10–20 days. If the effects are needed fairly promptly, a loading dose, traditionally called the digitalizing dose, is given.

For digoxin the oral digitalizing dose ranges from 1.0–2.5 mg and the intravenous dose from 0.5–1.0 mg. Usually the oral loading dose is given as two doses of 0.5 mg at an interval of 3–4 hr. If intravenous administration is needed and it is certain that the patient has *not* been taking any digitalis preparation, 1.0 mg of digoxin can be given over a period of 10–20 min. The digitalizing dose for digitoxin varies from 0.8–1.2 mg and, since absorption of oral drug is almost complete, the oral and intravenous doses are approximately the same.

In theory the loading or 'digitalizing' dose is the dose needed to bring the total body store and plasma level to the therapeutic range of concentrations. Obviously, this will vary with the age and size of the patient. In addition, there will be considerable variation depending on the condition of the heart and the desired end point. For the patient in failure the desired outcome is the restoration of compensation and for the patient with atrial fibrillation the desired end point is a suitable slowing of ventricular rate. The levels required will differ depending on the severity and perhaps the cause of failure; they also will vary among patients with atrial tachyarrhythmias. Since at the best the 'therapeutic' plasma level may not differ by much from the toxic level, and since digitalis toxicity often places the patient at risk, it is wise to err on the side of underestimating the size of the loading dose needed. As long as a significant effect is attained with the loading dose, further titration can be accomplished with subsequent maintenance doses. Also, instead of using the maximally tolerable plasma level, it is more reasonable to use other drugs, such as diuretics and drugs that reduce afterload, to achieve compensa-

tion and to employ beta-adrenergic blockade or verapamil to aid digitalis in slowing ventricular rate.

The loading dose is selected to result in a therapeutic plasma level and total body store. The daily maintenance dose must equal the daily loss. For digoxin this amounts to approximately 35% and for digitoxin 10%; variations in the rate of elimination of digoxin will modify this fraction considerably (see Table 1).

Drug interaction

A number of antiarrhythmic drugs have been shown to alter the serum concentration of digoxin when both the antiarrhythmic drug and digoxin are given concurrently. Less information is available for digitoxin. Interactions between quinidine and digoxin have been studied intensively in recent years.

Quinidine–digoxin interactions

If standard doses of quinidine are given to a patient taking maintenance doses of digoxin, in most cases the serum digoxin concentration will increase by 0.5 mg/ml or more [132–139], and usually the serum digoxin concentration will double when quinidine levels have reached a plateau. To some extent the magnitude of increase in digoxin levels is a function of the dose and serum level of quinidine. The two factors primarily responsible for the increase in digoxin levels are, first, a decrease in the volume of distribution of digoxin and, second, a decrease in renal and extra-renal elimination [139, 140]. Studies on rat and guinea pig heart have shown that quinidine does not modify ouabain binding to the Na^+, K^+-ATPase and does not influence the ouabain-induced inhibition of active transport or the sensitivity of the myocardium to ouabain [141]. Also, in cultured heart cells quinidine does not influence either the positive inotropic effect of digoxin or the inhibition of monovalent cation transport [142]. Since digoxin concentration in heart and other body tissues is much greater than in blood, a small decrease in tissue binding could cause a significant increase in serum level. The ability of quinidine to decrease renal clearance of digoxin is demonstrated in most patients and often amounts to a decrease of 40–50%. This most likely reflects a decrease in renal tubular secretion.

When concurrent administration of quinidine causes an increase in serum digoxin levels the likelihood of digitalis toxicity is increased. Even though completely satisfactory data are not yet available, it seems likely that when quinidine causes an increase in serum digoxin levels this is associated with an increased binding of digitalis to and inhibition of the myocardial Na^+, K^+-ATPase. This should result in more intense effects on electrical and mechanical activity. Whether or not levels of digoxin increase in different parts of the central nervous system during quinidine administration is uncertain. What is clear is that patients who begin to take therapeutic dose of quinidine during maintenance digoxin treatment are likely to show nausea, vomiting, and ventricular arrhythmias, and these toxic manifestations are relieved if the digoxin dose is reduced. Manifestations of increased digoxin effect may include an increase in P–R interval, a decrease in ventricular rate during fibrillation, and nonparoxysmal A–V junctional tachycardia. Effects of the interaction on mechanical activity of the heart are not clearly defined [143, 144].

Management of patients to prevent undesirable changes in digoxin levels and effects can be accomplished in several ways. The dose of digoxin can be reduced, but this may result in loss of control of congestive heart failure. An alternative digitalis preparation can be tried, but it is not certain that some interaction does not take place with digitoxin [145–150]. Probably the safest course is to employ an antiarrhythmic drug that does not interact with digoxin; no significant interactions have been reported for procainamide, mexilitine, and imipramine. Among the antiarrhythmic drugs aminodarone has been shown to increase serum digoxin levels, but data on the magnitude of and mechanisms for this effect are not available [151].

Interestingly, it has been reported that digoxin increased the antiarrhythmic effectiveness of disopyramide [152]. This interaction may result from the fact that the effect of disopyramide, like that of other local anesthetic antiarrhythmic drugs, is strongly dependent on the resting transmembrane potential. If digoxin causes some increase in plasma K^+ concentration, resting potential will decrease slightly.

Other interactions
Several other types of drugs have been reported to

cause significant modification of serum digoxin levels in humans. Verapamil has been studied fairly extensively and shown to cause a dose-dependent and gradual rise in serum digoxin level sufficient to require adjustment of digoxin dose. This effect is caused at least in part by a reduction in renal clearance of digoxin [153–155]. Nifedipine also has been reported to cause significant increases in the serum digoxin concentration [156], and so one might anticipate similar interactions with other drugs used to block slow inward channels.

There are indications that a number of other drugs may decrease the renal clearance of digoxin, including spironolactone, triamterene, and amiloride. Hypokalemia may have the same effect. Drugs which alter the serum concentration of K^+, Ca^{2+}, or Mg^{2+} will influence effect and likelihood of toxicity. Treatment of hypothyroidism can be expected to increase clearance of digoxin. Phenylbutazone, phenobarbital, and phenytoin may speed hepatic metabolism of digitoxin and thus modify both plasma levels and the elimination half-time.

Digitalis intoxication

Intoxication by digitalis is frequent and often can place the patient at risk of death. Withering (1785) was familiar with many of the major toxic effects of cardiac glycosides and commented: 'The floxglove when given in very large and quickly repeated doses occasions sickness, vomiting purging, giddiness, confused vision, objects appearing green or yellow; increased secretions of urine, with frequent motions to part with it; slow pulse, even as low as 35 in a minute, cold sweats, convulsions, syncope and death.' Since digitalis acts on all excitable cells, and probably all cells with a Na^+, K^+-ATPase of the cardiac type, it is not surprising that its toxic effects can involve almost all organ systems. Nevertheless, toxic effects on the heart and nervous system are the most characteristic, and cardiac toxicity is most important because of the associated risk. All clinically available digitalis preparations have comparable and low margins of safety; they differ in terms of the duration of toxicity because the half-times for elimination differ markedly among different preparations.

Cardiac toxicity

Even though excessive concentrations of digitalis can cause partial contracture and loss of contractility of cardiac preparations studied in vitro, it is most unlikely that excessive plasma levels resulting from therapeutic administration of digitalis cause a decrease in the force of cardiac contraction or significantly modify diastolic distensibility. The important toxic effects of digitalis consist of abnormalities of cardiac rhythm and A-V conduction. At the plasma levels usually attained in patients digitalis does not impair conduction in the His-Purkinje system or ventricles, and thus intoxication does not prolong the QRS complex during sinus rhythm. Very high levels may cause prolongation of the P wave and this most likely is due to impaired conduction in the atria.

Digitalis intoxication can cause depression of sinus impulse formation and severe bradycardia or partial or complete sino-atrial block. Toxic effects on the sinus node may be more likely in the presence of sinus node disease. The decrease in sinus rate and sino-atrial block probably result from both the enhancement of vagal activity and a direct depressant effect of digitalis. Recent studies employing sinus node electrograms to evaluate the function of the in situ canine sinus node [81] or intracellular microelectrodes to study transmembrane potentials of isolated tissues [80] have shown clearly that vagal activation can both block sino-atrial conduction and depress the sinus node action potential to a point at which impulse propagation fails. For the human heart there is evidence that digitalis causes much less enhancement of vagal activity than in canines [108] since effects of digitalis on sinus rate typically are not reversed by atropine. It seems likely, however, that, because digitalis can depress conduction between the right atrium and the sinus node, high concentrations will increase the likelihood of reentrant rhythms involving the sinus node. Toxic levels of digitalis have been shown to cause a variety of supraventricular arrhythmias including premature depolarizations and paroxysmal and sustained atrial tachycardias. The probable causes of these arrhythmias are delayed afterdepolarizations, which occur in atrial fibers exposed to toxic concentrations of digitalis, and reentrant excitation due to impaired conduction in either the A-V or, less commonly, the S-A node. Digitalis can enhance phase 4 depolarization in normally automatic tissues and thus also could cause automatic atrial rhythms.

The effects of excessive concentrations of digitalis on the A-V junction are typically the production of high grade A-V block and accelerated junctional rhythms which are manifested either as escape beats or as nonparoxysmal junctional tachycardia. Recent studies have demonstrated the probability that some accelerated junction rhythms caused by digitalis may be due to delayed afterdepolarizations [157]; others are likely caused by reentry or enhanced automaticity. The depression of conduction in the A-V node is due in part to the vagomimetic effect and in part to a direct depressant effect that cannot be reversed by atropine. With extreme intoxication that results in loss of K^+ from skeletal muscle, the increase in plasma potassium concentration will contribute both to the production of A-V block and the depression of sinus activity.

The ventricular arrhythmias most often seen during digitalis intoxication are premature depolarizations appearing as a bigeminal or trigeminal rhythm and ventricular tachycardia. Also, severe intoxication can result in ventricular fibrillation. The mechanisms for these ventricular arrhythmias in humans have not been demonstrated with certainty. It has been shown that digitalis decreases the effective refractory period of ventricular muscle more than that of the terminal Purkinje fibers [101], and thus a premature ventricular depolarization is more likely to result in reentrant excitation. Digitalis also can cause delayed afterdepolarizations in Purkinje fibers and ventricular muscle [65], and this mechanism could be responsible for the coupled premature depolarizations and runs of tachyarrhythmias. Finally, sustained ventricular tachycardia caused by digitalis excess probably results from enhanced automaticity in specialized ventricular fibers.

Toxic effects of digitalis on the heart are more likely in adults than in infants or children [158], and severely damaged hearts appear to be more sensitive than normal hearts to the toxic effects of glycosides. Studies on the transmembrane potentials of hearts from neonatal and young dogs show that digitalis causes less of a depression of membrane potential in fibers from young animals than those from adults and rarely causes an increase in phase 4 depolarization or DAD [159]. There thus may be an age-dependent basis for the differing incidence of

405

arrhythmias. When digitalis is ingested by individuals with normal hearts in attempts at suicide, arrhythmias usually are not prominent even in the presence of extremely high plasma level of drug. This may reflect differences in the sensitivity of the normal and abnormal hearts to digitalis or may result for the most part from the elevated plasma K^+ levels present in such patients. There is clear evidence that the likelihood that digitalis will cause premature depolarizations or ectopic junctional or ventricular rhythms is related to the simultaneous action of catecholamines on the cardiac tissues. Acute or chronic cardiac denervation [88, 89] changes the sensitivity of the heart to digitalis so that toxic concentrations cause only a decrease in heart rate, heart block, and asystole. The exact nature of the facilatatory effect of norepinephrine on digitalis-induced arrhythmias has not been demonstrated.

Factors influencing toxicity

The factors that are most important in relation to the likelihood of digitalis intoxication are listed in Table 2. The most frequent cause of toxicity, even in the absence of excessive plasma levels of digitalis, is a decrease in plasma K^+ concentration and depletion of body stores of potassium. This abnormality results most often from the concurrent administra-

Table 2. Conditions increasing the likelihood of digitalis toxicity.

I.   Other drugs
    1. Diuretics causing potassium depletion
    2. Quinidine
    3. Varapamil, nifedipine
    4. Spironactone
    5. Amiodarone
II. Increased cardiac sensitivity
    1. Hypokalemia
    2. Acute ischemia
    3. Increased sympathetic activity
    4. Hypercalcemia
    5. Hypomagnesemia
    6. Acute hypoxia
III. Excessive body stores
    1. Excessive dose
    2. Reduced elimination
      a) Decreased renal function (digoxin)
      b) Hypothyroidism
IV. Other conditions
    1. Cardiomyopathy
    2. Acute carditis

tion with digitalis of a kaliuretic diuretic. The relationship between plasma K^+ concentration and intensity of digitalis effect results from at least two factors. First, the binding of digitalis to the Na, K-ATPase is a function of the K^+ concentration [13]; second, it may be that an excessively low potassium concentration directly depresses the Na^+-K^+ pump. One study has shown that during potassium depletion in rats there is a marked decrease in ^3H ouabain binding sites and a reduced capacity for Na^+, K^+-ATPase-mediated K^+ uptake by skeletal muscle. This finding may explain in part the occurrence of digitalis toxicity during K^+ depletion. Toxicity also results from administration of an excessive dose; sometimes this may be caused by a change in the preparation ingested to one with greater bioavailability. A decrease in the rate of elimination of digitalis also can cause an excessive plasma level; this is more likely with digoxin, which is eliminated mainly in the urine, than with digotoxin. Since circulatory changes resulting from an increase in the severity of heart failure can reduce renal blood flow, a change in the degree of decompensation could reduce losses through glomerular filtration and increase reabsorption from tubular fluid; both effects would increase the plasma drug level.

Other extracellular ions can modify the intensity of effect of digitalis on the heart and thus influence the likelihood of toxicity. An elevated Ca^{2+} concentration can cause severe toxicity even in the presence of normal plasma levels of digitalis, and a reduction in Mg^{2+} concentration has effects similar to those of high calcium. Hypothyroidism is thought to enhance toxicity both by slowing elimination of digitalis and also by increasing sensitivity of the heart to the drug. Finally, it is important to remember that any change in the condition of the heart that is likely to depress the active membrane transport of Na^+ and K^+ will enhance digitalis toxicity. Thus ischemia or arterial hypoxia would be expected to increase the chance that previously nontoxic levels will cause arrhythmias. Acidosis probably sensitizes the heart to digitalis by a direct depressant effect of H^+ on the membrane transport system for Na^+ and K^+ [60]. An increase in the severity of heart failure will sensitize the heart to the toxic effects of digitalis both by causing an increase in heart rate, and thus in the need to transport Na^+ out of the myocardial cells, and also by augmenting activity of the sympathetic nervous system. Interactions between digitalis and other drugs to increase the likelihood of digitalis toxicity have been described.

The role of the central nervous system in cardiac toxicity

A large body of evidence implicates changes in neural activity in the genesis of arrhythmias due to digitalis intoxication and this evidence recently has been reviewed in detail [68]. The changes in autonomic activity result in part from sensitization of baroreceptors and in part from effects of digitalis on afferent terminals and autonomic ganglia. These have been described in some detail in an earlier section. In addition, it is clear that digitalis exerts direct effects on the central nervous system, and several studies have been directed toward demonstrating the importance of this site of action to arrhythmias. When a semisynthetic and highly polar cardiac glycoside was used to cause cardiac arrhythmias in dogs [93], arrhythmias were initiated without an accumulation of the glycoside in the cerebrospinal fluid. However, evidence was obtained that digitalis was exerting an effect on brain structures adjacent to the area postrema. As for the emetic effect of digitalis, the drug probably gains access to these brain structures because of the absence of a blood–brain barrier in this area [160].

Other toxic effects

The other major toxic effects of digitalis include anorexia, nausea, and vomiting; the latter is due to a direct effect of the glycoside on the chemoreceptor trigger zone in the area postrema [161] and not primarily to direct irritant effects on the gastrointestinal tract. Sometimes patients develop diarrhea or abdominal pain. Neurological abnormalities are common; these include headache, fatigue, and drowsiness. Infrequently, there may be neuralgic pain, disorientation, confusion, and even delerium. Visual disturbances also may occur including disturbances of color vision, ambylopia, diplopia, and scotomata. The contraction of ^{3}H-digoxin in the optic tract has been determined in dogs and a high concentration found in the choroid and retina [162]. This may be related to the effects of digitalis on vision. The treatment of digitalis intoxication is described in Chapter 14.

References

1. Gold H, Cattell M: Mechanism of digitalis action in abolishing heart failure. Arch Intern Med 65:263–278, 1940.
2. Ford LE: Effect of afterload reduction on myocardial energetics. Circ Res 46:161–166, 1980.
3. Wilbrandt W: Zum Wirkungsmechanismus des Herzglykoside. Schweiz Med Wochenschr 85:315–320, 1955.
4. Fozzard HA: Heart: excitation–contraction coupling. Ann Rev Physiol 39:201–210, 1977.
5. Gibbons WR, Fozzard HA: Relationships between voltage and tension in sheep cardiac Purkinje fibers. J Gen Physiol 65:345–365, 1975.
6. Reuter H: Exchange of calcium ions in the mammalian myocardium. Circ Res 34:599–605, 1974.
7. Blaustein MP: The interrelationship between sodium and calcium fluxes across cell membranes. Rev Physiol Biochem Pharmacol 70:33–82, 1974.
8. Caroni P, Carafoli E: An ATP-dependent Ca^{2+}-pumping system in dog heart sarcolemma. Nature 283:765–767, 1980.
9. Pitts BJR, Stoichiometry of sodium–calcium exchange in cardiac sarcolemmal vesicles. J Biol Chem 254:6232–6235, 1979.
10. Akera T, Brody TM: The role of Na^+, K^+-ATPase in the inotropic action of digitalis. Pharmacol Rev 29:187–188, 1977.
11. Akera T, Larsen FS, Brody TM: Correlation of cardiac sodium- and potassium-activated adenosine triphosphatase activity with ouabain-induced inotropic stimulation. J Pharmacol Exp Ther 173:145–151, 1970.
12. Besch HR Jr, Allen JC, Glick G, Schwartz A: Correlation between the inotropic action of ouabain and its effects on subcellular enzyme systems from canine myocardium. J Pharmacol Exp Ther 171:1–12, 1970.
13. Goldman RH, Coltart JD, Friedman JP, Nola GT, Berke DK, Schweizer E, Harrison DC: The inotropic effects of digoxin in hyperkalemia. Relation to Na^+, K^+ ATPase inhibition in the intact animal. Circulation 48:830–838, 1973.
14. Matsui H, Schwartz A: Mechanism of cardiac glycoside inhibition of the (Na^+-K^+)-dependent ATPase from cardiac tissue. Biochim Biophys Acta 151:655–663, 1968.
15. Michael LH, Schwartz A, Wallick ET: Nature of the transport adenosine triphosphatase-digitalis complex: XIV. Inotropy and cardiac glycoside interaction with Na^+, K^+-ATPase of isolated cat papillary muscles. Mol Pharmacol 16:134–146, 1979.
16. Hougen TJ, Smith TW: Inhibition of myocardial cation active transport by subtoxic doses of ouabain in the dog. Circ Res 42:856–863, 1978.
17. Miura DS, Rosen MR: The effects of ouabain on the transmembrane potentials and intracellular potassium activity of canine cardiac Purkinje fibers. Circ Res 42:333–338, 1978.
18. Deitmer JM, Ellis D: The intracellular sodium activity of cardiac Purkinje fibers during inhibition and reactivation of the Na-K pump. J Physiol 284:241–259, 1978.
19. Wier WG: Calcium transients during excitation-concen-

407

tration coupling in mammalian heart: aequorin signals of canine Purkinje fibers. Science 207:1085–1087, 1980.

20. Marban E: Regulation of Calcium Current and Calcium Activity in Heart Cells. PhD Dissertation, Yale Univ, 1981.

21. Lee CO, Kang DH, Sokol JH, Lee KS: Relation between intracellular Na ion activity and tension of sheep cardiac Purkinje fibers exposed to dihydro-ouabain. Biophys J 29:315–330, 1980.

22. Ellis D: The effects of external cations and ouabain on the intracellular sodium activity of sheep heart Purkinje fibers. J Physiol 273:211–240, 1977.

23. Tsien RY, Rink TJ: Neutral carrier ion-selective microelectrodes for measurement of intracellular free calcium. Biochim Biophys Acta 599:623–638, 1980.

24. Eisner DA, Lederer WJ: The relationship between sodium pump activity and twitch tension in cardiac Purkinje fibers. J Physiol 303:475–494, 1980.

25. Eisner DA, Lederer WH, Vaughan-Jones RD: The dependence of sodium pumping and tension on intracellular sodium activity in voltage-clamped sheep Purkinje fibers. J Physiol 317:163–187, 1981.

26. Eisner DA, Lederer WJ, Vaughan-Jones RD: Electrogenic sodium pumping in cardiac muscle: simultaneous measurement of intracellular sodium activity, membrane current and tension. J Physiol 300:42–43, 1980.

27. Michael L, Pitts BJR, Schwartz A: Is pump stimulation associated with positive inotropy of the heart? Science 200:1287–1289, 1978.

28. Grupp G, Grupp IL, Ghysel-Burton J, Godfraind T, Schwartz A: Effects of very low concentrations of ouabain on contractile force of isolated guinea-pig, rabbit and cat atria and right ventricular papillary muscles: an interinstitutional study. J Pharmacol Exp Ther 220:145–151, 1981.

29. Knight RG, Nosek TM: Effects of rubidium on contractility and sodium pump activity in guinea-pig ventricle. J Pharmacol Exp Ther 219:573–579, 1981.

30. Eisner DA, Lederer WJ, Vaughan-Jones RD: The effects of rubidium ions and membrane potential on the intracellular sodium activity of sheep Purkinje fibers. J Physiol 317:189–205, 1981.

31. Akera T, Bennett RT, Olgaard MK, Brody TM: Cardiac Na^+, K^+-adenosine triphosphatase inhibition by ouabain and myocardial sodium: a computer simulation. J Pharmacol Exp Ther 199:287–297, 1976.

32. Adams RJ, Schwartz A, Grupp G, Grupp I, Lee SW, Wallick ET: High-affinity ouabain binding site and low-dose positive inotropic effect in rat myocardium. Nature 296:167–171, 1982.

33. Huang W, Rhee HM, Chiu TH, Askari A: Re-evaluation of the relationship between the positive inotropic effect of ouabain and its inhibitory effect on $(Na^+ + K^+)$-dependent adenosine triphosphatase in rabbit and dog hearts. J Pharmacol Exp Ther 211:571–581, 1979.

34. Yamamoto S, Akera T, Kim DH, Brody TM: Tissue concentration of Na^+, K^+-adenosine triphosphatase and the positive inotropic action of ouabain in guinea-pig heart. J Pharmacol Exp Ther 217:701–707, 1981.

35. Hess P, Müller P: Extracellular versus intracellular digoxin action on bovine myocardium, using a digoxin antibody and intracellular glycoside application. J Physiol 322:197–210, 1982.

36. Kass RS, Tsien RW, Weingart R: Ionic basis of transient inward current induced by strophanthidin in cardiac Purkinje fibers. J Physiol 281:209–226, 1978.

37. Marban E, Tsien RW: Ouabain increases the slow inward calcium current in ventricular muscle of the ferret. J Physiol 292:72–73P, 1979.

38. Marban E, Tsien RW: Is the slow inward calcium current of heart muscle inactivated by calcium? Biophys J 33:143, 1981.

39. Vassalle M, Karis J, Hoffman BF: Toxic effects of ouabain on Purkinje fibers and ventricular muscle fibers. Am J Physiol 203:433–439, 1962.

40. Kassebaum DG: Electrophysiological effects of strophanthin in the heart. J Pharmacol Exp Ther 140:329–338, 1963.

41. Muller P: Ouabain effects on cardiac contraction, action potential and cellular potassium. Circ Res 17:46–56, 1965.

42. Rosen MR, Gelband H, Hoffman BF: Correlation between effects of ouabain on the cardiac electrocardiogram and transmembrane potentials of isolated Purkinje fibers. Circ Res 47:65–72, 1973.

43. Karagueuzian HS, Katzung BG: Relative inotropic and arrhythmogenic effects of five cardiac steroids in ventricular myocardium: oscillatory afterpotentials and the role of endogenous catecholamines. J Pharmacol Exp Ther 218:348–356, 1981.

44. Davis LD: Effect of changes in cycle length on diastolic depolarization produced by ouabain in canine Purkinje fibers. Circ Res 32:206–214, 1973.

45. Ferrier GR, Saunders JH, Mendez C: A cellular mechanism for the generation of ventricular arrhythmias by acetylstrophanthidin. Circ Res 32:600–609, 1973.

46. Rosen MR, Gelband H, Merker C, Hoffman BF: Mechanisms of digitalis toxicity: effects of ouabain on phase 4 of canine Purkinje fiber transmembrane potentials. Circ Res 47:681–689, 1973.

47. Rosen MR, Danilo P Jr: Digitalis-induced delayed afterdepolarizations. In: Zipes DP, Bailey JC, Elharrar V (eds) The Slow Inward Current and Cardiac Arrhythmias. Martinus Nijhoff, The Hague, 1980, pp 417–435.

48. Bassingthwaighte JB, Fry CH, McGuigan JAS: Relationship between internal calcium and outward current in mammalian ventricular muscle: a mechanism for the control of the action potential duration? J Physiol 262:15–37, 1976.

49. Baumgarten C, Isenberg G: Depletion and accumulation of potassium in the extracellular clefts of cardiac Purkinje fibers during voltage clamp hyperpolarization and depolarization. Pflugers Arch 368:19–31, 1977.

50. Attwell D, Eisner D, Cohen I: Voltage clamp and tracer flux data: effects of a restricted extra-cellular space. Q Rev Biophys 12:213–261, 1979.

51. Kunze DL: Rate-dependent changes in extracellular potassium in the rabbit atrium. Circ Res 41:122–127, 1977.

52. Kline RP, Morad M: Potassium efflux in heart muscle during activity: extracellular accumulation and its implications. J Physiol 280:537–558, 1978.

53. Tsien RW, Kass RS, Weingart R: Cellular and subcellular

mechanisms of cardiac pacemaker oscillations. J Exp Biol 81:205–215, 1979.

54. Lederer WJ, Tsien RW: Transient inward current underlying arrhythmogenic effects of cardiotonic steroids in Purkinje fibers. J Physiol 263:73–100, 1976.

55. Kass RS, Lederer WJ, Tsien RW, Weingart R: Role of calcium ions in transient inward currents and aftercontractions induced by strophanthidin in cardiac Purkinje fibers. J Physiol 281:187–208, 1978.

56. De Mello WC: Effect of intracellular injection of calcium and strontium on cell communication in heart. J Physiol 250:231–245, 1975.

57. Weingart R: The actions of ouabain on intracellular coupling and conduction velocity in mammalian ventricular muscle. J Physiol 264:341–365, 1977.

58. Schwartz A: Is the cell membrane Na^+, K^+-ATPase enzyme system the pharmacological receptor for digitalis? Circ Res 39:2–7, 1976.

59. Norgaard A, Kjeldsen K, Clausen T: Potassium depletion decreases the number of ^{3}H-ouabain binding sites and the active Na-K transport in skeletal muscle. Nature 293:739–741, 1981.

60. Brown RH, Cohen I, Noble D: The interactions of protons, calcium and potassium ions on cardiac Purkinje fibers. J Physiol 282:345–352, 1978.

61. Bonke FIM, Steinbeck G, Allessie MA, MacKaay AJC, Slenter VAJ: The electrophysiological effects of cardiac glycosides on the isolated sinus node of the rabbit. In: Paes de Carvalho A, Hoffman BF, Lieberman M (eds) Symposium on Normal and Abnormal Conduction in the Heart Beat. Futura Publ, New York, 1982.

62. Steinbeck G, Bonke FIM, Allessie MA, Lammers WJEP: The effect of ouabain on the isolated sinus node preparation of the rabbit studied with microelectrodes. Circ Res 46:406–414, 1982.

63. Hogan PM, Davis LD: Evidence for specialized fibers in the canine right atrium. Circ Res 23:387–396, 1968.

64. Hashimoto K, Moe GK: Transient depolarizations induced by acetylstrophanthidin in specialized tissues of dog atrium and ventricle. Circ Res 32:618–624, 1973.

65. Ferrier GR: The effects of tension and acetylstrophanthidin-induced transient depolarizations and aftercontractions in canine myocardial and Purkinje tissues. Circ Res 38:156–162, 1976.

66. Wit AL: Personal communication.

67. Wit AL, Cranefield PF, Gadsby DC: Electrogenic sodium extrusion can stop triggered activity in the canine coronary sinus. Circ Res 49:1029–1042, 1981.

68. Gillis RA, Quest JA: The role of the nervous system in the cardiovascular effects of digitalis. Pharmacol Rev 31:19–97, 1980.

69. Rosen MR: Interactions of digitalis with the autonomic nervous system and their relationship to cardiac arrhythmias. In: Abboud F, Fozzard H, Gilmore J, Reis D (eds) Disturbances in Neurogenic Control of the Circulation. Am Physiol Soc, Bethesda, 1981, pp 251–263.

70. Cook LS, Doherty JE, Straub KD, Nash CB, Caldwell RW: Digoxin uptake into peripheral autonomic cardiac nerves: possible mechanism of digitalis-induced antiar-

rhythmic and toxic electrophysiologic actions. Am Heart J 102:58–62, 1981.

71. Pace DG, Gillis RA: Neuroexcitatory effects of digoxin in the cat. J Pharmacol Exp Ther 199:583–600, 1976.

72. Saum RW, Brown AM, Tuley FH: An electrogenic sodium pump and baroceptor function in normotensive and spontaneously hypertensive rats. Circ Res 39:497–505, 1976.

73. Ayachi S, Brown AM: Hypotensive effects of cardiac glycosides in spontaneously hypertensive rats. J Pharmacol Exp Ther 213:520–524, 1980.

74. Chai CY, Wang HH, Hoffman BF, Wang SC: Mechanisms of bradycardia induced by digitalis substances. Am J Physiol 212:26–34, 1967.

75. Ten Eick RE, Hoffman BF: The effect of digitalis on the excitability of autonomic nerves. J Pharmacol Exp Ther 169:95–108, 1969.

76. Toda N, West TC: the action of ouabain on the function of the atrioventricular node in rabbits. J Pharmacol Exp Ther 169:287–297, 1969.

77. Horwitz LD, Atkins JM, Saito M: Effects of digitalis on left ventricular function in exercising dogs. Circ Res 41:744–749, 1977.

78. DiFrancesco D, Noma A, Trautwein W: Separation of current induced by potassium accumulation from acetylcholine-induced relaxation current in the rabbit S-A node. Pflugers Arch 387:83–90, 1980.

79. Paes de Carvalho A, Hoffman BF, de Paula Carvalho M: Two components of the cardiac action potential: 1. Voltage time course and the effect of acetylcholine on atrial and nodal cells of the rabbit heart. J Gen Physiol 54:607–635, 1969.

80. Woods WT, Urthaler F, James TN: Electrical activity in canine sinus node cells during arrest produced by acetylcholine. J Moll Cell Cardiol 13:349–357, 1981.

81. Hariman RJ, Hoffman BF: Effects of ouabain and vagal stimulation on sinus nodal function in conscious dogs. Circ Res 51:760–768, 1982.

82. Prokopczuk A, Lewartowski B, Czarnecka M: On the cellular mechanism of the inotropic action of acetylcholine on isolated rabbit and dog atria. Pflugers Arch 399:305–316, 1973.

83. Hoffman BF, Paes de Carvalho A, deMello WC, Cranefield PF: Electrical activity on single fibers on the atrioventricular node. Circ Res 7:11–18, 1959.

84. Cranefield PF, Hoffman BF, Paes de Carvalho A: Effects of acetylcholine on single fibers of the atrioventricular node. Circ Res 7:19–23, 1959.

85. Mendez C, Aceves J, Mendez R: Inhibition of adrenergic cardiac acceleration by cardiac glycosides. J Pharmacol Exp Ther 131:191–198, 1961.

86. Nadeau RA, James TN: Antagonistic effects on the sinus node of acetyl strophanthidin and adrenergic stimulation. Circ Res 13:388–391, 1963.

87. Tse WW, Han J: Interaction of epinephrine and ouabain on automaticity of canine Purkinje fibers. Circ Res 34:777–782, 1973.

88. Erlij D, Mendez R: The modification of digitalis intoxication by excluding adrenergic influences on the heart. J Pharmacol Exp Ther 144:97–103, 1964.

89. Ten Eick RE, Hoffman BF: Chronotropic effect of cardiac glycosides in cats, dogs and rabbits. Circ Res 25:365–378, 1969.

90. Berti F, Shore PA: A kinetic analysis of drugs that inhibit the adrenergic neuronal membrane amine pump. Biochem Pharmacol 16:2091–2096, 1967.

91. McLain PL: Effects of cardiac glycosides on spontaneous efferent activity in vagus and sympathetic nerves of cats. Int J Neuropharmacol 8:379–387, 1969.

92. Somberg JC, Risler T, Smith TW: Neural factors in digitalis toxicity: protective effect of C-I spinal cord transection. Am J Physiol 235:H531–H536, 1978.

93. Mudge GH, Lloyd BL, Greenblatt DJ, Smith TW: Inotropic and toxic effects of a polar cardiac glycoside derivative in the dog. Circ Res 43:847–854, 1978.

94. Thames MD: Acetylstrophanthidin-induced reflex inhibition of canine renal sympathetic nerve activity mediated by cardiac receptors with vagal afferents. Circ Res 44:8–15, 1979.

95. Mendez C, Mendez R: The action of cardiac glycosides on the excitability and conduction velocity of the mammalian atrium. J Pharmacol Exp Ther 121:402–413, 1957.

96. Trautwein W: Generation and conduction of impulses in the heart as affected by drugs. Pharmacol Rev 15:277–332, 1963.

97. Hoffman BF, Singer DH: Effects of digitalis on electrical activity of cardiac fibers. Prog Cardiovasc Dis 7:226–260, 1964.

98. Dhingra RC, Amat-y-Leon F, Wyndham C, Wu D, Denes P, Rosen K: The electrophysiological effects of ouabain on sinus node and atrium in man. J Clin Invest 56:555–562, 1975.

99. Moe GK, Mendez R: The action of several cardiac glycosides on conduction velocity and ventricular excitability in the dog heart. Circulation 4:729–734, 1951.

100. Swain HH, Weidner CL: A study of substances which alter intraventricular conduction in isolated dog heart. J Pharmacol Exp Ther 120:137–146, 1957.

101. Gomes JAC, Dhatt MS, Akhtar M, Carambas CR, Rubenson DS, Damato A: Effects of digitalis on ventricular myocardial and His-Purkinje refractoriness and reentry in man. Am J Cardiol 42:931–939, 1978.

102. Goodman DJ, Rossen RM, Cannom DS, Rider AK, Harrison DC: Effects of digoxin on atrioventricular conduction. Studies in patients with and without cardiac autonomic innervation. Circulation 51:251–256, 1975.

103. Wellens HJ, Durrer D: Effect of digitalis on atrioventricular conduction and circus movement tachycardias in patients with Wolff-Parkinson-White syndrome. Circulation 47:1229–1233, 1973.

104. Sellers TD Jr, Bashore TM, Gallagher JJ: Digitalis in the preexcitation syndrome: analysis during atrial fibrillation. Circulation 56:260–270, 1977.

105. Kosowsky BD, Haft JI, Stein E, Damato AN: The effects of digitalis on atrioventricular conduction in man. Am Heart J 75:736–742, 1968.

106. Paulay KL, Damato AN: Effect of digoxin on sinus nodal reentry in the dog. Am J Cardiol 35:370–375, 1975.

107. Zakauddin V, Miller RR, McMillin D, Mason DT: Effects of digitalis on sinus nodal function in patients with sick sinus syndrome. Am J Cardiol 41:318–375, 1978.

108. Reiffel JA, Bigger JT Jr, Cramer M: The effects of digoxin on sinus node function before and after vagal blockade in patients with sinus node dysfunction: a clue to the mechanisms of digitalis action on the sinus node. Am J Cardiol 43:983–989, 1970.

109. Margolis JR, Strauss HC, Miller HC, Gilbert M, Wallace AG: Digitalis and the sick sinus syndrome: clinical and electrophysiologic documentation of a severe toxic effect on sinus node function. Circulation 52:162–169, 1975.

110. Garan H, Powers ER, Ruskin JN, Powell WJ Jr: Neural effect of digitalis glycosides on gracilis vascular resistance in hypotension. Am J Physiol 238:H729–H739, 1980.

111. Ayachi S, Brown AM: Hypotensive effects of cardiac glycosides in spontaneously hypertensive rats. J Pharmacol Exp Ther 213:520–524, 1980.

112. Toda N: Mechanisms of ouabain-induced arterial muscle contraction. Am J Physiol 239:H199–H205, 1980.

113. Berlardinelli L, Harder D, Sperelakis N, Rubio R, Berne RM: Cardiac glycoside stimulation of inward Ca^{++} current in vascular smooth muscle of canine coronary artery. J Pharmacol Exp Ther 209:62–66, 1979.

114. Bing RJ, Maraist FM, Dammann JF, Draper A, Heimbecker R, Daley R, Gerard R, Calazel P: Effect of strophanthus on coronary blood flow and cardiac oxygen consumption of normal and failing human hearts. Circulation 2:513–516, 1950.

115. Vatner JF, Haig BW, Manders T, Murray PA: Effect of a cardiac glycoside on regional function, blood flow and electrograms in conscious dogs with myocardial ischemia. Circ Res 43:413–423, 1978.

116. McRitchie RJ, Vatner SF: The role of the arterial baroceptors in mediating cardiovascular responses to cardiac glycosides in conscious dogs. Circ Res 38:321–326, 1976.

117. Vatner SF, Braunwald E: Effects of chronic heart failure on the inotropic response of the right ventricle of the conscious dog to a cardiac glycoside and to tachycardia. Circulation 50:728–734, 1974.

118. Mason DT, Braunwald E: Studies on digitalis. X. Effects of ouabain on forearm vascular resistance and venous tone in normal subjects and in patients in heart failure. J Clin Invest 43:532–543, 1964.

119. Williams MH, Zohman LR, Ratner AC: Hemodynamic effects of cardiac glycosides on normal human subjects during rest and exercise. J Appl Physiol 13:417–421, 1958.

120. Smith TW, Haber E: Medical progress: digitalis. N Engl J Med 289:945–952, 1010–1015, 1063–1072, 1125–1129, 1973.

121. Braunwald E, Bloodwell RD, Goldberg LI, Morrow AG: Studies on Digitalis. IV. Observations in man on the effects of digitalis preparations on the contractility of the nonfailing heart and on total vascular response. J Clin Invest 40:52–59, 1959.

122. Dresdale PT, Yuceoglu YZ, Michton RJ, Schultz M, Lunger M: Effects of lanatoside C on cardiovascular hemodynamics – acute digitalizing doses in subject with normal hearts and with heart disease without failure. Am J Cardiol 4:88–99, 1959.

123. Selzer A, Hultgren HN, Ebnother CL, Bradley HW, Stone

410

AO: Effects of digoxin on the circulation in normal man. Br Heart J 21:335–342, 1959.

124. Lindenbaum J, Butler VP, Murphy JE, Cresswell RM: Correlation of digoxin-tablet dissolution rate with biological availability. Lancet 1:1215–1217, 1973.

125. Lindenbaum J, Mellow MH, Blackstone MO, Butler VP Jr: Variability in biological availability of digoxin from four preparations. N Engl J Med 285:1344–1347, 1971.

126. Wagner JG, Christensen M, Sakmar E, Blair D, Yates JD, Willis PW III, Sedman AH, Stall RG: Equivalence lack in digoxin plasma levels. J Am Med Assoc 224:199–204, 1973.

127. Harter JG, Skelly JP, Steers AW: Digoxin – the regulatory viewpoint. Circulation 49:395–398, 1974.

128. Lindenbaum J, Rund DG, Butler VP, Tse-Eng D, Saha JR: Inactivation of digoxin by the gut flora: reversal by antibiotic therapy. N Engl J Med 305:789–794, 1981.

129. Frazer G, Binnion P: ^{3}H-digoxin distribution in the nervous system in ventricular tachycardia. J Cardiovasc Pharmacol 3:1296–1305, 1981.

130. Cogan JJ, Humphreys MH, Carlson J, Benowitz NL, Rapaport E: Acute vasodilator therapy increases renal clearance of digoxin in patients with congestive heart failure. Circulation 64:973–976, 1981.

131. Risler T, Somberg JC, Blute RD Jr, Smith TW: The effect of altered renal perfusion pressure on clearance of digoxin. Circulation 61:521–525, 1980.

132. Leahey EB Jr, Reiffel JA, Drusin RE, Heissenbuttel RH, Lovejoy WP, Bigger JT Jr: Interaction between digoxin, quinidine. J Am Med Assoc 240:533–534, 1978.

133. Ejvinsson G: Effect of quinidine on plasma concentrations of digoxin. Br Med J 1:279–280, 1978.

134. Doering W, Konig E: Ansteig der digoxin Konzentration im Serum unter chinidin Medikation. Med Clin 73:1085–1088, 1978.

135. Doering W: Digoxin–quinidine interaction. N Engl J Med 301:400–405, 1979.

136. Leahey EB Jr, Reiffel JA, Giardina EGV, Bigger JT Jr: The effect of quinidine and other oral antiarrhythmic drugs on serum digoxin. A prospective study. Ann Intern Med 92:605–608, 1980.

137. Mungall DR, Robichaux RP, Perry W, Scott JW, Robinson A, Burelle T, Hurst D: Effects of quinidine on serum digoxin concentration. Ann Intern Med 93:689–693, 1980.

138. Pedersen KE, Hastrop J, Hvidt S: The effect of quinidine on digoxin kinetics in cardiac patients. Acta Med Scand 207:291–295, 1980.

139. Dahlqvist R, Ejvinsson G, Schenck-Gustafsson K: Effect of quinidine on plasma concentration and renal clearance of digoxin. A clinically important drug interaction. Br J Clin Pharmacol 9:412–418, 1980.

140. Leahey EB Jr, Bigger JT Jr, Bulter VP Jr, Reifer JA, O'Connell GC, Scaffidi LE, Rottman JN: Quinidine–digoxin interaction. Time course and pharmacokinetics. Am J Cardiol 48:1141–1146, 1981.

141. Kum DH, Akera T, Brody TM: Effects of quinidine on the cardiac-glycoside sensitivity of guinea-pig and rat heart. J Pharmacol Exp Ther 217:559–565, 1981.

142. Horowitz JD, Barry WH, Smith TW: Lack of interaction between digoxin and quinidine in cultured heart cells. J Pharmacol Exp Ther 220:488–493, 1982.

143. Hirsh PD, Weiner HJ, North RL: Further insights into digoxin–quinidine interaction: lack of correlation between serum digoxin concentration and inotropic state of the heart. Am J Cardiol 46:863–867, 1981.

144. Steiness E, Waldorff S, Hansen PB, Kjaergard H, Buch J, Edgblad H: Reduction of digoxin-induced inotropism during quinidine administration. Clin Pharmacol Ther 27:791–795, 1980.

145. Fenster PE, Powell JR, Graves PE, Conrad KA, Hager WD, Goldman S, Marcus FI: Digitoxin-quinidine interaction: pharmacokinetic evaluation. Ann Intern Med 93:698–701, 1980.

146. Garty M, Sood P, Rollins DE: Digitoxin elimination reduced during quinidine therapy. Ann Intern Med 94:35–37, 1981.

147. Ochs HR, Pabst J, Greenblatt DJ, Dengler HJ: Noninteraction of digitoxin and quinidine. N Engl J Med 303:672–674, 1980.

148. Peters U, Risler T, Grabensee B, Falkenstein U, Kroukou J: Interaktion von chinidin und digitoxin beim Menschen. Dtsch Med Wochenschr 105:438–442, 1980.

149. Storstein L, von der Lippe A, Amlie J, Storstein O: Is there an interaction between digitoxin and quinidine? Circulation 59–60 (Suppl II):II–230, 1979.

150. Keller F, Kreutz G: Chinidin Interaktion mit digitoxin. Dtsch Med Wochenschr 105:701–702, 1980.

151. Moysey JO, Jaggarao NSV, Grundy EN, Chamberlain DA: Amiodarone increases plasma digoxin concentrations. Br Med J 282:272–273, 1981.

152. Garcia-Barreto D, Groning E, Gonzalez-Gomez A, Perez A, Hernadez-Canero A, Toruncha A: Enhancement of the antiarrhythmic aciton of disopyramide by digoxin. J Cardiovasc Pharmacol 3:1236–1242, 1981.

153. Lang R, Klein HO, Weiss E, Libhaber C, Kaplinsky E: Effect of verapamil on blood level and renal clearance of digoxin. Circulation 62 (Suppl III):III–83, 1980.

154. Pedersen KE, Doph-Pedersen A, Hvidt S, Klitgaard NA, Nielsen-Kudsk F: Digoxin–verapamil interaction. Clin Pharmacol Ther 30:311–316, 1981.

155. Doering W: Quinidine–digoxin interaction (pharmacokinetics underlying mechanism and clinical implications). N Engl J Med 301:400–404, 1979.

156. Belz GG, Aust PE, Munkes R: Digoxin plasma concentrations and nifedipine. Lancet 1:844–845, 1981.

157. Rosen MR, Fisch C, Hoffman BF, Danilo P, Lovelace DE, Knoebel SB: Can accelerated atrioventricular junctional escape rhythms be explained by delayed afterdepolarizations? Am J Cardiol 45:1272–1284, 1980.

158. Irons GV Jr, Orgain ES: Digitalis-induced arrhythmias and their management. Prog Cardiovasc Dis 8:539–568, 1966.

159. Rosen MR, Hordof AJ, Hodess A, Verosky M, Vulliemoz L: Ouabain induced changes in electrophysiologic properties of neonatal, young and adult canine cardiac Purkinje fibers. J Pharmacol Exp Ther 194:255–263, 1973.

160. Somberg JC, Kuhlman JE, Smith TW: Localization of neurally mediated coronary vasoconstrictor properties of digitalis in the cat. Circ Res 49:226–233, 1981.

411

161. Chai CY, Hsu PL, Wang SC: Central locus of emetic action of digitalis substances in cats. Neuropharmacology 12: 1187–1193, 1973.

162. Binnion PF, Frazer G: [^{3}H] digoxin in the optic tract in digoxin intoxication. J Cardiovasc Pharmacol 2:699–706, 1980.

CHAPTER 12

The pharmacology of diuretics

PAUL J. CANNON

Introduction

The development of a variety of diuretic drugs during the past several decades has been a major advance in the therapy of cardiac failure and other
states characterized by edema formation. Diuretics
are drugs which increase urine volume. Most diuretics used clinically directly inhibit the renal tubular reabsorption of sodium and chloride resulting in
the excretion of a greater fraction of the glomerular
filtrate into the urine. Other agents (which will not
be discussed in this chapter) increase urinary volume by increasing the renal blood flow and the
glomerular filtration rate or by inhibiting the tubular reabsorption of water.

Chemical classes of diuretic agents

Figure 1 shows the chemical structure of compounds that are representative of the major classes
of diuretics which inhibit the tubular reabsorption
of electrolytes and water. Each class possesses some
features which are chemically unique and each class
exerts characteristic effects on the transport processes located in different segments of the nephron.
Even though the sites of action and the specific
effects on transport have been defined for many of
the diuretic agents, currently there is little definitive
knowledge concerning the mechanism of action of
diuretics at a biochemical or molecular level. Presumably they may interfere with electrolyte reabsorption: (a) by blocking entry of the ion into the
tubular cell at the luminal plasma membrane, (b) by
interfering with the production of energy to fuel the

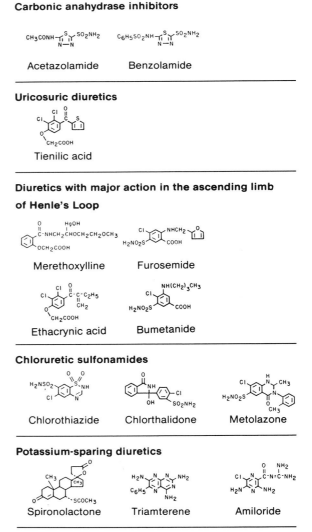

Carbonic anahydrase inhibitors

Acetazolamide   Benzolamide

Uricosuric diuretics

Tienilic acid

**Diuretics with major action in the ascending limb
of Henle's Loop**

Merethoxylline   Furosemide

Ethacrynic acid   Bumetanide

Chloruretic sulfonamides

Chlorothiazide   Chlorthalidone   Metolazone

Potassium-sparing diuretics

Spironolactone   Triamterene   Amiloride

Figure 1. Representatives of various chemical classes of diuretics.

Rosen, M. R. and Hoffman, B. F. (eds.), Cardiac Therapy. ISBN 0-89838-564-4.
© 1983, Martinus Nijhoff Publishers, Boston, The Hague, Dordrecht, Lancaster. Printed in the Netherlands.

413

transport pump, or (c) by interfering with the exit of the ion across the peritubular plasma membrane [1]. A consideration of how each class of diuretics influences transport in different nephron segments is appropriate to a discussion of the clinical use of these agents. Knowledge of these effects enables the physician to select and/or combine drugs more effectively and also to anticipate or forestall some of the disturbances of electrolyte or acid-base balance that may occur during diuretic therapy.

Functional subdivisions of the nephron

Figure 2 is a simplified schema of the major functional subdivisions of the nephron on which various sites of diuretic action are indicated. Details of nephron physiology have been treated more extensively in other reviews [2].

The glomerulus

In normal humans, the glomeruli of approximately 2,000,000 nephrons generate about 180 liters of an ultrafiltrate of plasma per 24 hr. About 99% of the glomerular filtrate is reabsorbed by the renal tubules; the remainder is excreted as urine. Diuretics may directly influence the renal blood flow and the glomerular filtration rate (GFR). Obviously the diuretic response to an agent which inhibits the tubular reabsorption of a given fraction of the glomerular filtrate will be larger if the GFR and the filtered load of sodium are also increased by the action of the drug. Diuretics also can influence the GFR indirectly. Any diuretic which induces a significant saliuresis and contraction of extracellular fluid volume may reduce plasma volume to such an extent that renal vasoconstriction occurs as a compensatory mechanism. If the renal vasoconstriction

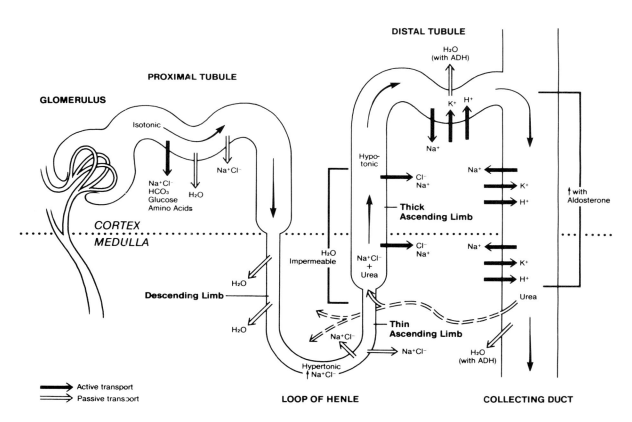

Figure 2. A simplified schema of functional subdivisions of a mammalian nephron.

414

(which is mediated in part by the sympathetic nervous system and in part by the vasoconstrictor action of angiotensin II) is sufficiently intense and involves the afferent arterioles, the GFR will fall.

The proximal tubules

The great bulk of the glomerular filtrate (i.e., about 50–65% of filtered sodium chloride and water and about 90% filtered HCO_3) is reabsorbed in the proximal tubules [2–5]. The reabsorption of sodium and its attendant anions in the proximal tubules is accompanied by isosmotic amounts of water; the tonicity of proximal tubular fluid does not change.

The fraction of the glomerular filtrate which is reabsorbed by the proximal tubules is not affected markedly by changes in GFR (this is called glomerulo-tubular balance) [2, 3, 5]. However, the fraction of the filtrate normally reabsorbed by proximal tubules is influenced significantly by expansion or contraction of the extracellular fluid (ECF) volume, i.e., in response to expansion of ECF volume, the fractional reabsorption of sodium and water by proximal tubules falls; in response to contraction of ECF volume, the fraction of filtrate reabsorbed in proximal tubules increases.

Normally in the proximal tubules there is a significant 'back leak' of electrolytes and water that have been reabsorbed by the tubular epithelium into the lumen (probably via the tight junctions from the intercellular spaces). The 'net' amount of salt and water reabsorbed in the proximal tubules is the difference between the quantity transported out of the tubular lumen and the amount that 'leaks' back. The important role of hemodynamic forces in the peritubular capillaries (the hydrostatic pressure and the colloid osmotic pressure) influencing the magnitude of the 'back leak' and hence of net reabsorption in the proximal nephron has been discussed elsewhere [5–7]. 'Back leak' diminishes and net tubular reabsorption increases in the proximal tubules when there is a reduction in the hydrostatic pressure and/or an increase in the colloid osmotic pressure in the peritubular capillaries. This pattern of hemodynamic change in peritubular capillaries occurs when there is an increase in the filtration fraction (i.e., the ratio of GFR/renal plasma flow) which is produced by vasoconstriction of the efferent arterioles distal to the glomeruli. Net tubular reabsorption falls when there is an increase in the hydrostatic pressure and/or a fall in the colloid osmotic pressure in the peritubular capillaries. This pattern of hemodynamic change occurs during renal vasodilation (when filtration fraction falls) or during infusion of an isotonic saline solution.

Recent micropuncture and tubular microperfusion studies have indicated that there are three anatomic and functional subdivisions of the proximal tubules – the early and the late portions of the proximal convoluted tubules and the straight portion [2, 5]. In the very first protions of the proximal tubule the transtubular potential difference is –3 mV, lumen negative. Active reabsorption of sodium at this site is coupled to the transport of bicarbonate, glucose, amino acids, and organic substrates such as lactate [2, 5, 8]. Sodium bicarbonate reabsorption, which is nonelectrogenic and dependent on tubular hydrogen ion transport and on intracellular and brush border carbonic anhydrase, occurs primarily in this segment. In later portions of the proximal convoluted tubule, the transtubular voltage is +1 to +3 mV with the lumen positive. Due to more proximal reabsorption of glucose and bicarbonate, the chloride concentration in the late proximal convoluted tubule is increased above that in blood. This favors the passive movement of chloride down its chemical gradient into peritubular blood; the resulting positive luminal charge favors passive sodium movement down the electrochemical gradient [9]. Thus in this nephron segment some of the chloride and sodium reabsorption is passive, driven by the chloride and bicarbonate concentration differences, the accompanying positive voltage and by bulk flow in response to osmotic gradients [2, 5, 9]. In the straight portion of the proximal tubule (transepithelial voltage –2 mV, lumen negative) active sodium reabsorption is not coupled to transfer of nonelectrolytes such as glucose or amino acids; chloride and water reabsorption are passive [2, 5].

The loop of Henle

The thin limb
Recent studies have not provided evidence to indicate that there is active salt transport in either the descending or ascending portions of the thin limb of Henle's loop [10, 11]. In the descending portion of the thin limb, the permeability of the tubular membranes is high to water and low to urea and sodium.

In this segment, water diffuses out of the tubule into the hypertonic medullary interstitium, and the tubular contents (particularly sodium and chloride) become concentrated at the tip of the loop. In the ascending portion of the thin limb, the permeability to water is very low [10, 11]. In this segment, the permeabilities of the tubular membranes to sodium and to urea are higher than in the descending limb; sodium chloride reabsorption in the ascending thin limb is passive, i.e., sodium (along with chloride) exits down its large concentration gradient. Since the ascending portion of the thin limb is impermeable to water, the hypertonicity of tubular fluid diminishes.

The thick ascending limb

The reabsorption of approximately 20–30% of the filtered sodium chloride occurs normally in the thick ascending limb of Henle's Loop [2, 11, 12]. The membranes of the medullary and cortical thick ascending limb are impermeable to water. Active salt reabsorption in the thick ascending limb renders the tubular fluid hypotonic. In the absence of antidiuretic hormone, this hypotonic tubular fluid is excreted as dilute urine. The sodium chloride which is transported out of the medullary portion of the thick ascending limb is deposited in the interstitial fluid of the renal medulla and is sequestered there by the vasa rectae in such a fashion that there is a progressively increasing solute concentration from renal cortex to the tip of the papilla. In the presence of ADH, water passes by diffusion from adjacent medullary collecting ducts into the hypertonic interstitium; this results in the excretion of a concentrated urine.

Microperfusion studies from several laboratories have indicated that there is active reabsorption of chloride in the thick ascending limb (which generates a transepithelial voltage of about +6 mV with lumen positive) [11–13]. The membranes of the ascending limb are quite permeable to sodium; sodium reabsorption and potassium reabsorption at this site are passive, driven by the positive voltage. As will be discussed subsequently, three major classes of diuretic agents, organomercurials, ethacrynic acid, and furosemide, induce saliuresis and diuresis by inhibiting active chloride transport in this nephron segment [14]. Interestingly, each of these drugs is more active on the luminal rather than the peritubular side of the tubule suggesting

that they may inhibit entry of the chloride into the cells.

Another important functional characteristic of the thick ascending limb of Henle's loop is that reabsorption of sodium chloride in this locus varies directly with the salt concentration in the tubular lumen. Thus reabsorption of sodium chloride in the ascending limb increases proportionately with the delivery of sodium and chloride to this segment. For this reason, a rise in the delivery of filtrate out of the proximal tubules (e.g., induced by a rise in GFR, by ECF volume expansion, or by administration of a diuretic which inhibits sodium reabsorption in the proximal tubules) may not result in a proportional increase of sodium excretion into the urine.

Distal convoluted tubules

The distal convoluted tubule which extends from the macula densa to the junction that forms the cortical collecting tubule is anatomically and functionally heterogeneous [2, 15]. Approximately 6–10% of filtered sodium is reabsorbed in the distal convoluted tubules and collecting ducts. In the beginning of the distal convoluted tubule the transepithelial voltage is lumen positive because there is active chloride reabsorption at this site, as in the ascending limb. In the major part of the distal convoluted tubule, however, the reabsorption of sodium is active and causes a large voltage (about −30 mV) with the lumen negative. Chloride reabsorption is passive and driven by the voltage. The reabsorption of sodium in the distal convoluted tubule is influenced directly by mineralocorticoids. At this locus aldosterone enhances sodium reabsorption and also promotes the secretion of potassium and of hydrogen ions into the tubular lumen. Water permeability is low in the distal convoluted tubules in the absence of ADH, so that reabsorption of salt may increase the hypotonicity of the tubular fluid. In the presence of ADH, water reabsorption increases at this site. Urea permeability is low in the distal convoluted tubules and the cortical collecting ducts so that the concentration of urea in tubular fluid rises as water is reabsorbed.

The collecting duct

The collecting ducts, (cortical, medullary, and papillary) are responsible for reabsorption of about 2–3% of filtered sodium [16]. The active transport of sodium, which in the collecting ducts is partially dependent on mineralocorticoid activity, produces a large transepithelial voltage with the lumen negative. Although it operates at a slow rate, collecting duct sodium transport is capable of generating a large sodium concentration difference across the tubular epithelium. Chloride reabsorption is passive and driven by the voltage. (Some studies, however, suggest that there is a component of active chloride reabsorption in the papillary portion of the collecting duct.) Sodium reabsorption in the collecting ducts is enhanced by aldosterone. In addition, aldosterone accelerates net secretion of potassium and hydrogen ions by the collecting duct cells into the tubular fluid. Aldosterone is thought to increase the permeability of the luminal membranes of the collecting duct cells to potassium which favors the secretion of potassium down its intracellular – luminal fluid concentration gradient. Hydrogen ion secretion in the collecting ducts participates in the regulation of bicarbonate reabsorption and in the process of urinary acidification. Collecting duct hydrogen ion secretion is increased by aldosterone and is reduced by inhibitors of carbonic anhydrase, by aldosterone antagonists, and by triampterene and amiloride.

The membranes of the collecting ducts are quite impermeable to water and urea in the absence of ADH. However, when ADH is present there is a large rise in water permeability and net reabsorption of water – which in the papillary portion of the collecting duct leads to the formation of a hypertonic urine. When ADH is present the papillary collecting duct is also permeable to urea. During hydropenia urea diffuses into the papillary interstitium and into the thin ascending limb. This recirculation of urea back into the medullary interstitum enables it to exert its osmotic effect in concentrating the urine in the descending limb of Henle's loop.

Recent studies by Stein et al. in rats have indicated that under conditions of varied sodium balance, the final regulation of urinary sodium excretion may occur in the collecting ducts [17, 18]. During expansion of ECF volume by infusion of saline or by infusion of hyperoncotic albumin, the delivery of filtered sodium beyond the distal tubules was not significantly different. However, in the saline-expanded animals, urinary sodium excretion was

higher than in the animals expanded with albumin. This augmented sodium excretion was not due to depressed collecting duct sodium reabsorption but to the addition of sodium rich fluid from deeper nephrons arriving in the papillary collecting duct [17, 18].

Potassium filtered by the glomerulus is reabsorbed in the proximal tubules ($\cong 70\%$) and in the ascending limb of the loop of Henle ($\cong 25\%$) and also in the distal nephron. It is the secretion of potassium into the tubular fluid in the distal convoluted tubules and cortical collecting ducts, however, that accounts for most of the urinary potassium excretion [19]. Sodium reabsorption is linked to potassium excretion in these nephron segments. However, the exact mechanism of the linkage between Na^+ and K^+ transport is unclear and the coupling ratio is quite variable (i.e., it may vary 10-fold). The secretion of potassium in the distal tubules and collecting ducts is directly related to the volume flow rate of fluid through these nephron segments, i.e., K^+ excretion increases with greater flow and falls with reduced flow.

Other factors which influence K^+ secretion in the distal nephron are the following: (a) the level of circulating aldosterone – a high aldosterone level stimulates K^+ secretion, provided that there is adequate delivery of fluid and sodium to the sites of K^+ secretion in the distal nephron; (b) the state of sodium delivery to the distal nephron – a low sodium diet reduces distal K^+ secretion and enhances K^+ reabsorption in the collecting duct, probably by reducing the volume of flow in these nephron segments; a high sodium diet has the opposite effect; (c) the state of K^+ balance (which probably influences distal tubular cell K^+ content) – a positive K^+ balance favors K^+ excretion, a negative K^+ balance favors K^+ retention; (d) the state of acid-base balance (which also influences distal tubular cell K^+ content) – alkalosis favors K^+ secretion, acidosis favors K^+ retention; (e) the anion composition of the tubular fluid. The electrical gradient (lumen negative) in the distal nephron provides a force that attracts K^+ into the urine; the magnitude of the electrical gradient increases if anions present in the tubular fluid (e.g., sulfate, nitrate) are impermeable and resist passive reabsorption as sodium is transported. The presence of impermeable anions in the tubular fluid in the presence of active sodium reabsorption (e.g., during sodium depletion) enhances

417

the electrical gradient and stimulates the distal secretion of potassium ions.

Mechanism of action of diuretic agents

The diuretics which exert their predominant action on transport systems of the proximal tubules

The carbonic acid inhibitors, e.g., acetazolamine and benzolamide, were the first effective oral diuretic agents [20]. They inhibit the enzyme carbonic anhydrase and thus inhibit the generation of hydrogen ions required for hydrogen ion transport in the proximal tubules and in the distal convoluted tubules and collecting ducts [20–23]. In the proximal tubules, the inhibition of carbonic anhydrase impairs the reabsorption of filtered bicarbonate; sodium and, to some extent, potassium are retained in the lumen to offset electrically the bicarbonate which is not reabsorbed. Interference with proximal bicarbonate reabsorption also reduces the chloride concentration gradient in the later portions of the proximal convoluted tubules, which normally promotes passive sodium chloride reabsorption. Following administration of an inhibitor of carbonic anhydrase, sodium, potassium, bicarbonate, and chloride are retained in the tubular lumen along with appropriate amounts of osmotically obligated water.

Because most of the sodium and chloride which escape reabsorption in the proximal tubules after administration of a carbonic anhydrase inhibitor are reabsorbed in the loop of Henle and distal convoluted tubules, these agents have little diuretic effect unless the more distal nephron has been blocked by administration of another diuretic agent such as furosemide or chlorothiazide [23, 24].

The carbonic anhydrase inhibitors have little effect on the glomerular filtration rate. In animals low doses did not influence the glomerular filtration rate, whereas high doses depressed it [25]. During diuresis caused by these agents, the urine is alkaline and contains an excess of sodium, bicarbonate, and potassium. There is generally little change in chloride excretion, and the urinary excretion rates of titratable acid and ammonium are low. Urinary potassium excretion increases because of increased secretion of potassium in the distal tubules and collecting ducts. The increased K^+ excretion results from a variety of factors including: increased delivery of fluid and sodium to the distal nephron, an increased distal transepithelial voltage produced by inhibition of carbonic anhydrase, the added effects of increased tubular bicarbonate concentration, and the alkaline pH of the tubular fluid [19].

The diuretic action of carbonic anhydrase inhibitors generally is self-limited. Metabolic acidosis results from reduced net urinary hydrogen ion excretion; and in the face of this acid-base disturbance (i.e., particularly the reduced filtered bicarbonate concentration) the compounds are no longer effective as diuretics. For this reason and also because of their low potency, carbonic anhydrase inhibitors are rarely used today as primary diuretics. They are more commonly used for the treatment of glaucoma (they reduce intraocular pressure by reducing the production of aqueous humor).

Carbonic anhydrase inhibitors, however, can be effective natriuretic agents in patients who have an elevated serum bicarbonate concentration (e.g., respiratory acidosis due to cor pulmonale or metabolic alkalosis induced by another diuretic). Although they diminish a mercurial diuresis, these drugs, however, may enhance or even potentiate the diuresis induced by diuretics which act more distally in the nephron such as furosemide or the thiazide diuretics through their action to impede proximal reabsorption. This feature may be particularly useful in the treatment of resistant edema. Because they reduce urinary acidification, carbonic anhydrase inhibitors may occasionally precipitate severe metabolic acidosis in patients with advanced renal or hepatic disease.

Two other drugs with predominant action on more distal nephron segments, furosemide and thiazide diuretics, have partial activity to inhibit carbonic anhydrase; a minor part of the diuresis induced by these agents results from their action to inhibit carbonic anhydrase in the proximal tubules.

Diuretics with a predominant action in the thick ascending limb of Henle's loop

Three chemical classes of diuretic agents have a predominant effect to inhibit salt reabsorption in the thick ascending limb of Henle's loop. These classes are represented by the organomercurials, ethacrynic acid, and furosemide [21]. All three classes of drugs inhibit active chloride transport in this nephron segment.

Organomercurials

The organic mercurial diuretics are the oldest class of diuretic agents. The natriuretic effect of these compounds was first discovered in 1919. During a mercurial diuresis the urine contains little or no bicarbonate and an amount of chloride which equals or exceeds that of sodium. For this reason early workers postulated that the organomercurials inhibited chloride reabsorption [26, 27]. Although this original theory was disregarded for many years, recently Burg and his collaborators demonstrated that mersalyl added to fluid perfusing the isolated thick ascending limb of the rabbit nephron caused the positive voltage and the net chloride transport in this nephron segment to decrease [21, 28]. The passive permeability to sodium and chloride was not affected. They concluded that the drug inhibited active chloride transport in the thick ascending limb by an action exerted primarily on the luminal membranes, and that diminished reabsorption of sodium and water were secondary events. They also showed that the effects of mersalyl on tubular transport could be reversed by p-chloromercuribenzoate, a substance known to prevent the diuretic effects of organomercurials in vivo. The latter findings suggest that the effect of the organomercurials on chloride transport in the ascending limb was directly related to the diuretic action of these compounds and was not a nonspecific toxic affect.

The organomercurials have little influence on renal hemodynamics. (There is some evidence, however, that organomercurials, thiazides and carbonic anhydrase inhibitors may decrease glomerular filtration rate by an intrarenal feedback mechanism which couples salt delivery to the macula densa with the rate of glomerular filtration in individual nephrons) [29]. The effects of organomercurials to increase urinary salt excretion are prolonged (12–24 hr) and substantial; about 15–20% of filtered sodium may be excreted. Urinary diluting and concentrating ability are reduced during the activity of mercurial diuretics. The mercurials also partially inhibit renal tubular potassium excretion in the distal tubules and collecting ducts [30]. Because this inhibition is only partial, potassium depletion may occur during a mercurial diuresis – possibly as a consequence of increased delivery of fluid and so-

dium to the sites of potassium secretion. Hydrogen ion secretion in the distal nephron is not inhibited by mercurials and may be accelerated during diuresis. As a consequence of these effects and the large chloride excretion, the patients develop a hypochloremic metabolic alkalosis following which the drugs are no longer effective as diuretics [27]. Diuretic responsiveness can be restored or enhanced by the administration of acidifying salts such as ammonium chloride or 1-lysine monohydrochloride. The mechanism of the restoration of the diuretic effect of organomercurials by acidifying salts has been disputed. Recently, it has been suggested that when the patient develops metabolic alkalosis urinary citrate concentration rises and that citrate may inactivate mercurials by chelation; acidifying salts would reverse this effect [31].

Organomercurials are ineffective after oral administration and must be given intramusculary. Reports of sudden death after intravenous doses contraindicate administration by this route. They induce hypersensitivity reactions in some patients and may be nephrotoxic in patients with renal insufficiency [32]. For these reasons use of the organomercurials has declined recently in favor of the newer drugs which also inhibit chloride transport in the ascending limb of the loop of Henle.

Ethacrynic acid

Ethacrynic acid, an aryloxyacetic acid derivative, can be administered intravenously or by mouth [33–35]. It has little effect on renal blood flow or glomerular filtration rate after administration to humans [34]. In dogs intravenous doses induced transient renal vasodilation [36]; in other studies reductions of GFR were observed despite replacement of diuretic-induced fluid losses [37]. Although the evidence concerning whether ethacrynic acid has effects on transport in the proximal tubule is not conclusive, clearance, micropuncture and tubular microperfusion studies indicate that ethacrynic acid inhibits salt reabsorption in the thick ascending limb of Henle's loop [21, 33–40]. It currently is believed that ethacrynic acid is converted to ethacrynic–cysteine, which is the active compound [21, 39]. This substance, which is bound to plasma proteins, probably reaches the tubular fluid via the organic acid secretory pathway in the proximal tubules. Both ethacrynic acid and ethacrynic–cysteine act on the luminal membranes of the thick ascending limb of Henle's loop to inhibit active chloride reabsorption [21, 40]. Both compounds have little effect on the permeability of the tubular membranes to sodium or chloride; their effects upon sodium and water reabsorption are secondary to inhibition of active chloride transport. The molecular basis for the effect of ethacrynic acid on transport, although extensively studied, is unknown. Studies implicating Na^+/K^+ ATPase activity, mitochondrial respiration, adenylate cyclase, or the renal prostaglandins are inconclusive [21, 41].

During diuresis with ethacrynic acid 20–25% of the filtered sodium chloride can be delivered into the urine along with osmotically obligated amounts of water [33–38]. The drug, by its action on transport in the thick ascending limb, reduces urinary dilution and impairs urinary concentrating ability. Studies in animals showed that the increasing solute concentration gradient in the renal medulla and papilla is reduced or abolished by this drug, an effect which enhances the excretion of water [42]. During diuresis with ethacrynic acid there is an increase in urinary potassium excretion [34]. This is due predominantly to the increased delivery of fluid and sodium to the K^+ secretory sites in the distal convoluted tubules and cortical collecting ducts. It may also, in part, be due to reduced passive K^+ reabsorption in the ascending limb as a consequence of the reduced positive voltage during drug action [21]. Urinary hydrogen ion secretion in the distal nephron increases during diuresis produced by ethacrynic acid [34]. These two effects, increased K^+ and H^+ secretion, plus the excretion of increased volumes of bicarbonate-free, chloride-rich urine may result in the development of hypokalemia and of a hypochloremic metabolic alkalosis [43]. In contrast to the mercurial diuretics, however, ethacrynic acid is still effective as a diuretic despite the presence of these disturbances of acid-base and electrolyte balance.

Furosemide

Furosemide is a sulfonamide derivative. Despite significant differences between furosemide and ethacrynic acid in chemical structure, the major diuretic actions of the two compounds are quite similar [21, 44–46]. Like ethacrynic acid, furosemide can be administered intravenously or by mouth. In therapeutic doses, furosemide does not depress renal blood flow or the glomerular filtration rate [44]. Large doses may produce renal vasodilation with selective increases in blood flow to the superficial renal cortex [36]. Because it is significantly bound to plasma proteins, it is thought that the drug reaches the tubular fluid not by filtration but by the organic acid secretory system in the proximal tubules. The effect of probenecid (which blocks the organic acid secretory pathway in proximal tubules) to inhibit a furosemide diuresis is consistent with this hypothesis [47]. Although furosemide in high doses partially inhibits carbonic anhydrase in the proximal tubules [44, 46–48], the major diuretic effect of furosemide is caused by inhibition of salt reabsorption in the thick ascending limb of Henle's loop [21, 49]. The drug acts on the luminal membranes of this segment to inhibit active tubular reabsorption of chloride which in turn retards sodium reabsorption. The molecular basis for the effect of furosemide on chloride transport is not understood [21]. Additional effects of furosemide to decrease sodium chloride and electrical conductance in the thick ascending limb are small and insufficient to account for the changes in salt reabsorption which are produced. During diuresis with furosemide, both urinary concentrating ability and urinary diluting ability are reduced; however, urinary dilution is impaired to a lesser extent than it is by ethacrynic acid.

Whether furosemide has an additional action to reduce salt reabsorption in the distal convoluted tubules is unsettled; major effects of furosemide on sodium reabsorption in the distal convoluted tubules are unlikely. Some micropuncture studies have even found increased net sodium reabsorption in the distal tubules during a furosemide diuresis. Furosemide has no effect on sodium transport in the collecting duct, but it, along with ethacrynic acid, has been reported to inhibit the action of vasopressin in isolated collecting tubules [50].

During a furosemide diuresis the distal tubular secretion of potassium rises; this appears to be a function of the increased volume flow and the rise in intratubular sodium concentration produced during diuresis [19]. The urinary excretion rates of titratable acid and ammonium also increase during a furosemide diuresis; however, these effects on net acid excretion are offset to some extent by carbonic anhydrase inhibition which may elevate urinary bicarbonate excretion during the initial period after the drug administration [44]. Eventually, however, the effects on K^+ and H^+ secretion, plus the high urinary chloride excretion lead to development of hypokalemia and a hypochloremic metabolic alkalosis.

Pharmacological features of diuresis with ethacrynic acid and furosemide

After intravenous administration, both ethacrynic acid and furosemide have a rapid onset of action, with peak effects at 15–30 min and a duration of action of 1–3 hr [44]. For this reason they are useful in the treatment of pulmonary edema. Recent studies have indicated that beneficial effects are observed after furosemide administration in patients with pulmonary edema prior to diuresis. An effect of the drug to diminish cardiac filling by causing venodilation has been postulated [51]. After oral doses of either drug, saliuresis peaks in about 1–2 hr and persists for 6–8 hr; hence the drugs may be administered from 1–4 times daily. The magnitude of salt and water excretion produced by the oral doses of the 'loop' diuretics may approach 20–40% of the filtered load; in some reports up to 18 pounds of edema have been mobilized in 24 hr [44]. Both drugs also remain effective diuretic agents in patients with significant disturbances of acid-base balance or electrolyte balance or with azotemia. Because excessive diuresis is potentially hazardous, institution of therapy should be cautious. Some investigators have advocated that low doses of ethacrynic acid or furosemide be administered initially so that the sensitivity of a patient to the natriuretic action of these drugs can be observed prior to institution of a chronic dosage schedule [35]. Many workers favor intermittent rather than daily administration of the drugs, so that homeostatic mechanisms during between-treatment periods can compensate for losses of potassium and hydrogen ions and obviate the development of acid-base or electrolyte abnormalities.

During diuresis with either ethacrynic acid or furosemide, urinary potassium losses may be significant and lead to depletion of potassium stores and hypokalemia. The magnitude of potassium excretion induced by both of the drugs (and other kaliuretic agents such as the thiazides) appears to be influenced greatly by the size and duration of the diuresis and also by the level of circulating aldosterone. Greater potassium losses for a given degree of natriuresis occur in patients that have a high circulating level of aldosterone (e.g., cirrhotics with ascites) [34, 44]. Combination of either drug with a potassium-sparing diuretic not only augments sodium excretion but may reduce concomitant potassium and hydrogen ion losses.

Both ethacrynic acid and furosemide inhibit calcium reabsorption in the thick ascending limb; the decline in the lumen-positive transepithelial voltage produced by inhibition of chloride transport reduces passive sodium and calcium reabsorption [21]. After intravenous administration of both drugs, urate excretion rises; however, intermittent oral therapy may be accompanied by hyperuricemia [34, 44]. Elevation of the serum uric acid occurs because both drugs compete with uric acid for secretion by the organic transport mechanism in the proximal tubules and because contraction of extracellular fluid volume induced by diuresis enhances passive reabsorption of urate in the proximal and distal nephron [52, 53].

Because ethacrynic acid and furosemide do not directly depress renal blood flow or GFR, they are frequently administered to mobilize edema in patients with parenchymal renal disease [54–56]. Because their powerful saliuretic effects persist in patients with azotemia or electrolyte or acidbase disturbances, caution to avoid over-diuresis is advisable.

Ethacrynic acid and furosemide are ototoxic; this possibly is related to their effect to inhibit chloride transport in cochlear membranes [57]. Ototoxicity has been observed following intravenous administration of large doses to patients with renal insufficiency. Permanent deafness has occurred in rare cases. Ethacrynic acid may produce abdominal pain and gastric intolerance. Furosemide may induce hemotological disturbances, rashes, and impaired carbohydrate tolerance in susceptible individuals.

Bumetanide

Bumetanide is another diuretic with a major action in the loop of Henle. Although a sulfonamide derivative, bumetanide contains a phenoxy group at the site occupied by chloride in furosemide (Figure 1). Bumetanide can be administered orally or intravenously [58–61]. Its onset and duration of action are similar to those of furosemide and ethacrynic acid; 20% of the filtered sodium may be delivered in the urine. The drug does not depress

Table 1. Representative classes of diuretics.

Generic name	Usual dosage	Onset	Peak	Duration
Carbonic anhydrase inhibitor				
Acetazolamide (diamox)	250–1,000 mg/day	1 hr	2–4 hr	8 hr
Thiazides and related agents				
Chlorothiazide (diuril)	500–2,000 mg/day	1 hr	4 hr	6–12 hr
Hydrochlorothiazide (esidrix)	25–100 mg/day	2 hr	4 hr	12 hr +
Chlorthalidone (hygroton)	100 mg/day	2 hr	6 hr	24 hr +
Trichlormethiazide (metahydrin, naqua)	4–8 mg/day	2 hr	6 hr	24 hr
Metolazone (zaroxolyn)	5–10 mg/day	1 hr	2–4 hr	24–48 hr
Mercurials				
Meralluride (mercuhydrin)	0.5–2.0 ml IM	2 hr	6–9 hr	12–24 hr
Mercaptomerin (thiomerin)	0.25–2.0 ml IM	2 hr	6–9 hr	12–24 hr
Loop diuretics				
Ethacrynic acid (edecrin)	50–200 mg/day	Oral, 30 min	Oral, 1–2 hr	Oral, 6–8 hr
		I.V., 15 min	I.V., 30–45 min	I.V., 2–3 hr
Furosemide (lasix)	40–120 mg/day	Oral, 1 hr	Oral, 1–2 hr	Oral, 6–8 hr
		I.V., 10–15 min	I.V., 30–45 min	I.V., 2–3 hr
Potassium-sparing diuretics				
Spironolactone (aldactone)	25–200 mg/day	Gradual	1–3 days	2–3 days after 1
Triampterene (dyrenium)	100–300 mg/day	2 hr	6–8 hr	12–16 hr

and may even increase the glomerular filtration rate and renal plasma flow [61]. Clearance studies suggest the major action of bumetanide is to inhibit sodium chloride reabsorption in the ascending limb of Henle's loop. Like other loop diuretics there is also an increased excretion of potassium, hydrogen, and calcium ions. Bumetanide appears to have some action in the proximal nephron. Since bicarbonate excretion rises only slightly, whereas phosphate excretion increases markedly, it has been postulated that bumetanide inhibits proximal sodium transport linked to phosphate reabsorption [61].

Diuretics with predominant action in the cortical diluting segment

Chlorothiazide, the first of the thiazides to be discovered, was introduced in 1958 [62]. The thiazide diuretics, sulfonamide derivatives with major effects to augment urinary chloride excretion, have become widely accepted as safe, effective oral diuretics of moderate potency. About 5–8% of the filtered sodium is excreted during peak diuresis with these drugs. A wide variety of thiazide compounds and also three nonthiazide compounds with similar actions (chlorthalidone, quinethazone, metolazone) have been developed (Table 1). The various compounds differ primarily in dosage required to achieve diuresis, the duration of natriuretic activ-

ity (e.g., natriuresis produced by chlorthalidone persists for more than 24 hr) and in the degree of carbonic anhydrase inhibition produced. Claims that they differ intrinsically in their relative abilities to promote potassium excretion are largely unsubstantiated.

Thiazide diuretics

The thiazide diuretics may depress GFR and renal blood flow moderately. They, therefore, can induce reversible mild azotemia in some patients, particularly those with parenchymal renal disease [63, 64]. Thiazides gain access to tubular fluid via the organic acid secretory pathway in the proximal tubules. If secretion of thiazides is blocked by probenecid, the diuretic effects of low doses of thiazides but not of high doses are blocked. During a thiazide-induced diuresis, the urine contains predominantly sodium and chloride along with lesser amounts of potassium and bicarbonate. Clearance studies indicated that the thiazides interfere with urinary dilution but have no effect on the renal concentrating mechanism [64, 65]. Because an action in the medullary thick ascending limb would have impaired both urinary concentration and dilution, it was postulated that thiazides impeded selective salt reabsorption in a cortical diluting segment.

Micropuncture studies have subsequently indicated that the thiazide diuretics inhibit carbonic anhydrase in the proximal tubules; this causes reduced reabsorption of sodium, chloride, bicarbonate, and water [22, 66]. However, this action in the proximal tubules is a minor component of the diuresis observed because there is concomitantly increased reabsorption of sodium and chloride in the loop of Henle [22]. There is uncertainly whether the thiazide diuretics inhibit chloride reabsorption in the late portion of the thick ascending limb of Henle's loop [21]; there is good evidence, however, that they inhibit sodium (and chloride) reabsorption in the distal convoluted tubules [66, 67]. Whether they act in the collecting duct is unclear. The molecular basis of thiazide action on renal transport is unknown. Because they are effective and have relatively mild side effects that are easily managed, the thiazide diuretics have been a mainstay in treatment of mild or moderate congestive heart failure and in the treatment of patients with mild hypertension. The lack of efficacy of thiazides in patients with severe heart failure or renal disease has led to the use of furosemide or ethacrynic acid in these situations.

During a thiazide diuresis, urinary potassium excertion increases. Urinary titratable acid and ammonium excretion also increase. However, because of the effect to inhibit carbonic anhydrase which impairs proximal bicarbonate reabsorption, net acid excretion (titratable acid plus ammonium minus bicarbonate) does not increase significantly during the first few days of thiazide diuresis [68]. The hypochloremic metabolic alkalosis observed in some patients after chronic administration is usually associated with hypokalemia [68].

As mentioned previously, the administration of thiazide diuretics impedes the capacity of the kidneys to dilute the urine by inhibiting selective salt reabsorption in the cortical diluting segment of the nephron. This effect may contribute to the pathogenesis of dilutional hypoosmolality in an edematous patient whose daily water intake is large. When administered chronically the thiazide diuretics also inhibit urinary dilution by another mechanism. In response to chronic thiazide administration, proximal tubular reabsorption of sodium and water increases in response to contraction of the extracellular fluid volume. Hence less sodium and water reach the diluting segments of the more distal nephron per unit of time. Because of the reduced delivery of sodium and water to the distal nephron, urinary

flow decreases and urinary osmolality increases even in the absence of ADH. This effect provides the basis for the use of thiazide diuretics in the treatment of nephrogenic diabetes insipidus [69]. A similar response can be produced by chronic dietary sodium depletion or by administration of other diuretics that reduce extracellular fluid volume.

In contrast to what is observed with the 'loop' diuretics, the administration of thiazide diuretics does not increase urinary calcium excretion [70–72]. Chronic administration of chlorothiazide results in a reduction of urinary calcium excretion, due to an increase in distal calcium reabsorption [66, 71]. This phenomenon may be associated with hypercalcemia in some patients [73, 74].

Urinary urate excretion rises after acute intravenous administration of thiazide diuretics; however, chronic administration of oral doses is associated with development of hyperuricemia (which may precipitate arthritis in susceptible gouty or hypertensive patients) [75]. Originally it was thought that low doses of thiazides inhibited urate secretion pharmacologically because they are secreted into the proximal tubules by the organic acid transport system [75, 76]; more recent evidence suggests that chronic sodium depletion and enhanced passive reabsorption of urate are primarily responsible for the diminished urate clearance and the increased serum urate concentration [52].

Tienilic acid
Investigators recently were interested in the new diuretic, tienilic acid (ticrynafen), which, although chemically related to ethacrynic acid, is similar in action, in many respects, to the thiazides (e.g., it inhibits salt reabsorption in the cortical diluting segment and it promotes urinary potassium excretion [77–79]). The drug is secreted by the proximal tubules, entering tubular fluid via this route. Natriuretic effects are correlated with urinary, not plasma, drug levels – and persist for 12–24 hr after an oral dose. Tienilic acid differs from thiazide diuretics in that it does not influence proximal bicarbonate reabsorption. More importantly, it is unique in that it reduces serum urate concentrations by inhibiting urate reabsorption at both pre- and post-secretory sites in the proximal tubules. Thus, urinary excretion rates of uric acid and of monosodium urate are increased. Interestingly, the hypouricemic effect of the drug occurs at doses which are lower

than those required to produce natriuresis. Initial enthusiasm for tienilic acid declined after the drug was released for clinical use because urate nephropathy and oliguria and hepatotoxicity occurred in a significant number of patients. Consequently the drug has been withdrawn from the market in most countries.

Metolazone

Metolazone is a quinethazone derivative which is somewhat similar to the thiazide diuretics in its site of action and potency [80–83]. Metolazone, in contrast to the thiazides, usually does not reduce and may increase the renal blood flow and the glomerular filtration rate. Because the drug is extensively bound to plasma proteins its duration of action may be 24–48 hr following a single dose. Metolazone has an effect to inhibit sodium reabsorption in the proximal tubules, not by carbonic anhydrase inhibition, but by inhibiton of sodium transport which is linked to phosphate reabsorption [82]. The drug also inhibits sodium and chloride reabsorption in the cortical diluting segment. Combination therapy of metolazone and furosemide has been effective in patients with refractory edema.

Diuretics with predominant action in the distal convoluted tubules and collecting ducts

Two types of compounds have been developed which increase sodium excretion and retard potassium losses in the distal nephron, spironolactone, a competitive antagonist of aldosterone, and two drugs which directly inhibit distal K^+ secretion, triamterene and amiloride. These are sometimes called the 'potassium-sparing' diuretics. The effects of all three compounds to augment sodium excretion are modest; about 2–3% of the filtered load of sodium is excreted during peak action.

Spironolactone

When aldosterone is administered to normal individuals, it causes (after a latent period of 45–60 min) a slight increase in the tubular reabsorption of sodium chloride in the distal nephron; it also increases urinary potassium and hydrogen ion excretion [84]. Spironolactone competitively inhibits the renal tubular actions of aldosterone and other mineralocorticoids; it is ineffective in adrenalectomized subjects [85, 86]. Spironolactone apparently binds to the cytoplasmic proteins which normally carry aldosterone from its surface membrane receptor to the nucleus of susceptible cells where it causes transcription of messenger RNA which in turn directs synthesis of proteins involved in sodium and potassium transport.

Spironolactone has little influence on GFR or renal blood flow. Although effects in the proximal tubules are not completely excluded, spironolactone acts predominantly in the distal convoluted tubules and collecting ducts. It is a weak diuretic whose full effects are observed only several days after administration. Nevertheless, the cumulative effects of chronic administration of spironolactone on sodium balance can be substantial. More importantly, spironolactone inhibits the kaliuresis and the increase in urinary hydrogen ion excretion caused by other diuretics.

Because it is a competitive antagonist of mineralocorticoids, spironolactone is more effective in clinical situations in which circulating aldosterone levels are high (e.g., cirrhosis with ascites, advanced right heart failure) [87]. In such situations high doses of the drug may be necessary to completely antagonize the mineralocorticoid.

Triamterene and amiloride

Triamterene, a pteridine derivative, and amiloride, a pyrazinoyl derivative, cause changes in urinary excretion similar to those induced by spironolactone, but these drugs are fundamentally different in mechanism of action. Although both drugs antagonize aldosterone, they are not competitive inhibitors and they also are effective in adrenalectomized subjects. After administration of either amiloride or triamterene there is a prompt increase in the urinary excretion of sodium and chloride and a decline in the excretion of potassium and in the net output of hydrogen ions [88–92]. Micropuncture studies have substantiated that amiloride inhibits potassium secretion and causes the electrical polarity of perfused cortical collecting cells to reverse from negative to positive [19, 93]. Additional work concerning mechanism of action is incomplete, but suggests that amiloride blocks the luminal entry of sodium into the tubular cells, making less sodium available for active transport across the contraluminal border of the cells [94, 95]. In microperfusion experiments triamterene, when introduced on the peritubular side, inhibited sodium transport in the collecting ducts but not in the distal convoluted tubules [96].

Triamterene and amiloride may depress renal blood flow and glomerular filtration rate substantially; therefore both drugs may induce azotemia, particularly in patients with renal disease. Both of the diuretics (and also spironolactone) may reduce urinary dilution slightly and thus contribute to hypoosmolality in the patient. Since all three of the potassium-sparing diuretics retard potassium excretion, potassium balance may become positive and hyperkalemia will result. Dangerous hyperkalemia has been reported occasionally when patients with intrinsic renal disease or patients receiving potassium supplements were treated with potassium-sparing drugs [97, 98]. Renal acidosis (due to reduced urinary hydrogen ion excretion) also has been induced by these agents (particularly triamterene and amiloride) in patients with renal disease.

Use of diuretics in the treatment of edema

Initial approaches to patients with edema

Prime focus upon the underlying disease
Because edema is a secondary manifestation of a primary disease, usually in the heart, liver, or kidneys, the major focus of therapy should be to remedy the underlying pathological process. In cardiac patients, the nature of the heart disease should be investigated thoroughly. A search should be made particularly for those forms of cardiac malfunction that can be remedied by specific treatment (e.g., mitral stenosis). Coexistent circulatory stresses should be remedied (e.g., anemia, infection, thyrotoxicosis). Other measures should also be undertaken to reduce the demands on the failing heart (e.g., antihypertensive treatment, reduction of afterload with vasodilating agents [99], restriction of physical activity or bed rest). When appropriate, ventricular performance should be augmented by administration of an inotropic agent such as digitalis. In patients with cirrhosis and ascites, the etiology of the hepatic disease should be investigated and specific treatment, together with nutritional and other supportive measures instituted. In patients with the nephrotic syndrome, the etiology of the nephrosis should be investigated. Specific treatment for certain forms (e.g., steroids or azothiaprine) should be administered in addition to dietary and other prophylactic measures.

Sodium restriction
Restriction of dietary or parenteral sodium intake is fundamental to most regimens for treatment of edema. In many patients with edema, the capacity of the kidneys to excrete the daily intake of sodium is only partially reduced [3]. In such patients, a moderate reduction of the dietary sodium content may reduce the daily sodium intake to an amount that the kidneys can excrete completely in 24 hr. Thus, in these patients diuretic treatment can be avoided.

Use of diuretics to treat edema

In more advanced cases of edema formation, the renal capacity to excrete sodium may be so reduced that the daily urinary sodium output falls below the daily sodium intake even when the salt in the diet has been reduced to unpalatable levels. Diuretic drugs are necessary adjuncts to treatment of such patients in order to promote renal losses of sodium and water and restoration of zero sodium balance.

Therapeutic objectives
In planning a diuretic regimen it is useful to recall that diuretic treatment of edema has two objectives: (a) to mobilize large surpluses of salt and water from the interstital fluid space and (b) to maintain a normal sodium balance in patients who have been rendered free from edema and in whom additional reductions of dietary sodium intake are not feasible due to the unpalatability or the high cost of a strict low sodium diet. Frequently the drug regimen chosen initially to achieve the first objective, mobilization of edema, is different from that required to maintain zero sodium balance in a more compensated patient. In general, a diuretic regimen should be individualized to the needs of each patient. The selection of specific drugs should be based on a secure understanding of the mechanism of action and of the effects of the different drugs on electrolyte and acid base balance.

Mild and resistant edema
In patients with mild disease and only slight amounts of edema, a moderate restriction of die-

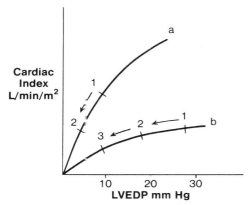

Figure 3. Left ventricular function curve: (a) normal subject; (b) patient with left ventricular failure.

tary sodium intake may be sufficient to induce a negative sodium balance which is followed by restoration of normal sodium balance but with lower total body sodium stores. In patients with more advanced disease, dietary sodium restriction combined with intermittent administration of one of the diuretics of intermediate potency, such as a thiazide, may be sufficient to achieve these objectives. Alternatively, intermittent low doses of a loop diuretic (e.g., every other day) or chronic administration of an antikaliuretic compound such as spironolactone may be used.

In treating patients with responsive edema, it is important not to produce excessive losses of extracellular fluid volume. Figure 3 shows two ventricular function curves, that of a normal subject (a) and that of a patient with moderately advanced congestive heart failure (b). Loss of extracellular fluid volume in a normal subject produces a drop in blood volume and venous return; the resulting decline in left ventricular end-diastolic filling pressure (LVEDP) is associated with a significant drop in cardiac output which may produce orthostatic hypotension. In the patient with depressed ventricular function and circulatory congestion, diuretic-induced losses of extracellular fluid volume improve symptoms and reduce LVEDP but are not initially associated with much change in cardiac performance. However when continued or excessive diuresis causes LVEDP to fall below normal levels, a drop in the already reduced cardiac output will result. This additional decline in ventricular function induced by excessive diuresis can produce renal vasoconstriction and more avid retention of sodium.

In patients with resistant edema the more potent diuretics such as ethacrynic acid or furosemide may be required. Alternatively, diuresis can be achieved with combinations of diuretics that inhibit transport in different nephron segments. For example, chronic administration of a potassium-sparing diuretic such as spironolactone may be combined with intermittent administration of a thiazide or furosemide or ethacrynic acid. In using the more powerful diuretics, it has been the experience of many investigators that intermittent administration of most diuretics (other than the potassium-sparing drugs) is more efficacious in promoting loss of edema fluid than continuous treatment with the same agents [34]. Another advantage of intermittent therapy is that the between-treatment intervals allow time for homeostatic mechanisms to compensate for losses of potassium, chloride, and hydrogen ions that occurred during diuresis.

Refractory edema
Patients with edema that does not respond to conventional therapy present a therapeutic challenge. Hospitalization may be required to reevaluate the basic disease, to ensure adequate control of sodium and water intake and to monitor serum electrolytes, acid-base status, and renal function. Several factors which may be involved in the pathogenesis of 'refractory' edema are listed here: (a) There may be a deterioration in the function of the organ with the primary disease, e.g., in a cardiac patient – additional myocardial damage or failure of the patient to take his digitalis preparation; (b) a new circulatory derangement may have developed – such as anemia, pulmonary infarction, or occult infection; (c) the patient may have increased his daily sodium intake; (d) the patient's renal function may have deteriorated (e.g., prerenal azotemia, pyelonephritis, ureteral obstruction; (e) the patient may have developed a significant electrolyte or acid-base balance disturbance as a consequence of previous diuretic therapy (e.g., dilutional hypoosmolality, hypochloremic-hypokalemic alkalosis); (f) the previous diuretic regimen of the patient may have been injudicious. Several examples of the latter may be mentioned.

In some patients with so called 'refractory' edema the excessive daily administration of diuretic drugs may have induced an unresponsive state which improves following a 'no-treatment' interval. For example, abrupt excessive diuresis (e.g., following very large doses of a 'loop' diuretic) may produce a rapid fall in plasma volume, LVEDP, and cardiac output; this in turn induces renal vasoconstriction with a fall in GFR and an increase in filtration fraction. Because these hemodynamic changes are associated with a reduction in peritubular hydrostatic pressure and a rise in peritubular oncotic pressure, net sodium and water reabsorption in the proximal tubules rises and less fluid is delivered to the distal nephron. Thus the patient becomes progressively refractory to the same dose of the 'loop' diuretic.

In other patients with 'refractory' edema, the doses of diuretic which are administered may be insufficient to accomplish the desired effect (e.g., spironolactone may be given in doses too low to compete effectively with high levels of circulating aldosterone). Finally, in some patients a particular drug regimen may have been ineffective because the selection of diuretics allowed sodium reabsorption to proceed unabated in other nephron segments. For example, when a carbonic anhydrase inhibitor is used as a primary diuretic, much of the sodium not reabsorbed by the proximal tubules will be reabsorbed in the ascending limb of Henle's loop. Similarly, when a 'loop' diuretic is administered to a patient with excessive circulating aldosterone (e.g., cirrhosis with ascites) much of the sodium not reabsorbed in the loop of Henle will be reabsorbed in association with potassium secretion more distally in the nephron to produce a urine rich in potassium and chloride but low in sodium content. In this setting administration of a combination of diuretics which inhibit sodium reabsorption in different nephron segments (e.g., a 'loop' diuretic and a potassium-sparing agent) may be required to achieve a negative sodium balance.

Pulmonary edema

Intravenous administration of furosemide or of ethacrynic acid has been found to be a useful adjunct in the treatment of acute pulmonary edema [33, 34, 100, 101]. Brisk increases in salt and water output peaking in 0.5–1 hr after administration of either drug relieve pulmonary congestion. Recent studies with furosemide in pulmonary edema indicate that beneficial effects are observed before the onset of diuresis as a consequence of venodilation and reduced cardiac filling pressure [51]. As mentioned previously, it is important to recall that an excessive decline in left ventricular filling pressure in patients with impaired left ventricular performance can produce a fall in cardiac output. In this manner, excessive diuresis in a patient with pulmonary edema due to an acute myocardial infarction can precipitate the syndrome of cardiogenic shock.

Use of diuretics in the treatment of hypertension

Diuretic drugs, particularly the thiazide diuretics, have long been used in the treatment of hypertension [102, 103]. They are very effective in lowering the systolic and diastolic blood pressures of one- to two-thirds of patients with mild and moderate essential hypertension. During the first few days following administration of diuretic drugs, there is a significant reduction of the systolic and diastolic blood pressures which is sustained during continued therapy. Diuretics are also used to enhance the antihypertensive action of other classes of drugs used to treat hypertension such as adrenergic blocking drugs, vasodilator drugs or drugs which inhibit the renin-angiotensin system. The precise mechanisms which underlie the antihypertensive action of diuretic drugs have not been defined. However, most investigators believe that the effect of diuretic drugs on blood pressure results from their action to produce a negative sodium balance. Diuretic drugs have a greater effect to lower blood pressure if the dietary sodium intake is reduced; the antihypertensive effect of diuretics can be overcome if the dietary sodium intake is increased markedly.

The most extensive studies of the effects of diuretics on cardiac and systemic hemodynamics were performed over a decade ago in patients receiving benzothiadiazines [104–107]. Initially, substantial urinary losses of salt and water induced by the drugs reduced plasma and extracellular fluid volumes. Venous filling pressures and cardiac output declined. Blood pressure also fell, even though total peripheral vascular resistance actually increased above normal in the initial stages. During the period of salt depletion plasma renin increased. In addition, the vasodepressor responses to adrenergic blocking agents were increased, while the blood pressure responses to pressor agents such as norepinephrine or angiotensin II were reduced. With continued administration of the drugs, the natriuretic effect declined and sodium balance returned to normal, albeit with a reduced total body sodium store. More recent studies indicate that in this stage plasma and ECF volumes remained below normal, and they increased acutely if the diuretic was stopped [108]. Cardiac output returned to normal as plasma and ECF volume increased. Total peripheral resistance however, fell during this late phase and the effect of treatment to depress the elevated blood pressure was maintained. The mechanism responsible for this late fall in total peripheral resistance is not known; the phenomenon has been called 'reverse autoregulation.' Because of these hemodynamic effects, which mimic the hemodynamic changes observed after drastic salt depletion, diuretics have remained one of the mainstays of the therapy of hypertension.

Special uses of diuretics

In addition to the treatment of edema and hypertension there are several special situations in which diuretics are used.

1. Because carbonic anhydrase inhibitors such as acetazolamide reduce the formation of aqueous humor, such drugs are used to treat patients with primary open angle glaucoma and other glaucomas that cannot be controlled by topical treatment alone.

2. Neither ethacrynic acid nor furosemide directly depress renal blood flow or glomerular filtration rate. Studies using inert gases have suggested that large doses of both drugs may acutely increase renal blood flow with a preferential increase in flow to the outer renal cortex [32]. In patients at risk for development of acute tubular necrosis (e.g., patients during surgery when the aorta is cross-clamped), it has been advocated that drugs such as furosemide may be administered intravenously to prevent the development of acute tubular necrosis. In such situations the rationale is to increase renal blood flow and to prevent tubular obstruction by increasing the intratubular flow rate. Obviously, adequate saline replacement to prevent plasma volume depletion is also necessary.

3. In patients with cardiovascular illness who develop oliguria, administration of large intravenous doses of furosemide has also been advocated by some investigators to distinguish 'pre-renal' causes of the oliguria from the development of acute tubular necrosis. If urine flow is significantly increased following administration of the drug, a 'pre-renal' cause has been inferred. A diuretic such as furosemide has no significant effect, however, to abort or ameliorate the oliguria associated with acute tubular necrosis [109, 110].

4. Furosemide and ethacrynic acid increase the urinary excretion of calcium and are useful in the emergency treatment of hypercalcemia [111]. Sodium chloride infusions must be given simultaneously, however; otherwise contraction of ECF volume may increase the proximal tubular reabsorption of calcium and reduce the therapeutic response.

5. The thiazides decrease urinary calcium excretion and are sometimes used to prevent the recurrence of calcium stones in patients with idiopathic hypercalciuria [112]. In a few patients, usually with primary or secondary hyperparathyroidism, the thiazides induce hypercalcemia. This results in part from an action of thiazides to release calcium from bone; this action is dependent on the presence of circulating parathyroid hormone (PTH) and is increased when PTH levels are excessive [73, 74].

6. The mechanism whereby sodium depletion induced by thiazide or mercurial diuretics reduces urinary volume and increases the urinary osmolality of patients with nephrogenic diabetes insipidus has been discussed elsewhere [69, 113].

Renal compensatory mechanisms during diuretic therapy

During diuretic therapy, a variety of compensatory mechanisms is set into operation as the patient's extracellular fluid volume is reduced by the action of the drug. If the salt and water excretion is so excessive that renal perfusion pressure falls, there will be a significant fall in the glomerular filtration rate. However, long before hypotension has developed, homeostatic adjustments occur which operate to reduce the excretion of salt and water and to limit the natriuretic effects of diuretic drugs. As ECF and plasma volumes shrink, the secretion of renin by the kidneys increases with a resulting rise in circulating angiotensin II. Angiotensin II stimulates secretion of aldosterone by the adrenal glomerulosa cells, and aldosterone acts to enhance sodium reabsorption in the distal nephron and to promote the secretion of potassium and hydrogen ions. As plasma volume declines below normal in response to diuresis, cardiac output falls, and there is a compensatory increase in peripheral and renal vascular resistance. Renal vasoconstriction, produced by angiotensin II and by the sympathetic nervous system, occurs first in the efferent arterioles and is associated with a rise in filtration fraction. The resulting alteration of intrarenal hemodynamics (reduced hydrostatic pressure and increased colloid osmotic pressure in peritubular capillaries) favors net tubular reabsorption of sodium and water particularly in the proximal tubules. If renal vasoconstriction is more intense, it can also involve the afferent arterioles and lead to a fall in the glomerular filtration rate.

Side effects of diuretic therapy

Two classes of side effects occur during diuretic treatment. The first class includes the disturbances of electrolyte and acid-base balance that are necessary consequences of the mechanism of action of the diuretic upon renal transport mechanisms in different segments of the nephron. The second class includes toxic and idiosyncratic drug reactions.

Electrolyte and acid-base disturbances

Table 2 lists ten electrolyte and acid-base disturbances that may occur during diuretic treatment.

1. In patients given the more potent saliuretic agents, such as ethyacrynic acid or furosemide, a true depletion of the extracellular fluid volume below normal may occur inadvertently. After excessively rapid and large diuresis, the depletion of arterial blood volume can produce orthostatic hypotension or shock. One must reemphasize that edema is an increase in the interstitial fluid volume. During diuretic therapy it is important to induce a negative sodium balance slowly in order to allow

Table 2. Electrolyte and acid-base disturbances during diuretic therapy.

1. Hypovolemia	6. Metabolic alkalosis
2. Hyponatremia	7. Metabolic acidosis
3. Dilutional hypoosomolity	8. Azotemia
4. Hypokalemia	9. Hyperuricemia
5. Hyperkalemia	10. Hypouricemia

time for salt and water to equilibrate between the interstitial and the intravascular fluid compartments.

2. When excessive amounts of diuretics are administered chronically (e.g., to patients with hypertension, or to female patients with idiopathic edema) a chronic depletion of total body sodium stores may result. In this setting of true sodium depletion, the patients may exhibit weakness, orthostatic hypotension, and hyponatremia in the absence of edema.

3. The syndrome of 'dilutional hypoosmolality' or 'dilutional hyponatremia' may occur spontaneously in patients with advanced cardiac failure or cirrhosis with ascites and, in this setting, often implies a poor prognosis. Dilutional hyponatremia occurs when there are increased total body stores of sodium and water (i.e., the patient is edematous), but the surplus of water is proportionately greater (i.e., the serum osmolality and sodium concentration are reduced). The capacity of the kidneys of patients with advanced heart failure or cirrhosis to dilute the urine is reduced in part because a diminished GFR and increased proximal tubular sodium reabsorption reduce the amount of salt presented to the diluting segments of the nephron [114]. In addition, some of these patients have inappropriately high circulating levels of ADH [115]. In those with increased plasma renin activity, thirst may be increased due to the dipsogenic action of angiotensin II. If patients are given diuretics which continuously block selective salt reabsorption in the ascending limb of Henle's loop or in the cortical diluting segment, the capacity of the kidneys to dilute the urine is reduced even more. Hence, if the water intake of the patient is high (i.e., substantially above insensible losses) the diuretic treatment may contribute to the pathogenesis of the electrolyte abnormality. Restriction of water intake below insensible and external losses is a fundamental component of the treatment of dilutional hypoosmolality. It also may be important to interrupt the administration of diuretics and to seek other measures to improve cardiac performance.

4. Diuretic therapy can induce significant disturbances of potassium balance [19]. However, this is much more common in the treatment of edema than in the treatment of patients with uncomplicated essential hypertension. During diuresis with agents that act proximal to the sites of potassium

secretion (carbonic anhydrase inhibitors, mercurials, furosemide, ethacrynic acid, thiazides), urinary potassium excretion rises because the increased delivery of fluid and the increased concentration of sodium in the tubular fluid stimulate potassium secretion in the distal convoluted tubules and collecting ducts. Diuretic treatment also tends to induce increases in circulating renin and aldosterone. As mentioned previously, greater amounts of potassium are lost into the urine for a given degree of sodium excretion in patients with elevated circulating levels of aldosterone. In addition, the presence of hypochloremic alkalosis also favors increased potassium excretion. The development of potassium depletion and hypokalemia during treatment with diuretics in turn may precipitate digitalis toxicity or produce lassitude, muscular weakness, gastrointestinal hypotonia, and impair reflexes and reduce urinary concentrating ability. One might note parenthetically that a coexisting hypochloremic alkalosis retards restoration of a normal potassium balance during potassium replacement therapy in hypokalemic patients [116]. If potassium supplements are administered, they are most effective if given as the chloride salt.

5. Conversely, hyperkalemia (with the attendant risk of cardiac arrest) may be induced when potassium-sparing diuretics such as spironolactone or triamterene or amiloride are administered to patients with renal disease or to patients that are receiving potassium supplements [97, 98].

6. The diuretics which enhance urinary sodium chloride excretion (ethacrynic acid, furosemide, mercurials; thiazides) and increase net urinary hydrogen ion excretion induce the development of hypochloremic alkalsis. Other mechanisms that may contribute to the development of alkalosis during therapy with these drugs are: (a) induced hyperaldosteronism, (b) hypokalemia, and (c) large rapid losses of relatively bicarbonate-free fluid from the extracellular fluid ('contraction' alkalosis) [43]. Studies by Schwartz and his colleagues have indicated that in sodium-retaining patients whose dietary intake of salt is restricted, a hypochloremic alkalosis induced by diuretics can persist for long periods (e.g., 1–2 weeks) even after drug treatment is discontinued. The administration of chloride facilitates the restoration of normal acid-base balance [117].

7. Two classes of diuretics induce metabolic aci-

dosis. Carbonic anhydrase inhibitors induce a hyperchloremic metabolic acidosis by promoting the urinary excretion of sodium bicarbonate. Metabolic acidosis of a lesser degree may be produced by the administration of spironolactone, amiloride, or triamterene which reduce hydrogen ion excretion in the distal nephron.

8. Reversible azotemia may be induced by diuretics such as chlorothiazide or triamterene which directly depress renal blood flow and glomerular filtration rate. Diuretic-induced azotemia occurs most frequently in patients with preexisting parenchymal renal disease. 'Pre-renal' azotemia may be brought about by any diuretic that produces excessively rapid or large urinary losses of sodium and water (particularly the more potent diuretics which inhibit salt reabsorption in the loop of Henle). When blood volume shrinks in response to urinary sodium chloride and water losses, increased activity of the sympathetic nervous system and of the renin-angiotensin II system may produce vasoconstriction of the afferent arterioles and a fall in the GFR [3]. This series of events frequently is observed in patients with advanced cirrhosis and ascites; brief periods of rapid diuresis deplete arterial blood volume and induce renal vasoconstriction before equilibration of salt and water has occurred between the intravascular compartment and the peritoneal space in which ascites has accumulated. As a result the GFR may fall and serum creatinine concentration may increase during diuretic treatment which is not successful in relieving the ascites.

9. Reduced renal clearance of urate and hypericemia may be induced by administration of thiazides, organomercurials, furosemide, and ethacrynic acid. As mentioned previously, the reduction of urinary urate output is in part a manifestation of sodium depletion and contraction of the extracellular fluid volume. The development of hyperuricemia after diuretic administration may occasionally be associated with an attack of gouty arthritis. There is little evidence that hyperuricemia induced in this way has deleterious effects upon the kidney, at least for plasma urate concentrations up to 10 mg/ 100 ml [118]. With higher levels of plasma urate, administration of allopurinol or of uricosuric drugs may be warranted. The potassium-sparing diuretics do not affect the serum urate concentration.

10. The new diuretic, tienilic acid, induces in-

creased urate excretion and hypouricemia in patients with hyperuricemia and in those with normal serum uric acid levels. The incidence of stone formation during the uricosuric effects of this drug, however, has been significant when the drug was administered to patients who had been rendered hyperuricemic by ECF volume depletion secondary to administration of other diuretic agents.

Toxic effects and modification of cardiovascular risk factors

Other side effects of diuretics are truly toxic manifestations. Rashes after thiazides, abdominal pain after ethacrynic acid, increases in blood sugar in some diabetics after thiazides or furosemide [119, 120], gynecomastia in males and menstrual disturbance in females, impotence or loss of libido in patients receiving spironolactone [121] and hepatotoxicity after tienilic acid are examples. In sensitive patients, organomercurials can produce fever, rash, or hypertension; large intravenous doses of furosemide or ethacrynic acid have produced ototoxicity in patients with advanced renal disease. Tests of auditory activity should be considered when such patients are given large doses of these drugs. Tienilic acid interferes with coagulation when patients are given coumadin [122].

A new question recently has been raised concerning the chronic use of diuretics that are sulfonamide derivatives in the treatment of hypertension – whether these drugs modify other cardiovascular risk factors adversely. Ames and Hill reported that serum cholesterol and triglyceride levels in a series of hypertensive patients were elevated following antihypertensive therapy with thiazide diuretics [123]. A similar elevation of triglyceride levels has been observed with administration of tienilic acid. Whether an adverse effect on one risk factor such as the serum lipid or glucose level counterbalances the beneficial effect of lowering blood pressure upon the atherosclerotic complications of hypertensive vascular disease is not known [124].

Conclusion

The physician today is fortunate to have an extensive variety of diuretics to use in the treatment of edema. An understanding of the mechanism of action of each of the classes of diuretics on the transport processes in different segments of the nephron benefits the physician in several ways: (a) It permits selection of the most appropriate drug to treat specific abnormalities of fluid and electrolyte homeostasis; (b) it enables one to anticipate and forestall many of the electrolyte and acid-base disturbances which may accompany diuresis; and (c) it enables one to combine diuretic agents which inhibit electrolyte transport in different segments of the nephron to mobilize so called 'refractory' edema fluid more efficaciously. Although much is known of the chemistry, pharmacology, and physiological actions of diuretic drugs, the molecular basis for the profound effects of these compounds on ion and water transport in different nephron segments remains to be discovered.

Acknowledgment

This work was supported in part by Grants HL 10182 and HL 14148 from the U.S.P.H.S.

References

1. Grantham JJ, Chonko AM: The physiological basis and clinical use of diuretics. In: Brenner BM, Stein JH (eds) Sodium and Water Homeostasis, vol 1. Churchill Livingston, New York, 1978, pp 178–211.
2. Burg M: The renal handling of sodium chloride. In: Brenner BM, Rector FC Jr (eds) The Kidney, vol 1. Saunders, Philadelphia, 1976, pp 272–298.
3. Cannon PJ: The kidney in heart failure. N Engl J Med 296:26–32, 1977.
4. Gottschalk GW, Lassiter WE, Mylle M: Localization of urine acidification in the mammalian kidney. Am J Physiol 98:581–585, 1960.
5. Giebisch G: The proximal nephron. In: Andreoli TE, Hoffman JF, Fanestil DD (eds) Physiology of Membrane Disorders. Plenum Publ, New York, 1978, p 629.
6. Earley L, Schrier, R: Intrarenal control of sodium excretion by hemodynamic and physical factors. In: Berne RM (ed) Handbook of Physiology. Section 8: Renal Physiology. Am Physiol Soc, Bethesda, 1973, pp 721–762.
7. Brenner B, Troy J, Daugherty T, MacInnes R: Quantitative importance of changes in post-glomerular colloid osmotic pressure in mediating glomerular tubular balance in the rat. J Clin Invest 52:190–197, 1973.
8. Kokko J: Proximal tubule potential difference. Dependence on glucose, HCO_3 and amino acids. J Clin Invest 52:1362–1367, 1973.
9. Rector FC, Martinez-Maldonado M, Brenner FP, Seldin W: Evidence of passive reabsorption of sodium chloride in the proximal tubule of rat kidney. J Clin Invest 45:1060, 1966.

431

10. Imai M, Kokko JP Sodium chloride urea and water transport in the thin ascending limb of Henle. J Clin Invest 53:383–402, 1974.

11. Burg MB, Stephenson JL: Transport characteristics of the loop of Henle. In: Andreoli TE, Hoffman JF, Fanestil DD (eds) Physiology of Membrane Disorders. Plenum Publ, New York, 1978, pp 661–679.

12. Burg MB, Green N Function of the thick ascending limb of Henle's loop. Am J Physiol 224:659–668, 1973.

13. Rocha AS, Kokko JP: Sodium chloride and water transport in the thick ascending limb of Henle. Evidence for active chloride transport. J Clin Invest 52:612–623, 1973.

14. Burg MB, Stoner L: Renal tubular chloride transport and mode of action of some diuretics. Ann Rev Physiol 38:37–45, 1976.

15. Windhager EE, Constanzo LS: Transport functions of the distal convoluted tubule. In: Andreoli TE, Hoffman JF, Fanestil DD (eds) Physiology of Membrane Disorders. Plenum Publ, New York, 1978, pp 681–706.

16. Shafer JA, Andreoli TE: The collecting duct. In: Andreoli TE, Hoffman JK, Fanestil DD (eds) Physiology of Membrane Disorders. Plenum Publ, New York, 1978, pp 707–737.

17. Stein JH, Reineck HJ: The role of the collecting duct in the regulation of excretion of sodium and other electrolytes. Kidney Int 6:1–9, 1974.

18. Osgood RW, Reineck HJ, Stein JH: Further studies on segmental sodium transport in the rat kidney during expansion of the extracellular fluid volume. J Clin Invest 62:311–320, 1978.

19. Giebisch G: Effects of diuretics on renal transport of potassium. In: Martinez–Maldonado M (ed) Methods in Pharmacology, vol 4A. Plenum Publ, New York, 1976, pp 121–164.

20. Maren TH: Carbonic anhydrase chemistry, physiology and inhibition. Physiol Rev 47:595–781, 1967.

21. Grantham JJ, Chonka M: The physiological basis and clinical use of diuretics. In: Brenner BM, Stein JH (eds) Sodium and Water Homeostasis, vol 1. Churchill Livingston, New York, 1978, pp 178–211.

22. Kunau R, Weller D, Webb H: Clarification of the site of action of chlorothiazide in the rat kidney. J Clin Invest 56:401–407, 1975.

23. Kunau R: The influence of the carbonic anhydrase inhibitor benzolamide (Cl-11 366) on the reabsorption of chloride. J Clin Invest 51:294–305, 1972.

24. Chou S, Porush JG, Slater PA, Flombaum CD, Shafi T, Fein PA: Effects on acetazolamide on proximal tubule Cl, Na, HCO_3 transport in normal and acidotic dogs during distal blockade. J Clin Invest 60:162–170, 1977.

25. Rector FC Jr, Selcin DW, Roberts AD Jr, Smith JS: The role of plasma CO_2 tension and carbonic anhydrase activity in the renal reabsorption of the bicarbonate. J Clin Invest 39:1706–1721, 1960.

26. Schwartz WB, Wallace NM: Electrolyte equilibrium during mercurial diuresis. J Clin Invest 30:1089–1104, 1951.

27. Axelrod DR, Pitts RF: The relationship of plasma pH and anion patterns to mercurial diuresis. J Clin Invest 31:171–174, 1952.

28. Burg MB, Green N: Effect of mersalyl on the thick ascending limb of Henle's loop. Kidney Int 4:245–251, 1973.

29. Wright FS: Intrarenal regulation of glomerular filtration rate. N Engl J Med 291:135–141, 1974.

30. Evanson RL, Lockhart EA, Dirks JH: Effect of mercurial diuretics on tubular sodium and potassium transport in dogs. Am J Physiol 222:282–289, 1974.

31. Nigrovic V, Cafruny EJ: Renal concentration of citrate as a negative modulator of diuretic response to mercurials. Nature 247:381–383, 1974.

32. Freeman RB, Maher JF, Schreiner GE, Mostofii FK: Renal tubular necrosis due to nephrotoxicity of organic mercurial diuretics. Ann Intern Med 57:34–43, 1962.

33. Cannon PJ, Ames RP, Laragh JH: Methylene butyryl phenoxyacetic acid. Novel potent natriuretic and diuretic agent. J Am Med Assoc 185:854–863, 1963.

34. Cannon PJ, Heinemann HO, Stason WB, Laragh JH: Ethacrynic acid-effectiveness and mode of diuretic action in man. Circulation 31:5–18, 1965.

35. Cannon PJ, Kilcoyne MM: Ethacrynic acid and furosemide. Renal pharmacology and clinical use. Prog Cardiovasc Dis 12:99–118, 1969.

36. Birtch AG, Zakheim RM, Jones LG, Barger AC: Redistribution of renal blood flow produced by furosemide and ethacrynic acid. Circ Res 21:869–878, 1967.

37. Clapp JR, Nottebohm GA, Robinson RR: Proximal site of action of ethacrynic acid: importance of filtration rate. Am J Physiol 220:1355–1360, 1976.

38. Goldberg M, McCurdy DK, Foltz EL, Bluemle LW Jr: Effects of ethacrynic acid (a new saluretic agent) on renal diluting and concentrating mechanisms: evidence for site of action in the loop of Henle. J Clin Invest 43:201–216, 1964.

40. Burg M, Green N: Effect of ethacrynic acid on the thick ascending limb of Henle's loop. Kidney Int 4:301–308, 1973.

41. Case D, Gunther S, Cannon PJ: Ethacrynate-induced depression of respiration in transport systems and kidney mitochondria. Am J Physiol 224:769–780, 1973.

42. Cannon PJ, Dell RB, Winters RW: Effects of diuretics on electrolyte and lactate gradients in dog kidney. J Lab Clin Med 72:192–203, 1968.

43. Cannon PJ, Heinemann HO, Albert MS, Laragh JH, Winters RW: 'Contraction' alkalosis after diuresis of edematous patients with ethacrynic acid. Ann Intern Med 62:979–990, 1965.

44. Stason WB, Cannon PJ, Heinemann HO, Laragh JH: Furosemide, a clinical evaluation of its diuretic action. Circulation 34:910–920, 1966.

45. Stein JH, Wilson CB, Kirkendall WM: Differences in the acute effects of furosemide and ethacrynic acid in man. J Lab Clin Med 71:654–665, 1968.

46. Puschett JB, Goldberg M: The acute effects of furosemide on acid and electrolyte excretion in man. J Lab Clin Med 71:666–677, 1968.

47. Hook JB, Williamson HE: Influence of probenecid and alterations in acid-balance on the saliuretic activity of furosemide. J Pharmacol Exp Ther 149:404–408, 1972.

48. Burke T, Robinson R, Clapp J: Determinants of the effect of furosemide on the proximal tubule. Kidney Int 1:12–18, 1972.

49. Burg M, Stoner L, Cardinal J, Green N: Furosemide effect on isolated perfused tubules. Am J Physiol 225:119–124, 1973.

50. Abramow M: Effects of ethacrynic acid on the isolated collecting tubule. J Clin Invest 53:796–804, 1974.

51. Dikshit K, Vyden JD, Forrester JS, Swan HJC: Renal and extra renal hemodynamic effects of furosemide in congestive heart failure after myocardial infarction. N Engl J Med 291:135–141, 1974.

52. Weinman EJ, Eknoyan G, Suki WN; The influence of extracellular fluid balance on the tubular transport of uric acid. J Clin Invest 55:283–291, 1975.

53. Engle JE, Steele TH: Variation of urate excretion with urine flow in normal man. Nephron 16:50–56, 1976.

54. Muth RG: Diuretic response to furosemide in the presence of renal insufficiency. J Am Med Assoc 195:1066–1069, 1966.

55. Berman LB, Ebrahimi A: Experiences with furosemide in renal disease. Proc Soc Biol Med 118:333–346, 1965.

56. Maher J, Schreiner GF: Studies on ethacrinc acid in patients with refractory edema. Ann Intern Med 62:15–29, 1965.

57. Schneider WJ, Becker EL: Acute transient hearing ions after ethacrynic acid therapy. Arch Intern Med 117:715–717, 1966.

58. Ashbury MJ, Gatenby PB, O'Sullivan S, Bourke E: 'Bumetanide' potent new 'loop' diuretic. Br Med J 1:211–213, 1972.

59. Olesen KH, Sigurd B, Steiness E, Leth A: Bumetanide, a new potent diuretic. Acta Med Scand 193:119–131, 1973.

60. Carriere S, Dandavino R: Bumetanide, a new loop diuretic. Clin Pharmacol Ther 20:424–438, 1976.

61. Jayakumar S, Puschett JB: Study of the sites and mechanisms of action of bumetanide in man. J Pharmacol Exp Ther 201:251–258, 1977.

62. Beyer K, Baer J: Physiologic basis for the action of newer diuretic agents. Pharmacol Rev 13:517–564, 1961.

63. Pitts R, Kruch F, Lozano R, Taylor D, Heidenreich O, Kessler R: Studies on the mechanism of diuretic action of chlorothiazide. J Pharmacol Exp Ther 123:89–97, 1958.

64. Heinemann HO, Demartini EE, Laragh JH: The effect of chlorothiazide on renal excretion of electrolytes and free water. Am J Med 26:853–861, 1959.

65. Earley LE, Kahn M, Orloff J: Effects of infusions of chlorothiazide on urinary dilution and concentration in the dog. J Clin Invest 40:857–866, 1961.

66. Edwards F, Baer P, Sutton R, Dirks J: Micropuncture study of diuretic effects on sodium and calcium reabsorption in the dog nephron. J Clin Invest 52:2418–2427, 1978.

67. Ullrich K, Baumann K, Loeschke K, Ramrich G, Stolte H: Micropuncture experiments with saluretic sulfonamides. Ann NY Acad Sci 139:416–423, 1966.

68. Goldring RM, Cannon PJ, Heinemann HO, Fishman AP: Respiratory adjustment to chronic metabolic alkalosis in man. J Clin Invest 47:188–202, 1968.

69. Earley L, Orloff J: The mechanism of antidiuresis associated with the administration of hydrochlorothiazide to patients with vasopressin-resistant diabetes mellitus. J Clin Invest 41:1988–1997, 1962.

70. Lamberg BA, Kuhlback G: Effect of chlorothiazide and hydrochlorothiazide on the excretion of sodium in the urine. Scand J Clin Lab Invest 11:351–357, 1959.

71. Costanzo LS, Windhager EE: Distal reabsorption of calcium: effect of load and chlorothiazide (CTZ). Fed Proc 35:466, 1976.

72. Brickman A, Wassry S, Coburn J: Changes in serum and urinary calcium during treatment with hydrochlorothiazide. J Clin Invest 51:945–954, 1972.

73. Parfitt AM: The interactions of thiazide diuretics with parathyroid hormone and vitamin D. Studies in patients wiht hypoparathyroidism. J Clin Invest 51:1879–1888, 1972.

74. Popoutzer MM, Subryan VL, Alfey AC, Reeve EB, Schrier RM: The acute effect of chlorothiazide on serum-ionized calcium: evidence for a parathyroid hormone-dependent mechanism. J Clin Invest 55:1295–1302, 1975.

75. DeMartini FE, Wheaton, EA, Healy LA, Laragh JH: Effect of chlorothiazide on renal excretion of uric acid. Am J Med 32:572–577, 1962.

76. Steele TH, Oppenheimer S: Factors affecting urate excretion following diuretic administration in man. Am J Med 47:564–574, 1969.

77. Stote RM, Dubb JW, Familiar RG, Alexander F: Ticrynafen, a uricosuric antihypertensive diuretic. Clin Pharmacol 23:456–460, 1978.

78. Nemati M, Kyle MC, Fries ED: Clinical study of ticrynafen, a new diuretic antihypertensive and uricosuric agent. J Am Med Assoc 237:652–657, 1977.

79. Wood AJ, Bolli P, Waal-Manning HJ, Simpson FD: Ticrynafen: kinetics, protein binding, and effects on serum and urinary uric acid. Clin Pharmacol Ther 23:697–702, 1978.

80. Beck P, Asseher AW: Clinical evaluating metolazone (zaroxolyn): a new quinazoline diuretic. Clin Trials J 8:13–18, 1971.

81. Steinmuller SR, Puschett JB: Effects of metolazone in man: comparison with chlorothiazide. Kidney Int 1:169–181, 1972.

82. Fernandez PC, Puschett JB: Proximal tubular actions of metolazone and chlorothiazide. Am J Physiol 225:954–961, 1973.

83. Bennett WM, Porter GA: Efficacy and safety of metolazone in renal failure and the nephrotic syndrome. J Clin Pharmacol 13:357–364, 1973.

84. Sonnenblick EH, Cannon PJ, Laragh JH: The nature of the action of intravenous aldosterone: evidence for a role of the hormone in urinary dilution. J Clin Invest 40:903–913, 1961.

85. Kagawa C, Sturterant F, VanArman C: Pharmacology of a new steroid that blocks salt activity of aldosterone and desoxycorticosterone. J Pharmacol Exp Ther 126:123–130, 1959.

86. Liddle G: Specific and non-specific inhibiton of mineralocorticoid activity. Metabolism 10:1021–1030, 1961.

87. Coppage WS Jr, Liddle GW: Mode of action and clinical usefulness of aldosterone antagonists. Ann NY Acad Sci 88:815–821, 1960.

88. Baba W, Tudhope G, Wilson G: Triampterene, a new

diuretic drug. Br Med J 2:756–760, 1962.

89. Crosley AP Jr, Ronquille LM, Strickland WH, Alexander F: 'Triampterene', a natriuretic agent. Preliminary observations in man. Ann Intern Med 56:241–251, 1962.

90. Weibelhaus V, Weinstock J, Maass A, Brennan F, Sosnowski G, Larsen T: The diuretic and natriuretic activity of triampterene and several related pteridines in the rat. J Pharmacol Exp Ther 149:397–403, 1965.

91. Baba W, Lant A, Smith A, Townsend M, Wilson G: Pharmacological effects in animals and normal human subjects of the diuretic amiloride hydrochloride (MK-870). Clin Pharmacol Ther 9:318–327, 1968.

92. Bull MD, Laragh JH: 'Amiloride' a potassium-sparing natriuretic agent. Circulation 37:45–53, 1968.

93. Duarte CG, Chomety F, Giebisch G: Effect of amiloride, ouabain and furosemide on distal tubular function in the rat. Am J Physiol 221:632–640, 1972.

94. Bentley P: Amiloride, a potent inhibitor of sodium transport across toad bladder. J Physiol 195:317–330, 1968.

95. Crabbe J: A hypothesis concerning the mode of action of amiloride and triampterene. Arch Intern Pharmacodyn Ther 173:474–477, 1968.

96. Stoner LC, Burg MB, Orloff J: Ion transport in cortical collecting tubule; effect of amiloride. Am J Physiol 227: 453–459, 1974.

97. Greenblatt DJ, Koch-Weser J: Adverse reactions to spironolactone. J Am Med Assoc 225:40–43, 1973.

98. Schultze RG: Recent advances in the physiology and pathophysiology of potassium excretion. Arch Intern Med 131:885–897, 1973.

99. Cohn JH, Franciosa JA: Vasodilator therapy of cardiac failure. N Engl J Med 297:27–31, 254–261, 1977.

100. Iff NW, Flenley DC: Blood–gas exchange after furosemide in acute pulmonary edema. Lancet 1:616–618, 1971.

101. Scheinman M, Brown M, Rapaport E: Hemodynamic effects of ethacrynic acid in patients with refractory acute left ventricular failure. Am J Med 50:291–296, 1971.

102. Freis ED, Wanko A, Wilson IM, Parrish AE: Chlorothiazide in hypertensive and normotensive patients. Ann NY Acad Sci 71:450–455, 1958.

103. Hollander W, Chobanian AV: Mode of action of chlorothiazide and mercurial diuretics as antihypertensive agents. J Clin Invest 37:902, 1958.

104. Wilson IM, Freis ED: Relationship between plasma and extracellular fluid volume depletion and antihypertensive effect of chlorothiazide. Circulation 20:1028–1036, 1959.

105. Alexsandrow D, Wysznacka W, Gajewski J: Studies on mechanisms of hypertensive action of chlorothiazide. N Engl J Med 260:51–55, 1959.

106. Frolich ED, Schnaper HW, Wilson IM, Freis ED: Hemodynamic alterations in hypertensive patients due to chlorothiazide. N Engl J Med 262:1261–1263, 1960.

107. Conway J, Lauwers P: Hemodynamic and hypotensive effect of long-term treatment with hydrochlorothiazide. Circulation 21:21–27, 1960.

108. Tarazi RC, Dustan HP, Frolich ED: Long-term thiazide in essential hypertension. Evidence for persistent alteration in plasma volume and renin activity. Circulation 41:709–717, 1970.

109. Minuth AN, Terrell JB Jr, Suki WN: Acute renal failure in study of the course and prognosis of 104 patients and the role of furosemide. Am J Med Sci 271:317–324, 1976.

110. Epstein ME, Schneider NS, Befeler B: Effect of intrarenal furosemide on renal function and intrarenal hemodynamics in acute renal failure. Am J Med 58:510–516, 1975.

111. Suki WN, Yium JJ, VonMinden M, Saller-Herbert C, Ekkoyan G, Martinez Maldonado M: Acute treatment of hypercalcemia with furosemide. N Engl J Med 283:836–840, 1970.

112. Yendt ER, Guay GF, Garcia DA: The use of thiazides in the prevention of renal calculi. Can Med Assoc J 102: 614–620, 1970.

113. Crawford JD, Kennedy GC, Hill LE: Clinical results of treatment of diabetes insipidus with drugs of the chlorothiazide series. N Engl J Med 262:737–743, 1960.

114. Bell NH, Schedl HP, Bartter FC: An explanation of abnormal water retention and hypoosmolality in congestive heart failure. Am J Med 36:351–360, 1964.

115. Verney EV: Croonian lecture: the antidiuretic hormone and the factors which determine its release. Proc R Soc Lond (Series B) 135:25–106, 1947.

116. Kassirer JP, Berkman PM, Lawrenz DR, Schwartz WB: Critical role of chloride in the correction of hypokalemic alkalosis in man. Am J Med 38:172–189, 1965.

117. Kassirer JP, Schwartz WB: Correction of metabolic alkalosis in man without repair of potassium deficiency. Am J Med 40:19–26, 1966.

118. Berger L, Yu T: Renal function in gout. IV. An analysis of 524 gouty subjects including long-term follow-up studies. Am J Med 59:605–613, 1975.

119. Breckenridge A, Welbern TA, Dollery CT, Fraser TR: Glucose tolerance in patients on long-term diuretic therapy. Lancet 1:61–64, 1967.

120. Glodner MG, Zarowitz H, Akgun F: Hyperglycemia and glucosuria due to thiazide derivatives administered in diabetes mellitus. N Engl J Med 262:403–405, 1960.

121. Loreauz L, Menard R, Taylor A, Patpita JC, Sauten R: Spironolactone and endocrine dysfunction. Ann Intern Med 85:630–636, 1976.

122. Potter H, Destaing F, Chauve L: Potentialization de l'effet des anticoagulants coumariniques par l'acid tienilique: use nouvelle observation. Nouv Presse Med 6:468, 1977.

123. Ames RP, Hill P: Elevation of serum lipids during diuretic therapy of hypertension. Am J Med 61:748–757, 1976.

124. Freis E, et al: Study group on antihypertensive agents. Effects of treatment in morbidity in hypertension. J Am Med Assoc 202:1028–1034, 1967; 213:1143–1152, 1970.

434

CHAPTER 13

The pharmacolgy of vasodilator and antianginal drugs

ALAN S. NIES and GWYNNE NEUFELD

Vasodilator therapy of congestive heart failure

The treatment of congestive heart failure with vasodilators is one of the most profound changes in cardiac pharmacologic therapy of recent years. Traditional therapy with salt and water restriction, diuretics, and digitalis has been adequate in controlling the symptoms of most patients with mild to moderate congestive heart failure. However, there remains a group of patients with severe congestive heart failure that will not respond adequately to traditional therapy. This latter group has provided the impetus for investigation of newer treatment modalities.

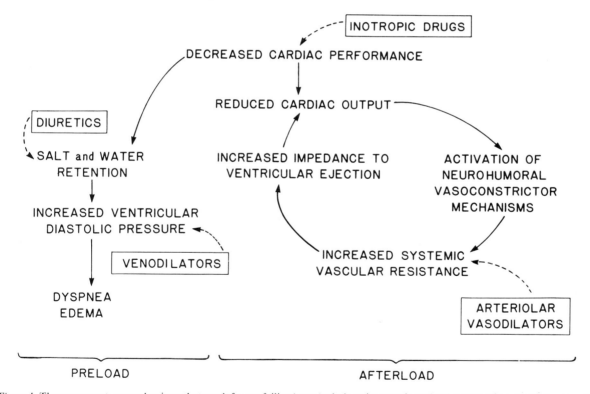

Figure 1. The compensatory mechanisms that result from a failing heart include an increase in preload (on the left) and afterload (on the right). Vasodilators counteract the compensatory mechanisms. Afterload-reducing drugs allow the failing heart to pump more effectively, and preload-reducing drugs improve the symptom of dyspnea.

Rosen, M. R. and Hoffman, B. F. (eds.), Cardiac Therapy. ISBN 0-89838-564-4.
© 1983, Martinus Nijhoff Publishers, Boston, The Hague, Dordrecht, Lancaster. Printed in the Netherlands.

Congestive heart failure is a complex clinical syndrome that results from an impaired ability of the heart to pump an adequate quantity of blood to maintain body requirements. Compensatory mechanisms in heart failure produce an increase in cardiac preload, due to renal salt and water retention, and an increase in cardiac afterload, due to an activation of the sympathetic nervous system, the renin-angiotensin system, vasopressin release, and possibly other mechanisms. These compensatory mechanisms, although geared for short-term benefit, may produce deleterious long-term effects. The increase in preload can result in symptoms of dyspnea and edema, and the increase in afterload appears to limit the ability of the damaged heart to supply an adequate cardiac output (Figure 1). The pathophysiology of heart failure is discussed in detail in Chapter 3.

Vasodilator therapy of heart failure is an attempt to counteract the changes in preload and afterload produced by the body's compensatory mechanisms without altering cardiac contractility. This approach to therapy is in contrast to traditional therapy with digitalis where cardiac contractility is improved, and the compensatory mechanisms may no longer be required. Vasodilators act primarily on either the veins (capacitance vessels) to increase venous pooling, the arterioles (resistance vessels) to decrease systemic arterial resistance, or both. Venodilatation reduces the return of blood to the heart and thus reduces the left ventricular end-diastolic pressure and volume. Venodilators, therefore, can add to the effects of diuretics to reduce cardiac preload. Venodilators have very little effect on the cardiac output unless cardiac filling is reduced sufficiently to cause a drop in cardiac output due to the Frank-Starling mechanism. Symptomatic improvement from systemic venodilation is related to relief of pulmonary congestion and dyspnea at rest and during exercise. Arteriolar dilators, on the other hand, facilitate ventricular emptying with a resultant increase in stroke volume and cardiac output due to reduced impedance to left ventricular ejection. This improvement in cardiac output can usually be accomplished with little change in arterial pressure or reflex increase in heart rate. In fact, the plasma concentration of norepinephrine, an index of sympathetic nervous activity, often decreases with succesful vasodilator therapy of heart failure [1] in contrast to the situation in normal individuals in which arteriolar dilation results in a decrease in arterial pressure and a reflex rise in heart rate and plasma norepinephrine concentration. Myocardial oxygen consumption is generally unchanged or reduced during therapy with vasodilators unless the agent used has intrinsic inotropic properties.

The hemodynamic effects of the vasodilators that have been evaluated vary as to the balance of venous and arteriolar vasodilation produced, with some agents acting primarily as venous dilators and others acting primarily as arteriolar dilators. This division of agents into those which act primarily to cause venous pooling and those which act primarily to reduce arterial resistance is helpful in choosing a particular agent in the clinical setting. If a patient's symptoms are related to an increased preload, such as dyspnea, but cardiac output is adequate, venodilators will be most helpful. However, if an inadequate cardiac output is a prominent feature as manifested by fatigue or prerenal azotemia, reduction of the afterload with arteriolar dilators will be most beneficial. The majority of patients with severe heart failure will require both preload and afterload reduction for optimum benefit.

Venous dilator drugs

Nitrates

Glyceryl trinitrate (nitroglycerin) is the prototype organic nitrate vasodilator. The principal action of the nitrates is direct relaxation of venous smooth muscle with much less effect on systemic arterioles [2]. This action results primarily in reduction of preload secondary to venous pooling with little change in total peripheral vascular resistance or cardiac output [3, 4] except in the setting of severe cardiac dysfunction in which a small decrease in peripheral vascular resistance may be accompanied by an increase in cardiac output [5]. The reduction in preload by nitroglycerin and resultant fall in wall tension and left ventricular chamber size results in a decrease in myocardial oxygen consumption [4]. In addition, the reduced end-diastolic pressure within the left ventricle may allow increased diastolic coronary blood flow to ischemic subendocardium resulting in improved contraction of the previously ischemic myocardium with further enhancement of cardiac function.

The mechanism whereby the organic nitrates produce their vascular effect is unknown. The generally accepted theory is that the nitrates interact with a sulfhydryl-containing receptor to produce nitrite ion, the sulfhydryl is oxidized to a disulfide, and relaxation of the smooth muscle occurs [6]. According to this hypothesis, tolerance to the nitrates reflects a lack of sulfhydryl groups at the receptor site. Recently, data have been presented that do not support the postulate that nitroglycerin must be metabolized to nitrite prior to vascular relaxation, but imply that the nitroglycerin molecule is required for activity [7].

The steps leading to smooth muscle relaxation following nitrate interaction with the receptor are also not well understood. One hypothesis relates relaxation to increases in intracellular cyclic GMP [8, 9]. However, more data are required to determine whether the correlations observed between an increase in cGMP and relaxation have any causal relationship.

Nitroglycerin is well absorbed across mucus membranes and can be absorbed through the skin. Recently described assays for the organic nitrates in plasma indicate that patients with congestive heart failure vary in their responsiveness to the same plasma concentration of nitroglycerin. The minimum effective concentration of nitroglycerin was 1.2 ng/ml achieved with an intravenous infusion rate of 15 μg/min, but some patients with very severe heart failure had little response at blood levels of 18 ng/ml [10]. Nitroglycerin is rapidly metabolized by the liver and other organs with a half-life of 1–3 min and a total body clearance of 1–20 l/min.

When given sublingually, nitroglycerin is rapidly absorbed and achieves an average peak plasma concentration of about 2 ng/ml at 2 min after a 0.6-mg dose [11, 12]. The vasodilation produced by sublingual nitroglycerin lasts approximately 30 min. A reduction of cardiac preload for up to 8 hr may be produced by sustained release oral nitroglycerin (6.5–19.5 mg) or by transcutaneous absorption from 2% nitroglycerin ointment (1–3 in) [4, 13, 14]. Differences in response to the nitroglycerin ointment do not seem to be related entirely to variation in absorption across the skin since nonresponders achieved the same blood concentrations as did the responders. Administration of small doses (0.6 mg) of nitroglycerin by mouth will not produce an effect because of extensive metabolism of the drug by the liver during absorption with none appearing in the systemic circulation.

Other nitrates have been formulated to provide a longer duration of action. Isosorbide dinitrate given sublingually (5–10 mg) can produce effects for 1–2 hr, whereas orally administered isosorbide dinitrate (10–60 mg) or pentaerythrityl tetranitrate (40–50 mg) can reduce left ventricular end-diastolic pressure for 4–6 hr [15].

Side effects are infrequent during the administration of the nitrates with one group reporting no adverse reactions after an average of seven months of chronic treatment with isosorbide dinitrate [16]. Headache is seen frequently with initiation of nitrate therapy, but these headaches usually disappear after one to two weeks of treatment. Reduction of filling pressures to below ideal levels can lead to lowered cardiac output, hypotension, or syncope if improper patient selection is made or overdosage occurs.

Tolerance to the effects of the organic nitrates has received considerable attention. In experimental animals, tolerance to the vascular effects of nitrates can be produced easily, and one nitrate can produce tolerance to another, a phenomenon called 'cross-tolerance' [6]. In normal individuals exposed to nitroglycerin in the munitions industry, tolerance to the headaches develops during a few days and disappears over a weekend giving rise to the syndrome of 'Monday head' [17]. In the clinical literature, the importance of nitrate tolerance and cross-tolerance is unresolved. In a recent study correlating hemodynamic effects of isosorbide dinitrate with plasma drug concentration, partial tolerance to isosorbide dinitrate was demonstrated to occur within 24–48 hr [18]. Moreover, the tolerance was not related to enhanced metabolism since the patients responded less to doses that produced the same or higher concentrations of the nitrate. Cross-tolerance to nitroglycerin has also been shown to occur during therapy with isosorbide dinitrate [18] and pentaerythrityl tetranitrate [19]. In spite of these convincing demonstrations of tolerance and cross-tolerance of the organic nitrates, sustained effects of nitrates when used for heart failure or angina have been reported. Probably the tolerance is only partial allowing these sustained effects to occur.

Arteriolar dilator drugs

Hydralazine

Hydralazine is a direct systemic vasodilating agent with action confined almost totally to the arterial tree with very little effect on veins [20, 21]. This action results in a return of the depressed cardiac output towards normal with only a small reduction of left ventricular filling pressures in patients with heart failure [20, 22]. Reflex tachycardia occurs occasionally but is much less common in patients with normotensive congestive heart failure than in normal or hypertensive individuals without heart failure [22]. Patients that respond best to hydralazine alone have the largest left ventricular chamber size prior to drug administration [23]. In addition to reducing afterload, hydralazine has inotropic effects, most likely due to reflex and direct release of catecholamines resulting in beta-adrenergic stimulation [24]. This inotropic effect has a tendency to increase myocardial oxygen consumption, but the net effect on myocardial oxygen consumption is probably to lower it because of the marked reduction in ventricular impedance and the resultant reduction in wall tension needed for ventricular ejection. Sustained improvement in hemodynamics and symptoms follows administration of hydralazine at doses from 25 to 150 mg four times per day [24] with beneficial effects seen for several months [25]. Some patients are resistant to the effects of these doses of hydralazine and may require 150–800 mg as single oral doses in order to have a response [26]. Long-term use of such large doses probably will produce a higher incidence of side effects (see below).

The metabolism of hydralazine has proven to be more complicated than initially suspected. The drug is, in part, acetylated, and this metabolic pathway affects the bioavailability of the parent compound. Genetically 'slow' acetylators achieve higher plasma hydralazine concentrations than genetically 'fast' acetylators following oral administration [27]. This probably is the result of a slower metabolism of the drug during absorption by the intestinal mucosa and/or liver of slow acetylators, thereby allowing a greater fraction of the orally administered dose to reach the systemic circulation. Other metabolic pathways also seem to be important for hydralazine, and metabolism may occur in sites other than the liver [27–29]. Intravascular conversion of hydralazine to an active metabolite, hydralazine pyruvic acid hydrazone, has been described. The half-life of the parent drug is short (< 1 hr), but the duration of action is at least 6 hr and is longer than 12 hr when the drug is used as an antihypertensive agent. The usual explanation for the long duration of action is that hydralazine may be localized in vascular tissues where it produces a prolonged effect [30]. However, the recent discovery of active metabolites of hydralazine with longer half-lives offers an alternative explanation.

Hydralazine is usually well tolerated by patients with heart failure. Headache may occur on institution of therapy. The tachycardia and palpitations frequently seen in normals or hypertensive patients are much less of a problem in patients with heart failure, and heart rate usually is unchanged. In 10–20% of hypertensive patients receiving 400 mg/day or more for a year, hydralazine has produced a drug-induced lupus erythematosus syndrome [31]. This syndrome occurs predominantly in Caucasian slow acetylators and rarely in fast acetylators or Blacks regardless of acetylator phenotype. Although the mechanism of lupus production is unknown, the syndrome is reversible with cessation of the drug, and persistent sequelae are rare [31]. Other side effects include nausea, fluid retention, and a rare pyridoxine responsive peripheral neuropathy primarily in slow acetylators.

Minoxidil

Minoxidil, a potent direct arteriolar smooth muscle relaxant, has recently been marketed for the treatment of hypertension refractory to conventional therapy [32]. It has been evaluated for the treatment of congestive heart failure much less thoroughly than hydralazine but appears to have similar hemodynamic effects [33]. Minoxidil is 90% metabolized by the liver and has a reported half-life of about 4 hr and a duration of action up to 24 hr. Like hydralazine, minoxidil has been found to persist in arteriolar smooth muscle, perhaps accounting for its prolonged action. The side effects of minoxidil include significant and sometimes massive fluid retention and cosmetically disturbing hypertrichosis. Its role, if any, in the treatment of normotensive congestive heart failure is unclear and will require further evaluation.

Mixed venous and arteriolar dilator drugs

Nitroprusside

The hypotensive action of nitroprusside is the result of a balanced relaxation of resistance and capacitance vessels independent of sympathetic tone [34, 35]. As measured by plethysmography, nitroprusside increases venous capacitance and reduces arteriolar resistance, thus producing a relatively greater effect on resistance vessels than the nitrates. This reduction in afterload produced by nitroprusside allows the ejection fraction of the left ventricle to increase in ischemic heart disease and congestive cardiomyopathies [36] in contrast to the nitrates, which reduce preload but frequently do not increase ejection fraction. No inotropic properties have been ascribed to nitroprusside, and thus the major beneficial hemodynamic effects of nitroprusside as compared to the nitrates appear to result from afterload reduction that is balanced with preload reduction [26].

The reduction in ventricular preload resulting from pooling of blood in the capacitance vessels affects the failing ventricle variably depending on the left ventricular end-diastolic pressure present at initiation of therapy and the magnitude of reduction in left ventricular end-diastolic pressure that results from nitroprusside therapy [36]. When left ventricular filling pressure is decreased below 12 mmHg by nitroprusside therapy, cardiac output does not increase or may even decline because the beneficial effects of impedance reduction are counteracted by the negative effects of the decreased preload placing the ventricle on the ascending limb of the Frank-Starling curve [36]. Maximal enhancement of cardiac output by nitroprusside probably occurs when the left ventricular end-diastolic pressure is maintained in the range of 15–18 mmHg [25].

Nitroprusside decreases myocardial oxygen consumption since ventricular wall tension is reduced while heart rate and contractile state remain relatively constant. This is in direct contrast to the inotropic drugs, which increase myocardial oxygen consumption significantly as they increase cardiac output. Perfusion of ischemic myocardium in patients with coronary artery disease appears to be maintained during nitroprusside therapy as long as mean arterial blood pressure is preserved [37, 38].

However, in contrast to nitroglycerin, nitroprusside does not appear to redistribute the coronary blood flow to ischemic areas [39]. This has been interpreted to indicate that nitroprusside affects primarily the resistance vessels in the coronary circulation, whereas nitroglycerin has a major effect on larger conductance vessels and on collaterals.

Nitroprusside must be administered intravenously and has an immediate effect by this route. Its half-life is very short with all demonstrable action gone in a few minutes following cessation of therapy. The dosage of nitroprusside must be determined in each patient by titration, with an average dose of 75 μg/min. The major side effect relates to hypotension produced by an excessive dose. Other side effects relate to the metabolism of nitroprusside. The drug is metabolized in the blood to cyanide, which is further metabolized to thiocyanate, a compound slowly cleared by the kidneys. In patients with normal renal function, thiocyanate has a half-life of four days, but this is prolonged in patients with renal failure. When nitroprusside is infused for several days, thiocyanate can accumulate and produce toxicity. At concentrations of 10 mg/dl, thiocyanate can produce weakness, nausea, tinnitus, muscle spasms, disorientation, and psychosis. Very high infusion rates of nitroprusside (usually $>$ 15 μg/kg/min) even for a few hours may result in cyanide toxicity presenting with lactic acidosis, lack of tissue oxygen extraction, refractory hypotension, and death. Cyanide toxicity is not a problem at the low infusion rates ($<$ 10 μg/kg/min) usually required for the treatment of congestive heart failure [40].

Nitroprusside is light sensitive and unstable in aqueous solution. As it decomposes, nitroprusside solution darkens. The solutions should therefore be made fresh and shielded from light.

When nitroprusside is abruptly discontinued, patients can undergo hemodynamic deterioration rapidly with a rise in systemic vascular resistance and left ventricular end-diastolic pressure associated with fall in cardiac output to levels below those existing prior to the nitroprusside [41]. A similar rebound has been described in hypertensive patients in whom the blood pressure can overshoot following discontinuation of nitroprusside [42]. Although the mechanism of this transient rebound is not entirely certain, it seems likely to be related to reflex vasoconstrictor mechanisms, such as an increase in plasma renin activity, resulting from the hemodynamic effects produced by the nitroprusside [43]. In any event, nitroprusside infusions should not be discontinued abruptly, and other drugs should be given as the nitroprusside is tapered to maintain the hemodynamic benefits of preload and afterload reduction.

Alpha-adrenergic blocking drugs

Drugs blocking alpha-adrenergic receptors in the vasculature can reverse adrenergically mediated arteriolar and venous constriction. These vascular alpha-adrenergic receptors are subclassified as alpha$_1$-adrenergic receptors. Alpha$_2$-adrenergic receptors exist on adrenergic nerve endings and when stimulated result in a decrease in norepinephrine release. If these alpha$_2$-adrenergic receptors are blocked, norepinephrine release is enhanced. The classic alpha-adrenergic-blocking drugs, phentolamine and phenoxybenzamine, block both the alpha$_1$- and alpha$_2$-adrenergic receptors. Prazosin, however, has a higher affinity for alpha$_1$-adrenergic receptors, and so the alpha$_2$-adrenergic receptors remain responsive to norepinephrine maintaining the negative feedback response for norepinephrine release. As a result, prazosin produces less tachycardia than phentolamine or phenoxybenzamine for equivalent blockade of vascular alpha$_1$-receptors [44].

Prazosin

Prazosin is the most thoroughly studied of the alpha-adrenergic-blocking drugs that have been used in the management of chronic congestive heart failure. Given acutely, prazosin produces hemodynamic effects resembling those of nitroprusside, i.e., a balanced dilation of resistance and capacitance vessels. These effects result in a lowering of the left ventricular filling pressure due to venous pooling of blood and improved cardiac output with enhanced ventricular ejection due to reduced vascular impedance. The reduction of blood pressure in patients with severe congestive heart failure is modest and the heart rate is unchanged. Indirect evidence suggests that myocardial oxygen consumption is reduced, and no direct inotropic properties of prazosin have been discovered. The effects of a single dose of prazosin persists for at least 6 hr [45, 46].

Tolerance to the effects of prazosin develops rapidly with repeated dosing [47–50]. The mechanism of the development of tolerance is unknown. It is not related to reduction in the plasma concentration of the drug during chronic therapy, but rather is related to insensitivity of the vasculature to the drug. The rapid development of tolerance in patients with chronic congestive heart failure is analogous to the 'first-dose' phenomenon described in hypertensive patients given prazosin [51]. In the hypertensive patients, the initial dose of prazosin has a much more potent effect than subsequent doses. However, in both the hypertensive patients and in congestive heart failure patients, long-term therapy with prazosin can produce persistent beneficial effects but requires doses of 16–24 mg/day in many patients [52–54]. Because of the sensitivity to initial doses, prazosin should be begun with a 1-mg dose, and the patient cautioned not to stand up quickly for several hours because of the possibility of orthostatic hypotension. Subsequent doses can be increased depending on the patient's response.

Although originally developed as a drug that would cause vasodilation by inhibiting phosphodiesterase, prazosin is now known to produce its major effects by blocking the alpha$_1$-adrenergic receptor. The drug does have the ability to inhibit phosphodiesterase but only at concentrations several orders of magnitude higher than achieved clinically [51].

Prazosin is nearly entirely metabolized by the liver with less than 10% excreted unchanged in the urine. In normal individuals, prazosin has a half-life of 2.5 hr and a total body clearance of 200–300 ml/min. In patients with heart failure, the half-life is prolonged to 4–6 hr [55, 56]. Renal failure does not seem to alter the kinetics of prazosin [57].

Side effects of prazosin therapy are few. Fluid retention may occur during long-term therapy [53]. Orthostatic hypotension is frequent after the first dose in hypertensive patients but is less common in patients in heart failure with high left ventricular end-diastolic pressure. Headache, weakness, and nausea are uncommon [51]. In rare cases, prazosin therapy has been associated with priapism [58].

Phentolamine and Phenoxybenzamine

Limited data are available on the use of the classical alpha-adrenergic-blocking drugs phentolamine and phenoxybenzamine. Both drugs produce arteriolar and venous dilation, but the arteriolar dilation seems to predominate. This is particularly true with phentolamine, which can produce direct arteriolar vasodilation as well as alpha-adrenergic blockade [59]. When compared to nitroprusside, phentolamine produces less of a change in preload for a given reduction in afterload [45].

Phentolamine has been primarily administered intravenously by constant infusion at rates of 0.3–2 mg/min [26]. Because the drug is very expensive, (marketed as a test substance in 5-mg vials) its prolonged use is impractical. There has been very little experience with long-term oral use of phentolamine and little is known about its metabolism and pharmacokinetics.

Phenoxybenzamine (10–40 mg each 8–12 hr) produces a long-lasting alpha-adrenergic blockade, but experience with its oral administration is limited. One study combined phenoxybenzamine with oral isosorbide dinitrate with apparent benefit, although the contribution of the alpha-adrenergic blockade to the overall response was not assessed directly [60]. The metabolic fate of phenoxybenzamine has not been studied adequately.

Side effects of alpha-adrenergic blockade include orthostatic hypotension, nasal congestion, and inhibition of ejaculation.

Combination therapy

A variety of drug combinations has been given to patients with acute or chronic congestive heart failure. During acute studies a vasodilator, such as nitroprusside, has been combined with an inotropic agent, such as dopamine or dobutamine. The combination has the effects predicted by adding the effects of each agent. In this way, greater increases in cardiac output can be obtained at any given left ventricular end-diastolic pressure than with either a vasodilator or inotropic drug alone [61–63]. Such a combination has its greatest utility in patients with severe cardiac failure in whom a vasodilator alone produces hypotension and cannot increase cardiac output sufficiently, and an inotropic agent alone is insufficiently effective, or concern about augmented myocardial oxygen consumption with worsening myocardial ischemia dictates the use of as little inotropic drug as possible [64].

For chronic therapy, oral inotropic drugs and vasodilators could be combined. The limitation is the lack of available oral inotropic drugs other than the cardiac glycosides, which have limited efficacy. In the future, new inotropic drugs may be marketed to fill this void.

Oral therapy with combinations of vasodilators has been attempted to produce a balanced arteriolar and venous dilation similar to that produced by nitroprusside. Prazosin alone has a balanced effect but long-term effects, although demonstrable, may be insufficient to provide symptomatic relief. Several encouraging studies have been reported with the combination of the arteriolar dilator hydralazine and a long-acting nitrate. Such a combination does appear to produce a balanced decrease in preload and afterload and offers symptomatic improvement [33, 65–67].

The mortality rate for patients with severe heart failure is high. In one study of patients with severe pump failure following a myocardial infarction, 24 of 43 patients survived with parenteral vasodilator therapy and were discharged on oral vasodilators. Fourteen of these 24 patients died within two years of discharge [68]. In another group of patients with chronic congestive failure followed long term on hydralazine (eight patients) or hydralazine/nitrate combination (50 patients) the mortality in the first year was 37%. Those patients that improved clinically had a lower mortality rate than the nonresponders [69]. In no study is it certain that vasodilator therapy has improved survival, but symptomatic relief is produced by vasodilator therapy in some patients. The use of vasodilator therapy in mild to moderate congestive heart failure is yet to be evaluated in comparison with traditional therapy with digitalis and diuretics.

Converting enzyme inhibitors

Plasma renin activity is high in many patients with severe heart failure, and increased levels of angiotensin II may contribute to the elevated systemic vascular resistance in this setting. Inhibition of the formation or action of angiotensin II should reduce the peripheral resistance, decrease cardiac afterload, and improve ventricular performance. Initial experiments with intravenous saralasin, a competitive antagonist of the angiotensin II receptor, and with intravenous teprotide, an inhibitor of the enzyme converting angiotensin I to angiotensin II, indicated that afterload reduction could be accomplished with agents affecting the renin-angiotensin system [70–73]. Since the development of the orally active converting enzyme inhibitor, captopril, chronic treatment of heart failure by inhibiting angiotensin II formation has been accomplished [74–78]. The results to date are very encouraging even in patients who have been resistant to nonspecific vasodilators. Sustained improvement for several months has been documented with chronic captopril treatment. It appears that both preload and afterload are reduced with converting enzyme inhibition [1], although formal comparison of captopril with other agents has not been reported. With teprotide, forearm venous capacitance does not appear to be increased [73], although it is with captopril [74].

The response to captopril is not entirely correlated with the initial plasma renin activity implying that there may be mechanisms of action other than inhibition of converting enzyme [77, 78]. In fact, patients who have low plasma renin activity may respond to captopril. A similar phenomenon has been described in the hypertension literature. These findings indicate that the vasodilation produced by captopril may not be as specific as originally thought [79]. Another known possibility for the action of captopril is that the drug may increase the concentration of the vasodilator, bradykinin, since angiotensin-converting enzyme is the same enzyme that destroys bradykinin.

Only limited data on the pharmacokinetics and metabolism of captopril in humans are available. The drug has been given in doses of 25–150 mg each 8 hr for the treatment of heart failure. In normal volunteers about 75% of an oral dose is absorbed. The drug is a thiol and is metabolized by oxidation to mixed disulfides. The half-life is probably less than 4 hr.

Although usually well tolerated, captopril does have both trivial and serious side effects, and the profile of adverse effects resembles that of penicillamine, another sulfhydryl-containing drug [79]. Rashes are reported in up to 15% of patients. Serum sickness may occur with fever and rash. Persistant metallic or salty taste occurs in about 6% of patients. Leukopenia or agranulocytosis has occurred and appears to be reversible unless patients become septic and expire. Nephrotic syndrome or proteinuria has been reported in about 2% of cases treated for eight months or more, but most of these patients were hypertensive with preexisting renal disease, and the relation to drug therapy is uncertain. A recent report indicates that captopril may be associated with immune complex deposits along the glomerular basement membrane in patients without any proteinuria or renal symptoms [80].

In view of the experimental nature of the drug and the occasional severe side effects, captopril therapy should be reserved for patients who do not respond to other therapy for heart failure. Nonetheless, the drug has opened a heretofore unexplored area, and newer converting enzyme inhibitors that do not produce severe side effects would seem to offer high promise.

Drug therapy of angina pectoris

Angina pectoris is a syndrome of chest pain due to myocardial ischemia that is produced when myocardial oxygen demands exceed the available supply. The syndrome usually occurs in patients with fixed coronary lesions and is precipitated by increases in oxygen demands because of increases in heart rate, wall tension, or contractility. Since the heart has little ability to operate anaerobically, and the extraction of oxygen from coronary arterial blood is near maximum, the only way the heart can receive more oxygen during periods of increased demand is by an increase in coronary blood flow. When coronary stenosis occurs, the resistance vessels distal to the stenosis dilate to keep coronary flow normal. When stenosis is severe, however, the resistance vessels cannot dilate further, and any increase in oxygen demand will result in ischemia.

Although most cases of angina pectoris are due to fixed critical coronary artery stenoses, some cases are due, at least in part, to a reduction in oxygen delivery to the myocardium rather than an increased oxygen demand. Coronary artery spasm has been increasingly recognized as a cause of angina pectoris. Platelet plugging, hypoxemia, or a reduction in oxygen carrying capacity of the blood, such as by carbon monoxide or methemoglobinemia produced by smoking, may also be important in a few patients.

When the myocardium becomes ischemic, it contracts less well and the left ventricular end-diastolic pressure rises. Angina pectoris, therefore, is associated with a transient, reversible period of acute heart failure that further increases wall tension and myocardial oxygen demands at the same time as the high diastolic filling pressures of the ventricle reduce the pressure gradient for coronary blood flow to the subendocardium. It is the subendocardium, therefore, that is most vulnerable to ischemia. Classical angina pectoris occurs at a similar heart rate–systolic blood pressure product indicating the crucial level of work load where myocardial oxygen demands exceed the supply. Medical management of angina pectoris generally is intended to reduce myocardial oxygen demand, although in some instances an increase in oxygen supply is important.

Nitrates

Nitroglycerin has been the primary treatment of angina pectoris for over 100 years [81]. It was originally thought to act as a coronary dilator and increase oxygen delivery to the myocardium since it will increase total coronary blood flow in normal individuals. However, total coronary blood flow is not increased by nitroglycerin in patients with angina pectoris due to fixed coronary obstruction, and the major beneficial effect of the drug appears to be venodilation with a reduction of cardiac preload and a resultant reduction in left ventricular size, wall tension, and myocardial oxygen demands [82]. The small reduction of systemic vascular resistance and thus afterload produced by nitroglycerin also reduces left ventricular wall stress and

contributes to the reduced myocardial oxygen consumption and the relief of ischemia. Frequently the heart rate is slightly increased by nitroglycerin, probably due to reflex sympathethic activation. The increase in heart rate may increase myocardial oxygen demand, but the overall effect of the nitroglycerin is to reduce oxygen demand (Table 1).

The most convincing demonstration that an increase in total coronary blood flow is not the important factor in response of classical angina pectoris to nitroglycerin was the finding that intracoronary administration of nitroglycerin did not relieve angina pectoris induced by pacing even though total coronary blood flow increased. Intravenous nitroglycerin, on the other hand, did relieve the pacing-induced angina at a time when total coronary blood flow was actually decreased [83].

Although an increase in total coronary blood flow is not the explanation for the beneficial effect of nitroglycerin in angina, there is evidence that nitroglycerin administration redistributes coronary blood flow to favor the ischemic subendocardial region, improves contraction of ischemic areas of myocardium, and increases the ejection of blood from the left ventricle, which contributes to the reduced ventricular volume [84–87]. There are two possible explanations for this redistribution of coronary blood flow. It could be due to an increased pressure gradient for coronary perfusion of the ischemic subendocardium because of a reduction in left ventricular end-diastolic pressure. This effect is indirect and results from the peripheral action of nitroglycerin to reduce preload [88, 89]. The other

Table 1. Drug effects in angina pectoris.

| | Nitrates | Beta-adrenergic blockers | Calcium channel blockers | |
			Verapamil	Nifedipine
Heart rate				
Rest	↑	↓↓	±↓	↑
Exercise	0	↓↓	0	0
Wall tension				
Ventricular volume	↓↓	±↑	±	↓
Systolic pressure	↓	↓	↓	↓
Contractility	±↑	↓	↓	±
Coronary spasm	Block	±? Increase	Block	Block
Myocardial oxygen demands	↓	↓	↓	↓

443

possibility for the redistribution of coronary blood flow is that nitroglycerin dilates conductance (large coronary) vessels to increase flow through a stenotic area or through collaterals supplying an ischemic area. Nitroglycerin clearly seems to have effects to dilate larger coronary vessels [90, 91] and experimentally can redistribute coronary blood flow in the absence of changes in heart size, hemodynamic parameters, or total coronary flow [92]. Intracoronary injections of nitroglycerin in patients with coronary artery disease recently have been shown to directly increase the diameter of the coronary arteries without improving left ventricular function, left ventricular volume, or left ventricular end-diastolic pressure [93]. These data imply that the major salutary actions of nitroglycerin in relieving cardiac ischemia are indirect in spite of the demonstrable effects on the coronary vessels.

Although the debate continues regarding the therapeutic importance of the direct coronary vascular effects of nitroglycerin in patients with classical angina pectoris, there is no question that the direct coronary vascular effects are important for those patients in whom coronary spasm produces the angina pectoris [94].

Long-acting nitrates have been shown to increase significantly the amount of exercise performed before angina occurs in patients with coronary artery disease [95–98] presumably on the basis of the beneficial alterations of hemodynamics discussed in the section on unloading therapy of congestive heart failure. It is important that adequate and frequent dosages be administered to provide around-the-clock hemodynamic improvement. Representative doses are: sublingual isosorbide dinitrate 5–20 mg every 4 hr, oral isosorbide dinitrate 10–40 mg orally every 4–6 hr, nitroglycerin ointment 1–3″ every 4–6 hr, sustained-release oral nitroglycerin 6.5–13 mg every 6–8 hr.

Although partial tolerance to some of the hemodynamic effect of nitrates has been demonstrated as discussed in the previous section, the antianginal effects of nitrates are not greatly reduced during chronic nitrate therapy, and repeated efficacy of nitroglycerin can be demonstrated even after a month of isosorbide dinitrate, 40 mg each 8 hr [99].

An unusual syndrome of nonocclusive coronary disease has been reported in normal individuals exposed to high concentrations of nitrates in industry [100, 101]. It is postulated that nitrate dependence is produced such that coronary vasospasm may occur when the workers are rapidly removed from the nitrate exposure. In view of these reports, high-dose, long-term nitrate therapy probably should not be abruptly discontinued.

Beta-adrenergic-blocking drugs

The initial impetus for the discovery of drugs that block beta-adrenergic receptors was that such drugs might be useful for the treatment of angina pectoris. The reasoning was that myocardial oxygen demands were increased by sympathetically mediated increases in heart rate and contractility, and drugs that blocked the cardiac effects of sympathetic stimulation might therefore be beneficial [102]. The reasoning has proven to be correct, and the beta-adrenergic-blocking drugs are now firmly established along with the nitrates as a major medical therapy for angina pectoris.

The principal mode of action of the beta-adrenergic-blocking drugs in angina pectoris is to reduce the tachycardia, the increased force of contraction and the blood pressure response to stresses, such as exercise, that increase myocardial oxygen demands. The patients can therefore perform more exercise with a lower heart rate–pressure product and hence with a lower myocardial oxygen demand while taking a beta-adrenergic-blocking drug. Since sympathetic activity is minimal at rest, the beta-adrenergic-blocking drugs have relatively little effect on resting myocardial consumption. Beta-adrenergic blockade can result in an increase in ventricular size and an increase in systolic ejection time, both of which may increase myocardial oxygen demands. The overall effect of beta-adrenergic blockade, however, clearly is to decrease oxygen demands (Table 1). Patients who have angina pectoris produced by coronary vasospasm frequently are not improved with beta-adrenergic-blocking drugs, and some patients may actually deteriorate.

As described in Chapter 6, the available beta-adrenergic-blocking drugs may be nonselective blockers (such as propranolol, timolol, and nadolol), or they may be relatively selective for cardiac beta-adrenergic receptors (such as metoprolol and atenolol). There does not appear to be any difference in antianginal efficacy between the two types of beta-adrenergic-blocking drugs [103]. Beta-adrenergic-blocking drugs also may have membrane stabilizing properties, or they may directly stimulate beta-adrenergic receptors, the so-called intrinsic sympathetic activity. Membrane stabilization is unimportant in antianginal efficacy as indicated by the finding that d-propranolol, which possesses membrane stabilizing activity but produces little beta-adrenergic blockade, is ineffective in angina pectoris [104]. Intrinsic sympathomimetic activity does not seem to reduce or enhance the effectiveness of beta-adrenergic-blocking drugs in the treatment of exercise-induced angina [103]. However, because resting heart rate is reduced little or not at all by beta-adrenergic-blocking drugs with intrinsic sympathomimetic activity, angina occurring at rest in the absence of coronary spasm may benefit more from drugs without this property [105].

The doses of beta-adrenergic-blocking drugs required for adequate therapy of angina pectoris are variable but generally modest and within the range needed to block exercise-induced tachycardia in normal individuals. For propranolol, the blood levels that are needed for improvement of angina pectoris vary from 10–100 ng/ml, which corresponds to concentrations necessary to produce 50–100% inhibition of sympathetically mediated exercise tachycardia in normals [106]. Because of the wide interindividual variability in antianginal response, plasma concentrations of the beta-blocking drugs cannot predict the dose at which maximum improvement will occur. Therefore, when beginning therapy in patients with angina pectoris, low doses of beta-adrenergic blockers should be used. Most patients have maximal improvement in exercise tolerance at some dose, and that improvement may be diminished if the dose is increased. The deterioration with too high a dose may be related to reduction in exercise tolerance due to fatigue. The optimum dose is best determined by blockade of exercise tachycardia during treadmill testing; resting heart rate is a relatively poor way to judge dose [107]. It now appears that the duration of action of propranolol and other beta-adrenergic-blocking drugs is sufficiently long to allow twice daily dosing [103, 108]. For nadolol, once daily dosing should suffice.

Propranolol has been found to produce two other effects that in theory could improve angina pectoris. One group of investigators has found that chronic propranolol therapy shifts the oxyhemo- globin dissociation curve to the right, indicating that the affinity of hemoglobin for oxygen is reduced, oxygen can be more easily given up to the tissues, and therefore oxygen delivery to ischemic myocardium may be increased [109]. Whether this effect is produced by beta-adrenergic-blocking drugs other than propranolol is unknown. There is probably little importance to this effect in any event since exercise-induced angina pectoris is produced in patients taking propranolol at a heart rate–blood pressure product that is similar to, or even less than, the heart rate–pressure product prior to beta-adrenergic blockade, implying no enhancement of oxygen delivery to ischemic myocardium [110]. The second potentially beneficial effect described for propranolol is suppression of platelet aggregation. Some patients with coronary artery disease have hyperaggregable platelets that will revert to normal during propranolol administration in therapeutic doses [111, 112]. It is postulated that platelet aggregation may be contributing to the inadequate oxygen supply in patients with angina pectoris. However, for the reasons outlined above, it seems unlikely that an enhancement of oxygen delivery is an important effect of beta-adrenergic blockade in the therapy of angina pectoris.

The pharmacokinetics, metabolism, and side effects of beta-adrenergic-blocking drugs have been discussed in Chapter 6. It is important to realize that nitrates and beta-adrenergic-blocking drugs act by entirely different mechanisms to reduce myocardial oxygen demand, and the effect of the drugs are additive (Table 1). Beta-adrenergic blockade can reduce the tachycardia sometimes produced by reflex sympathetic activation during nitrate therapy, and nitrates can reduce the left ventricular size and systolic ejection time that is a consequence of beta-adrenergic blockade. Digoxin has also been used to reduce cardiac size in patients on propranolol who develop an enlarged left ventricle [113].

There is considerable clinical and investigative interest in the potential problems that occur when therapy with beta-adrenergic-blocking drugs is discontinued. The initial reports suggested that a high percentage of patients were at risk for for the development of unstable or crescendo angina pectoris, myocardial infarction, arrhythmias, or sudden death when therapy was stopped abruptly [114, 115]. Recently, it appears that only 1–5% of patients with angina pectoris have problems when beta-adrenergic blockade is terminated. The patients who develop the problems are generally those who have had considerable benefit from beta-adrenergic blockade and in whom the drug has been withdrawn while they are ambulatory. If therapy with beta-adrenergic blockade is to be discontinued, it is prudent to hospitalize the patient and/or use a gradually tapering regimen and caution patients to reduce their activity.

The mechanisms whereby propranolol withdrawal may produce problems is not entirely understood [116]. Effective beta-adrenergic blockade decreases platelet aggregability, plasma renin activity, and the cardiac response to exercise. When propranolol is discontinued these effects disappear quickly. Patients accustomed to a certain level of activity may rapidly find they are unable to perform as well off therapy as on therapy. Progression of the coronary disease may have been masked during beta-adrenergic blockade producing an apparent rebound effect upon propranolol withdrawal. In addition, some investigators have described hyperresponsiveness to beta-sympathomimetic drugs shortly after withdrawal of propranolol in normal volunteers or hypertensive patients [117, 118], and plasma renin activity overshoots in the first few days after propranolol withdrawal [119]. Experimental studies in animals and humans have suggested that the density of beta-adrenergic receptors in the tissues increases during propranolol treatment, and this increase persists for a short time following drug elimination [120, 121]. These findings might explain an increased response to sympathomimetics following propranolol withdrawal. However, since not all investigators find an increased responsiveness to catecholamines during the withdrawal period, the mechanism and even the existence of the withdrawal phenomenon remain topics for continued investigation [122].

Calcium channel blocking agents

Several drugs have been developed to inhibit the slow inward flux of positive ions into cardiac and vascular smooth muscle cells. These agents called 'calcium channel blocking' agents are being developed as antiarrhythmic, antianginal, and antihypertensive drugs. Calcium is required for contraction of muscle and also has important effects on the electrophysiology of cardiac cells (see Chapter 1).

Blockade of calcium entry into the cardiac cells can reduce cardiac contractility, slow impulse generation in the sinoatrial node, and reduce impulse conduction and prolong the effective refractory period of atrioventricular nodal tissue. Although these cardiac effects resemble the effects of beta-adrenergic-blocking drugs, the actions of the calcium channel blockers are not mediated by the autonomic nervous system. In vascular smooth muscle, the calcium channel blocking agents reduce the amount of calcium available to initiate contraction. The vasodilation thus produced is in contrast to the effects of beta-adrenergic-blocking drugs. Also, the calcium channel blockers do not increase bronchiolar resistance and therefore are not contraindicated in asthma or chronic lung disease, a distinct advantage over the beta-adrenergic blockers.

The potential beneficial effects of the calcium channel blocking drugs in angina pectoris are several. The drugs may reduce myocardial oxygen consumption by reducing heart rate and contractility due to their cardiac effects. In addition, they can relieve coronary spasm and produce coronary and peripheral vasodilation thus reducing afterload and, in some cases, improving oxygen delivery to the myocardium. In this way, these drugs possess the potential to achieve effects similar to those produced by a combination of beta-adrenergic-blocking drugs and nitrates. The peripheral vascular effects of the calcium channel blockers differ from those of nitrates, however, in that the calcium channel blockers have a predominant effect on arterioles and little effect on veins so that preload is relatively unchanged.

Of the drugs being investigated, verapamil, nifedipine, and diltiazem have been investigated most thoroughly. A detailed description of these drugs may be found in one of the several recent reviews and symposia dealing with calcium channel blockade [123–128]. Although they are grouped together, it is clear that the various calcium channel blocking drugs are quite different. The drugs are structurally dissimilar and have different relative potencies for their cardiac and vascular effects. Additionally, the vasodilation produced by some of the drugs may activate reflex mechanisms that can counteract the direct cardiac effects. Finally, it is not at all certain that blockade of calcium channels is the only way in which these drugs exert their effects.

As a result of these differences, the net hemodynamic effects of the various calcium channel blocking drugs show great variation. Nifedipine produces arteriolar dilation at doses that produce little depression of cardiac contractility or heart rate. Because of the decrease in peripheral resistance, the sympathetic nervous system is activated and counteracts the small, direct, negative inotropic, chronotropic and dromotropic effects. Verapamil, on the other hand, produces much greater cardiac effects for the same degree of peripheral vasodilation. Therefore, whereas nifedipine produces effects resembling those of the arteriolar vasodilators, the net hemodynamic effects of verapamil include a negative dromotropic effect, particularly at the AV node, and can produce negative inotropic and chronotropic effects especially if the cardiac beta-adrenergic receptors are blocked. Diltiazem has been studied less than the other two drugs but seems to produce effects intermediate between them.

The calcium channel blockers seem to be ideal for the treatment of angina pectoris due to coronary artery spasm in contrast to the beta-adrenergic blockers that do little for spasm-induced ischemia and may actually make it worse. Nifedipine in doses of 40–160 mg/day has proven to be effective in nearly 90% of patients with spasm-induced angina [129]. Verapamil in doses of 120–320 mg/day has also produced encouraging results [125]. Although less well studied, diltiazem at 120 mg/day has been effective in a small number of patients [129]. The effectiveness of all these agents in classical angina pectoris has also been shown in an ever increasing number of studies. The calcium channel antagonists reduce the pressure–rate product at submaximal exercise indicating a reduction of myocardial oxygen demands. At the onset of angina, however, the pressure–rate product is similar during treatment and control periods indicating that for classical angina the drugs are beneficial by decreasing myocardial oxygen demand rather than increasing oxygen delivery to ischemic areas. In general, the calcium channel blockers are about as effective as nitrates or beta-adrenergic-blocking drugs for classical angina pectoris although the data for diltiazem are too scanty to make a judgement at this time.

Combination therapy with nifedipine and beta-adrenergic blockers has been evaluated. Because nifedipine acts similarly to a vasodilator, the combination is rational and has been shown to produce effects greater that either drug alone. Little is known about combinations with verapamil or diltiazem. Because verapamil exhibits considerable negative dromotropic and inotropic effects relative to peripheral vascular effects, the addition of beta-adrenergic blockade can result in deleterious cardiac depression.

The pharmacokinetics of the drugs differ [123–128]. Nifedipine is well absorbed and can be administered orally or sublingually. Most of the drug is metabolized with a half-life of about 4 hr. The dose range is 30–120 mg daily in three to six divided doses. Verapamil can be given orally or intravenously. When given orally, verapamil is well absorbed by the gut, but 80–90% of the oral dose is metabolized in the first pass through the liver. The clearance of the drug approximates liver blood flow, and the half-life is 3–4 hr in normals. In patients with liver disease the clearance is reduced and the half-life is prolonged to 13 hr [131]. The I.V. dose is 5–10 mg, and the oral dose is 80–160 mg. Diltiazem is rapidly and completely absorbed from the intestine and has a half-life of about 4 hr. It usually is given orally in doses of 30–90 mg every 8 hr.

Side effects of these drugs include headache, flushing, and hypotension. Verapamil in particular can produce atrioventricular conduction disturbances, and bradycardia or asystole may occur if verapamil is combined with a beta-adrenergic blocker. Only rarely is cardiac failure produced by these drugs, and some patients with cardiac failure may be improved because of the afterload reduction produced, particularly by nifedipine.

References

1. Vrobel TR, Cohn JN: Comparative hemodynamic effects of converting enzyme inhibitor and sodium nitroprusside in severe heart failure. Am J Cardiol 45:331–336, 1980.
2. MacKenzie JE, Parratt JR: Comparative effects of glyceryil trinitrate on venous and arterial smooth muscle in vitro: relevance to antianginal activity. Br J Pharmacol 60:155–160, 1977.
3. Gray R, Chatterjee J, Vyden JK, Gana W, Forrester JS, Swan HJC: Hemodynamic and metabolic effects of isosorbide dinitrate in chronic congestive heart failure. Am Heart J 90:346–352, 1975.
4. Awan NA, Miller RR, Maxwell KS, Mason DT: Cardiocirculatory and antianginal actions of nitroglycerin oint-

ment. Evaluation by cardiac catheterization, forearm plethysmography and treadmill stress testing. Chest 73:14–18, 1978.

5. Franciosa JA, Blank RC, Cohn JN: Nitrate effects on cardiac output and left ventricular outflow resistence in chronic congestive heart failure. Am J Med 64:207–213, 1978.

6. Needleman P, Johnson EM: Mechanism of tolerance development for organic nitrates. J Pharmacol Exp Ther 184:709–715, 1973.

7. Armstrong JA, Marks GS, Armstrong PW: Absence of metabolite formation during nitroglycerin induced relaxation of isolated blood vessels. Mol Pharmacol 18:112–116, 1980.

8. Katsuk S, Murad F: Regulation of adenosine cycle 3′,5′-monophosphate and guanosine cyclic 3′, 5′-monophosphate levels and contractility in bovine tracheal smooth muscle. Mol Pharmacol 13:330–341, 1977.

9. Axelsson KL, Wikberg JES, Andersson RGG: Relationship between nitroglycerin, cyclic GMP and relaxation of vascular smooth muscle. Life Sci 24:1779–1786, 1979.

10. Armstrong PW, Armstrong JA, Marks GS: Pharmacokinetic-hemodynamic studies of intravenous nitroglycerin in congestive cardiac failure. Circulation 62:160–166, 1980.

11. Wei J, Reid PR: Quantitative determination of trinitroglycerin in human plasma. Circulation 59:588–592, 1979.

12. Armstrong PW, Armstrong JA, Marks GS: Blood levels after sublingual nitroglycerin. Circulation 59:585–588, 1979.

13. Armstrong PW, Armstrong JA, Marks GS: Pharmacokinetic-hemodynamic studies of nitroglycerin ointment in congestive heart failure. Am J Cardiol 46:670–676, 1980.

14. Strumza P, Regand M, Mechmeche R, Rocha P, Baudet M, Bardet J, Bourdarias JP: Prolonged hemodynamic effects (12 hours) of orally administered sustained release nitroglycerin. Am J Cardiol 43:272–277, 1979.

15. Thadani U, Fung H-L, Darke AC, Parker JO: Oral isosorbide dinitrate in the treatment of angina pectoris. Dose-response relationship and duration of action during acute therapy. Circulation 62:491–502, 1980.

16. Williams DO, Bommer WJ, Miller RR, Amsterdam EA, Mason DT: Hemodynamic assessment of oral peripheral vasodilator therapy in chronic congestive heart failure: prolonged effectiveness of isosorbide dinitrate. Am J Cardiol 39:84–90, 1977.

17. McGuinness BW, Harris EL: 'Monday head'. An interesting occupational disorder. Br Med J 2:745–747, 1961.

18. Thadani U, Manyari D, Parker JP, Fung H-L: Tolerance to the circulatory effect of oral isosorbide dinitrate. Rate of development and cross-tolerance to glyceryl trinitrate. Circulation 61:526–535, 1980.

19. Schelling J, Lasagna L: A study of cross tolerance to circulating effects of organic nitrates. Clin Pharmacol Ther 8: 256–260, 1967.

20. Mehta J, Iacona M, Pepine CJ, Conti CR: Comparison of haemodynamic effects of oral prazosin, oral hydralazine, and intravenous nitroprusside in same patients with chronic heart failure. Br Heart J 42:664–670, 1979.

21. Chatterjee K, Perts TA, Arnold S, Brundage B, Parmley W: Comparison of haemodynamic effects of oral hydralazine and prazosin hydrochloride in patients with chronic congestive heart failure. Br Heart J 42:657–663, 1979.

22. Chatterjee K, Parmley WW, Massie B, Greenberg B, Werner J, Klausner S, Norman A: Oral hydralzine therapy for chronic refractory heart failure. Circulation 54:879–883, 1976.

23. Packer M, Meller J, Medina N, Gorlin R, Herman MV: Importance of left ventricular chamber size in determining the response to hydralazine in severe chronic heart failure. N Engl J Med 303:250–255, 1980.

24. Khatri I, Uemura N, Notargiacomo A, Freis ED: Direct and reflex cardio stimulating effects of hydralazine. Am J Cardiol 40:38–42, 1977.

25. Mason DT: Afterload reduction and cardiac performance. Physiologic basis of systemic vasodilators as a new approach in treatment of congestive heart failure. Am J Med 65:106–125, 1978.

26. Packer M, Meller J, Medina N, Gorlin R, Herman MV: Dose requirements of hydralazine in patients with severe chronic heart failure. Am J Cardiol 45:655–660, 1980.

27. Shepherd AMM, Ludden TM, McNay JL, Lin M-S: Hydralazine kinetics after single and repeated oral doses. Clin Pharmacol Ther 28:804–811, 1980.

28. Ludden TM, Shepherd AMM, McNay JL, Lin M-S: Hydralazine kinetics in hypertensive patients after intravenous administration. Clin Pharmacol Ther 28: 736–742, 1980.

29. Reece PA, Cozamanis I, Zacest R: Kinetics of hydralazine and its main metabolites in slow and fast acetylators. Clin Pharmacol Ther 28:769–778, 1980.

30. Moore-Jones D, Perry HM: Radioautographic localization of hydralazine I-C^{14} in arterial wall. Proc Soc Exp Biol Med 122:576–579, 1966.

31. Perry HM: Late toxicity to hydralazine resembling systemic lupus erythematosus or rheumatoid arthritis. Am J Med 54:58–72, 1973.

32. Linas SL, Nies AS: Minoxidil. Ann Intern Med 94:61–65, 1981.

33. Chatterjee K, Drew D, Parmley WW, Klausner SC, Polonsky J, Zacherle MD: Combination vasodilator therapy for severe chronic congestive heart failure. Ann Intern Med 85:467–470, 1976.

34. Bhatia SK, Froehlich ED: Hemodynamic comparison of agents useful in hypertensive emergencies. Am Heart J 85: 367–373, 1973.

35. Miller RR, Vismira LA, Williams DO, Amsterdam EA, Mason DT: Pharmacologic mechanisms for left ventricular unloading in clinical congestive heart failure. Differential effects of nitroprusside, phentolamine and nitroglycerin on cardiac function and peripheral circulation. Cir Res 39:127–133, 1976.

36. Miller RR, Mason DT, Zelis R, Amsterdam EA, Mason DT: Clinical use of sodium nitroprusside in chronic ischemic heart disease: effects on peripheral vascular resistance and venous tone and on ventricular volume, pump and mechanical function. Circulation 51:328–336, 1975.

37. Daluz PL, Forrester JS, Wyatt HL, Tyberg JV, Chagrasulis R, Parmley WW, Swan HJC: Hemodynamic and metabolic sodium nitroprusside on the performance and metabolism of regional ischemic myocardium. Circulation

52:400–407, 1975.

38. Miller RR, Awan NA, Kamiyima T, Mason DT: Relations between systemic pressure, coronary blood flow, regional myocardial ischemia and energetics with impendence reduction by nitroprusside in experimental coronary stenosis. Circulation 56 (Suppl 3):150, 1977.

39. Mann T, Cohn PF, Holman L, Green LH, Markis JE, Phillips DA: Effect of nitroprusside on regional myocardial blood flow in coronary artery disease. Results in 25 patients and comparison with nitroglycerin. Circulation 57:732–738, 1978.

40. Cohn JN: Nitroprusside. Ann Intern Med 91:752–757, 1979.

41. Packer M, Meller J, Medina N, Gorlin R, Herman MV: Rebound hemodynamic events after the abrupt withdrawal of nitroprusside in patients with severe chronic heart failure. N Engl J Med 301:1193–1197, 1979.

42. Cottrell JE, Illner P, Kittay MJ, Steele JM, Lowenstein J, Turndorf H: Rebound hypertension after sodium nitroprusside-induced hypotension. Clin Pharmacol Ther 27:32–36, 1980.

43. Gerber JG, Nies AS: Abrupt withdrawal of cardiovascular drugs. N Engl J Med 301:1234–1235, 1979.

44. Brogden RN, Heel RC, Speight TM, Avery GS: Prazosin: a review of its pharmacological properties and therapeutic efficacy in hypertension. Drugs 14:163–197, 1977.

45. Awan NA, Miller RR, Mason DT: Comparison of effects of nitroprusside and prazosin on left ventricular function and the peripheral circulation in chronic refractory congestive heart failure. Circulation 57:152–159, 1978.

46. Mehta J, Iacona M, Feldman R, Pepine CJ, Conti CR: Comparative hemodynamic effects of intravenous nitroprusside and oral prazosin in refractory heart failure. Am J Cardiol 41:925–930, 1978.

47. Elkayam U, Lejemtel TH, Mathew M, Rebner HS, Frishman WH, Strom J, Sonnenblick EH: Marked early attenuation of hemodynamic effects of oral prazosin therapy in chronic congestive heart failure. Am J Cardiol 44:540–545, 1979.

48. Packer M, Meller J, Gorlin R, Herman MV: Hemodynamic and clinical tachyphylaxis to prazosin-mediated afterload reduction in severe chronic congestive heart failure. Circulation 59:531–539, 1979.

49. Desch CE, Magorien RD, Triffon DW, Blanford MF, Unverferth DV, Leier CV: Development of pharmacodynamic tolerance to prazosin in congestive heart failure. Am J Cardiol 44:1178–1182, 1979.

50. Arnold SB, Williams RL, Ports TA, Baughman RA, Benet LZ, Parmley WW, Chatterjee K: Attenuation of prazosin effect on cardiac output in chronic heart failure. Ann Intern Med 91:345–349, 1979.

51. Graham RM, Pettinger WA: Prazosin. N Engl J Med 300:232–235, 1979.

52. Aronow WS, Lurie M, Turbow M, Whittaker K, Van Camp S, Hughes D: Effect of prazosin vs placebo on chronic left ventricular heart failure. Circulation 59:344–350, 1979.

53. Goldman SA, Johnson LL, Escala E, Cannon PJ, Weiss MB: Improved exercise ejection fraction with long-term prazosin therapy in patients with heart failure. Am J Med

68:36–42, 1980.

54. Colucci WS, Wynne J, Holman BL, Braunwald E: Long-term therapy of heart failure with prazosin: a randomized double blind trial. Am J Cardiol 45:337–344, 1980.

55. Jaillon P, Rubin P, Yee Y-G, Ball R, Kates R, Harrison D, Blaschke T: Influence of congestive heart failure on prazosin kinetics. Clin Pharmacol Ther 25: 790–794, 1979.

56. Jaillon P: Clinical pharmacokinetics of prazosin. Clin Pharmacokinet 5:365–376, 1980.

57. Lowenthal DT, Hobbs D, Affrime MB, Twomey TM, Martinez EW, Onesti G: Prazosin kinetics and effectiveness in renal failure. Clin Pharmacol Ther 27:779–783, 1980.

58. Bhalla AK, Hoffbrand BI, Phatak PS, Reuben SR: Prazosin and priapism. Br Med J 2:1039, 1979.

59. Taylor SH, Sutherland GR, MacKenzie GJ, Staunton HP, Donald KW: The circulatory effects of intravenous phentolamine in man. Circulation 31:741–754, 1965.

60. Kovick RB, Tillich JH, Berens SC, Bramowitz AD, Shine KI: Vasodilator therapy for chronic left ventricular failure. Circulation 59:322–328, 1976.

61. Mikulic E, Cohn JN, Franciosa JA: Comparative hemodynamic effects of inotropic and vasodilator drugs in severe heart failure. Circulation 56:528–533, 1977.

62. Miller RR, Awan NA, Joyce JA, Maxwell KS, DeMaria AN, Amsterdam EA, Mason DT: Combined dopamine and nitroprusside therapy in congestive heart failure. Greater augmentation of cardiac performance by addition of inotropic stimulation to afterload reduction. Circulation 55:881–884, 1977.

63. Stemple DR, Kleiman JH, Harrison DC: Combined nitroprusside-dopamine therapy in severe chronic congestive heart failure. Dose-related hemodynamic advantages over single drug infusions. Am J Cardiol 42:267–275, 1978.

64. Cohn JN, Franciosa JA: Selection of vasodilator, inotropic or combined therapy for the management of heart failure. Am J Med 65:181–188, 1978.

65. Franciosa JA, Cohn JN: Immediate effects of hydralazine-isosorbide dinitrate combination on exercise capacity and exercise hemodynamics in patients with left ventricular failure. Circulation 59:1085–1091, 1979.

66. Massie B, Chatterjee K, Werner J, Greenberg B, Hart R, Parmley WW: Hemodynamic advantage of combined administration of hydralazine orally and nitrates non-parenterally in the vasodilator therapy of chronic heart failure. Am J Cardiol 40:794–801, 1977.

67. Chatterjee K, Massie B, Rubin S, Gelberg H, Brundage BH, Ports TA: Long-term outpatient vasodilator therapy of congestive heart failure. Consideration of agents at rest and during exercise. Am J Med 65:134–145, 1978.

68. Chatterjee K, Swan HJC, Kaushik VS, Jobin G, Magnuson P, Forrester JS: Effects of vasodilator therapy for severe pump failure in acute myocardial infarction on short-term and late prognosis. Circulation 53:797–802, 1976.

69. Massie B, Ports T, Chatterjee K, Parmley W, Ostland J, O'Young J, Hanghom F: Long-term vasodilator therapy for heart failure: clinical response and its relationship to hemodynamic measurements. Circulation 63:269–278, 1981.

449

70. Curtiss C, Cohn JN, Vrobel T, Franciosa JA: Role of the renin-angiotensin system in the systemic vasoconstriction of chronic congestive heart failure. Circulation 38:763–770, 1978.

71. Gavras H, Faxon DP, Berkoben J, Brunner HR, Ryan TJ: Angiotensin converting enzyme inhibition in patients with congestive heart failure. Circulation 58:770–776, 1978.

72. Gavras H, Flessas A, Tyan TJ, Brunner HR, Flaxon DP, Gavras I: Angiotensin II inhibition. Treatment of congestive heart failure in a high-renin hypertension. J Am Med Assoc 238:880–882, 1977.

73. Faxon DP, Creager MA, Halperin JL, Gavras H, Coffman JD, Ryan TJ: Central and peripheral hemodynamic effects of angiotensin inhibition in patients with refractory congestive heart failure. Circulation 61:925–930, 1980.

74. Awan NA, Evenson MK, Needham KE, Win A, Mason DT: Efficacy of oral angiotensin converting enzyme inhibition with captopril therapy in severe chronic normotensive congestive heart failure. Am Heart J 101:22–31, 1981.

75. Ader R, Chatterjee K, Ports T, Brundage B, Hiramatsu B, Parmley W: Immediate and sustained hemodynamic and clinical improvement in chronic heart failure by an oral angiotensin-converting enzyme inhibitor. Circulation 61:931–937, 1980.

76. Dzau VJ, Colucci WS, Williams GH, Curfman G, Meggs L, Hollenberger NK: Sustained effectiveness of converting-enzyme inhibition in patients with severe congestive heart failure. N Engl J Med 302:1373–1379, 1980.

77. Levine TB, Franciosa JA, Cohn JN: Acute and long-term response to an oral converting-enzyme inhibitor, captopril, in congestive heart failure. Circulation 62:35–41, 1980.

78. Davis R, Rebner HS, Keung E, Sonnenblick EH, LeJemtel TH: Treatment of chronic congestive heart failure with captopril, an oral inhibitor of angiotensin-converting enzyme. N Engl J Med 301:117–121, 1979.

79. Heel RC, Brogden RN, Speight TM, Avery GS: Captopril: a preliminary review of its pharmacological properties and therapeutic efficacy. Drugs 20:409–452, 1980.

80. Hoorntje SJ, Kallenberg CGM, Weening JJ, Donker ABJM, The TH, Hoedemacker PJ: Immune-complex glomerulopathy in patients treated with captopril. Lancet 1:1212–1215, 1980.

81. Lead article, Nitroglycerin – the first hundred years. Lancet 2:1340–1341, 1979.

82. Greenberg H, Dwyer EM Jr, Jameson AG, Pinkerneys VH: Effects of nitroglycerin on the major determinants of myocardial oxygen consumption. Angiographic and hemodynamic assessment. Am J Cardiol 36:426–432, 1975.

83. Ganz W, Marcus HS: Failure of intracoronary nitroglycerin to alleviate pacing-induced angina. Circulation 46:880–889, 1972.

84. Cohn PF, Maddox D, Holma BL, Markis JE, Adams DF, See JR: Effect of sublingually administered nitroglycerin on regional myocardial blood flow in patients with coronary artery disease. Am J Cardiol 39:672–678, 1977.

85. Sharma B, Hodges M, Asinger RW, Goodwin JF, Francis GD: Left ventricular function during spontaneous angina pectoris: effect of sublingual nitroglycerin. Am J Cardiol 46:34–41, 1980.

86. Helfant RH, Pine R, Meister SG, Feldman MS, Traut RG, Vanka VS: Nitroglycerin to unmask reversible asynergy: correlation with post coronary bypass ventriculography. Circulation 50:108–113, 1974.

87. Mehta J, Pepine CJ: Effect of sublingual nitroglycerin on regional flow in patients with and without coronary disease. Circulation 58:803–807, 1978.

88. Parratt JR: Recent advances in the pathophysiology and pharmacology of angina. Gen Pharmacol 6:247–251, 1979.

89. Gross GJ, Warltier DC: Intracoronary versus intravenous nitroglycerin on the transmural distribution of coronary blood flow. Cardiovasc Res 11:499–506, 1977.

90. Feldman RL, Pepine CJ, Curry RC, Conti CR: Coronary arterial responses to graded doses of nitroglycerin. Am J Cardiol 43:91–97, 1979.

91. Vatner SF, Pagani M, Manders WT, Pasipoularides AD: Alpha-adrenergic vasoconstriction and nitroglycerin vasodilation of large coronary arteries in the conscious dog. J Clin Invest 65:5–14, 1980.

92. Swain JL, Parker JP, McHald PA, Greenfield JC Jr: Effects of nitroglycerin and propranolol on the distribution of transmural myocardial blood flow during ischemia in the absence of hemodynamic changes in the unanesthetized dog. J Clin Invest 63:947–953, 1979.

93. Hood WP Jr, Amende I, Simon R, Lichtlen PR: The effects of intracoronary nitroglycerin on left ventricular systolic and diastolic function in man. Circulation 60:1098–1104, 1980.

94. Hillis LD, Braunwald E: Coronary spasm. N Engl J Med 299:695–702, 1978.

95. Danahy DT, Aranow WS: Hemodynamics and antianginal effects of high dose oral isosorbide dinitrate after chronic use. Circulation 56:205–212, 1977.

96. Markis JE, Gorlin R, Mills RM, Williams RA, Schweitzer P, Ransil BJ: Sustained effect of orally administered isosorbide dinitrate on exercise performance of patients with angina pectoris. Am J Cardiol 43:265–271, 1979.

97. Abrams J: Nitroglycerin and long-acting nitrates. N Engl J Med 302:1234–1237, 1980.

98. Reichek N, Goldstein RE, Redwood DR, Epstein SE: Sustained effects of nitroglycerin ointment in patients with angina pectoris. Circulation 50:348–352, 1974.

99. Lee G, Mason DT, De Maria AN: Effects of long-term oral administration of isosorbide dinitrate on the antianginal response to nitroglycerin. Absence of nitrate cross-tolerance and self tolerance shown by exercise testing. Am J Cardiol 41:82–87, 1978.

100. Lange RL, Reid MS, Tresch DD, Keelan MH, Bernhard VM, Coolidge G: Nonatheromatous ischemic heart disease following withdrawal from chronic industrial nitroglycerin exposure. Circulation 46:666–678, 1972.

101. Klock JC: Nonocclusive coronary disease after chronic exposure to nitrates: evidence for physiological nitrate dependence. Am Heart J 89:510–513, 1975.

102. Black JW, Stephenson JS: Pharmacology of a new adrenergic β-receptor blocking compound (nethalide). Lancet 2:311–314, 1962.

103. Thadani J, Davidson C, Singleton W, Taylor SH: Comparisons of fine beta-adrenoceptor antagonists with different ancillary properties during sustained twice daily therapy in angina pectoris. Am J Med 68:243–250, 1980.

104. Wilson AG, Brooke OG, Lloyd HJ, Robinson BF: Mechanism of action of β-adrenergic receptor blocking agents in angina pectoris: comparison of the actions of propranolol with dextropropranolol and practolol. Br Med J 4:399–401, 1969.

105. Frishman W, Kostis J, Strom J, Hossler M, Elkayam U, Goldner S, Silverman R, Davis R, Weinstein J, Sonnenblick E: Clinical pharmacology of the new beta-adrenergic blocking drugs. Part 6. A comparison of pindolol and propranolol in treatment of patients with angina pectoris. The role of intrinsic sympathomimetic activity. Am Heart J 98:526–535, 1979.

106. Chidsey C, Pine M, Favrot L, Smith S, Leonetti G, Morselli P, Zanchetti A: The use of drug concentration measurements in studies of the therapeutic response to propranolol. Postgrad Med J 52(Suppl 4):26–32, 1976.

107. Jackson G, Atkinson L, Oram S: Reassessment of failed β-blocker treatment in angina pectoris by peak exercise heart rate measurements. Br Med J 3:616–618, 1975.

108. Thadani U, Parker JD: Propranolol in angina pectoris: comparison of therapy given two and four times daily. Am J Cardiol 46:117–123, 1980.

109. Schrumpf JD, Sheps DS, Wolfson S, Aronson AL, Cohen LS: Altered hemoglobin-oxygen affinity with long-term propranolol therapy in patients with coronary artery disease. Am J Cardiol 40:76–82, 1977.

110. Robinson BF: Mechanism of action of β-blocking drugs in angina pectoris. Postgrad Med J 52(Suppl 4):43–45, 1976.

111. Frishman WH, Weksler BB, Christodoulou JP, Smithen C, Killip T: Reversal of abnormal platelet aggregability and change in exercise tolerance in patients with angina pectoris following oral propranolol. Circulation 50:887–896, 1974.

112. Mehta J, Mehta P, Pepine CJ: Platelet aggregation in aortic and coronary venous blood in patients with and without coronary disease. 3. Role of tachycardia stress and propranolol. Circulation 58:881–886, 1978.

113. Crawford MH, LeWinter MM, O'Rourke RA, Karliner JS, Ross J Jr: Combined propranolol and digoxin therapy in angina pectoris. Ann Intern Med 83:449–455, 1975.

114. Alderman EL, Coltart DJ, Wettach GE, Harrison DC: Coronary artery syndromes after sudden propranolol withdrawal. Ann Intern Med 81:625–627, 1974.

115. Miller RR, Olson HG, Amsterdam EA, Mason DT: Propranolol withdrawal rebound phenomenon. N Engl J Med 293:416–418, 1975.

116. Shand DG, Wood AJJ: Propranolol withdrawal syndrome – why? Circulation 58:202–203, 1978.

117. Boudoulas H, Lewis RP, Kates RE, Dalamangas G: Hypersensitivity to adrenergic stimulation after propranolol withdrawal in normal subjects. Ann Intern Med 87:433–436, 1977.

118. Nattel S, Rangno RE, Van Loon G: Mechanism of propranolol withdrawal phenomenon. Circulation 59:1158–1164, 1979.

119. Garrett BN, Kaplan NM: Plasma renin activity suppression. Duration after withdrawal from β-adrenergic blockade. Arch Intern Med 140:1316–1318, 1980.

120. Glaubiger G, Lefkowitz RJ: Elevated β-adrenergic receptor number after chronic propranolol treatment. Biochem Biophys Res Commun 78:720–725, 1977.

121. Aarons RD, Nies AS, Gal J, Hegstrand LR, Molinoff PB: Elevation of β-adrenergic receptor density in human lymphocytes after propranolol administration. J Clin Invest 65:949–959, 1980.

122. Lindenfeld J, Crawford JH, O'Rourke MH, Levine SP, Montiel MM, Horwitz LD: Adrenergic responsiveness after abrupt propranolol withdrawal in normal subjects and in patients with angina pectoris. Circulation 62:704–711, 1980.

123. Ellrodt G, Chew CYC, Singh BN: Therapeutic implications of slow channel blockade in cardiocirculatory disorders. Circulation 62:669–679, 1980.

124. Antman EM, Stone PH, Miller JE, Braunwald E: Calcium channel blocking agents in the treatment of cardiovascular disorders. Part I. Basic and clinical electrophysiologic effects. Ann Intern Med 93:875–885, 1980.

125. Stone PH, Antman EM, Miller JE, Braunwald E: Calcium channel blocking agents in the treatment of cardiovascular disorders. Part II. Hemodynamic effects and clinical applications. Ann Intern Med 93:886–904, 1980.

126. Seminar on calcium channel blockers. Part I. Am J Cardiol 46:1045–1067, 1980.

127. Seminar on calcium channel blockers. Part II. Am J Cardiol 47:157–184, 1981.

128. Symposium: calcium, calcium antagonists, and cardiovascular disease. Chest 78 (Suppl 1):121–248, 1980.

129. Antman E, Muller J, Goldberg S, Mac Alpin R, Rubenfire M, Tabatznik B, Liang CS, Heupler F, Achuff S, Reichek N, Geltman E, Kerin NZ, Neff RK, Braunwald E: Nifedipine therapy for coronary artery spasm. N Engl J Med 302:1269–1273, 1980.

130. Rosenthal SJ, Ginsburg R, Lamb IH, Baim DS, Schroeder JS: Efficacy of diltiazem for control of symptoms of coronary arterial spasm. Am J Cardiol 46:1027–1032, 1980.

131. Woodcock BG, Rietbrock I, Vöhringer HF, Rietbrock N: Verapamil disposition in liver disease and intensive-care patients: kinetics clearance and apparent blood flow relationships. Clin Pharmacol Ther 29:27–34, 1981.

CHAPTER 14

Treatment of cardiac failure

ERIC S. WILLIAMS and CHARLES FISCH

Introduction

Cardiac failure is the clinical syndrome that results
when the heart is unable to pump blood in an
amount that adequately meets the metabolic needs
of the body. It is the end result of a heterogeneous
group of disorders that, in most cases, directly or
indirectly impair myocardial contractility. Cardiac
failure also can occur when the normal myocardium is presented suddenly with a load that exceeds
its capacity and when ventricular filling is restricted. Implicit in the definition of cardiac failure is the
requirement that an abnormality of cardiac function induces the basic hemodynamic consequences
of reduction of cardiac output and increase in venous pressure behind one or both ventricles. This is
in contrast to the low-output states due to diminished systemic venous return and the congestive
states that accompany primary renal and hepatic
disorders. The recognition of heart failure rests on
the identification of a group of characteristic clinical findings that vary greatly depending on whether
the failure is acute or chronic, predominantly left or
right sided and low or high output in nature. The
variability of the clinical features arises in large part
from the fact that they result both from the underlying hemodynamic abnormality and from the compensatory mechanisms that are invoked when myocardial performance is impaired.

The above statements serve to emphasize the
number and diversity of the factors responsible for
the development and clinical manifestations of
heart failure. Moreover, they provide the rationale
for an individualized therapeutic program for each
patient. In this chapter, we present the principles of
an integrated approach to the treatment of patients,
focusing on the low-output failure state that occurs
in most forms of heart disease. The overall goals of
the therapy are: (a) identification and removal of
the causes of cardiac failure; (b) improvement of the
heart's pumping performance; and (c) reversal of
the congested state. The achievement of these goals
may require changes in the patient's dietary habits
and physical activity, surgical therapy, or the use of
drugs that increase the inotropic state of the myocardium, promote the renal excretion of sodium
and water or alter vascular tone (Figure 1). To
choose and properly use these measures, the clinician first must acquire a thorough understanding of
the factors that regulate cardiac function and the
mechanisms by which heart failure can develop. In
addition, he must recognize the role of the major
compensatory mechanisms of ventricular hypertrophy, dilation, and autonomic nervous system
stimulation in the hemodynamic changes associated
with cardiac failure.

Regulation of cardiac function

In the intact heart the pumping performance of the
ventricle is regulated by four major control mechanisms: (a) the length of the muscle fibers at the onset
of contraction (preload); (b) the myocardial wall
tension developed during contraction (afterload);
(c) contractility; and (d) the heart rate [1, 2]. The
manner in which these factors affect cardiac output
in normal individuals and in patients with cardiac
failure is depicted in Figure 2.

In the normal heart, an increase in preload

Rosen, M. R. and Hoffman, B. F. (eds.), Cardiac Therapy. ISBN 0-89838-564-4.
© 1983, Martinus Nijhoff Publishers, Boston, The Hague, Dordrecht, Lancaster. Printed in the Netherlands.

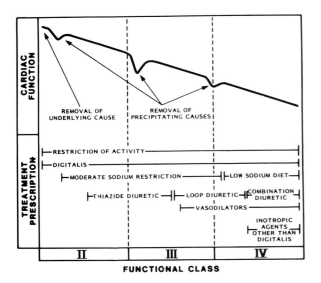

Figure 1. Example of the overall therapeutic approach to patients with chronic congestive heart failure (New York Heart Association classification). The upper curve depicts the change in intrinsic cardiac pumping function over time. The treatment prescription serves as a guide to the use of the individual components of therapy but is not intended to indicate a rigid treatment schedule. The timing of institution and the emphasis of each component is determined also by the specific causes and chronicity of the cardiac failure. The term 'loop diuretic' refers to furosemide and ethacrinic acid.

through increased venous return to the ventricle leads to the ejection of an augmented stroke volume (Frank-Starling principle). In panel A of Figure 2 this is represented as the relationship of stroke volume and left ventricular filling pressure (similar to the left atrial pressure). It is important to recognize, however, the central role of ventricular distensibility or compliance in determining the diastolic wall tension at any given volume of venous return. The utilization of this Frank-Starling mechanism to improve stroke volume is one of the compensatory changes invoked during heart failure. The increase in venous return results from selective vasoconstriction (mediated by humoral mechanisms and reflex sympathetic nervous system stimulation) as well as from sodium and water retention. Unfortunately, the decrease in contractility of the failing ventricle results in a ventricular function curve that is not only displaced downward but is also less steep [3]. Thus, the increase in stroke volume elicited by the increased venus return is attenuated. This often occurs at the expense of lung congestion as the left atrial and pulmonary venous pressures rise.

Figure 2 also depicts the potential beneficial effects of inotropic and diuretic agents on the ventricular function curve. In patients with heart fail-

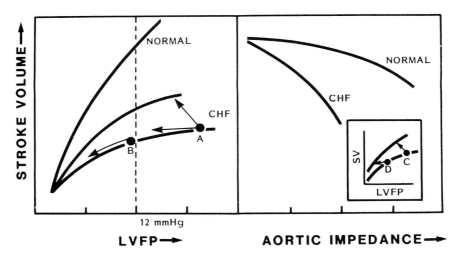

Figure 2. Determinants of cardiac pumping function. The ventricular function curve shown on the left depicts the relationship of stroke volume and left ventricular filling pressure (LVFP) or preload in normal individuals and in patients with cardiac failure. When LVFP is high, pulmonary congestion and dyspnea are the major clinical manifestations. When diminished cardiac output is the major hemodynamic change, fatigue is the predominant symptom. The use of digitalis at point A shifts the curve upward, the use of diuretic agents at A reduces the LVFP (toward B). The use of diuretics with normal or low initial LVFP (B) reduces stroke volume. The right panel depicts the relationship of stroke volume and aortic impedance. In patients with cardiac failure, stroke volume is reduced as the resistance to ventricular ejection is increased. The ventricular function curve in the insert shows the effect of reducing impedance (upper curve) by vasodilators. These drugs increase stroke volume when LVFP remains satisfactory (C) but reduce it when LVFP is low (D).

ure, the magnitude of the improvement in cardiac performance caused by inotropic drugs is limited by the myocardial contribution to the cardiac failure and by the residual capacity of muscle to respond to the inotropic stimulus. Effective digitalis action shifts the ventricular function curve upward and to the left. The increase in cardiac output also promotes salt and water excretion thereby lowering left ventricular filling pressure and the degree of pulmonary congestion. It is important to emphasize that successful therapy with diuretic drugs decreases pulmonary congestion but does not directly improve cardiac output. In fact, stroke volume is diminished if the filling pressure is reduced below the plateau of the ventricular function curve. This is particularly important in disorders, such as acute myocardial infarction, in which a decrease in ventricular compliance is a major pathophysiologic change [4]. In this situation, a higher than normal filling pressure may be required to maintain optimal stroke volume, and excessive diuresis can lead to a precipitous fall in cardiac output. Ventricular filling is also lowered by drugs that act directly on the capacitance vessels to increase venous pooling [5]. These venodilators exert effects on the ventricular function curve that are similar to those of diuretic drugs.

The magnitude of ventricular afterload is determined by several factors [6] including ventricular chamber size and wall thickness. An important component of afterload is the aortic impedance or dynamic resistance to ventricular ejection. The aortic impedance, in turn, is largely determined by the systemic vascular resistance. In the normal heart, stroke volume is decreased only slightly as the aortic impedance is increased. By contrast, the damaged ventricle often is exquisitely sensitive to changes in outflow resistance [7]. A substantial reduction in stroke volume and increase in end-systolic volume of the ventricle ensue when the aortic impedance is increased. Such a situation occurs in patients with advanced heart failure in whom the level of systemic vascular resistance is characteristically increased, presumably as a result of heightened sympathetic nervous system activity and in some patients, activation of the renin-angiotensin system [8, 9]. This compensatory change, which acts to maintain blood pressure and perfusion of critical organs, may exert deleterious effects in the patient with myocardial failure [10]. Conversely, vasodilat-

ing drugs that act directly to reduce peripheral vascular resistance can improve ventricular function as long as satisfactory perfusion pressure is maintained [5, 11–13]. The application of this concept is a major recent advance in cardiovascular therapy. It is particularly advantageous since it offers a means of improving cardiac output without relying on an increase in the intrinsic contractile function, and thus oxygen consumption, of the heart muscle.

The heart rate exerts direct and indirect effects on cardiac function and, along with contractility and ventricular wall tension, is a major determinant of myocardial oxygen demand [14]. An increase in heart rate through sympathetic nervous system stimulation is an important mechanism by which cardiac output is increased during short periods of exercise or stress [15]. An increase in heart rate also can act to restore or maintain cardiac output in patients whose stroke volume is limited by cardiac disease. This compensatory change is often more prominent in the setting of acute cardiac failure [16]. During the arrhythmias that result in very rapid heart rates, the cardiac output falls as stroke volume is limited by the shortened diastolic ventricular filling time. Since ventricular filling occurs primarily in early diastole, satisfactory inflow usually is maintained in resting individuals without cardiac disease until the heart rate exceeds 160 beats/min [17]. Compensatory mechanisms (including peripheral vasoconstriction) contribute to the maintenance of cardiac output at these rapid heart rates by supporting an adequate level of systemic venous return. In patients with myocardial damage or impaired compensatory mechanisms due to drugs or disease, the cardiac output can decrease as a consequence of lesser degrees of tachycardia.

A progressive increase in heart rate also affects cardiac function independently of its action on the ventricular filling time. In anesthetized animals [18], an acceleration of the frequency of contraction regularly enhances myocardial contractility (Bowditch effect). Although a similar effect may occur in conscious humans, its magnitude appears to be slight and its significance is questioned by some investigators [19–21]. In patients with coronary artery disease, an inordinate increase in heart rate can worsen cardiac function if the myocardial oxygen requirement is increased to levels that precipitate myocardial ischemia and ventricular dyssynergy [22].

455

Table 1. Causes of cardiac failure.

I.   Myocardial damage or disease
     A. Infarction/Ischemia
         1. Atherosclerotic coronary artery obstruction
         2. Coronary artery spasm
         3. Coronary artery thrombosis or embolism
         4. Coronary artery vasculitis
     B. Myocarditis (e.g., viral; associated with collagen disease; idiopathic)
     C. Congestive, restrictive, or hypertrophic cardiomyopathy.
         1. Secondary to toxic agents (e.g., ethanol; adriamycin)
         2. Due to infiltrative disorders (e.g., amyloidosis; sarcoidosis)
         3. Due to nutritional deficiency (e.g., thiamine) or endocrine disorder (e.g. thyrotoxicosis; myxedema; diabetes mellitus)
         4. Genetic (e.g., hypertrophic cardiomyopathy with or without obstruction)
         5. Idiopathic
     D. Myocardial contusion
II. Excess load on the ventricle
     A. Volume overload
         1. Valve regurgitation
         2. Shunt
     B. Pressure overload
         1. Systemic or pulmonary arterial hypertension
         2. Outflow tract obstruction (subvalvular, valvular, supravalvular)
III. Resistance to flow into the ventricle
     A. Mitral or tricuspid stenosis
     B. Pericardial tamponade/constriction
IV. Cardiac arrhythmias or altered conduction sequence
     A. Marked bradycardia or tachycardia
     C. Conduction disturbance

Mechanisms of cardiac failure

Cardiac failure commonly results from disease or damage of the myocardium (Table 1). This can be a consequence of the loss of functioning muscle (e.g., myocardial infarction), or inflammation (e.g., viral myocarditis), or infiltration of the myocardium (e.g., amyloidosis). Not infrequently, the precise etiology of the myocardial damage cannot be identified.

Cardiac failure can also result from disorders, often mechanical, that subject the ventricle to an excess load. In patients with aortic stenosis or systemic hypertension, for example, the ejection of the blood must be carried out against high resistance, and this produces a pressure overload of the ventricle and hypertrophy as a major compensatory change. In patients with mitral or aortic regurgitation, the ventricle is presented with a volume overload and ventricular dilation predominates as a compensatory mechanism. The effects of the volume and pressure overloads on cardiac function are dependent both on the magnitude of the excess load and the rapidity with which it develops. For example, acute mitral regurgitation due to ruptured chordae tendinae frequently results in fulminant heart failure, whereas chronic mitral regurgitation due to rheumatic valvular disease is often tolerated for years because of the development of effective compensatory mechanisms. However, the chronic increase in cardiac work associated with the excess load eventually leads to myocardial damage that persists after repair of the mechanical lesion. In patients with chronic valvular disease, the development of heart failure usually indicates that substantial reduction of contractility has occurred [23]. The therapy of patients with these disorders, therefore, involves measures both to reduce the excess load and to improve myocardial contractility.

Arrhythmias can be a primary cause of heart failure but more commonly contribute to the cardiac dysfunction of patients with myocardial or mechanical disorders. In addition to the underlying status of the myocardium, the hemodynamic consequences of arrhythmia depend on the ventricular rate, the regularity of cardiac rhythm, and the presence or absence of effective atrial contraction. The loss of the atrial contribution to stroke volume, e.g., as a result of atrial fibrillation or a junctional or ventricular rhythm (Figure 3) is most damaging in disorders in which filling of the ventricle is further limited by atrioventricular valvular stenosis or by a decrease in ventricular compliance. The importance of effective atrial contraction also must be considered when pacemaker therapy is contemplated for patients with cardiac failure and coexistent bradycardia. Increasing the heart rate to a range of 80–100 beats/min can improve cardiac function in some patients with underlying bradycardia. However, it is not unusual to see individuals whose effective cardiac output is greater with a sinus rate of 50 beats/min than with an artificial ventricular pacemaker-induced rate of 80 beats/min. This circumstance largely attests to the importance of the atrial contraction, but the alteration in the sequence of depolarization of the ventricular muscle also likely contributes to the decrease in stroke volume

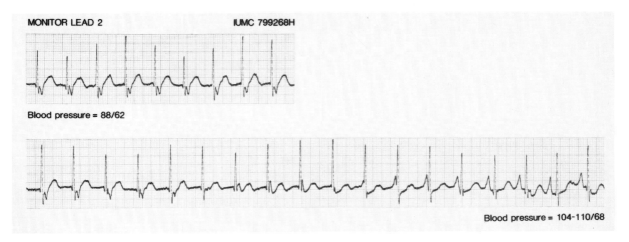

MONITOR LEAD 2   IUMC 799268H

Blood pressure = 88/62

Blood pressure = 104-110/68

Figure 3. Rhythm strip of a patient with acute myocardial infarction. The upper tracing shows an accelerated junctional rhythm. In the bottom panel, the restoration of sinus rhythm (and effective atrial contraction) results in an 18–20-mm Hg increase in blood pressure despite a minimal change in the ventricular rate. Fusion p waves are visible in the middle portion of the lower panel.

[24] during this rhythm. In selected cases, utilization of atrioventricular sequential pacing may overcome the drawback of loss of effective atrial action.

Clinical approach to the therapy of patients with cardiac failure

Identification and removal of the causes of cardiac failure

The most direct and potentially successful therapy in the treatment of patients with cardiac failure is the removal of its underlying cause. Thus, accurate diagnosis of the heart disease is the first goal in the clinical evaluation of patients. Although this usually can be accomplished by a careful medical history, physical examination, and noninvasive laboratory tests, cardiac catheterization often is required to investigate fully the underlying etiology. Removal of the underlying cause of cardiac failure is possible for some disorders in which myocardial function is directly impaired. More commonly, it can be achieved when the ventricle is subjected to an excess load such as occurs with systemic hypertension and many congenital and acquired valvular heart lesions. For some congenital disorders (e.g., atrial septal defect or patent ductus arteriosus with significant left to right shunt), the knowledge of the natural history of the lesion permits surgical therapy to

be carried out electively before the development of symptoms or complications [25]. When acquired valvular disease is present, the patient's symptoms and functional capacity are important determinants in the choice of surgical therapy [26]. Successful treatment of these disorders serves not only to prevent progression of heart failure but can restore cardiac function toward normal levels if completed before the myocardium is substantially damaged [27, 28]. Unfortunately, when mechanical lesions are responsible for the excess load, their removal requires surgical procedures that carry their own risks and complications. The placement of an artificial valve to relieve aortic stenosis, for example, can be complicated by prosthesis malfunction, infection, and systemic embolization [29]. Lifelong anticoagulation is frequently required. Thus, the timing of surgical repair of a congenital or acquired valvular defect requires consideration of the anticipated natural history of the lesion, the functional status of the patient and the risks and benefits of the specific surgical procedure. Obviously, the age and general health of the patient are also important factors.

The decision to recommend valve replacement is often easier in situations in which the ventricle is subjected to a pressure rather than volume overload. When syncope, angina pectoris or the symptoms of heart failure develop in patients with significant aortic stenosis, the projected mortality rate with medical therapy is about 50% over the succeeding four years [30]. Thus, prompt surgical interven-

457

tion is recommended for the symptomatic individual with a calculated aortic orifice area of less than 0.75 cm^2 (or a peak systolic gradient greater than 50 mmHg with a normal cardiac output). Left ventricular function can improve after surgery for aortic stenosis, even if it has been markedly depressed preoperatively [27, 31]. Patients with chronic aortic or mitral regurgitation, on the other hand, form a more heterogeneous group with regard to prognosis and the rate of progression of myocardial damage, which is usually gradual even after the onset of symptoms [32, 33]. Surgery is often elected when the patient's ordinary activity is limited by symptoms or when there is objective evidence of progression of cardiomegaly or ventricular dysfunction. Unfortunately, with this approach heart failure persists postoperatively in some patients because of myocardial damage [34, 35]. The ability of radionuclide and other noninvasive studies to identify patients with subtle myocardial damage or reduced cardiac reserve from chronic volume overload currently are being evaluated [26, 35, 36]. These studies may result in the earlier use of valve replacement in some patients as the emphasis of therapy shifts from relief of symptoms to preservation of ventricular function.

From an epidemiologic standpoint, systemic hypertension is the most important cause of cardiac failure resulting from excess ventricular load. Effective treatment of hypertension reduces the risk of developing heart failure as well as other cardiovascular complications [37] and improves ventricular function when coexistent myocardial damage is present. The long-term benefits of antihypertensive treatment extend to those with only mild elevation of diastolic blood pressure [38]. In the presence of malignant or severe acute exacerbations of hypertension, the use of parenteral vasodilators, such as sodium nitroprusside, permits minute-by-minute adjustment of therapy to control the blood pressure during the early stages of treatment [39] while a program of oral antihypertensive drugs is instituted or adjusted.

Chronic congestive heart failure is rarely associated with a slow progressive decline in ventricular function. Rather, the course usually is punctuated by periods of exacerbation when the compensatory mechanisms and therapy no longer maintain satisfactory cardiac pumping function (Figure 1). The identification removal (and, when possible, prevention) of the factors that precipitate acute episodes of decompensation are important parts of the treatment. One of the major precipitating causes of heart failure is lack of compliance with the therapeutic plan [40]. This applies not only to drug therapy but also to dietary prescriptions and activity limitation. The metabolic and hemodynamic stresses produced by systemic infection and pulmonary embolism also can lead to acute cardiac decompensation in patients with heart disease. Other extracardiac disorders, such as thyroid disease and anemia, can similarly exacerbate cardiac dysfunction. Arrhythmias are common complications in all forms of heart disease and can precipitate heart failure because of ventricular rates that are too slow or too fast. As previously noted, the arrhythmias that result in loss of effective atrial contraction impose a further limitation of ventricular filling. The importance of these factors is illustrated dramatically in some previously well-compensated patients with mitral valve disease when the onset of atrial fibrillation with a rapid and irregular ventricular rate results in acute heart failure and pulmonary edema. In this circumstance, the primary therapy is directed toward control of the ventricular rate by digitalis and, when feasible, the restoration of sinus rhythm.

A consideration of the factors that precipitate or exacerbate cardiac failure must include the adverse and unintended effects of medications as well as the untoward actions that result from the interaction of various components of the treatment plan. The negative inotropic effect of the beta-adrenergic-blocking drugs can contribute to the development of heart failure when these drugs are administered to patients with significant left ventricular dysfunction [41] since reflex sympathetic stimulation may be required to maintain satisfactory cardiac output. The risk of propranolol-induced heart failure is greatest when the drug is administered by the intravenous route to patients with acute cardiac failure. The use of digitalis and diuretics by patients with hypertrophic obstructive cardiomyopathy can lead to a worsening of cardiac function. In this condition, an increase in contractility induced by digitalis or a decrease in cardiac filling (and chamber size) due to excessive diuresis can heighten the outflow tract obstruction and further limit effective stroke volume [42]. Many antiarrhythmic drugs, e.g., quinidine and procainamide, depress myocardial contractility [43, 44] in laboratory animals.

Nevertheless, these commonly used antiarrhythmic agents usually are tolerated by patients with cardiac dysfunction if administered in appropriate dosages [43, 45]. Disopyramide may be an exception to this statement since the potential for this drug to impair myocardial function appears to be greater than that of other conventional antiarrhythmic agents. In one series, acute congestive heart failure developed in 16 of 100 patients following treatment with disopyramide [45]. The precipitation of cardiac failure by drug-induced arrhythmias or heart block is a final example of the manner in which pharmacologic therapy can contribute to clinical decompensation. This situation can occur, for example, following the addition of quinidine to the medical regimen of patients receiving digoxin [46]. Quinidine increases blood levels of the glycoside [47] and can thereby evoke arrhythmias and conduction disturbances due to digitalis intoxication. Even in the absence of concomitant therapy, antiarrhythmic drugs can lead to a worsening of ventricular ectopy and the emergence of life-threatening arrhythmias in some patients [48].

Improvement of the heart's pumping performance

After efforts to remove the underlying and precipitating causes, the next goal in the treatment of cardiac failure is to decrease the disparity between the heart's pumping performance and the metabolic needs of the patient. This is done most simply by limitation of physical activity. Although adequate rest and restriction of undue exertion are important components of therapy at each stage of heart failure, they frequently are overlooked, and patients often do not understand the rationale for their prescription. The degree of activity limitation is dependent on the extent of ventricular dysfunction. The symptoms of chronic heart failure initially occur only with greater-than-usual levels of activity, and, at this stage, only vigorous exertion need be avoided. As myocardial damage progresses, the cardiac reserve is diminished along with activity tolerance. As a general rule, activities that result in symptoms should be avoided. Short of this, patients with chronic heart failure should be encouraged to remain active. A regular program of walking, for example, helps not only to maintain a satisfactory level of cardiovascular conditioning but may also reduce the anxiety and depression that frequently accompany this disorder. Conditioning may be particularly beneficial for patients with ischemic heart disease. In this setting, the increase in exercise tolerance is due largely to the ability to perform a greater degree of work for a given amount of cardiac oxygen consumption. Although the issue is not fully resolved [49], training does not appear to enhance significantly the intrinsic ventricular function of patients with preexistent cardiac dysfunction [50].

Digitalis glycosides for chronic cardiac failure
The ability of digitalis to improve the heart's pumping performance was recognized by Withering in 1785, and for almost two hundred years it has been the most commonly prescribed cardiotonic drug for patients with chronic heart failure. The modest increase in contractility that follows the initiation of digitalis therapy enhances cardiac output, promotes diuresis, and the subsequent reduction of ventricular filling pressure decreases pulmonary congestion [51–53]. These hemodynamic changes are manifested clinically by improved exercise tolerance and a decrease in dyspnea and orthopnea. Despite the documentation of these beneficial effects of acute digitalis treatment, and the extensive clinical experience supporting its chronic use, the utility of maintenance digitalis therapy in patients with chronic heart failure has been somewhat controversial [54, 55]. This controversy stems from questions about the magnitude and duration of the improvement in cardiac function in patients who have normal sinus rhythm and from the risk of drug toxicity, which may be present in greater than 10% of patients taking digitalis [56]. Obviously, the potential benefit of an inotropic agent depends on the myocardial contribution to the heart failure state as well as the residual capacity of the heart muscle to increase contractility in response to the drug. Patients with very advanced ventricular dysfunction, e.g., those with end-stage congestive cardiomyopathy, may have little or no demonstrable response to the drug [57]. The difficulty in objectively demonstrating the benefit of maintenance digitalis therapy in some clinical studies is due, in part, to limitations of the commonly used indices of cardiac pumping function in the intact individual and to methodologic problems that arise when one attempts to use acute hemodynamic measurements as an indicator of the effectiveness of a chronically

administered agent. Furthermore, objective evidence of improvement may be demonstrable only if the studies are carried out following exercise or other forms of stress. Such a study [58] recently has confirmed the effectiveness of long-term digitalis treatment in a group of patients with chronic heart failure due to ischemic and hypertensive cardiovascular diseases.

An additional concern has been raised. In the presence of chronic coronary artery disease, a digitalis-induced increase in myocardial contractility could enhance oxygen demand of the heart muscle and thereby precipitate myocardial ischemia and angina pectoris. Moreover, there is clinical evidence that ventricular function deteriorates when digitalis is administered to some patients with coronary artery disease without overt cardiac failure, presumably due to aggravation of ischemia-mediated wall motion abnormalities [59]. When digitalis is used to treat patients with heart failure, however, the increase in oxygen demand due to the stimulation of contractility is opposed by a reduction in ventricular wall tension (decreased chamber size) and heart rate as the degree of cardiac failure diminishes [60]. Thus, in most patients with chronic cardiac failure, digitalis improves pumping performance without untoward effects on the overall oxygen demand–supply balance.

It is our belief that digitalis therapy should be employed in patients with objective evidence of congestive heart failure resulting from myocardial dysfunction even if they experience symptoms only with more-than-usual levels of activity (functional class II). The drug is of potential benefit when the myocardial function is directly impaired, as in ischemic heart disease and cardiomyopathy, and when contractility is secondarily impaired by hypertension and valvular or congenital heart diseases. It is not recommended for patients with congestive heart failure due to mitral stenosis unless right ventricular failure has resulted from associated pulmonary hypertension [61]. The use of digitalis must, of course, include a consideration of the general health of the patient and the presence of factors, such as renal or hepatic disorders, that enhance the risk of drug toxicity [62]. Although it has been demonstrated clearly that digitalis can increase contractility in the nonfailing heart [63], it does not significantly enhance cardiac output in this setting. This presumably results, in part, from

the direct effect of digitalis to heighten arteriolar tone and peripheral vascular resistance. We do not recommend the use of digitalis for its inotropic effect in patients with cardiac disease until there is objective evidence of heart failure. It must be emphasized, however, that the recognition of the earliest stages of failure may be difficult, and physical signs may be detectable only during exertion. The evaluation of patients with suspected ventricular dysfunction should usually include examination following some form of exercise. In some cases, this may simply involve a short walk or a brief period of flexing and extending one leg while in bed. At times, structured exercise treadmill examination provides the first objective evidence of heart failure [64].

The choice of a specific digitalis preparation usually is based on the clinical setting in which it is to be used and the physician's familiarity with the drug. Digoxin is the most commonly used glycoside for patients with cardiac failure. Its popularity stems from the flexibility of routes of administration and its intermediate duration of action. This latter characteristic may be of particular importance in situations in which the risk of drug toxicity is high. Conversely, its duration of action may not always be advantageous in the out-patient setting. As noted previously, strict compliance with the therapeutic program is a problem for many individuals with chronic illnesses. Omission of digoxin by a patient for one or two days substantially reduces the body stores of the medication. For this reason, some authorities prefer digitoxin, with an effective half-life of about five days, for patients with chronic heart failure [65]. In the past, digitoxin ususally was chosen for patients with chronic renal failure because of the central role of the kidney in the elimination of digoxin. The relationship between renal function, as reflected by the creatinine clearance, and digoxin excretion is now well established, and digoxin can be administered to patients with kidney disease after the appropriate reduction in dosage [62].

The recommended dosages, metabolism, and pharmacokinetics of the digitalis preparations have been reviewed in detail in Chapter 11. The importance of an understanding of this material for the clinician cannot be overemphasized. Ogilvie and Reedy reported a 50% decrease in the incidence of digitalis intoxication in patients cared for by physicians who had completed an educational program in the clinical pharmacology of digitalis [66]. Unfortunately, some potential for drug toxicity exists even after proper consideration of the drug's pharmacologic characteristics and, in the study cited above, the incidence of digitalis intoxication was about 10% after the educational program. Continued close observation of the patient is required when chronic digitalis therapy is undertaken.

The optimal use of digitalis for chronic heart failure is limited by the absence of clear-cut therapeutic end-points in patients who have sinus rhythm. The physician must be guided by the 'average' initial and maintenance dosages of digitalis, but the key to successful therapy is appropriate modification of these average dosages based on an appreciation of the wide variation of individual response and the presence or absence of factors that alter digitalis effectiveness and tolerance. Furthermore, it is important to recognize that the inotropic effect of digitalis is dose- and plasma concentration-dependent [67], and it may not be necessary to achieve the maximal tolerated level of the drug to obtain a satisfactory clinical response. In light of the availability of potent diuretics and other modalities of therapy, the treatment of chronic cardiac failure need not rest solely on attaining a maximal digitalis effect.

Whenever possible, the oral route of digitalis administration is preferred. The rapidity with which it is initially administered ('digitalization') is dependent on the severity of the clinical failure. When digoxin is chosen, the loading dose can be given in divided doses over a 24-hr period. Digitalization also can be achieved over a period of about one week in patients with normal renal function by giving the daily maintenance dose without any loading dose. This method is preferable for many patients with chronic cardiac failure, particularly in the outpatient setting. Gradual digitalization can be carried out with digitoxin but because of its longer half-life, an interval of three to four weeks is required to reach steady-state conditions. Thus, when digitoxin is chosen for patients with chronic heart failure, the calculated loading dose is usually administered over a period of several days. The availability of radioimmunoassay techniques to monitor digitalis blood levels provides a means of confirming that the patient is taking and absorbing the preparation and is particularly helpful for patients with altered metabolism of the glycoside. However, the variability both of individual response and susceptibility to toxicity has precluded the use of this test to identify the optimal dose of the medication for most patients [68]. Digitalis intoxication can occur in the presence of 'therapeutic' blood levels, and, as studies of patients with atrial fibrillation have revealed, concentrations that exceed the 'therapeutic' levels may be found in many patients with no clinical evidence of drug intoxication.

In addition to renal and hepatic dysfunction (which alter the metabolism and excretion of digoxin and digitoxin, respectively), a number of clinical conditions appear to place some patients at increased risk for the development of digitalis intoxication. These conditions include pulmonary and thyroid disorders [69] and advanced age. The latter is likely the result of an associated decrease in renal function. The etiology and severity of the heart failure state are similarly important considerations. Clinical studies suggest that patients with myocarditis and some types of cardiomyopathy are more likely to develop digitalis intoxication with usual dosages of the medication [70]. Regardless of the etiology, heart failure of severe degree raises the risk of drug toxicity as liver and renal function are indirectly impaired by the low cardiac output and elevated venous pressure.

For several decades, there has been a widely held clinical impression that the risk of digitalis intoxication is increased in patients with advanced pulmonary disease [71]. Data from epidemiologic studies [56, 72] support this tenet although the magnitude and significance of the enhanced risk is difficult to assess precisely. The correct diagnosis of digitalis intoxication in this setting is complicated by the fact that the arrhythmias commonly observed with digitalis excess also occur independently, as a consequence of respiratory insufficiency [73]. The toxic effects of catecholamine and theophylline preparations used to treat the pulmonary disease can lead to supraventricular and ventricular arrhythmias similar to those caused by digitalis [74, 75].

The mechanism of the proposed susceptibility to digitalis intoxication in patients with pulmonary disease is unknown. There is no evidence that the pharmacokinetics of digitalis are altered in this setting [76]. The manifestations of intoxication can occur with lower-than-usual doses and serum levels

461

of the digitalis preparations [77]. Hypoxia and sympathetic neuroexcitory effects likely contribute to the heightened digitalis sensitivity but do not explain it fully, especially in the setting of chronic respiratory insufficiency [78].

Although treatment of the underlying lung disorder is important, digitalis remains the drug of choice for certain supraventricular arrhythmias, including atrial fibrillation, atrial flutter, and atrial tachycardia (not due to digitalis excess). Digitalis is also beneficial for patients with coexistent left ventricular failure but must be administered cautiously to the patient with severe pulmonary disease. It often is wise to arbitrarily reduce the dose. The role of digitalis in the treatment of cor pulmonale remains controversial [76]. It is established that digitalis exerts an inotropic effect on right ventricular myocardium [79, 80], but the clinical value of this effect is uncertain. Pulmonary artery systolic pressure (and pulmonary vascular resistance) may actually increase in some patients following the acute administration of digitalis [81, 82]. The treatment of respiratory failure with cor pulmonale and right heart failure should focus on measures to correct the reversible component of the elevated resistance to right ventricular outflow, including oxygen and bronchodilators. Our approach is to administer digitalis cautiously to patients who continue to exhibit overt right heart failure despite intensive therapy of the underlying pulmonary disease. The need to continue digitalis treatment after resolution of a bout of acute decompensation must be reassessed frequently with consideration of the long-term risk: benefit ratio.

The diagnosis of digitalis intoxication requires the recognition of characteristic symptoms and clinical findings. Since the early evidence is often subtle and nonspecific, e.g., anorexia and nausea, a high index of suspicion is most important. Digitalis intoxication frequently is manifested by rhythm and conduction disorders [83], and the diagnosis of drug toxicity may be suspected by their detection at the bedside or on the electrocardiogram. These arrhythmias can occur before and in the absence of extracardiac manifestations of drug intoxication. Although digitalis excess has been associated with almost every type of disturbance of cardiac rhythm, certain arrhythmias (e.g., atrial tachycardia with block, accelerated junctional rhythm) are characteristic of intoxication. They are not specific, however, and also can result at times from the underlying cardiac disease rather than digitalis excess. The emergence of rhythm and conduction abnormalities during carotid massage may provide an early clue to digitalis excess. However, in this situation carotid massage is not without risk and can result in transient but symptomatic atrioventricular heart block.

Temporary withdrawal of digitalis is the most important step when drug intoxication is suspected, and resolution of the accompanying symptoms and findings supports the clinical diagnosis of digitalis excess. For many patients, it is the only 'treatment' that is required and the drug can be reinstituted subsequently at lowered doses, if needed. The recognition and correction of hypokalemia are important measures for patients with suspected digitalis excess, particularly if the toxicity is manifested by arrhythmias arising from enhanced automaticity [84]. The manner and rapidity with which supplemental potassium is given is determined by the serum potassium level, the serum pH and the extent of the total body potassium depletion. In most cases, replacement can be carried out with oral potassium chloride. When serious arrhythmias and hypokalemia coexist, or when nausea and vomiting complicate the clinical state, the intravenous route may be required. Administration by this route must be performed cautiously and with close observation of the patient (including electrocardiographic monitoring) because of the risk of hyperkalemia and life-threatening cardiac toxicity that can accompany the rapid administration of potassium [85]. It is generally recommended that the rate of intravenous administration of potassium not exceed 30–40 mEq/hr, although higher rates may be required in emergencies. The potassium chloride in the fluid to be administered must be diluted adequately, usually to a concentration of 30–40 mEq/liter. Unless extenuating circumstances are present, the maximum recommended concentration is 80 mEq/liter. It must be recognized also that hyperkalemia, particularly if induced rapidly, can cause conduction disturbances in the presence of digitalis intoxication [84]. This effect involves both atrioventricular and intraventricular conduction. Fortunately, the level of hyperkalemia required to induce atrioventricular block usually is in excess of that necessary to decrease automaticity. Nevertheless, potassium must be administered with great caution (if at all) in the presence of advanced conduction disturbances (i.e., second- or third-degree heart block).

Complex ventricular arrhythmias induced by digitalis that produce symptoms or are potentially life-threatening also can be treated with lidocaine or diphenylhydantoin [86]. These drugs appear to be preferable to procainamide. Propranolol also may be effective, but the risks of bradycardia and heart block are greater than with the other antiarrhythmic agents. It is important to recognize the substantial risk of cardioversion in patients with digitalis intoxication [87]. This procedure should be used only as a last resort after failure of the above measures to control life-threatening ventricular tachycardia or supraventricular tachycardia with hemodynamic decompensation. The lowest effective energy level should be employed if cardioversion is required.

Moderate digitalis-induced atrioventricular conduction disturbances, e.g., the Wenckebach phenomenon, do not require specific therapy other than temporary discontinuation of the digitalis. If high-degree atrioventricular block is present administration of atropine may reduce this, but temporary transvenous pacemaker placement may be required. Electrical pacing is not without hazard in this setting and should not be utilized unless the heart block results in symptoms or hemodynamic impairment.

Digitalis for acute cardiac failure due to myocardial infarction

Considerable controversy also has centered about the role of digitalis in the treatment of heart failure complicating acute myocardial infarction [88]. The controversy exists despite documentation that digitalis exerts an inotropic effect in this setting [89] and results from the apparently limited improvement in overall cardiac function caused by digitalis, the potential for extension of the myocardial infarction and, as above, the risks of drug toxicity [90]. The digitalis-induced increase in contractility may be blunted immediately after infarction [91, 92] and be opposed by enhanced dyskinetic bulging of the ischemic or infarcted myocardium. Overall, the administration of digitalis to patients with acute myocardial infarction and mild to moderate heart failure has been estimated to increase cardiac ejection fraction by about 10% [93].

The effects of digitalis acting to increase myocar-

dial oxygen demand and their attenuation when the use of the drug is restricted to patients with overt cardiac failure were reviewed above. An additional caution involves the route and rapidity of digitalis administration. The likelihood that digoxin's direct effect to heighten coronary and peripheral arterial resistances will predominate is increased when the drug is given by rapid intravenous infusion. These changes adversely affect the myocardial oxygen supply: demand ratio. If a parenteral route of digoxin usage is required, the drug should be given by slow intravenous infusion over 10–20 min. When assessed by use of thallium-201 perfusion and the study of regional wall motion, infarct size is not increased by the administration of digitalis to patients with myocardial infarction and cardiac failure [93].

The question of increased risk of drug toxicity, i.e., drug-induced arrhythmias, in this setting stems largely from studies on animals that utilize experimentally induced myocardial infarction and large doses of digitalis. These experiments demonstrated that ventricular arrhythmias in animals subjected to coronary artery ligation predictably occur after they are given less than half the dose of digitalis required to induce similar arrhythmias prior to the coronary artery ligation [94]. Clinical data about this point are not consistent [95] and clear-cut evidence that myocardial irritability is significantly increased by the acute administration of appropriate dosages of digitalis to patients hospitalized for myocardial infarction is not available.

In addition to the possibility of adverse digitalis effects in the acute setting, Moss and colleagues [96] have recently reported that, in some patients, digitalis treatment is associated with an increase in the early posthospitalization mortality following myocardial infarction. In this large retrospective study, the increased risk in patients taking digitalis was limited to those with cardiac failure during the acute stage and complex ventricular arrhythmias detected by Holter monitoring prior to discharge. The mechanism underlying the effect is not clear. Congestive heart failure [97] and ventricular arrhythmias [98] following acute infarction are recognized adverse prognostic signs. In the study sited above, congestive heart failure and ventricular arrhythmias were also present in the control patients, but the severity of the underlying cardiac disease appeared to be greater in the digitalis-treated group. Additional data, including those from controlled prospective studies, will be required to clarify the contribution of digitalis in this setting.

All things considered, we currently use the following guidelines for the administration of digitalis in the coronary care unit. In the first 36–48 hr after infarction, patients with mild to moderate heart failure manifested by pulmonary congestion are treated cautiously with diuretic drugs rather than digitalis. If evidence of heart failure persists, digitalis then is added, but the loading dose is arbitrarily reduced (e.g., digoxin 0.5 mg p.o. or I.V. over 10–20 min followed by 0.25 mg/day). For patients with moderately severe heart failure, we usually consider hemodynamic monitoring and the use of vasodilating or inotropic drugs other than digitalis. Although digitalis is not employed in these patients as an initial form of therapy, it is often added later. We continue digitalis treatment in patients who required the drug prior to infarction unless there is evidence of drug toxicity. Digitalis is not used for the acute treatment of cardiogenic shock since it is of limited value in this condition, and its inotropic effect is less potent than that of dobutamine and other sympathomimetic drugs. Digitalis remains the drug of choice for the recurrent or sustained supraventricular arrhythmias, e.g., atrial fibrillation, that not infrequently complicate the course of acute myocardial infarction. The antiarrhythmic actions of the drug and the improvement in cardiac failure (underlying the development of the arrhythmia) combine to restore satisfactory heart rate and rhythm.

Relief of congestion

The above measures to improve the heart's pumping performance promote diuresis in patients with congestive heart failure since decreased renal perfusion is central to the disturbed salt regulation in this disorder [99]. Further therapy of the congested state involves sodium restriction and drugs that affect renal function directly to enhance water and sodium excretion. Dietary sodium restriction is prescribed when the first evidence of fluid retention becomes manifest. Initially, this simply involves removal of the saltshaker from the dining table, unless the heart failure is severe. This measure alone can reduce the sodium intake from greater than 5 g/day to about 3 g/day. If congestion recurs, an oral diuretic of mild to moderate potency, such as a thiazide, is added. Strict sodium restriction is not employed at this stage, in order to permit the patient to receive a palatable and nutritous diet. Moreover, it is likely that specially prepared low-sodium foods are as expensive as daily diuretic therapy. In patients with severe heart failure, and in those with glomerular filtration rates below 30 ml/min, the thiazides are less effective [100] and a diuretic that acts on the loop of Henle, e.g., furosemide, is employed instead. Ethacrinic acid is an alternative, particularly for patients who cannot take furosemide because of an allergy to sulfonamides. The 'loop' diuretics, ethacrinic acid and furosemide, are structurally distinct but of equivalent potency.

If fluid retention cannot be controlled by the above measures, dietary sodium is further limited by use of a low-sodium diet (0.5–2.0 g sodium/day). Combination therapy with diuretics that act at different sites or by different mechanisms can be employed since their effects may be additive. Moreover, the combination of two agents can reduce some of the undesirable effects of diuretic therapy. The addition of spironolactone to patients taking furosemide or thiazide drugs, for example, not only enhances diuretic action but also diminishes the urinary potassium loss. Another combination that is frequently effective in patients with severe congestive heart failure is furosemide and metolazone, an agent that acts on the distal renal tubule. Although related to the thiazides, metolazone appears to maintain diuretic efficacy at low glomerular filtration rates [101].

The chronic administration of diuretic drugs is not without complications [100, 102] and can lead to elevation of the serum levels of uric acid, glucose, calcium and lipids [103]. Perhaps the most common clinically significant problem is hypokalemia, a development of particular concern in the patient who is also receiving digitalis. Metabolic alkalosis is common and develops by two mechanisms: increased hydrogen ion secretion (in light of decreased intracellular potassium content) and increased resorption of filtered bicarbonate in the proximal tubule. When metabolic alkalosis and hypokalemia coexist, treatment with oral potassium chloride is effective. Diuretic therapy can contribute to dilutional hyponatremia, particularly in patients with advanced heart failure who are susceptible to excessive antidiuretic hormone secretion

[104]. Free water restriction usually results in improvement. For patients with severe symptomatic hyponatremia, some authors [100] recommend parenteral treatment with furosemide and a moderately hypertonic saline infusion at a rate of 50–75% of the urine flow rate. However, this procedure demands intensive bedside monitoring of the patient's fluid balance and cardiac function.

Finally, it must be recognized that excessive diuresis results in intravascular volume depletion and a fall in cardiac output because of suboptimal preload. This complication can be avoided in most patients with chronic heart failure by frequent clinical evaluation (including documentation of weight change, presence or absence of edema or rales, and development of orthostatic blood pressure changes) and laboratory studies (including chest X-ray and indices of renal function). However, these findings may be difficult to interpret in the sedentary patient with advanced heart disease, particularly if there is coexistent pulmonary, hepatic, renal, or peripheral venous disease. The question of excessive diuresis is also commonly encountered in the patient receiving potent intravenous diuretics for acute heart failure. The problem is compounded by the fact that there may be a lag between the decrease in the intravascular volume and the corresponding changes in some of the physical findings and chest X-ray.

When the clinical signs indicate that mild intravascular volume depletion is present, the temporary interruption of diuretic therapy may be the only 'treatment' required, assuming the patient can take oral fluids. When intravascular volume depletion is suspected in the compromised patient, the cautious intravenous administration of a 'fluid challenge' with saline solution or colloid preparation coupled with close observation of the patient's cardiovascular status can resolve the question. Stabilization of blood pressure, reduction in resting heart rate, and improvement of renal function in the absence of worsening of pulmonary status following fluid administration support the impression that the ventricular filling pressure was inadequate. When the clinical indicators of intravascular volume are inconsistent or when the risk of fluid challenge is increased (e.g., coexistent renal insufficiency) bedside hemodynamic monitoring with the triple-lumen, balloon-tip catheter [106] provides a means of directly assessing the left ventricular filling pressure (see below).

Vasodilators

Although the rationale for the use of vasodilator therapy for heart failure has been recognized for more than two decades [107, 108], this form of treatment was not systematically applied to patients with cardiac failure due to myocardial dysfunction until the early 1970s [8, 109]. Since then, a number of clinical trials [9, 110–113] have confirmed that dramatic short-term hemodynamic improvement can occur in some patients following administration of vasodilator drugs. These studies have focused attention on the important role of the peripheral circulation in the heart failure state [114], and the limitation of function of the damaged left ventricle by excessive aortic impedance. The physician is now offered an alternative to the use of intravenous inotropic drugs for severe acute heart failure and an additional means of oral therapy for the patient with refractory chronic cardiac failure.

The clinical use of the vasodilators involves the consideration of three questions, the answers to which are only partly available at present: (a) By what criteria should patients be selected for this treatment? (b) Which vasodilator should be prescribed for individual patients? and (c) What are the long-term clinical benefits of vasodilator therapy, including their effect on mortality?

The nature and severity of the underlying cardiac disease, the levels of ventricular filling pressure and peripheral vascular resistance, and the systemic blood pressure are major determinants in the decision to employ vasodilator therapy. The goals of therapy of advanced cardiac failure are to increase cardiac output and decrease the excessively elevated left ventricular filling pressure while maintaining an adequate arterial pressure to perfuse the coronary arteries and other vital vascular beds. Effective therapy should also reduce the excess load that contributes to the impairment of ventricular function. When these goals cannot be met by conventional treatment, sympathomimetic or vasodilator drugs are usually administered. One general approach [115] is to use the vasodilators for patients with severe or refractory heart failure when the initial blood pressure is maintained at normal levels by high peripheral vascular resistance, but to select

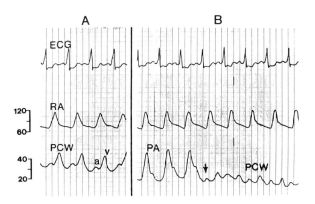

Figure 4. Bedside hemodynamic data for a patient with acute myocardial infarction complicated by cardiac failure and mitral regurgitation. Panel A is a tracing obtained before the institution of drug therapy. The PCW is elevated and a prominent v wave is present. The tracing in Panel B was obtained during treatment with sodium nitroprusside (75 μg/min I.V.). The catheter balloon was inflated at the arrow. The PCW pressure has been reduced and the v wave is less prominent: ECG = electrocardiogram (monitor lead); RA = radial artery pressure curve; PA = pulmonary artery tracing; PCW = pulmonary capillary wedge pressure; pressures are in mmHg.

sympathomimetic drugs for patients whose cardiac failure is complicated by hypotension. The presence of certain mechanical lesions provides an additional reason to consider vasodilator therapy (Figure 4). In patients with mitral or aortic regurgitation and in those with ventricular septal defect, the regurgitant or shunt flow is a direct function of the systemic vascular resistance. The use of a vasodilator to lower aortic impedance favors forward flow [116, 117].

The selection of a specific vasodilator is largely determined by the acuteness and severity of the cardiac failure and by the relative contributions of vascular congestion and decreased perfusion to the clinical state. The presence of extracardiac disease that alters the metabolism or heightens the risk of toxicity of a specific agent as well as the ability of the patient to comply with the requirements of the individual dosage regimens also are important considerations. When pulmonary congestion is the major manifestation, an agent that acts primarily to increase venous capacitance offers the greatest potential value. When decreased perfusion due to an inadequate cardiac output predominates, a drug that dilates the arteriolar bed to reduce aortic impedance and thereby facilitate ventricular emptying and increase stroke volume is preferred. Commonly, evidence both of pulmonary congestion and diminished cardiac output is present, indicating the need for a drug (or combination of drugs) that exerts balanced vasodilating effects on the venous and arteriolar vascular beds (Table 2). For patients with severe acute heart failure, a short-acting drug that can be administered by the intravenous route is most useful. Patients with chronic cardiac failure that has become refractory to conventional therapy also may respond to a short course of intravenous vasodilator treatment. Sodium nitroprusside is the parenteral agent with which there is the greatest experience [8, 110, 111]. Nitroprusside acts directly to dilate both venous and arteriolar vascular beds. Nitroglycerin can be administered by continuous intravenous infusion [118] and may offer additional advantages when the cardiac failure is a consequence of acute ischemic heart disease (see page 470). Nitroglycerin acts primarily on the venous (capacitance) vessels and is most effective in decreasing ventricular preload and pulmonary congestion.

Table 2. Vasodilator drugs in adult patients with cardiac failure.

Drug	Site(s) of action	Frequently used dosage range
Parenteral		
Sodium nitroprusside	Arterial & venous	10–500 μg/min intravenously
Nitroglycerin	Venous > arterial	10–60 μg/min (or higher) intravenously
Nonparenteral		
Isosorbide dinitrate	Venous > arterial	10–60 mg orally every 4–6 hr
2% Nitroglycerin ointment	Venous > arterial	0.5–2″ applied to skin every 4–6 hr
Prazosin	Arterial & venous	1–6 mg orally every 8 hr
Hydralazine	Arterial	25–100 mg orally every 6–8 hr
Captopril	Arterial & (probably) venous	25–100 mg orally every 8 hr
Trimazosin	Arterial & venous	50–300 mg orally every 8 hr

Phentolamine and trimethaphan are effective when administered intravenously. Because of side effects, however, these vasodilators are less desirable than sodium nitroprusside for the acute treatment of myocardial failure [119, 120]. Phentolamine is more likely than nitroprusside to induce sinus tachycardia. Trimethaphan treatment can be associated with severe orthostatic hypotension. Respiratory arrest has been reported as a consequence of trimethaphan treatment.

The principle sites of action of the orally active vasodilators are listed in Table 2. Although this classification is useful, the designation of veno- or arteriolar dilator is often relative rather than absolute. Also, a significant change in one vascular compartment is frequently accompanied by indirect changes in other compartments as well. The reduction of ventricular preload by a venodilator leads to a decrease in ventricular size, which along with aortic impedance is an important determinant of ventricular afterload. Moreover, as the cardiac function improves, the resultant decrease in sympathetic nervous system-mediated vasoconstriction reduces aortic impedance to further reduce afterload and improve the heart's pumping action.

The answer to the third question posed in the introduction to this section remains unclear. It is established [10, 121, 122] that certain regimens of vasodilator therapy can result in sustained hemodynamic effects (at least for months) in some patients and that many patients experience sustained symptomatic improvement during administration of these drugs. Nevertheless, some patients do not respond to vasodilator treatment or experience limiting side effects, and a variable degree of tolerance to the beneficial hemodynamic effects of most of the vasodilator agents has been reported [123–125]. The likelihood that a given patient will obtain long-term improvement in exercise capacity and the degree of improvement are difficult to predict precisely even if the initial effectiveness of the vasodilator regimen is confirmed by hemodynamic monitoring [121, 122, 126]. Bedside hemodynamic monitoring during the institution of chronic vasodilator therapy can serve to identify individuals who do not respond to certain vasodilating agents [127] and can aid in the estimation of an effective initial drug dosage while preventing excessive lowering of the ventricular filling pressure. That vasodilator treatment for cardiac failure alters the natural history of

the underlying cardiac disorder or reduces the mortality in any group or subgroup of patients has not yet been demonstrated conclusively.

In the remainder of this section we will review the use of vasodilators in specific clinical situations. The indications and choice of individual drugs will be guided by the principles outlined above. Controversy persists regarding the timing of the institution of vasodilator therapy. Some investigators have suggested that vasodilators be used early in the treatment of chronic heart failure since they act to reverse one of the underlying mechanisms for its development. Because long-term effects of this form of treatment largely remain to be established, we prefer at the present time to limit their use in this setting to patients who do not respond adequately to conventional therapy.

Vasodilator therapy for acute cardiac failure
Perhaps the most straightforward application of vasodilator therapy is in the treatment of acute cardiac failure due to uncontrolled hypertension [39, 128]. In patients with this disorder, pulmonary edema can occur despite normal or near-normal cardiac output. Intravenous nitroprusside, through its direct relaxation of vascular smooth muscle, reduces the abnormally elevated total peripheral resistance underlying the elevation in blood pressure and reduces pulmonary congestion as well. Careful monitoring of arterial pressure is required as the drug is administered by infusion pump. The recommended initial dosage is $0.5–1.0 \, \mu g/kg/min$ which is titrated upward to achieve satisfactory control of the blood pressure. The average maintenance dosage is about $3 \, \mu g/kg/min$. If high doses or prolonged treatment with nitroprusside is required, the patient must be observed closely for signs of toxicity due to accumulation of the nitroprusside metabolites thiocyanate and cyanide. Thiocyanate blood levels can be monitored to aid in the prevention of this complication [129]. Oral antihypertensive medications are begun (or their dosage adjusted) during this acute treatment period. Effective oral therapy usually requires a combination of drugs and often includes an oral vasodilator along with a diuretic agent. Propranolol (or other beta-adrenergic-blocking drugs) also can be given to many of these patients since the cardiac failure is secondary to the marked elevation in blood pressure, and, after its control, myocardial function is

satisfactory.

Sodium nitroprusside has proven to be effective in the treatment of severe left heart failure due to acute myocardial infarction [11, 112]. The resulting decreases in preload and peripheral vascular resistance are accompanied by a reduction in myocardial oxygen demand because of the decrease in ventricular wall tension. As the elevated diastolic ventricular pressure declines, its action to perhaps impede subendocardial blood flow is lessened. Heart rate, although usually unchanged, may decrease [110] if there is significant hemodynamic improvement and care is taken to avoid excessive lowering of the systemic arterial and left ventricular filling pressures. The above actions favorably influence the myocardial oxygen demand: supply ratio and, theoretically, could limit ischemia. However, the balance of myocardial oxygen demand and supply is governed by a complex interaction of hemodynamic variables [130], and the net effect of a vasodilator on this balance must include consideration of the attendant changes in collateral blood flow and coronary perfusion pressure (in the setting of acute ischemia due to obstructive coronary artery disease, the myocardial blood flow is perfusion-pressure dependent). Some studies of experimentally induced myocardial ischemia have indicated that nitroprusside reduces transmural blood flow in the ischemic area [131]. This effect may result from a reduction of collateral blood flow (coronary steal).

At the present time, sodium nitroprusside is used in patients with acute myocardial infarction to reduce symptoms and signs resulting from the hemodynamic changes of severe heart failure. But the intensive research to determine the effects of vasodilators in the setting of acute myocardial infarction is also in response to the recognition of the central role of ventricular function in determining prognosis. For hospitalized patients with acute myocardial infarction, the major cause of death is cardiac failure, and Forrester and colleagues have confirmed the close relationship of mortality with the extent of pump failure [132] which, in turn, is related to the amount of the myocardium damaged by infarction. Even for the patients who initially respond favorably to vasodilators, the long-term prognosis remains poor, attesting to the extent of myocardial damage underlying the cardiac failure [133]. Controlled prospective studies to assess the effect of vasodilator treatment on mortality from acute myo-

cardial infarction complicated by cardiac failure are limited. The Veterans Administration Cooperative Study [134] of the use of sodium nitroprusside in acute myocardial infarction with left ventricular failure found that overall mortality at 21 days and 13 weeks was not significantly affected by treatment. In this randomized double-blind placebo-controlled trial, there appeared to be a beneficial effect on mortality in the subgroup in which the drug treatment was initiated more than 9 hr after the onset of pain. In the group in which treatment was started within 9 hr, the drug appeared to adversely affect mortality. The significance of the subgroup mortality data has been questioned because of methodological problems [135], and the central conclusion is that overall mortality was not altered by nitroprusside. Durrer and colleagues [136] studied the effect of sodium nitroprusside on 163 randomly selected patients with acute myocardial infarction. The patients were not selected because of cardiac failure, and, in fact, a majority did not exhibit clinical evidence of elevated left ventricular filling pressure (hemodynamic monitoring was not performed). In this study, short-term mortality was significantly reduced by nitroprusside treatment. Peak levels of myocardial creatine kinase (MB isoenzyme) were reduced, possibly reflecting a decrease in infarct size. Although these results are encouraging, additional studies confirming this effect are required before the routine treatment with nitroprusside in this setting can be recommended. Such studies may permit the identification of selected patients or subgroups likely to respond favorably with regard to mortality.

The use of sodium nitroprusside to reduce symptoms and improve hemodynamics in patients with severe heart failure due to acute myocardial infarction requires bedside hemodynamic monitoring. This serves, first, to exclude relative or absolute hypovolemia in patients who exhibit decreased perfusion as the major manifestation of heart failure. Even in patients with obvious pulmonary congestion, the clinical assessment of optimal ventricular filling pressure can be difficult since the patients often have received potent diuretics. Some clinical indices of intravascular volume, e.g., congestive changes seen on the chest X-ray, may lag behind the changes in ventricular filling pressures in their response to treatment. It also is important to recognize that, because of the decrease in ventricular compliance brought about by the infarction, a higher-than-normal filling pressure may be required to obtain the optimal stroke volume. In patients with initially normal left ventricular filling pressure, sodium nitroprusside use can lead to a fall in the stroke volume as ventricular preload becomes limiting. This change elicits a greater degree of sinus tachycardia. As noted previously, the difficulties in estimating the optimal level of the left ventricular filling pressure can be obviated by the use of the percutaneously inserted, balloon-tip triple-lumen catheter introduced by Swan, Ganz, and colleagues [106]. This monitoring technique can be performed in the Intensive Care Unit with low risk to allow continuous measurement of right atrial and pulmonary artery pressures. Inflation of the balloon permits measurement of the pulmonary wedge (or left ventricular filling) pressure. A thermistor on the tip of the catheter permits serial determination of cardiac output by the thermodilution method [137]. From these measurements, the following parameters can be calculated: cardiac index (cardiac output/body surface area); stroke volume index (cardiac index/heart rate); systemic vascular resistance ($80 \times$ (mean arterial pressure–right atrial pressure)/cardiac output); pulmonary vascular resistance (mean pulmonary artery pressure–mean pulmonary wedge pressure/cardiac output $\times$ 80 (dynes $\cdot$ sec $\cdot$ cm^{-5}). The normal values for these parameters are listed in Table 3. Blood samples can be obtained readily for measurement of mixed venous oxygen content. The initial data from the bedside hemodynamic measurements not only aid in the use of vasodilator treatment but also provide short-term prognostic indices [132]. Hemodynamic monitoring is helpful in the recognition of associated right ventricular infarction and mechanical lesions, such as ventricular septal defect and mitral regurgitation. The finding of a right atrial pressure

equal to or greater than the left ventricular filling pressure in the setting of acute myocardial infarction suggests that right ventricular dysfunction, such as results from right ventricular infarction, is present [138]. A characteristic right-atrial pressure wave contour also is present in some patients with this disorder which usually is a complication of inferior or posterior infarction. Postinfarction ventricular septal defect results in a step-up of blood oxygen content when samples of blood from the right-atrial and the pulmonary-artery ports of the balloon catheter are compared. Significant mitral regurgitation is suggested by the presence of large 'V' waves in the wedge pressure tracing [139] (Figure 4). This finding, however, is not specific for mitral regurgitation. The risks of Swan-Ganz catheterization include conduction disturbance and arrhythmia [140, 141], vascular or valve trauma [142, 143], thrombosis [106], and pulmonary infarction [144]. The latter complication occurs when spontaneous advancement of the catheter occludes the distal pulmonary artery. It can be avoided by prompt action (i.e., cautious catheter withdrawal) when the characteristic pulmonary artery waveform is lost. Knotting and entrapment of the catheter are rare complications that, at times, can be corrected by nonsurgical means [145]. Obviously, proper use of the technique requires well maintained and frequently calibrated monitoring equipment. A multichannel strip chart recorder facilitates analysis of the data by allowing temporal correlation of electrocardiographic and pressure recordings.

For the patient with severe myocardial failure and satisfactory blood pressure, nitroprusside is administered intravenously by infusion pump, beginning with 10–20 μg/min. The dose is increased every 10–15 min until the filling pressure is reduced to 16–18 mmHg and perfusion is enhanced to ac-

Table 3. Normal values for hemodynamic parameters.

Pressures (mmHg)		Resistances (dynes $\cdot$ sec $\cdot$ cm^{-5})	
	0–8		
Right atrium	15–30	Systemic vascular resistance	900–1,400
Pulmonary artery	———	Pulmonary vascular resistance	150–250
	5–12		
LVFP[a]	5–12[b]	Cardiac index (liter/min/m²)	2.7–4.3

[a] LVFP = left ventricular filling (pulmonary capillary wedge) pressure.
[b] Although the normal value is 12 mmHg, left ventricular filling pressures of 16–18 mmHg are frequently required to achieve optimal stroke volume in patients with cardiac disease. Levels greater than 20 mm Hg are unlikely to further increase stroke volume significantly but can lead to pulmonary congestion.

469

ceptable levels. This often occurs with a dosage of 50–100 μg/min, but the optimal dosage varies considerably. For many patients, the dose of nitroprusside is limited, ultimately, by a drop in systemic arterial pressure. Careful and continuous monitoring of the blood pressure is required to avoid hypotension which can occur precipitously. In the presence of reduced blood flow to the arm and marked vasoconstriction, the auscultatory method of blood pressure determination can be artifactually low [146]. For this reason, arterial cannulation is often required. The minimum safe level of blood pressure is not known precisely and probably is different in individual patients [147] As a general rule, systolic blood pressure should not be allowed to drop below 100 mmHg, although at times patients with borderline pressure and intense peripheral vasoconstriction will respond favorably to nitroprusside treatment without a further drop in the arterial blood pressure. Since coronary perfusion of the left ventricle occurs primarily during diastole, some authorities have focused on the diastolic pressure, not permitting it to drop below 60 mmHg [5]. If sodium nitroprusside treatment lowers the ventricular filling pressure to less than 14 mm Hg and evidence of hypoperfusion persists, the cautious administration of saline or colloid in 50–100 ml aliquots may further improve cardiac output. For patients with hypoperfusion despite treatment with sodium nitroprusside, dobutamine (2–10 μg/kg/min) or dopamine (1–4 μg/kg/min) can be added to further increase cardiac output. The beneficial effects of vasodilator and inotropic drugs result from independent mechanisms and the combination of the two forms of therapy provides the most potent pharmacologic means of improving cardiac function in patients with severe heart failure [120].

An attempt to wean the patient from nitroprusside and institute oral vasodilator drug therapy usually is made after the ventricular filling pressure has decreased to 16–18 mmHg and the cardiac index has risen to greater than 2 liter/min/m². For many patients, this can be accomplished after 48–72 hr of nitroprusside therapy, but the vasodilator infusion can be continued for seven to ten days if necessary. Thiocyanate levels should be monitored during prolonged treatment. This metabolite is excreted by the kidney and the risk of toxicity is enhanced by the presence of renal insufficiency. The abrupt withdrawal of nitroprusside can result

in adverse rebound phenomena, including marked sinus tachycardia [148]. These changes probably result from vasodilator-induced reflex sympathetic nervous and renin-angiotensin system activation. They are most likely to occur in patients with initially less severe depression of cardiac function. The administration of nitroprusside to patients with congestive heart failure can result in a decrease in arterial blood oxygen saturation [149], presumably as a consequence of dilation (and enhanced perfusion) of previously constricted pulmonary arterioles supplying poorly ventilated areas of the lung. Because of this increase in ventilation–perfusion mismatch, adjustment of oxygen therapy and drug dosage may be required, especially in the initial stages of treatment of patients with marked hypoxemia.

Intravenous nitroglycerin has been used to treat cardiac failure due to acute myocardial infarction. Moreover, the results of some studies suggest that nitroglycerin, in contrast to nitroprusside, acts directly to increase perfusion of ischemic myocardium [131]. The disparate actions of nitroglycerin and nitroprusside on ischemic blood flow may result from nitroglycerin's predominant effect on large coronary arteries (including collaterals) rather than the smaller coronary resistance vessels. Nitroglycerin decreases left ventricular filling pressure to a greater extent than it lowers systemic vascular resistance [150], and, consequently, the drug is most commonly used in patients with heart failure to provide relief from pulmonary congestion. Cardiac output usually improves following nitrate therapy, particularly if the initial left ventricular filling pressure is significantly elevated [118]. However, for a given degree of preload reduction, there is a smaller reduction of aortic impedance (and lesser increase in cardiac output) with parenteral nitroglycerin than with sodium nitroprusside [5]. As with the other vasodilators, it is essential that left ventricular filling pressure remain satisfactory. The vigorous administration of nitroglycerin to patients with initially normal or low filling pressures is followed by reflex tachycardia and hypotension, changes that act to worsen myocardial ischemia. These points emphasize the need for careful observation and heart rate monitoring when this drug is used to treat acute cardiac failure due to myocardial infarction. The intravenous infusion of nitroglycerin is usually begun at 10–15 μg/min and gradually increased in 5–10 μg/ min increments every 10–15 min until the desired hemodynamic changes occur or the treatment is limited by a drop in blood pressure.

Unloading of the ventricle also can be accomplished by use of the intraaortic balloon pump [151]. This technique, which can be performed percutaneously, not only reduces aortic impedance during systole but also enhances diastolic perfusion pressure and coronary flow. Because of its potential to limit infarct size, some authorities recommend the early use of the balloon pump in patients with significant heart failure due to acute myocardial infarction. The effect of this form of therapy on mortality from severe heart failure is not yet clear. Early reports [151] indicated that it improved survival only if followed by surgical procedures to restore coronary blood flow or repair associated mechanical lesions. More recent studies [152] suggest that mortality may be reduced in some groups of patients in the absence of lesions amenable to surgical therapy. The risks of intraaortic balloon pumping include thrombosis and embolism as well as vascular trauma. Not infrequently, the patients have coexistent peripheral vascular disease and the further reduction in lower extremity blood flow by the balloon catheter can precipitate acute ischemia. In some cases, the catheter cannot be inserted because of the intrinsic vascular disease.

Vasodilator therapy for chronic cardiac failure
The acute improvement in cardiac performance elicited by intravenous nitroprusside has led to an investigation of the use of oral vasodilators by ambulatory patients with chronic heart failure. The initial studies to assess the benefit of oral unloading therapy focused on the short-term administration of nitrates [113], hydralazine [12], and prazosin [153]. Although the results of these studies were favorable, caution was properly advised regarding their long-term use because the beneficial hemodynamic changes were measured only at rest (in the supine position) and because of the potential for the development of tolerance and side effects to the medications. Recently, reports of the more prolonged use of oral vasodilators in ambulatory patients both at rest [121, 122, 124, 127, 154, 155] and following exercise [156–159] have become available, confirming their sustained hemodynamic effectiveness in some clinical situations. It appears that sustained improvement in symptoms also

occurs in many patients [127, 155–157]. Unfortunately, the relationship of the initial measured hemodynamic response to the vasodilator therapy and the subsequent clinical response is not close [121, 122, 155]. At least with some regimens (e.g., hydralazine-nitrates), a lack of any acute hemodynamic improvement following the administration of these vasodilators makes subsequent clinical improvement unlikely, but for patients who do respond acutely, the subsequent change in symptoms and functional classification cannot be accurately predicted by the magnitude of the objectively measured initial hemodynamic improvement [155]. The longer-term studies have also demonstrated that side effects [154], and tolerance to the hemodynamic effects of the vasodilators [124, 125] limit their effectiveness in some patients.

The choice and proper use of oral vasodilator drugs requires a thorough understanding of the mechanisms of their actions and an appreciation of their limitations and risks (Chapter 13). Drugs that share the ability to dilate arterioles may exert different effects on the distribution of regional blood flow [159] and evoke reflex circulatory changes to different degrees. Although the vasodilators share some side effects, each agent is associated with unique problems. In all cases, the ventricular filling pressure must remain satisfactory and care must be taken to avoid hypotension, particularly in patients with coronary artery disease. Since the patients are ambulatory, this caution must include checks for orthostatic changes in blood pressure. Although heart rate usually is unchanged when vasodilators are used to treat patients with advanced cardiac failure, an acceleration of the sinus rate can occur. Peripheral edema often accompanies chronic vasodilator therapy and necessitates an increase in diuretic dosage. It has been proposed that fluid retention, resulting in reduced vascular responsiveness, contributes to the tolerance to chronic vasodilator therapy [125].

Nitrates [122, 158] and hydralazine [9, 121, 127, 156] are among the most commonly used unloading agents for the treatment of chronic cardiac failure. The combination of the two drugs produces hemodynamic effects that are qualitatively similar to those of intravenous nitroprusside [160]. A number of nitrate preparations are available, including isosorbide dinitrate, nitroglycerin ointment and pentaerythral tetranitrate [161]. Nitroglycerin also can

471

be administered by a recently developed transdermal delivery system designed to provide controlled release of the drug for up to 24 hr.

There is considerable variability in the response of individual patients to the hemodynamic effects of the nitrates, and usually it is best to begin treatment with a low dose that is then titrated upward with frequent determination of blood pressure in the recumbent and upright positions. All nitrate preparations can produce headache, a side effect that is often self-limited. If bothersome or persistent it can be controlled by decreasing the dose.

When oral isosorbide dinitrate is chosen, doses of 20–40 mg or more every 4–6 hr may be required to achieve the optimal clinical response because of 'first-pass' hepatic metabolism. Nitroglycerin ointment is often substituted for the bedtime dose of isosorbide dinitrate. Although the ointment offers an alternative to isosorbide dinitrate for the daytime treatment of chronic heart failure, it is disliked by some patients for cosmetic reasons. The hemodynamic effects of the ointment persist for 4–6 hr after application [161]. The sustained-release transdermal nitroglycerin preparations are easier to apply and appear to be cosmetically superior to the standard nitroglycerin ointment. Although there is no obvious reason to suspect that they would not be similarly effective in the treatment of cardiac failure, there are only limited data about their use in this setting.

The acute administration of oral hydralazine, through its selective vasodilation of the arteriolar bed [162], lowers systemic vascular resistance and raises stroke volume with lesser (or no) effect on ventricular filling pressure [9]. The heart rate is not substantially changed in most patients with advanced heart failure. The potential for sinus rate acceleration does exist, and this untoward effect can occur in some patients in the absence of a change in arterial pressure. Because of the reduction in impedance to forward flow, the drug is particularly beneficial when mitral regurgitation contributes to the development of the heart failure [116, 163]. In this case, hydralazine reduces both regurgitant flow and ventricular filling pressure.

Hydralazine is also useful for patients with cardiac failure due to chronic aortic regurgitation, either in preparation for valve replacement or for individuals who decline surgery [156]. Arteriolar dilation enhances forward stroke volume at the expense of the regurgitant flow. In some patients, ejection fraction is improved as well. Although systemic arterial pressure is often unchanged or only slightly decreased during hydralazine treatment of heart failure, it must be measured frequently to assure adequate coronary perfusion pressure. This is especially important in patients with aortic regurgitation since the circulatory runoff lowers the diastolic coronary perfusion pressure.

Hydralazine therapy is usually initiated with a 25-mg dose, although in patients with borderline blood pressure a 10-mg dose may be preferred. The dose is then gradually increased. Most patients require 25–100 mg three to four times daily. The magnitude of the response varies and for some patients higher doses are required to obtain optimal hemodynamic effect [164]. Side effects are not uncommon during hydralazine therapy [154, 163] and can necessitate discontinuation of the drug in the early or late stages of treatment. In addition to orthostatic hypotension, the side effects include anorexia, nausea, and drug fever. The lupus syndrome has also been reported as a complication of hydralazine treatment of cardiac failure [154]. Experience in patients with hypertension indicates that this adverse effect is related both to the duration of treatment and the drug dosage (rarely occurring with dosages less than 200 mg/day). The individuals with rapid acetylation rates are at increased risk for this complication [162]. Several studies have demonstrated that the hemodynamic and clinical improvement evoked by hydralazine persists during the chronic treatment of heart failure [121, 127, 154, 155]. However, tolerance to the hemodynamic effects of hydralazine (accompanied by symptomatic deterioration) has been reported [125]. The mechanism of the tolerance is not clear, but it appears to be drug specific.

The postsynaptic alpha-adrenergic-blocking agent, prazosin [13, 165], offers an alternative to the combination of nitrates and hydralazine since it exerts balanced effects on the venous and arteriolar vascular beds. It is administered every 6–8 hr, beginning with a 1-mg dose. Therapy is frequently initiated at bedtime to reduce the likelihood of the 'first-dose phenomenon' in which exaggerated postural hypotension can lead to dizziness and other symptoms. The dose is gradually adjusted upward with frequent checks of supine and upright blood pressure. The end-points of therapy include adequate clinical response, symptomatic orthostatic hypotension (or other side effects), or a maximal dose of 20 mg/day. Frequent reevaluation is necessary to detect evidence of increased fluid retention and tolerance to the vasodilator effect. These changes often can be reversed by increasing the doses of diuretic or prazosin, respectively. Although prazosin treatment can lead to sustained improvement of exercise tolerance and hemodynamics [13, 157], the development of drug tolerance is a particularly important problem with this agent [124], and the blunting of the beneficial hemodynamic effects can occur in some patients shortly after the initiation of therapy. This effect may be due, in part, to an increase in plasma norepinephrine levels following prazosin treatment [166]. Such a change could act to attenuate the competitive alpha-adrenergic blockade that underlies the prazosin-induced vasodilation.

The oral antihypertensive agent, captopril [167], can provide effective arterial and venous dilation in many patients with advanced congestive heart failure by reducing systemic vascular resistance and ventricular filling pressure while increasing cardiac index [168]. Renal function is improved, a change that may result in part from favorable redistribution of regional blood flow [169]. The beneficial hemodynamic effects and clinical improvement appear to be sustained during chronic treatment [170].

The effectiveness of captopril treatment further supports the important role, in some patients [8, 171], of the renin-angiotensin system in the excessive systemic vascular resistance that can accompany and contribute to the heart failure state [172]. By blocking the formation of the potent vasopressor, angiotensin II, captopril may act to limit also the reactive vasoconstriction that can reduce the chronic effectiveness of arterial dilators and contribute to rebound hemodynamic changes following the cessation of vasodilator therapy [148, 173]. Furthermore, the tendency for vasodilator-induced sodium retention is counteracted by a decrease in the secretion of aldosterone from the adrenal gland. Renal potassium loss is decreased [167]. The magnitude of the acute hemodynamic effects appears to be related directly to pretreatment levels of plasma renin activity, but some patients with low pretreatment levels respond favorably to the drug. A beneficial chronic clinical response to captopril treatment does not appear to be dependent on a good

acute response to the drug [168].

Experience with captopril, thus far, suggests that oral angiotensin-converting enzyme inhibitors may play an important role in the treatment of advanced heart failure. However, the experience is still limited, and the factors that will favor their selection, alone or in combination with other agents, over other vasodilators remain to be established. The use of captopril by patients with hypertension has been associated with a number of allergic and toxic reactions, including rash, proteinuria, and neutropenia [167]. Although the incidence of these effects is small, it may limit the usefulness of the drug. Studies of analogues of captopril that may be less likely to induce allergic phenomena currently are underway.

Other inotropic agents

Catecholamines and other sympathomimetic amines offer an alternative or additional approach to the treatment of severe acute cardiac failure. In the presence of significant hypotension, they constitute the medical treatment of choice. These agents also can benefit the patient with chronic heart failure who has experienced acute decompensation or whose symptoms remain refractory despite optimal treatment with conventional agents. In this setting, a several-day course of an appropriate intravenously administered catecholamine (or combination of catecholamine and vasodilator) may restore hemodynamic compensation and stabilization.

The pharmacologic properties of the sympathomimetic drugs have been reviewed in Chapter 6. The net hemodynamic effects of the sympathomimetic agents in patients with cardiac failure are the result of the interaction of their myocardial and peripheral vascular actions as well as the reflex circulatory changes that follow the administration of the drugs. In the setting of coronary artery disease, the decision to use a specific catecholamine to increase contractility must include consideration of its potential to induce sinus tachycardia and increase systemic-vascular resistance: changes that increase myocardial oxygen demand and can worsen ischemia or extend infarct size [174]. Largely because of these considerations, dopamine [175] and dobutamine [176] have become the catecholamines used most commonly for the treatment of cardiac failure, unless a strong vasoconstrictor effect is required to maintain systemic arterial (and coronary perfusion) pressure. In the latter circumstance, norepinephrine may be preferred.

Although dopamine produces less vasoconstriction than norepinephrine and less tachycardia than isoproterenol, it does exert dose-dependent effects on the sinus node and peripheral vascular beds. When administered in low doses (< 5 μg/kg/min), dopamine increases cardiac output and renal blood flow with little change in heart rate and vascular resistance. At higher doses, alpha- adrenergic vascular effects begin to predominate and systemic vascular resistance increases. The heart rate increases as well with higher doses. For patients with refractory cardiac failure but satisfactory blood pressure, dopamine treatment is initiated with a low dose (1.0–3.0 μg/kg/min) intravenous infusion. The dose is gradually increased until a satisfactory response has occurred or until the heart rate or indices of systemic vascular resistance increase. In patients with hypotension, higher initial doses may be required. Dopamine (and dobutamine) therapy can result in supraventricular and ventricular cardiac arrhythmias. Their emergence requires reduction in dosage or discontinuation of the drug.

Dobutamine is less likely than dopamine to increase heart rate when given in dosages that enhance myocardial contractility [177]. Ventricular arrhythmias also may occur less frequently during dobutamine infusion than with dopamine. Although dobutamine lacks dopamine's direct vasodilator action on the renal vasculature, the alpha-adrenergic vasoconstrictor effect seen with higher doses of dopamine also is less prominent. Dobutamine offers the additional advantage of reducing left ventricular filling pressure [177, 178]. In patients with cardiac failure, the systemic vascular resistance is often reduced by dobutamine, likely due to attenuation of the reflex sympathetic nervous system-mediated vasoconstriction. The usual dose of dobutamine is 2.5–10 μg/kg/min.

The use of drugs that directly enhance cardiac contractility carries the risk of precipitating myocardial ischemia since contractility is a major determinant of myocardial oxygen demand. However, when used in the patient with significant heart failure, the net oxygen demand may be unchanged or actually reduced if the improvement in cardiac pumping function is not accompanied by a direct action of the drug to accelerate the heart rate or

increase aortic impedance to any appreciable degree. Taken together, the actions of dobutamine should limit myocardial oxygen demand to a greater extent than dopamine. When used to treat normotensive patients with cardiac failure due to ischemic heart disease, it is often preferred over dopamine [179]. It appears that the cautious administration of dobutamine to patients with acute myocardial infarction can result in favorable hemodynamic effects without a change in the estimated infarct size or the incidence of ventricular arrhythmias [178, 180].

It has been proposed that the combination of dopamine and dobutamine can offer additional benefits for some patients with refractory heart failure. Dopamine is given in low doses (1.5–3.0 μg/kg/min) to elicit selective vasodilation in the renal and mesenteric vascular beds and dobutamine is used to ensure optimal inotropic stimulation. Dopamine is preferred over dobutamine for hypotensive patients who require peripheral vascular constriction to obtain a satisfactory perfusion pressure. When marked hypotension is present, norepinephrine infusion (2–8 μg/min) may be required to maintain adequate perfusion pressure. The lowest effective dose of the drug should be used in order to avoid excessive vasoconstriction and the emergence of ventricular arrhythmias.

At the present time, digitalis glycosides are the only readily available orally active inotropic drugs of established value in the treatment of chronic congestive heart failure. The identification and synthesis of new inotropic agents is an area of intensive research. Preliminary data are available concerning the oral beta-adrenergic agonist, pirbuterol [182]. When administered as a single dose to ten patients with refractory chronic cardiac failure due to ischemic heart disease, pirbuterol led to an increase in cardiac index and decreases in left ventricular filling pressure and systemic vascular resistance. These beneficial hemodynamic changes persisted for several hours with only a slight decrease in mean systemic blood pressure and a slight increase in heart rate. Long-term studies to confirm the potential benefits and to identify the limitations and side effects of the use of pirbuterol in patients with cardiac failure remain to be completed.

Considerable experimental data are available about the effects of the bipyridine derivative, amrinone, on cardiac pumping function [183, 184]. The mechanism of its inotropic action is not fully understood but is dissimilar to that of digitalis. Amrinone does not inhibit sodium, potassium ATPase activity. Recent studies suggest that it may act through the cyclic nucleotide system, although via a mechanism not involving the beta-receptor. Its actions are not blocked by propranolol. Oral and intravenous preparations of amrinone have been evaluated in small groups of patients with advanced cardiac failure [185–187]. When administered acutely, amrinone increases cardiac output and decreases ventricular filling pressure and systemic vascular resistance. These effects are not associated with significant changes in systemic blood pressure or heart rate. The acute hemodynamic benefits of amrinone appear to be similar in magnitude to those of dobutamine (titrated to achieve optimal effects) [188]. In patients with chronic cardiac failure due to coronary artery disease, amrinone can improve the heart's pumping function without clinical evidence of myocardial ischemia, despite a measured decrease in coronary blood flow and an estimated increase in contractility [185]. Presumably, the reduction in oxygen requirement resulting from reduced ventricular wall tension offsets an increased oxygen need due to enhanced contractility. Net myocardial oxygen demand may actually decrease. Amrinone can worsen experimentally induced cardiac ischemia [185], however, and thus may be detrimental to some patients with acute myocardial infarction or ischemia. The incidence of other reported side effects including nausea and premature ventricular beats during amrinone infusion [184] and thrombocytopenia and nephrogenic diabetes insipidus during oral amrinone treatment [185] as well as the overall effectiveness and risk: benefit ratio during long-term treatment remain to be established.

References

1. Braunwald E, Ross J Jr, Sonnenblick EH: Mechanisms of Contraction of the Normal and Failing Heart. Little, Brown, Boston, 1968, p 77.
2. Mason DT et al: Clinical determination of left ventricular contractility by hemodynamics and myocardial mechanics. In: Yu PN, Goodwin JF (eds) Progress in Cardiology. Lea and Febiger, Philadelphia, 1972, p 121.
3. Ross J Jr et al: Left ventricular performance during muscular exercise in patients with and without cardiac dysfunction. Circulation 34:597, 1966.
4. Diamond G, Forrester JS: Effects of coronary artery disease and acute myocardial infarction on left ventricular compliance in man. Circulation 45:11, 1972.
5. Chatterjee K, Parmley WW: The role of vasodilator therapy in heart failure. Prog Cardiovasc Dis 19:310, 1977.
6. Mason DT et al: Alterations of hemodynamics and myocardial dynamics in patients with congestive heart failure. Pathophysiologic mechanisms and assessment of cardiac function and ventricular contractility. Prog Cardiovasc Dis 12:507, 1970.
7. Cohn JN: Physiologic basis of vasodilator therapy for heart failure. Am J Med 71:135, 1981.
8. Levine TB et al: Activity of the sympathetic nervous system and renin-angiotensin system assessed by plasma hormone levels and their relation to hemodynamic abnormalities in congestive heart failure. Am J Cardiol 49:1659, 1982.
9. Grancis GS et al: Response of plasma norepinephrine and epinephrine to dynamic exercise in patients with congestive heart failure. Am J Cardiol 49:1152, 1982.
10. Ross J Jr: Afterload mismatch and preload reserve: a conceptual framework for the analysis of ventricular function. Prog Cardiovasc Dis 18:255, 1976.
11. Franciosa JA et al: Improved left ventricular function during nitroprusside infusion in acute myocardial infarction. Lancet 1:650, 1972.
12. Chatterjee K et al: Oral hydralazine for chronic refractory heart failure. Circulation 54:879, 1976.
13. Colucci WS et al: Chronic therapy of heart failure with prazosin: a randomized double-blind trial. Am J Cardiol 45:337, 1980.
14. Braunwald E: Control of myocardial oxygen consumption: physiologic and clinical considerations. Am J Cardiol 27:416, 1971.
15. Braunwald E et al: An analysis of the cardiac response to exercise. Circ Res 20:44, 1962.
16. Goldstein RE et al: Impairment of autonomically mediated heart rate control in patients with cardiac dysfunction. Circ Res 36:571, 1975.
17. Corday E, Lang FW: Altered physiology associated with cardiac arrhythmias. In: Hurst JW (ed) The Heart. McGraw Hill, New York, 1978, pp 630–631.
18. Boerth RC, Covell JW, Pod PE, Ross J Jr: Increased myocardial oxygen consumption and contractile state associated with increased heart rate in dogs. Circ Res 24:725, 1969.
19. Ricci D et al: Role of tachycardia as an inotropic stimulus in man. J Clin Invest 63:695, 1979.
20. DeMaria A et al: Systematic correlation of cardiac chamber size and ventricular performance determined with echocardiography and alterations in heart rate in normal persons. Am J Cardiol 43:1, 1979.
21. Vatner SF, Braunwald E: Cardiac frequency-control and adjustments to alterations. Prog Cardiovasc Dis 14:431, 1972.
22. Moraski RR et al: Left ventricular function in patients with and without myocardial infarction and one, two or three vessel coronary artery disease. Am J Cardiol 35:1010, 1975.
23. Mason DT et al: Comparison of the contractile state of the normal, hypertrophied and failing heart in man. In: Alpert

NR (ed) Cardiac Hypertrophy. Academic Press, New York, 1971, p 433.

24. Escher DJW: Types of pacemakers and their complications. Circulation 47:119, 1973.

25. Dalen JE, Haynes FW, Dexter L: Life expectancy with atrial septal defect. J Am Med Assoc 200:442, 1967.

26. Ross J Jr: Left ventricular function and the timing of surgical treatment in valvular heart disease. Ann Intern Med 94:498, 1981.

27. Henry WL et al: Evaluation of aortic valve replacement in patients with valvular aortic stenosis. Circulation 61:814, 1980.

28. Schuler G et al: Serial noninvasive assessment of left ventricular hypertrophy and function after surgical correction of aortic regurgitation. Am J Cardiol 44:585, 1979.

29. Kloster FE: Diagnosis and management of complications of prosthetic heart valves. Am J Cardiol 35:872, 1975.

30. Frank S, Johnson A, Ross J Jr: Natural history of valvular aortic stenosis. Br Heart J 35:41, 1973.

31. Smith N, McAnulty JH, Rahimtoola SH: Severe aortic stenosis with impaired left ventricular function and clinical heart failure: results of valve replacement. Circulation 58:255, 1978.

32. Segal J, Harvey WP, Hufnagel C: A clinical study of one hundred cases of severe aortic insufficiency. Am J Med 21:200, 1956.

33. Rapaport E: Natural history of aortic and mitral valve disease. Am J Cardiol 35:221, 1975.

34. Gault JH, Covell JW, Braunwald E, Ross J Jr: Left ventricular performance following correction of free aortic regurgitation. Circulation 42:773, 1970.

35. Schuler G et al: Temporal response of left ventricular performance to mitral valve surgery. Circulation 59:1218, 1979.

36. Borer JS et al: Exercise-induced left ventricular dysfunction in symptomatic and asymptomatic patients with aortic regurgitation: assessment with radionuclide cineangiography. Am J Cardiol 42:351, 1978.

37. Veterans Administration Cooperative Study Group on Antihypertensive Agents: Effects of treatment on morbidity in hypertension. J Am Med Assoc 202:1028, 1967.

38. Hypertension Detection and Follow-up Program Cooperative Group: Five year findings of the Hypertension Detection and Follow-up Program. I. Reduction in mortality of persons with high blood pressure, including mild hypertension. J Am Med Assoc 242:2562, 1979.

39. Schlant RC, Tsagaris TS, Robertson RJ Jr: Studies on the acute cardiovascular effects of intravenous sodium nitroprusside. Am J Cardiol 9:51, 1962.

40. Kleiger JH, Dirks JF: Medication compliance in chronic asthmatic patients. J Asthma Res 16:93, 1979.

41. Stephen SA: Unwanted effects of propranolol. Am J Cardiol 18:463, 1966.

42. Braunwald E et al: Idiopathic hypertrophic subaortic stenosis. Circulation 29/30 (Suppl IV):1, 1964.

43. Markiewicz W et al: Normal myocardial contractile state in the presence of quinidine. Circulation 53:101, 1976.

44. Kayden HJ, Brodie BB, Steele JM: Procainamide: a review. Circulation 15:118, 1952.

45. Podrid PJ, Schoeneberger A, Lown B: Congestive heart failure caused by oral disopyramide. N Engl J Med 302:614, 1980.

46. Leahoy EJ Jr et al: Interaction between digoxin and quinidine. J Am Med Assoc 240:533, 1978.

47. Mungall DR et al: Effects of quinidine on serum digoxin concentration. Ann Intern Med 93:689, 1980.

48. Koster RW, Wellens HJJ: Quinidine-induced ventricular flutter and fibrillation without digitalis therapy. Am J Cardiol 38:519, 1976.

49. Jensen D et al: Improvement in ventricular function during exercise studied with radionuclide ventriculography after cardiac rehabilitation. Am J Cardiol 46:770, 1980.

50. Verani MS et al: Effects of exercise training on left ventricular performance and myocardial perfusion in patients with coronary artery disease. Am J Cardiol 47:797, 1981.

51. Harvey RM et al: Some effects of digoxin upon the heart and circulation in man: digoxin in left ventricular failure. Am J Med 7:439, 1949.

52. Ferrer MI, Convoy RJ, Harvey RM: Some effects of digoxin on the heart and circulation in man: digoxin in combined ventricular failure. Circulation 21:372, 1960.

53. Bloomfield RA et al: The effects of cardiac glycosides upon the dynamics of the circulation in congestive heart failure. J Clin Invest 27:588, 1948.

54. Hull SM, Mackintosh A: Discontinuation of maintenance digoxin therapy in general practice. Lancet 2:1054, 1977.

55. Johnston GD, McDevitt DG: Is maintenance digoxin necessary in patients with sinus rhythm? Lancet 1:567, 1979.

56. Beller GA et al: Digitalis intoxication. A prospective clinical study with serum level correlations. N Engl J Med 284:989, 1971.

57. Cohn K et al: Variability of hemodynamic responses to acute digitalization in chronic cardiac failure due to cardiomyopathy and coronary artery disease. Am J Cardiol 35:461, 1975.

58. Arnold SB et al: Long-term digitalis therapy improves left ventricular function in heart failure. N Engl J Med 303:1443, 1980.

59. Kleiman JH et al: Effect of digitalis on normal and abnormal left ventricular segmental dynamics. Am J Cardiol 43:1001, 1979.

60. Covell JW et al: Studies on digitalis. Effects on myocardial oxygen consumption. J Clin Invest 1535, 1966.

61. Beiser GD et al: Studies on digitalis XVII. Effects of ouabain on the hemodynamic response to exercise in patients with mitral stenosis in normal sinus rhythm. N Engl J Med 278, 1968.

62. Doherty JE: Digitalis glycosides. Ann Intern Med 79:229, 1973.

63. Braunwald E et al: Studies on digitalis: observations in man on the effects of digitalis preparations on the contractility of the non-failing heart and on total peripheral resistance. J Clin Invest 40:52, 1961.

64. McHenry PL: Exercise stress testing: methods, protocols, measurements and new indices. In: Advances in Heart Disease, vol II. Grune and Stratton, New York, 1978, pp 273–306.

65. Silber EN, Katz LM: The treatment of heart failure. In: Silber EN, Katz LN (eds) Heart Disease. Macmillan, New

York, 1975, pp 1145.

66. Ogilvie R, Reedy J: An educational program in digitalis therapy. J Am Med Assoc 222:50, 1972.

67. Williams JF Jr, Klocke FJ, Braunwald E: Studies on digitalis XIII. A comparison of the effects of potassium on the inotropic and arrhythmia-producing actions of ouabain. J Clin Invest 45:346, 1966.

68. Koch-Weser J: Serum drug concentrations as therapeutic guides. N Engl J Med 287:227, 1972.

69. Doherty JE, Perkins WH: Digoxin metabolism in hypo and hyperthyroidism. Studies with titrated digoxin in thyroid disease. Ann Intern Med 64:489, 1966.

70. Surawicz B, Mortelman S: Factors affecting individual tolerance to digitalis. In: Fisch C, Surawicz B (eds) Digitalis. Grune and Stratton, New York, 1969, p 127.

71. Baum GL et al: Digitalis toxicity in chronic cor pulmonale. South Med J 49:1037, 1956.

72. Rodensky PL, Wasserman F: Observations on digitalis intoxication. Arch Intern Med 108:171, 1961.

73. Hudson LD et al: Arrhythmias associated with acute respiratory failure in patients with chronic airway obstruction. Chest 63:661, 1973.

74. Collins JM et al: The cardiotoxicity of isoprenaline during hypoxia. Br J Pharmacol 36:35, 1969.

75. Camarata SJ, Weil MH, Hanashiro PK: Cardiac arrest in the critically ill. A study on predisposing causes in 132 patients. Circulation 44:688, 1971.

76. Green LH, Smith TW: The use of digitalis in patients with pulmonary disease. Ann Intern Med 87:459, 1977.

77. Klein MD et al: Comparison of serum digoxin level measurement with acetylstrophanthidin tolerance testing. Circulation 49:1053, 1974.

78. Beller GA et al: Cardiac and circulatory effects of digitalis during chronic hypoxia in intact conscious dogs. Am J Physiol 229:270, 1975.

79. Ferrer MI et al: Some effects of digoxin upon the heart and circulation in man: digoxin in chronic cor pulmonale. Circulation 1:161, 1950.

80. Cattell M, Gold H: The influence of digitalis glycosides on the force of contraction of mammalian cardiac muscle. J Pharmacol Exp Ther 62:116, 1938.

81. Jozek V, Schrizen F: Hemodynamic effect of deslanoside at rest and during exercise in patients with chronic bronchitis. Br Heart J 35:2, 1973.

82. Linde LM et al: Pulmonary and systemic hemodynamic effects of cardiac glycosides. Am Heart J 76:356, 1968.

83. Fisch C, Knoebel SB: Recognition and therapy of digitalis intoxication. Prog Cardiovasc Dis 12:71, 1970.

84. Fisch C: Relation of electrolyte disturbances to cardiac arrhythmias. Circulaton 47:408, 1973.

85. Whang R: Hyperkalemia: diagnosis and treatment. J Med Sci 272:19, 1976.

86. Helfant RH, Scherlag BJ, Damato AN: The electrophysiological properties of diphenylhydantoin sodium as compared to procainamide in the normal and digitalis-intoxicated heart. Circulation 34:108, 1967.

87. Resnekov L: Present status of electroversion in the management of cardiac dysrhythmias. Circulation 47:1356, 1973.

88. Marcus FI: Use of digitalis in acute myocardial infarction. Circulation 62:17, 1980.

89. Rahimtoola SH et al: Effects of ouabain on impaired left ventricular function in acute myocardial infarction. N Engl J Med 287:527, 1972.

90. Rahimtoola SH, Gunnar RM: Digitalis in acute myocardial infarction: help or hazard? Ann Intern Med 82:234, 1974.

91. Kumar R et al: Experimental myocardial infarction. VI. Efficacy and toxicity of digitalis in acute and healing phase in intact conscious dogs. J Clin Invest 49:358, 1970.

92. Kerber RE et al: Effect of inotropic agents on the localized dyskinesis of acutely ischemic myocardium. Circulation 49:1038, 1974.

93. Morrison J et al: Digitalis and myocardial infarction in man. Circulation 62:8, 1980.

94. Ku DD, Lucchesi BR: Ischemic-induced alterations in cardiac sensitivity to digitalis. Eur J Pharmacol 57:135, 1979.

95. Lown B et al: Sensitivity to digitalis drugs in acute myocardial infarction. Am J Cardiol 30:388, 1972.

96. Moss AJ et al: Digitalis-associated cardiac mortality after myocardial infarction. Circulation 64:1150, 1981.

97. Humphries JP: Survival after myocardial infarction: prognosis and management. Mod Concepts Cardiovasc Dis 46: 51, 1977.

98. Schulze RA, Strauss HW, Pi HB: Sudden death in the year following myocardial infarction: relation to ventricular premature contractions in the late hospital phase and left ventricular ejection fraction. Am J Med 62:192, 1977.

99. Cannon PJ: The kidney in heart failure. N Engl J Med 296:26, 1977.

100. Porter GA: The role of diuretics in the treatment of heart failure. J Am Med Assoc 244:1614, 1980.

101. Bennett WM, Porter GA: Efficacy and safety of metolazone in renal failure. J Clin Pharmacol 13:357, 1973.

102. Frazier HS, Yager H: The clinical use of diuretics. N Engl J Med 288:200, 1973.

103. Grimm RH Jr et al: Effects of thiazide diuretics on plasma lipids and lipoproteins in mildly hypertensive patients. Ann Intern Med 94:7, 1981.

104. Humes HD: The kidney in congestive heart failure. In: Brenner BM, Stein JH (eds) Sodium and Water Homeostasis. Churchill Livingstone, New York, 1978.

105. Ramo BW et al: Hemodynamic findings in 123 patients with acute myocardial infarction on admission. Circulation 42:567, 1970.

106. Swan HJC et al: Catheterization of the heart in man with use of a flow-directed balloon tipped catheter. N Engl J Med 283:447, 1970.

107. Burch GE: Evidence for increased venous tone in chronic congestive heart failure. Arch Intern Med 98:750, 1956.

108. Judson WE, Hollander W, Wilkins RW: The effects of intravenous hydralazine on cardiovascular and renal function in patients with and without congestive heart failure. Circulation 8:664, 1956.

109. Majid PA, Sharma B, Taylor SH: Phentolamine for vasodilator treatment of severe heart failure. Lancet 2:719, 1971.

110. Guiha NA et al: Treatment of refractory heart failure with infusion of nitroprusside. N Engl J Med 291:587, 1974.

111. Cohn JN et al: Chronic vasodilator therapy in the management of cardiogenic shock and intractable left ventricular failure. Ann Intern Med 81:777, 1974.

112. Chatterjee J et al: Hemodynamic and metabolic responses to vasodilator therapy in acute myocardial infarction. Circulation 48:1183, 1973.

113. Taylor WR et al: Hemodynamic effects of nitroglycerin ointment in congestive heart failure. Am J Cardiol 38:469, 1976.

114. Cohn JN et al: Role of vasoconstrictor mechanisms in the control of left ventricular performance of the normal and damaged heart. Am J Cardiol 44:1019, 1979.

115. Cohn JN, Franciosa JA: Selecton of vasodilator, inotropic or combined therapy for the management of heart failure. Am J Med 65:181, 1978.

116. Greenberg BH et al: Beneficial effects of hydralazine in severe mitral regurgitation. Circulation 58:273, 1978.

117. Greenberg BH et al: Beneficial effects of hydralazine on rest and exercise hemodynamics in patients with chronic severe aortic insufficiency. Circulation 62:49, 1980.

118. Flaherty JT et al: Effect of intravenous nitroglycerin on left ventricular function and ST segment changes in acute myocardial infarction. Br Heart J 38:612, 1976.

119. Kelly DT et al: Use of phentolamine in acute myocardial infarction associated with hypertension and left ventricular failure. Circulation 47:723, 1973.

120. Cohn JN, Franciosa JA: Vasodilator therapy of cardiac failure. N Engl J Med 297:27. 1977.

121. Chatterjee K et al: Oral hydralazine in chronic heart failure: sustained beneficial hemodynamic effects. Ann Intern Med 92:600, 1980.

122. Franciosa JA, Cohn JN: Sustained hemodynamic effects without tolerance during long-term isosorbide dinitrate treatment of chronic left ventricular failure. Am J Cardiol 45:648, 1980.

123. Thadani U et al: Tolerance to the circulatory effects of oral isosorbide dinitrate: rate of development and cross-tolerance to glyceryl trinitrate. Circulation 61:526, 1980.

124. Packer M et al: Hemodynamic and clinical tachyphylaxis to prazosin-mediated afterload reduction in severe chronic congestive heart failure. Circulation 59:531, 1979.

125. Packer M et al: Hemodynamic characterization of tolerance to long-term hydralazine therapy in severe chronic heart failure. N Engl J Med 306:57, 1982.

126. Franciosa JA, Ziesche S, Wilen M: Functional capacity of patients with chronic left ventricular failure. Relationship of bicycle exercise performance to clinical and hemodynamic characterization. Ann J Med 67:460, 1979.

127. Massie B et al: Long-term vasodilatory therapy for heart failure: clinical response and its relationship to hemodynamic measurements. Circulation 63:269, 1981.

128. Cohn JN, Rodriguera E, Guiha NH: Left ventricular function in hypertensive heart disease. In: Onesti G, Kim KE (eds) Hypertension Mechanisms and Management. Grune and Stratton, New York, 1973, p 191.

129. Cohn JN, Burke LP: Nitroprusside. Ann Intern Med 91:752, 1979.

130. Hoffman JIE: Determinants and prediction of transmural myocardial perfusion. Circulation 58:381, 1978.

131. Chiariello M et al: Comparison between the effects of nitroprusside and nitroglycerin on ischemic injury during acute myocardial infarction. Circulation 54:766, 1976.

132. Forrester JS et al: Medical therapy of acute myocardial infarction by application of hemodynamic subsets. N Engl J Med 295:1356, 1976.

133. Chatterjee MB et al: Effects of vasodilator therapy for severe pump failure in acute myocardial infarction on short-term and late prognosis. Circulation 53:797, 1976.

134. Cohn JN et al: Effect of short-term infusion of sodium nitroprusside on mortality rate in acute myocardial infarction complicated by left ventricular failure. N Engl J Med 306:1129, 1982.

135. Wayman SM: Nitroprusside in myocardial infarction. N Engl J Med 306:1168, 1982.

136. Durrer JD et al: Effect of sodium nitroprusside on mortality in acute myocardial infarction. N Engl J Med 306:1121, 1982.

137. Ganz W, Swan HJC: Measurement of blood flow by thermodilution. Am J Cardiol 29:241, 1972.

138. Lopez-Sendon J, Coma-Canella I, Gamallo C: Sensitivity and specificity of hemodynamic criteria in the diagnosis of acute right ventricular infarction. Circulation 64:515, 1981.

139. Friedman AM, Stern L: Identification of mitral regurgitation following acute myocardial infarction by hemodynamic monitoring. Chest 79:252, 1980.

140. Abernathy WS: Complete heart block caused by the Swan-Ganz catheter. Chest 65:349, 1974.

141. Castellanos A et al: Left fascicular blocks during right-heart catheterization using the Swan-Ganz catheter. Circulation 64:1271, 1981.

142. Smith WR, Glauser FL, Jemison P: Ruptured chordae of the tricuspid valve. The consequence of flow-directed Swan-Ganz catheterization. Chest 70:790, 1976.

143. Pape LA et al: Fatal pulmonary hemorrhage after use of the flow-directed balloon-tipped catheter. Ann Intern Med 90:344, 1979.

144. Foote GA, Schabel SI, Hodges M: Pulmonary complications of the flow-directed balloon-tipped catheter. N Engl J Med 290:927, 1974.

145. Voei G et al: Retrival of entrapped and knotted balloon-tipped catheters from the right heart. Ann Intern Med 92:638, 1980.

146. Cohn JN: Blood pressure measurement in shock. Mechanism of inaccuracy in auscultatory and palpatory methods. J Am Med Assoc 199:972, 1967.

147. Bodenheimer MM et al: Effect of progressive pressure reduction with nitroprusside on acute myocardial infarction in humans. Ann Intern Med 94:435, 1981.

148. Packer M et al: Rebound hemodynamic events after abrupt withdrawal of nitroprusside in patients with severe chronic heart failure. N Engl J Med 301:1193, 1979.

149. Pierpont G et al: Effects of vasodilators on pulmonary hemodynamics and gas exchange in left ventricular failure. Am Heart J 88:256, 1980.

150. Miller RR, Vismara LA, Williams DA: Pharmacological mechanisms for left ventricular unloading in clinical congestive heart failure. Circ Res 39:127, 1976.

151. Dunkman WB et al: Clinical hemodynamic results of intraaortic balloon pumping and surgery for cardiogenic shock. Circulation 46:465, 1972.

152. Hagemeijer F et al: Effectiveness of intraaortic balloon pumping without cardiac surgery for patients with severe

heart failure secondary to a recent myocardial infarction. Am J Cardiol 40:951, 1977.

153. Awan NA et al: Efficacy of ambulatory systemic vasodilator therapy with oral prazosin in chronic refractory heart failure. Circulation 56:346, 1977.

154. Walsh WF, Greenberg BH: Results of long-term vasodilator therapy in patients with refractory congestive heart failure. Circulation 64:499, 1981.

155. Massie BM, Kramer B, Haughom F: Acute and long-term effects of vasodilator therapy on resting and exercise hemodynamic and exercise tolerance. Circulation 64:1218, 1981.

156. Hindman MC et al: Rest and exercise hemodynamic effects of oral hydralazine in patients with coronary artery disease and left ventricular dysfunction. Circulation 61:751, 1980.

157. Aronow WS et al: Effect of prazosin vs. placebo on chronic left ventricular heart failure. Circulation 59:344, 1979.

158. Hecht HS et al: Improvement in supine bicycle exercise performance in refractory congestive heart failure after isosorbide dinitrate: radionuclide and hemodynamic evaluation of acute effects. Am J Cardiol 49:133, 1982.

159. Leier CV, Magorien RD, Desch CE: Hydralazine and isosorbide dinitrate: comparative central and regional hemodynamic effects when administered alone or in combination. Circulation 63:102, 1981.

160. Massie B et al: Hemodynamic advantage of combined administration of hydralazine orally and nitrates non-parenterally in the vasodilator therapy of chronic heart failure. Am J Cardiol 40:794, 1977.

161. Abrams J: Nitroglycerin and long-acting nitrates. N Engl J Med 302:1234, 1980.

162. Koch-Weser J: Hydralazine. N Engl J Med 295:320, 1976.

163. Greenberg BH, DeMots H, Murphy E: Arterial dilators in mitral regurgitation: effects on rest and exercise hemodynamics and long-term clinical follow-up. Circulation 65:181, 1982.

164. Packer M et al: Dose requirements of hydralazine in patients with severe chronic congestive heart failure. Am J Cardiol 46:655, 1980.

165. Mehta J et al: Comparative hemodynamic effects of intravenous nitroprusside and oral prazosin in refractory heart failure. Am J Cardiol 41:925, 1978.

166. Colucci WS, Williams GH, Braunwald E: Increased plasma norepinephrine levels during prazosin therapy for severe congestive heart failure. Ann Intern Med 93:452, 1980.

167. Koch-Weser J: Captopril. N Engl J Med 306:214, 1982.

168. Levine TB, Franciosa JA, Cohn JN: Acute and long-term response to an oral converting-enzyme inhibitor, captopril, in congestive heart failure. Circulation 62:35, 1980.

169. Creager MA, Halperin JL, Bernard DB: Acute regional circulatory and renal hemodynamic effects of converting-enzyme inhibition in patients with congestive heart failure. Circulation 64:483, 1981.

170. Dzau VJ et al: Sustained effectiveness of converting-enzyme inhibition in patients with severe congestive heart failure. N Engl J Med 302:1373, 1980.

171. Kluger J, Cody RJ, Laragh JH: The contributions of sympathetic tone and the renin-angiontensin system to severe chronic congestive heart failure: response to specific inhibitors (prazosin and captopril). Am J Cardiol 49:1667, 1982.

172. Curtiss C et al: Role of the renin-angiotensin system in the systemic vasoconstriction of chronic congestive heart failure. Circulation 58:763, 1978.

173. Packer M et al: Determinants of drug response in severe chronic heart failure. I. Activation of avasoconstrictor forces during vasodilator therapy. Circulation 64:506, 1981.

174. Maroko PR et al: Factors influencing infarct size following experimental coronary artery occlusions. Circulation 43:67, 1971.

175. Goldberg LI, Hsieh Y-Y, Resnekov L: Newer catecholamines for treatment of heart failure and shock: an update on dopamine and a first look at dobutamine. Prog Cardiovasc Dis 19:327, 1977.

176. Sonnenblick EH, Frishman WH, LeJemtel TH: Dobutamine: a new synthetic cardioactive sympathetic amine. N Engl J Med 300:17, 1979.

177. Leier CV, Heban PT, Huss P: Comparative systemic and regional hemodynamic effects of dopamine and dobutamine in patients with cardiomyopathic heart failure. Circulation 58:466, 1978.

178. Goldstein RA, Pasamani ER, Roberts R: A comparison of digoxin and dobutamine in patients with acute infarction and cardiac failure. N Engl J Med 303:846, 1980.

179. Loeb HS, Bredakis J, Gunnar RM: Superiority of dobutamine over dopamine for augmentation of cardiac output in patients with chronic low output cardiac failure. Circulation 55, 375, 1977.

180. Gillespie TA et al: Effects of dobutamine in patients with acute myocardial infarction. Am J Cardiol 39: 588, 1977.

181. Miller RR et al: Combined dopamine and nitroprusside therapy in congestive heart failure. Circulation 55:881, 1977.

182. Awan NA, Evenson MK, Needham KE: Hemodynamic effects of oral pirbuterol in chronic severe congestive heart failure. Circulaton 63:96, 1981.

183. Alousi AA et al: Cardiotonic activity of amrinone. Circ Res 45:666, 1979.

184. Benotti JR et al: Hemodynamic assessment of amrinone: a new inotropic agent. N Engl J Med 299:1373, 1978.

185 Benotti JR et al: Effects of amrinone myocardial energy metabolism and hemodynamics in patients with severe congestive heart failure due to coronary artery disease. Circulation 62:28, 1980.

186. Wynne J et al: Oral amrinone in refractory congestive heart failure. Am J Cardiol 45:1245, 1980.

187. Weber KT, Andrews V, Janicki JS: Amrinone and exercise performance in patients with chronic heart failure. Am J Cardiol 48:164, 1981.

188. Klein NA et al: Hemodynamic comparison of intravenous amrinone and dobutamine in patients with chronic congestive heart failure. Am J Cardiol 48:170, 1981.

CHAPTER 15

Medical management of ischemic heart disease

DAVID W. SNYDER and BURTON E. SOBEL

Introduction

The underlying process responsible for the large majority of cases of ischemic heart disease (IHD) is coronary atherosclerosis. This entity, the leading cause of death of American men of middle age, is responsible for more than 600 000 deaths annually in the United States alone [1]. Its manifestations include angina pectoris, congestive heart failure, myocardial infarction, and sudden cardiac death. Approaches to the modification of IHD include primary prevention of atherosclerosis, early intervention to forestall development of symptomatic IHD, and medical and surgical therapy of specific manifestations.

Primary prevention of coronary atherosclerosis has the greatest public health potential. Between 1968 and 1976, the age-adjusted IHD mortality rate in the United States declined by 24%. This unprecedented change has resulted in an estimated sparing of more than 100 000 deaths annually [2]. Accurate estimates of the total incidence of IHD during the past decade are not available. Nevertheless, it appears likely that at least some of the decline in mortality is a reflection of primary prevention or retardation of progression of occlusive coronary disease.

Unfortunately, however, despite rapidly increasing understanding of atherogenesis, progress in primary prevention has been slow and difficult to validate. Modification of identified coronary risk factors such as hyperlipidemia may reduce the incidence of IHD or slow the progression of asymptomatic coronary disease, but intervention trials have not yet demonstrated this conclusively. Therapeu-

tic modalities employed in the management of symptomatic IHD, such as beta-adrenergic blockade [3] or antiplatelet agents [4], may delay the development of overt manifestations of asymptomatic coronary artery disease. However, methods for detection of asymptomatic disease are too insensitive and nonspecific to make routine screening practical. Therefore, the major thrust of medical management of IHD remains the therapy of its complications. Treatment is directed not only toward symptomatic relief but also toward preventing sequelae and reducing mortality associated with critical coronary events, such as myocardial infarction. Accordingly, in the material to follow we shall consider primary prevention only briefly, and focus instead on treatment of the specific manifestations of IHD. Important aspects of therapy such as surgical intervention and external circulatory assist will not be reviewed because of the selective focus of the material on clinical pharmacology.

Prevention of ischemic heart disease

Studies of the pathophysiology of atherogenesis have implicated circulating low density lipoproteins and their receptors [5, 6], vascular smooth muscle cell mitogens and hyperplasia [7], and platelet factors such as thromboxane and mitogens [8, 9] as potential contributing etiological factors. However, prevention has been focused primarily on modification of risk factors identified through epidemiological observations.

The most salient risk factor in the United States is hypercholesterolemia, in part a manifestation of

Rosen, M. R. and Hoffman, B. F. (eds.), Cardiac Therapy. ISBN 0-89838-564-4.
© 1983, Martinus Nijhoff Publishers, Boston, The Hague, Dordrecht, Lancaster. Printed in the Netherlands.

the American diet [2]. Populations with a low incidence of IHD such as inhabitants of Japan, who move to the United States and adopt a western diet, acquire a risk of IHD typical of native Americans [10, 11]. In populations with diets low in cholesterol and saturated fat, IHD is rare despite the presence of hypertension or cigarette smoking [2]. Laboratory studies of atherogenesis in cholesterol-fed monkeys confirm these demographic observations. Furthermore, regression of the disease induced in the laboratory has been achieved by resumption of low fat diets [12]. In addition to the atherogenic, normal American diet, other major risk factors have been identified including hypertension [13], cigarette smoking [14], and diabetes mellitus [15]. Physical inactivity [16] and emotional stress [17] have been associated with a high risk of IHD as well.

Despite the acknowledged association of risk factors with IHD, more fundamental questions are whether the factors cause the disease and whether their modification will result in reduced incidence or severity of disease. Unfortunately, with only a few exceptions, definitive conclusions are not established. Some trials designed to examine effects of interventions implemented to modify risk factors (intervention trials) have been encouraging. The Finnish Mental Hospital Study demonstrates that dietary habits and body lipid composition can be altered markedly among subjects in a confined setting and that coronary heart disease (CHD) mortality can be reduced substantially by the intervention [18]. However, although dietary modification in free living populations has produced comparable reductions in serum cholesterol [19], consistent effects on mortality have not been discernible. The Veterans Administration trial clearly demonstrated that systemic arterial blood pressure can be reduced in a sustained fashion in ambulatory subjects with a significant associated reduction in cardiovascular mortality [20, 21]. However, most of the impact was not on IHD per se. Cessation of smoking in individuals susceptible to coronary artery disease reduces the incidence of coronary events and mortality even in those who have suffered prior myocardial infarction [22]. However, the impact on the progression or severity of underlying coronary vascular disease is less striking.

Widespread recognition of coronary risk factors and subsequent efforts by physicians and the population at large to modify them may well account for the recent reduction of IHD mortality in the United States. During the past two decades, polyunsaturated fat consumption has increased and cholesterol content has decreased in the American diet [23, 24]. Concomitantly, average serum cholesterol has declined by >10 mg % [25]. Between 1964 and 1975, the percentage of male Americans who smoke cigarettes fell from 53% to 37%, with a more modest decline among females [26]. Hypertension has been more vigorously controlled – approximately 50% of all Americans with hypertension are now being adequately treated [27]. Judging from the apparent contributions of individual risk factors to the overall incidence of IHD in the Framingham study, these changes in national coronary risk factors may account for a large fraction of the decline in coronary mortality observed since 1968 [1].

Early detection of asymptomatic ischemic heart disease

The encouraging reduction in IHD mortality suggests that comparable measures could be effective in arresting or possibly reversing the progression of established atheromatous lesions. Unfortunately, objective validation of this hypothesis has been elusive. Identification of patients with asymptomatic early coronary disease is difficult. Noninvasive tests such as electrocardiographic or radionuclide exercise testing or radionuclide perfusion scintigraphy are neither sufficiently sensitive nor specific for use as screening procedures [28–30], although markedly positive responses provide grounds for increased suspicion of significant occlusive disease [31]. Cardiac catheterization can identify early disease, but the procedure entails some risk (albeit slight) and substantial cost. Thus, definitive evaluation in large groups of subjects of the efficacy of secondary prevention on coronary vascular disease itself is not yet practical.

Treatment of manifestations of IHD - acute myocardial infarction

One of the most dramatic consequences of IHD is acute myocardial infarction. It is now clear that this phenomenon is not a discrete event in which the sole goal of therapy should be support of the circulation but rather that it is a dynamic phenomenon in which maintenance of myocardial viability is an important focus of therapy as well.

Therapy of all manifestations of IHD entails efforts to maintain a favorable balance of myocardial oxygen demand and supply while at the same time maintaining ventricular performance, supporting hemodynamics, preventing malignant dysrhythmia, and forestalling catastrophic complications. These considerations are inherent in the principles underlying the therapy of acute infarction.

Since myocardial infarction is a dynamic process with disparate clinical manifestations dominant at different intervals after its onset, therapy appropriate during the first hours after the onset of infarction may be inappropriate later. The opportunities to favorably alter the patient's course may be lost if definitive treatment is delayed. Accordingly, management during the acute and convalescent phases will be considered separately.

General supportive measures

During the hours early after the onset of infarction, jeopardized ischemic myocardium may be potentially salvageable, judging from results in experimental animals and some clinical studies [32]. Pain and anxiety with their reflex and humoral sequelae may augment myocardial oxygen demands by augmenting heart rate, peripheral vascular resistance, and catecholamine-stimulation of the heart. Accordingly, measures such as reassurance, mild sedation, and effective analgesia play an important role in early management. Morphine sulfate remains the agent of choice for relief of pain and should be given intravenously in initial doses ranging from 3 to 15 mg with further titration to achieve satisfactory analgesia. Meperidine is an alternative, but its vagolytic effect may potentiate undesirable tachycardia in patients with high intrinsic sympathetic tone [33]. Pentazocine is contraindicated since it increases systemic arterial blood pressure and left ventricular end-diastolic pressure and thus myocardial oxygen requirements (MVO_2) [34]. Phenothiazine antiemetics are useful to counter the nausea that may result from administration of narcotics. Bradycardia and hypotension occasionally induced by morphine are usually readily reversible by prompt administration of 0.5–2 mg of atropine intravenously (see section below on prehospital

phase of infarction). Significant respiratory depression does not generally occur when morphine is used judiciously or in the face of persistent pain [34].

An alternative to narcotic analgesia is the administration of nitrous oxide by inhalation, in concentrations of 40–50% with adequate precautions to maintain the oxygen fraction in inspired gas above 20% and to avoid hypoxemia. This agent frequently provides rapid pain relief with a fall in heart rate, systemic pressure, and left ventricular volume secondary to reduction of the reflex responses to pain [35]. It has virtually no direct effects on ventricular or systemic vascular function in conventionally used doses.

The use of supplemental oxygen has become a common component in the initial therapy of acute infarction [36]. In dogs with coronary occlusion, infarct size determined by myocardial CK depletion and by epicardial ST-segment mapping is reduced by inhalation of 40% and 100% oxygen [37]. Mild arterial blood hemoglobin desaturation is almost universal in patients with infarction, but saturations less than 90% are seen only rarely in uncomplicated cases [38, 39]. The use of high flow oxygen in such patients adds little to arterial blood oxygen content and may adversely increase MVO_2 by elevating systemic valular resistance and arterial pressure [40]. Nonetheless, reductions of ST-segment elevation have been observed in patients with acute infarction [38], and protection against pacing induced angina by administration of oxygen has been demonstrated [41]. Thus, it seems prudent to administer low flow oxygen to all patients in the acute phase of infarction, to monitor the adequacy of oxygenation by arterial blood gas determinations, and to employ more aggressive oxygen supplementation in complicated patients with demonstrable refractory hypoxemia. Early initiation of assisted ventilation is particularly helpful in patients with pulmonary edema not only to improve arterial PO_2 but also to reduce the augmented work of breathing and its deleterious effects on circulatory requirements and hemodynamics.

During the very early hospital phase of acute myocardial infarction, patients should be at bed rest. However, prolonged bed rest is undesirable because of the rapid deconditioning effect it has on skeletal muscle and vascular tone as well as the risk of deep vein thrombosis. Hemodynamically stable patients should be encouraged to assume a bed–chair regimen within 24–48 hr, although ambulation should be delayed for several days. Avoidance of prolonged bed rest has reduced complications [42] and appears to facilitate earlier ambulation and hospital discharge [43]. However, for patients with continued or recurrent chest pain, congestive heart failure, hypotension, persistent tachycardia, or other complications of infarction, more prolonged bed rest is necessary. Such patients are at particularly high risk (>40%) [42, 44] for deep vein thrombosis and require prophylactic anticoagulation [45]. Full-dose anticoagulation with heparin and coumadin markedly reduces the incidence of deep vein thrombosis [46], pulmonary emboli, and arterial embolization secondary to mural thrombi [47]. Bleeding complications of this therapy are rare when patients lacking specific contraindications are selected [47]. Furthermore, heparin may limit ultimate infarct size by its antithrombotic and antiplatelet actions or other mechanisms [48]. In complicated situations anticoagulation should be continued for several weeks so that organization of mural thrombi and endothelialization of the infarct zone can be completed without induction of additional thrombus. Patients with contraindications to full-dose anticoagulation and those who are at low risk for thrombotic complications should be treated with small doses of heparin (5,000 units subcutaneously every 8–12 hr). This regimen activates antithromin III, inhibiting activation of factor X [49]. In patients recovering from infarction, this regimen reduces the incidence of deep vein thrombosis by nearly 90% [50, 51]. However, its efficacy in preventing pulmonary and arterial embolic events has not been established definitively. In addition to anticoagulation, physical therapy and well-fit elastic stockings may contribute to prevention of deep vein thrombosis.

The role of antiplatelet agents in patients with acute myocardial infarction has not been established. Under some conditions aspirin and dipyridamole appear to exert synergistic effects on platelets [52], and their combined use reduces the incidence of postoperative deep vein thrombosis [53]. The two drugs appear to limit infarct size in experimental animals, but clarification of their utility in patients with infarction awaits results of additional research (see section below on additional approaches to limiting infarct size).

Prevention and treatment of dysrhythmia

Disruption of normal cardiac rhythm is a potentially lethal but eminently treatable complication of acute infarction. Effective therapy for dysrhythmias accounts in large measure for the reduction in hospital mortality that resulted from the advent of coronary care units (CCUs). The prevalence of specific dysrhythmias encountered depends markedly on the interval after onset and the locus of infarction. A particularly critical phase is that of the earliest hours after the onset of myocardial injury.

Prehospital phase of infarction
Although implementation of coronary care units has substantially diminished overall hospital mortality associated with infarction, two-thirds of all coronary deaths occur suddenly or before a patient can be hospitalized [54]. In the United States only 20% of patients with evolving infarction are admitted to the CCU within 4 hr. In contrast, 60% of all coronary deaths occur within 1 hr [55]. To reduce early mortality substantially, intensive care must be available not only in the hospital but also in the community, ideally in the form of mobile intensive care units.

During the initial hours after onset of infarction, an imbalance of autonomic tone is common [56]. Parasympathetic hyperactivity (vagotonia) is frequently dominant in patients with inferior infarction. Thus, sinus bradycardia often associated with hypotension and varying degrees of atrioventricular (AV) block is prevalent. Among patients with anterior infarction, either sympathetic or parasympathetic tone may predominate. Only approximately 25% of all patients with infarction in progress manifest a normal heart rate and normal blood pressure [55].

Ventricular extrasystoles are virtually universal during the initial hours after onset of infarction. Seventy-five percent of patients with infarction who are destined to suffer primary ventricular fibrillation (i.e., fibrillation without preceding heart failure or shock) do so within the first 2 hr [56]. In this hyperacute phase of infarction, ventricular premature complexes (VPCs) occurring during the vulnerable period of the cardiac cycle (early VPCs) appear to be particularly prone to initiate ventricular fibrillation [57]. Accordingly, suppression with lidocaine is indicated.

The optimal initial therapy for patients with excess parasympathetic activity has been debated, in part because of lack of differentiation of the implications of bradycardia in patients with infarcts at disparate loci (inferior versus anterior) and the implications of bradycardia at different intervals after the onset of infarction. In dogs with experimentally induced acute anterior infarction, rapid heart rates have been associated with serious ventricular dysrhythmia. Acceleration of heart rate in this preparation with atropine aggravated ventricular irritability [58]. In some patients, administration of atropine intravenously may induce undesirable tachycardia, augment myocardial oxygen demands, and apparently precipitate ventricular dysrhythmia [59, 60]. On the other hand, hypotension with relative or absolute sinus bradycardia or impaired AV conduction may compromise myocardial perfusion, ventricular performance, and cardiac output, and thereby further aggravate myocardial ischemia. Under these conditions, atropine (0.5–2 mg in 0.4–0.6-mg aliquots) often corrects hemodynamics, reverses ST-segment elevation, and abolishes bradycardia-dependent ventricular dysrhythmia [54]. Since lower doses can paradoxically slow heart rate [61], and higher initial doses may increase the risk of excessive tachycardia [60], titration should be aggressive yet judicious.

In contrast to the atropine-responsive vagotonia during the first hours after onset of infarction, bradycardia several hours or more after symptom onset or bradycardia without hypotension carries different implications. Vagotonia is less likely to be its cause, and treatment, if necessary to maintain an adequate cardiac output, should rely on the use of artifical pacemakers. Asymptomatic sinus bradycardia or bradycardia with first-degree AV block, unassociated with hypotension, precipitation of VPCs, or compromised cardiac output, requires only vigilant monitoring.

Sympathetic hyperactivity during the early phase of acute myocardial infarction is manifested often by systemic arterial hypertension and tachyarrhythmia. Other causes of a hyperdynamic circulation or tachycardia such as hypoxemia, hypovolemia, or covert left ventricular failure must, of course, be excluded or treated specifically. Analgesia, reassurance, and sedation frequently suffice in controlling sympathetic hyperactivity. Occasionally however, therapy with beta-adrenergic-receptor-blocking agents is required to slow an accelerated sinus rhythm and reduce myocardial oxygen demands [55]. Administration of beta-adrenergic-blocking agents may reduce myocardial oxygen requirements not only directly via receptor blockade, but also indirectly by lowering intrinsic sympathetic activity and circulating levels of catecholamines, presumably via effects on presynaptic beta-receptors [62].

High grade ventricular dysrhythmia, common during the first hour of infarction, may be refractory to lidocaine [56]. This phenomenon is particularly evident in patients with heightened sympathetic activity. Among such patients, lidocaine reduces ectopic activity in only approximately one-third [55]. Thus, if three bolus doses of lidocaine (total of 2 mg/kg in 15 min) followed by an infusion (2 mg/kg/min intravenously) are ineffective, the addition of a beta-adrenergic antagonist such as propranolol (to a maximum of 0.1 mg/kg in graded doses) may alleviate the dysrhythmia [63, 64].

For the majority of patients seen before hospitalization during the hyperacute phase of infarction, constant monitoring and intravenous infusion of drugs are not yet practical. Prophylactic administration of lidocaine (300 mg im) appears to be beneficial in this setting although its efficacy has not been established unequivocally [64, 65].

Early hospital phase of infarction
Despite the fact that most patients reach an intensive care setting several hours after the onset of infarction, malignant dysrhythmia remains the major threat requiring therapeutic alteration. The 50% reduction of hospital mortality from 30% to approximately 15% has been due primarily to prompt detection and treatment of dysrhythmia [64]. Even electrophysiologically benign dysrhythmia may be poorly tolerated if it involves marked tachycardia or impairment of the physiological atrial transport of blood during ventricular diastole (atrial kick). Excessive myocardial oxygen demand with exacerbation of ischemia, compromise of ventricular performance, or possibly potentiation of intracardiac thrombosis and peripheral embolization may result.

The incidence of supraventricular dysrhythmia with acute myocardial infarction is approximately 40%, excluding sinus tachycardia or bradycardia. Factors potentially underlying these disturbances

485

include: (a) atrial or sinus node ischemia; (b) increased atrial pressure and distension due to pump failure; (c) pericarditis; (d) autonomic nervous system imbalance; (e) drug effects; and (f) electrolyte abnormalities [66, 67]. The occurrence of new onset atrial fibrillation is associated with a two- to threefold increase in mortality rate [68], probably a reflection of the severity of the underlying myocardial damage rather than a direct consequence of the dysrhythmia [66]. Even atrial premature contractions (APCs) alone are associated with a 25% incidence of mortality [66].

Sinus tachycardia and sinus bradycardia generally reflect responses to other factors perturbing autonomic balance. Thus, they should rarely be considered as primary dysrhythmias. Nevertheless, alterations of cardiac rate can have deleterious consequences and require appropriate and vigorous therapeutic intervention directed at the inciting cause.

Sinus tachycardia is common early in the course of infarction. Often it is a response to pain, anxiety, hypoxia, hypovolemia, left ventricular dysfunction, fever, electrolyte imbalance, drug effect (especially catecholamines), or pericarditis. In such instances, correction of the underlying disturbance is essential rather than misdirected attempts to manipulate cardiac rate directly. In some instances, persistent sympathetic hyperactivity is responsible [69]. When other factors can be excluded and when additional evidence of sympathetic hypertonus is present such as hypertension, loud heart tones, or bounding pulse, appropriate therapy consists of beta-adrenergic blockade, generally with intravenous propranolol. Propranolol can be given safely in the setting of myocardial infarction, usually without significant reduction of cardiac output or elevation of left ventricular filling pressures, even in patients with compromised left ventricular function [70]. With slowing of the heart rate, myocardial ischemia is often reduced, and a fall in left atrial pressure may ensue. Propranolol should be given in divided doses, with the actual dosage modified by heart rate, blood pressure, and pulmonary artery occlusive pressure in patients with hemodynamic complications. The usual maximal loading dose is 0.1 mg/kg. Maintenance therapy can generally be continued with oral medication. Progressive AV block, bronchospasm, or decompensation of left ventricular function are indications for discontinuation of the drug.

Sinus bradycardia during the early CCU course is generally due to vagotonia and often associated with inferior infarction. In the absence of hypotension, high grade AV block, or bradycardia-dependent ventricular dysrhythmia, it does not require therapy. Intravenous atropine in carefully titrated doses is the treatment of choice for symptomatic bradycardia indicative of vagotonia. Caution identical to that required in the prehospital phase must be exercised to avoid tachycardia due to atropine excess. If the response to 2 mg of atropine is not satisfactory, consideration should be given to pacemaker therapy. When bradycardia or AV block occurs later in the hospital course, after the initial 12–24 hr, it is unlikely to be due to vagotonia. It may reflect ischemic insult to the SA or AV node or drug toxicity. Under these conditions atropine is rarely beneficial [54] and should not be employed indiscriminately since the therapy of choice is insertion of a temporary transvenous pacemaker.

Atrial fibrillation is the most common supraventricular tachyarrhythmia associated with acute myocardial infarction. It occurs in 7–11% of patients [68]. Most episodes begin during the first 48 hr and persist for less than 4 hr. Higher mortality rates are associated with rapid ventricular rates (>120) and persistence of the dysrhythmia. Therapy is dictated by the hemodynamic status of the patient. If the ventricular rate is relatively slow and the patient is asymptomatic, optimal control of rate should be achieved with intravenous digoxin in anticipation of reversion (usually spontaneous) to sinus rhythm. Alternatively, or in addition to digitalization, low-dose beta-adrenergic blockade or intravenous verapamil may be used to effectively slow the ventricular response. Embolization is rare except when fibrillation is sustained. Thus, anticoagulation need not be instituted acutely. If hypotension, congestive heart failure, pain, or an excessively rapid ventricular rate that jeopardizes myocardial oxygenation are present, DC cardioversion should be implemented to restore sinus rhythm expeditiously. Surprisingly high energy discharges (>200 Joules) may be required, however. Intense shocks may of course induce myocardial damage reflected by modest release of macromolecules such as MB CK into the circulation [71].

Atrial flutter is much less common, occurring in less than 5% of patients with infarction and virtual-

486

ly exclusively in patients with congestive heart failure or shock [67]. This dysrhythmia is tolerated poorly not only because of the severity of underlying myocardial damage it reflects, but also because of its predilection to give rise to rapid ventricular rates difficult to control with pharmacologic agents. When left ventricular failure is not prominent, verapamil may be administered intravenously in a dose of 5–10 mg to depress AV nodal conduction. In as many as 50% of patients, conversion occurs to sinus rhythm or to atrial fibrillation with a slower ventricular response. DC cardioversion or intraatrial electrical stimulation is indicated to restore sinus rhythm. DC cardioversion is often the method of choice because of its availability, simplicity and speed. Low energy discharges (as little as 5–10 Joules) generally are successful and are not likely to induce biologically significant myocardial damage. MM CK release from chest wall musculature is common and may be misleading if diagnostic enzyme determinations are being performed without isoenzyme analysis [71].

In patients with suspected sinus node disease, digitalis intoxication, or severe hypotension countermanding anesthesia employed for DC shock, cardioversion by rapid atrial pacing is safe and effective. In 90% of cases atrial flutter is converted either directly to sinus rhythm or to atrial fibrillation with a slower ventricular rate, followed by spontaneous conversion to sinus rhythm within minutes to 24 hr [72, 73]. An advantage of this technique is its potential for repeated treatment of recurrent episodes with a pacing wire left in place or advanced into the ventricle if treatment of bradycardia or prophylaxis for progressive AV block is required.

Paroxysmal supraventricular tachycardia (PSVT) is rare in patients with acute myocardial infarction (<5%). It is almost always transient, lasting for only a few minutes [67]. When vagal maneuvers such as Valsalva or carotid sinus massage are ineffective, resistant PSVT can be treated with intravenous verapamil in a dose of 5–10 mg over 2–5 min. Ninety-five percent of patients with reentrant PSVT will revert to sinus rhythm within minutes after the 10-mg dose [74–76]. This is in contrast to patients with atrial flutter or fibrillation in whom slowing of the ventricular response may be induced by verapamil but generally without reversion sinus rhythm [75–77]. Verapamil is contraindicated in patients with severe depression of left ventricular function, in those with sinus node or AV node dysfunction, as well as in patients treated with parenteral propranolol. In such instances, termination of PSVT by low energy DC cardioversion or rapid atrial pacing should be considered.

Simple APCs occur in approximately one-third of patients with myocardial infarction. Though they may cause no hemodynamic compromise directly, they often are harbingers or reflections of more serious complications such as congestive heart failure, pericarditis, or drug toxicity [66]. Moreover, since 50% of supraventricular tachyarrhythmias are pressaged by APCs, administration of digitalis may be indicated not only to suppress the APC, but also to induce AV block and preclude an excessively rapid ventricular response to ensuing atrial fibrillation or flutter.

Ventricular ectopic activity (VEA) occurs in virtually all patients hospitalized with acute myocardial infarction [78]. Paroxysmal ventricular tachycardia (six consecutive beats or more) occurs in over 10% [79], and primary ventricular fibrillation (VF) in approximately 8% [80]. VEA may require treatment because it may compromise ventricular performance. Generally, however, when treatment is initiated in patients with infarction and VEA, the treatment is designed to prevent VF. Since VEA and VF may have different underlying electrophysiological precipitants and progenitors, abolition of VEA provides no assurance of an adequate antifibrillatory regimen on the one hand, and adequate prophylaxis for VF may be achieved with regimens that fail to abolish VEA on the other. From a clinical point of view the only consistant conclusion that can be drawn from suppression of VEA by a specific regimen is that the dosage is sufficient to achieve a pharmacological response. Several classification schemes have been suggested to stratify the severity of VEA based on the view that patients with higher grades of VEA are more apt to develop ventricular tachycardia or fibrillation [81]. Unfortunately, routine monitoring is of limited effectiveness in identifying such warning arrhythmias [78]. Moreover, in the majority of cases of primary VF during the early hospital phase, preceding warning arrhythmias either are not present or do not occur sufficiently in advance to allow adequate antiarrhythmic therapy before fibrillation ensues [80, 82]. 'Warning arrhythmias' are present in an equal fraction of patients who do, compared to those who do not, develop VF [83, 84]. With a few notable exceptions, early VPCs (complexes exhibiting the 'R on T' phenomenon), which are assigned the highest severity grade in the Lown classification [81], have no greater significance than late VPCs as predictors of primary VF [84–86]. In fact, high-grade VEA during the hospital phase of acute myocardial infarction is more closely associated with late rather than early VPCs [86].

In view of these considerations, limiting antiarrhythmic therapy to patients who display 'warning arrhythmias' would leave many untreated who were destined to suffer primary VF. In a well-staffed CCU, ventricular tachycardia and fibrillation can be promptly detected and rapidly corrected, with little change in demonstrable mortality [80]. However, transient tachyarrhythmia and hypotension may aggravate underlying ischemia and may therefore be undesirable. In the community hospital setting, primary VF even in a CCU has been associated with 47% mortality [87]. Thus, enthusiasm for an effective regimen for prophylaxis of ventricular fibrillation appears justified.

Many drugs have been evaluated as potential prophylactic agents for patients with acute myocardial infarction. The most extensive experience involves the use of lidocaine [64]. When given in full intravenous doses (2.5–3 mg/min after a loading dose), lidocaine markedly decreases the incidence of ventricular tachycardia and primary fibrillation during the first 48 hr after onset of infarction [88, 89]. Unfortunately, however, it is not clear that ventricular tachycardia or fibrillation complicating severe heart failure or shock is similarly responsive to lidocaine prophylaxis. The lack of a demonstrable reduction in mortality induced by prophylaxis is not surprising, in view of the efficacy of prompt defibrillation and the low overall incidence of death in patients hospitalized with infarction, and hence the large number of patients that would be required for detection of a small improvement in overall survival.

The incidence of toxicity when lidocaine is administered according to this full-dose regimen is relatively high (15%). Although toxic manifestations are reversible and generally mild, coma and seizures may occur [88]. Cardiac complications such as clinically significant depression of myocardial contractility or impaired SA or AV node func-

tion are rare [64]. On the other hand, in patients with disease of the distal conduction system, lidocaine may increase HV conduction time further or precipitate complete heart block. With block distal to the AV node, subsidiary pacemaker function may be inhibited by lidocaine and result in asystole [90].

Given these considerations it seems prudent to administer lidocaine prophylactically to patients with acute myocardial infarction, especially if they cannot be monitored rigorously in a well-staffed CCU. The incidence of primary ventricular fibrillation is higher in young patients in contrast to the incidence of lidocaine toxicity which is more prevalant in the elderly. Accordingly, routine prophylaxis is not recommended for patients more than 65 years of age [89]. Since serious dysrhythmias occur primarily during the first hours after the onset of infarction and since lidocaine elimination slows with prolonged infusions, prophylactic infusion should be limited to 24 hr. A full-dose regimen (100-mg loading dose followed by an infusion of 2.5 mg/min) is appropriate for patients with uncomplicated infarction, but dosage must be reduced to compensate for decreased hepatic metabolism in patients with congestive heart failure, hypotension, or primary liver disease. The efficacy of prophylaxis is suggested by an observed fall in the incidence of primary ventricular fibrillation from 6.5% to 0.3% in the community hospital setting [91].

For patients with acute myocardial infarction hospitalized in a nonintensive care setting, prophylaxis is essential but adequate monitoring of continuous intravenous infusions may be impractical. Orally administered disopyramide may reduce the incidence of ventricular tachycardia and fibrillation in the early and late hospital phases of infarction, reduce the incidence of extension of infarction, and reduce hospital mortality [92, 93]. In doses of 100 mg four times daily, infrequent urinary retention was the only recognized side effect, and negative inotropic effects were not observed. These encouraging results however, have not yet been confirmed, and negative inotropic effects have been encountered with increasing frequency [94].

Reduction in the incidence of high grade VEA, ventricular tachycardia, and ventricular fibrillation have been achieved with oral procainamide. Dysrhythmia-related mortality decreased and minimal side effects were encountered when plasma drug levels were maintained within the therapeutic range [95]. A commonly recommended dose schedule includes a loading dose as large as 1 g followed by daily maintenance therapy of 2–4 g, depending on body weight, for at least three days. For this purpose the drug must be given at 3-hr intervals to avoid wide swings in plasma levels. When toxic levels occur, significant depression of myocardial function may occur.

Evidence is inconclusive regarding the efficacy of prophylaxis with quinidine [96], but propranolol [97] and bretylium [98] are not effective and frequently elicit undesirable complications. Thus, they are contraindicated for prophylaxis.

In patients not treated prophylactically or those for whom prophylaxis is inadequate, frequent VPCs, especially multiform VPCs or runs, should prompt a search for initiating and aggravating factors as well as implementation of specific antiarrhythmic therapy. Correction of hypoxia, electrolyte imbalance or drug toxicity, treatment of congestive heart failure or pericarditis, and removal of irritating intracardiac devices may occasionally diminish or preclude otherwise refractory dysrhythmia. In the vast majority of instances, when dysrhythmia is a direct consequence of myocardial ischemia, drug therapy is indicated. Exceptions include infrequent single VPCs or accelerated idioventricular rhythm. Although episodes of ventricular tachycardia have been associated with accelerated idioventricular rhythm [99, 100], the clinical course and the prognosis of this dysrhythmia are generally benign. Specific therapy is rarely indicated unless hemodynamic stability is compromised [101, 102].

The antiarrhythmic drug of choice for VEA is intravenous lidocaine. This agent is effective in suppressing VPCs in 90% of cases [103]. In high doses it is an effective antifibrillatory agent [89, 104]. Therapeutic plasma levels of 1.2–5.5 μg/ml can be achieved in patients with normal hemodynamics by an initial slow injection of 2 mg/kg followed by a maintenance infusion of 55 μg/kg/min. Since most patients with infarction exhibit moderately reduced cardiac output, the loading dose should be reduced to 1.5 mg/kg and the maintenance to 30 μg/kg/min to avoid depression of already compromised contractility. In patients with pulmonary edema or shock, doses should be reduced further to 0.75 mg/kg loading and 10–20 μg/kg/min maintenance [105]. In patients with severe liver disease the maintenance infusion rate should be reduced by 50% without a change in loading dose [106]. The elimination half-life of lidocaine after a 24-hr infusion is prolonged compared with that after a 12-hr infusion. Thus, the maintenance infusion rate should be reduced after 12 hr to avoid late toxicity [107].

Toxicity, aside from common and usually mild central nervous system effects, is unusual. However, large bolus injections of lidocaine can produce bradycardia and hypotension due to myocardial depression. In patients with preexisting sinus node disease or infraHis conduction system disease, toxic blood levels of lidocaine may cause sinus arrest and/or second- and third-degree AV block [105]. Cardioacceleration may be a problem in patients with atrial fibrillation or flutter due to facilitation of impulse transmission through the AV node [108]. The efficacy of lidocaine is enhanced by hyperkalemia and markedly curtailed by hypokalemia.

If ventricular dysrhythmias persist despite adequate doses of lidocaine, a second drug must be added or substituted. Procainamide is the most suitable conventionally available drug for acute intravenous therapy. The simplest regimen calls for a loading infusion of 15 mg/kg over a 60-min interval followed by a maintenance infusion of 2.8 mg/kg/hr (12 mg/kg and 1.4 mg/kg/hr for patients with heart failure). This regimen provides therapeutic drug levels within 15 min and steady-state levels within 2 hr [109]. Maintenance can be continued with oral medication whenever desired. A 50% reduction of maintenance dosage is necessary in patients with renal failure. Clinical trials with this regimen demonstrate that 75% of lidocaine-resistant ventricular dysrhythmias are controlled and that toxicity is rare even when relatively high plasma levels occur [110].

An alternative agent is disopyramide. However, because marked negative inotropic and coronary and peripheral vasoconstrictor effects may occur after intravenous administration, this agent may be less suitable for use in the acute phase of infarction [111, 112].

Aprindine, an antiarrhythmic agent used widely in Europe, has local anesthetic properties and inhibits the fast sodium current, slows conduction, and lengthens myocardial refractory periods [113].

When given intravenously, a loading dose of 200 mg is infused over 30–60 min. Blood pressure and PR and QRS intervals should be monitored. Repeated 100-mg doses are given 1 and 4–10 hr later to complete the loading process. Maintenance doses of 25–50 mg every 8–12 hr can be given intravenously or orally to maintain therapeutic blood levels of 1–2 μg/ml. Aprindine is highly effective in controlling ventricular dysrhythmia, even dysrhythmia refractory to more standard agents [113]. However, it has a low toxic:therapeutic ratio. GI intolerance, tremor, ataxia, vertigo, and occasionally seizures complicate therapy. Mild depression of left ventricular function may result from therapeutic levels. Prolonged therapy has been associated rarely with agranulocytosis and cholestatic jaundice [114].

Occasionally malignant dysrhythmia persists or recurs despite maximum doses of lidocaine and the other aforementioned drugs. Bretylium, an agent with striking antifibrillatory efficacy [115], may be useful in this setting [116–118]. Given intravenously or intramuscularly in an initial dose of 5–20 mg/kg, bretylium may elicit significant cardioacceleration and hypertension initially because it releases norepinephrine from sympathetic nerve terminals. The same mechanism may exacerbate dysrhythmias especially when due to digitalis excess. These potentially deleterious early effects may exacerbate myocardial ischemia [119, 120]. Subsequently the drug induces partial adrenergic blockade due to depletion of norepinephrine. Hypotension, bradycardia, and enhanced sensitivity to exogenous catecholamine drugs may result. The antiarrhythmic effect of bretylium is delayed, generally occurring no sooner than 30 min to 2 hr after the first dose, although antifibrillatory activity may be conferred much more rapidly [121–124]. The delay in onset of antiarrhythmic actions and the potentially deleterious physiological consequences early after initiation of treatment with bretylium detract somewhat from its value as a first-line antifibrillatory agent. Prolonged administration is not practical because of a high incidence of disabling parotitis [117].

Other antiarrhythmic agents are only rarely indicated in treatment of ventricular dysrhythmia during the acute phase of myocardial infarction. However, beta-adrenergic blockade may be useful in the prevention of recurrent ventricular tachycardia, especially in patients with augmented intrinsic sympathetic tone [63]. Propranolol has been used most widely, but cardioselective agents such as metoprolol, atenolol, or acebutolol, and agents with some intrinsic sympathomimetic activity such as pindolol or alprenolol may be advantageous and appear to be of comparable efficacy [125, 126]. Phenytoin is often beneficial when digitalis intoxication is responsible for dysrhythmia but is otherwise generally of limited value [127, 128]. Several investigational (in the United States) antiarrhythmic agents, such as mexilitine, tocainide, and encainide, are used chiefly in chronic oral therapy. They have not yet been thoroughly evaluated for treatment of malignant dysrhythmia during the hospital phase of acute myocardial infarction.

When recurrent ventricular tachycardia or fibrillation persists despite aggressive drug therapy and correction of identifiable predisposing factors, underdrive or overdrive pacemaker therapy may be helpful. Pacing the heart from the right ventricle at rates between 90 and 150 may successfully suppress ventricular ectopic activity. At shorter cycle lengths, the extrastimuli may reduce the inhomogeneity of refractory periods within the left ventricle, thus inhibiting a reentry circuit [129]. Alternatively, overdrive suppression of a spontaneously depolarizing focus may inhibit dysrhythmia dependent upon enhanced automaticity. An important observation is that the pacing cycle length need not necessarily be shorter than the sinus-to-ectopic beat interval to be effective. Thus, occasionally VPCs which closely follow a sinus beat may be overdriven by electrical pacing. Unfortunately, however, competitive chamber pacing (i.e., from a chamber in which a ventricular tachycardia is not initiated or sustained via a reentry circuit) may precipitate ventricular fibrillation. Thus, RV pacing may be hazardous in patients with VEA initiated or sustained by reentry within the left ventricle and should be initiated only under conditions providing adequate electrophysiological surveillance facilities and expertise.

Late hospital phase of infarction
Sudden death during hospitalization for acute MI is unfortunately a common event. It occurs in 8% of apparently stable patients who have been discharged from a CCU [130]. Patients with high-grade ventricular dysrhythmia, impaired AV or intraventricular conduction, persistent sinus tachycardia or other evidence of congestive heart failure

while in the CCU, and extensive infarction are at particularly high risk [131]. Because of the potential for prophylaxis, patients with persistent dysrhythmia after the acute ischemic episode subsides should be treated aggressively with oral therapy designed to prevent ventricular fibrillation. High risk patients without overt dysrhythmia should be observed closely, preferably with telemetry, because of the risk of late development of ventricular dysrhythmia and fibrillation [132]. Antiarrhythmic therapy is initiated in the hospital and therapeutic and nontoxic drug levels assured. Efficacy should be documented by telemetry or ambulatory monitoring, even though partial or complete suppression is not necessarily tantamount to effective prophylaxis of VF. Therapy should be maintained for at least six months, an interval during which the incidence of sudden death is greatest [133]. Since there is no predictable diminution of the frequency of VPBs with time after infarction and since interruption of therapy may intensify dysrhythmia, patients should be evaluated with sequential ambulatory ECG recording (Holter tapes) when drug therapy is modified or stopped [134]. Complex VEA late after infarction is a risk factor for sudden death. Despite the absence of proof that treatment of VEA modifies the risk for primary VF, we believe that complex VEA late in the course should be suppressed [135].

Conduction disorders associated with acute myocardial infarction

Disordered AV and intraventricular conduction represent frequent complications of acute myocardial infarction. First-degree AV block and Mobitz I second-degree block are commonly associated with inferior infarction. Early after the onset of infarction they are often due to enhanced vagal tone [54]. When associated with significant hypotension or bradycardia, the early AV block should be managed by administration of intravenous atropine. Electrical pacing is only rarely required and should be initiated only when hemodynamic deterioration occurs due to an excessively slow ventricular rate. Later in the course, vagal influences are less prevalent and AV block is most frequently due to ischemic damage to the AV node. Often, Mobitz I block ensues, and rarely it progresses to high grade second-degree or third-degree AV block. Even with complete heart block however, an AV junctional

escape focus usually drives the ventricle resulting in narrow QRS complexes, a heart rate of 50–60 beats/min and uncompromised hemodynamics. Inferior infarction associated with complete AV block results in an average mortality of 20% [136]. Atropine is generally not effective hours to days after the onset of the acute ischemic episode. Instead, electrical pacing should be employed when the heart rate is extremely slow. Normal AV conduction generally returns within 72 hr. When it does, pacing can be discontinued.

Bundle branch block occurs in approximately 20% of patients; and, in the setting of anterior infarction, it is associated with important prognostic significance. Right bundle branch block, with or without associated anterior or posterior fascicular block, progresses to complete heart block in 40% of patients. Left bundle branch block evolves to bilateral bundle branch block less often in only 20% of cases [137]. Even without evolution to complete heart block, bundle branch block is associated with a mortality increase of two- to three-fold compared to that among comparable patients without intraventricular conduction block [137–139].

Mobitz II AV block is uncommon, accounting for only 10% of second-degree AV block in the setting of acute infarction [140]. This type of block (also called bilateral bundle branch block) is generally seen in patients with extensive anterior infarction, is associated with block below the His bundle, and is generally preceded by conduction block in one of the bundle branches. The development of Mobitz II block is ominous, as the block may proceed abruptly to complete AV block. Since bilateral bundle branch block is a result of extensive myocardial necrosis, left ventricular reserve is usually poor. The slow ventricular escape rhythm that emerges frequently is not sufficient to support the circulation because stroke volume is restricted by poor ventricular performance. Ventricular asystole occurs commonly and without warning. Patients with infarction complicated by bilateral bundle branch block exhibit a mortality of 80–90% [137].

Because of the high incidence and frequently sudden onset of complete heart block in patients with anterior infarction and Mobitz II block or right bundle branch block, insertion of a prophylactic temporary transvenous pacemaker is recommended. Since left bundle branch block with a normal PR interval leads to third-degree heart block less often, routine prophylactic pacemaker insertion is not indicated [137, 141]. Similarly, unifascicular block, bundle branch block with inferior infarction, or bundle branch block arising late (more than 72 hr) after anterior infarction is not an indication for prophylactic pacemaker therapy. Although definitive data are not available, at least in the case of right bundle block, chronic bundle branch block preceding anterior infarction carries at least as high a risk of evolution to complete heart block as does acute bundle branch block. Prophylactic pacing is appropriate for both [142, 143]. Unfortunately, however, even with a pacemaker in place, 80% of patients who develop complete heart block will die because of the hemodynamic consequences of the large extent of underlying necrosis responsible for interruption of all three major conduction fascicles.

In those rare patients who survive anterior infarction associated with complete heart block, permanent damage to the bundle branch system is likely. Even among those who return to normal or near normal intraventricular conduction, the subsequent rate of sudden death is high (65% in 12 months). Recurrent heart block appears to be at least partly responsible since 90% of such patients who are treated with a permanent pacemaker survive for one year. Thus, survivors of complete heart block associated with anterior infarction should be treated with insertion of a pacemaker before discharge [137, 138, 144, 145].

Left ventricular failure associated with acute myocardial infarction

Two-thirds of patients with acute myocardial infarction exhibit significant left ventricular dysfunction reflecting loss of functional myocardial contractile elements [69]. The impairment of the pumping function of the heart can lead to pulmonary congestion, hypoperfusion, or, in its most severe form, cardiogenic shock. The increased left ventricular end-diastolic volume and heart rate augment myocardial oxygen demands. Increased end-diastolic pressure reduces effective coronary perfusion pressure and, coupled with the accelerated heart rate which abbreviates total diastolic time available for coronary perfusion, decreases oxygen supply to the ischemic left ventricle. Both effects exacerbate ischemia, aggravate dysrhythmia, and appear to augment ultimate infarct size.

Conventional clinical evaluation identifies many patients with incipient or overt left ventricular failure. Clinical classification based on estimates of pulmonary congestion and peripheral hypoperfusion provide prognostic information and help to define therapeutic decisions [146, 147]. However, exclusive reliance on pulmonary rales, ventricular gallops, or chest X-ray abnormalities to define left ventricular performance is fraught with uncertainties due to the insensitivity and nonspecificity of signs as well as phase lags between changes in pulmonary hemodynamics and fluid volumes and the indices monitored [147, 148]. Therefore in patients with hemodynamically or clinically complicated infarction, bedside hemodynamic monitoring with a flow-directed balloon catheter should be implemented [149]. The indications for catheterization include persistent or recurrent chest pain, persistent or recurrent sinus tachycardia, hypoxemia, hypotension, pulmonary congestion, and refractory dysrhythmia. Invasive monitoring provides not only diagnostic information needed for identifying potentially correctable contributors to these manifestations, but also the data needed for rational selection of therapy.

Hemodynamic subsets

As discussed in detail later, prognosis after infarction is inversely dependent on the cumulative extent of injury sustained. Based on results in experimental animals, it appears that appropriate physiological and pharmacological interventions can favorably influence the evolution of infarction, protect ischemic tissue, and limit the ultimate effect of injury sustained. Although proof of benefits of such an approach in humans remains inferential, it appears likely that the same principles apply.

Accordingly, judicious manipulations of ventricular loading factors can favorably influence the balance between myocardial oxygen supply and demand, facilitating protection of jeopardized ischemic myocardium while maintaining systemic hemodynamics. Identification of specific hemodynamic subsets of patients and monitoring of physiological responses to therapy have become essentials in management of patients with complicated myocardial infarction.

Hyperdynamic hemodynamics

Among all patients with acute myocardial infarction, 5% have increased cardiac output with normal or low left ventricular filling pressures. Such patients are often hypertensive, and tachycardia and recurrent chest pain are common. If other causes of excess sympathetic tone, such as drug effects, are excluded and if other factors underlying the circulatory response such as hypoxia or fever are absent or corrected first, then beta-adrenergic blockade is useful. Propranolol is the drug most often used, in divided doses up to a total loading dose of 0.1 mg/kg intravenously. Anticipated results include a slowing of heart rate, relief of chest pain, and little or no change in left ventricular filling pressure [69]. With relief of ischemia, left ventricular contractility often improves and filling pressures may fall.

Hypovolemia

A frequent cause of tachycardia and mild hypotension in patients with acute infarction is a suboptimal left ventricular filling pressure. The hypovolemia responsible may be absolute, reflecting volume depletion attributable to preexisting or concomitant anorexia, diaphoresis, or occult blood loss. On the other hand it may be relative since the noncompliant left ventricle requires a high filling pressure for maintenance of performance. Because diminished compliance is characteristic of acute infarction [150], optimal left ventricular stroke volume is often achieved only with preload augmented by a filling pressure in the range of 15–20 mmHg [151, 152]. Effective therapy for patients with tachycardia or other manifestations of hypovolemia there-

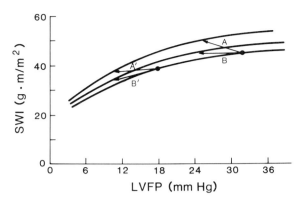

Figure 2. Left ventricular function curves demonstrating the effects on preload and stroke work index (SWI) induced by nitroprusside (A, A′) and by nitroglycerin (B, B′). With equivalent effects on left ventricular filling pressure (LVFP), nitroprusside is less likely to diminish SWI.

fore entails expansion of volume, preferably with a colloid solution such as low molecular weight dextran [153] in order to avoid crystaloid-induced pulmonary edema (Figure 1).

Elevated left ventricular filling pressure and pulmonary vascular congestion with or without pulmonary edema

Patients with a left ventricular filling pressure in excess of 18–20 mmHg and a cardiac index >2.2 l/min/m² fit into this category. Hospital mortality of this group is approximately 10% [148]. Treatment employs reduction of preload with diuretics. In patients with symptoms of pulmonary edema a head-up tilt and occasionally the application of tourniquets or phlebotomy will immediately lower venous return to the heart. Furosemide is the preferred diuretic agent for acute treatment since, in addition to its renal effects, it dilates the pulmonary and systemic venous capacitance beds and causes a rapid decline of diastolic left ventricular and pulmonary venous pressures [154].

Vasodilators can be used in conjunction with diuretics to reduce preload (Figure 2). They are especially useful if hypertension, mitral regurgitation, left ventricular aneurysm, or ventricular septal rupture are present or when impaired renal function limits the efficacy of diuretics. Because of its rapid onset of action and short half-life, intravenous nitroprusside (10–200 μg/min) is the drug most often used to decrease systemic arterial resistance.

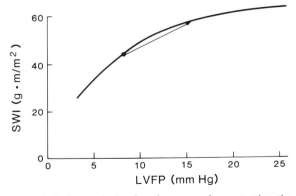

Figure 1. Left ventricular function curve demonstrating the increase in stroke work index (SWI) resulting from augmentation of left ventricle preload (LVFP) by volume expansion.

493

In conventional doses it also exerts modest dilator effects on veins. Although its mode of action is not known, its stimulation of cyclic GMP synthesis has been thought by some to mediate vasodilation. When the infusion rate is adjusted so that pulmonary artery occlusive pressure declines to no less than 15–16 mmHg, significant tachycardia and systemic arterial hypotension can be avoided despite reduction of pulmonary congestion and left ventricular end-diastolic volume. Unfortunately, nitroprusside may produce 'coronary steal' by dilating coronary resistance vessels in nonischemic zones [155, 156] and may augment ST-segment elevation in patients by precipitating hypotension or tachycardia [157]. On the other hand, a carefully titrated nitroprusside infusion reduces manifestations of severe ischemia in experimental animals [158] and in patients with left ventricular dysfunction [159–161].

Toxicity from nitroprusside is usually a reflection of its pharmacological actions and a result of injudicious administration. However, prolonged use can result in accumulation of cyanate with elevated levels in plasma and impairment of tissue oxidative metabolism reflected clinically by central nervous system depression and obtundation.

In contrast to nitroprusside, nitroglycerin (NTG), in conventional therapeutic doses (20–100 μg/min) preferentially dilates the systemic venous capacitance bed with relatively little effect on arterial vessels [162]. Since NTG increases prostaglandin synthesis in vitro, its effects have been attributed by some to mediation by prostaglandins. However, conclusive evidence such as antagonism by aspirin is not available. Since it dilates large coronary conductance vessels rather than resistance vessels, NTG is less likely than nitroprusside to produce 'coronary steal' [156]. The use of intravenous NTG to reduce preload in patients decreases pulmonary congestion, decreases MVO_2, and reduces manifestations of ischemia such as the intensity of ST-segment elevation, impairment of left ventricular ejection fraction, and lactate production [163, 164]. However, injudicious administration of nitrates by oral, sublingual, transcutaneous, or intravenous routes is hazardous in the setting of acute infarction, since excessive lowering of left ventricular filling pressures (to values <15 mmHg) may result in a decline in cardiac output, reflex tachycardia, systemic hypotension, exacerbation of impaired

coronary perfusion, increased myocardial ischemia, and bradycardia due to intensification of ischemia [165–167] (Figure 2).

Both nitroglycerin and nitroprusside dilate pulmonary arterial vessels. Thus, pulmonary ventilation-perfusion mismatching can occur with consequent systemic arterial hypoxemia [168, 169].

Phentolamine is an effective vasodilator in patients with acute infarction. It exerts a balanced effect on the arterial and venous vessels similar to that of nitroprusside, resulting generally in a decrease in left ventricular filling pressure and an increase in cardiac output [170]. However, it is prone to cause tachycardia more than other generally available vasodilators because it elicits overflow beta-adrenergic stimulation as a result of presynaptic alpha-2 receptor blockade [171]. Blockade of the alpha-2 receptors leads to inhibition of the physiological negative feedback mechanisms which normally blunt endogenous catecholamine synthesis. Accordingly, endogenous catecholamines are released in excess and stimulate the unblocked, postsynaptic beta-receptors causing acceleration of heart rate. Moreover, phentolamine is extremely expensive. For these two reasons it is not a first line drug.

Trimethaphan, a ganglionic blocking agent used in doses of 0.1–2 mg/min, is a vasodilator with the advantage of blocking reflex tachycardia as well as reducing preload and afterload. It has been shown to reduce enzymatically estimated infarct size in hypertensive patients with evolving infarction [172]. However, urinary retention and complications such as adynamic ileus preclude its prolonged or routine use.

Other vasodilators, such as hydralazine, prazosin, and trimazosin are generally administered orally and employed for prolonged therapy of congestive heart failure rather than in the treatment of acute myocardial infarction. They will be discussed in the section on chronic ischemic heart disease – congestive heart failure. Recently, two new classes of vasodilator drugs for patients with congestive heart failure and/or myocardial infarction have been explored and have aroused considerable interest. These include the calcium channel-blocking drugs such as nifedipine and verapamil and angiotensin-converting enzyme inhibitors such as captopril.

Before the advent and extensive evaluation of vasodilators, pulmonary congestion was classically treated by administration of agents with positive inotropic effects, such as digitalis glycosides. In addition to the slow onset and unpredictability of the response encountered, several theoretical objections have led to markedly circumscribed reliance on such agents in the acute setting. First, in contrast to reduction of preload with diuretics or vasodilators which decreases cardiac work and MVO_2, agents with positive inotropic effects may increase MVO_2 in the absence of left ventricular failure [173, 174]. Second, the zone of already completed infarction cannot respond to agents with inotropic effects and the surrounding viable tissue is already markedly stimulated by endogeneous catecholamines. Accordingly, patients with extensive infarction and severe failure tend to respond poorly to exogenous agents with positive inotropic effects [175]. In contrast, favorable hemodynamic changes in response to vasodilator therapy are particularly marked in those patients with more severe left ventricular dysfunction [69].

In some patients with significant heart failure, agents with positive inotropic effects decrease left ventricular end-diastolic volume by increasing contractility. Consequently, the oxygen utilization stimulated by the drug may be offset by decreased oxygen demand resulting from decreased wall tension. Under these circumstances, exacerbation of manifestations of ischemia is not a common problem [176–178]. Agents with positive inotropic effects may be particularly useful in the acute phase of infarction when hypotension or tachycardia limit the use of vasodilators.

Systemic hypoperfusion without elevated left ventricular filling pressure or pulmonary congestion
Patiens with a cardiac index of $<2.2\,l/min/m^2$, but with pulmonary artery occlusive pressures <18 mmHg, have a hospital mortality rate of nearly 25% [148]. The poor cardiac output may be attributable to several potential causes. In some patients it reflects inadequate left ventricular filling pressure and will respond to volume expansion. In others, marked bradycardia and a relatively fixed stroke volume are responsible. If so, cardiac output can be increased by accelerating heart rate either by removing an initiating cause of the bradycardia such as propranolol or by implementing pacemaker therapy. In a third group of patients, those with inferior infarction, concomitant right ventricular infarction

may be a major cause of reduced cardiac output. Associated right ventricular involvement in such patients is remarkably common. Such patients exhibit low output failure and engorged neck veins, but no signs of pulmonary edema [179]. Right ventricular filling pressure is elevated disproportionately to left ventricular filling pressure. Right atrial pressure recordings may demonstrate prominent X and Y descents (in contrast to the blunted Y descent seen with hemopericardium) and a 'square root sign' may be evident on right ventricular pressure tracings indicative of diminished right ventricular compliance. Equalization of right and left atrial pressures and pulsus paradoxus may be seen and mimic signs of pericardial tamponade [179–181]. Patients with extensive right ventricular dysfunction and infarction have proximal occlusion of the right coronary artery evident at postmortem and frequently exhibit infarction of the lateral and posterior right ventricular walls, posterior interventricular septum and left ventricular inferior wall [182]. The syndrome of profound right ventricular dysfunction has a high incidence among patients selected on the basis of autopsy series, but is clinically manifest in less than 5% of patients with acute infarction [180]. Treatment of marked right ventricular dysfunction resulting in diminished cardiac output includes volume expansion to provide adequate left ventricular filling and administration of agents with positive inotropic effects. Vasodilator therapy can be employed to reduce systemic arterial resistance, left ventricular afterload and end-diastolic pressure, and hence indirectly to reduce right ventricular afterload [179, 180]. Since heart block is quite common in these patients (due to the locus and extent of infarction), pacemaker therapy is often necessary as well.

The majority of patients with systemic hypoperfusion and pulmonary artery occlusive pressure <18 mmHg fall into a different category. Their left ventricular failure is attributable to relatively flat left ventricular function curves due to impaired left ventricular contractility. Thus, volume expansion does not augment cardiac output substantially and entails the risk of precipitating pulmonary edema [147]. In these patients, systemic arterial vasodilator therapy may be helpful, especially if peripheral vascular resistance is elevated and left ventricular filling pressure is adequate. However, since pulmonary congestion is not present, nitrates are not indicated and may reduce cardiac output by excessively lowering left ventricular filling pressure. Nitroprusside can increase cardiac output by reducing afterload. With judicious titration of dosage, it rarely lowers preload excessively and reflex tachycardia and aggravation of myocardial ischemia can be avoided [157]. Pulmonary arterial occlusive pressure should be maintained at or above 15 mmHg while nitroprusside is being administered. Theoretically, phentolamine may be a more ideal agent, since it reduces afterload even more preferentially with less venodilating effect compared to nitroprusside [171]. However, cost and its propensity to elicit tachycardia detract from its value.

In this subset of patients, hypotension may preclude the use of vasodilator therapy. Mechanical assist devices to support the circulation (such as intraaortic balloon counterpulsation) and, alternatively, agents with positive inotropic effects may be particularly helpful. Catecholamines and their congeners continue to be the primary pharmacological agents used in the peri-infarction setting. Isoproterenol, although a potent beta-1 agonist, stimulates beta-2 adrenoceptors resulting in peripheral vasodilation, excessive reflex and directly induced tachycardia, and aggravation of dysrhythmia. Epinephrine and norepinephrine are nonspecific agonists with undesirable positive chronotropic and vasopressor effects respectively. One of the most promising congeners developed recently, dopamine (in doses of 3–20 μg/kg/min), is a somewhat more cardioselective beta-1 agonist. However, it exhibits some potentially deleterious beta-2 and alpha agonistic properties, especially at high doses, with resulting augmentation of peripheral vascular resistance, ventricular afterload and myocardial oxygen requirements. Phentolamine is useful as an antagonist to offset these manifestations. Dopaminergic receptor stimulation mediates dilation of the renal arteries and may facilitate diuresis.

Dobutamine is a potent catecholamine with positive inotropic effects and with little positive chronotropic or arrhythmogenic effects when infused at a maximal dose of 10–15 μg/kg/min [178, 183]. At very high doses, dobutamine may elicit tachycardia or augmented systemic blood pressure. However, acceleration of heart rate even at low doses can occur in patients with atrial fibrillation [184]. When dobutamine is administered in doses sufficient to increase cardiac output, peripheral resistence falls

initially, and blood pressure remains essentially unaltered. The relative distribution of flow to the coronary and skeletal muscle beds is increased, whereas that to the renal and splanchnic beds is decreased. Absolute renal blood flow is generally unchanged [185]. In contrast to dopamine, dobutamine is a direct acting beta-1 agonist and therefore not dependent on release of endogeneous catecholamines or characterized by tachyphylaxis. Nevertheless, with prolonged use responsiveness to all adrenergic agents may decline because of down regulation of receptor number. Thus, prolonged dobutamine infusions require a gradual increase in dose to elicit a constant hemodynamic response [186]. Dobutamine, when titrated judiciously, does not aggravate manifestations of ischemia [178]. In dogs it appears to exert a protective effect on tissue rendered ischemic, probably by favorably altering the overall cardiac oxygen supply–demand balance [187].

Dopamine appears to be somewhat less useful than dobutamine in this setting. At a dose of 5 μg/kg/min, it is less effective in increasing cardiac output or natriuresis. At higher doses, it often increases mean arterial pressure, pulmonary artery occlusive pressure, heart rate, and the frequency of VPCs [188, 189]. Moreover, the positive inotropic effects of dopamine are highly dependent on endogeneous catecholamine stores and release: this accounts for the rapid onset of tachyphylaxis encountered clinically [188, 190]. However, the vasopressor (alpha-1 mediated) effects of dopamine are occasionally helpful and the drug may be particularly useful in hypotensive patients without elevated peripheral vascular resistance.

In patients with heart failure, indiscriminate use of dopamine should be avoided because of several considerations:

(a) Peripheral resistance in most patients with cardiac failure is spontaneously elevated, and further vasoconstriction and increased afterload will therefore augment MVO$_2$ and reduce cardiac output [177];

(b) The critical perfusion pressure for the heart is difficult to define accurately in each patient, especially in the face of a diseased coronary circulation. It is undoubtedly markedly variable from patient to patient;

(c) With vasopressor doses, dopaminergic, and selective renal artery vasodilation is counteracted by alpha-adrenergic-mediated constriction. Furthermore dopamine may lead to undesirable increases in heart rate and dysrhythmia.

If hypotension and evidence of hypoperfusion (chest pain, altered mental status, or oliguria) persist despite augmentation of cardiac output with dobutamine, then cautious use of vasopressor therapy must be considered. One alternative is dopamine. Another is the addition to dobutamine of an alpha agonist such as phenylephrine (5–30 μg/min I.V.) to increase peripheral vascular resistance. This regimen minimizes the risks of tachycardia and ventricular dysrhythmia that may complicate high-dose infusions of dopamine.

Digoxin and other cardiac glycosides are no longer used routinely in the peri-infarction period. Delayed onset of action, relatively weak positive inotropic effect [191], and the potential for aggravating or initiating ventricular dysrhythmia and conduction disturbances account for the change in practice. However, the arrhythmogenicity of digitalis glycosides in patients with infarction may be overrated [192]. Although not as powerful as catecholamines [191], digitalis glycosides exert positive inotropic effects in patients with acute infarction with modest beneficial effects on cardiac output and left ventricular filling pressure [176, 193]. The likelihood that glycosides will increase infarct size by augmenting myocardial oxygen requirements [194] or by increasing coronary and peripheral vascular resistance is probably low. Slow (15 min) intravenous infusions avoid the alpha-adrenergically mediated coronary vasoconstriction [195] that may result from bolus injections. When digitalis is used in the setting of heart failure, it improves myocardial oxygen balance [196]. Thus, digitalis glycosides may be of use in the treatment of mild heart failure in patients with acute infarction. Their main utility in the setting of infarction is, however, slowing the ventricular rate in patients with atrial fibrillation.

Glucagon, another agent with prolonged positive inotropic effects after bolus injection (3–5 mg I.V.), is used only rarely in the peri-infarction setting. Although it stimulates myocardial cyclic AMP production without dependence on beta-receptors and is therefore capable of accelerating heart rate and stimulating contractility in the presence of propranolol, its major toxicity, nausea and vomiting, is troublesome. Pretreatment with phenothiazine antiemetics may be helpful in precluding these untoward effects. Arrhythmogenicity has not been prominent. Glucagon is hypothetically useful for treatment of heart failure induced or exacerbated by beta-adrenergic blockade [197, 198].

A new class of compounds that appears to be particularly promising for augmentation of cardiac contractility is represented by amrinone, currently an investigational drug in the United States. Amrinone exerts its effects through mechanisms independent of adrenergic receptors, adenyl cyclase, or sodium-potassium ATPase, apparently by augmenting calcium flux [199]. Although clinical experience is limited, potentiation of contractility occurs without arrhythmogenicity or marked effects on peripheral vasodilation. Like digitalis, amrinone may exacerbate myocardial injury in ischemic zones [200].

Pulmonary congestion and peripheral hypoperfusion

The combined presence of elevated pulmonary venous pressure (>18 mmHg) and reduced cardiac output (cardiac index <2.2 l/min/m^2) results from extensive myocardial damage and portends a mortality rate of 50% [148]. In combination with clinical manifestations of hypoperfusion (systolic blood pressure less than 90 mmHg, oliguria, and altered mental status), the full syndrome of cardiogenic shock is present and a mortality of 90% or more is the rule [201–203]. Aggressive therapy to reverse abnormal hemodynamics may improve the dismal prognosis [159], but conclusive evidence is lacking that medical interventions change the outlook more than temporarily.

Vasodilator therapy alters the course of severe heart failure acutely, whether or not it favorably influences long-term survival. The hemodynamic response to vasodilators generally follows a three-step progression. With low doses, peripheral resistance falls and cardiac output improves with little change in systemic blood pressure. At higher doses, cardiac output increases further, but blood pressure begins to decline. With excessively high doses, left ventricular preload is markedly reduced, cardiac output falls, and marked tachycardia and hypotension ensue. Thus, in patients with cardiogenic shock, extreme caution must be used in the initiation and maintenance of vasodilator therapy to avoid exacerbating hypotension. Hemodynamic monitoring including pulmonary pressure recordings and serial determinations of cardiac output is essential, as is accurate assessment of systemic blood pressure, preferably with an intraarterial catheter. If peripheral perfusion pressure begins to fall or if systolic pressure is below 90 mm Hg initially, a cardiotonic agent such as dobutamine may augment cardiac output and blood pressure and decrease pulmonary congestion [196]. Once an adequate systemic perfusion pressure is obtained, vasodilators can be initiated (Figure 3). In contrast, if systolic blood pressure remains less than 90 mm Hg and clinical evidence of hypoperfusion persists, a vasoconstrictor such as phenylephrine or norepinephrine (1–10 μg/min) may improve coronary perfusion, myocardial metabolism, and hemodynamics as well as ventricular performance [204, 205].

Recently, considerable enthusiasm has developed for the use of intraaortic balloon counterpulsation in the treatment of cardiogenic shock. By providing augmentation of diastolic pressure and hence of coronary perfusion pressure and by reducing systolic pressure and left ventricular afterload, this technique can increase myocardial oxygen supply and decrease demand while improving cardiac output and left ventricular function. The hospital mortality rate in patients treated with counterpulsation for cardiogenic shock has been reported to be as low as 60%. However, such series include patients with surgically remedial mechanical lesions such as rupture of the ventricular septum or papillary muscle [206, 207]. Unfortunately, among patients without surgically correctable lesions, both short- and long-term results of counterpulsation are poor [207, 208]. Complications of the intraarterial balloon are not rare, and balloon dependency is a frequent result with the ensuing ethical and medical dilemma of whether and how to terminate a supportive procedure without which the patient cannot survive [209, 210]. Externally applied counterpulsation offers some of the hemodynamic advantages of the intraaortic balloon and avoids some of its complications [211]. However, it cannot be tolerated for prolonged intervals by patients who are alert.

It is clear that continuous mechanical circulatory assist can be extremely useful in temporarily reversing the hemodynamic manifestations of extensive infarction with shock. It can provide support required for left ventricular and coronary angio-graphy with increased safety in those patients potentially harboring a surgically correctable lesion. However, for those with shock due to extensive myocardial injury, counterpulsation provides no long-term solution. Our current view is that it should be initiated in the treatment of shock in patients with acute myocardial infarction only when immediate invasive diagnostic studies are contemplated for detection of surgically correctable lesions.

Treatment of complications of acute myocardial infarction: pain

Chest pain is, of course, an almost universal presenting symptom. Severe, persistent, and refractory pain must be controlled aggressively to provide comfort to the patient and to prevent the deleterious consequences that physiological responses to pain impose on the circulation and the jeopardized left ventricle. In addition to the vigorous use of analgesics outlined above in the section on general supportive measures in the treatment of acute myocardial infarction, several other measures should be considered. Intensive efforts should be made to detect and treat aggravating factors such as hyper- or hypotension; hypoxemia; congestive heart failure; mechanical lesions such as left ventricular aneurysm, papillary muscle rupture or ventricular septal rupture; dysrhythmia including tachycardia

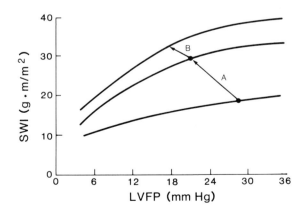

Figure 3. Left ventricular function curves demonstrating the combined efficacy of dobutamine (A) plus nitroprusside (B). Although both agents will increase cardiac output and lower left ventricular filling pressure (LVFP), dobutamine has a more favorable influence on stroke work index (SWI) since it maintains or augments systemic blood pressure.

due to anxiety, fever, or occult blood loss; pericarditis; or pulmonary emboli. Invasive monitoring is indicated often to characterize hemodynamics and identify occult states such as ventricular failure or a hyperdynamic circulatory response. Specific therapy of underlying factors will often alleviate the pain. Thus, propranolol should be used in hemodynamically hyperdynamic patients during monitoring of left ventricular function. With reduction of the intensity of myocardial ischemia, propranolol may lower left ventricular end-diastolic pressure [70, 212]. Nitrates are useful in the setting of mild heart failure or hypertension but may aggravate hypoxemia and can produce tachycardia and hypotension if left ventricular filling pressure is lowered below approximately 15 mmHg.

In patients with smouldering or refractory chest pain without identifiable aggravating features, anticoagulation has been recommended by some but without proof of efficacy [45]. Intraaortic balloon counterpulsation can effectively relieve pain and is occasionally useful in patients with pain refractory to other measures. It has been suggested that coronary artery bypass surgery should be attempted in these patients before cessation of counterpulsation, but objective proof of the utility and long-term benefit of this approach is not available.

Hypertension

Systemic arterial hypertension is common during the first hours after the onset of infarction, especially among patients with anterior infarction. It often accompanies other evidence of heightened sympathetic tone. Blood pressure generally declines with alleviation of anxiety, analgesia, or sedation. However, persistently elevated blood pressure imposes a significant burden on the heart. In its presence, specific therapy directed toward reduction of peripheral arterial resistence diminishes the extent of infarction [172].

Presently, nitroprusside is considered by most to be the antihypertensive agent of choice since it is effective immediately and can be titrated easily based on results of hemodynamic monitoring. However, a predilection to produce coronary steal [155] and to aggravate electrocardiographic ST-segment shifts even in mildly hypertensive patients [157] has been reported, suggesting that therapy with nitroprusside is indicated only when hyperten-

sion is at least moderate and persistent. Hemodynamic monitoring to assure maintenance of adequate left ventricular filling pressure ($>$15 mmHg) will avoid excessive tachycardia in response to nitroprusside and favor a reduction of myocardial ischemia [160, 161]. In patients with less severe hypertension, oral antihypertensive therapy should be initiated cautiously. Propranolol may be appropriate since cardioacceleration is blunted and efficacy of diuretics enhanced due to inhibition of renin release that might occur otherwise. Long-term beta blockade may be particularly helpful in hypertensive patients with severe coronary disease, since beta blockade is well tolerated, effective, and likely to decrease the reinfarction and sudden death rate [3].

Pericarditis

Pericardial friction rubs are audible in as few as 10% of patients with infarction even though symptoms of pericarditis are evident in as many as half [213–215]. When pain occurs, it usually appears during the first week after the onset of transmural infarction and persists for a few hours to several days. Late pericarditis may be a reflection of reinfarction or Dressler's syndrome [216]. When pain is severe, nonsteroidal antiinflammatory agents such as aspirin (600–900 mg six times daily) or indomethacin (25–50 mg three times daily) are usually helpful. Corticosteroids are effective also but at least hypothetically may impair reparative processes in the injured heart [217]. When a pericardial rub is detected, anticoagulation may be contraindicated because of the risk of hemopericardium [214]. Low-dose subcutaneous heparin is unlikely to precipitate bleeding and may be continued.

Surgically correctable lesions

Mechanical complications of infarction such as mitral regurgitation secondary to papillary muscle rupture, ventricular septal defect, or left ventricular aneurysm can be palliated by afterload reduction with vasodilators and support of the circulation with intraaortic balloon counterpulsation. Prompt definitive diagnostic studies and surgical correction are indicated. Rupture of the heart is generally a catastrophic and terminal event but rarely may result in a false aneurysm which can be treated surgically as soon as the diagnosis has been established. These aspects of therapy are discussed in Chapter 16.

Limitation of infarct size

Results from studies of experimentally induced infarction in animals subjected to coronary ligation and from clinical studies suggest that the evolution of myocardial infarction is a dynamic process developing over several hours after critical reduction of myocardial perfusion. Although the center of the ischemic zone undergoes irreversible injury within 30 min to 1 hr, epicardial tissue and regions near the periphery of the ischemic zone may remain viable for longer intervals. These regions of jeopardized tissue are potentially salvageable depending on the ratio of myocardial oxygen supply to demand, among other factors. Physiological or pharmacological interventions that exacerbate the balance between supply and demand will potentiate injury and may extend the infarct. Those that favorably modify the ratio may result in salvage of some myocardium. However, it appears likely that appreciable salvage can be engendered only during the first 6–8 hr after the onset of infarction, since subsequently the process of infarction may be virtually complete. Thus, many patients who come to medical attention only after substantial delay following the onset of symptoms may not be candidates for effective salvage of jeopardized tissue. A significant subset of patients exhibits persistent or recurrent chest pain and prolonged elevation of plasma MB CK suggestive of progressive infarction. Such patients may be particularly likely to benefit from appropriate protective interventions [218], even if intervention is relatively delayed.

An additional potential value of intervention therapy is the prevention of early recurrent infarction, often called extension of infarction. The incidence of this phenomenon is reported as ranging from 13% to 86%, depending on the diagnostic criteria employed for its recognition or definition [219–223]. Based on appearance of new plasma peaks of enzymes released from the heart, its incidence is approximately 20%. Patients with subendocardial infarction appear to be at particularly high risk of early recurrence [223]. Since early recurrent infarction is a major complication and since it contributes approximately 25% of the cumulative

infarct size in patients exhibiting the phenomenon, it may contribute markedly to left ventricular dysfunction, dysrhythmia, and overall mortality [220, 221, 223]. On the other hand, interventions designed to protect jeopardized ischemic myocardium may be particularly effective in reducing the incidence and severity of early recurrent infarction since they can be implemented *before* the process begins. If ischemic myocardium can be preserved for several days, collateral flow may increase sufficiently to adequately subserve oxygen requirements [224].

The ultimate extent of infarction is now recognized to be a major determinant of prognosis. Impairment of left ventricular function [225], reduction of ventricular fibrillation threshold [226], the severity and incidence of ventricular dysrhythmia during the hospital phase and the late recovery phase of acute myocardial infarction [227, 228], as well as overall mortality are closely correlated with infarct size [228, 229]. When 40% or more of the left ventricle becomes necrotic, cardiogenic shock is likely to supervene [230].

Despite these considerations, limitation of evolution of ischemic injury ('reduction of infarct size') has not yet been shown objectively to improve prognosis. In fact, it is possible that residual myocardium at risk may be particularly arrhythmogenic and therefore a risk factor for sudden death or reinfarction [223, 231]. On the other hand, 'preserved myocardium' may become extensively revascularized [224].

In view of its potential benefit, limitation of infarct size has become one focus of investigation in ischemic heart disease and an important goal of therapy. Most methods proposed for protecting jeopardized myocardium are aimed at decreasing myocardial oxygen requirements by reducing cardiac work or altering myocardial metabolism. Some have been aimed at increasing myocardial perfusion and oxygen supply in the ischemic zone (Table 1). Furthermore, in addition to the specific therapeutic approaches that have been suggested, it has become clear that meticulous attention to all aspects of patient care may offer particular promise in effecting myocardial salvage. Thus, consideration of effects on myocardial metabolism enters into decisions regarding oxygen therapy, treatment of hypertension or pain, management of stress and tachycardia, use of antiarrhythmic drugs, and he-

Table 1. Interventions proposed to limit infarct size – hypothetical mechanisms.

Intervention	Increase perfusion	Increase O_2 supply	Improve substrate transport	Decrease MVO_2	Decrease inflamation	Decrease circulating free fatty acids	Increase anaerobic metabolism
Recanalization	++	++					
Thrombolytics	++	++					
Nitroglycerin	+	+		++			
Hyaluronidase	±	±	±				
Propranolol		±		++		+	
Antilipolytic agents				+		++	+
Glucose – insulin – potassium				+		++	++
Calcium antagonists	+	+		++			
Antiplatelet agents	++	+					
Corticosteroids					++		
Hyperosmolar mannitol	+	+					
Hyperbaric oxygen		++					
Counterpulsation	+	+		++			

++ = major effect, + = minor effect, ± = putative but not established effect.

modynamic manipulations including the administration of diuretics, vasodilators, agents with positive inotropic effects, or augmentation of vascular volumes.

Augmentation of myocardial perfusion
Conceptually, the most direct approach to improving myocardial oxygenation involves restoration of coronary perfusion, either surgically [232], by percutaneous transluminal coronary angioplasty [233], by pharmacologically opening the occluded coronary with thrombolytic agents with or without associated mechanical recanalization [234], by overcoming coronary spasm with nitroglycerin [235], or by facilitating maintenance of perfusion with antiplatelet agents that hypothetically may reduce coronary vasospasm and/or platelet aggregation [236, 237]. In experimental animals, the most effective preservation of myocardial viability by reperfusion results when flow is restored as early as possible. Salvage is seen in only some animals when revascularization is delayed for 3 hr. Hemorrhagic infarction and extension of myocardial damage occur as a consequence of loss of microvascular integrity in others [238, 239]. These time constraints may seriously limit the applicability of direct surgical and other revascularization techniques to patients with evolving infarction. Furthermore, until the relative importance of thrombosis [240–242], platelet microaggregation [236–243], coronary spasm [244–

247], or other factors in initial or early recurrent infarction have been clarified, selection and documentation of potentially promising pharmacological approaches to reperfusion will be difficult. Unfortunately, preliminary clinical trials of all such approaches have been difficult to interpret. The necessity to act as early as possible has marred several studies in which interventions were initiated so early that definitive enzymatic confirmation of infarction was not possible – even retrospectively. Thus, it has not been clear whether the intervention prevented infarction or whether it was simply applied in patients with threatened infarction that would not otherwise have occurred regardless. Among patients with already evolving irreversible injury, reperfusion may exacerbate the process indirectly by inducing reperfusion dysrhythmia or directly by increasing local concentrations of calcium which in turn mediate explosive irreversible injury to cells with increased calcium permeability.

A less direct approach to augmentation of myocardial perfusion has included administration of hyaluronidase, a hydrolytic enzyme that degrades a major constituent of connective tissue ground substance, hyaluronic acid. Hyaluronidase limits morphologically defined infarct size in experimental animals subjected to coronary occlusion and appears to reduce electrocardiographic ST-segment elevation and Q-wave evolution in patients [248–252]. When given as late as 6 hr after occlusion,

501

hyaluronidase preserves jeopardized ischemic myocardium in experimental animals judging from electrocardiographic, histologic, and enzymatic analyses [249]. When given in doses of 500 NF units/kg intravenously every 6 hr to patients with infarction of less than 8 hr duration, hyaluronidase decreases ST-segment elevation and preserves R-wave amplitude compared to findings in conventionally treated controls [248, 252]. Significant toxicity or hemodynamic alterations have been observed only rarely and consist almost exclusively of infrequent urticarial allergic reactions. The mechanism of action of hyaluronidase is not clear. The drug may reduce myocardial edema and thereby maintain microvascular function. As a result, nutrient and collateral blood flow may be improved and promote enhanced oxygen delivery and washout of noxious metabolites [253].

Reduction of myocardial oxygen demand
Other agents, such as nitroglycerin, have been reputed to limit infarction at least in part by increasing coronary perfusion. However, it appears that beneficial effects reported are more correctly attributable to reduction of oxygen demand. Contradictory reports of nitroglycerin-induced changes in myocardial blood flow are difficult to interpret. When the drug is given systemically to animals without coronary occlusion in doses that avoid hypotension and tachycardia, intravenous nitroglycerin augments coronary flow by direct vasodilatory actions on the coronary arterial circulation. When given to dogs without diffuse coronary arterial lesions but with an experimentally induced occlusion, it increases collateral blood flow to the ischemic zone and increases the endocardial-to-epicardial ratio of perfusion [254–257]. However, the magnitude of these changes is small, and they are unlikely to fully explain the protective effect of the drug. Systemically administered nitroglycerin exerts effects predominantly on venous capacitance vessels. Thus, nitroglycerin reduces MVO_2 by reducing ventricular volume and decreasing afterload [163, 164]. In excessive doses or in the presence of low left ventricular filling pressures, nitroglycerin can promote hypotension and tachycardia with deleterious effects that outweigh the potential benefits of the drug on collateral blood flow and MVO_2. In contrast, judicious doses reduce ischemia in patients with diffuse coronary atherosclerosis [258].

Intracoronary administration to achieve the same coronary arterial concentration is not effective; this clearly implicates the primary role of systemic as opposed to coronary vascular actions in mediating its beneficial effects [259].

Results in studies with animals given nitroglycerin demonstrate the importance of maintenance of normal systemic blood pressure. When systemic arterial resistence is sustained with methoxamine, tachycardia is precluded and beneficial effects of nitroglycerin on electrocardiographic manifestations of ischemia are promoted [256, 260]. Administration of nitroglycerin to dogs for 5 hr after coronary occlusion results in a reduction in infarct size based on assessment of CK depletion and morphometry [261]. In addition, nitroglycerin increases the threshold to ventricular fibrillation and reduces spontaneous ventricular dysrhythmia in animals with experimental myocardial infarction [262–264].

Studies of patients given nitroglycerin demonstrate reduction of ST-segment elevation [265–268]. In patients with elevated filling pressures, hypotension and tachycardia can be avoided by monitoring the infusion carefully; and regression of electrocardiographic manifestations of ischemic injury is the rule [265]. In patients with low left ventricular filling pressure, however, the use of methoxamine to maintain arterial blood pressure may be required to avoid tachycardia and aggravation of ischemia [267, 268]. Preliminary findings in additional studies report not only regression of electrocardiographic changes but a reduction of hospital mortality in patients treated with nitroglycerin [269].

Although nitroglycerin is effective orally or sublingually, the intravenous route of administration is preferred for patients with threatened or evolving myocardial infarction to facilitate titration in response to results of hemodynamic monitoring. Initial doses of 10 μg/min should be increased gradually until systolic arterial blood pressure has declined by a maximum of 20 mmHg or heart rate has increased by 10 beats/min. Even when the drug is titrated carefully, however, hypotension can occur suddenly, especially early in the course of treatment or when patients assume or are placed in an upright posture. Because of this risk, hemodynamic monitoring is desirable to detect those patients with low filling pressures who are particularly prone to develop hypotension and reduced cardiac output. A fall in blood pressure should be treated by prompt cessation of nitroglycerin, elevation of the legs, expansion of vascular volume, and administration of vasopressors when required.

Beta-adrenergic blockade

Propranolol and other beta-adrenergic-blocking agents may be useful in limiting infarct size. By reducing heart rate, contractility, and systemic arterial blood pressure while changing left ventricular filling pressure only modestly, these agents markedly decrease determinants of myocardial oxygen demand [270]. On the other hand, they may increase oxygen supply by augmenting collateral blood flow and improving the endocardial-to-epicardial flow ratio [271, 272]. The increase in perfusion may reflect reduction in left ventricular diastolic pressure and hence augmentation of the diastolic pressure gradient for coronary perfusion, decreased heart rate with augmented diastolic perfusion time [70, 273] or possibly reduction of paradoxical, beta-mediated constriction of coronary arterial vessels within ischemic zones. Additional benefit on the balance between myocardial oxygen supply and demand may result from effects of propranolol on fatty acid metabolism. Beta-adrenergic blockade reduces arterial free fatty acid (FFA) concentrations and consequently decreases fatty acid uptake by the heart; this uptake is known to be linearly related to arterial FFA. Fatty acids have been implicated in the alleged oxygen-wasting effects of catecholamines. Thus, reduction of myocardial FFA uptake may reduce futile oxygen consumption and favor myocardial viability. Furthermore, myocardial fatty acids and fatty acid metabolites have been implicated in arrhythmogensis and as mediators of ischemic injury [274–278]. The net effects of reduced work load, improved regional blood flow, and a shift from FFA to carbohydrate catabolism are manifested by decreased myocardial oxygen utilization, reversal of lactate production to extraction, and a relative maintenance of intracellular high energy phosphate stores [270, 279–281].

Effects of propranolol in experimental animals with coronary occlusion include reduction of electrocardiographic ST-segment shifts indicative of ischemia, diminished Q-wave evolution, prevention of myocardial CK depletion, and reduction of morphometric infarct size when administered as late as 3 hr after occlusion [120, 272, 282, 283]. In pilot studies in patients, administration of propranolol

appears to reduce pain and dysrhythmia due to ischemia as well as to decrease MVO_2 and lactate production, electrocardiographic manifestations of ischemia, and infarct size estimated enzymatically [212, 270, 281, 284–286]. Preliminary results of the initiation of beta-adrenergic blockade within 12 hr after the onset of chest pain (5 mg of atenolol intravenously with 50 mg orally immediately and 50 mg every 12 hr thereafter) have demonstrated a reduction in infarct size judging from analysis of plasma CK activity and enhanced preservation of R-wave amplitude, and apparent prevention of infarction in some patients with threatened myocardial infarction and unstable angina [287].

Propranolol and other beta blockers are well tolerated in most patients. In addition to exerting direct effects on the heart, beta blockers lower endogenous sympathetic tone reflected by circulating levels of norepinephrine, presumably by presynaptic effects that increase negative feedback on neural release [62]. In the clinical setting, hemodynamic and electrocardiographic monitoring is desirable to detect potential exacerbation of congestive heart failure, sinus bradycardia, or AV conduction block. Heart failure is precipitated only rarely in hemodynamically stable patients. However, preexistent failure may be aggravated [70]. On the other hand, among patients with infarction and elevated pulmonary artery occlusive pressure, propranolol often lowers left ventricular filling pressure moderately, presumably by improving contractility secondary to a favorable oxygen supply and demand balance. Hypothetically, agents with mild intrinsic sympathomimetic activity such as alprenolol or pindolol may be less likely to aggravate congestive heart failure, and cardioselective agents such as metoprolol and atenolol may be less likely to increase perpherial resistance and hence left ventricular afterload. However, the clinical relevance of these considerations has not been established. Based on promising results in several pilot studies, large scale prospective, double-blind, randomized clinical trials employing several beta-adrenergic-blocking agents in patients with acute myocardial infarction are in progress.

Modification of myocardial metabolism

An additional approach to limitation of infarct size entails modification of myocardial FFA metabolism. Free fatty acids are the physiologically preferred substrate for the heart, but their utilization is highly oxygen-dependent. Aerobic carbohydrate utilization, on the other hand, is a physiologically minor energy source, though carbohydrate oxidation provides a higher ratio of high energy phosphate synthesis per mole of oxygen consumed. In ischemic tissue, continued FFA uptake results in the accumulation of intermediate metabolites such as acyl carnitine and acyl CoA which appear to exert potentially deleterious effects on membrane integrity and hence electrophysiological stability and cellular viability [288–291]. High levels of circulating FFAs are virtually universal in patients early after the onset of infarction. Under such conditions, FFAs increase MVO_2, depress contractility, and promote ventricular dysrhythmia [275]. Inhibition of lipolysis with nicotinic acid or beta-pyridyl carbinol prior to experimental coronary occlusion reduces the subsequent magnitude of epicardial ST-segment shifts, CK depletion, and severity of ventricular dysrhythmia [274, 292]. In patients, nicotinic acid analogs reduce cardiac FFA metabolism and promote carbohydrate utilization, thus increasing the myocardial respiratory quotient and decreasing MVO_2 [278, 293]. The duration of exercise in patients with chronic stable angina prior to precipitation of pain is prolonged and ventricular dysrhythmia in patients with infarction is reduced [276].

Infusion of glucose-insulin-potassium (GIK) (300 g glucose, 50 U insulin, and 80 meq KCl/l) markedly decreases plasma FFA levels and myocardial FFA uptake while glucose uptake and metabolism are enhanced and oxygen utilization decreased [294]. Studies of animals with coronary occlusion demonstrate preservation of high energy phosphate stores, elevation of ventricular fibrillation threshold, and limitation of infarct size judging from analysis of ST-segment elevation and myocardial CK depletion [295–297]. In patients, infusion of glucose at rates of 0.25–0.5 g/kg/hr suppresses circulating FFA levels below the 350 $\mu g/l$ threshold generally required for myocardial uptake [298]. Preliminary studies demonstrate a reduction in ventricular dysrhythmia without a detectable change in infarct size in a small group of patients, and a reduction of in-hospital mortality compared to that of historic controls [298, 299]. However, despite these encouraging observations some negative reports have appeared [300]. Furthermore,

conclusions regarding GIK and other regimens as well require prospective, randomized, double-blind studies with sufficiently large numbers of patients to assure adequate sensitivity and accuracy of analysis of results. Definitive evidence that GIK preserves myocardial viability, improves long-term survival, or both is not yet available. Since complications of GIK infusions are not rare, including hyper- and hypoglycemia, intravascular volume overload, and life-threatening hyperklemia even after discontinuation of the infusion [300], routine implementation of this still experimental regimen is not justified presently.

Calcium antagonists

Calcium channel-blocking drugs were utilized initially in patients with ischemic heart disease because of their physiological effects on arterial smooth muscle and myocardial cell function, manifested by peripheral and coronary dilation, and decreased cardiac contractility with a consequent reduction of myocardial oxygen requirements and potential facilitation of myocardial perfusion. However, metabolic considerations may provide an even more cogent rationale regarding limitation of infarct size. In addition to inducing afterload reduction, diminished contractility, and enhanced regional myocardial blood flow, these agents exert effects on myocardial metabolism directly attributable to the inhibition of inward calcium flux [301, 302]. In several systems, calcium has been shown to be a mediator of cell death, presumably acting in part by activating calcium-dependent degradative enzymes such as phospholipases, by inhibiting mitochondrial production of high energy phosphate compounds, and by activating calcium-dependent systems hydrolyzing ATP such as myosin ATPase [303]. Thus, liver cells rendered permeable to calcium by exposure to a variety of toxins retain viability until they are exposed to calcium in the medium after which they promptly manifest stigmata of irreversible injury [304]. Similarly, normoxic cardiac muscle cells, rendered permeable to calcium by brief exposure to calcium-free media, undergo irreversible injury when reexposed to calcium [305]. A clinical counterpart of this phenomenon may be reperfusion injury with the initial ischemia rendering myocardium excessively permeable to calcium and reperfusion delivering sufficient calcium to mediate injury. Preliminary results in animals with experimentally induced infarction treated with nifedipine, a calcium channel blocker, have demonstrated preservation of high energy phosphate stores, potentiation of mitochondrial respiratory function, and reduction of infarct size based on morphometric and enzymatic estimates [301, 302, 306]. Despite the direct depressant effect of calcium channel blockers on contractility, left ventricular function and exercise tolerance generally improve with therapeutic doses of nifedipine, verapamil, or diltiazem as a result of the dominant effects of decreased afterload on ventricular performance and the oxygen supply:demand ratio [307–310].

Additional approaches

High-dose corticosteroid therapy has been reported to limit infarct size in experimental animals [311, 312] but not consistently [313, 314]. Corticosteroids delay healing and can therefore potentiate myocardial rupture or aneurysm formation. In patients, despite some favorable early reports [315], high-dose corticosteroid therapy may increase mortality by impairing reparative processes and predisposing to ventricular rupture [217].

External counterpulsation has been employed to preserve jeopardized ischemic myocardium. Available data are conflicting [316, 317], and the use of this modality may be limited by patient discomfort and inapplicability to patients with severe peripheral vascular disease or marked disturbances of rhythm.

Hyperosmolar solutions of mannitol or glucose have been employed to reduce myocardial cell and endothelial cell swelling to promote collateral flow to the ischemic zone and limit the extent of infarction [318–320]. However, volume overload is a complication that, coupled with the inconclusive demonstration of benefit, leaves us with limited enthusiasm for widespread application of this approach.

Coronary platelet microthrombi are frequently associated with acute transmural infarction and are evident at autopsy in victims of sudden cardiac death. Platelet thrombi may be deleterious not only because of the mechanical effects of occlusion but also because of deleterious vasoconstrictor and platelet aggregating effects of thromboxane elaborated [321, 322]. Antiplatelet drugs have been considered to be potentially protective agents. Aspirin pretreatment (inhibiting thromboxane synthesis)

reduces platelet accumulation in coronary vasculature in the infarct zone, increases collateral flow, and reduces ventricular dysrhythmia in dogs with coronary occlusion [237, 323, 324]. Similarly, ibuprofen, a reversible cyclooxygenase inhibitor, reduces the extent of necrosis after experimental coronary occlusion [325]. However, contrary results have been reported. For example, large doses of indomethacin increase infarct size in the dog [326]. Disparate consequences of administration of agents of this type may be due to opposing effects on the progress of infarction as a whole mediated by thromboxane (which aggregates platelets, constricts coronary vessels, and may therefore exacerbate ischemia), and prostacyclin (PGI_2) (which prevents aggregation and dilates coronaries, thereby facilitating regional perfusion) [327]. All these inhibitors of prostaglandin synthesis can affect synthesis of thromboxane, PGI_2, or both, depending on the dose of each specific agent. Thus, the negative findings with indomethacin may be a reflection of a dominant effect of inhibition on endothelial cell prostaglandin and particularly PGI_2 synthesis with consequent exacerbation of ischemia.

Other antiplatelet agents such as dipyridamole are potent coronary as well as peripheral vasodilators. Reported efficacy of such agents in reducing the extent of experimental infarction may reflect the benefit of reduction of afterload, coronary dilation, or both [328, 329]. However, the possibility that coronary steal will result in patients with multivessel coronary artery disease is not adequately explored in experiments in which ligation is the cause of infarction in dogs with otherwise normal coronary vessels. Furthermore, clinical efficacy has not been established.

Because of a lack of definitive evidence establishing efficacy for any of these agents or approaches, we do not believe that nicotinic acid analogs, GIK, calcium channel blockers, corticosteroids, or antiplatelet drugs should generally be employed presently as conventional therapy for patients with evolving myocardial infarction in the absence of other specific indications.

Treatment of unstable angina

Unstable angina – often referred to as the intermediate syndrome, coronary insufficiency, crescendo or preinfarction angina – comprises a syndrome of relatively precipitous deterioration or change in the pattern of angina such as increased frequency, ease of provocation, prolonged duration, and/or increased severity. Patients with angina of recent onset or slowly progressive exertional angina, included in some studies of unstable angina, have a different and better prognosis compared to those with the 'intermediate syndrome.' Our discussion concerns this type of unstable angina which is characterized by severe, prolonged chest pain that may occur at rest and is accompanied by repolarization abnormalities on the electrocardiogram, but no elevations of plasma enzymes diagnostic of infarction [330]. Patients of this type have an in-hospital infarction rate of approximately 25% and a one-year infarction rate of 35% [330, 331]. The one-year mortality rate is between 10% and 22% [331–336]. These figures are remarkably similar to the recognized incidence of in-hospital extension or late reinfarction among patients presenting initially with acute myocardial infarction and emphasize the need for aggressive therapy.

The principles underlying therapy of unstable angina are essentially identical to those that apply to therapy of patients with evolving acute myocardial infarction. It is necessary to identify and correct unsuspected provoking factors such as arrhythmia, occult congestive heart failure, hypertension, hypoxemia, anemia, occult blood loss, thyrotoxicosis, and noncompliance with drug therapy or use of outdated nitroglycerin. Medical management for patients in whom such factors are not responsible comprises hospitalization, preferably in a CCU or other facility with monitoring capabilities, bed rest, administration of oxygen, analgesia, and sedation. Pain unresponsive to nitrates should be treated vigorously with morphine. In the absence of specific contraindications, beta blockade with propranolol or other beta-blocking agent should be initiated, preferably with intravenous administration of the drug, and titrated to achieve a heart rate near 60 and a blunted chronotropic response to sympathetic stimulation [337]. Treatment with beta-blocking agents often controls chest pain, reverses electrocardiographic changes indicative of ischemia, and may reduce the subsequent in-hospital infarction rate [287, 338, 339]. Long-acting nitrates such as isosorbide dinitrate should be initiated concomitantly, initially at low doses (5 mg p.o.q.

4–6 hr) and increased rapidly (to 120 mg/day or more) using the patient's tolerance and hemodynamic response as guides (see the section above on elevated left ventricular filling pressure and pulmonary vascular congestion with or without pulmonary edema). These measures alone will generally alleviate pain and stabilize the patient's condition. Although the use of anticoagulants has been supported enthusiastically as a means of prevention of infarction in high risk patients, completed clinical studies suffer from serious design flaws [340]. No prospective, well-controlled trial is available establishing the benefit of anticoagulants for this purpose. Low-dose heparin, administered to prevent deep vein thrombosis, is justified for patients subjected to prolonged bed rest or for those with overt congestive failure.

Recently, calcium channel-blocking drugs have been evaluated in the treatment of unstable angina [341]. Their apparent efficacy may reflect a reduction of MVO_2 secondary to decreased afterload and diminished contractility, as well as possible enhancement of myocardial perfusion due to reduction of physiologically inappropriately elevated coronary tone (spasm) in ischemic zones. Although most patients with unstable angina have severe occlusive coronary artery disease [342], 10–20% exhibit angiographically normal coronary arteries [340, 343]. The syndrome in such patients may epitomize unstable angina due to coronary artery spasm [344]. In some patients refractory to conventional therapeutic measures, nifedipine has been successful in controlling manifestations of recurrent ischemia [345].

In patients with unstable angina who fail to respond promptly to medical management, stabilization of hemodynamics and reduction of pain can be achieved with intraaortic balloon counterpulsation. Coronary angiography and sometimes urgent surgery is indicated. This approach is associated with 1% early and 1% late mortality, 5% perioperative infarction rate, and attainment of late functional class I or II in 90% of patients [346]. These impressive results have stimulated early surgical intervention [347]. However since most patients can be stabilized medically, aggressive medical management appears to be the primary treatment of choice, with urgent angiography and surgery reserved for patients with medically refractory symptoms [348]. Among patients with symptoms successfully controlled without surgery, approximately 40% will be in functional class I after 48 months of medical therapy [349]. For those whose symptoms are not controlled satisfactorily, elective surgery can be planned along guidelines similar to those that apply to patients with stable angina.

Treatment of chronic stable ischemic heart disease

The medical management of chronic IHD differs from treatment of emergencies such as myocardial infarction and unstable angina only in terms of temporal sequences of initiation and duration of specific regimens and priorities or primary focus; the basic principles are the same. In the case of chronic IHD, more emphasis can be placed on modification of life style, physical rehabilitation, and preventive measures. The specific major syndromes of chronic IHD – angina pectoris, congestive heart failure, and sudden cardiac death due most often to ventricular fibrillation – are analogous to the major life-threatening complications of infarction. Thus, it is not surprising that the principles and many of the specifics of therapy are similar in the two settings.

The patient with chronic IHD must be educated thoroughly to reduce established risk factors that accelerate atherogenesis or precipitate clinical consequences of underlying coronary artery disease. Cessation of cigarette smoking decreases the subsequent risk of infarction, heart failure, angina, and cardiac mortality by as much as 50% compared to that in persistent smokers within 1.5 years [22]. Reduction of serum cholesterol may retard or reverse atherosclerotic plaque formation [350, 351]. Weight reduction, control of blood pressure, and avoidance of emotional stress reduce symptoms by decreasing the work load placed on the heart. Atherogenesis may be slowed as well, especially by preclusion of hypertension.

Regular physical exercise, preferably initiated under medical supervision, can reduce cumulative stress on the circulation by slowing heart rate and reducing cardiac output and blood pressure at rest and by improving peripheral oxygen delivery and extraction. The frequently attendant weight loss may be symptomatically beneficial, carbohydrate intolerance in diabetic patients is often improved, plasma LDL cholesterol and triglycerides often fall,

and HDL cholesterol may increase [352, 353]. These changes potentially are capable of contributing to a decreased rate of atherogenesis. Effective exercise training can be accomplished safely in patients with angina or prior infarction if care is taken to ensure that isotonic exercise is performed only after a gradual warm-up, that cardio-acceleration is limited to no more than 85% of the patient's maximal tolerated heart rate on treadmill testing and that the accelerated heart rate is maintained for 20–30 min during at least three exercise sessions weekly [354].

Prophylactic pharmacological measures to reduce the likelihood of sudden cardiac death should be considered for all patients with chronic IHD, though firm evidence of prolongation of life is not yet available. Most experience has been gathered with chronic beta-adrenergic blockade in the treatment of patients surviving myocardial infarction. After two preliminary trials of chronic alprenolol therapy (400 mg daily) demonstrated a significant reduction in sudden death and reinfarction [355, 356], results in a multicenter trial of practolol (200 mg twice daily) in postinfarction patients demonstrated a 38% reduction in overall one-year mortality and sudden death with benefits confined virtually exclusively to patients with prior transmural anterior infarction [3, 357]. When practolol was discontinued, there was no discernible increase in mortality or 'rebound phenomenon' (see following section). More recently, a third study of alprenolol therapy initiated while patients were still hospitalized in the CCU demonstrated a nearly 50% reduction in one-year mortality in patients with coronary insufficiency or confirmed myocardial infarction [358]. However, treated patients over 65 years of age had a significantly higher in-hospital mortality rate than controls. Whether propranolol can favorably affect long-term prognosis is not yet clear. This question should be resolved by several ongoing clinical trials.

Large scale studies designed to evaluate the efficacy of antiplatelet agents in prolonging life among patients with chronic IHD have produced inconsistent results. Platelet turnover is accelerated in patients with coronary artery disease, platelet aggregation has been documented within the coronary circulation in patients who succumb, platelet aggregation is intensified by exercise stress, and aggregation can be blocked with aspirin [237, 359,

360]. Release of thromboxane A_2 from platelets undergoing aggregation may reduce coronary blood flow by eliciting coronary constriction and thereby may exacerbate or precipitate angina, ventricular dysrhythmia, or infarction. Repetitive platelet release of mitogenic factors capable of stimulating vascular smooth muscle proliferation *in vitro* has been implicated as a factor capable of accelerating atherogenesis *in vivo* [9]. Nevertheless, clinical studies with aspirin, administered to inhibit platelet aggregation and thromboxane synthesis, have failed to provide conclusive positive results. Favorable trends suggesting a reduction in mortality have been noted in several trials with aspirin, but none has yielded statistically significant results [361–365]. Others have failed to show even favorable trends [366, 367]. A recently completed study with dipyridamole and aspirin alone or in combination has reported favorable results [365]. Another antiplatelet drug, sulfinpyrazone, at a dose of 800 mg/day, has been reported to reduce mortality due to sudden cardiac death during the first eight months of therapy after infarction [4]. However, the classification of patients regarding mode of death has been seriously questioned and deemed inadequate by the FDA, overall mortality was not reduced, and the trial was flawed by exclusion of patients who were randomized but subsequently withdrawn from the study. This may result in serious bias because factors leading to withdrawal may be related to unrecognized factors contributing to death.

It is difficult to be arbitrary regarding prophylaxis in view of the conflicting and inconclusive data. However it seems likely that prophylactic therapy with beta-adrenergic-blocking agents should be considered in high risk patients under the age of 65. As cardioselective drugs and agents designed to be excluded by the blood–brain barrier are now available in the United States, it should be possible to achieve beta blockade with fewer side effects and possibly more unequivocal efficacy.

Stable angina pectoris

The natural history of survival among patients with exertional angina is not qualitatively dissimilar to that of patients with acute myocardial infarction. The annual mortality rate is estimated to be 4% with half of the deaths being sudden. Five percent per year suffer acute myocardial infarction. Patients with left ventricular dysfunction, rhythm disturbances, and hypertension have a more grave prognosis [368, 369]. On the other hand, more than one-third of patients with angina can expect spontaneous remission of pain lasting for two years or more [370]. Aggressive medical therapy can markedly improve symptoms in at least 90% of patients [371].

General measures including risk factor modification and supervised exercise training can be particularly helpful to patients with exertional angina. Augmented carboxyhemoglobin levels, caused by heavy freeway traffic, proximity to cigarette smokers, or especially cigarette smoking itself, aggravate angina pectoris [372, 373]. Accordingly, deleterious exposure should be avoided and smoking precluded. Excessive alcohol ingestion is proscribed because of its adverse effect on heart rate and blood pressure and on tolerance of exercise duration prior to the onset of pain [374]. Medical problems such as anemia, thyrotoxicosis, pulmonary disease with hypoxia, occult or overt heart failure, or ventricular aneurysm all can aggravate angina. They should be identified and treated specifically. In patients with cardiomegaly, covert heart failure presenting as nocturnal angina, or overt heart failure, digoxin can be a potent antianginal drug [375]. However, in the nonfailing heart, the positive inotropic effect of cardiac glycosides can increase MVO_2. Therefore these agents may occasionally aggravate angina.

Specific treatment of angina pectoris with organic nitrates remains the cornerstone of modern therapy. Nitroglycerin is a potent coronary vasodilator that can increase blood flow to an ischemic zone and preferentially direct flow to the subendocardium in animals subjected to coronary ligation in which the remainder of the coronary vasculature is normal [254–257]. This effect is relatively unimportant in the relief of exertional angina, however, which instead is attributable primarily to the drug's peripheral hemodynamic effects [259]. The reduction in preload, left ventricular chamber size, and afterload diminish MVO_2. Oxygen supply is unchanged or modestly increased because of the coronary vasodilation or increased myocardial perfusion due to diminished left ventricular diastolic pressure. In patients, coronary obstructive lesions are distributed diffusely in contrast to the case in experimental animal preparations studied in the laboratory. Accordingly, coronary vasodilation is less likely to augment perfusion to ischemic zones. It is therefore not surprising that intracoronary nitroglycerin does not increase the threshold to pacing-induced angina although systemically administered nitroglycerin does [259]. Rarely, patients with angina develop marked tachycardia or hypotension after taking nitroglycerin, thus increasing MVO_2 and reducing coronary perfusion pressure [376]. This can be prevented by advising the patient to sit or lie down or by concomitantly administering beta-adrenergic-blocking agents to blunt the tachycardia.

Nitroglycerin (0.3–0.6 mg) administered sublingually provides prompt relief of pain in most patients with angina. The drug is effective also when taken prophylactically before any activity that regularly induces an attack. Sublingual nitroglycerin alone is adequate for most patients with infrequent chest pain. However, its therapeutic effect is brief, lasting less than 0.5 hr. Therefore, to achieve a more prolonged antianginal effect, several long-acting nitrate preparations have been introduced. Nitroglycerin ointment (2%) can be applied cutaneously in strips of 0.5–2 in (5–25 mg of nitroglycerin); this results in sustained hemodynamic and antianginal effects that persist for at least 3 hr [377, 378]. The response is directly influenced by the area of skin to which a given amount of ointment is applied. The ointment should be kept refrigerated to preserve activity. Unfortunately, however, refrigeration makes it difficult to express the material from its container. This mode of therapy is cosmetically unacceptable for many physically active patients.

Several sublingual and orally administered long-acting nitrates are available. The advantage of sublingual administration of these agents is that absorption occurs into the systemic venous circulation, the liver is bypassed, and the drug escapes the marked first-pass hepatic degradation seen after oral administration. However, the onset of action after sublingual administration is abrupt, limiting the total dose that can be tolerated. The duration of the antianginal effects of sublingual isosorbide dinitrate (5–10 mg), erythrityl tetranitrate (10 mg), and pentaerythritol trinitrate (10 mg) is approximately 1 hr, an interval not significantly longer than that after sublingual nitroglycerin [379, 380].

Orally administered nitrates have a more gradual onset and more prolonged duration of action, though relatively large doses are required to overwhelm hepatic organic nitrate reductase activity. Oral isosorbide dinitrate in doses of 15–60 mg protects against exertional angina for 4–8 hr [381–383]. Sustained release oral nitroglycerin in doses of 2.5–9 mg exerts hemodynamic and antianginal effects for up to 8 hr [384]. Maximal doses of these drugs, titrated to avoid excessive hypotension or tachycardia and to minimize nitrate headaches, can be given at 6–8-hr intervals with sustained antianginal efficacy [385]. The major reservations regarding chronic high-dose nitrate therapy include the possible development of tolerance to nitrates analagous to the well-recognized tolerance to nitrate headaches, and the possibility of a withdrawal rebound syndrome similar to that manifested by the onset of angina or acute myocardial infarction in munition workers removed from chronic nitrate exposure. However, extensive clinical experience and carefully designed drug trials have failed to demonstrate substantial tolerance to the antianginal effects of either isosorbide dinitrate or oral nitroglycerin therapy [385, 386]. Nevertheless, the potential for nitrate dependence must be considered when prescribing chronic high-dose nitrates. Nitrate therapy should be tapered gradually when discontinuation is planned.

In addition to nitrates, beta-adrenergic-receptor blockade has proven to be an effective approach to the treatment of angina. Beta blockers improve cardiac function in ischemic heart disease dy decreasing MVO_2 secondary to decreased contractility, heart rate, and systemic arterial blood pressure (mediated in part by inhibition of renin release from the kidney). Combined therapy with nitrates and beta-adrenergic-blocking agents is particularly effective, since propranolol alone may increase left ventricular end-diastolic volume and prolong ejection time, and thereby undesirably add to myocardial oxygen demands. Nitrate-induced preload and afterload reduction counteract these effects. On the other hand, beta blockade will blunt the otherwise deleterious tachycardia that may occur in response to nitrates [387]. The direct cardiodepressant effects and antiplatelet effects of membrane active beta blockers (propranolol, oxprenolol, and pindolol) may contribute to antianginal effects, although agents without these 'local anesthetic' properties have similar therapeutic efficacy.

Table 2. Beta-adrenoceptor-blocking agents.

Drug	Cardio-selectivity[a]	Intrinsic sympatho-mimetic effect	Membrane depressant effect independent of blockade	Lipid solubility[b]	Potency compared to l-propranolol	Average daily dose (mg)	Plasma half-life (hr)	Therapeutic plasma level (ng/ml)
Acebutolol	+	+	+	++	0.3	600–1,200	8	200–2,000
Alprenolol	0	++	+	+++	0.3	400	2–3	50–100
Atenolol	+	0	0	+	1	100	6–9	200–500
Metoprolol	+	0	±	++	1	150–300	3–4	50–100
Nadolol	0	0	0	+	2–4	80–240	17–24	50–150
Oxprenolol	0	++	+	++	0.5–1	120–400	2	80–100
Pindolol	0	+++	+	++	6	7.5–22.5	3–4	50–150
Practolol	+	++	0	+	0.3	400	6–8	1,500–5,000
Propranolol	0	0	++	+++	1	120–400	3.5–6	50–100
Sotalol	0	0	0	+	0.3	240–480	5–13	500–4,000
Timolol	0	±	0	++	6	15–45	4–5	5–10

0 = no effect, ± = possible effect, + = weak effect, +++ = potent effect.
[a] Cardioselectivity is less evident at higher doses.
[b] Penetration across the blood–brain barrier is proportional to lipid solubility.

The choice of which beta blocker is best for a given patient is becoming more and more important as additional drugs are becoming available. The agents differ in cardioselectivity, membrane stabilizing activity, intrinsic adrenergic agonistic activity, ability to penetrate the blood–brain barrier and pharmacokinetics (Table 2). In the United States, propranolol, metoprolol, nadolol, atenolol, and timolol have been released for oral administration. Pindolol may soon be approved as well. Metoprolol and atenolol are relatively selective for beta-1 blockade and are, therefore, the currently preferred agents of choice for use in the treatment of patients with concomitant lung disease, insulin-dependent diabetes, or peripheral vascular disease (to avoid unmasked alpha stimulation and peripheral vasoconstriction). None of the beta blockers currently available in the United States has significant intrinsic sympathomimetic activity, the presence of which in some studies appears to limit cardiodepressant and undesirable beta-2-blocking effects of such agents as oxprenolol, alprenolol, or pindolol[388–391]. However, even practolol, which is both cardioselective and has intrinsic sympathomimetic activity, can precipitate bronchospasm or heart failure in patients predisposed to these complications, and no agent retains cardioselectivity at high doses. Atenolol and nadolol have a potential advantage over propranolol in that they have a longer plasma half-life and can be administered once daily. However, the physiologic effects of beta blockers long outlast the maintenance of 'therapeutic' plasma levels. Thus, all of the available agents can be quite effective when used in a twice daily dosage regimen [392–394]. Propranolol is highly lipid soluble and therefore readily penetrates the blood–brain barrier. For patients bothered by vivid dreams, hallucinations, or depression, a change to a poorly lipid soluble agent such as nadolol or atenolol may be helpful.

Regardless of which beta-adrenoceptor antagonist is used, the dose must be titrated on an individual basis. With agents metabolized extensively in the liver such as propranolol, dosages required to achieve adequate plasma levels and desired physiologic effects vary widely from one patient to another. Most commonly, therapy is initiated at a low dose and increased until a resting heart rate of 50–60 is obtained, although additional antianginal efficacy may be gained by pushing the dose to tolerance [395]. To date, careful clinical studies have revealed no significant difference in the ability of individual beta-adrenergic-blocking drugs to prevent angina [394, 396].

Most beta blockers are generally well tolerated by patients with uncomplicated angina pectoris.

Table 3. Properties of calcium channel blocking drugs.

Property[a]	Verapamil[b]	Diltiazem	Nifedipine
Coronary and peripheral vasodilation	++	++	+++
Depression of myocardial contractility	++	+	±
Depression of AV conduction	+++	++	0
Noncompetitive sympathetic antagonism	+	++	0
Inhibition of fast channel	±	+	0
Oral dose	80–160 mg q 8 hr	60–90 mg q 6 hr	10–20 mg q 8 hr
Plasma half-life	5 hr	4 hr	4 hr
Side effects	Rare precipitation of left ventricular failure, AV conduction block, nausea, flushing	Rare precipitation of left ventricular failure, AV conduction block, bradycardia, hypotension, flushing	Palpitations, hypotension, nausea, flushing

0 = no effect, + = weak effect, +++ = potent effect.
[a] Effects at conventional therapeutic doses.
[b] Contrary to nifedipine, verapamil-effects on the heart are rate dependent and more evident when cardioacceleration is present.

However, uncompensated left ventricular failure, heart block, severe bronchial asthma or chronic obstructive lung disease, depression, and severe peripheral vascular disease are contraindications to beta blockade. Complications or side effects, observed in approximately 10% of patients, generally occur early after initiation of therapy and are not dose dependent [397]. When heart failure is aggravated by propranolol, therapy with digitalis and diuretics is often sufficiently effective to permit continued beta blockade and maintenance of antianginal effects [398]. Use of a cardioselective drug in this setting is desirable to decrease beta-2 antagonistic effects that otherwise may result in enhanced peripheral vascular resistance, increased left ventricular afterload and exacerbation of failure [399]. Therapeutic failures among patients with angina treated with beta antagonists are generally due to poor compliance, insufficient dosage, or occult left ventricular failure.

An uncommon but life-threatening complication may occur with sudden cessation of beta blocker therapy. This so called 'rebound phenomenon' [400], manifested within two weeks of discontinuation of therapy, entails exacerbation of angina and dysrhythmia, precipitation of unstable angina, and sometimes provocation of acute myocardial infarction. The phenomenon is probably due to supersensitivity to beta-receptor stimulation as a result of 'up regulation' of the number of beta receptors during therapy [401, 402]. Termination of beta block-

ade therefore requires gradual reduction of dose rather than sudden withdrawal. For patients undergoing cardiac or other surgery, beta blockade should be continued until the time of surgery and resumed promptly thereafter [403].

A new noncardioselective beta antagonist is labetalol, which has the unusual property of blocking alpha-adrenergic receptors as well as beta receptors, and in addition exerts direct vasodilating effects [404, 405]. Labetalol decreases peripheral vascular resistance and increases coronary blood flow. By decreasing left ventricular afterload, labetalol is likely to be particularly well tolerated in patients with congestive heart failure. Its effect on coronary vasculature may be particularly important in those patients in whom coronary vasospasm plays a pathogenetic role underlying angina [406, 407]. Preliminary results of treatment of hypertensive as well as normotensive patients with angina confirm the drug's efficacy [405, 408], but further study is required to determine whether labetalol has clinically significant advantages over more conventional beta blockers.

A third class of agents offering promise in the treatment of angina is that of the calcium antagonists, including verapamil, nifedipine, diltiazem, and perhexiline. These drugs share the property of blocking slow channel calcium influx into myocytes and vascular smooth muscle cells but differ extensively with respect to the kinetics of blockade, the predominant target tissue, and the presence or

511

absence of ancillary membrane active properties (Table 3). Verapamil, a racemic mixture whose d and l stereoisomers have vastly different electrophysiologic effects, blocks sodium channels as well as calcium channels, prolongs the refractory periods of action potentials dependent on the slow inward current, depresses SA and AV node function, and exerts a prominent negative inotropic effect [409]. Although verapamil has been highly effective in the treatment of effort angina [410, 411], it is contraindicated in patients with heart failure and concomitant conduction system disease. It should be used cautiously in patients treated concomitantly with beta-blocking agents because of potentially additive effects on AV conduction and contractility.

Nifedipine is a calcium channel blocker with predominant effects on coronary and peripheral arterial smooth muscle. It reduces the intensity of ischemic insults by decreasing MVO_2 secondary to reduction of afterload [412, 413]. It also may increase regional myocardial blood flow secondary to direct effects on coronary arterial smooth muscle [414, 415]. The antianginal efficacy of nifedipine compares favorably to that of sublingual nitrates, verapamil, and propranolol [416]. The drug can be used safely in conjunction with beta blockers because it lacks appreciable cardiac depressant effects in conventional therapeutic doses and does not interfere with atrioventricular conduction [416, 417]. Its potent coronary vasodilator effects explain its utility in the relief of Prinzmetal's angina and are probably important in many patients with effort angina with associated superimposed spasm [406, 418].

Perhexiline and diltiazem have not yet been as well characterized clinically as verapamil and nifedipine. Perhexiline has a long plasma half-life. It appears to be effective in the relief of angina due to either coronary spasm or fixed obstruction presumably because of peripheral as well as coronary vascular effects [419, 420]. However, its use is associated with frequent and sometimes severe side effects including hepatitis, peripheral neuropathy, myopathy, and vision loss. Diltiazem has characteristics similar to those of verapamil. It is, like verapamil, an effective antiarrhythmic useful in the conversion of supraventricular and AV nodal reentry tachycardias by virtue of its effects on AV nodal conduction. In addition it exhibits potent coronary and peripheral arterial vasodilator properties [421,

422]. Its sympathetic antagonistic effect prevents reflex tachycardia common to most vasodilators [423].

The mode of action and efficacy of calcium channel-blocking drugs suggest that they will become mainstays in the treatment and chronic prophylaxis of pain. Used in conjunction with beta blockers, the coronary and peripheral vasodilating properties of nifedipine would counter the tendency of beta blockade to increase left ventricular volume and coronary and peripheral vascular resistance. Furthermore, reflex tachycardia generally seen with nifedipine therapy may be blunted by concomitantly administered beta-blocking agents. Both verapamil and diltiazem display intrinsic sympatholytic effects and thus offer hemodynamic advantages similar to those obtained with nitrate-beta-blocker combination therapy. Furthermore, in contrast to the beta blockers, these agents can be used in subjects with bronchospasm or peripheral vascular disease. Despite these promising yet still somewhat hypothetical considerations, rigorously controlled clinical trials will be required to determine whether these agents will be more effective or better tolerated than conventional approaches such as the use of sustained action nitrates.

Another antianginal agent currently not available in the United States is amiodarone, a potent antifibrillatory drug, which decreases MVO_2, produces coronary vasodilation, and increases coronary blood flow. Positive chronotropic and inotropic responses to isoproterenol and to glucagon are blunted by this drug, as are the vasoconstrictor responses to alpha-adrenergic-receptor stimulation [424]. Thus, although it is not an adrenergic-receptor blocker, amiodarone exerts many effects on the heart and circulation resembling those induced by propranolol and particularly labetalol. In clinical studies, its antianginal efficacy is comparable to that of propranolol. No appreciable decrease in cardiac output or aggravation of congestive heart failure has been observed [425]. Although chronic use of this drug may be limited due to the development of cutaneous pigmentary deposition, corneal microdeposits and rarely reported pulmonary fibrosis and chemical hepatitis, it has few other side effects and may serve as a prototype for a new generation of antianginal and antiarrhythmic drugs.

Numerous vasodilator drugs have been suggested for use in the therapy of angina pectoris. Agents such as dipyridamole, papaverine, prenylamine, and ethaverine have been employed; but conclusive data documenting their efficacy are lacking [426]. Thus, although progress is being made with development of newer antianginal drugs, the primary cornerstone of treatment in the United States presently remains the use of nitrates and beta-adrenergic-receptor antagonists. These agents, when used in optimal dose regimens and after thorough attention to and correction of contributory medical illness and daily stresses, provide satisfactory symptomatic relief in more than 90% of patients [371]. Medically refractory patients, or those suspected of having severe three-vessel coronary disease or left main coronary artery stenosis, should undergo diagnostic coronary angiography with a view towards possible surgical revascularization [427, 428]. In rare cases of angina (10%) of recent onset attributable to a single proximal uncalcified partially obstructing lesion, percutaneous transluminal coronary angioplasty may be elected, though the long-term results of this procedure have not yet been defined [233, 429].

Vasospastic angina

In its pure form, variant (or Prinzmetal's) angina due to coronary artery spasm occurs with the patient at rest and in patients with angiographically normal coronary arteries. Such angina is characterized electrocardiographically by ST elevation, generally evident in the inferior leads [430, 431]. In the United States, angina of this type is rare. However coronary vasospasm is now recognized frequently in other settings and frequently coexists with significant atherosclerotic occlusive disease. Thus, angina at rest [432, 433], nocturnal angina [418], exertional angina [407, 434], unstable angina [435], myocardial infarction [246, 247], and sudden death [436] have all been associated with coronary spasm superimposed on macroscopic, occlusive coronary lesions.

The frequent association between vasospasm and atheromatous lesions is unlikely to be accidental. It has been suggested by some that recurrent vasospasm in a normal coronary artery will potentiate formation of atherosclerotic plaques due to local trauma [437]. On the other hand, atherosclerotic vessels appear to be exquisitely sensitive to vasospastic stimuli of diverse nature [438], presumably because of membrane alterations in vascular smooth muscle which alter receptor density, accessibility, or affinity. Thus, vessels exposed to cholesterol in vitro become supersensitive to stimulation with ergonovine and serotonin, as do vessels from hypercholesterolemic rabbits. Clinically, the enhanced constriction of coronary vessels in response to the cold presser test in patients with atherosclerotic coronary artery disease may be an analogous phenomenon [406, 439].

In patients with angiographically normal coronary arteries, vasospastic angina can be suspected from a history of angina at rest, often with diurnal variation in its occurrence, ST elevation at the time of occurrence of pain (although depression may occur instead) and frequent episodes of conduction block or high-grade ventricular dysrhythmia at the time of angina [431]. The diagnosis is confirmed angiographically when the patient experiences spontaneous chest pain or pain induced by provocative maneuvers such as the cold presser test [440], administration of methacholine [441], or administration of ergonovine [442–444]. The use of ergonovine in 0.05 mg intravenous doses at 5-min intervals to a total dose of not more than 0.3 mg is thought to provide a sensitive and reasonably specific test for detection of vasospasm [442, 445]. In this dose regimen, it is unlikely to precipitate vasospasm refractory to prompt reversal with nitroglycerin [446]. Ergonovine testing must be performed under conditions of maximum surveillance, generally in the catheterization laboratory. Angiographic documentation of spasm is essential. Intracoronary vasodilator therapy (nitroglycerin or nitroprusside) should be implemented promptly as necessary to relieve induced spasm. Repeated testing has been advocated by some to assess the adequacy of a therapeutic regimen [445], although this probably is not necessary. Significant atherosclerotic coronary artery disease is a contraindication to provocative testing because of the risk of excessive or uncontrollable interruption of myocardial perfusion.

The prognosis of variant angina is generally benign, and long periods of spontaneous remission occur. However, unstable angina, myocardial infarction, and sudden death are encountered occasionally [430–432]. Nitrates are generally effective in relieving attacks. Sustained therapy with long-acting nitrates frequently reduces the incidence of recurrent attacks. However, it is not always successful in completely controlling pain [447]. Beta-adrenergic-receptor blockade is generally not of benefit. Furthermore, it may precipitate spasm because of unopposed alpha-adrenergic vasoconstriction. Because excessive adrenergic tone has been implicated as a pathogenetic factor in variant angina [448], alpha-adrenergic blockade has been employed, but with only limited success [447]. Potent antianginal protection is afforded, however, by calcium channel-blocking drugs such as nifedipine [447, 449–452], perhexiline [419], or verapamil [453] (preceding section). Nifedipine has been used most widely and is generally well tolerated in a dose of 10–40 mg four times daily [447].

Among patients with fixed, occlusive coronary artery disease, superimposed spasm may aggravate ischemia. Propranolol may increase angina in some patients with ischemic heart disease [454], although direct evidence documenting enhanced vasospasm is lacking. The successful use of calcium channel blockers for the treatment of both effort angina and unstable angina may in part reflect relief to vasospasm. However, their failure to increase the double product (heart rate multiplied by systolic blood pressure) at the onset of angina induced by exercise suggests that their primary effect in prolonging exercise duration prior to pain is peripheral vasodilation [412, 416, 417]. The possible efficacy of calcium channel blockers in limiting ischemic injury in patients with acute myocardial infarction is currently under study.

Chronic ischemic heart disease – arrhythmias

Among the 600,000 annual deaths due to ischemic heart disease, two-thirds occur before the victim can be hospitalized. Most appear to be a result of sudden circulatory collapse accompanying ventricular fibrillation [455]. Effective prophylaxis requires prospective delineation of a subset of the population at greatest risk. Although almost all individuals with symptomatic IHD have some ventricular ectopic activity (VEA) [456], the presence of high-grade VEA is one predictor of sudden death [135]. However, since high-grade VEA correlates well with severe underlying coronary artery disease and severely impaired left ventricular function, it might be related to sudden death only indirectly [457, 458]. Nevertheless, specific antifibrillatory

therapy may be prophylactically effective and life saving [459, 460].

Other factors associated with sudden cardiac death, the presence of which may suggest the need for antiarrhythmic therapy, include recent myocardial infarction, congestive heart failure, conduction defects, electrocardiographic repolarization abnormalities, and diffuse coronary artery disease [461, 462].

Antiarrhythmic therapy is discussed in detail in Chapter 5. However, several important considerations regarding the general approach to management of arrhythmia deserve emphasis.

Effective prophylaxis for patients at high risk of sudden death depends mainly on early detection of dysrhythmia and definition of its nature, prompt implementation and documentation of efficacy of antifibrillatory measures, and continued follow-up. Detection and quantification of dysrhythmia is best accomplished with 24-hr ambulatory electrocardiographic recordings. Rarely, treadmill testing elicits ectopy not demonstrable at rest. Thus, it may be indicated in some patients with IHD and symptoms which appear with exertion. If high-grade VEA (multiform VPCs, couplets, salvos, or more than 30 VPC/hr) is detected, if the patient has documented IHD, and if no aggravating cause of dysrhythmia such as drug toxicity, metabolic or electrolyte abnormality, decompensated heart failure or hypoxia is present, then pharmacologic suppression of the VEA should be attempted. Its goal is two-fold: (a) provision of an antifibrillatory level of the drug selected that may or may not be accompanied by suppression of VEA; and (b) reduction of VEA during episodes of ischemia when the threshold for ventricular fibrillation declines and a single ventricular premature depolarization may be sufficient to initiate ventricular fibrillation.

Drugs generally are tested empirically in individual patients, using repeated ambulatory monitoring to assess drug efficacy.

In practice, drug selection for an individual patient is limited by the need to avoid toxicity and is further determined by convenience of administration rather than exclusively by considerations of specific electrophysiologic properties (Table 4). A thorough knowledge of drug pharmacokinetics, metabolism, and toxicities is therefore essential. In considering drug therapy, several important caveats apply: (a) Only a dramatic reduction in VPC

Table 4. Orally administered antiarrhythmic agents.

Drug	Reference	Oral dose (mg)	Plasma half life (hr)	Therapeutic blood level (μg/ml)	Elimination[a]	Metabolites	Toxicity
Quinidine	[469–76]	300–600 q 6–8 hr	6	3–5	liver	inactive	Vagolytic effect. Direct depression of AV conduction. GI intolerance. Cinchonism, thrombocytopenia
Procainamide	[468, 477]	250–1 000 q 4 hr	2.5–4.5	4–10	kidney liver	active	Vagolytic effect. Pacemaker suppression. Lupus syndrome (20%), GI intolerance; agranulocytosis
N-acetyl procainamide	[478–80]	500–1 500 q 6 hr	6–8	10–25	kidney	–	GI intolerance, insomnia, blurred vision
Disopyramide phosphate	[481, 482]	100–400 q 6 hr	6	2–8	kidney (liver)	inactive	Vagolytic and negative inotropic effects on heart, anticholinergic effects
Encainide	[489, 490]	25–100 q 8 hr	2–4	0.01–0.1	liver	? active	Ataxia, diplopia
Aprindine	[113]	50–100 q 12 hr	20–30	1–2	liver	active	QRS prolongation, AV block, tremor, dizziness, cholestatic jaundice, agranulocytosis
Ethmozin	[114, 491]	200–250 q 8 hr	5–10	0.5–1	liver	–	Headache, dizziness, nausea, vomiting
Tocainide	[495, 497]	400–800 q 8 hr	10–15	6–10	liver	active	Lightheadedness, tremor, vertigo, ataxia
Mexilitine	[492–94]	250–500 q 8–12 hr	10–24	0.75–2	liver	–	Nausea, vomiting, nystagmus, tremor, seizures
Phenytoin	[128, 476]	300–400 q d	20–26 (highly variable)	10–16	liver	inactive	Pacemaker suppression, cerebellar toxicity, megaloblastic anemia, neuropathy
Propranolol	[483–88]	20–240 q 6 hr	2–3.5	0.04–0.085	liver	active	Pacemaker suppression, AV block, heart failure, bronchospasm, peripheral vasoconstriction
Amiodarone	[498–500]	200–800 q d	>30 d	–	–	–	Thyroid imbalance, constipation, photodermatosis, corneal microdeposits, intraventicular or AV block, pacemaker suppression, hepatitis, ? pulmonary fibrosis

[a] The organ system primarily responsible for drug-elimination is noted.

frequency (approximately 90%) on a 24-hr tape can be accepted as firm evidence of drug efficacy rather than chance variation [463]; (b) adequate therapeutic blood levels of a drug must be documented before that drug can be dismissed as being ineffective; (c) although one drug from a particular class of antiarrhythmic agents is ineffective, another from the same class may be effective; (d) complete abolition of VEA or even of high grade VEA may not be possible or even necessary for the prevention of sudden death. Indeed the drug most effective in suppressing VPCs is not necessarily the one that will most successfully prevent recurrent ventricular tachycardia or ventricular fibrillation.

In patients with life-threatening arrhythmias, a prolonged empirical approach may not be satisfactory. Acute drug testing, with either continuous ECG monitoring to characterize rhythm [464] or with invasive electrophysiologic testing [459, 465–467] should be performed. Valuable lessons derived from invasive electrophysiological studies include recognition that: (a) a drug that prevents reinitiation of ventricular tachycardia is very likely to be effective in the long-term prevention of cardiac arrest [459, 466, 467]; (b) very high doses of a drug are often required for control of arrhythmia and may be well tolerated chronically [468]; (c) a decline in blood levels of a drug below that required for efficacy in acute drug testing may result not only in loss of efficacy but may potentiate dysrhythmia [468]; (d) dysrhythmia refractory to drugs in the acute setting pressages failure of empirical drug therapy and necessitates consideration of alternative approaches. Such alternative approaches include implantation of a pacemaker and the use of surgical techniques in patients unresponsive to pharmacologic therapy. The pacemaker techniques include overdrive suppression with a permanent pacemaker [501], automatic defibrillation with an implanted defibrillator [502], and patient-activated, programmed ventricular stimulation to interrupt reentrant ventricular tachycardia [503–505]. Surgical resection of ventricular aneurysms coupled with coronary revascularization has been successful in approximately 50% of patients [506–510]. A greater success rate may be achieved when the site of origin or pathway of a reentrant dysrhythmia has been determined with the use of endocardial and epicardial mapping techniques, thereby facilitating more selective surgical ablation [511, 512].

Chronic ischemic heart disease – congestive heart failure

Chronic congestive heart failure among patients with IHD is generally the result of loss of contractile tissue and its replacement by fibrotic tissue. Obviously, the scar itself is not functional. However, surviving myocardium can be stimulated to contract more vigorously with agents having positive inotropic effects. Contributing phenomena such as elevated peripheral vascular resistance, dyskinetic wall segments, or a regurgitant mitral valve can be modified with the use of arterial vasodilators. Symptomatic pulmonary congestion can be relieved with the use of diuretics with or without appropriate vasodilator therapy. The importance of ensuring optimal ventricular function is perhaps greater in patients with ischemic heart disease than those with other conditions since decompensation aggravates angina and may induce lethal dysrhythmia.

In general, the discussion of therapy of heart failure presented in Chapter 14 applies well to patients with chronic IHD. Nevertheless, some considerations deserve special emphasis. Agents with

positive inotropic effects are most useful in patients with mild left ventricular dysfunction. They are relatively ineffective when loss of contractile elements is already substantial or when effective ventricular ejection is severely compromised by a regurgitant mitral valve or paradoxical systolic filling of a ventricular aneurysm. Agents with positive inotropic effects such as cardiac glycosides or beta-adrenergic agonists such as terbutaline or salbutamol are particularly apt to elicit severe ventricular dysrhythmia in the setting of intermittent ischemia.

Vasodilators provide several potential advantages in the treatment of failure associated with IHD. Myocardial oxygen balance may be improved, toxicity is generally readily controllable or preventable, and peripheral blood flow may be improved. However, caution is necessary since coronary perfusion pressure is dependent on diastolic blood pressure and can therefore be severely compromised by drug-induced postural hypotension. The effects of vasodilators on the coronary circulation have been insufficiently characterized, and coronary steal is a risk associated with several commonly used agents such as nitroprusside. The same homeostatic mechanisms that initially led to elevated peripheral vascular resistance in patients with congestive heart failure may persist and partially counteract the desired effects of any vasodilator. If the drug is then withdrawn suddenly, compensatory vasoconstrictor mechanisms including increased catecholamine release, up-regulation of alpha receptors, and augmented activity of the renin-angiotension system may cause a rebound increase in afterload, thus aggravating left ventricular dysfunction and exacerbating myocardial ischemia [513].

The same principles and considerations that guide therapeutic decisions for patients hospitalized in a coronary care unit apply, although on a less immediate scale, to patients with chronic IHD. Specific drug therapy generally is limited to orally active drugs. Titration of dose is generally modulated on the basis of changes in symptoms, physical findings, and noninvasive criteria of cardiac function. It is only rarely necessary to hospitalize a patient for hemodynamic study or titration of therapy based on analysis of central pressure and cardiac output.

In patients with moderate left ventricular dysfunction, reduction of preload with the use of diuretic therapy coupled with moderate doses of a

Table 5. Vasodilators used for treatment of chronic heart failure.

Drug	Dose (mg)	Responses				Comments
		Preload	Afterload	Cardiac output	Heart rate	
Isosorbide dinitrate (oral)	20–40 q 4–6 hr	+++	+	±	±	
Nitroglycerin oral, sustained action	6.5–19.5 q 8–12 hr	+++	+	±	±	Question of tolerance and nitrate dependence unresolved. May be ineffective with very high central venous pressure. May cause postural hypotension.
Nitroglycerin 2% ointment	1–2 in q 6 hr	+++	+	±	±	
Hydralazine	50–100 q 6–8 hr	+	+++	+++	++	Large doses may be needed. Lupus syndrome occurs in 10–20%. Increases natriuresis. Pyridoxine-dependent neuropathy.
Prazosin	5–10 tid	++	++	++	±	First-dose syncope. Some tachyphylaxis with chronic use. Alpha-1 receptor specific.
Trimazosin	100–150 tid	++	++	++	±	Not currently available in U.S. Similar to prazosin but no first-dose syncope reported.
Captopril	25–150 q 8 hr	++	++	++	±	Advantages include diminution of Angiotensin II and inhibition of aldosterone release. Risk of proteinuria, agranulocytosis.
Nifedipine	10–20 q 8–12 hr	+	+++	++	±	Postural hypotension, flushing.

± = inconstant effect, + = weak effect, +++ = consistent effect.

digitalis glycoside remain standard therapy. Since long-term efficacy of digitalis in this setting is somewhat controversial and since alternative approaches are available, elevation of plasma levels to potentially toxic ranges is unwarranted [514, 515]. If a compliant patient does not respond adequately to diuretics and agents with positive inotropic effects, vasodilator therapy may be helpful. The choice of a specific vasodilator is usually dictated by the extent to which pulmonary congestion compared to decreased cardiac output contributes to symptoms (Table 5).

For patients with paroxysmal nocturnal dyspnea, the bedtime use of a long-acting nitrate preparation substituted for a second diuretic dose may avoid nocturnal diuresis. Oral nitrate therapy may effectively reduce left ventricular filling pressure and, as in patients with acute myocardial infarction, may compromise cardiac output or induce sudden hypotension and tachycardia if preload is lowered excessively. In patients refractory to diuretics, however, symptoms of congestive failure

often respond well to nitrate therapy. Moreover, exercise hemodynamics, exercise tolerance, and peripheral oxygen consumption all improve with chronic nitrate therapy [516]. Only partial hemodynamic tolerance is likely to develop [517–519]. It appears, however, that responsiveness to nitrates in some patients, particularly those with marked peripheral edema, may be curtailed severely [520, 521].

Among the many preparations available, oral controlled-release nitroglycerin [384, 522] and oral isosorbide dinitrate [523] have been studied most thoroughly and appear to be most suitable for long-term use. The propensity of nitrates to aggravate pulmonary ventillation:perfusion mismatch with consequent reduction of peripheral arterial oxygen saturation presents a potential hazard for patients with angina [168, 524]. When long-term nitrate therapy is discontinued, withdrawal should be gradual to avoid potential rebound coronary vasoconstriction [386].

Another vasodilator, hydralazine, has little direct effect on preload [525]. However, it markedly increases cardiac output and improves renal blood flow, facilitating diuresis and thereby reducing pulmonary venous pressure [526–528]. Disproportionate tachycardia due to cardiac catecholamine release is generally not a problem in patients with chronic failure. Combination therapy with hydralazine and nitrates may be helpful in providing balanced effects on preload and afterload. On the other hand, hydralazine plus conventional therapy with diuretics often will suffice. Initially, relatively high doses of hydralazine may be required in patients with significant right heart failure and poor absorption [529]. Such patients must be followed closely so that doses can be reduced as hemodynamics and hence alimentary tract perfusion and absorption improve.

Balanced effects on preload and afterload are produced with the alpha-1-adrenergic-receptor-blocking agents, prazosin [530] and trimazosin [531]. Sustained use of prazosin has been associated with rapid but only partial tolerance to its hemodynamic effects [532–535]. Both stimulation of the renin-angiotension system with resultant hyperaldosteronism and salt retention [532] and augmented norepinephrine release [533] have been documented and may explain this physiological tachyphylaxis. Despite the precipitious early diminution of hemodynamic response, however, prolonged therapy with prazosin leads to sustained effects on preload, afterload, and cardiac output [536, 537], especially during exercise [538, 539]. Both prazosin and trimazosin improve exercise hemodynamics, increase exercise duration, and augment peripheral oxygen utilization [538–541].

Captopril, an oral angiotension converting enzyme inhibitor, is another agent that appears to exert a balanced effect on preload and afterload [542–544]. In clinical trials, it has been well tolerated without exhibiting substantial tachyphylaxis [545, 546]. Its aldosterone-synthesis inhibiting effects may counter the salt retention that often accompanies vasodilator therapy. However, reports of proteinuria and agranulocytosis in some patients given captopril have limited initial enthusiasm for widespread use of this drug, though conclusive characterization of the incidence of toxicity is not yet available [547, 548].

Several other modes of therapy require consideration. Unfortunately, vasodilators such as mi-noxidil and sustained-release phentolamine commonly elicit major side effects [549]. However, calcium channel blockers such as nifedipine are generally well tolerated, reduce afterload more markedly than preload, reduce the frequency and severity of angina, and mollify congestive heart failure [310, 550]. A recently developed agent with positive inotropic effects, amrinone, increases contractility without altering sodium-potassium-dependent ATPase activity, cyclic AMP levels, or phosphodiesterase activity [199]. It acts through mechanisms independent of catecholamines and does not interact with other agents such as digitalis glycosides. It has modest direct vasodilatory effects, and its potent positive inotropic effects persist despite long-term use [551, 552]. Although this drug may never become available for clinical use in the United States due to its potential to induce thrombocytopenia, safer agents of the same type are likely to become available soon.

Conclusions

Although preventive measures such as modification of coronary risk factors hold the greatest potential for public health benefit, management of advanced, symptomatic coronary artery disease is a frequent therapeutic challenge. Recently available treatment modalities, as well as improved understanding of the hemodynamic and metabolic derangements accompanying ischemic heart disease, have led to more effective and more specific therapeutic intervention. A thorough familiarity with the cardiovascular consequences of each intervention considered, including its effects on electrophysiology, left ventricular loading conditions and contractility, and myocardial oxygen supply and demand, is a prerequisite for rational therapy. Whether directed toward treatment of acute myocardial infarction, unstable angina, or chronic stable IHD, such considerations of the physiologic consequences of an intervention should precede its implementation. Based on such considerations, judiciously selected therapy may not only palliate symptoms, but possibly reduce the progression or recurrence of ischemic insults as well.

References

1. Stern MP: The recent decline in ischemic heart disease mortality. Ann Intern Med 91:630–640, 1979.
2. Stamler J: Research related to risk factors. Circulation 60:1575–1587, 1979.
3. Multicentre International Study: Reduction in mortality after myocardial infarction with long-term beta-adreno-ceptor blockade: supplemental report. Br Med J 2:419–421, 1977.
4. The Anturane Reinfarction Trial Research Group: Sulfin-pyrazone in the prevention of sudden death after myocardial infarction. N Engl J Med 302:250–256, 1980.
5. Goldstein JL, Brown MS: The low density lipoprotein pathway and its relation to atherosclerosis. In: Snell E, Boyer P, Meister A, Richardson C (eds) Annual Review of Biochemistry. Annual Reviews Inc, Palo Alto, 1977, pp 897–930.
6. Steinberg D: Research related to underlying mechanisms in atherosclerosis. Circulation 60:1559–1565, 1979.
7. Ross R, Glomset JA: The pathogenesis of atherosclerosis. N Engl J Med 295:369–377, 420–427, 1976.
8. Samuelsson B, Hamberg, M, Malmsten C, Svensson J: The role of prostaglandin endoperoxides and thromboxanes in platelet aggregation. Adv Prostaglandin Thromboxane Res 2:737–746, 1976.
9. Rutherford BR, Ross R: Platelet factors stimulate fibroblasts and smooth muscle cells quiescent in plasma-sera to proliferate. J Cell Biol 69:196–204, 1976.
10. Robertson TL, Kato H, Gordon T, Kagan A, Rhoads GG, Land CE, Worth RM, Belsky JL, Dock DS, Myanishi M, Kawamoto SP: Epidemiologic studies of coronary heart disease and stroke in Japanese men living in Japan, Hawaii, and California: coronary heart disease risk factors in Japan and Hawaii. Am J Cardiol 39:244–249, 1977.
11. Kagan A, Harris BR, Winkelstein W Jr, Johnson KG, Kato H, Syme SL, Rhoads GG, Gay ML, Nichaman MZ, Hamilton HB, Tillotson J: Epidemiologic studies of coronary heart disease and stroke in Japanese men living in Japan, Hawaii, and California: demographic, physical, dietary, and biochemical characteristics. J Chronic Dis 27:345–351, 1974.
12. Wissler RW, Vesselinovitch D: The effect of feeding various dietary fats on the development and regression of hypercholesterolemia and atherosclerosis. In: Sirtori C, Ricci G, Gorini S (eds) Diet and Atherosclerosis. Plenum Press, New York, 1975, pp 65–78.
13. Rabkin SW, Mathewson FAL, Tate RB: Predicting risks of ischemic heart disease and cerebrovascular disease from systolic and diastolic blood pressures. Ann Intern Med 88:342–345, 1978.
14. Vlietstra RE, Frye RL, Kronmal RA, Sim DA, Phil M, Tristani FE, Killip T III, the Coronary Artery Surgery Study Group: Risk factors and angiographic coronary artery disease: a report from the Coronary Artery Surgery Study (CASS). Circulation 62:254–261, 1980.
15. Kannel WB, McGee DL: Diabetes and cardiovascular risk factors: the Framingham Study. Circulation 59:8–13, 1979.
16. Paffenbarger RS, Hale WE: Work activity and coronary heart disease. N Engl J Med 292:545–550, 1975.
17. Blumenthal JA, Williams RB, Kong Y, Schamberg SM, Thompson LW: Type A behavior pattern and coronary atherosclerosis. Circulation 58:634–639, 1978.
18. Turpeinen O: Effect of cholesterol-lowering diet on mortality from coronary heart disease and other causes. Circulation 59:1–7, 1979.
19. National Diet-Heart Study Group: The National Diet-Heart Study final report. Circulation 37 (Suppl I):I-1-I-428, 1968.
20. Veterans Administration Cooperative Study on Antihypertensive Agents: Effects of treatment on morbidity in hypertension – results in patients with diastolic blood pressures averaging 115 through 129 mmHg. J Am Med Assoc 202:1028–1034, 1967.
21. Veterans Administration Cooperative Study on Antihypertensive Agents: Effects of treatment on morbidity in hypertension. II. Results in patients with diastolic blood pressures averaging 90 through 114 mmHg. J Am Med Assoc 213:1143–1152, 1970.
22. The Coronary Drug Project Research Group: Cigarette smoking as a risk factor in men with a prior history of myocardial infarction. J Chronic Dis 32:415–425, 1979.
23. Gortner WA: Nutrition in the United States, 1900–1974. Cancer Res 35:3246–3253, 1975.
24. Page L, Friend B: The changing United States diet. Bio Sci 28:192–202, 1978.
25. Taylor HL, Romo M, Jacobs DR, Blackburn H: Secular changes in coronary heart disease risk factors. Circulation 52 (Suppl II):II-96, 1975 (abstract).
26. Bureau of Health Education. Adult Use of Tobacco, 1975, Center for Disease Control, Atlanta, 1976.
27. Hypertension Detection and Follow-Up Program Cooperative Group: Blood pressures from fourteen communities: a two-stage screen for hypertension. J Am Med Assoc 237:2385–2391, 1977.
28. Froelicher VF, Thompson AJ, Longro MR Jr, Triebwasser JH, Lancaster ML: Value of exercise testing for screening asymptomatic men for latent coronary artery disease. Prog Cardiovasc Dis 18:265–276, 1976.
29. Borer JS, Brensike JF, Redwood DR, Itscoitz SB, Passamani ER, Stone NJ, Richardson JM, Levy RI, Epstein SE: Limitations of the electrocardiographic response to exercise in predicting coronary artery disease. N Engl J Med 293:367–371, 1975.
30. Ritchie JL, Trobaugh GB, Hamilton GW: Myocardial imaging with thallium-201 at rest and during exercise. Circulation 56:66–71, 1977.
31. Rifkin RD, Hood WB Jr: Bayesian analysis of electrocardiographic exercise stress testing. N Engl J Med 297:681–686, 1977.
32. Maroko PR, Braunwald E: Modification of myocardial infarction size after coronary occlusion. Ann Intern Med 79:720–733, 1973.
33. Harvey WP, Berkman F, Leonard J: Caution against the use of meperidine hydrochloride (Isomipecaine, Demerol) in patients with heart disease, particularly auricular flutter. Am Heart J 49:758–769, 1955.
34. Lee G, DeMaria AN, Amsterdam EA, Realyvasquez F, Angel J, Morrison S, Mason DT: Comparative effects of morphine, meperidine, and pentazocine on cardiocircula-

tory dynamics in patients with acute myocardial infarction. Am J Med 60:949-955, 1976.

35. Wynne J, Mann T, Alpert JS, Grossman W: Beneficial effects of nitrous oxide in patients with ischemic heart disease. Circulation 56 (Suppl III):III-8, 1977 (abstract).

36. Gunnar RM, Loeb HS, Scanlon PJ, Moran JF, Johnson SA, Pifarre R: Management of acute myocardial infarction and accelerating angina. Prog Cardiovasc Dis 22:1-30, 1979.

37. Maroko PR, Radvany P, Braunwald E, Hale SL: Reduction of infarct size by oxygen inhalation following acute coronary occlusion. Circulation 52:360-368, 1975.

38. Madias JE, Madias NE, Hood WB: Precordial ST-segment mapping. 2. Effects of oxygen inhalation on ischemic injury in patients with acute myocardial infarction. Circulation 53:411-417, 1976.

39. Sukumalchantra Y, Levy S, Danzig R, Rubin S, Alpern H, Swan HJC: Correcting arterial hypoxemia by oxygen therapy in patients with acute myocardial infarction: effects on ventilation and hemodynamics. Am J Cardiol 24:838-852, 1969.

40. Thomas M, Malmcrona R, Shillingford J: Haemodynamic effect of oxygen in patients with acute myocardial infarction. Br Heart J 27:401-407, 1965.

41. Horvat M, Yoshida S, Prakash R, Marcus HS, Swan HJC, Ganz W: Effect of oxygen breathing on pacing-induced angina pectoris and other manifestations of coronary insufficiency. Circulation 45:837-844, 1972.

42. Miller RR, Lies JE, Carretta RF, Wampold DB, DeNardo GL, Kraus JF, Amsterdam EA, Mason DT: Prevention of lower extremity venous thrombosis by early mobilization. Ann Intern Med 84:700-703, 1976.

43. Hayes MJ, Morris GK, Hampton JR: Comparison of mobilization after two days and nine days in uncomplicated myocardial infarction. Br Med J 3:10-13, 1974.

44. Maurer BJ, Wray R, Shillingford JP: Frequency of venous thrombosis after myocardial infarction. Lancet 2:1385-1387, 1971.

45. Frishman WH, Ribner HS: Anticoagulation in myocardial infarction: modern approach to an old problem. Am J Cardiol 43:1207-1213, 1979.

46. Wray R, Maurer B, Shillingford J: Prophylactic anticoagulant therapy in the prevention of calf-vein thrombosis after myocardial infarction. N Engl J Med 288:815-817, 1973.

47. Veterans Administration Study Group: Anticoagulation in acute myocardial infarction: results of a cooperative clinical trial. J Am Med Assoc 225:724-729, 1973.

48. Saliba MJ, Kuzman WJ, Marsh DG, Lasry JE: Effect of heparin in anticoagulant doses on the electrocardiogram and cardiac enzymes in patients with acute myocardial infarction. Am J Cardiol 37:605-607, 1976.

49. Biggs R, Denson KWE, Akman N, Borrett R, Hadden M: Antithrombin III, antifactor X_a, and heparin. Br J Haematol 19:283-305, 1970.

50. Warlow C, Beattie AG, Terry G, Ogston D, Kenmure ACF, Douglas AS: A double-blind trial of low doses of subcutaneous heparin in the prevention of deep vein thrombosis after myocardial infarction. Lancet 2:934-936, 1973.

51. Gallus AS, Hirsh J, Tuttle RJ, Trebilcock R, O'Brien SE, Carroll JJ, Minden JH, Hudecki SM: Small subcutaneous doses of heparin in prevention of venous thrombosis. N Engl J Med 288:545-551, 1973.

52. Harker LA, Slichter SJ: Studies of platelet and fibrinogen kinetics in patients with prosthetic heart valves. N Engl J Med 283:1302-1305, 1970.

53. Renny JTG, O'Sullivan EF, Burke PF: Prevention of postoperative deep vein thrombosis with dipyridamole and aspirin. Br Med J 1:992-994, 1976.

54. Adgey AAJ, Geddes JS, Mulholland HC, Keegan DAJ, Pantridge JF: Incidence, significance, and management of early bradyarrhythmias complicating acute myocardial infarction. Lancet 2:1097-1101, 1968.

55. Pantridge JF, Webb SW, Adgey AAJ, Geddes JS: The first hour after the onset of acute myocardial infarction. In: Yu PN, Goodwin JF (eds) Progress in Cardiology, vol 3. Lea and Febiger, Philadelphia, 1974, pp 173-188.

56. Adgey AAJ, Allen JD, Geddes JS, James RGG, Webb SW, Zaidi SA, Pantridge JF: Acute phase of myocardial infarction. Lancet 2:501-504, 1971.

57. Moss AJ, Goldstein S, Greene W, DeCamilla J: Prehospital precursors of ventricular arrhythmias in acute myocardial infarction. Arch Intern Med 129:756-762, 1972.

58. Epstein SE, Goldstein RE, Redwood DR, Kent KM, Smith ER: The early phase of acute myocardial infarction: pharmacologic aspects of therapy. Ann Intern Med 78:918-936, 1973.

59. Richman S: Adverse effects of atropine during myocardial infarction. J Am Med Assoc 228:1414-1416, 1974.

60. Scheinman MM, Thorburn D, Abbott JA: Use of atropine in patients with acute myocardial infarction and sinus bradycardia. Circulation 52:627-633, 1975.

61. Das G, Talmers FN, Weissler AM: New observations on the effects of atropine on sinoatrial and atrioventricular nodes in man. Am J Cardiol 36:281-285, 1975.

62. Mueller HS, Ayres SM: Propranolol decreases sympathetic nervous activity reflected by plasma catecholamines during evolution of myocardial infarction in man. J Clin Invest 65:338-346, 1980.

63. Lemberg L, Castellanos A, Arcebal AG: The use of propranolol in arrhythmias complicating acute myocardial infarction. Am Heart J 80:479-487, 1970.

64. Ribner HS, Isaacs ES, Frishman WF: Lidocaine prophylaxis against ventricular fibrillation in acute myocardial infarction. Prog Cardiovasc Dis 21:287-310, 1979.

65. Valentine PA, Frew JL, Mashford ML, Sloman JG: Lidocaine in the prevention of sudden death in the pre-hospital phase of acute infarction. N Engl J Med 291:1327-1331, 1974.

66. Cristal N, Szwarcberg J, Gueron M: Supraventricular arrhythmias in acute myocardial infarction. Ann Intern Med 82:35-39, 1975.

67. Liberthson RR, Salisbury KW, Hutter AM, DeSanctis RW: Atrial tachyarrhythmias in acute myocardial infarction. Am J Med 60:956-960, 1976.

68. Klass M, Haywood LJ: Atrial fibrillation associated with acute myocardial infarction: a study of thirty-four cases. Am Heart J 79:752-760, 1970.

69. Forrester JA, Chatterjee K, Jobin G: A new conceptual approach to the therapy of acute myocardial infarction. Adv Cardiol 15:111–123, 1975.
70. Mueller HS, Ayres SM: The role of propranolol in the treatment of acute myocardial infarction. Prog Cardiovasc Dis 19:405–412, 1977.
71. Ehsani A, Ewy GA, Sobel BE: Effect of electric countershock on serum creatine phosphokinase (CPK) isoenzyme activity. Am J Cardiol 37:12–18, 1976.
72. Haft JI: Treatment of arrhythmias by intracardiac electrical stimulation. Prog Cardiovasc Dis 16:539–568, 1974.
73. Pittman DE, Makar JS, Kooros KS, Joyner CR: Rapid atrial stimulation: successful method of conversion of atrial flutter and atrial tachycardia. Am J Cardiol 32:700–706, 1973.
74. Krikler DM: Verapamil in cardiology. Eur J Cardiol 2:3–10, 1974.
75. Schamroth L, Krikler DM, Garrett C: Immediate effects of intravenous verapamil in cardiac arrhythmias. Br Med J 1:660–662, 1972.
76. Singh BN, Ellrodt G, Peter CT: Verapamil: a review of its pharmacological properties and therapeutic use. Drugs 15:169–177, 1978.
77. Hagemeijer F: Verapamil in the management of supraventricular tachyarrhythmias occurring after a recent myocardial infarction. Circulation 57:751–755, 1978.
78. Romhilt DW, Bloomfield SS, Chou T-C, Fowler NO: Unreliability of conventional electrocardiograph monitoring for arrhythmia detection in coronary care units. Am J Cardiol 31:457–461, 1973.
79. Rothfield EL, Parsonnet J, McGorman W, Linden S: Harbingers of paroxysmal ventricular tachycardia in acute myocardial infarction. Chest 71:142–145, 1977.
80. Lawrie DM, Higgins MR, Godman MJ, Oliver MF, Julian DG, Donald KW: Ventricular fibrillation complicating acute myocardial infarction. Lancet 2:523–528, 1968.
81. Lown B, Calvert AF, Armington R, Ryan M: Monitoring for serious arrhythmias and high risk of sudden death. Circulation 51–52 (Suppl III):III-189–III-198, 1975.
82. Bennett MA, Pentecost BL: Warning of cardiac arrest due to ventricular fibrillation and tachycardia. Lancet 1:1351–1352, 1972.
83. Lie KI, Wellens HJT, Downar E, Durrer D: Observations on patients with primary ventricular fibrillation complicating acute myocardial infarction. Circulation 52:755–759, 1975.
84. El-Sherif N, Myerburg RJ, Scherlag BJ, Befeler B, Aranda JM, Castellanos A, Lazzara R: Electrocardiographic antecedents of primary ventricular fibrillation: value of the R-on-T phenomenon in myocardial infarction. Br Heart J 38:415–422, 1976.
85. Engel TR, Meister SG, Frankl WS: The 'R-on-T' phenomenon: an update and critical review. Ann Intern Med 88:221–225, 1978.
86. Roberts R, Ambos HD, Loh CW, Sobel BE: Initiation of repetitive ventricular depolarization by relatively late premature complexes in patients with acute myocardial infarction. Am J Cardiol 41:678–683, 1978.
87. Wyman MG, Swan HJC, Rapaport E, Rockwell M: Arrhythmia deaths in 15 000 acute myocardial infarctions.

Circulation 47–48 (Suppl IV):IV-30, 1973 (abstract).
88. Pitt A, Lipp H, Anderson ST: Lignocaine given prophylactically to patients with acute myocardial infarction. Lancet 1:612–615, 1971.
89. Lie KI, Wellens HJ, van Capelle FJ, Durrer D: Lidocaine in the prevention of primary ventricular fibrillation: a double blind, randomized study of 212 consecutive patients. N Engl J Med 291:1324–1326, 1974.
90. Gupta PK, Lichstein E, Chadda KD: Lidocaine-induced heart block in patients with bundle branch block. Am J Cardiol 33:487–492, 1974.
91. Wyman MG, Hammersmith L: Comprehensive treatment plan for the prevention of primary ventricular fibrillation in acute myocardial infarction. Am J Cardiol 33:661–667, 1974.
92. Jennings G, Model DG, Jones MBS, Turner PP, Besterman EMM, Kidner PH: Oral disopyramide in prophylaxis of arrhythmias following myocardial infarction. Lancet 1:51–54, 1976.
93. Zainal N, Carmichael DJS, Griffiths JW, Besterman EMM, Kidner PH, Gillham AD, Summers GD: Oral disopyramide for the prevention of arrhythmias in patients with acute myocardial infarction admitted to open wards. Lancet 2:887–889, 1977.
94. Wilcox RG, Rowley JM, Hampton JR, Mitchell JRA, Roland JM, Banks DC: Randomized placebo-controlled trial comparing oxprenolol with disopyramide phosphate in immediate treatment of suspected myocardial infarction. Lancet 2:765–769, 1980.
95. Koch-Weser J, Klein SW, Foo-Canto LL, Kastor JA, DeSanctis RW: Antiarrhythmic prophylaxis with procainamide in acute myocardial infarction. N Engl J Med 281:1253–1260, 1969.
96. Jones DT, Kostuk WJ, Gunton RW: Prophylactic quinidine for the prevention of arrhythmias after acute myocardial infarction. Am J Cardiol 33:655–660, 1974.
97. Balcon R, Jewitt DE, Davies JPH, Oram S: A controlled trial of propranolol in acute myocardial infarction. Lancet 2:917–920, 1966.
98. Taylor SH, Saxton C, Davies PS, Stoker JB: Bretylium tosylate in prevention of cardiac dysrrhythmias after myocardial infarction. Br Heart J 32:326–329, 1970.
99. deSoyza N, Bissett JK, Kane JJ, Murphy ML, Doherty JE: Association of accelerated idioventricular rhythm and paroxysmal ventricular tachycardia in acute myocardial infarction. Am J Cardiol 34:667–670, 1974.
100. Lichstein E, Ribas-Menecleir C, Gupta PK, Chadda KD: Incidence and description of accelerated ventricular rhythm complicating acute myocardial infarction. Am J Med 58:192–198, 1975.
101. Rothfeld EL, Zucker IR, Parsonnet V, Alinsonorin CA: Idioventricular rhythm in acute myocardial infarction. Circulation 37:203–209, 1968.
102. Norris RM, Mercer CJ: Significance of idioventricular rhythms in acute myocardial infarction. Prog Cardiovasc Dis 16:455–468, 1974.
103. Chopra MP, Thadani U, Portal RW, Aber CP: Lignocaine therapy for ventricular ectopic activity after acute myocardial infarction: a double blind trial. Br Med J 3:668–670, 1971.

104. Lown B, Fakhro AM, Hood WB Jr, Thorn GW: The coronary care unit. J Am Med Assoc 199:188–198, 1967.

105. Collinsworth KA, Kalman SM, Harrison DC: The clinical pharmacology of lidocaine as an antiarrhythmic drug. Circulation 50:1217–1230, 1974.

106. Thompson PD, Melmon KL, Richardson JA, Cohn K, Steinbrunn W, Cudihee R, Rowland M: Lidocaine pharmacokinetics in advanced heart failure, liver disease, and renal failure in humans. Ann Intern Med 78:499–508, 1973.

107. LeLorier J, Grenon D, Latour Y, Caillé G, Dumont G, Brosseau A, Solignac A: Pharmacokinetics of lidocaine after prolonged intravenous infusions in uncomplicated myocardial infarction. Ann Intern Med 87:700–702, 1977.

108. Danahy DT, Aronow WS: Lidocaine-induced cardiac rate change in atrial fibrillation and atrial flutter. Am Heart J 95:474–482, 1978.

109. Lima JJ, Conti DR, Goldfarb AL, Golden LH, Jusko WJ: Pharmacokinetic approach to intravenous procainamide therapy. Eur J Clin Pharmacol 13:303–308, 1978.

110. Lima JJ, Goldfarb AL, Conti DR, Golden LH, Bascomb BL, Benedetti GM, Jusko WJ: Safety and efficacy of procainamide infusions. Am J Cardiol 43:98–105, 1979.

111. Kötter V, Linderer T, Schröder R: Effects of disopyramide on systemic and coronary hemodynamics and myocardial metabolism in patients with coronary artery disease: comparison with lidocaine. Am J Cardiol 46:469–475, 1980.

112. Jensen G, Sigurd B, Uhrenholt A: Hemodynamic effect of intravenous disopyramide in heart failure. Eur J Clin Pharmacol 8:167–173, 1975.

113. Fasola AF, Nobel RJ, Zipes DP: Treatment of recurrent ventricular tachycardia and fibrillation with aprindine. Am J Cardiol 39:903–909, 1977.

114. Zipes DP, Troup PJ: New antiarrhythmic agents. Am J Cardiol 41:1005–1024, 1978.

115. Bacaner MB: Quantitative comparison of bretylium with other antifibrillatory drugs. Am J Cardiol 21:504–512, 1968.

116. Terry G, Vellani CW, Higgins MR, Doig A: Bretylium tosylate in treatment of refractory ventricular arrhythmias complicating myocardial infarction. Br Heart J 32:21–25, 1970.

117. Heissenbuttel RH, Bigger JT: Bretylium tosylate: a newly available antiarrhythmic drug for ventricular arrhythmias. Ann Intern Med 91:229–238, 1979.

118. Bernstein JG, Koch-Weser J: Effectiveness of bretylium tosylate against refractory ventricular arrhythmias. Circulation 45:1024–1034, 1972.

119. Gillis RA, Clancy MM, Anderson RJ: Deleterious effects of bretylium in cats with digitalis-induced ventricular tachycardia. Circulation 47:974–983, 1973.

120. Maroko PR, Kjekshus JK, Sobel BE, Watanabe T, Covell JW, Ross J Jr, Braunwald E: Factors influencing infarct size following experimental coronary artery occlusions. Circulation 43:67–82, 1971.

121. Anderson JL, Patterson E, Conlon M, Pasyk S, Pitt B, Lucchesi BR: Kinetics of antifibrillatory effects of bretylium: correlation with myocardial drug concentrations. Am J Cardiol 46:583–592, 1980.

122. Bacaner MB: Treatment of ventricular fibrillation and other acute arrhythmias with bretylium tosylate. Am J Cardiol 21:530–543, 1968.

123. Sanna G, Arcidiacono R: Chemical ventricular defibrillation of the human heart with bretylium tosylate. Am J Cardiol 32:982–987, 1973.

124. Holder DA, Sniderman AD, Fraser G, Fallen EL: Experience with bretylium tosylate by a hospital cardiac arrest team. Circulation 55:541–544, 1977.

125. Aronow WS, Turbow M, Lurie M, Whittaker K, vanCamp S: Treatment of premature ventricular complexes with acebutolol. Am J Cardiol 43:106–108, 1979.

126. Amsterdam EA, Lee G, Morrison S, Tonkin MJ, DeMaria AN, Mason DT: Efficacy of beta-selective adrenergic blockade with intravenously administered tolamolol in the treatment of cardiac arrhythmias. Am J Cardiol 38:195–199, 1976.

127. Lown B, Wolf M: Approaches to sudden death from coronary heart disease. Circulation 44: 130–142, 1971.

128. Stone N, Klein M, Lown B: Diphenylhydantoin in the prevention of recurring ventricular tachycardia. Circulation 43:420–427, 1971.

129. Han J, Millet D, Chizzonnitti B, Moe GK: Temporal dispersion of recovery of excitability in atrium and ventricle as a function of heart rate. Am Heart J 71:481–487, 1966.

130. Thompson P, Sloman G: Sudden death in hospital after discharge from coronary care unit. Br Med J 4:136–139, 1971.

131. Graboys TB: In-hospital sudden death after coronary care unit discharge. Arch Intern Med 135:512–514, 1975.

132. Vismara LA, DeMaria AN, Hughes JL, Mason DT, Amsterdam EA: Evaluation of arrhythmias in the late hospital phase of acute myocardial infarction compared to coronary care unit ectopy. Br Heart J 37:598–603, 1975.

133. Moss AJ, DeCamilla J, Davis H: Cardiac death in the first 6 months after myocardial infarction: potential for mortality reduction in the early post-hospital phase. Am J Cardiol 39:816–820, 1977.

134. Moss AJ, DeCamilla JJ, Davis HP, Bayer L: Clinical significance of ventricular ectopic beats in the early post-hospital phase of myocardial infarction. Am J Cardiol 39:635–640, 1977.

135. Kotler MN, Tabatznik B, Mower MM, Tominaga S: Prognostic significance of ventricular ectopic beats with respect to sudden death in the late postinfarction period. Circulation 47:959–966, 1973.

136. Biddle TL, Ehrich DA, Yu PN, Hodges M: Relation of heart block and left ventricular dysfunction in acute myocardial infarction. Am J Cardiol 39:961–966, 1977.

137. Mullins CB, Atkins JM: Prognosis and management of conduction blocks in acute myocardial infarction. Mod Concepts Cardiovasc Dis 45:129–133, 1976.

138. Atkins JM, Leshin SJ, Blomqvist G, Mullins CB: Ventricular conduction blocks and sudden death in acute myocardial infarction: potential indications for pacing. N Engl J Med 288:281–284, 1973.

139. Lie KI, Wellens HJ, Schuilenburg RM, Becker AE, Durrer D: Factors influencing prognosis of bundle branch block complicating acute anteroseptal infarction: the value of His recordings. Circulation 50:935–941, 1974.

140. Meltzer LE, Cohen HE: The incidence of arrhythmias associated with acute myocardial infarction. In: Meltzer

522

LE, Dunning AJ (eds) Textbook of Coronary Care. Charles Press, Philadelphia, 1972, pp 107–133.

141. Gould L, Ramana CV, Gomprecht RF: Left bundle branch block – prognosis in acute myocardial infarction. J Am Med Assoc 225:625–627, 1973.

142. Gann D, Balachandran PK, El-Sherif N, Samet P: Prognostic significance of chronic versus acute bundle branch block in acute myocardial infarction. Chest 67: 298–303, 1975.

143. Nimetz AA, Shubrooks SJ Jr, Hutter AM Jr, DeSanctis RW: Significance of bundle branch block during acute myocardial infarction. Am Heart J 90:439–444, 1975.

144. Waugh RA, Wagner GS, Haney TL, Rosati RA, Morris JJ Jr: Immediate and remote prognostic significance of fascicular block during acute myocardial infarction. Circulation 47:765–775, 1973.

145. Hindman MC, Wagner GS, JaRo M, Atkins JM, Scheinman MM, DeSanctis RW, Hutter AH, Yeatman L, Rubenfire M, Pujura C, Rubin M, Morris JJ: The clinical significance of bundle branch block complicating acute myocardial infarction. 2. Indications for temporary and permanent pacemaker insertion. Circulation 58:689–699, 1978.

146. Killip T, Kimball JT: A survey of the coronary care unit: concept and results. Prog Cardiovasc Dis 11:45–51, 1968.

147. Forrester JS, Diamond G, Chatterjee K, Swan HJC: Medical therapy of acute myocardial infarction by application of hemodynamic subsets. N Engl J Med 295:1356–1362, 1404–1413, 1976.

148. Forrester JS, Diamond GA, Swan HJC: Correlative classification of clinical and hemodynamic function after acute myocardial infarction. Am J Cardiol 39:137–145, 1977.

149. Swan HJC, Ganz W, Forrester J, Marcus H, Diamond G, Chonetti D: Catheterization of the heart in man with use of a flow-directed balloon-tipped catheter. N Engl J Med 283:447–451, 1970.

150. Broder MI, Cohn JN: Evolution of abnormalities in left ventricular function after acute myocardial infarction. Circulation 46:731–743, 1972.

151. Crexells C, Chatterjee, K, Forrester JS, Dikshit K, Swan HJC: Optimal level of filling pressure in the left side of the heart in acute myocardial infarction. N Engl J Med 289:1263–1266, 1973.

152. Russell RO Jr, Rackley CE, Pombo J, Hunt D, Potanin C, Dodge HT: Effects of increasing left ventricular filling pressure in patients with acute myocardial infarction. J Clin Invest 49:1539–1549, 1970.

153. Stein L, Beraud J-J, Morissette M, daLuz P, Weil MH, Shubin H: Pulmonary edema during volume infusion. Circulation 52:483–489, 1975.

154. Dikshit K, Vyden JK, Forrester JS, Chatterjee K, Prakash R, Swan HJC: Renal and extrarenal hemodynamic effects of furosemide in congestive heart failure after acute myocardial infarction. N Engl J Med 288:1087–1090, 1973.

155. Mann T, Cohn PF, Holman BL, Green LH, Markis JE, Phillips DA: Effects of nitroprusside on regional myocardial blood flow in coronary artery disease. Circulation 57:732–737, 1978.

156. Warltier DC, Gross GT, Brooks HL: Coronary steal-induced increase in myocardial infarct size after pharmacologic vasodilation. Am J Cardiol 46:83–90, 1980.

157. Chiariello M, Gold HK, Leinbach RC, Davis MA, Maroko PR: Comparison between the effects of nitroprusside and nitroglycerin on ischemic injury during acute myocardial infarction. Circulation 54:766–773, 1976.

158. daLuz PL, Forrester JS, Wyatt HL, Tyberg JV, Chagrasulis R, Parmley WW, Swan HJC: Hemodynamic and metabolic effects of sodium nitroprusside on the performance and metabolism of regional ischemic myocardium. Circulation 52:400–407, 1975.

159. Chatterjee K, Parmley WW, Ganz W, Forrester J, Walinsky P, Crexells C, Swan HJC: Hemodynamic and metabolic response to vasodilator therapy in acute myocardial infarction. Circulation 48:1183–1193, 1973.

160. Awan NA, Miller RR, Vera Z, DeMaria AN, Amsterdam EA, Mason DT: Reduction of ST-segment elevation with infusion of nitroprusside in patients with acute myocardial infarction. Am J Cardiol 38:435–439, 1976.

161. Mukherjee D, Feldman MS, Helfant RH: Nitroprusside therapy: treatment of hypertensive patients with recurrent resting chest pain, ST-segment elevation, and ventricular arrhythmias. J Am Med Assoc 235:2406–2407, 1976.

162. Armstrong PW, Walker DC, Burton JR, Parker JO: Vasodilator therapy in acute myocardial infarction: a comparison of sodium nitroprusside and nitroglycerin. Circulation 52:1118–1122, 1975.

163. Flaherty JT, Come PC, Baird MG, Rouleau J, Taylor DR, Weisfeldt ML, Greene HL, Becker LC, Pitt B: Effects of intravenous nitroglycerin on left ventricular function and ST-segment changes in acute myocardial infarction. Br Heart J 38:612–621, 1976.

164. Awan NA, Amsterdam EA, Vera Z, DeMaria AN, Miller RR, Mason DT: Reduction of ischemic injury by sublingual nitroglycerin in patients with acute myocardial infarction. Circulation 54:761–765, 1976.

165. Williams DO, Amsterdam EA, Mason DT: Hemodynamic effects of nitroglycerin in acute myocardial infarction: decrease in ventricular preload at the expense of cardiac output. Circulation 51:421–427, 1975.

166. Come P, Pitt B: Nitroglycerin-induced severe hypotension and bradycardia in patients with acute myocardial infarction. Circulation 54:624–628, 1976.

167. Cottrell JE, Turndorf H: Intravenous nitroglycerin. Am Heart J 96:550–553, 1978.

168. Hales CA, Westphal D: Hypoxemia following the administration of sublingual nitroglycerin. Am J Med 65:911–918, 1978.

169. Mookherjee S, Keighly JFH, Warner RA, Bowser MA, Obeid AI: Hemodynamic, ventilatory and blood gas changes during infusion of sodium nitroprusside: studies in patients with congestive heart failure. Chest 72:273–278, 1977.

170. Gould L, Reddy CVR, Kalanithi P, Espina L, Gomprecht RF: Use of phentolamine in acute myocardial infarction. Am Heart J 88:144–148, 1974.

171. Kötter V, von Leitner ER, Wunderlich J, Schröder R: Comparison of hemodynamic effects of phentolamine, sodium nitroprusside, and glyceryl trinitrate in acute myocardial infarction. Br Heart J 39:1196–1204, 1977.

172. Shell WE, Sobel BE: Protection of jeopardized ischemic

myocardium by reduction of ventricular afterload. N Engl J Med 291:481–486, 1974.

173. Franciosa JA, Notargiacomo AV, Cohn JN: Comparative hemodynamic and metabolic effects of vasodilator and inotropic agents in experimental myocardial infarction. Cardiovasc Res 12:294–302, 1978.

174. Stephens J, Ead H, Spurrell R: Haemodynamic effects of dobutamine with special reference to myocardial blood flow: a comparison with dopamine and isoprenaline. Br Heart J 42:43–50, 1979.

175. Hood WB, McCarthy B, Lown B: Myocardial infarction following coronary artery ligation in dogs: hemodynamic effects of isoproterenol and acetylstrophanthidin. Circ Res 21:191–199, 1967.

176. Mason DT, Amsterdam EA, Miller RR, Williams DO: What is the role of positive inotropic agents in the treatment of acute myocardial infarction? Cardiovasc Clin 8:113–122, 1977.

177. Watanabe T, Covell JW, Maroko PR, Braunwald E, Ross J Jr: Effects of increased arterial pressure and positive inotropic agents on the severity of myocardial ischemia in the acutely depressed heart. Am J Cardiol 30:371–377, 1972.

178. Gillespie TA, Ambos HD, Sobel BE, Roberts R: Effects of dobutamine in patients with acute myocardial infarction. Am J Cardiol 39:588–594, 1977.

179. Cohn JN, Guiha NH, Broder MI, Limas CJ: Right ventricular infarction: clinical and hemodynamic features. Am J Cardiol 33:209–214, 1974.

180. Lorell B, Leinbach RC, Pohost GM, Gold HK, Dinsmore RE, Hutter AM Jr, Pastore JO, DeSanctis RW: Right ventricular infarction: clinical diagnosis and differentiation from cardiac tamponade and pericardial constriction. Am J Cardiol 43:465–471, 1979.

181. Coma-Canella I, Lopez-Sendon J: Ventricular compliance in ischemic right ventricular dysfunction. Am J Cardiol 45:555–561, 1980.

182. Ratliff NB, Hackel DB: Combined right and left ventricular infarction: pathogenesis and clinicopathologic correlation. Am J Cardiol 45:217–221, 1980.

183. Leier CV, Webel J, Bush CA: The cardiovascular effects of the continuous infusion of dobutamine in patients with severe cardiac failure. Circulation 56: 468–472, 1977.

184. Sonnenblick EH, Frishman WH, Le Jemtel TH: Dobutamine: a new synthetic cardioselective sympathetic amine. N Engl J Med 300:17–22, 1979.

185. Vatner SF, McRitchie RJ, Braunwald E: Effects of dobutamine on left ventricular performance, coronary dynamics, and distribution of cardiac output in conscious dogs. J Clin Invest 53:1265–1273, 1974.

186. Unferferth DV, Blanford M, Kates RE, Leier CV: Tolerance to dobutamine after a seventy-two hour infusion. Am J Med 69:262–266, 1980.

187. Tuttle RR, Pollock GD, Todd G, MacDonald B, Tust R, Dusenberry W: The effect of dobutamine on cardiac oxygen balance, regional blood flow, and infarction severity after coronary artery narrowing in dogs. Circ Res 41: 357–364, 1977.

188. Leier CV, Heban PT, Huss P, Bush CA, Lewis RP: Comparative systemic and regional hemodynamic effects of dopamine and dobutamine in patients with cardiomyopathic heart failure. Circulation 58: 466–475, 1978.

189. Beregovich J, Bianchi C, Rubler S, Lomnitz E, Cagin N, Levitt B: Dose-related hemodynamic and renal effects of dopamine in congestive heart failure. Am Heart J 87: 550–557, 1974.

190. Tuttle RR, Mills J: Dobutamine: development of a new catecholamine to selectively increase cardiac contractility. Circ Res 36:185–196, 1975.

191. Goldstein RA, Passamani ER, Roberts R: A comparison of digoxin and dobutamine in patients with acute infarction and cardiac failure. N Engl J Med 303:846–850, 1980.

192. Lown B, Klein MD, Barr I, Hagemeijer F, Kosowsky BD, Garrison H: Sensitivity to digitalis drugs in acute myocardial infarction. Am J Cardiol 30:388–395, 1972.

193. Rahimtoola SH, Sinno MZ, Chuquimia R, Loeb HS, Rosen KM, Gunnar RM: Effects of ouabain on impaired left ventricular function in acute myocardial infarction. N Engl J Med 287:527–531, 1972.

194. Varonkov Y, Shell WE, Smirnov V, Gukovsky D, Chazov EI: Augmentation of serum creatine phosphokinase activity by digitalis in patients with acute myocardial infarction. Circulation 55:719–727, 1977.

195. DeMots H, Rahimtoola SH, McAnulty JH, Porter GA: Effects of ouabain on coronary and systemic vascular resistance and myocardial oxygen consumption in patients without heart failure. Am J Cardiol 41:88–93, 1978.

196. Morrison J, Coromilas J, Robbins M: Digitalis and myocardial infarction in man. Circulation 62:8–16, 1980.

197. Williams JF Jr: Glucagon and the cardiovascular system. Ann Intern Med 71:419–423, 1969.

198. Kosinski EJ, Malindzak GS Jr: Glucagon and isoproterenol in reversing propranolol toxicity. Arch Intern Med 132:840–843, 1973.

199. LeJemtel TH, Keung E, Sonnenblick EH, Ribner HS, Matsumoto M, Davis R, Schwartz W, Alousi AA, Davolos D: Amrinone: a new non-glycosidic, non-adrenergic cardiotonic agent effective in the treatment of intractable myocardial failure in man. Circulation 59:1098–1104, 1979.

200. Rude RE, Kloner RA, Maroko PR, Khuri S, Karaffa S, Deboer LWV, Braunwald E: Effects of amrinone on experimental acute myocardial ischaemic injury. Cardiovasc Res 14:419–427, 1980.

201. Weil MH, Shubin H: Shock following acute myocardial infarction: current understanding of hemodynamic mechanisms. Prog Cardiovasc Dis 11:1–17, 1968.

202. Ratshin RA, Rackley CE, Russell RO Jr: Hemodynamic evaluation of left ventricular function in shock complicating myocardial infarction. Circulation 45:127–139, 1972.

203. Scheidt S, Ascheim R, Killip T III: Shock after acute myocardial infarction. Am J Cardiol 26:556–564, 1970.

204. Mueller H, Ayres SM, Giannelli S Jr, Conklin EF, Mazzara JT, Grace WJ: Effect of isoproterenol, ℓ-norepinephrine, and intraaortic counterpulsation on hemodynamics and myocardial metabolism in shock following acute myocardial infarction. Circulation 45:335–351, 1972.

205. Kerber RE, Abboud FM: Effect of alterations of arterial blood pressure and heart rate on segmental dyskinesis during acute myocardial ischemia and following coronary reperfusion. Circ Res 36:145–155, 1975.

206. Johnson SA, Scanlon PJ, Loeb HS, Moran JM, Pifarre R, Gunnar RM: Treatment of cardiogenic shock in myocardial infarction by intraaortic balloon counterpulsation and surgery. Am J Med 62:687–692, 1977.

207. Baron DW, O'Rourke MF: Long-term results of arterial counterpulsation in acute severe cardiac failure complicating myocardial infarction. Br Heart J 38:285–288, 1976.

208. Cohen LS: Current status of circulatory assist devices. Am J Cardiol 33:316–318, 1974.

209. Pace PD, Tilney NL, Lesch M, Couch NP: Peripheral arterial complications of intraaortic balloon counterpulsation. Surgery 82:685–688, 1977.

210. Lefemine AA, Kosowsky B, Madoff I, Black H, Lewis M: Results and complications of intraaortic balloon pumping in surgical and medical patients. Am J Cardiol 40:416–420, 1977.

211. Parmley WW, Chatterjee K, Charuzi Y, Swan HJC: Hemodynamic effects of noninvasive systolic unloading (nitroprusside) and diastolic augmentation (external counterpulsation) in patients with acute myocardial infarction. Am J Cardiol 33:819–825, 1974.

212. Waagstein F, Hjalmarson AC: Effect of cardioselective beta-blockade on heart function and chest pain in acute myocardial infarction. Acta Med Scand (Suppl) 587:193–200, 1976.

213. Lichstein E, Liu H-M, Gupta P: Pericarditis complicating acute myocardial infarction: incidence of complications and significance of electrocardiogram on admission. Am Heart J 87:246–252, 1974.

214. Niarchos AP, McKendrick CS: Prognosis of pericarditis after acute myocardial infarction. Br Heart J 35:49–54, 1973.

215. Thadani U, Chopra MP, Aber CP, Portal RW: Pericarditis after acute myocardial infarction. Br Med J 2:135–137, 1971.

216. Dressler W: The post-myocardial infarction syndrome: a report of forty-four cases. Arch Intern Med 103:28–42, 1959.

217. Kloner RA, Fishbein MC, Lew H, Maroko PR, Braunwald E: Mummification of the infarcted myocardium by high dose corticosteroids. Circulation 57:56–63, 1978.

218. Essen RV, Merx W, Doerr R, Effert S, Silny J, Rau G: QRS mapping in the evolution of acute myocardial infarction. Circulation 62:266–276, 1980.

219. Reid PR, Taylor DR, Kelley DT, Weisfeldt ML, Humphries JO, Ross RS, Pitt B: Myocardial infarct extension detected by precordial ST-segment mapping. N Engl J Med 290:123–128, 1974.

220. Mathey D, Bleifeld W, Buss H, Hanrath P: Creatine kinase release in acute myocardial infarction: correlation with clinical, electrocardiographic, and pathological findings. Br Heart J 37:1161–1168, 1975.

221. Fraker TD Jr, Wagner GS, Rosati RA: Extension of myocardial infarction: incidence and prognosis. Circulation 60:1126–1129, 1979.

222. Rothkopf M, Boerner J, Stone MJ, Smitherman TC, Buja LM, Parkey RW, Willerson JT: Detection of myocardial infarction extension by CK-B radioimmunoassay. Circulation 59:268–274, 1979.

223. Marmor A, Sobel BE, Roberts R: Prospective characterization of extension of infarction detected with plasma MB CK. Circulation 62 (Suppl III):III–81, 1980 (abstract).

224. Bishop SP, White FC, Bloor CM: Regional myocardial blood flow during acute myocardial infarction in the conscious dog. Circ Res 38:429–438, 1976.

225. Rogers WJ, McDaniel HG, Smith LR, Mantle JA, Russell RO, Rackley CE: Correlation of angiographic estimates of myocardial infarct size and accumulated release of creatine kinase MB isoenzyme in man. Circulation 56:199–205, 1977.

226. Bloor CM, Ehsani A, White FC, Sobel BE: Ventricular fibrillation threshold in acute myocardial infarction and its relation to myocardial infarct size. Cardiovasc Res 9:468–472, 1975.

227. Roberts R, Husain A, Ambos HD, Oliver GC, Cox JR, Sobel BE: Relation between infarct size and ventricular arrhythmias. Br Heart J 37:1169–1175, 1975.

228. Geltman EM, Ehsani AA, Campbell MK, Schectman K, Roberts R, Sobel BE: The influence of location and extent of myocardial infarction on long-term ventricular dysrrhythmias and mortality. Circulation 60:805–814, 1979.

229. Thompson PL, Fletcher EE, Katavatis V: Enzymatic indices of myocardial necrosis: influence on short- and long-term prognosis after myocardial infarction. Circulation 59:113–119, 1979.

230. Alonso DR, Scheidt S, Post M, Killip T: Pathophysiology of cardiogenic shock – quantification of necrosis: clinical, pathologic, and electrocardiographic correlations. Circulation 48:588–596, 1973.

231. Cannom DS, Levy W, Cohen LS: The short- and long-term prognosis of patients with transmural and non-transmural myocardial infarction. Am J Med 61:452–458, 1976.

232. Roberts R, Sobel BE: Coronary revascularization during evolving myocardial infarction – the need for caution. Circulation 50:867–870, 1974.

233. Grüntzig AR, Senning A, Siegenthaler WE: Nonoperative dilation of coronary artery stenosis: percutaneous transluminal coronary angioplasty. N Engl J Med 301:61–68, 1979.

234. European Cooperative Study Group for streptokinase treatment in acute myocardial infarction: Streptokinase in acute myocardial infarction. N Engl J Med 301:797–802, 1979.

235. Mathey D, Kuck K-H, Tilsner V, Bleifeld W: Non-surgical coronary artery recanalization in acute myocardial infarction. Circulation 62 (Suppl III):III–160, 1980 (abstract).

236. Haft JI, Gershengorn K, Kranz PD, Oestreicher R: Protection against epinephrine-induced myocardial necrosis by drugs that inhibit platelet aggregation. Am J Cardiol 30:838–843, 1972.

237. Ruf W, McNamara JJ, Suehiro A, Suehiro G, Wickline SA: Platelet trapping in myocardial infarction in baboons: therapeutic effect of aspirin. Am J Cardiol 46:405–412, 1980.

238. Ginks WR, Sybers HD, Maroko PR, Covell JW, Sobel BE, Ross J Jr: Coronary artery reperfusion. II. Reduction of myocardial infarct size at one week after the coronary occlusion. J Clin Invest 51:2717–2723, 1972.

239. Lang T-W, Corday E, Gold H, Meerbaum S, Rubins S, Costantini C, Hirose S, Osher J, Rosen V: Consequences of

reperfusion after coronary occlusion – effects on hemodynamics and regional myocardial metabolic function. Am J Cardiol 33:69–81, 1974.

240. Chandler AB, Chapman J, Erhardt LR, Roberts WC, Schwartz CJ, Sinapius D, Spain DM, Sherry S, Ness PM, Simon TL: Coronary thrombosis in myocardial infarction: report of a workshop on the role of coronary thrombosis in the pathogenesis of acute myocardial infarction. Am J Cardiol 34:823–832, 1974.

241. Silver MD, Baroldi G, Mariani F: The relationship between acute occlusive coronary thrombi and myocardial infarction studied in one hundred consecutive patients. Circulation 61:219–227, 1980.

242. DeWood MA, Spores J, Notske R, Mouser LT, Burroughs R, Golden MS, Lang HT: Prevalence of total coronary occlusion during early hours of transmural myocardial infarction. N Engl J Med 303:897–902, 1980.

243. Mehta P, Mehta J; Platelet function studies in coronary artery disease. V. Evidence for enhanced platelet microthrombus formation activity in acute myocardial infarction. Am J Cardiol 43:757–760, 1979.

244. Maseri A, Mimmo R, Chierchia S, Marchesi C, Pesola A, L'Abbate A: Coronary artery spasm as a cause of acute myocardial ischemia in man. Chest 68:625–633, 1975.

245. Hellstrom HR: Coronary artery vasospasm: the likely immediate cause of acute myocardial infarction. Br Heart J 41:426–432, 1979.

246. Oliva PB, Breckinridge JC: Arteriographic evidence of coronary arterial spasm in acute myocardial infarction. Circulation 56:366–374, 1977.

247. Maseri A, L'Abbate A, Baroldi G, Chierchia S, Marzilli M, Ballestra AM, Severi S, Parodi O, Biagini A, Distante A, Pesola A: Coronary vasospasm as a possible cause of myocardial infarction. N Engl J Med 299:1271–1277, 1978.

248. deOliveira JM, Carballo R, Zimmerman HA: Intravenous injection of hyaluronidase in acute myocardial infarction: preliminary report of clinical and experimental observations. Am Heart J 57:712–713, 1959.

249. Hillis LD, Fishbein MC, Braunwald E, Maroko P: The influence of the time interval between coronary artery occlusion and the administration of hyaluronidase on salvage of ischemic myocardium in dogs. Circ Res 41:26–31, 1977.

250. Maroko PR, Libby P, Bloor CM, Sobel BE, Braunwald E: Reduction by hyaluronidase of myocardial necrosis following coronary artery occlusion. Circulation 46:430–435, 1972.

251. Maclean D, Fishbein MC, Maroko P, Braunwald E: Hyaluronidase-induced reduction in myocardial infarct size. Science 194:199–200, 1976.

252. Maroko PR, Hillis LD, Muller JE, Tavazzi L, Heyndrickx GR, Ray M, Chiariello M, Distante A, Askenazi J, Salerno J, Carpentier J, Reshetnaya NI, Radvany P, Libby P, Raabe DS, Chazov EI, Bobba P, Braunwald E: Favorable effects of hyaluronidase on electrocardiographic evidence of necrosis in patients with acute myocardial infarction. N Engl J Med 296:898–903, 1977.

253. Askenazi J, Hillis LD, Diaz PE, Davis MA, Braunwald E, Maroko P: The effects of hyaluronidase on coronary blood flow following coronary artery occlusion in the dog. Circ Res 40:566–571, 1977.

254. Cribier A, Nair R, Totten G, Ganz W: Effect of nitroglycerin on collateral flow early and late post coronary occlusion. Circulation 55–56 (Suppl III):III–109, 1977 (abstract).

255. Swain J, Parker JP, McHale PA, Greenfield JC Jr: Effects of nitroglycerin and propranolol on the distribution of transmural myocardial blood flow during ischemia in the absence of hemodynamic changes in the unanesthetized dog. J Clin Invest 63:947–953, 1979.

256. Capurro NL, Kent KM, Smith HJ, Aamodt R, Epstein SE: Acute coronary occlusion; prolonged increase in collateral flow following brief administration of nitroglycerin and methoxamine. Am J Cardiol 39:679–683, 1977.

257. Bache RJ: Effects of nitroglycerin and arterial hypertension on myocardial blood flow following acute coronary artery occlusion in the dog. Circulation 57:557–562, 1978.

258. Goldstein R, Stinson EB, Scherer JL, Seningen RP, Grehl TM, Epstein SE: Intraoperative coronary collateral function in patients with coronary occlusive disease: nitroglycerin responsiveness and angiographic correlations. Circulation 49:298–308, 1974.

259. Ganz W, Marcus HS: Failure of intracoronary nitroglycerin to alleviate pacing-induced angina. Circulation 46: 880–889, 1972.

260. Myers RW, Scherer JL, Goldstein RA, Goldstein RE, Kent KM, Epstein SE: Effects of nitroglycerin and nitroglycerin-methoxamine during acute myocardial ischemia in dogs with pre-existing multivessel coronary occlusive disease. Circulation 51:632–640, 1975.

261. Hirshfeld JW Jr, Borer JS, Goldstein RE, Barrett MJ, Epstein SE: Reduction in severity and extent of myocardial infarction when nitroglycerin and methoxamine are administered during coronary occlusion. Circulation 49:291–297, 1974.

262. Kent KM, Smith ER, Redwood DR, Epstein SE: Beneficial electrophysiologic effects of nitroglycerin during acute myocardial infarction. Am J Cardiol 33:513–516, 1974.

263. Borer JS, Kent KM, Goldstein RE, Epstein SE: Nitroglycerin-induced reduction in the incidence of spontaneous ventricular fibrillation during coronary occlusion in dogs. Am J Cardiol 33:517–520, 1974.

264. Stockman MB, Verrier RL, Lown B: Effect of nitroglycerin on vulnerability to ventricular fibrillation during myocardial ischemia and reperfusion. Am J Cardiol 43: 233–238, 1979.

265. Come PC, Flaherty JT, Baird MG, Rouleau JR, Weisfeldt ML, Greene HL, Becker L, Pitt B: Reversal by phenylephrine of the beneficial effects of intravenous nitroglycerin in patients with acute myocardial infarction. N Engl J Med 293:1003–1007, 1975.

266. Flaherty JT, Reid RR, Kelley DT, Taylor DR, Weisfeldt ML, Pitt B: Intravenous nitroglycerin in acute myocardial infarction. Circulation 51:132–139, 1975.

267. Borer JS, Redwood DR, Levitt B, Cagin N, Bianchi C, Vallin H, Epstein SE: Reduction in myocardial ischemia with nitroglycerin or nitroglycerin plus phenylephrine administered during acute myocardial infarction. N Engl J Med 293:1008–1012, 1975.

268. Miller RR, Awan NA, DeMaria AN, Amsterdam EA, Mason DT: Importance of maintaining systemic blood pressure during nitroglycerin administration for reducing

ischemic injury in patients with coronary artery disease. Am J Cardiol 40:504–508, 1977.

269. Chiche P, Baligadoo SJ, Derrida JP: A randomized trial of prolonged nitroglycerin infusion in acute myocardial infarction. Circulation 59–60 (Suppl II):II–165, 1979 (abstract).

270. Mueller HS, Ayres SM, Religa A, Evans RG: Propranolol in the treatment of acute myocardial infarction: effect on myocardial oxygenation and hemodynamics. Circulation 49:1078–1086, 1974.

271. Becker LC, Fortuin NJ, Pitt B: Effects of ischemia and antianginal drugs on the distribution of radioactive microspheres in the canine left ventricle. Circ Res 28:263–269, 1971.

272. Fox KM, Selwyn AP, Welman E: The effects of propranolol on myocardial perfusion and metabolism during acute regional ischemia. Clin Cardiol 3:47–50, 1980.

273. Gross GT, Warltier, DC, Hardman HF: Beneficial action of N-dimethyl propranolol on myocardial oxygen balance and transmural perfusion gradient distal to a severe coronary artery stenosis in the canine heart. Circulation 58: 663–669, 1978.

274. Kjekshus JK, Mjos OD: Effect of inhibition of lipolysis on infarct size after experimental coronary artery occlusion. J Clin Invest 52:1770–1778, 1973.

275. Opie LH: Metabolism of free fatty acids, glucose, and catecholamines in acute myocardial infarction: relation to myocardial ischemia and infarct size. Am J Cardiol 36:938–953, 1975.

276. Oliver MF, Rowe MJ, Luxton MR, Miller NE, Neilson JM: Effect of reducing circulating free fatty acids on ventricular arrhythmias during myocardial infarction and on ST-segment depression during exercise-induced ischemia. Circulation 53 (Suppl I):I-210–I-212, 1976.

277. Shrago E, Shug, AL, Sul H, Bittar N, Folts JD: Control of energy production in myocardial ischemia. Circ Res 38 (Suppl I):75–78, 1976.

278. Simonsen S, Kjekshus JK: The effect of free fatty acids on myocardial oxygen consumption during atrial pacing and catecholamine infusion in man. Circulation 58:484–491, 1978.

279. Obeid A, Spear R, Mookherjee S, Warner R, Eich R: The effects of propranolol on myocardial energy stores during myocardial ischemia in dogs. Circulation 49 (Suppl II): II–159, 1976 (abstract).

280. Kligfield P, Horner H, Smithen C, Brachfeld N: Metabolic effect of propranolol on ischemic myocardium. Circulation 51–52 (Suppl II):II–26, 1975 (abstract).

281. Mueller HS, Rao PS, Fletcher J, Evans R, Hertelendy F, Stickley L, Walter K: Propranolol during the evolution and subsequent ten days of myocardial infarction in man: hemodynamic, initial cardiac energetics, and neurohumoral response. Clin Cardiol 2:393–403, 1979.

282. Ergin MA, Dastgir G, Butt KMH, Stuckey JH: Prolonged epicardial mapping of myocardial infarction: the effects of propranolol and intraaortic balloon pumping following coronary artery occlusion. J Thorac Cardiovasc Surg 72:892–899, 1976.

283. Rassmussen MM, Reimer KA, Kloner RA, Jennings RB: Infarct size reduction by propranolol before and after coronary ligation in dogs. Circulation 56:794–798, 1977.

284. Gold HK, Leinbach RC, Maroko PR: Propranolol-induced reduction of signs of ischemic injury during acute myocardial infarction. Am J Cardiol 38:689–695, 1976.

285. Pelides LJ, Reid DS, Thomas M, Shillingford JP: Inhibition by β-blockade of the ST-segment elevation after acute myocardial infarction in man. Cardiovasc Res 6:295–301, 1972.

286. Peter T, Norris RM, Clarke ED, Heng MK, Singh BN, Williams B, Howell DR, Ambler PK: Reduction of enzyme levels by propranolol after acute myocardial infarction. Circulation 57:1091–1095, 1978.

287. Yusuf S, Ramsdale D, Peto R, Furse L, Bennett D, Bray C, Slight P: Early intravenous atenolol treatment in suspected acute myocardial infarction. Lancet 2:273–276, 1980.

288. Pitts BJR, Tate CA, van Winkle WB, Wood JM, Entham ML: Palmitylcarnitine inhibition of the calcium pump in cardiac sarcoplasmic reticulum: a possible role in myocardial ischemia. Life Sci 23:391–402, 1978.

289. Wood JM, Bush B, Pitts BJR, Schwartz A: Inhibition of bovine heart Na^+, K^+-ATPase by palmitylcarnitine and palmityl Co-A. Biochem Biophys Res Commun 74:677–684, 1977.

290. Idell-Wenger JA, Grotyohann LW, Neely JR: Coenzyme A and carnitine distribution in normal and ischemic hearts. J Biol Chem 253:4310–4318, 1978.

291. Corr PB, Snyder DW, Cain ME, Crafford WA Jr, Gross RW, Sobel BE: Electrophysiological effects of amphiphiles on canine Purkinje fibers: implications for dysrrhythmia secondary to ischemia. Circ Res 49:354–363, 1981.

292. Smith ER, Duce BR: Anti-arrhythmic and serum free fatty acid lowering effects of 5-fluoro-nicotinyl alcohol following experimentally-induced myocardial infarction in the dog. Cardiovasc Res 8:550–561, 1974.

293. Atkinson L, Bergman G, Jackson N, Jewitt DE, Metcalfe JM: Potential protective value of enhanced myocardial carbohydrate utilization with reduced free fatty acid uptake after UK25842 in patients with coronary artery disease. Br J Pharmacol 66:444P, 1979.

294. Russell RO Jr, Rogers WJ, Mantle JA, McDaniel HG, Rackley CE: Glucose-insulin-potassium, free fatty acids, and acute myocardial infarction in man. Circulation 53 (Suppl I):I-207–I-211. 1976.

295. Opie LH, Bruyneel K, Owen P: Effects of glucose, insulin, and potassium infusion on tissue metabolic changes within the first hour of myocardial infarction in the baboon. Circulation 52:49–57, 1975.

296. Obeid AI, Verrier RL, Lown B: The effect of glucose, insulin, and potassium on vulnerability to ventricular fibrillation in dogs. Circulation 56 (Suppl III):III–159, 1977 (abstract).

297. Maroko PR, Libby P, Sobel BE, Bloor CM, Sybers HD, Shell WE, Covell JW, Braunwald E: Effect of glucose-insulin-potassium infusion on myocardial infarction following experimental coronary artery occlusion. Circulation 45: 1160–1175, 1972.

298. Rogers WJ, Stanley AW Jr, Breinig JB, Prather JW, McDaniel HG, Moraski RE, Mantle JA, Russell RO Jr,

Rackley CE: Reduction of hospital mortality rate of acute myocardial infarction with glucose-insulin-potassium infusion. Am Heart J 92:441–454, 1976.

299. Rogers WJ, Segall PH, McDaniel HG, Mantle JA, Russell RO Jr, Rackley CE: Prospective randomized trial of glucose-insulin-potassium in acute myocardial infarction: effects on myocardial hemodynamics, substrates, and rhythm. Am J Cardiol 43: 801–809, 1979.

300. Heng MK, Norris RM, Singh BN, Barratt-Boyes C: Effects of glucose and glucose-insulin-potassium on haemodynamics and enzyme release after acute myocardial infarction. Br Heart J 39:748–757, 1977.

301. Henry PD, Shuchleib R, Borda LJ, Roberts R, Williamson JR, Sobel BE: Effects of nifedipine on myocardial perfusion and ischemic injury in dogs. Circ Res 43:372–380, 1978.

302. Nayler WG, Ferrari R, Williams A: Protective effect of pretreatment with verapamil, nifedipine and propranolol on mitochondrial function in the ischemic and reperfused myocardium. Am J Cardiol 46:242–248, 1980.

303. Sobel BE: Mechanisms of action and clinical implications of calcium antagonists. Prac Cardiol 13:31–40, 1981.

304. Schanne FAX, Kane AB, Young EE, Farber JL: Calcium dependence of toxic cell death. Science 206:700–702, 1979.

305. Nayler WG, Poole-Wilson PA. Williams A: Hypoxia and calcium. J Mol Cell Cardiol 11:683–706, 1979.

306. Reimer KA, Lowe FE, Jennings RE: Effect of the calcium antagonist verapamil on necrosis following temporary coronary artery occlusion in dogs. Circulation 55:581–587, 1977.

307. Henry PD, Shuchleib R, Clarke RE, Perez JE: Effect of nifedipine on myocardial ischemia: analysis of collateral flow, pulsatile heat, and regional muscle shortening. Am J Cardiol 44:817–824, 1979.

308. Ferlinz J, Easthope JL, Aronow WS: Effects of verapamil on myocardial performance in coronary disease. Circulation 59:313–319, 1979.

309. Walsh R, Badke F, O'Rourke R: Differential effects of diltiazem and verapamil on left ventricular performance in conscious dogs. Circulation 59–60 (Suppl II)II–15, 1979 (abstract).

310. Polese A, Florentini C, Olivari MT, Guazzi MD: Clinical use of a calcium antagonistic agent (nifedipine) in acute pulmonary edema. Am J Med 66:825–830, 1979.

311. Spath JA Jr, Lane DL, Lefer AM: Protective action of methylprednisolone on the myocardium during experimental myocardial ischemia in the cat. Circ Res 35:44–51, 1974.

312. Libby P, Maroko PR, Bloor CM, Sobel BE, Braunwald E: Reduction of experimental myocardial infarct size by corticosteroid administration. J Clin Invest 52:599–607, 1973.

313. Osher J, Lang T-W, Meebaum S, Hashimoto K, Farcot J-C, Cordau E: Methylprednisolone treatment in acute myocardial infarction: effect on regional and global myocardial function. Am J Cardiol 37:564–571, 1976.

314. deMello VR, Roberts R, Sobel BE: Deleterious effects of multiple dose methylprednisolone on evolving myocardial infarction. Circulation 51–52 (Suppl II):II–104, 1975 (abstract).

315. Morrison J, Reduto L, Pizzarello R, Geller K, Maley T,

Gulotta S: Modification of myocardial injury in man by corticosteroid administration. Circulation 53 (Suppl I):I-200–I-203, 1976.

316. Amsterdam EA, Banas J, Criley JM, Loeb HS, Mueller H, Willerson JT, Mason DT: Clinical assessment of external pressure circulatory assistance in acute myocardial infarction. Am J Cardiol 45:349–356, 1980.

317. Gowda S, Gillespie TA, Byrne JD, Ambos HD, Sobel BE, Roberts R: Effects of external counterpulsation on enzymatically estimated infarct size and ventricular arrhythmias. Br Heart J 40:308–314, 1978.

318. Powell WJ Jr, DiBona DR, Flores J, Leaf A: The protective effect of hyperosmotic mannitol in myocardial ischemia and necrosis. Circulation 54:603–615, 1976.

319. Powell WJ Jr, DiBona DR, Flores J, Frega N, Leaf A: Effects of hyperosmolar mannitol in reducing ischemic cell swelling and minimizing mycardial necrosis. Circulation 53 (Suppl I):I-45–I-49, 1976.

320. Willerson JT, Watson JT, Platt MR: Effect of hypertonic mannitol and intraaortic counterpulsation on regional myocardial blood flow and ventricular performance in dogs during myocardial ischemia. Am J Cardiol 37:514–519, 1976.

321. Jorgensen L, Roswell HC, Hovig T, Glynn MR, Mustard JG: Adenosine diphosphate-induced platelet aggregation and myocardial infarction in swine. Lab Invest 17:616–644, 1967.

322. Needleman P, Kulkarni PS, Raz A: Coronary tone modulation: formation and actions of prostaglandins, endoperoxides, and thromboxanes. Science 195:409–412, 1977.

323. Moschos CB, Lahiri K, Lyons M, Weisse AB, Oldewurtel HA, Regan TJ: Relation of microcirculatory thrombosis to thrombus in the proximal coronary artery: effect of acetyl salicylic acid, dipyridamole, and thrombolysis. Am Heart J 86:61–68, 1973.

324. Cappuro NL, Marr KC, Aamodt R, Goldstein RE, Epstein SE: Aspirin-induced increase in collateral flow after acute coronary occlusion in dogs. Circulation 59:744–747, 1979.

325. Jugdutt BI, Hutchins GM, Buckley BH, Becker LC: Salvage of ischemic myocardium by ibuprofen during infarction in the conscious dog. Am J Cardiol 46:74–82, 1980.

326. Jugdutt BI, Hutchins GM, Buckley BH, Pitt B, Becker LC: Effect of indomethacin on collateral blood flow and infarct size in the conscious dog. Circulation 59:735–743, 1979.

327. Berger HJ, Zaret BL, Speroff L, Cohen LS, Wolfson S: Cardiac prostaglandin release during myocardial ischemia induced by atrial pacing in patients with coronary artery disease. Am J Cardiol 39:481–486, 1977.

328. Roberts AJ, Jacobstein JG, Cipriano PR, Alonso DR, Combes JR, Gay WA Jr: Effectiveness of dipyridamole in reducing the size of experimental myocardial infarction. Circulation 61:228–236, 1980.

329. Rees JR, Redding VJ: Effects of dipyridamole on anastomotic blood flow in experimental myocardial infarction. Cardiovasc Res 1:179–183, 1967.

330. Bertolasi CA, Tronge JE, Riccitelli MA, Villamayor RM, Zuffardi E: Natural history of unstable angina with medical and surgical therapy. Chest 70:596–605, 1976.

331. Gazes PC, Mobley EM Jr, Faris HM Jr, Duncan RC, Humphries GB: Preinfarction (unstable) angina: a pros-

pective study – ten year follow-up. Circulation 48:331–337, 1973.

332. Schroeder JS, Lamb IH, Harrison DC: Patients admitted to the coronary care unit for chest pain: high risk subgroup for subsequent cardiovascular death. Am J Cardiol 39:829–832, 1977.

333. Krauss KR, Hutter AM Jr, DeSanctis RW: Acute coronary insufficiency: course and follow-up. Arch Intern Med 129:808–813, 1972.

334. Schroeder JS, Lamb IH, Hu M: Do patients in whom myocardial infarction has been ruled out have a better prognosis after hospitalization than those surviving infarction? N Engl J Med 303:1–5, 1980.

335. Vakil RJ: Preinfarction syndrome: management and follow-up. Am J Cardiol 14:55–63, 1964.

336. Wood P: Acute and subacute coronary insufficiency. Br Med J 1:1779–1782, 1961.

337. Sobel BE: Propranolol and treatment of myocardial infarction. N Engl J Med 300:191–193, 1979 (editorial).

338. Norris RM, Sammel NL, Clarke ED, Smith WM: Protective effect of propranolol in threatened myocardial infarction. Lancet 2:907–909, 1978.

339. Fischl SF, Herman MV, Gorlin R: The intermediate coronary syndrome. N Engl J Med 288:1193–1198, 1973.

340. Cairns JA, Fantus IG, Klassen GA: Unstable angina pectoris. Am Heart J 92:373–386, 1976.

341. Parodi O, Maseri A, Simonetti I: Management of unstable angina at rest by verapamil: a double blind cross-over study in the coronary care unit. Br Heart J 41:167–174, 1979.

342. Roberts WC, Virmani R: Quantification of coronary artery narrowing in clinically-isolated unstable angina pectoris. Am J Med 67:792–799, 1979.

343. Pugh B, Platt MR, Mills LJ, Crumbo D, Poliner LR, Curry GC, Blomqvist GC, Parkey RW, Buja LM, Willerson JT: Unstable angina pectoris: a randomized study of patients treated medically and surgically. Am J Cardiol 41:1291–1298, 1978.

344. Neill WA, Ritzmann LW, Selden R: The pathophysiologic basis of acute coronary insufficiency: observations favoring the hypothesis of intermittment reversible coronary obstruction. Am Heart J 94:439–444, 1977.

345. Moses J, Feldman MS, Helfant RH: Efficacy of nifedipine in the intermediate syndrome refractory to propranolol and nitrate therapy. Am J Cardiol 45:390, 1980 (abstract).

346. Weintraub RM, Aroesty JM, Paulin S, Levine FH, Markis JE, LaRaia PJ, Cohen SI, Kurland GF: Medically refractory unstable angina pectoris. I. Long-term follow-up of patients undergoing intraaortic balloon counterpulsation and operation. Am J Cardiol 43:877–882, 1979.

347. Olinger GN, Bonchek LI, Keelan MH Jr, Tresch DD, Siegel R, Bamrah V, Tristani FE: Unstable angina: the case for operation. Am J Cardiol 42:634–640, 1978.

348. National Cooperative Study Group: Unstable angina pectoris: national cooperative study group to compare surgical and medical therapy. III. Results in patients with ST-segment elevation during pain. Am J Cardiol 45: 819–824, 1980.

349. Plotnick GD, Conti CR: Unstable angina: angiography, short- and long-term morbidity, mortality, and sympto-

matic states of medically treated patients. Am J Med 63:870–873, 1977.

350. Blankenhorn DH, Brooks SH, Selzer RH, Barndt R Jr: The rate of atherosclerotic changes during treatment of hyperlipoproteinemia. Circulation 57:355–361, 1978.

351. Kuo PT, Hayase K, Kostis JB, Moreyra AE: Use of combined diet and colestipol in long-term (7–7½ years) treatment of patients with type II hyperlipoproteinemia. Circulation 59:199–211, 1979.

352. Scheuer J, Greenberg MA: Exercise training in patients with coronary artery disease. Mod Concepts Cardiovasc Dis 47:85–90, 1978.

353. Kellerman JJ: Rehabilitation of patients with coronary heart disease. Prog Cardiovasc Dis 17:303–328, 1975.

354. Hellerstein HK, Franklin BA: Exercise testing and prescription. In: Wenger NK, Hellerstein HK (eds) Rehabilitation of the Coronary Patient. John Wiley, New York, 1978, pp 149–202.

355. Wilhelmsson C, Vedin JA, Wilhelmsen L, Werkö L: Reduction of sudden deaths after myocardial infarction by treatment with alprenolol. Lancet 2:1157–1160, 1974.

356. Ahlmark G, Saetre H, Korsgren M: Reduction of sudden death after myocardial infarction. Lancet 2:1563–1564, 1974.

357. Multicentre International Study: Improvement in prognosis of myocardial infarction by long-term beta-adrenoreceptor blockade using practolol. Br Med J 3:735–740, 1975.

358. Andersen MP, Frederiksen J, Jürgensen HJ, Pedersen F, Bechsgaard P, Hansen DA, Nielsen B, Pedersen-Bjergaard O, Rasmussen SL: Effect of alprenolol on mortality among patients with definite or suspected acute myocardial infarction. Lancet 2:865–868, 1979.

359. Kumpuris AG, Luchi RJ, Waddell CC, Miller RR: Production of circulating platelet aggregates by exercise in coronary patients. Circulation 61:62–65, 1979.

360. Steele PP, Weily HS, Davies H, Genton E: Platelet function studies in coronary artery disease. Circulation 48: 1194–1200, 1972.

361. Elwood PC, Cochrane AL, Burr ML, Sweetnam PM, Williams G, Welsby E, Hughes SJ, Renton R: A randomized controlled trial of acetyl salicylic acid in the secondary prevention of mortality from myocardial infarction. Br Med J 1:436–440, 1974.

362. Boston Collaborative Drug Surveilance Group: Regular aspirin intake and acute myocardial infarction. Br Med J 1:440–443, 1974.

363. Coronary Drug Project Research Group: Aspirin in coronary artery disease. J Chronic Dis 29:625–642, 1976.

364. Elwood PC, Sweetnam PM: Aspirin and secondary mortality after myocardial infarction. Lancet 2:1313–1315, 1979.

365. The Persantine-Aspirin Reinfarction Study Research Group: Persantine and aspirin in coronary heart disease. Circulation 62:449–461, 1980.

366. Hammond EC, Garfinkel L: Aspirin and coronary heart disease: findings of a prospective study. Br Med J 2:269–271, 1975.

367. Aspirin Myocardial Infarction Study Research Group: A randomized, controlled trial of aspirin in persons recov-

ered from myocardial infarction. J Am Med Assoc 243: 661–667, 1980.

368. Frank CW, Weinblatt E, Shapiro S: Angina pectoris in men: prognostic significance of selected medical factors: Circulation 47:509–516, 1973.

369. Kannel WB, Feinleib M: Natural history of angina pectoris in the Framingham Study: prognosis and survival. Am J Cardiol 29:154–163, 1972.

370. Kannel WB, Sorlie PD: Remission of clinical angina pectoris: the Framingham Study. Am J Cardiol 42:119–123, 1978.

371. Russek HI: The 'natural' history of severe angina pectoris with intensive medical therapy alone: a five year prospective study of 133 patients. Chest 65:46–51, 1974.

372. Aronow WS: Effect of passive smoking on angina pectoris. N Engl J Med 299:21–24, 1978.

373. Rabinowitz BD, Thorp K, Huber GL, Abelman WH: Acute hemodynamic effects of cigarrette smoking in man assessed by systolic time intervals and echocardiography. Circulation 60:752–760, 1979.

374. Orlando J, Aronow WS, Cassidy J, Prakash R: Effect of ethanol on angina pectoris. Ann Intern Med 84:652–655, 1976.

375. Harding PR, Aronow WS, Eisenman J: Digitalis as an antianginal agent. Chest 64:439–443, 1973.

376. Aronow WS: Clinical use of nitrates. I. Nitrates as antianginal drugs. Mod Concepts Cardiovasc Dis 48:31–35, 1979.

377. Reichek N, Goldstein RE, Redwood DR, Epstein SE: Sustained effects of nitroglycerin ointment in patients with angina pectoris. Circulation 50:348–352, 1974.

378. Hardarson T, Henning H, O'Rourke RA: Prolonged salutary effect of isosorbide dinitrate and nitroglycerin ointment on regional left ventricular function. Am J Cardiol 40:90–98, 1977.

379. Opie LH: Drugs and the heart. II. Nitrates. Lancet 1:750–753, 1980.

380. Klaus AP, Zaret BL, Pitt BL, Ross RS: Comparative evaluation of sublingual long-acting nitrates. Circulation 48:519–525, 1973.

381. Markis JE, Gorlin R, Mills RM, Williams RA, Schweitzer P, Ransil RJ: Sustained effects of orally administered isosorbide dinitrate on exercise performance in patients with angina pectoris. Am J Cardiol 43:265–271, 1979.

382. Danahy DT, Burwell DT, Aronow WS, Prakash R: Sustained hemodynamic and antianginal effect of high dose oral isosorbide dinitrate. Circulation 55:381–387, 1977.

383. Thadani U, Fung H-L, Darke AC, Parker JO: Oral isosorbide dinitrate in the treatment of angina pectoris: dose–response relationship and the duration of action during acute therapy. Circulation 62:491–502, 1980.

384. Strumza P, Rigaud M, Mechmeche R, Rocha P, Baudet M, Bardet J, Bourdarias J-P: Prolonged hemodynamic effects (12 hours) of orally administered sustained-release nitroglycerin. Am J Cardiol 43:272–277, 1979.

385. Lee G, Mason DT, DeMaria AN: Effects of long-term oral administration of isosorbide dinitrate on the antianginal response to nitroglycerin: absence of nitrate cross-tolerance and self-tolerance shown by exercise testing. Am J Cardiol 41:82–87, 1978.

386. Abrams J: Nitrate tolerance and dependence. Am Heart J 99:113–123, 1980.

387. Steele PP, Maddoux G, Kirch DL, Vogel RA: Effects of propranolol and nitroglycerin on left ventricular performance in patients with coronary artery disease. Chest 73:19–23, 1978.

388. Rivier J-L, Nissiotis E, Jaeger M: Comparison of the immediate haemodynamic effects of three beta-adrenergic blocking agents. Postgrad Med J (Suppl):44–48, 1970.

389. Majid PA, Sharma B, Saxton C, Stoker JB, Taylor SH: Haemodynamic effects of oxprenolol in hypertensive patients. Postgrad Med J (Suppl):67–72, 1970.

390. Imhof PR: Characterization of beta blockers as antihypertensive agents in the light of human pharmacologic studies. In: Schweizer W (ed) Beta-Blockers – Present Status and Future Prospects. Hans Huber Publ, Bern, 1974, pp 40–50.

391. Giudicelli JF, Lhoste F, Bossier JR: β-adrenergic blockade and atrioventricular conduction impairment. Eur J Pharmacol 31:216–225, 1975.

392. Thadani U, Parker JO: Propranolol in the treatment of angina pectoris: comparison of duration of action in acute and sustained oral therapy. Circulation 59:571–579, 1979.

393. Thadani U, Parker JO: Propranolol in angina pectoris: comparison of therapy given two and four times a day. Am J Cardiol 46:117–123, 1980.

394. Thadani U, Davidson C, Singleton W, Taylor SH: Comparison of five beta-adrenoreceptor antagonists with different ancillary properties during sustained twice daily therapy in angina pectoris. Am J Med 68:243–250, 1980.

395. Prichard BNC, Gillam PMS: Assessment of propranolol in angina pectoris: a clinical dose response curve and the effect on the electrocardiogram at rest and on exercise. Br Heart J 33:473–480, 1971.

396. Thadani U, Davidson C, Chir B, Singleton W, Taylor SH: Comparison of the immediate effects of five β-adrenoreceptor-blocking drugs with different ancillary properties in angina pectoris. N Engl J Med 300:750–755, 1979.

397. Greenblatt DJ, Koch-Weser J: Adverse reactions to propranolol in hospitalized medical patients: a report from the Boston Collaborative Drug Surveillance Project. Am Heart J 86:478–484, 1973.

398. Crawford MH, LeWinter MM, O'Rourke RA, Karliner JS, Ross J Jr: Combined propranolol and digoxin therapy in angina pectoris. Ann Intern Med 83:449–455, 1975.

399. Bourdillon PD, Canepa-Anson R, Rickards AF: Hemodynamic effects of intravenous metoprolol. Am J Cardiol 44:1195–1200, 1979.

400. Miller RR, Olson HG, Amsterdam EA, Mason DT: Propranolol-withdrawal rebound phenomenon: exacerbation of coronary events after abrupt cessation of antianginal therapy. N Engl J Med 293:416–418, 1975.

401. Boudoulas H, Lewis RP, Kates RE, Dalamangas G: Hypersensitivity to adrenergic stimulation after propranolol withdrawal in normal subjects. Ann Intern Med 87:433–436, 1977.

402. Nattel S, Rangno RE, Van Loon G: Mechanism of propranolol withdrawal phenomenon. Circulation 59:1158–1164, 1979.

403. Oka Y, Frishman W, Becker RM, Kadish A, Strom J,

Matsumoto M, Orkin L, Frater R: Clinical pharmacology of the new beta-adrenergic blocking drugs. Part 10. Beta-adrenoceptor blockade and coronary artery surgery. Am Heart J 99:255–269, 1980.

404. Brittain RT, Levy GP: A review of the animal pharmacology of labetalol: a combined α- and β-adrenoceptor-blocking drug. Br J Clin Pharmacol 3 (Suppl 3):681–694, 1976.

405. Halprin S, Frishman W, Kirschner M, Strom J: Clinical pharmacology of the new beta-adrenergic blocking drugs. Part II. Effects of oral labetalol in patients with both angina pectoris and hypertension: a preliminary experience. Am Heart J 99:388–396, 1980.

406. Mudge GH Jr, Grossman W, Mills RM Jr, Lesch M, Braunwald E: Reflex increase in coronary vascular resistance in patients with ischemic heart disease. N Engl J Med 295:1333–1337, 1976.

407. Yasue H, Omote S, Takizawa A, Nagao M, Miwa K, Tanaka S: Exertional angina pectoris caused by coronary arterial spasm: effects of various drugs. Am J Cardiol 43:647–652, 1979.

408. Brevetti G, Chiariello M, Renyo F, Chiariello L, Paudice G, Laracetta G, Condorelli M: Labetalol in coronary artery disease. Abstracts VIII World Cong Cardiol 1:194, 1978.

409. Henry PD: Comparative pharmacology of calcium antagonists: nifedipine, verapamil and diltiazem. Am J Cardiol 46:1047–1058, 1980.

410. Livesley B, Catley PF, Campbell RC, Oram S: Double-blind evaluation of verapamil, propranolol, and isosorbide dinitrate against a placebo in the treatment of angina pectoris. Br Med J 1:375–378, 1973.

411. Subramanian B, Bowles M, Lahiri A: Long-term antianginal action of verapamil assessed with quantitated serial treadmill stress testing. Am J Cardiol 48:529–535, 1981.

412. Atterhög J-H, Ekelund L-G, Melin A-L: Effect of nifedipine on exercise tolerance in patients with angina pectoris. Eur J Clin Pharmacol 8:125–130, 1975.

413. Moskowitz RM, Piccini PA, Nacarelli GV, Zelis R: Nifedipine therapy for stable angina pectoris: preliminary results of effects on angina frequency and treadmill exercise response. Am J Cardiol 44:811–816, 1979.

414. Lichtlen PR, Engel HJ, Wolf R, Hundeshagen H: Effect of nifedipine on regional myocardial blood flow at rest and in pacing-induced ischemia. Circulation 59–60 (Suppl II):II-249, 1979 (abstract).

415. Henry PD, Clark RE: Protection of ischemic myocardium with nifedipine. In: Winbury, Katz (eds) Perspective in Cardiovascular Research. Raven Press, New York (in press).

416. dePonti C, Mauri F, Ciliberto GR, Caru B: Comparative effects of nifedipine, verapamil, isosorbide dinitrate and propranolol on exercise-induced angina pectoris. Eur J Cardiol 10:47–58, 1979.

417. Ekelund L-G, Orö L: Antianginal efficiency of nifedipine with and without a beta-blocker, studied with exercise testing: a double-blind, randomized study. Clin Cardiol 2:203–211, 1979.

418. Figueras J, Singh BN, Phil D, Ganz W, Charuzi Y, Swan HJC: Mechanism of rest and nocturnal angina: observations during continuous hemodynamic and electrocardio-graphic monitoring. Circulation 59:955–968, 1979.

419. Curry RC Jr, Pepine CJ, Conti CR: Refractory variant angina treated with perhexiline maleate: results in fourteen patients. Circulation 58 (Suppl II):II-179, 1978 (abstract).

420. Wright GJ, Leeson GA, Zeiger AV, Lang JF: The absorption, excretion, and metabolism of perhexiline maleate by the human. Postgrad Med J 49 (Suppl III):8–15, 1973.

421. Sato M, Nagao T, Yamaguchi I, Kakajima H, Kiyomoto A: Pharmacological studies on a new 1,5-benzothiazepine derivative (CRD-401). Arzneimittelforsch 21:1338–1343, 1971.

422. Zsoter TT: Calcium antagonists. Am Heart J 99:805–810, 1980.

423. Ellrodt G, Chew CYC, Singh BN: Therapeutic implications of slow-channel blockade in cardiocirculatory disorders. Circulation 62:669–679, 1980.

424. Charlier R: Cardiac actions in the dog of a new antagonist of adrenergic excitation which does not produce complete blockade of adrenoceptors. Br J Pharmacol 39:668–674, 1970.

425. Singh BN, Jewitt DE, Downey JM, Kirk ES, Sonnenblick EH: Effects of amiodarone and L8040, novel antianginal and antiarrhythmic drugs, on cardiac and coronary haemodynamics and on cardiac intracellular potentials. Clin Exp Pharmacol Physiol 3:427–442, 1976.

426. Aronow WS: Medical treatment of angina pectoris. VIII. Miscellaneous antianginal drugs. Am Heart J 85:132–137, 1973.

427. Takaro T, Hultgren HN, Lipton MJ, Detre KM: The VA cooperative randomized study of surgery for coronary arterial occlusive disease. II. Subgroup with significant left main lesions. Circulation 54: (Suppl III):III-107–III-117, 1976.

428. Hurst JW, King SB III, Logue RB, Hatcher CR Jr, Jones EL, Craver JM, Douglas JS Jr, Franch RH, Dorney ER, Cobbs BW Jr, Robinson PH, Clements SD Jr, Kaplan JA, Bradford JM: Value of coronary bypass surgery: controversies in cardiology: part 1. Am J Cardiol 42:308–329, 1978.

429. Hamby RI, Katz S: Percutaneous transluminal coronary angioplasty: its potential impact on surgery for coronary artery disease. Am J Cardiol 45:1161–1166, 1980.

430. Heupler FA: Syndrome of symptomatic coronary artery spasm with nearly normal coronary arteriograms. Am J Cardiol 45:873–881, 1980.

431. Selzer A, Langston M, Ruggeroli C, Cohn K: Clinical syndrome of variant angina with normal coronary arteriogram. N Engl J Med 295:1343–1347, 1976.

432. Severi S, Davies G, Maseri A, Marzullo P, L'Abbate A: Long-term prognosis of 'variant' angina with medical treatment. Am J Cardiol 46:226–232, 1980.

433. Chierchia S, Brunelli C, Simonetti I, Lazzari M, Maseri A: Sequence of events in angina at rest: primary reduction in coronary flow. Circulation 61:759–768, 1980.

434. Yasue H, Omote S, Takizawa A, Nagao M, Miwa K, Tanaka S: Circadian variation of exercise capacity in patients with Prinzmetal's variant angina: role of exercise-induced coronary artery spasm. Circulation 59:938–948, 1979.

435. Scanlon PJ, Nemickas R, Moran JF, Talano JV, Amirparviz F, Pifarre R: Accelerated angina pectoris: clinical, he-

modynamic, arteriographic, and therapeutic experience in 85 patients. Circulation 47:19–26, 1973.

436. Weaver WD, Lorch GS, Alvarez HA, Cobb LA: Angiographic findings and prognostic indications in patients resuscitated from sudden death. Circulation 54:895–900, 1976.

437. Marzilli M, Goldstein S, Trivella MG, Palumbo C, Maseri A: Some clinical considerations regarding the relation of coronary vasospasm to coronary atherosclerosis: a hypothetical pathogenesis. Am J Cardiol 45:882–886, 1980.

438. Yokoyama M, Henry PD: Sensitization of isolated canine coronary arteries to calcium ions after exposure to cholesterol. Circ Res 45:479–486, 1979.

439. Gunther S, Green L, Muller JE, Mudge GH, Grossman W: Inappropriate coronary vasoconstriction in patients with coronary artery disease: a role for nifedipine? Am J Cardiol 44:793–797, 1979.

440. Raizner AE, Chahine RA, Ishimori T, Verani MS, Zacca N, Jamal N, Miller RR, Luchi RJ: Provocation of coronary artery spasm by the cold pressor test: hemodynamic, arteriographic, and quantitative angiographic observations. Circulation 62:925–932, 1980.

441. Endo M, Hirosawa K, Kaneko N, Hase K, Inoue Y, Konno S: Prinzmetal's variant angina: coronary arteriogram and left ventriculogram during angina attack induced by methacholine. N Engl J Med 294:252–255, 1976.

442. Curry RC Jr, Pepine CJ, Sabom MB, Feldman RL, Christie LG, Varnell JH, Conti CR: Hemodynamic and myocardial metabolic effects of ergonovine in patients with chest pain. Circulation 58:648–654, 1978.

443. Curry RC Jr, Pepine CJ, Sabom MB, Conti CR: Similarities of ergonovine-induced and spontaneous attacks of variant angina. Circulation 59:307–312, 1979.

444. Cipriano PR, Guthaner DF, Orlick AE, Ricci DR, Wexler L, Silverman JF: The effects of ergonovine maleate on coronary artery size. Circulation 59:82–89, 1979.

445. Théroux P, Waters DD, Affaki GS, Crittin J, Bonan R, Mizgala HF: Provocative testing with ergonovine to evaluate the efficacy of treatment with calcium antagonists in variant angina. Circulation 60:504–510, 1979.

446. Buxton A, Goldberg S, Hirshfeld JW, Wilson J, Mann T, Williams DO, Overlie P, Oliva P: Refractory ergonovine-induced coronary vasospasm: importance of intracoronary nitroglycerin. Am J Cardiol 46:329–334, 1980.

447. Antman E, Muller J, Goldberg S, MacAlpin R, Rubenfire M, Tabatznik B, Liang C-S, Heupler F, Achuff S, Reichek N, Geltman E, Kerin NZ, Neff RK, Braunwald E: Nifedipine therapy for coronary artery spasm: experience in 127 patients. N Engl J Med 302:1269–1273, 1980.

448. Ricci DR, Orlick AE, Cipriano PR, Guthaner DF, Harrison DC: Altered adrenergic activity in coronary arterial spasm: insight into mechanisms based on study of coronary hemodynamics and the electrocardiogram. Am J Cardiol 43:1073–1079, 1979.

449. Muller JE, Gunther SJ: Nifedipine therapy for Prinzmetal's angina. Circulation 57:137–139, 1978.

450. Previtali M, Salerno JA, Tavazzi L, Ray M, Medici A, Chimienti M, Specchia G, Bobba P: Treatment of angina at rest with nifedipine: a short-term controlled study. Am J Cardiol 45:825–830, 1980.

451. Goldberg S, Reichek N, Wilson J, Hirshfeld JW Jr, Muller J, Kastor JA: Nifedipine in the treatment of Prinzmetal's (variant) angina. Am J Cardiol 44:804–810, 1979.

452. Heupler FA Jr, Proudfit WL: Nifedipine therapy for refractory coronary arterial spasm. Am J Cardiol 44:798–803, 1979.

453. Hansen JF, Sandøe E: Treatment of Prinzmetal's angina due to coronary artery spasm using verapamil: a report of three cases. Eur J Cardiol 7:327–335, 1978.

454. Aronow WS: The medical treatment of angina pectoris. VI. Propranolol as an antianginal drug. Am Heart J 84:706–709, 1972.

455. Klein RC, Vera Z, Mason DT, DeMaria AN, Awan NA, Amsterdam EA: Ambulatory holter monitor documentation of ventricular tachyarrhythmias as mechanism of sudden death in patients with coronary artery disease. Clin Res 27:7A, 1979 (abstract).

456. Ryan M, Lown B, Horn H: Comparison of ventricular ectopic activity during 24-hour monitoring and exercise testing in patients with coronary heart disease. N Engl J Med 292:224–229, 1975.

457. Calvert A, Lown B, Gorlin R: Ventricular premature beats and anatomically defined coronary heart disease. Am J Cardiol 39:627–634, 1977.

458. Snyder DW, Sheridan DJ, Sobel BE: Premature ventricular complexes: therapeutic dilemmas and decisions. Adv Cardiol 27:322–342, 1980.

459. Ruskin JN, DiMarco JP, Garan H: Out-of-hospital cardiac arrest: electrophysiologic observations and selection of long-term antiarrhythmic therapy. N Engl J Med 303:607–613, 1980.

460. Myerburg RJ, Conde C, Sheps DS, Appel RA, Kiem I, Sung RJ, Castellanos A: Antiarrhythmic drug therapy in survivors of prehospital cardiac arrest: comparison of effects on chronic ventricular arrhythmias and recurrent cardiac arrest. Circulation 59:855–863, 1979.

461. Chiang BN, Perlman LV, Fulton M, Ostrander LD Jr, Epstein FH: Predisposing factors in sudden cardiac death in Tecumseh, Michigan: a prospective study. Circulation 41:31–37, 1970.

462. Margolis JR, Hirshfeld JW Jr, McNeer JF, Starmer CF, Rosati RA, Peter RH, Behar VS, Kong Y: Sudden death due to coronary artery disease: a clinical, hemodynamic, and angiographic profile. Circulation 51–52 (Suppl III): III-180–III-188, 1975.

463. Winkle RA: Antiarrhythmic drug effect mimicked by spontaneous variability of ventricular ectopy. Circulation 57:1116–1120, 1978.

464. Lown B, Graboys TB: Management of patients with malignant ventricular arrhythmias. Am J Cardiol 39:910–918, 1977.

465. Horowitz LN, Josephson ME, Farshidi A, Spielman SR, Michelson EL, Greenspan AM: Recurrent sustained ventricular tachycardia. 3. Role of electrophysiologic study in selection of antiarrhythmic regimens. Circulation 58:986–997, 1978.

466. Mason JW, Winkle RA: Electrode-catheter arrhythmia induction in the selection and assessment of antiarrhythmic drug therapy for recurrent ventricular tachycardia. Circulation 58:971–985, 1978.

467. Mason JW, Winkle RA: Accuracy of the ventricular tachycardia-induction study for predicting long-term efficacy and inefficacy of antiarrhythmic drugs. N Engl J Med 303:1073–1077, 1980.

468. Greenspan AM, Horowitz LN, Spielman SR, Josephson ME: Large dose procainamide therapy for ventricular tachyarrhythmia. Am J Cardiol 46:453–462, 1980.

469. Conrad KA, Molk BL, Chidsey CA: Pharmacokinetic studies of quinidine in patients with arrhythmias. Circulation 55:1–7, 1977.

470. Doering W: Quinidine-digoxin interaction: pharmacokinetics, underlying mechanism and clinical implications. N Engl J Med 301:400–404, 1979.

471. Doherty JE, Straub KD, Murphy ML, deSoyza N, Bissett JK, Kane JJ: Digoxin-quinidine interaction: changes in canine tissue concentration from steady state with quinidine. Am J Cardiol 45:1196–1200, 1980.

472. Mungall DR, Robichaux RP, Perry W, Scott JW, Robinson A, Burelle T, Hurst D: Effects of quinidine on serum digoxin concentration: a prospective study. Ann Intern Med 93:689–693, 1980.

473. Leahy EB Jr, Reiffel JA, Giardina E-GV, Bigger JT Jr: The effect of quinidine and other oral antiarrhythmic drugs on serum digoxin. Ann Intern Med 92:605–608, 1980.

474. Ochs HR, Pabst J, Greenblatt DJ, Dengler HJ: Noninteraction of digitoxin and quinidine. N Engl J Med 303:672–674, 1980.

475. Fenster PE, Powell JR, Graves PE, Conrad KA, Hager WD, Goldman S, Marcus FI: Digitoxin-quinidine interaction: pharmacokinetic evaluation. Ann Intern Med 93:698–701, 1980.

476. Data JL, Wilkinson GR, Nies AS: Interaction of quinidine with anticonvulsant drugs. N Engl J Med 294:699–702, 1976.

477. Roden DN, Reele SB, Higgins SB, Wilkinson GR, Smith RF, Oates JA, Woosley RL: Antiarrhythmic efficacy, pharmacokinetics, and safety of N-acetyl procainamide in human subjects: comparison with procainamide. Am J Cardiol 46:463–468, 1980.

478. Jaillon P, Winkle RA: Electrophysiologic comparative study of procainamide and N-acetyl procainamide in anesthetized dogs: concentration–response relationships. Circulation 60:1385–1394, 1979.

479. Kluger J, Drayer D, Reidenberg M, Ellis G, Lloyd V, Tyberg T, Hayes J: The clinical pharmacology and antiarrhythmic efficacy of acetylprocainamide in patients with arrhythmias. Am J Cardiol 45:1250–1287, 1980.

480. Lee W-K, Strong JM, Kehoe RF, Dutcher JS, Atkinson AJ Jr: Antiarrhythmic efficacy of N-acetyl procainamide in patients with ventricular premature contractions. Clin Pharmacol Ther 19:512–514, 1976.

481. Vismara LA, Vera Z, Miller RR, Mason DT: Efficacy of disopyramide phosphate in the treatment of refractory ventricular tachycardia. Am J Cardiol 39:1027–1034, 1977.

482. Podrid PJ, Schoenenberger A, Lown B: Congestive heart failure caused by oral disopyramide. N Engl J Med 302:614–617, 1980.

483. Woosley RL, Kornhauser D, Smith R, Reele S, Higgins SB, Nies AS, Shand DG, Oates JA: Suppression of chronic ventricular arrhythmias with propranolol. Circulation 60:819–827, 1979.

484. Koppes GM, Beckmann CH, Jones FG: Propranolol therapy for ventricular arrhythmias two months after acute myocardial infarction. Am J Cardiol 46:322–328, 1980.

485. Nixon JV, Pennington W, Ritter W, Shapiro W: Efficacy of propranolol in the control of exercise-induced or augmented ventricular ectopic activity. Circulation 57:115–122, 1978.

486. Fors WJ Jr, Vanderark CR, Reynolds EW Jr: Evaluation of propranolol and quinidine in the treatment of quinidine-resistant arrhythmias. Am J Cardiol 27:190–194, 1971.

487. Frishman W, Silverman R: Clinical pharmacology of the new beta-adrenergic blocking drugs. Part 3. Comparative clinical experience and new therapeutic applications. Am Heart J 98:119–131, 1979.

488. Frishman W, Silverman R: Clinical pharmacology of the new beta-adrenergic blocking drugs. Part 2. Physiologic and metabolic effects. Am Heart J 97:997–1007, 1979.

489. Sami M, Mason JW, Peters F, Harrison DC: Clinical and electrophysiologic effects of encainide, a newly developed antiarrhythmic agent. Am J Cardiol 44:526–532, 1979.

490. Roden DM, Reele SB, Higgins SB, Mayol RF, Gammans RE, Oates JA, Woosley RL: Total suppression of ventricular arrhythmias by encainide. N Engl J Med 302:877–882, 1980.

491. Podrid PJ, Lyakishev A, Lown B, Mazur N: Ethmozin, a new antiarrhythmic drug for suppression of ventricular premature contractions. Circulation 61:450–457, 1980.

492. Campbell NPS, Pantridge JF, Adgey AAJ: Long-term oral antiarrhythmic therapy with mexilitine. Br Heart J 40:796–801, 1978.

493. Talbot RG, Julian DG, Prescott LF: Long-term treatment of ventricular arrhythmias with oral mexilitine. Am Heart J 91:58–65, 1976.

494. Campbell NPS, Pantridge JF, Adgey AAJ: Mexilitine in the management of ventricular dysrrhythmias. Eur J Cardiol 6:245–258, 1977.

495. Winkle Ra, Meffin PJ, Harrison DC: Long-term tocainide therapy for ventricular arrhythmias. Circulation 57:1008–1016, 1978.

496. Woosley RL, McDevitt DG, Nies AS, Smith RF, Wilkinson GR, Oates JA: Suppression of ventricular ectopic depolarizations by tocainide. Circulation 56:980–984, 1977.

497. LeWinter MM, Engler RL, Karliner JS: Tocainide therapy for treatment of ventricular arrhythmias: assessment with ambulatory electrocardiographic monitoring and treadmill exercise. Am J Cardiol 45:1045–1052, 1980.

498. Rosenbaum MB, Chiale PA, Halpern MS, Nau GJ, Przybylski J, Levi RJ, Lazzari JO, Elizari MV: Clinical efficacy of amiodarone as an antiarrhythmic agent. Am J Cardiol 38:934–944, 1976.

499. Lubbe WF, McFadyen ML, Worthington M, Opie LH: Protective action of amiodarone against ventricular fibrillation in the isolated perfused rat heart. Am J Cardiol 43:533–540, 1979.

500. Côté, P, Bourassa MG, Delaye J, Janin A, Froment R, David P: Effects of amiodarone on cardiac and coronary hemodynamics and on myocardial metabolism in patients

with coronary artery disease. Circulation 59:1165–1172, 1979.

501. Johnson RA, Hutter AM, DeSanctis RW, Yurchak PM, Leinbach RC, Harthorne JW: Chronic overdrive pacing in the control of refractory ventricular arrhythmias. Ann Intern Med 80:380–383, 1974.

502. Mirowski M, Reid PR, Mower MM, Watkins L, Gott VL, Schauble JF, Langer A, Heilman MS, Kolenik SA, Fischell RE, Weisfeldt ML: Termination of malignant ventricular arrhythmias with an implanted automatic defibrillator in human beings. N Engl J Med 303:322–324, 1980.

503. Fisher JD, Mehra R, Furman S: Termination of ventricular tachycardia with bursts of rapid ventricular pacing. Am J Cardiol 41:94–102, 1978.

504. Ruskin JN, Garan H, Poulin F, Harthorne JW: Permanent radiofrequency ventricular pacing for management of drug-resistant ventricular tachycardia. Am J Cardiol 46:317–321, 1980.

505. Hartzler GO: Treatment of recurrent ventricular tachycardia by patient-activated radiofrequency ventricular stimulation. Mayo Clin Proc 54:75–82, 1979.

506. Gallagher JJ: Surgical treatment of arrhythmias: current status and future directions. Am J Cardiol 41:1035–1044, 1978.

507. Ricks WB, Winkle RA, Shumway NE, Harrison DC: Surgical management of life-threatening ventricular arrhythmias in patients with coronary artery disease. Circulation 56:38–42, 1977.

508. Sami M, Chaitman BR, Bourassa MG, Charpin D, Chabot M: Long-term follow-up of aneurysmectomy for recurrent ventricular tachycardia or fibrillation. Am Heart J 96:303–308, 1978.

509. deSoyza N, Murphy ML, Bissett JK, Kane JJ, Doherty JE III: Ventricular arrhythmias in chronic stable angina pectoris with surgical or medical treatment. Ann Intern Med 89:10–14, 1978.

510. Lehrman KL, Tilkian AG, Hultgren HN, Fowles RE: Effect of coronary artery bypass surgery on exercise-induced ventricular arrhythmias. Am J Cardiol 44:1056–1061, 1979.

511. Horowitz LN, Harken AH, Kastor JA, Josephson ME: Ventricular resection guided by epicardial and endocardial mapping for recurrent ventricular tachycardia. N Engl J Med 302:589–593, 1980.

512. Guiraudon G, Fontaine G, Frank R, Escande G, Etievent P, Cabrol C: Encircling endocardial ventriculotomy: a new surgical treatment of life-threatening ventricular tachycardias resistant to medical treatment following myocardial infarction. Ann Thorac Surg 26:438–443, 1978.

513. Packer M, Meller J, Medina N, Gorlin R, Herman MV: Rebound hemodynamic events after the abrupt withdrawal of nitroprusside in patients with severe chronic heart failure. N Engl J Med 301:1193–1197, 1979.

514. O'Rourke RA, Henning H, Theroux P, Crawford MH, Ross J Jr: Favorable effects of orally administered digoxin on left heart size and ventricular wall motion in patients with previous myocardial infarction. Am J Cardiol 37:708–715, 1976.

515. Firth BG, Dehmer GJ, Corbett JR, Lewis SE, Parkey RW, Willerson JT: Effect of chronic oral digoxin therapy on ventricular function at rest and peak exercise in patients with ischemic heart disease: assessment with equilibrium gated blood pool imaging. Am J Cardiol 46:481–490, 1980.

516. Franciosa JA, Goldsmith SR, Cohn JN: Contrasting immediate and long-term effects of isosorbide dinitrate on exercise capacity in congestive heart failure. Am J Med 69:559–566, 1980.

517. Danahy DT, Aronow WS: Hemodynamic and antianginal effects of high dose oral isosorbide dinitrate after chronic use. Circulation 56:205–212, 1977.

518. Thadani U, Manyari D, Parker JO, Fung H-L: Tolerance to the circulatory effects of oral isosorbide dinitrate. Circulation 61:526–535, 1980.

519. Franciosa JA, Cohn JN: Sustained hemodynamic effects without tolerance during long-term isosorbide dinitrate treatment of chronic left ventricular failure. Am J Cardiol 45:648–654, 1980.

520. Armstrong PW, Armstrong JA, Marks GS: Pharmacokinetic-hemodynamic studies of intravenous nitroglycerin in chronic cardiac failure. Circulation 62:160–166, 1980.

521. Magrini F, Niarchos AP: Ineffectiveness of sublingual nitroglycerin in acute left ventricular failure in the presence of massive peripheral edema. Am J Cardiol 45:841–847, 1980.

522. Amsterdam EA, Awan NA, DeMaria AN, Miller RR, Williams DO, Mason DT: Sustained salutary effects of oral controlled-release nitroglycerin on ventricular function in congestive heart failure. Clin Cardiol 2:19–25, 1979.

523. Franciosa JA, Mikulic E, Cohn JN, Jose E, Fabie A: Hemodynamic effects of orally administered isosorbide dinitrate in patients with congestive heart failure. Circulation 50:1020–1024, 1974.

524. Mookherjee S, Fuleihan D, Warner RA, Vardan S, Obeid AI: Effects of sublingual nitroglycerin on resting pulmonary gas exchange and hemodynamics in man. Circulation 57:106–115, 1978.

525. Chatterjee K, Parmley WW, Massie B, Greenberg B, Werner J, Klausner S, Norman A: Oral hydralazine therapy for chronic refractory heart failure. Circulation 54:879–883, 1976.

526. Cogan JJ, Humphreys MH, Carlson CJ, Rapaport E: Renal effects of nitroprusside and hydralazine in patients with congestive heart failure. Circulation 61:316–323, 1980.

527. Pierpont GL, Brown DC, Franciosa JA, Cohn JN: Effect of hydralazine on renal failure in patients with congestive heart failure. Circulation 61:323–327, 1980.

528. Fitchett DH, Neto JAM, Oakley CM, Goodwin JF: Hydralazine in the management of left ventricular failure. Am J Cardiol 44:303–309, 1979.

529. Packer M, Meller J, Medina N, Gorlin R, Herman MV: Dose requirements of hydralazine in patients with severe chronic congestive heart failure. Am J Cardiol 45:655–660, 1980.

530. Awan NA, Miller RR, Mason DT: Comparison of effects of nitroprusside and prazosin on left ventricular function and the peripheral circulation in chronic refractory congestive heart failure. Circulation 57:152–159, 1978.

531. Awan NA, Hermanovich J, Whitcomb C, Skinner P, Ma-

son DT: Cardiocirculatory effects of afterload reduction with oral trimazosin in severe chronic congestive heart failure. Am J Cardiol 44:126–131, 1979.

532. Colucci WS, Wynne J, Holman BL, Braunwald E: Long-term therapy of heart failure with prazosin: a randomized double blind trial. Am J Cardiol 45:337–344, 1980.

533. Colucci WS, Williams GH, Braunwald E: Increase plasma norepinephrine levels during prazosin therapy for severe congestive heart failure. Ann Intern Med 93:452–453, 1980.

534. Elkayam U, LeJemtel TH, Mathur M, Ribner HS, Frishman WH, Strom J, Sonnenblick EH: Marked early attenuation of hemodynamic effects of oral prazosin therapy in chronic congestive heart failure. Am J Cardiol 44:540–545, 1979.

535. Arnold SB, Williams RL, Ports TA, Baughman RA, Benet LZ, Parmley WW, Chatterjee K: Attenuation of prazosin effects on cardiac output in chronic heart failure. Ann Intern Med 91:345–349, 1979.

536. Awan NA, Miller RR, DeMaria AN, Maxwell KS, Neumann A, Mason DT: Efficacy of ambulatory systemic vasodilator therapy with oral prazosin in chronic refractory heart failure. Circulation 56:346–354, 1977.

537. Aronow WS, Lurie M, Turbow M, Whittaker K, Van Kamp S, Hughes D: Effect of prazosin versus placebo on chronic left ventricular heart failure. Circulation 59:344–350, 1979.

538. Rubin SA, Chatterjee K, Gelberg HJ, Ports TA, Brundage BH, Parmley WW: Paradox of improved exercise but not resting hemodynamics with short-term prazosin in chronic heart failure. Am J Cardiol 43:810–815, 1979.

539. Goldman SA, Johnson LL, Escala E, Cannon PJ, Weis MB: Improved exercise ejection fraction with long-term prazosin therapy in patients with heart failure. Am J Med 68:36–42, 1980.

540. Weber KT, Kinasewitz GT, West JS, Janicki JS, Reichek N, Fishman AP: Long-term vasodilator therapy with trimazosin in chronic cardiac failure. N Engl J Med 303:242–250, 1980.

541. Aronow WS, Greenfield RS, Alimadadian H, Danahy DT: Effect of the vasodilator trimazosin versus placebo on exercise performance in chronic left ventricular failure. Am J Cardiol 40:789–793, 1977.

542. Davis R, Ribner HS, Keung E, Sonnenblick EH, LeJemtel TH: Treatment of chronic congestive heart failure with captopril, an oral inhibitor of angiotensin-converting enzyme. N Engl J Med 301:117–121, 1979.

543. Vrobel TR, Cohn JN: Comparative hemodynamic effects of converting enzyme inhibition and sodium nitroprusside in severe heart failure. Am J Cardiol 45:331–336, 1980.

544. Ader R, Chatterjee K, Ports T, Brundage B, Hiramatsu B, Parmley W: Immediate and sustained hemodynamic and clinical improvement in chronic heart failure by an oral angiotensin-converting enzyme inhibitor. Circulation 61:931–937, 1980.

545. Levine TB, Franciosa JA, Cohn JN: Acute and long-term response to an oral angiotensin-converting enzyme inhibitor, captopril, in congestive heart failure. Circulation 62:35–41, 1980.

546. Dzau VJ, Colucci WS, Williams GH, Curfman G, Meggs L, Hollenberg NK: Sustained effectiveness of converting-enzyme inhibition in patients with severe congestive heart failure. N Engl J Med 302:1373–1379, 1980.

547. Prins EJL, Hoorntje SJ, Weening JJ, Donker AJM: Nephrotic syndrome in a patient on captopril. Lancet 2:306–307, 1979.

548. vanBrummelen P, Willenze R, Tau WD, Thompson J: Captopril-associated agranulocytosis. Lancet 1:150, 1980.

549. Bleifeld W, Kupper W, Hanrath P, Mathey D: New and traditional therapy of congestive heart failure: a European view. Am J Med 65:203–207, 1978.

550. Matsumoto S, Ito T, Sada T, Takahashi M, Su K-M, Ueda A, Okabe F, Sato M, Sekine I, Ito Y: Hemodynamic effects of nifedipine in congestive heart failure. Am J Cardiol 46:476–480, 1980.

551. LeJemtel TH, Keung E, Ribner HS, Davis R, Wexler J, Blaufox MD, Sonnenblick EH: Sustained beneficial effects of oral amrinone on cardiac and renal function in patients with severe congestive heart failure. Am J Cardiol 45:123–129, 1980.

552. Wynne J, Malacoff RF, Benotti JR, Curfman GD, Grossman W, Holman BL, Smith TW, Braunwald E: Oral amrinone in refractory congestive heart failure. Am J Cardiol 45:1245–1249, 1980.

CHAPTER 16

Cardiac surgical therapy of atherosclerosis and angina

RICHARD O. RUSSELL, Jr., CHARLES E. RACKLEY,
and NICHOLAS T. KOUCHOUKOS

Introduction

Although there is almost universal agreement that coronary artery bypass grafting has been a major advance for therapy of the patient moderately or severely symptomatic with angina pectoris, there is less agreement and often controversy over its use in certain groups of patients with coronary artery disease. For example, it is unclear whether to advise revascularization surgery for the patient minimally symptomatic with angina pectoris; for the asymptomatic patient with a positive exercise test and coronary artery disease; for the asymptomatic patient with calcification in the coronary arteries seen at fluoroscopy, and subsequently proven coronary disease [1]; for the patient with proven coronary artery spasm, mild to moderate, and fixed coronary artery restrictive disease; for the patient symptomatic with angina but with single-vessel coronary disease; and for the patient with recurrent angina despite one or two prior coronary bypass operations. A dilemma which is as yet unanswered is what role will calcium-blocking agents play in decisions for surgery in the presence of known coronary artery disease. Yet another and different focus of concern is the economic impact that coronary artery bypass surgery would have if advised in all patients with coronary artery disease [2, 3]. Unfortunately, the tabulation of these areas of uncertainty does not imply that we shall provide solutions to them in this chapter. It does signify that coronary artery bypass surgery is a useful form of therapy but should not be advised routinely as we face therapeutic options at any given point in the life history of a patient with coronary artery disease.

Existing studies do not lend support to a staunch position on the questions listed, but it is relevant to consider data from studies which clarify our understanding of the natural history of unoperated patients with angina pectoris. There are no studies of the survival of patients with angina pectoris left untreated, but certainly the nonoperative treatment of these patients has varied over the years. Moreover, based on longevity studies of patients having had coronary arteriography, there is the suggestion that perhaps in the last sveral years the unoperated patient with angina pectoris has an improved prognosis over that which might have been expected [4]. Thus, perhaps medical therapy itself has improved and may have improved somewhat the prognosis of patients with angina pectoris due to coronary artery disease. This possibility may heighten rather than resolve our therapeutic uncertainties.

We shall consider the natural history of patients with angina pectoris both from earlier studies as well as from studies with coronary arteriography; the surgical management of coronary artery disease; then prospective randomized studies of medical, or surgical plus medical, therapy of angina pectoris. This will be followed by our current recommendations for treatment.

Natural history of angina pectoris

To evaluate newer methods of treatment for angina pectoris, be they surgical or medical, it is incumbent on clinicians to have some appreciation of the course of patients with this syndrome. Although

Rosen, M. R. and Hoffman, B. F. (eds.), Cardiac Therapy. ISBN 0-89838-564-4.
© 1983, Martinus Nijhoff Publishers, Boston, The Hague, Dordrecht, Lancaster. Printed in the Netherlands.

knowledge of coronary artery anatomy and left ventricular function from angiographic studies has contributed greatly to our understanding of the prognosis for the patient with angina, early studies conducted prior to angiography helped establish a framework for prognosis.

Mortality was found to be higher in the first year after onset or diagnosis of angina pectoris than in subsequent years. In a large series from the Mayo Clinic (6,882 patients) the greatest mortality rate, about 15%, occurred in the first year after diagnosis whereas the mortality rate was about 9% annually thereafter [5]. From studies of 456 patients with angina pectoris over a period of 25 years, Richards, Bland, and White found an average duration of survival of 9.4 years (11.0 years for females and 8.9 years for males) [6]. The higher survival rate for females after the diagnosis of angina pectoris was substantiated in the Framingham Study [7]. However, an overall better prognosis in men as well was found in the Framingham Study in which angina was attended by a 4% mortality per year [7]. Interestingly, the length of survival after diagnosis of angina pectoris was not influenced by age [5, 7]. However, the survival rate over several years was clearly worse for patients with angina than for the normal population [5, 6]. From these early studies, factors which worsened the prognosis of patients with angina pectoris included hypertension, myocardial infarction, cardiac enlargement, an abnormal electrocardiogram, and congestive heart failure [5, 6]. However, Kannel and Feinlieb found that survival in patients having angina with a history of a myocardial infarction was approximately the same as those with uncomplicated angina [6]. Thus the presence of angina had implications, with regard to survival, similar to those for patients surviving the acute period of a myocardial infarction [7].

Reeves et al. have reviewed the natural history of angina pectoris, highlighting the contributions of coronary arteriography to our understanding of the mortality of unoperated patients with angina [8]. Several excellent studies have been performed wherein patients with angina pectoris have had coronary anteriography without operation and have been followed for several years [9-17]. Significant coronary artery obstructive disease was usually considered to be a 50% or greater narrowing by selective coronary arteriography. The investigators followed patients for a period of one to five years and three studies reported data for 10-12-year unoperated survival. Annual mortalities have ranged from 4% to 19% averaging 8.9% for the total series (Table 1). However, subcategorization by extent of coronary artery disease in terms of numbers of vessels diseased refines the mortality risk considerably. Left main coronary artery disease was not delineated for separate analysis in all studies. Patients having single-vessel disease exhibited an avery annual mortality of 3.8% with a range from 1.9% to 6.5%. Isolated left anterior descending disease had a worse prognosis than isolated involvement of right or left circumflex coronary arteries [9, 11, 12]. In patients with two-vessel disease the annual mortality averaged 9.6% and ranged from 4.1% to 19.0%. Three-vessel disease had the highest annula mortality with a mean of 13.0% and a range of 6.0%-25%. Thus as the extent of coronary artery disease increased from one- to two- and three-vessel disease, the average annual mortality increased from 3.8% to 9.6% and 13.0% respectively.

Despite the relative severity and risk as assessed by knowledge of coronary artery disease, other factors including ventriculography and clinical and laboratory data contributed to our knowledge of the degree of risk in patients with coronary artery disease. As the ventriculogram showed progressive damage when judged by categories of normal, local scar, aneurysm, and diffuse scar, prognosis worsened beyond that predicted based on coronary disease alone [18]. Thus a patient with single-vessel disease and a normal ventricle had a cumulative five-year mortality of approximately 8%, whereas a patient with single-vessel disease and diffuse scar had a cumulative five-year mortality of approximately 56%. If three-vessel disease and diffuse scar were present the five-year mortality approached 90%. When ventricular function was characterized in terms of left ventricular ejection fraction the variation in mortality was further delineated; e.g., patients with three-vessel coronary artery disease and a normal ejection fraction (> 0.50) had a lower mortality (12%) than did patients with three-vessel disease and a reduced ejection fraction (33%) [19].

Other significant clinical determinants of mortality were history (mortality rose with severity as well as duration of symptoms), abnormal electrocardiogram particularly with conduction disturbances, congestive heart failure, and presence of diabetes

Table 1. Coronary arteriographic series, average follow-up, and mortality rates (natural history studies of patients having coronary arteriography for ischemic heart disease).

Series	Number of patients	Average follow-up (months)	Annual Mortality % (approx)
Total series			
Bruschke et al., 1974 [9]	590	60	6.9
Bruschke, 1977 [10]	601	120	5.9
Oberman et al., 1972 [11]	148	21	11.5
Lichtlen & Moccetti, 1972 [12]	231	32.5	7.7
Slagle et al., 1972 [13]	94	15	19.0
Burggraf & Parker, 1975 [14]	259	51	5.3
Parker, 1977 [15]	259	120	4.1
Amsterdam et al., 1970 [16]	66	26	11.0
Average			8.9
One-vessel disease			
Bruschke et al., 1974 [9]	202	60	2.9
Bruschke, 1977 [10]	-	120 (first 4 yrs)	2.4
		(next 6 yrs)	5.2
Oberman et al., 1972 [11]	46	20	2.6
Lichtlen & Moccetti, 1972 [12]	83	32.5	3.5
Slagle et al., 1972 [13]	20	15	5.0
Burggraf & Parker, 1975 [14]	101	51	1.9
Parker, 1977 [15]	101	120	3.9
Amsterdam et al., 1970 [16]	21	26	6.5
Average			3.8
Two-vessel disease			
Bruschke et al., 1974 [9]	233	60	7.5
Bruschke et al., 1977 [10]	-	120	5.5
Oberman et al., 1972 [11]	50	22.7	13.7
Lichtlen & Moccetti, 1975 [12]	62	32.5	6.6
Slagle et al., 1972 [13]	26	15	19.0
Burggraf & Parker, 1975 [14]	94	51	8.2
Parker, 1977 [15]	94	120	4.1
Amsterdam et al., 1970 [16]	11	26	12.4
Average			9.6
Three-vessel disease			
Bruschke et al., 1974 [9]	118	60	10.7
Bruschke, 1977 [10]	-	120	7.6
Oberman et al., 1972 [11]	52	19.3	18.0
Lichtlen & Moccetti 1975 [12]	86	32.5	12.5
Slagle et al., 1972 [13]	48	15.0	25.0
Burggraf & Parker, 1975 [14]	64	51	10.5
Parker, 1977 [15]	64	120	6.0
Amsterdam et al., 1970 [16]	34	26	13.4
Average			13.0

(Note: In the One-vessel disease section, the values 2.4 and 5.2 are bracketed together with ">3.8" to the right.)

mellitus [18]. Determined to be independent predictors of mortality were heart size, disease (> 50% obstruction) of distal anterior descending artery, dyspnea on exertion accompanied by paroxysmal nocturnal dyspnea or orthopnea, resting heart rate, disease of the main left coronary artery, distal circumflex, and proximal right coronary artery disease [11]. These factors represent two basic determinants of prognosis: presence of congestive heart failure (even if not overt) and multiple vessel coronary artery disease.

Thus it is important, in our judgment, in assessing overall risk in patients with angina pectoris to include coronary arteriography and left ventriculography in the evaluation. Whereas left ventricular function may be determined by radionuclide studies, it is not presently possible to assess the extent and severity of the coronary artery disease without coronary arteriography.

Surgical management of coronary artery disease – clinical syndromes in which it may be useful

When one refers to coronary artery surgery, one usually means bypass grafting of obstructing coronary lesions using reversed segments of the patient's own saphenous veins. For analysis of results it is important to compare patients with comparable symptoms, comparable degrees of atherosclerotic coronary artery disease and comparable left ventricular function treated with and without operation. Preoperative evaluation includes, in addition to coronary arteriography and left ventriculography, thoughtful analysis of symptoms such as presence of serum enzymes (although this can be misleading), and an objective examination including a resting electrocardiogram and frequently an exercise stress test with or without accompanying radionuclide studies of perfusion or wall motion, or elevation and roentgenography of the chest, often including cardiac fluoroscopy.

In addition to coronary artery bypass grafting, surgery on the myocardium itself, such as left ventricular aneurysmectomy, may be performed as indicated to treat complications of coronary artery disease. The reversed segment of autogenous saphenous vein is sewn to the aorta and then end-to-side to a single coronary artery. When several branches of coronary arteries require bypassing, the graft proceeds from aorta attaching side-to-side to one or more coronary artery branches sequentially and then end-to-side for the final graft site to the several branches. Myocardial preservation techniques employing cardiopulmonary extracorporeal circulation during the surgery are vitally important and have improved greatly, providing a high degree of safety.

Resection of segments of myocardium including ventricular aneurysms or, less commonly, segments of dyskinesia is possible. These scars result from transmural myocardial infarction and most commonly occur anteriorly following occlusion of the anterior descending coronary artery and, less frequently, posteriorly or inferiorly, as a result of occlusion of left circumflex or right coronary arteries. Ventricular septal rupture may follow myocardial infarction and usually involves the inferior portion of the muscular septum adjacent to anterior or posterior necrosis. The defect is best approached through the adjacent anterior or posterior scars and can be closed with or without the use of a synthetic patch. Mitral imcompetence may follow myocardial infarction with rupture of a papillary muscle or chordae tendineae or result from myocardial damage with papillary muscle dysfunction. Mitral valve replacement is usually required if the incompetence is severe. Coronary artery bypass grafting may be performed along with any of the procedures on the myocardium.

During the postoperative period the cardiac output is usually normal in the absence of impaired ventricular function. With current techniques occurrence of perioperative myocardial infarction has been reduced to 5% or less. The intraaortic balloon-assist device is used in patients in whom cardiopulmonary bypass cannot be discontinued without hemodynamic deterioration and in patients who deteriorate later in the postoperative period.

The standard indication for direct coronary revascularization has been the presence of disabling angina pectoris refractory to optimal medical therapy in patients with high-grade proximal lesions in major coronary arterial segments demonstrated angiographically, but without severe left ventricular dysfunction. However, there are subsets of patients at varying risk of death from coronary artery disease, and, in these patients, the indications for operation have been extended to the prolongation of life and, possibly, reduction of the incidence of myocardial infarction.

In stable angina pectoris the risk of coronary artery bypass grafting is more directly related to the degree of left ventricular function present preoperatively than to the number of vessels diseased, the number of grafts inserted, the severity of symptoms, the presence of previous myocardial infarctions or age though the risk rises after the age of 70. In general the hospital mortality for experienced surgical teams varies between 1% and 3%. For patients with congestive heart failure with or without angina or with significant impairment of ventricular function, hospital mortality ranged between 10% and 50% [20–23]. Thus patients with cardiomegaly, predominant symptoms of congestive failure, diffuse contraction abnormalities, elevated left ventricular end-diastolic pressure, and depressed ejection fraction are at greater risk for surgery.

In an assessment of current operative risk of coronary bypass grafting, Kouchoukos et al. reviewed the experience with isolated bypass grafting (3,057 patients) and bypass grafting combined with excision of left ventricular aneurysm or scars (141 patients) during an eight-year interval (1970–1977) at the University of Alabama in Birmingham [24]. In period 1 (1970–1973), the 30-day mortality for the two procedures was 2.7% and 16.7% respectively. In period 2 (1974–1977) this mortality was 1.2% and 2.7% respectively (p < 0.01).

The incidence of definite or probable myocardial infarction among the patients with isolated bypass grafting procedures decreased from 11.4% (45 of 395 patients with available data) in period 1 to 2.4% (28 of 1,178) in period 2 (p < 0.001).

The mortality was no different for the patients who received two or three grafts (1.3%) than for those receiving four to seven grafts (1.4%). There were 44 deaths among the 2,814 males (1.6%) and ten among the 384 females (2.6%), a difference which was not significant. The highest mortality occurred in patients younger than 40 years and older than 70 years of age. The majority of deaths were cardiac related, resulting from pump failure, arrhythmias, and myocardial infarction. Left main coronary artery disease had an over all 30-day mortality rate of 2.5% and a rate of 1.7% for 360 patients in period 2 [24].

The reduction in mortality for coronary bypass surgery is doubtless the result of many factors. Patients with unstable angina pectoris were admitted to a coronary care unit with suspected myocardial infarction and were allowed to stabilize with medical therapy. An operation was performed if no evidence of myocardial necrosis developed in seven to ten days. Improved coronary arteriography has allowed more precise delineation of obstructive lesions in major coronary arterial branches, allowing more complete revascularization. Modifications of anesthetic management are also important. These include systematic control of factors known to increase myocardial oxygen requirements during induction and in the interval between induction and the onset of cardiopulmonary bypass. This has resulted in a reduced incidence of perioperative in-farction and early mortality. Newer methods for intraoperative myocardial protection using cold cardioplegia have had beneficial results. Increasing surgical experience and improved techniques, particularly the use of sequential grafts, have allowed more complex procedures to be performed without unduly prolonging the duration of myocardial ischemia and cardiopulmonary bypass [24].

The reduction of early mortality has an important effect on long-term survival after bypass grafting. The differences in survival among patients with two- and three-vessel disease between earlier and more recent mortality results have been related almost exclusively to reduced early mortality. Thus the greatest potential for improving long-term survival appears to be the reduction of early (hospital) mortality [24].

Relief of angina following coronary artery bypass occurs in 70–80% of patients in the early years after operation. However, with continued follow-up, the percentage of patients totally free of angina has declined. The cause of this may be graft failure, progression of coronary atherosclerosis, or both. Thus coronary artery bypass has been more effective in controlling angina pectoris in the early years following surgery than current medical therapy. Objective assessment with exercise testing after operation has demonstrated improvement in the majority of patients but the percentage of patients experiencing subjective improvement is even greater. Data demonstrating improvement in left ventricular function and symptoms of left ventricular failure remain inconclusive. Prevention of further deterioration of myocardial function after operation has been demonstrated and may be a major indication for operation [21–23].

Approximately 80–85% of vein grafts are patent at one year after operation but an additional 5% become occluded in the period between one and three years. Long-term function of the bypass grafts has not been studied extensively.

Effects of surgical therapy on survival remains under scrutiny, but it is essential that either retrospective or prospective comparisons of patients be made among comparable groups. In patients with left main coronary artery disease, consistently improved survival has been demonstrated in surgically treated patients in retrospective and prospective studies. Retrospective studies have compared surgically treated patients with patients considered operative candidates but treated nonoperatively for a variety of reasons. In patients with triple-vessel disease retrospective studies comparing operated patients to operative candidates in the same institution have shown significant improvement in survival of surgical patients at 36 months [25]. Similarly in patients with double-vessel disease, retrospective studies of comparable patients in the same institution have shown a statistically significant improvement in survival in surgically treated patients at 43 months [25]. With the possible exception of patients with lesions in the proximal left anterior descending coronary artery, increased survival has not been clearly demonstrated by surgical therapy in patients with single-vessel disease in the five to seven years after diagnosis.

Unstable angina pectoris, including recent onset of angina, pain at rest, pain with less activity but with increasing frequency and duration, is known also as acute coronary insufficiency, intermediate syndrome, or preinfarction angina. Usually to fulfill this diagnosis transient electrocardiographic ST- and/or T-wave changes are required with pain, but other electrocardiographic or enzymatic changes of infarction should be absent. Although urgent coronary artery bypass grafting has been advised to prevent death or myocardial infarction as well as to relieve pain, results often have indicated a higher operative mortality rate and a higher incidence of perioperative myocardial infarction than for patients with stable angina operated on in the same institution. Results of randomized trials (as indicated subsequently) comparing medical and surgical therapy in patients with unstable angina have demonstrated comparable early mortality rates and myocardial infarction rates [4]. Thus surgical therapy has not been shown to reduce the incidence of myocardial infarction even if performed soon after the diagnosis of unstable angina pectoris.

Coronary artery bypass grafting has been used for patients in some centers without shock in the very early hours after acute myocardial infarction. The rationale for immediate revascularization in such patients is the assumption that, even though irreversible myocardial necrosis may have occurred, improvement in oxygen delivery to adjacent areas of myocardium will minimize or prevent subsequent necrosis in these areas. The majority of these patients are those having infarction which occurred during or early after coronary arteriography with the bypass operation being performed within a very few hours of the onset of symptoms. Whether this hypothesis is correct, i.e., that surgical therapy is more effective than medical therapy in reducing the extent of necrosis in patients with comparable degrees of coronary atherosclerosis and ischemic myocardium, is uncertain. In limited experience with such patients with documented acute myocardial infarction without hemodynamic abnormalities, the operative mortality has been under 5% [26]. The results of myocardial revascularization with coronary artery bypass in patients who sustain an in-hospital myocardial infarction cannot be extrapolated to patients with acute myocardial infarction admitted to a coronary care unit with chest pain of over 6–8 hr.

In patients with acute myocardial infarction with left ventricular failure and shock, without an associated lesion (such as severe mitral regurgitation or ventricular septal rupture), coronary artery bypass has been performed often with infarctectomy, but such an operation has followed a period of intraaortic balloon support. Patients with cardiogenic shock and infarction (new plus old) of 40% or more of the left ventricular myocardium will be unlikely to benefit from the coronary artery bypass grafting even after a period of circulatory support.

In patients with acute myocardial infarction with left ventricular failure and cardiogenic shock and associated lesions such as rupture of the ventricular septum, repair is generally advisable since a minority survive more than two months with conservative management. If possible, four to six weeks should elapse prior to operation to allow fibrous healing of the septum adjacent to the defect to permit more effective closure without recurrence. Use of drugs that modify preload and afterload, in addition to the use of the intraaortic balloon pump to stabilize the patient during this period, has been an important therapeutic adjunct and has resulted in significant clinical and hemodynamic improvement. Coronary arteriography and left ventriculography prior to surgery will delineate not only the septal defect but an associated myocardial scar or ventricular aneurysm which may need excision at surgery.

Acute mitral regurgitation in patients with myocardial infarction may result from rupture of a papillary muscle or from dysfunction of the left ventricular free wall and the papillary muscle at its mooring. Operation is advisable in these patients to treat the severe mitral regurgitation, cardiac failure, and shock.

Coronary bypass grafting previously has been advised for patients with chronic congestive failure as the predominant manifestation of their coronary artery disease when such patients have areas of noncontracting ventricular myocardium. Operations might also consist of mitral valve replacement or annuloplasty for papillary muscle dysfunction causing chronic mitral regurgitation. Results have been disappointing; there has been little or no improvement in left ventricular contractility, reduction of elevated end-diastolic pressure or increase in reduced cardiac output. Operation is not advised currently for these patients.

Operative treatment in patients with lesser left ventricular dysfunction and with angina pectoris despite optimal medical therapy may be somewhat better, although with slightly increased operative risk. With improved intraoperative techniques and postoperative management including use of the intraaortic balloon, patients with a moderately reduced ejection fraction (0.2–0.4) can be operated on with an operative and hospital mortality of approximately 10–15%. Although left ventricular function may not be restored to normal, such patients may anticipate an improved survival and possibly reduction in further deterioration [21–23].

Life-threatening ventricular arrhythmias refractory to medical therapy have been treated with coronary bypass grafting, resection of left ventricular aneurysm, or infarctectomy either in the chronic stage of ischemic heart disease or during healing of a myocardial infarction; success has been variable. Newer and more promising surgical therapy has involved localization of arrhythmogenic foci with mapping techniques at open intracardiac operation. Use of cryotherapy, stripping of an area of ventricular endocardium, and encircling myotomy have been utilized with success in the control of recalcitrant ventricular arrhythmias (for further discussion, see Chapter 10).

Results of prospective randomized trials of medical or surgical plus medical therapy for angina pectoris

Although controversy has existed over the 'best' therapy for symptomatic coronary disease in patients with stable or unstable angina pectoris, most clinicians recognize that utilization of either or both modes of therapy will probably be necessary at some stage in the course of these patients. Both retrospective and prospective approaches to compare these modes of therapy, i.e., medical or surgical, have been proposed [27]. However, prospective randomized clinical trials provide the best opportunity for such comparisons [28]. It is useful to review the results of these prospective randomized clinical trials some of which have been cooperative from several institutions, whereas others have been performed at a single institution.

Results in studies of unstable angina pectoris

For uniformity we shall analyze numbers of patients studied, length of follow-up, in-hospital and late mortality, and nonfatal myocardial infarction rate; plus prevalence of severe angina during follow-up. Bertolasi and colleagues [29, 30] from Argentina reported on their experience in two groups of patients: those having the intermediate syndrome and those having progressive angina. In those with the intermediate syndrome the angina was prolonged, severe, recurrent, and unrelated to exercise. There were no extracardiac accessory factors, no significant enzyme elevations, and no severe pump failure or prolonged arrhythmias. The patients in this group had at least two of the following: little or no response to nitrates, transitory electrocardiographic ST or T changes with pain, transitory arrhythmias, and a history of less than one month between the onset of angina and admission into the study. In this group there were 24 medical patients and 28 surgical patients, randomly allocated. During the initial hospitalization among medical patients there was a 21% mortality and among surgical patients an 11% mortality. During an average of 32 months of follow-up, 25% of medical patients died, whereas no surgical patients died. With regard to myocardial infarction 25% of medical patients and 14% of surgical patients sustained a myocardial infarction during the initial hospitalization, whereas during follow-up 12% of medical patients and no surgical patients sustained a myocardial infarction. During follow-up approximately 17% of medical patients had severe angina as compared to approximately 4% of surgical patients.

The progressive group as defined by Bertolasi and colleagues contained patients who had experienced a change in the pattern of their angina during the preceding three months with an increase in the intensity, duration, and frequency of angina but without the requirements for the intermediate syndrome. In the progressive group there were 27 medical patients and 34 surgical patients again randomly allocated. There was a 4% initial medical and 9% initial surgical mortality, with an additional 4% mortality during the 32-month follow-up period in medical patients as compared to no deaths among the surgical patients. Four percent of medical and 12% of surgical patients had a myocardial infarction during initial hospitalization, and during follow-up 4% of medical patients and no surgical patients sustained a myocardial infarction. Approximately 18% of medical patients experienced severe angina while no surgical patients had severe angina during follow-up.

Another prospective randomized study of unstable angina was performed at the University of Oregon by Selden and colleagues [31]. There were 19 medical patients and 21 surgical patients, with no medical and 5% surgical mortality during initial hospitalization. No deaths occurred in any group during follow-up. No medical patients had a myocardial infarction during the initial hospitalization, whereas 14% of surgical patients had. During follow-up 10% of medical patients and no surgical patients had a myocardial infarction. However, severe angina occurred in 63% of medical patients and in 5% of surgical patients during a mean follow-up period of 21 months.

A third prospective randomized study of unstable angina has been reported from Southwestern University in Dallas by Pugh and colleagues [32]. In this study there were 14 medical patients and 13 surgical patients, with no medical and 8% surgical mortality during the initial hospitalization. The follow-up period was 18–19 months and 7% of medical patients died, whereas no surgical patients did so during this interval. During initial hospitalization no medical patients and 15% of surgical patients had a myocardial infarction but no infarction occurred in any group during follow-up. Thirty-six percent of medical patients had severe angina, whereas no surgical patients experienced severe angina during follow-up.

In the cooperative study sponsored by the National Heart, Lung, and Blood Institute, the unstable angina pectoris study group reported on 147 medical patients and 141 surgical patients for a mean follow-up of 30 months [4]. Mortality during initial hospitalization was 3% among medical and 5% among surgical patients; and, during follow up, 7% among medical and 5% among surgical patients. Myocardial infarction occurred in 8% of medical and 17% of surgical patients during initial hospitalization, and 11% of medical and 13% of surgical patients had a myocardial infarction during follow-up. However, 40% of medical patients experienced severe angina during follow-up, whereas only 14% of surgical patients had this degree of angina. In this study 35% of medically treated patients later underwent bypass surgery for unacceptable angina pectoris. The mortality in this latter subgroup was comparable to that in patients having early surgery after randomization. The relatively large numbers of these medical patients having later surgery prevents definite conclusions about the long-term effect of medical therapy on survival.

With regard to these prospective randomized trials of unstable angina, we would feel, based on the latter three studies, that acute intensive medical management seems to be an acceptable alternative to emergency or semiurgent bypass surgery. Most patients with unstable angina can be improved symptomatically with a maximal medical program and their course usually stabilized. Administration of propranolol, 80 or 160 mg daily (and occasionally up to 320 mg), as well as long-acting nitrates used throughout the 24-hr period usually achieve relief of symptoms and therapeutic control of blood pressure. If the symptoms seem to be exacerbated by propranolol, the presence of coronary spasm should be considered and the dosage of beta blocker reduced or even eliminated under careful observation in the hospital. Our experience has been that most patients will become clinically stable on this regimen. The patient should then undergo coronary arteriography within two to four days: this procedure is probably safer when the patient is more stable. The patient can undergo elective bypass surgery if indicated. The role of calcium blockers in the syndrome of unstable angina appears promising but is undefined in large numbers of patients. We believe the lessons that have been learned from the randomized trials are that in the majority of cases it is not necessary to perform emergency bypass

Table 2. Unstable angina: randomized studies (prospective randomized trials of medical or surgical therapy in patients with unstable angina pectoris).

Study	No. of patients	Mortality init hosp	Mortality follow-up	Myocardial inf init hosp	Myocardial inf follow-up	Severe angina follow-up
Medical						
Bertolasi [29, 30]						
Intermed	24	5	6	6	3	(16.6%)
Progress	27	1	1	1	1	(18.5%)
Selden [31]	19	0	0	0	2	(63%)
Pugh [32]	14	0	1	0	0	(36%)
NHLBI [4]	147	4	10	12	16	(40%)
	231	10 (4.3%)	18 (7.8%)	19 (8.2%)	22 (9.5%)	(34.8%)
Surgical						
Bertolasi [29, 30]						
Intermed	28	3	0	4	0	(3.5%)
Progress	34	3	0	4	0	(0%)
Selden [31]	21	1	0	3	0	(5%)
Pugh [32]	13	1	0	2	0	(0%)
NHLBI [4]	141	7	7	24	18	(14%)
	237	15 (6.3%)	7 (3.0%)	37 (15.6%)	18 (7.6%)	(4.5%)

Init hosp = initial hospitalization; Inf = infarction; Intermed = intermediate; Progress = progressive; NHLBI = National Heart Lung and Blood Institute.

surgery for unstable angina pectoris with the goal of preventing acute death or imminent myocardial infarction and that surgery can be performed more safely after the patient has been stabilized on medication (Table 2).

Randomized studies of chronic stable angina pectoris

For the prospective randomized studies of stable angina pectoris in medical and surgical patients, we shall analyze mortality, both operative and total for the entire study, cumulative survival, and nonfatal myocardial infarction for the entire study, as well as severe angina during follow-up.

In the Veterans Administration Hospital Cooperative Study of the medical or surgical treatment of stable angina pectoris, the subgroup of patients with left main coronary disease consisted of 53 medical and 60 surgical patients [33]. There was a 14% operative mortality. The total mortality for the entire study was 36% for medical and 20% for surgical patients during the mean follow-up of 30 months. The cumulative survival for the entire study was approximately 65% of medical and 82% of surgical patients. Among medical patients 35%

required no subsequent hospitalization, whereas 66% of surgical patients required no subsequent hospitalization. This subgroup of patients with significant lesions in the left main coronary artery survived longer when they were treated surgically than when they were treated medically.

In the overall Veterans Administration prospective study, there were 310 medical and 286 surgical patients [34]. The operative mortality was 5.6% for the entire study and the cumulative survival for the mean follow-up of 36 months was 87% for medical and 88% for surgical patients.

In a separate study, not part of the cooperative study, Mathur and Guinn from the Houston Veterans Administration Hospital randomly allocated 60 patients to medical treatment and 56 patients to surgical treatment [35–38]. There was a 5.3% surgical mortality, and a total mortality for the study of 18% of medical and 9% of surgical patients. Nonfatal myocardial infarction during the entire study occurred in 17% of medical and 11% of surgical patients, and severe angina during follow-up occurred in 48% of medical and 18% of surgical patients. Follow-up was reported for 52 months.

A study of stable angina from the University of Oregon Health Sciences Center by Kloster included 49 medical and 51 surgical patients [39]. There was a 2% operative mortality and the total mortality for the entire study was 10% in medical and 8% in surgical patients. Nonfatal myocardial infarction was 16% for medical and 30% for surgical patients during the entire study. Among medical patients, 31% had severe angina, whereas 12% of surgical patients sustained severe angina during follow-up of approximately 37 months.

In another collaborative effort, the European Coronary Surgery Group performed a randomized study of 373 medical and 395 surgical patients with stable angina [40–42]. The follow-up period was three years for all patients, four years for 60%, and five years for 25% of all patients. There was a 3.5% overall operative mortality for the entire study, and the cumulative survival for the entire study (60 months) was 84.1% for the medical and 93.5% for the surgical group. The surgical regimen was associated with significantly better five-year survival than the nonsurgical ($p < 0.001$). The subgroups of patients with left main coronary artery disease and three-vessel disease benefited most from surgery with values of significance <0.037 and <0.001 respectively. The survival rate at 60 months was 61.7% for medical and 92.9% for surgical patients with left main disease. The corresponding values for medical and surgical patients with three-vessel disease were 84.8% and 94.9% respectively. No significant difference between the two survival curves was found in the subgroup of patients with two-vessel disease, $p = 0.0668$. The cumulative survival rate at 60 months was 87.5% for medical and 91.6% for surgical patients. To evaluate the possible prognostic role of proximal left anterior descending disease (defined as 50% or greater obstruction located in the proximal third of the left anterior descending artery), survival in medical patients with two-vessel disease was evaluated. In 40% of these patients, the proximal left anterior descending was not obstructed. This was associated with a survival rate of 96% at 60 months. In the remaining 60% of these patients with coexistent proximal left anterior descending disease survival was 82%. The prognostic effect of proximal left anterior descending obstruction in medical patients with three-vessel disease was markedly less important with the survival rate at 60 months, being 87.8% for those without and 83.9% for those with proximal left anterior descending narrowing. The proportion of asymptomatic patients at one, two, and three years was 58%,

55%, and 49% for the surgical group and 15%, 16%, and 20% for the medical group respectively.

The Coronary Artery Surgery Study (CASS), a large cooperative study in the United States, is still underway and has a registry of over 20,000 patients and a smaller subgroup of randomly allocated patients [43–46].

Among these randomized trials of medical and surgical treatment of stable angina pectoris, there seems to be no overall difference in mortality for the follow-up period of two to three years when all degrees of severity of disease are considered. It seems apparent that patients with significant left main coronary artery disease from the Veterans Administration Study had an improved longevity when treated surgically as compared to medically. The subgroup of patients with left main and with three-vessel disease in the European trial had a greater survival at five years with surgery than with medical care [42]. Also in the Veterans Administration Hospital Study, those patients having three-vessel disease and abnormal left ventricular function had a somewhat greater survival at 54 months, though this was not statistically significant [47]. It is apparent that more patients are asymptomatic with surgical than with medical therapy. There is no difference in the incidence of nonfatal myocardial infarction between the two modes of therapy. Patients treated medically in these studies have a greater incidence of angina, and they require more frequent hospitalizations than do patients treated surgically (Table 3).

It is of interest that patients with two- or three-vessel coronary disease who are asymptomatic or mildly symptomatic have an average annual mortality of only about 2% during a mean follow-up of two years in a study by Epstein et al. [48]. In most of the prospective studies of unstable angina and stable angina, medical therapy has shown better results with regard to mortality and myocardial infarction than might have been expected from previous natural history studies. Earlier natural history studies of patients with angina pectoris found the annual mortality rate to be approximately 8–9%. The improvement in mortality rates of patients with coronary artery disease may be due to many factors including better diagnosis and earlier treatment of acute myocardial infarction, better definition of groups of patients with angina pectoris and coronary artery disease by coronary arteriography, and

Table 3. Stable angina: randomized studies* (prospective randomized trials of medical or surgical therapy in patients with stable angina pectoris).

Study	No. of patients	Mortality (operative)	Mortality (total for entire study)	Cumulative survival (entire study)	Nonfatal myocardial infarction (entire study)	Severe angina follow-up
Medical						
Murphy (VA) [34]	310		-	(87%)	-	-
Mathur [35, 38]	60		(18%)	-	(17%)	(48%)
Kloster [39]	49		(10%)	-	(16%)	(31%)
Europ SG [40–42]	373		-	(84.1%)	-	(52%)
	792		(14%)	(85.5%)	(16.5%)	(44%)
Surgical						
Murphy (VA) [34]	286	(5.6%)	-	(88%)	-	-
Mathur [35, 38]	56	(5.3%)	(9%)	-	(11%)	(18%)
Kloster [39]	51	(2%)	(8%)	-	(30%)	(12%)
Europ SG [40–42]	395	(3.5%)	-	(93.5%)	-	(20%)
	788	(4.1%)	(8.5%)	(90.8%)	(20.5%)	(17%)

* Excluding left main study of Takaro et al.; SG = Study group; VA = Veterans Administration.

perhaps improved treatment of angina pectoris with round-the-clock nitrates and liberal use of beta-blocking agents.

Current recommendations

From these data and our own experience it would seem that the indications for saphenous vein bypass graft surgery may be similar, if not the same, for both unstable and stable angina pectoris. Our own current recommendations are based on considerations of anatomy as well as symptoms and manifestations of coronary artery disease.

With regard to coronary anatomy we believe that definite indications for bypass surgery include left main coronary disease greater than 50% and triple-vessel disease with two or more 90% stenoses or total occlusions, particularly if the right and left anterior descending coronary are involved. Less compelling indications would be lesser degree of triple-vessel disease, and double-vessel or, rarely, single-vessel disease.

With regard to symptoms in patients having *unstable* angina we believe that definite indications for surgery would include patients with left main coronary stenosis, patients with persistent pain or other evidence of ischemia despite intensive medical treatment and failure of medical therapy following hospital discharge. We also believe that patients with three- and two-vessel disease and unstable angina pectoris should have surgery. Similarly, the patient with high-grade single-vessel disease, especially in the left anterior descending location, with continuing angina despite a medical program should be advised to have surgery. The use of percutaneous transluminal coronary angioplasty and also the addition of calcium antagonists to medical therapy may reduce the number of patients requiring coronary bypass surgery. Indications for surgery in these patients would be the high probability of continued anginal symptoms despite medical therapy and the need to undergo other major surgical procedures.

In patients with *stable* angina pectoris, definite indications for saphenous vein bypass would include continued pain and/or cardiac disability despite appropriate medical therapy or the inability to tolerate medical therapy. Relative indications would include externally imposed limitations on work status and life style.

There are other groups of patients whose symptoms suggest bypass surgery is indicated. These include patients with cardiac failure without mechanical complications such as ventricular aneurysm, ventricular septal rupture, or papillary muscle dysfunction, but who have reversibly ischemic myocardium and an ejection fraction greater than 15% or 20%. They also include patients with life-threatening arrhythmias such as exercise-induced ventricular arrhythmias, and survivors of 'sudden-death' (here, surgery on the myocardium based on preoperative and intraoperative mapping techniques should be considered along with bypass surgery), those with an acute myocardial infarction occurring in the hospital following catheterization or coronary artery balloon dilatation, and patients with acute myocardial infarction having persistent pain or other evidence of ischemia despite intensive medical therapy.

In the asymptomatic or minimally symptomatic group the indications for surgery may be controversial. However, we believe that patients having left main coronary disease of greater than 50% or triple-vessel disease with two or more 90% lesions, or total occlusion involving the right and left anterior descending coronary should be considered candidates for bypass. Areas of uncertainty that remain include the desirability of surgery for asymptomatic patients with a positive exercise test or other evidence of reversible ischemia with triple-, double-, or single-vessel disease and patients with a previous history of myocardial infarction.

Also influencing us would be considerations of left ventricular function. Granted that the coronary arteries are acceptable for grafting, we would consider as suitable for surgery any degree of left ventricular dysfunction less than severe. Severe left ventricular dysfunction would be considered diffuse generalized hypokinesis with an ejection fraction below 15% or 20%. A relatively less compelling indication for surgery with regard to left ventricular function includes severe impairment of contractility with evidence of reversible myocardial ischemia manifest as angina and a positive exercise test with or without the thallium portion being positive.

Further implications for bypass operation in patients with coexisting heart disease include mechanical complications of ischemic heart disease such as ventricular aneurysm, rupture of the ventricular septum, and papillary muscle rupture or dysfunction. Other indications include patients with valvular heart disease, congenital heart disease, and ascending aortic disease with associated significant coronary artery disease.

In summary, on the basis of the information presented, we advise operation for all patients with severe and disabling stable angina pectoris who do not respond to adequate medical therapy and who do not have severe left ventricular dysfunction, regardless of the extent of the disease. Asymptomatic or minimally symptomatic patients with lesions of the left main coronary artery or triple-vessel disease without severe impairment of ventricular function also are advised to undergo operation because of the beneficial effect of coronary artery bypass on these subgroups. In patients with double-vessel disease, we advise bypass grafting if there are no major contraindications to operation since retrospective studies have shown that longevity may be improved in this subgroup. Asymptomatic or minimally symptomatic patients with lesions in only a single coronary artery are not advised to undergo surgery at the present time. For patients with unstable angina pectoris, we attempt to stabilize the patient using a medical regimen, and follow this with coronary arteriography and bypass grafting on a less urgent basis, usually during the same hospitalization. Patients with persistent and prolonged episodes of chest pain despite intensive medical therapy are advised to have more immediate operation.

These recommendations represent our current thinking with regard to indications for surgery and may very well change with availability of further data. Clearly we try to approach each patient by individualizing his or her circumstances and to make a decision based on these considerations plus available data from other reported studies of coronary artery disease.

Acknowledgment

This research was supported in part by the National Heart, Lung, and Blood Institute (Specialized Center of Research for Ischemic Heart Disease Contract 5P50 HL1776-06, program project grant HL11310, and the Clinical Research Unit Grant MO-RR0001-3, General Clinical Research Centers Program, Division of Research Resources) of the National Institutes of Health, Bethesda, MD 20014

References

1. Souza AS Jr, Bream PR, Elliott LP: Chest film detection of coronary artery calcification. The value of the CAC triangle. Radiology 129:7–10, 1978.
2. Charles ED, Kronenfeld JJ, Wayne JB, Kouchoukos NT, Oberman A, Rogers WJ, Mantle JA, Rackley CE, Russell RO Jr: Unstable angina pectoris: a comparison of the costs of medical and surgical treatment. Am J Cardiol 44:112–117, 1979.
3. Charles ED, Kronenfeld JJ: In: Charles ED, Kronenfeld JJ (eds) Social and Economic Impacts of Coronary Artery Disease. Lexington Books, Lexington, Mass, 1980, pp 1–41.
4. Unstable Angina Pectoris Study Group: Unstable Angina Pectoris: National Cooperative Study Group to compare surgical and medical therapy. II. In-hospital experience and initial follow-up results in patients with one, two and three vessel disease. Am J Cardiol 42:839–848, 1978.
5. Block WJ Jr, Crumpacker EL, Dry TJ, Gage RP: Prognosis of angina pectoris: observations in 6,882 cases. J Am Med Assoc 150:259–264, 1952.
6. Richards DW, Bland EF, White PD: A completed twenty-five year follow-up study of 456 patients with angina pectoris. J Chronic Dis 4:423–433, 1956.
7. Kannel WB, Feinleib M: Natural history of angina pectoris in the Framingham Study. Prognosis and survival. Am J Cardiol 29:154–163, 1972.
8. Reeves TJ, Oberman A, Jones WB, Sheffield LT: Natural history of angina pectoris. Am J Cardiol 33:423–430, 1974.
9. Bruschke AVG, Proudfit WL, Sones FM Jr: Progress study of 590 consecutive nonsurgical cases of coronary disease followed 5–9 years. I. Arteriographic correlations. Circulation 47:1147–1153, 1973.
10. Bruschke AVG: Ten-year follow-up of 601 nonsurgical cases of angiographically documented coronary disease. Arteriographic correlations. Cleve Clin Q (The First Decade of Bypass Graft Surgery for Coronary Artery Disease – An International Symposium) 45:143–144, 1977.
11. Oberman A, Jones WB, Riley CP, Reeves TJ, Sheffield LT, Turner ME: Natural history of coronary artery disease. Bull NY Acad Med 48:1109–1125, 1972.
12. Lichtlen PR, Moccetti T: Prognostic aspects of coronary angiography. Circulation 46 (Suppl II):7, 1972 (abstract).
13. Slagle RC, Bartel AG, Behar VS, Peter RH, Rosati RA, Kong Y: Natural history of angiographically documented coronary artery disease. Circulation 46 (Suppl II):60, 1972.
14. Burggraf GW, Parker JO: Prognosis in coronary artery disease. Angiographic, hemodynamic and clinical factors. Circulation 51:146–156, 1975.
15. Parker JO: Prognosis in coronary artery disease. Arteriographic, ventriculographic, and hemodynamic factors. Cleve Clin Q (The First Decade of Bypass Graft Surgery for Coronary Artery Disease – An International Symposium) 45:145–146, 1977.
16. Amsterdam EA, Most AS, Wolfson S, Kemp H, Gorlin R: Relation of degree of angiographically documented coronary artery disease to mortality. Ann Intern Med 72:780, 1970 (abstract).
17. Humphries J O'N, Kuller L, Ross RS, Friesinger GC, Page EE: Natural history of ischemic heart disease in relation to arteriographic findings. A twelve year study of 225 patients. Circulation 49:489–497, 1974.
18. Bruschke AVG, Proudfit WL, Sones FM Jr: Progress study of 590 consecutive nonsurgical cases of coronary disease followed 5–9 years. II. Ventriculographic and other correlations. Circulation 47:1154–1163, 1973.
19. Nelson GR, Cohn PF, Gorlin R: Prognosis in medically treated coronary artery disease. Influence of ejection fraction compared to other parameters. Circulation 52:408–412, 1975.
20. Kouchoukos NT, Kirklin JW: Surgical treatment of coronary atherosclerotic heart disease. In: Hurst JW, Logue RB, Schlant RC, Wenger NK (eds) The Heart, Arteries and Veins. McGraw Hill, New York, 1978, pp 1295–1303.
21. Lefemine AA, Moon HS, Flessas A, Ryan TJ: Myocardial resection and coronary artery bypass for left ventricular failure following myocardial infarction. Results in patients with ejection fraction of 40% or less. Ann Thorac Surg 17:1–15, 1974.
22. Isom OW, Spencer FC, Glassman E, Dombrow JM, Pasternack BS: Long-term survival following coronary bypass surgery in patients with significant impairment of left ventricular function. Circulation 52 (Suppl I):141–147, 1975.
23. Manley JC, King JF, Zeft HJ, Johnson WD: The 'bad' left ventricle – results of coronary surgery effect on late survival. J Thorac Cardiovasc Surg 72:841–848, 1976.
24. Kouchoukos NT, Oberman A, Kirklin JW, Russell RO Jr, Karp RB, Pacifico AD, Zorn GL: Coronary bypass surgery: analysis of factors affecting hospital mortality. Circulation 62 (Suppl I):84–89, 1980.
25. Oberman A, Kouchoukos NT, Holt JH, Russell RO Jr: Long term results of the medical treatment of coronary artery disease. Angiology 28:160–168, 1977.
26. De Wood MA, Spores J, Notske RN, Lang HT, Shields JP, Simpson CS, Rudy LW, Grunwald R: Medical and surgical management of myocardial infarction. Am J Cardiol 44:1356–1364, 1979.
27. Hurst JW, King SB, Logue RB, Hatcher CR, Jones EL, Craver JM, Douglas JS, Franch RH, Dorney ER, Cobbs BW Jr, Robinson PH, Clements SD Jr, Kaplan LA, Bradford JM: Value of coronary bypass surgery. Am J Cardiol 42:308–329, 1976.
28. Conti CR: Influence of myocardial revascularization on survival. Am J Cardiol 42:330–332, 1978.
29. Bertolasi CA, Tronge JE, Carreno CA, Jalon J, Ruda Vegas M: Unstable angina – prospective and randomized study of its evolution with and without surgery. Preliminary report. Am J Cardiol 33:201–208, 1974.
30. Bertolasi CA, Tronge JE, Riccitelli MA, Villamayor RM, Zuffardi E: Natural history of unstable angina with medical or surgical therapy. Chest 70:596–605, 1976.
31. Selden R, Neill WA, Ritzmann LW, Oakies JE, Anderson RP: Medical versus surgical therapy for acute coronary insufficiency – a randomized study. N Engl J Med 26:1329–1333, 1975.
32. Pugh B, Platt MR, Mills LJ, Crumbo D, Poliner LR, Curry GC, Blomqvist GC, Parkey RW, Buja LM, Willerson JT: Unstable angina pectoris: a randomized study of patients treated medically and surgically. Am J Cardiol 41:1291–1298, 1978.

549

33. Takaro T, Hultgren HN, Lipton MJ, Detre KM, Participants in the Study Group: The VA cooperative randomized study of surgery for coronary arterial occlusive disease. II. Subgroup with significant left main lesions. Circulation 54 (Suppl III):107–117, 1976.

34. Murphy ML, Hultgren HN, Detre K, Thompson J, Takaro T, Participants in the Veterans Administration Cooperative Study: Treatment of chronic stable angina – a preliminary report of survival data of the randomized Veterans Administration Cooperative Study. N Engl J Med 277:621–627, 1977.

35. Mathur VS, Guinn GA: Prospective randomized study of coronary bypass surgery in stable angina. Circulation 52 (Suppl I):133–140, 1975.

36. Guinn GA, Mathur VS: Surgical versus medical treatment for stable angina pectoris: prospective randomized study with a 1- to 4-year follow-up. Ann Thorac Surg 22:524–527, 1976.

37. Mathur VS, Guinn GA, Anastassiades LC, Chahine RA, Korompai FL, Montero AC, Luchi RJ: Surgical treatment for stable angina pectoris – prospective randomized study. N Engl J Med 292:709–713, 1975.

38. Mathur VS, Guinn GA: Sustained benefit from aortocoronary bypass surgery demonstrated for 5 years: a prospective randomized study. Circulation 56 (Suppl III):190, 1977.

39. Kloster FE, Kremkau EL, Ritzmann LW, Rahimtoola SH, Rosch H, Kanarek PH: Coronary bypass for stable angina – a prospective randomized study. N Engl J Med 300:149–157, 1979.

40. European Coronary Surgery Study Group: Coronary artery bypass surgery in stable angina pectoris. Survival at two years. Lancet 1:889–892, 1979.

41. Varnauskas E, Olsson SB: The European multicenter CABG trial. In: Yu PN, Goodwin JF (eds) Progress in Cardiology. Lea & Febiger, Philadelphia, 1977, pp 83–89.

42. European Coronary Surgery Study Group: Prospective randomized study of coronary artery bypass surgery in stable angina pectoris. Second interim report. Lancet II:491–495, 1980.

43. Kronmal RA, Davis K, Fisher LD, Jones RA, Gillespie MJ: Data management for a large collaborative clinical trial (CASS: Coronary Artery Surgery Study). Comput Biomed Res 11:553–556, 1979.

44. Davis J, Kennedy JW, Kemp HC Jr, Judkins MP, Gosselin AJ, Killip T: Complications of coronary arteriography from the collaborative study of coronary artery surgery. Circulation 59:1105–1112, 1979.

45. Vliestra RE, Frye RL, Kronmal RA, Sim D, Tristani FE, Killip T III, Participants in the Coronary Artery Surgery Study: Risk factors and angiographic coronary artery disease: a report from the Coronary Artery Surgery Study (CASS). Circulation 62:254–260, 1980.

46. Chaitman BR, Rogers WJ, Davis K, Tyras DH, Berger R, Bourassa M, Fisher L, StoverHertzberg V, Judkins MP, Mock MB, Killip T: Operative risk factors in patients with left main coronary disease. N Engl J Med 303:953–957, 1980.

47. Read RC, Murphy ML, Hultgren HN, Takaro T: Survival of men treated for chronic stable angina pectoris – a cooperative randomized study. J Thorac Cardiovasc Surg 75:1–12, 1978.

48. Epstein SE, Kent KM, Goldstein RE, Borer JS, Rosing DR: Strategy for evaluation and surgical treatment of the asymptomatic or mildly symptomatic patient with coronary artery disease. Am J Cardiol 43:1015–1025, 1979.

Subject index

552

553

555

556

562

adrenergic-receptor activity of, 145
for cardiac failure, 474
for cardiogenic shock, 146
hemodynamic responses to, 145
interaction with beta-receptors, 85
interaction with digitalis, 396
necrosis of tissue caused by, 146
parasympathetic regulation of, 103

Oliguria, furosemide for, 428
Organomercurial diuretics, pharmacokinetics of, 419
side effects of, 430
Ouabain, 10, 387
Overdrive suppression, defined, 304
effects on abnormal automaticity, 10–11
mechanics of, 5
use of cardiac pacing to induce, 304–05
Oxotremorine, properties of, 126
Oxprenolol, administration and absorption of, 198
antianginal effects of, 509
as nonselective beta-blocking agent, 194
Oxygen, supplemental, in treatment of acute myocardial infarction, 483
Oxygen consumption, myocardial, 439
Oxygen demand, in coronary circulation, 26–27
Oxygen-hemoglobin dissociation curve, shift in, as compensatory mechanism in congestive heart failure, 36

Pacemaker. *See also* Cardiac pacing
temporary transvenous, in treatment of myocardial infarction, 486, 491–92
Pacemaker therapy, for ventricular tachycardia or fibrillation in acute myocardial infarction, 490
Paget's disease, and elevated cardiac output, 35
Pain, treatment of,
in acute myocardial infarction, 498–99
in angina pectoris, 512
Papillary duct, role in diuresis, 416–17
Parasympathetic nervous system, effect of digitalis on, 395–96
effect on cardiac function by, 97–102
evidence supporting vagus innervation of ventricles, 95–96
impulse transmission by, 96
interneuronal interaction with sympathetic nervous system, 102–04
intracellular interaction with sympathetic nervous system, 104–07
structure of, 73–74
Parasympathetic tone, effect on antimuscarinic agents, 131–32
Parasystole, 15
Pentaerythral tetranitrate, use of, for chronic cardiac failure, 471
Pentaerythritol trinitrate, antianginal effects of, 509
Pentazocine, contraindications for use in acute myocardial infarction, 481
Perhexiline, antianginal effects of, 512
Pericardium, structure and function of, 25
Pericarditis, constrictive, 25
treatment of, in acute myocardial infarction, 499
Peripheral vascular disease, as adverse effect of beta-blockade, 160

Phenobarbital, interaction with digoxin, 404
interaction with quinidine, 176
Phenoxybenzamine, alpha-receptor blockade with, 149
vasodilating effects of, 440–41
Phentolamine, administration of, 149
alpha-receptor blockade with, 149
as test for pheochromocytoma, 149
for cardiac failure, 467
for pulmonary vascular congestion, 494
vasodilating effects of, 440–41
Phenytoin, antiarrhythmic use of, 246
chemical structure of, 172, 190
circulatory effects of, 192
combination therapy with, 247
contraindications for use of, 248
dosage and administration of, 192, 247
drug interactions with, 176, 246, 247, 404
electrophysiologic effects of, 190–92
for digitalis-induced dysrhythmia, 490
pharmacokinetics of, 192–93, 246–47
plasma levels of, 247–48
Phenylbutazone, interaction with digoxin, 404
Phenylephrine, adrenergic-receptor activity of, 145
effect of atropine on, 8
for cardioversion of paroxysmal atrial tachycardia, 146
for testing baroreceptor sensitivity, 89
peak plasma levels of, 146
pressor effects of, 145
Pheochromocytoma, fluid management in, 146
hypotension in, 146
phentolamine as test for, 149
propranolol for ventricular arrhythmia in, 163
Phlebotomy, for treatment of acute cardiogenic pulmonary edema, 41
Physostigmine, cardiovascular effects of, 129
Pilomotor muscle, norepinephrine stimulation of, 145
Pindolol, as nonselective beta-blocking agent, 194
elimination of, 198
Pirbuterol, for treatment of chronic cardiac failure, 474
Platelet aggregation, suppression of, with propranolol, 445
Posterior septal bypass tract, 339
surgical ablation of, 347–48
Postextrasystolic potentiation, effects of, following acute coronary occlusion, 58, 59
Potassium, effect of diuretics on balance of, 421, 429–30
reabsorption of, in diuresis, 416, 417
supplemental, for digitalis intoxication, 462
Potassium equilibrium potential, Nernst equation for, 1
Potassium ion gradient, 1–2
"Power failure" syndrome, in acute myocardial infarction, 47
Practolol, as cardioselective beta-blocking agent, 194
elimination of, 198
prophylactic use of, 507, 164
Prazosin, as alpha-adrenergic blocking agent, 8
alpha-receptor blockade with, 149–50
for chronic heart failure, 471, 472–73
for congestive heart failure, 150, 440, 518
side effects of, 150
Pregnancy, and elevated cardiac output, 35
Preload, defined, 27

indices of, 27
reduction of,
    in acute cardiogenic pulmonary edema, 40
    with diuretics, 38
    with nitroglycerin, 436
    with nitroprusside, 439
Pressor amine therapy, 146
Pressure development, as determinant of oxygen demand, 26
Prinzmetal's (variant) angina, characteristics of, 513
    ergonovine testing for, 513
    prevention of, with verapamil, 201
    treatment of, 512, 514
Probenecid, 420
Procainamide, antiarrhythmic use of, 252
    as precipitating cause of heart failure, 458
    chemical structure of, 172
    circulatory effects of, 178
    combination therapy with, 253
    dosage and administration of, 178–79, 253
    electrophysiologic and hemodynamic effects of, 177–78, 252
    for ventricular dysrhythmia, in acute myocardial infarction, 489
    pharmacokinetics of, 179–80, 252–53
    plasma levels of, 253
    prophylactic use of, 279, 488–89
    toxicity of, 180, 253–54
Procaine, 177
Propranolol: administration of, oral vs. intravenous, 157
    age-related resistance to, 153
    and reduction of sudden death following myocardial infarction, 163–64, 280
    antiarrhythmic effects of, 162, 261–63
    as precipitating cause of heart failure, 458
    beta-adrenergic blockade by, 153
    blood levels of, 263
    chemical structure of, 172
    circulatory effects of, 162, 261–63
    combined with isoproterenol, 154
    contraindications for use in diabetes mellitus, 155
    development of suicidal depression from, 163
    dosage of, 263
    effect of, during acute coronary occlusion, 56–57
    effect of, in acute partial coronary stenosis, 59–60
    effect of withdrawal from, 160–61, 446
    effect on hemodynamic function following acute myocardial infarction, 57
    effect on monophasic action potential, 154
    electrophysiologic effects of, 194–96
    for acute heart failure, 467
    for angina pectoris, 64, 445, 509, 510
    for cyanotic attacks associated with tetralogy of Fallot, 164
    for digitalis-induced arrhythmias, 163
    for dysrhythmias in acute myocardial infarction, 490
    for exercise-induced arrhythmias, 163
    for hyperdynamic hemodynamics in acute myocardial infarction, 493
    for hypertension, 161–62, 499
    for hypertrophic obstructive cardiomyopathy, 164
    for limitation of infarct size, 503
    for sinus tachycardia, 486

for unstable angina, 506, 544
for ventricular arrhythmias in pheochromocytoma, 163
in combination therapy
    with digoxin, 263
    with isoproterenol, 154
    with nitroprusside, 164
    with quinidine, 264
interaction with lidocaine, 185
interaction with quinidine, 177
pharmacokinetics of, 156–57, 197–98, 263
toxicity of, 199, 264
Proximal tubule, inhibition of carbonic anhydrase in, 418
role in diuresis, 415
Pulmonary capillary wedge pressure, as prognostic indicator, 43
    defined, 27
    elevated, in heart failure, 36
    measurement of, 27
Pulmonary congestion, and peripheral hypoperfusion, in acute myocardial infarction, 497–98
    symptoms of, 21
Pulmonary disease, and increased risk of digitalis intoxication, 461–62
Pulmonary edema, acute digitalization for, 41–42
    clinical symptoms of, 40
    cough in, 40
    diuretic therapy for, 427
    furosemide for, 40, 493
    morphine sulphate for, 40
    sublingual nitroglycerin for, 40
Pulmonary embolism, as precipitating cause of congestive heart failure, 40
Pulmonary fibrosis, diffuse interstitial, as adverse effect of amiodarone therapy, 272
Pulmonary hyperventilation, induced by arterial chemoreceptor stimulation, 90
Pulmonary vascular congestion, treatment of, in acute myocardial infarction, 493–94
Pulsus alternans, as indication of left ventricular dysfunction, 35
Purkinje fiber(s), abnormal automaticity in, 211
    action potential in, 81
    effect of beta-adrenergic stimulation on, 8
    effect of catecholamines on, 82
    electrophysiologic properties of, 2–3
        effect of ethmozin on, 209
    generation of automatic impulse in, 4, 5
    ionic basis for slow diastolic depolarization in, 75
    normal automaticity in, 9
    refractoriness in, 4
        effect of digitalis on, 398
    resting potential in, 1, 4
    summation in, 15

Quinethazone, as diuretic, 422
Quinidine, antiarrhythmic use of, 248–50
    anticholinergic effects of, 135–36
    as precipitating cause of heart failure, 458, 459
    chemical structure of, 172
    circulatory effects of, 174
    combined with propranolol, for atrial and ventricular fibrillation, 264